AF598409

FUNCTIONAL NEUROLOGIC DISORDERS

HANDBOOK OF CLINICAL NEUROLOGY

Series Editors

MICHAEL J. AMINOFF, FRANÇOIS BOLLER, AND DICK F. SWAAB

VOLUME 139

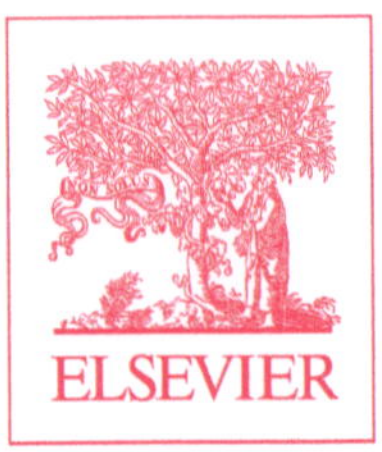

AMSTERDAM BOSTON HEIDELBERG LONDON NEW YORK OXFORD
PARIS SAN DIEGO SAN FRANCISCO SINGAPORE SYDNEY TOKYO

FUNCTIONAL NEUROLOGIC DISORDERS

Series Editors

MICHAEL J. AMINOFF, FRANÇOIS BOLLER, AND DICK F. SWAAB

Volume Editors

MARK HALLETT, JON STONE, AND ALAN CARSON

VOLUME 139

3rd Series

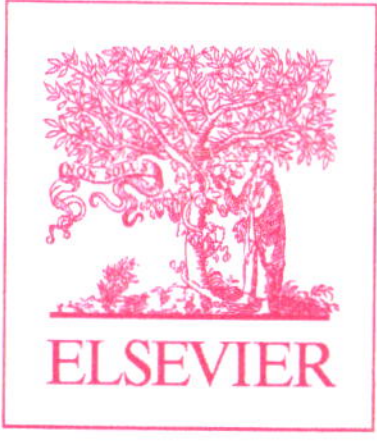

AMSTERDAM BOSTON HEIDELBERG LONDON NEW YORK OXFORD
PARIS SAN DIEGO SAN FRANCISCO SINGAPORE SYDNEY TOKYO

ELSEVIER
Radarweg 29, PO Box 211, 1000 AE Amsterdam, Netherlands
The Boulevard, Langford Lane, Kidlington, Oxford OX5 1GB, United Kingdom
50 Hampshire Street, 5th Floor, Cambridge, MA 02139, United States

Notices
Knowledge and best practice in this field are constantly changing. As new research and experience broaden our understanding, changes in research methods, professional practices, or medical treatment may become necessary.

Practitioners and researchers must always rely on their own experience and knowledge in evaluating and using any information, methods, compounds, or experiments described herein. In using such information or methods they should be mindful of their own safety and the safety of others, including parties for whom they have a professional responsibility.

With respect to any drug or pharmaceutical products identified, readers are advised to check the most current information provided (i) on procedures featured or (ii) by the manufacturer of each product to be administered, to verify the recommended dose or formula, the method and duration of administration, and contraindications. It is the responsibility of practitioners, relying on their own experience and knowledge of their patients, to make diagnoses, to determine dosages and the best treatment for each individual patient, and to take all appropriate safety precautions.

To the fullest extent of the law, neither the Publisher nor the authors, contributors, or editors, assume any liability for any injury and/or damage to persons or property as a matter of products liability, negligence or otherwise, or from any use or operation of any methods, products, instructions, or ideas contained in the material herein.

British Library Cataloguing-in-Publication Data
A catalogue record for this book is available from the British Library

Library of Congress Cataloging-in-Publication Data
A catalog record for this book is available from the Library of Congress

ISBN: 978-0-12-801772-2

For information on all Elsevier publications
visit our website at https://www.elsevier.com/

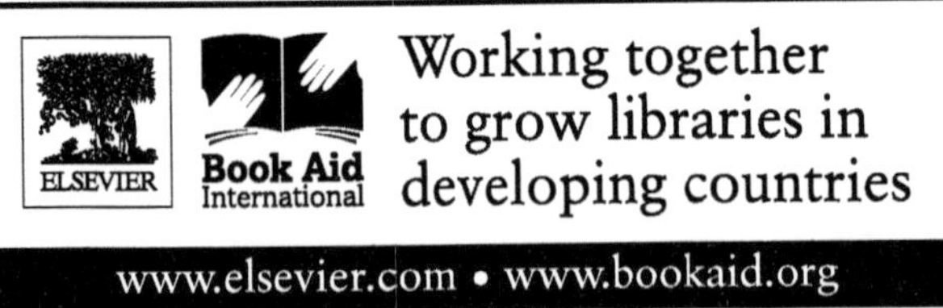

Publisher: Mara Conner
Editorial Project Manager: Kristi Anderson
Production Project Manager: Sujatha Thirugnana Sambandam
Cover Designer: Alan Studholme

Typeset by SPi Global, India

Handbook of Clinical Neurology 3rd Series

Available titles

Vol. 79, The human hypothalamus: basic and clinical aspects, Part I, D.F. Swaab, ed. ISBN 9780444513571
Vol. 80, The human hypothalamus: basic and clinical aspects, Part II, D.F. Swaab, ed. ISBN 9780444514905
Vol. 81, Pain, F. Cervero and T.S. Jensen, eds. ISBN 9780444519016
Vol. 82, Motor neurone disorders and related diseases, A.A. Eisen and P.J. Shaw, eds. ISBN 9780444518941
Vol. 83, Parkinson's disease and related disorders, Part I, W.C. Koller and E. Melamed, eds. ISBN 9780444519009
Vol. 84, Parkinson's disease and related disorders, Part II, W.C. Koller and E. Melamed, eds. ISBN 9780444528933
Vol. 85, HIV/AIDS and the nervous system, P. Portegies and J. Berger, eds. ISBN 9780444520104
Vol. 86, Myopathies, F.L. Mastaglia and D. Hilton Jones, eds. ISBN 9780444518996
Vol. 87, Malformations of the nervous system, H.B. Sarnat and P. Curatolo, eds. ISBN 9780444518965
Vol. 88, Neuropsychology and behavioural neurology, G. Goldenberg and B.C. Miller, eds. ISBN 9780444518972
Vol. 89, Dementias, C. Duyckaerts and I. Litvan, eds. ISBN 9780444518989
Vol. 90, Disorders of consciousness, G.B. Young and E.F.M. Wijdicks, eds. ISBN 9780444518958
Vol. 91, Neuromuscular junction disorders, A.G. Engel, ed. ISBN 9780444520081
Vol. 92, Stroke – Part I: Basic and epidemiological aspects, M. Fisher, ed. ISBN 9780444520036
Vol. 93, Stroke – Part II: Clinical manifestations and pathogenesis, M. Fisher, ed. ISBN 9780444520043
Vol. 94, Stroke – Part III: Investigations and management, M. Fisher, ed. ISBN 9780444520050
Vol. 95, History of neurology, S. Finger, F. Boller and K.L. Tyler, eds. ISBN 9780444520081
Vol. 96, Bacterial infections of the central nervous system, K.L. Roos and A.R. Tunkel, eds. ISBN 9780444520159
Vol. 97, Headache, G. Nappi and M.A. Moskowitz, eds. ISBN 9780444521392
Vol. 98, Sleep disorders Part I, P. Montagna and S. Chokroverty, eds. ISBN 9780444520067
Vol. 99, Sleep disorders Part II, P. Montagna and S. Chokroverty, eds. ISBN 9780444520074
Vol. 100, Hyperkinetic movement disorders, W.J. Weiner and E. Tolosa, eds. ISBN 9780444520142
Vol. 101, Muscular dystrophies, A. Amato and R.C. Griggs, eds. ISBN 9780080450315
Vol. 102, Neuro-ophthalmology, C. Kennard and R.J. Leigh, eds. ISBN 9780444529039
Vol. 103, Ataxic disorders, S.H. Subramony and A. Durr, eds. ISBN 9780444518927
Vol. 104, Neuro-oncology Part I, W. Grisold and R. Sofietti, eds. ISBN 9780444521385
Vol. 105, Neuro-oncology Part II, W. Grisold and R. Sofietti, eds. ISBN 9780444535023
Vol. 106, Neurobiology of psychiatric disorders, T. Schlaepfer and C.B. Nemeroff, eds. ISBN 9780444520029
Vol. 107, Epilepsy Part I, H. Stefan and W.H. Theodore, eds. ISBN 9780444528988
Vol. 108, Epilepsy Part II, H. Stefan and W.H. Theodore, eds. ISBN 9780444528995
Vol. 109, Spinal cord injury, J. Verhaagen and J.W. McDonald III, eds. ISBN 9780444521378
Vol. 110, Neurological rehabilitation, M. Barnes and D.C. Good, eds. ISBN 9780444529015
Vol. 111, Pediatric neurology Part I, O. Dulac, M. Lassonde and H.B. Sarnat, eds. ISBN 9780444528919
Vol. 112, Pediatric neurology Part II, O. Dulac, M. Lassonde and H.B. Sarnat, eds. ISBN 9780444529107
Vol. 113, Pediatric neurology Part III, O. Dulac, M. Lassonde and H.B. Sarnat, eds. ISBN 9780444595652
Vol. 114, Neuroparasitology and tropical neurology, H.H. Garcia, H.B. Tanowitz and O.H. Del Brutto, eds. ISBN 9780444534903
Vol. 115, Peripheral nerve disorders, G. Said and C. Krarup, eds. ISBN 9780444529022
Vol. 116, Brain stimulation, A.M. Lozano and M. Hallett, eds. ISBN 9780444534972
Vol. 117, Autonomic nervous system, R.M. Buijs and D.F. Swaab, eds. ISBN 9780444534910
Vol. 118, Ethical and legal issues in neurology, J.L. Bernat and H.R. Beresford, eds. ISBN 9780444535016
Vol. 119, Neurologic aspects of systemic disease Part I, J. Biller and J.M. Ferro, eds. ISBN 9780702040863
Vol. 120, Neurologic aspects of systemic disease Part II, J. Biller and J.M. Ferro, eds. ISBN 9780702040870
Vol. 121, Neurologic aspects of systemic disease Part III, J. Biller and J.M. Ferro, eds. ISBN 9780702040887
Vol. 122, Multiple sclerosis and related disorders, D.S. Goodin, ed. ISBN 9780444520012
Vol. 123, Neurovirology, A.C. Tselis and J. Booss, eds. ISBN 9780444534880

Vol. 124, Clinical neuroendocrinology, E. Fliers, M. Korbonits and J.A. Romijn, eds. ISBN 9780444596024
Vol. 125, Alcohol and the nervous system, E.V. Sullivan and A. Pfefferbaum, eds. ISBN 9780444626196
Vol. 126, Diabetes and the nervous system, D.W. Zochodne and R.A. Malik, eds. ISBN 9780444534804
Vol. 127, Traumatic brain injury Part I, J.H. Grafman and A.M. Salazar, eds. ISBN 9780444528926
Vol. 128, Traumatic brain injury Part II, J.H. Grafman and A.M. Salazar, eds. ISBN 9780444635211
Vol. 129, The human auditory system: Fundamental organization and clinical disorders, G.G. Celesia and G. Hickok, eds. ISBN 9780444626301
Vol. 130, Neurology of sexual and bladder disorders, D.B. Vodušek and F. Boller, eds. ISBN 9780444632470
Vol. 131, Occupational neurology, M. Lotti and M.L. Bleecker, eds. ISBN 9780444626271
Vol. 132, Neurocutaneous syndromes, M.P. Islam and E.S. Roach, eds. ISBN 9780444627025
Vol. 133, Autoimmune neurology, S.J. Pittock and A. Vincent, eds. ISBN 9780444634320
Vol. 134, Gliomas, M.S. Berger and M. Weller, eds. ISBN 9780128029978
Vol. 135, Neuroimaging Part I, J.C. Masdeu and R.G. González, eds. ISBN 9780444534859
Vol. 136, Neuroimaging Part II, J.C. Masdeu and R.G. González, eds. ISBN 9780444534866
Vol. 137, Neuro-otology, J.M. Furman and T. Lempert, eds. ISBN 9780444634375
Vol. 138, Neuroepidemiology, C. Rosano, M.A. Ikram and M. Ganguli, eds. ISBN 9780128029732

Foreword

The purpose of a foreword is to introduce the readers of a book to both its subject matter and its authors. While this is generally a worthwhile endeavor, in the present instance the subject matter is explained with great clarity in the preface written by the authors themselves. Indeed, if ever a justification was needed for such a volume, they have provided it most eloquently and cogently. Whether designated as "hysterical," "psychogenic," or "functional," these disorders have intrigued, puzzled, or frustrated neurologists from the very early days of the specialty and they continue to do so. To affected patients, whether limited by pain, subjective sensory complaints, abnormal movements, seizures, or some other disturbance of neurologic function that is difficult to explain, their complaints are as distressing or disabling as when they arise from some recognizable organic cause – indeed, these patients have the added burden of coping with medical ignorance, physician intolerance, the stigma often associated with a disorder "that is in the mind," and the insecurity that results from the absence of a specific diagnosis with a recognized treatment. If this volume helps to educate physicians about this group of disorders, it will have provided an immensely valuable service both to them and to the patients they serve. We believe that it may also stimulate advances in the field, for possible neurobiologic mechanisms underlying certain of these disorders can be glimpsed in some of the chapters.

The editors of the volume are all well known in their respective fields. Mark Hallett is a past president of the Movement Disorders Society and the current president of the International Federation of Clinical Neurophysiology, a senior investigator in the Human Motor Control Section of the National Institute of Neurological Disorders and Stroke in Bethesda, Maryland, and has had a long interest in psychogenic movement disorders. Jon Stone, a consultant neurologist and honorary reader in neurology at the University of Edinburgh, specializes in functional disorders in neurological practice. Alan Carson, his colleague in Edinburgh, is a consultant neuropsychiatrist and reader at the university there, and has focused his work on disorders on the borderland between clinical psychiatry and neurology. We are delighted that they accepted our invitation to put together this volume. Together, they have been an impressive editorial team that has brought together a multidisciplinary group of authors to develop a comprehensive volume that we are delighted to include as part of the *Handbook of Clinical Neurology*. We are grateful to them and to all the contributors to this volume.

As series editors, we have reviewed and commented on each of the chapters. This has encouraged our belief that clinicians in a multitude of different specialties, as well as basic scientists, will find this volume of considerable interest and a valuable resource. The availability of the volume electronically on Elsevier's Science Direct site should ensure its ready accessibility and facilitate searches for specific information.

We are grateful to Elsevier, our publishers, for their continued support of the *Handbook* series, and extend our thanks especially to Michael Parkinson in Scotland and to Mara Conner and Kristi Anderson in California for their unfailing assistance in the development and production of this volume.

Michael J. Aminoff
François Boller
Dick F. Swaab

Preface

It is remarkable that this is the first book devoted completely to functional neurologic disorders in the history of the *Handbook of Clinical Neurology* series, which began in 1968 and is now in its third series. Patients with functional disorders represent about 15% of patients seen by neurologists, and the recognition that hysteria, the original term for these disorders, is a medical condition has been appreciated for at least 3000 years, as noted in Chapter 1 of this volume. Interest peaked at the time of Charcot and Freud, and for various reasons then declined through the mid 20th century, as described in Chapters 2–4.

The absence of functional disorders in textbooks and teaching, until recently, reflects generations of lack of interest from neurologists and psychiatrists in the second half of the 20th century and a failure to develop research and knowledge about these patients. Recognition of these disorders has been poor and many neurologists have been taught to regard patients with functional disorders with distrust as exaggerating, malingering, or just not having a "real" condition within the proper boundaries of neurology. There have also been problems within psychiatry, where it was commonly taught that such disorders were largely historic anachronisms and that when the diagnosis was made it was likely erroneous and would prove to have a pathophysiologic cause in the fullness of time. For the patient in the middle, a common experience was to feel dismissed by the neurologist as having something "all in the mind," often accompanied by not so subtle suggestions of malingering, and to be sent to the psychiatrist who would respond, equally unhelpfully, "this patient has nothing psychiatric wrong" or even "are you sure the diagnosis is correct?" Whilst we recognize there were many isolated areas of good practice on both sides of the divide during this period, this caricature has been all too prevalent, and the consequent neglect has resulted in many patients receiving substandard assessment and poor standards of care.

There is now increasing recognition of functional neurologic disorders. Two international meetings were organized in 2003 and 2009 dealing with "psychogenic" movement disorders, each of which produced a book (Hallett et al., 2006, 2011). Conferences and books have now also dealt with dissociative seizures (psychogenic nonepileptic seizures), perhaps the most common type of functional neurologic disorder (Schacter and LaFrance, 2010). On the other hand, while many other types of functional symptoms and disorders involving the voluntary motor and sensory nervous system have been long recognized, there has been little written in a comprehensive fashion. The current book attempts to cover the whole field, bringing all aspects up to date. The authorship includes neurologists and psychiatrists but also neuroscientists, physiotherapists, psychologists, pediatric neurologists, gastroenterologists, audiologists, urologists, speech and language therapists, and ophthalmologists.

The book begins with the history and epidemiology. The next broad section tackles the difficult area of pathophysiology, and to a certain extent takes the assumption that most, or all, functional disorders may have similar underlying factors. We deal with psychologic issues, social factors, genetics, clinical physiology, and neuroimaging, the latter being relatively more recent perspectives on the subject. The next set of chapters deals with general principles of assessment, scales, and formal classifications. Chapters 18–42 deal with the different types of functional neurologic disorders. In the remaining chapters, we deal with treatment. For many patients this seems to be the most difficult aspect, and there is certainly more work to be done to fashion better therapies, but there has been significant progress in evidence for both physical and psychologic therapies in recent years.

A word about terminology. Hysteria had been the common term for centuries, but in the 20th century the term psychogenic became popular. Like conversion disorder and somatization, it derived in part from the concept that the disorders are a consequence of a psychologic, or psychiatric, disorder. The term "functional disorder," popularized in the late 19th and early 20th century, has had a renaissance as a label which does not presuppose etiology and simply accepts there is a disorder of function of the nervous system. There are contemporary debates in the literature about terminology which are rehearsed in Chapter 44 on "Explanation of the diagnosis." As editors we view "functional disorders," although imperfect, as our preferred term, for reasons we outline in that chapter, but we have allowed authors in this volume to use whichever term they are comfortable with. However, via keywords, we have linked each article to both terms. As we learn more about the pathophysiology, the terminology may continue to evolve.

We hope that this volume will increase interest in the field as well as augment knowledge of practitioners. In the future, functional disorders might even develop as a subspecialty of neurology. The approach must be multidisciplinary but the patients are primarily sent to neurologists who are usually tasked with making the diagnosis and are in the best position to provide initial treatment. There are certainly enough patients to warrant a subspecialty and, as these chapters illustrate, a large amount of knowledge to digest on the topic. When one of us, as a junior neurologist, presented our first platform presentation on functional disorders to a neurologic audience, a colleague leant over afterwards and said, "Interesting, I didn't think you could make science out of nonorganic things." It turns out you can – as the many fascinating scientific approaches to this topic in this volume show.

Better research on functional disorders is arguably the best way to change attitudes and improve training. Changes in training curricula, classifications, and information for patients can all change practice. We are all doing better, especially in the last 10–15 years, but much more progress is needed. What would be the prize for neurology and all the other specialties working with these patients? A healthcare system equipped to treat all patients with neurologic symptoms, and not just those in whom we can identify a disease process; healthcare professionals interested in parts of their job they previously regarded as irrelevant or beyond their expertise; and satisfied patients who experience and benefit from good treatment.

This book defines the state of the art at the time of publication. The editors are very grateful to the contributing authors who have done outstanding work creating new syntheses on many topics, some, like hearing and urologic disorders, for the first time. We hope and expect this field to continue to grow, and that our understanding will increase. We have many patients waiting for us to help them.

Mark Hallett
Jon Stone
Alan Carson

References

Hallett M, Fahn S, Jankovic J et al. (2006). Psychogenic Movement Disorders. Neurology and Psychiatry, Lippincott Williams & Wilkins, Philadelphia, PA.

Hallett M, Lang AE, Jankovic J et al. (2011). Psychogenic Movement Disorders and Other Conversion Disorders, Cambridge University Press, Cambridge.

Schacter SC, LaFrance Jr WC (2010). Gates and Rowan's Nonepileptic Seizures, 3rd edn. Cambridge University Press, Cambridge.

Contributors

S. Aybek
Neurology Service, Geneva University Hospitals and Laboratory for Behavioural Neurology and Imaging of Cognition, University of Geneva-Campus Biotech, Geneva, Switzerland

D.M. Baguley
Department of Audiology, Cambridge University Hospitals, Cambridge, UK

J. Baker
Speech Pathology and Audiology, School of Health Sciences, Flinders University, Adelaide, Australia

C. Bass
Department of Psychological Medicine, John Radcliffe Hospital, Oxford, UK

A. Baumann
Department of Internal Medicine, Albert Einstein Medical Center, Philadelphia, PA, USA

F. Benedetti
Department of Neuroscience, University of Turin Medical School, Turin, Italy and Plateau Rosa Labs, Breuil-Cervinia, Italy and Zermatt, Switzerland

K.P. Bhatia
Sobell Department of Motor Neuroscience and Movement Disorders, National Hospital for Neurology and Neurosurgery, Queen Square, London, UK

V. Biousse
Departments of Ophthalmology and Neurology, Emory University Hospital, Emory University School of Medicine, Atlanta, GA, USA

A.S. Blum
Department of Neurology, Rhode Island Hospital, Brown University, Providence, RI, USA

T. Brandt
German Center for Vertigo and Balance Disorders, Ludwig-Maximilians-University Munich, Klinikum Grosshadern, Munich, Germany

A.M. Bronstein
Division of Brain Sciences, Department of Neuro-otology, Imperial College London and Department of Neuro-otology, The National Hospital for Neurology and Neurosurgery, London, UK

R.J. Brown
Division of Psychology and Mental Health, University of Manchester, Manchester, UK

B.B. Bruce
Department of Ophthalmology and Department of Neurology, Emory University Hospital, Emory University School of Medicine, and Department of Epidemiology, Rollins School of Public Health, Emory University, Atlanta, GA, USA

E. Carlino
Department of Neuroscience, University of Turin Medical School, Turin, Italy

A. Carson
Departments of Clinical Neurosciences and of Rehabilitation Medicine, NHS Lothian and Centre for Clinical Brain Sciences, University of Edinburgh, Edinburgh, UK

D.C. Cath
Department of Clinical and Health Psychology, Utrecht University/Altrecht, Utrecht, The Netherlands

T.E. Cope
Department of Neurology, Cambridge University Hospitals, Cambridge, UK

R.C. Dale
Department of Neurology, Westmead Children's Hospital, Sydney, Australia

M. Dattilo
Department of Ophthalmology, SUNY Downstate Medical Center, Brooklyn, NY, USA

Q. Deeley
Department of Forensic and Neurodevelopmental Sciences, Institute of Psychiatry, Kings College, London, UK

C. Derry
Department of Clinical Neurosciences, Western General Hospital, Edinburgh, UK

G. Deuschl
Department of Neurology, University Hospital Schleswig-Holstein, Campus Kiel, Kiel, Germany

M. Dieterich
Department of Neurology and German Center for Vertigo and Balance Disorders, Ludwig-Maximilians-University Munich, Klinikum Grosshadern, Munich, Germany

Y.E.M. Dreissen
Department of Neurology, University Medical Centre Groningen, Groningen, The Netherlands

J.R. Duffy
Division of Speech Pathology, Mayo Medical School, Rochester, MN, USA

R. Duncan
Department of Neurology, University of Otago and Department of Neurology, Christchurch Hospital, Christchurch, New Zealand

M.J. Edwards
Department of Molecular and Clinical Sciences, St George's University of London and Atkinson Morley Regional Neuroscience Centre, St George's University Hospitals NHS Foundation Trust, London, UK

A.J. Espay
Gardner Family Center for Parkinson's Disease and Movement Disorders, Department of Neurology, University of Cincinnati, Cincinnati, OH, USA

S. Fahn
Department of Neurology, Columbia University Medical Center, New York, NY, USA

A. Fasano
Morton and Gloria Shulman Movement Disorders Clinic and the Edmond J. Safra Program in Parkinson's Disease, Toronto Western Hospital and Division of Neurology, University of Toronto and Krembil Research Institute, Toronto, Ontario, Canada

T. Frodl
Department of Psychiatry and Psychotherapy, Otto von Guericke University of Magdeburg, Germany and Department of Psychiatry, Trinity College, Dublin, Ireland

V.S.C. Fung
Movement Disorders Unit, Department of Neurology, Westmead Hospital and Sydney Medical School, University of Sydney, Sydney, Australia

C. Ganos
Sobell Department of Motor Neuroscience and Movement Disorders, National Hospital for Neurology and Neurosurgery, Queen Square, London, UK and Department of Neurology, University Medical Center Hamburg-Eppendorf (UKE), Hamburg, Germany

C. Gasca-Salas
Morton and Gloria Shulman Movement Disorders Clinic and the Edmond J. Safra Program in Parkinson's Disease, University Health Network, Toronto Western Hospital, Toronto, Ontario, Canada and HM CINAC-Hospital Universitario HM Puerta del Sur, Móstoles, Universidad CEU San Pablo, Madrid, Spain

J. Gelauff
Department of Neurology, University Medical Center Groningen, University of Groningen, Groningen, The Netherlands

C.G. Goetz
Department of Neurology and Department of Pharmacology, Rush University Medical Center, Chicago, IL, USA

L.H. Goldstein
Department of Psychology, Institute of Psychiatry, Psychology and Neuroscience, King's College London, De Crespigny Park, London, UK

P.J. Grattan-Smith
Department of Neurology, Westmead Children's Hospital, Sydney, Australia

J. Griem
Institute of Psychiatry, Psychology and Neuroscience, King's College London, London, UK

P. Haggard
Institute of Cognitive Neuroscience, London, UK

M. Hallett
Human Motor Control Section, National Institute of Neurological Disorders and Stroke, Bethesda, MD, USA

P. Halligan
School of Psychology, Cardiff University, Cardiff, UK

I. Hoeritzauer
Centre for Clinical Brain Sciences, University of Edinburgh, UK

J. Jankovic
Parkinson's Disease Center and Movement Disorders Clinic, Department of Neurology, Baylor College of Medicine, Houston, TX, USA

R.A.A. Kanaan
Department of Psychiatry, University of Melbourne, Austin Hospital, Heidelberg, Australia

D. Kaski
Division of Brain Sciences, Department of Neuro-otology, Imperial College London and Department of Neuro-otology, The National Hospital for Neurology and Neurosurgery, London, UK

P.O. Katz
Division of Gastroenterology, Albert Einstein Medical Center, Philadelphia, PA, USA

M.D. Kopelman
Institute of Psychiatry, Psychology and Neuroscience, King's College London, London, UK

K. LaFaver
Movement Disorders Clinic, University of Louisville, Louisville, KY, USA

W.C. LaFrance Jr.
Division of Neuropsychiatry and Behavioral Neurology, Rhode Island Hospital, Providence, RI, USA

A.E. Lang
Morton and Gloria Shulman Movement Disorders Clinic and the Edmond J. Safra Program in Parkinson's Disease, University Health Network, Toronto Western Hospital, Toronto, Ontario, Canada

A. Lehn
Department of Neurology, Princess Alexandra Hospital and School of Medicine, University of Queensland, Brisbane, Australia

J.L. Levenson
Department of Psychiatry, Virginia Commonwealth University School of Medicine, Richmond, VA, USA

L. Ludwig
Departments of Clinical Neurosciences and of Rehabilitation Medicine, NHS Lothian and Centre for Clinical Brain Sciences, University of Edinburgh, Edinburgh, UK

H.J. Markowitsch
Department of Physiological Psychology, University of Bielefeld, Bielefeld, Germany

D.J. McFerran
Department of Otolaryngology, Colchester Hospital University, Colchester, UK

L. McWhirter
Department of Clinical Neurosciences, Western General Hospital, Edinburgh, UK

J.D.C. Mellers
Department of Neuropsychiatry, Maudsley Hospital, South London and Maudsley NHS Foundation Trust, Denmark Hill, London, UK

N.J. Newman
Department of Ophthalmology, Department of Neurology, and Department of Neurological Surgery, Emory University Hospital, Emory University School of Medicine, Atlanta, GA, USA

T.R.J. Nicholson
Section of Cognitive Neuropsychiatry, Institute of Psychiatry, Psychology and Neuroscience, King's College London, London, UK

G. Nielsen
Sobell Department of Motor Neuroscience and Movement Disorders, UCL Institute of Neurology and Therapy Services, National Hospital for Neurology and Neurosurgery, Queen Square, London, UK

J.N. Panicker
Department of Uro-Neurology, The National Hospital for Neurology and Neurosurgery and UCL Institute of Neurology, Queen Square, London

J. Pasman
Behavioural Science Institute, Radboud University Nijmegen, Nijmegen, The Netherlands

A. Piedimonte
Department of Neuroscience, University of Turin Medical School, Turin, Italy

V. Phé
Department of Uro-Neurology, The National Hospital for Neurology and Neurosurgery, London, UK and Department of Urology, Pitié-Salpêtrière Academic Hospital, Paris, France

R. Ranieri
Department of Psychiatry, Università degli Studi di Milano, Ospedale San Paolo, Milan, Italy

G.H. Rawlings
Academic Neurology Unit, University of Sheffield, Sheffield, UK

M. Reuber
Academic Neurology Unit, University of Sheffield, Sheffield, UK

E.H. Reynolds
Institute of Epileptology, King's College, Denmark Hill, London, UK

K. Roelofs
Behavioural Science Institute, Radboud University Nijmegen and Donders Institute for Brain Cognition and Behaviour, Nijmegen, The Netherlands

K.S. Rommelfanger
Department of Neurology, Department of Psychiatry and Neuroethics Program, Center for Ethics, Emory University, Atlanta, GA, USA

D.A. Schmerler
Gardner Family Center for Parkinson's Disease and Movement Disorders, Department of Neurology, University of Cincinnati, Cincinnati, OH, USA

P. Schwingenschuh
Department of Neurology, Medical University of Graz, Graz, Austria

M. Sharpe
Department of Psychiatry, University of Oxford, Oxford, UK

J.P. Staab
Department of Psychiatry and Psychology, Mayo Clinic, Rochester, MN, USA

A. Staniloiu
Department of Physiological Psychology, University of Bielefeld, Bielefeld, Germany and Department of Psychiatry, Sunnybrook Hospital, Toronto, ON, Canada

M.-P. Stenner
Wellcome Trust Centre for Neuroimaging, Institute of Neurology, London, UK and Department of Neurology, Otto-von-Guericke-University Magdeburg, Magdeburg, Germany

J. Stone
Department of Clinical Neurosciences, Centre for Clinical Brain Sciences, University of Edinburgh, Edinburgh, UK

M.A. Thenganatt
Parkinson's Disease Center and Movement Disorders Clinic, Department of Neurology, Baylor College of Medicine, Houston, TX, USA

M. Tinazzi
Department of Neurological and Movement Sciences, University of Verona, Italy

M.A.J. Tijssen
Department of Neurology, University Medical Centre Groningen, Groningen, The Netherlands

M. Trimble
Institute of Neurology, Queen Square, London, UK

M. Vermeulen
Department of Neurology, Academic Medical Center, Amsterdam, The Netherlands

V. Voon
Department of Psychiatry, Behavioural and Clinical Neurosciences Institute, University of Cambridge, Cambridge, UK

P. Vuilleumier
Laboratory for Behavioural Neurology and Imaging of Cognition, Department of Neuroscience, University of Geneva-Campus Biotech, Geneva, Switzerland

K. Welch
Departments of Clinical Neurosciences and of Rehabilitation Medicine, NHS Lothian and Centre for Clinical Brain Sciences, University of Edinburgh, Edinburgh, UK

D.T. Williams
Movement Disorders Division, Columbia University Medical Center and Department of Psychiatry, Columbia College of Physicians and Surgeons, New York, NY, USA

S. Williams
Department of Clinical Neurosciences, Western General Hospital, Edinburgh, UK

Contents

Section 1

History

Handbook of Clinical Neurology, Vol. 139 (3rd series)
Functional Neurologic Disorders
M. Hallett, J. Stone, and A. Carson, Editors
http://dx.doi.org/10.1016/B978-0-12-801772-2.00001-1

Chapter 1

A brief history of hysteria: From the ancient to the modern

M. TRIMBLE[1]* AND E.H. REYNOLDS[2]
[1]*Institute of Neurology, Queen Square, London, UK*
[2]*Institute of Epileptology, King's College, Denmark Hill, London, UK*

Abstract

In this paper we discuss the history of hysteria from the Babylonian and Assyrian texts through to the situation as it appears to us at the end of the 19th century. We note the shifting emphasis on causation, earlier ideas being linked to uterine theories, later speculations moving to the brain, and then the mind. We note the persistence of the condition referred to as hysteria over the millennia and the fascination that the condition has held for physicians, neurologists, and psychiatrists since the origins of known medical texts.

INTRODUCTION

For various reasons it is impracticable to begin this article with a definition of hysteria. However familiar the name and the disease there is difference of opinion as to the precise connotation of the term and as to its clinical limitations. Our ideas on hysteria are in a state of flux, due in part to the fact that rival theories of its nature hold the field and show little sign of harmonising themselves (Kinnier Wilson, 1919).

This quotation from Kinnier Wilson's review nearly a century ago is as appropriate today as it was for many centuries before it was written. It is doubtful if there is any word in the medical vocabulary, other than hysteria, that has changed its meaning and associated clinical phenomena more often in the two and a half millennia since it was first coined in the *Corpus Hippocraticum* around 400 BC.

As foreshadowed by Kinnier Wilson, there has been a litany of synonymous diagnostic labels in the 20th century, reflecting fluctuations in clinical concepts and interpretations. These include hysterical neurosis, conversion disorder, somatoform disorder, dissociative disorder, posttraumatic stress disorder, psychogenic disorder and, as in the title of this *Handbook*, functional neurologic disorder. The one thing they all have in common is that they converge in some way on the mysterious relationship between brain and mind. But in the long history of hysteria this focus on the brain and mind is a relatively recent phenomenon in the last 500 years.

As is widely acknowledged, the English word "hysteria" is of Greek origin, linked in various ways to the womb. Recent scholarship, for example, Veith (1965) and King (1993), has led to considerable debate about the meaning of *hysterikos* and its derivatives, which can be and have been variously translated in several volumes of the *Corpus*, especially the three known as "Diseases of Women," as "all diseases of the womb," "from the womb," "connected with the womb," "liable to disorders of the womb," "suffocation of the womb," as well as "movement or wandering of the womb." We need not concern ourselves with these various nuances now, not least because since the 17th century the focus has moved or wandered from the womb to the brain. However, three general points from the *Corpus* are worth stressing: (1) the Greek word or words never described a specific clinical diagnostic entity, but only an explanation for a multitude of symptoms or diseases, many of them gynecologic or related to pregnancy and its complications, but also symptoms related to pressure or influence on other organs of the abdominal or thoracic cavities; (2) this led to the subsequent view that

*Correspondence to: Professor Michael Trimble, The National Hospital for Neurology and Neurosurgery, Queen Square, London WC1N 3BG, UK. Tel: +44-20-3456-7890, E-mail: mtrimble@ion.ucl.ac.uk

"hysteria" as a diagnostic concept was a disorder of women; and (3) although Littré (1849) in his 19th-century French translation of the *Corpus* tried to distinguish between "imaginary" and "real" movements of the uterus, King (1993) is certain that this is a retrospective and erroneous application of 19th-century concepts to ancient texts. King is clear that all the symptoms described in the *Corpus*, gynecologic or otherwise, were viewed by Greek physicians as "real" or "organic."

Early in the 17th century, the focus of attention gradually switched from the uterus to the brain as the organ of hysteria, although initially the uterus was thought to influence the brain by "sympathetic" mechanisms involving blood vessels or nerves (e.g., Harvey, 1651). At the same time it dawned that males could also suffer from hysteria, which became linked to hypochondria and melancholy by some authorities, such as Burton (1621) and Sydenham (1682). Throughout the 18th and 19th centuries hysteria was widely classified as one of the neuroses in the original sense of the word as a disorder of function of the nervous system (Whytt, 1751; Cullen, 1777). Increasingly "the mind," in addition to the body, was also viewed as an important source or trigger of hysteric symptoms.

"Animal spirits" and "passions" in the 17th century were gradually replaced in the 18th and 19th centuries by emotions, imagination, ideas, and attention to social and cultural influences acting on the brain. With the increasing development of neuropathology in the 19th century, some continued to look for a pathologic explanation in the nervous system for hysteria. The failure of this search was associated with increasing awareness that the neurologic symptoms of hysteria often mimicked so-called "organic" nervous system disorders but could be clinically distinguished by careful attention to the characteristic neurologic symptoms and signs (e.g., Paget, 1873; Charcot, 1881). This in turn gave rise to the concept feigning of neurologic disease. Finally, in the late 19th and early 20th centuries new psychologic theories evolved invoking subconscious concepts such as "dissociation," "conversion," intrapsychic conflict, repression, and secondary gain (e.g., Freud, 1894; Janet, 1907).

Modern understanding of hysteria continues to be dominated by these psychologic concepts but, as will be apparent from this *Handbook*, some have not yet given up hope of identifying disorders of function in the nervous system that may explain the symptoms and signs. Thus, the title of this book, *Functional Neurologic Disorders*, may be viewed as ambiguous. The word "functional" is widely used to imply a psychologic disorder but can be used in the sense of a disorder of function of the nervous system, a physiologic connotation. Perhaps this ambiguity is fair in our present state of relative ignorance and uncertainty in the continuing state of flux of our understanding of hysteria over the centuries.

If many now view hysteria as neurologic symptoms and signs which cannot be explained by our present understanding of nervous system structure or function, can we detect evidence of hysteria, as currently conceived, in ancient or more recent accounts of so-called hysteria (or other diseases)?

BABYLON AND ASSYRIA

The earliest descriptions of what we now call neurologic and psychiatric disorders date from the Old Babylonian Dynasty of the first half of the second millennium BC. In cuneiform tablets located in museums in London, Paris, Berlin, Istanbul, and elsewhere, Reynolds and Kinnier Wilson (2014) have studied detailed descriptions of what are now termed epilepsy, stroke, facial palsy, psychoses, obsessive-compulsive disorder, psychopathic behavior, depression, and anxiety. The Babylonians were remarkably acute and objective observers of medical disorders and human behavior, but they had no knowledge of the brain or of psychologic function. They simply documented the clinical features of many of the common neuropsychiatric disorders we recognize today, most of which they viewed as supernatural in origin, although some forms of paralysis might have a physical basis, for example after a snake bite or scorpion sting.

The Babylonian descriptions are entirely objective without any account of subjective phenomena such as obsessional thoughts or ruminations in obsessive-compulsive disorder or sadness in depression. They do recognize disturbances of behavior such as the liar, the thief, the trouble maker, the sexual offender, the immature, the violent, and the social misfit, which they mostly viewed as a mystery yet to be resolved. Reynolds and Kinnier Wilson have not yet encountered any descriptions which might be recognizable in modern terms as hysteria. This is hardly surprising, as the Babylonians were only documenting for the first time neuropsychiatric disorders without any knowledge of neuropathology or psychopathology. At that time they would almost certainly have found it impossible to distinguish mimicry of the disorders they were first describing, even if it existed, which is questionable.

A later possible link to hysteria in the late second millennium or early first millennium BC in Assyria are three possible examples of posttraumatic stress disorder in military casualties which are referred to in the textbook on Assyrian and Babylonian medicine by Scurlock and Andersen (2005) and which have been extracted and amplified by Abdul-Hamid and Hughes (2014). Symptoms included: "If his words are unintelligible for three days"; "He experiences wandering about for three days";

"A roaming ghost afflicts him"; and, "If in the evening, he sees either a living person or a dead person or someone known to him or someone not known to him or anybody or anything and becomes afraid; he turns around, but like one who has [been hexed with?] rancid oil, his mouth is seized so that he is unable to cry out to one who sleeps next to him, 'hand' of ghost."

Scurlock and Andersen also include the words "mentation" and "depression" in their translations, but no such words existed in the Mesopotamian languages and are retrospective projections from modern medicine and psychology. The Assyrians and Babylonians had no knowledge or concept of brain or mind, but they did observe and document behavior. Abdul-Hamid and Hughes conclude that generally the clinical features are compatible with posttraumatic stress disorder, especially nocturnal sleep disorder, fear, mutism, and possibly nightmares. "Ghosts" were a common explanation for Babylonian/Assyrian medical and behavioral disorders and in this instance they may have been the "ghosts" of enemy killed in battle. The authors acknowledged that they could not exclude the possibility that some of the symptoms were due to traumatic brain injury.

A possible example of hysteria has been suggested for the speech disturbance of King Mursili II of the Hittites around 1200 BC. The Hittites occupied areas of modern Turkey and Syria to the north of Assyria. The clinical details of the King's affliction are sketchy. The King was caught out in a thunderstorm. The Storm God was immensely important to the Hittites. The King was terrified and experienced a temporary speech disturbance, possibly mutism. He recovered but many years later had frequent nightmares about the incident, in one of which he awoke with a temporary disturbance of his speech or his "mouth." Most of the text was taken up with methods of appeasing the Storm God. This account was first translated by Goetze and Pedersen in 1934 and interpreted by Oppenheim (1956) as hysteric aphonia, a view endorsed by Kinnier Wilson (1967).

ANCIENT EGYPT

According to York and Steinberg (2009), we cannot say that the ancient Egyptians had any meaningful neurology. These authors noted that modern specialists are especially attracted to Ancient Egypt with its own specialization and strict ranks of social order for various physicians, but it would be wrong to read too much into Egyptian medical practices. We know little of their theories, values, or perspectives, and our knowledge of their medicine is so fragmentary that we dare not assert a certain understanding of it.

Like Babylonian and Assyrian medicine, Egyptian medicine was a compound of rational, magical, and religious elements. It seems probable, however, that less of the more fragile Egyptian medical papyri have survived than Mesopotamian cuneiform clay tablets. In a textbook on *Ancient Egyptian Medicine* (Nunn, 1996) there is no mention of the brain, or what we might view as neurologic disorder. Like the Babylonians and Assyrians, the Egyptians appear to have had no understanding of the brain or of psychologic function. Emotion and knowledge were related to the heart, as much later attested also by Aristotle. There is no certain evidence of stroke in ancient Egyptian texts (Reynolds and Kinnier Wilson, 2004). This may be because the relevant documents are yet to be found. The nearest the Egyptians came to a possible link between the brain and motor function is case 8 of the Edwin Smith papyrus, in which a comminuted skull fracture was associated with limping on the same side of the body. It is by no means certain that the limping was linked in the ancient mind to the brain (York and Steinberg, 2009). In case 22 of the same papyrus head trauma is described in the temple region with extracranial bleeding, loss of consciousness, and neck stiffness, but there is no record of paralysis (Reynolds and Kinnier Wilson, 2004).

None of the above considerations deterred Veith (1965) from detecting "hysteria" in ancient Egypt or in linking it to a "wandering womb." Based on interpretations of the Kahun papyrus (1900 BC) and the Ebers papyrus (1600 BC), the clinical symptoms were mainly pain in various parts of the body, including eye sockets, teeth, jaws, neck, and limbs, which, it is claimed, were related to the position of the womb. However, later study of the same two papyri by Merskey and Potter (1989) cast great doubt on Veith's view. In particular, when these texts blamed the uterus for a symptom at a distance it is never said to be mobile, and when it is said to be out of its place (usually by prolapse), symptoms at a distance are not described. Thus there is no warrant for the fanciful view that the ancient Egyptians believed that a variety of bodily complaints were due to an animate (wandering) womb (Merskey and Potter, 1989). Likewise, it seems that Veith's suggestion that the Greek concept of the "wandering womb" was transmitted from Egyptian medicine is doubtful.

GREECE AND ROME

As already noted, the word hysteria originated in the *Corpus Hippocraticum* in the fourth/third centuries BC as an explanation for a multitude of gynecologic and medical symptoms suspected in the Greek mind to be linked to the womb. Searching in this literature for "modern" examples of hysteria, i.e., linked to brain and mind, is a difficult task as Greek descriptions of illness or disease were frequently brief or fragmentary and overridden with much more detailed accounts of interpretation and treatment, whether natural, as in the influence of the womb (or brain), or supernatural, associated with numerous gods (Simon, 1978).

Micale (1989) states that the *Corpus* contains "no coherent clinical syndrome in the modern sense but only the most casual enumeration of symptoms, including laboured breathing, loss of voice, neck pain, heart palpitations, dizziness, vomiting and sweating." On the other hand, Veith (1965) suggests that in the book on epidemics there is a convincing account of hysteric mutism in the wife of Polemarchus. Veith also suggests a hysteric motor disorder in a woman in whom: "Following a short and insignificant cough she experienced a paralysis of the right upper limb and the left lower limb, nothing in the face, nothing affecting her intelligence. This woman began to improve on the 20th day."

As will be discussed in more detail in later centuries and sections of this review, the differential diagnosis between epilepsy and hysteric convulsions has always been difficult. Already Hippocrates was suggesting for the first time that "The Sacred Disease" arose in the brain, but did he and some of his colleagues distinguish genuine convulsions of cerebral origin from hysteric convulsions influenced by the womb? It is difficult to say, but both Veith (1965) and Merskey (1995) referred to the example of convulsions from which the patient can be awoken if the abdominal skin is pressurized or pinched.

The concept of a wandering womb causing medical havoc by behaving like an animal within an animal seems to have been influential over the next 500 years, from Plato to Aretaeus of Cappadocia. Among the many isolated symptoms attributed to this behavior are choking, and difficulties with breathing or speech. Whether any such symptoms were hysteric in the modern sense is impossible to discern.

By the second century AD both Soranus of Ephasus and Galen of Pergamon and Rome denied that the womb can wander, but both accepted that a diseased or dysfunctional womb can have remote medical influences. Soranus, for example, refers to symptoms of obstructed respiration, loss of voice, and a "seizure of the senses."

Galen (*c.*130–*c.*201 AD) was the most influential physician of his era and, among other achievements, he understood the influence of emotion on the body, for example, the pulse (Veith, 1965). He was perhaps the earliest exponent of what is now sometimes called psychosomatic medicine. In his treatise on "That the mental faculties follow the bodily constitution" he develops a theory of reciprocal influences of mind and body on each other (Galen, 1929). And yet he did not apply this to hysteria.

According to Veith (1965), Galen recognized three categories of hysteric symptoms in women: (1) episodes of lost consciousness; (2) collapse from weakness and breathing difficulties without loss of consciousness; and (3) contractures of the limbs. Recognizing that these symptoms more commonly occurred in the absence of sexual relations, especially in widows, Galen developed a unique uterine theory of his own in which he assumed that the healthy active uterus produced a secretion analogous to semen in males. Retention or repression of the seminal secretion resulted in hysteric symptoms through corruption of the blood or irritation of the nerves. A corollary of his hypothesis was that hysteric symptoms could also occur in males by a similar mechanism.

It is a remarkable fact that, although Galen had an early understanding of emotional influences on the body and he observed the link between sexual abstinence and hysteric symptoms, he developed a modified physical uterine theory of his own which, such was his influence, perpetuated the concept of hysteria as a disorder of the womb for more than a further millennium.

MIDDLE AGES

The Middle Ages, with its neo-Platonic theologic stranglehold on developing scientific thought, and thus on the medical sciences, often conflated the manifestations that we would now view as hysteria with those of witchcraft. The book *Malleus Maleficarium* was used from the late 1400s as a text on the identification of the signs of witchcraft, which included the presence of seizures (Institoris et al., 1948). Witchcraft first became a statutory crime in 1541, a date which heralded 200 years of witch hunting and persecution. The detection of witches became paramount, and stigmata were identified. In particular, "witches' patches", i.e., areas of sensory anesthesia, were recorded, but the muscular contortions and convulsions of the afflicted were also well documented. King James I of England and VI of Scotland in 1597 published *Daemonologie, in the Forme of a Dialogue,* an attempt to re-emphasize the dangers of witchcraft. This increased the enthusiasm for witch hunting, with more and more witches being identified, especially by the anesthetic patches, and brought before the courts.

Edward Jorden (1603), a physician of London and Bath, wrote a treatise called *A Brief Discourse of a Disease Called the Suffocation of the Mother* to counteract the prevailing view, which was to attribute such symptoms to possession by some supernatural power (Trimble, 1982). His view was that the so-thought stigmata of hysteria were in fact signs of mental illness, thus reclaiming, for the first time since Hippocrates and Galen, the essentially medical, somatic nature of the phenomena. He considered the passions of the body to have natural causes, and, while the uterus was the seat of the pathology, "sympathy" explained distant effects.

Jorden recognized the polymorphous nature of the symptoms, its link to the female sex, and the importance of "perturbations of the mind" in the cause of the disorder.

With Jorden's account we had not only the first English book on hysteria, including hysteric convulsions, but another example of medical opinion breaking down supernatural theories of causation. Here were also the beginnings of ideas of conversion of symptoms from one part of the body to another, with sympathetic reactions between one organ and another, and hints at a psychotherapeutic treatment. Jorden opined that the brain was involved, the animal faculty becoming disturbed, accounting for sensory and motor symptoms, the beginning of a shift of psychiatric symptoms away from the uterus to the brain.

Jorden was not alone in his beliefs. The Dutch physician Johann Weyer was one of the first whose major interest was in mental disorders, especially in women, and published in 1563 De Praestigiis Daemonum et Incantationibus ac Venificiis [*On the Deceptions of the Demons and on Spells and Poisons*]. This was an attack on the *Witches' Hammer* (*Malleus Maleficarium*). He examined a number of the accused himself, and reported his findings, which were early examples of the psychiatric method of examination. He discussed differences between medical illness and malingering, which he discovered in certain patients.

MASS HYSTERIA

Outbreaks of mass hysteria, in which groups of people manifested mainly motor abnormalities, were well described in the Middle Ages, and culminated in the grand chorea epidemics of Europe. Outbursts of St. Vitus' dance, tarantism, *convulsionnaires,* and the like referred to groups of people, from half a dozen to several hundred, who would display exaggerated movements, dance, and convulse until they dropped exhausted (Waller, 2008). Many episodes were noted in relation to natural disasters, for example, after the spread of the great plague, but other outbreaks came in closely knit social groups, often united by some strong religious belief. These phenomena emphasized the imitative nature of many hysteric afflictions, and the powerful role of social and cultural pressure, and contagion in their pathogenesis.

WILLIS (1621–1675) AND THE BEGINNINGS OF NEUROLOGY

Concepts of etiology slowly moved from the supernatural to the natural. The uterus remained popular, but several other shifts of emphasis occurred. The uterine theories slowly gave way to two interpenetrating themes, namely that the main organ involved in hysteria was the brain, and that somehow emotions were highly relevant. The English neurologist Thomas Willis was one of the first to espouse the central importance of the brain. He reflected that "this passion comes not from the vapours rising into the head from the uterus or spleen, nor from a rapid flow of blood into the pulmonary vessels, but has its origin in the brain itself" (Dewhurst, 1980). He was led to this conclusion, not only following postmortem examinations and by his clinical observations of the disorder in prepubertal and senile women, but by the irreconcilable fact that he observed hysteria in men! For Willis the condition was primarily convulsive: "the distemper named from the womb is chiefly and primarily convulsive, and chiefly depends on the brain and nervous stock being affected" (Willis, 1684). Hysteric fits were caused by "spirits inhabiting the brain, now being prepared for explosions." Since, in further studies, Willis came to the conclusion that it was the animal spirits in the middle part of the brain that were disturbed in epilepsy, he must have thought that both epileptic and nonepileptic convulsions have a similar basis.

The emphasis on the emotions was taken up by several writers, including Sydenham (1682), who opined that, of all chronic medical conditions, next to infections, hysteria in his practice was the commonest, afflicting one-sixth of patients. Not only did Sydenham suggest the chronic nature of the condition, but he hinted at personality contributions. Patients were prone to irritability and anger outbursts; they were capricious, and labile in their moods and affections. He firmly placed the origins of hysteria in the mind, referring to "over-ordinate commotions of the mind," with a "faulty disposition of the animal spirits" (Payne, 1900). In an analysis of the diagnosis of hysteria by several well-reputed doctors of the 17th century in England, 6–10% of patients were so diagnosed. Further, its form and characteristics were inscribed into the popular lay health manuals and it was a part of everyday doctor–patient discourse (Williams History of Psychiatry).

Associations with what we may now refer to as depression were noted in Burton's *The Anatomy of Melancholy* (1621), and the concept that the mind could influence the body, a precursor of 20th-century psychosomatic concepts, became well accepted. The Scottish physician Whytt, discoverer of reflex activity in the nervous system, and one who recognized that the mind could cause actions not appreciated by consciousness, discussed the newly invented term "nervous disorders," namely those "which, on account of an unusual delicacy, or unnatural state of the nerves, are produced by causes, which, in people of a sound constitution, would either have no such effects, or at least in a much less degree." In a passage which antedated the later importance given to psychologically traumatic events, he opined: "Thus doleful or moving stories, horrible or unexpected sights, great grief, anger, terror and other passions, frequently occasion the most sudden and violent nervous symptoms" (Whytt, 1751).

18th AND 19th CENTURIES

A close link between hysteria and epilepsy continued throughout the 18th and 19th centuries. Boerhaave felt that hysteria could degenerate into epilepsy and Cheyne (1733), in his book, *The English Malady or a Treatise of Nervous Diseases of All Kinds as Spleen, Vapours, Lowness of Spirits, Hypochondriacal and Hysterical Distempers,* noted few differences between epilepsy and hysteria, saying that the former

> *differs very little or not at all, or at most in a few circumstances only, from Hypochondriacal and Hysteric Fits: which last when violent, terminate always in these Epileptik Fits, as they, on the other hand, when they become weak, dwindle into the Hysterik Kind.*

Themes of either sexual frustration or sexual excess in hysteria inherent in names such as *hysteria libidinosa* or *furor uterinus,* while tending to wane in the 18th century, continued to resurface. Laycock (1840), teacher of Hughlings Jackson (1835–1911), wrote about the reciprocal relationships between the body and mind, developing a biologically oriented scientific psychology. He believed that the nervous system was implicated in hysteria, which disorder was seen in the majority of cases in females of child-bearing ages, and therefore the generative organs were involved in the pathogenesis. The condition often came on following grief, terror, fear, or disappointment in love; these emotional events excited deranged actions in the generative system and thence the hysteric phenomena.

Laycock's investigations led him to speculate into the nature of the mind, and on the role of consciousness in these phenomena. Following on from Whytt's studies of reflex activity and Marshall Hall's (1833) demonstration in animals of the spinal reflex arc, Laycock suggested that the cerebrum (cranial ganglia) was also a reflex center like the spinal ganglia, and he developed his law of the unconscious functional activity of the brain. This was several decades before the Freudian elaboration.

The general practitioner, later ophthalmologist, Carter (1853) divided hysteria into two main forms: simple, which manifest essentially as hysteric seizures, and complicated. The latter, foreshadowing the later Briquet's form, "generally involves much moral and intellectual, as well as physical derangement, and when it is fully established, the primary convulsion, the *fons et origo mali* is sometimes suffered to fall into obeyance … being arrested by the urgency of new maladies." He implicated sexual emotions as causative, and shifted the whole debate away from pathology of the sexual organs to inhibited sexual passions. This was, according to Veith (1965), the first theory of repression. Emotions led to physical disorders by somatic discharge, affects provoking the wide range of motor and sensory states seen in the condition. Interestingly, Carter also observed the factitious nature of the illness in many patients, some using leeches in the mouth to produce bleeding, or bandages to cause limb swellings and the like. Since the time of Sydenham in the 17th century, when the chameleon-like and simulative nature of hysteria was recognized, this seems one of the first texts to raise the question of the patient's motives and actions more directly.

Thus, summarizing the history of hysteria from the 17th to the mid 19th century, several new concepts emerged. The condition "hysteria" had been recognized for millennia, and had always been the source of much speculation regarding etiology and pathogenesis. It is not clear how many patients given this diagnosis by earlier physicians were in reality suffering from now-recognized neurologic disorders. Many nosologic and diagnostic confusions continued to exist. Causation had now shifted away from the uterus to the brain, and then to the mind. Psychosomatic concepts were readily accepted, for example, emotions, especially sexual, discharging through the somatic apparatus to provoke the polymorphous, often bizarre symptomatology, recognized as hysteria. The potential chronicity of the condition was well recorded, as was its occurrence in males. Certain personality types seemed more susceptible, and external exciting causes such as accidents could be relevant. Convulsions were often specifically discussed as an emblem of hysteria.

As the 19th century progressed, there was an explosion of interest in hysteria, although the main writings came not from England, but from France. Not only did the sexual theme become revived, but also the concept of posttraumatic hysteria crystallized. Some of the early-19th-century French physicians, such as Pinel, Louyer-Villermay, and Landouzy reverted to uterine theories, challenging the concept of male hysteria. However, cerebral origins of hysteria found increasing support through Georget and Briquet. The latter was chief physician to the Paris *Charité* hospital, and he admitted that he undertook to study hysteria as a matter of duty, on account of the frequency of cases that he reluctantly had to examine. His book, *Traité Clinique et Therapeutique de l'Hystérie* (Briquet, 1859), was based on personal examinations of nearly 450 patients, and stands as the 19th-century landmark in hysteria studies, having a considerable influence on Charcot and his school.

Briquet firmly rejected uterine theories, and described a series of cases in males. He outlined the multifarious symptoms, including the spasms, anesthesias, convulsions, paralyses, and contractures, which, by then had become familiar in descriptions of patients diagnosed as hysteria. He emphasized the potential chronicity of the disorder. Of 418 patients, 179 had the condition for between 6 months and 4 years, 81 between 5 and 10 years, and of the rest, in 59 patients the disorder lasted longer than 20 years, in 5 patients for 55 years. These patients were polysymptomatic, "des troubles permanents qui portent sur presque tous les organes." The latter were clearly examples of what was later called Briquet's hysteria.

As to pathogenesis, Briquet was clear that it was a condition of that portion of the brain which received sensations and affective impressions. He described hysteria as a nervousness (neurosis) of the encephalon. However, he recognized many interacting factors. These included heredity, emotional predisposition and lability, and impressionability. He described several antecedents, including physical and emotional trauma or abuse. Incidentally, Briquet was critical of the term hysteria, but felt it should be continued to be used because it had been in use so long and everyone understood its meaning. The hysteria mantle than fell to Charcot, the doyen of mid to late-19th-century French neurology, and his school of successors, taken up in Chapter 2.

CONCLUSIONS

The history of hysteria is long, complicated, fluctuating, and central to the history of medicine and neuropsychiatry, especially epilepsy. Patients with medically unexplained syndromes have been recognized in many different cultures for up to 4000 years, and the term hysteria has been used with various meanings to describe many such patients for approximately 2500 years. In the last 500 years the focus has gradually shifted, firstly, from uterine theories in females to brain and mind explanations in males and females; and, more recently, from theoretic concepts to a greater emphasis on detailed clinical descriptions, especially neurologic and psychologic, as illustrated in this *Handbook*.

The history of hysteria provides a perspective of medical practice and social commentary over many centuries. It has appeal and relevance well beyond the field of clinical medicine to psychology, sociology, history, and literature. It is intimately linked to concepts of causality involving cerebral anatomy and physiology, personality, deception, unconscious forces, social influences, and continuing attempts to understand brain–mind relationships. No agreed definition of hysteria has ever been possible and its meaning has changed with historic epochs. It has probably always been with us. Some view it as a snare and a delusion (Slater, 1965). Others point out that it has always outlived its obituarists (Lewis, 1975). We can agree with Kinnier Wilson (1919), a century ago, that hysteria remains in a state of flux.

References

Abdul-Hamid WK, Hughes JH (2014). Nothing new under the sun: post-traumatic stress disorders in the ancient world. Early Sci Med 19: 549–557.

Briquet P (1859). Traité Clinique et Therapeutique de l'Hystérie. J-B Balliere, Paris.

Burton R (1621). The Anatomy of Melancholy, Longman, Rees, London.

Carter RB (1853). On the Pathology and Treatment of Hysteria, Churchill, London.

Charcot JM (1881). In: P Richer (Ed.), Etudes Cliniques sur la Grande Hystérie ou Hystéro-épilepsie. Delahaye et Lecrosnier, Paris.

Cheyne G (1733). The English Malady; or a Treatise of Nervous Diseases of All Kinds, as Spleen, Vapours, Lowness of Spirit, Hypochondriacal and Hysterical Distempers etc, Strahan and Leake, London.

Cullen W (1777). First lines of the Practice of Physic, Creech, Edinburgh.

Dewhurst K (1980). Thomas Willis' Oxford Lectures, Sanford Publications, Oxford.

Freud S (1894). The psycho-neuroses of defence. In: J Strachey (Ed.), The Complete Psychological Works, Vol. 3. Hogarth, London.

Galen C (1929). That the mental faculties follow the bodily constitution. In: AJ Brock (Ed.), Greek Medicine, JM Dent, London, p. 233.

Goetze A, Pedersen H (1934). Muršilis Sprachlähmung, Levin and Munksgaard, Copenhagen.

Hall M (1833). On the reflex function of the medulla oblongata and medulla spinalis. Phil Trans Roy Soc 123: 635–665.

Harvey W (1651). Exertionates de generatione animalium. In: R Willis (Ed.), The Works of William Harvey, 1847, The Sydenham Society, London.

Institoris H, Sprenger J, Sommers H (1948). Malleus Maleficarium, Pushkin, London.

Janet P (1907). The Major Symptoms of Hysteria, Macmillan, London.

Jorden E (1603). A Disease Called the Suffocation of Mother, John Windet, London.

King H (1993). Once upon a text: hysteria from Hippocrates. In: SL Gilman, H King, R Porter et al. (Eds.), Hysteria beyond Freud, University of California Press, Berkeley, CA.

King James I of England and VI of Scotland (1597). Daemonologie, in the forme of a dialogue.

Kinnier Wilson SA (1919). Hysteria. In: JW Ballentyne (Ed.), Encylopedia Medica, VI. Edinburgh, W Green, pp. 315–351.

Kinnier Wilson JV (1967). Mental diseases of ancient Mesopotamia. In: D Brothwell, AT Sandison (Eds.),

Diseases in Antiquity: A Survey of the Diseases, Injuries and Surgery of Early Populations, Springfield, IL, Charles C Thomas, pp. 723–733.

Laycock T (1840). An Essay on Hysteria, Barrington and Haswell, Philadelphia.

Lewis A (1975). The survival of hysteria. Psychol Med 5: 9–12.

Littré E (1849). Hippocrate: Oeuvres Completès, 10 Volumes. JB Baillière, Paris.

Merskey H (1995). The Analysis of Hysteria, 2nd edn. Gaskell, London.

Merskey H, Potter P (1989). The womb lay still in ancient Egypt. Br J Psychiatry 154: 751–753.

Micale M (1989). Hysteria and its hysteriography. A review of past and present writings. Hist Sci 27: 223–261, 319–351.

Nunn JF (1996). Ancient Egyptian Medicine, British Museum Press, London.

Oppenheim AL (1956). The interpretation of dreams in the ancient Near East. Trans Am Phil Soc 46: 230.

Paget J (1873). Nervous mimicry of organic diseases. Lancet 11: 511–513, 547–549, 619–621.

Payne JF (1900). Thomas Sydenham, T. Fisher Unwin, London.

Reynolds EH, Kinnier Wilson JV (2004). Stroke in Babylonia. Arch Neurol 61: 597–601.

Reynolds EH, Kinnier Wilson JV (2014). Neurology and psychiatry in Babylon. Brain 137: 2611–2619.

Scurlock JA, Andersen BR (2005). Diagnoses in Assyrian and Babylonian Medicine. Ancient Sources, Translations and Modern Medical Analyses, University of Illinois Press, Urbana.

Simon B (1978). Mind and Madness in Ancient Greece: The Classical Roots of Modern Psychiatry, Cornell University Press, Ithaca.

Slater E (1965). Diagnosis of hysteria. Br Med J 1: 1395–1399.

Sydenham T (1682). The Works of Thomas Sydenham, Sydenham Society, London.

Trimble MR (1982). Functional Diseases. BMJ 285: 1768–1770.

Veith I (1965). Hysteria: The History of a Disease, The University of Chicago Press, Chicago, IL.

Waller J (2008). A time to dance, a time to die: The extraordinary story of the dancing plague of 1518, Icon Books, Cambridge.

Weyer J (1563). De Praestigiis Daemonum et Incantationibus ac Verificiis. Libri V, Basileae: Ioannem Oporinum.

Whytt R (1751). Observations on the Nature, Causes and Cure of those Disorders which have been called Nervous, Hypochondiac or Hysteric, to which are Prefixed some Remarks on the Sympathy of the Nerves. Becket and Du Hodt, Edinburgh.

Williams History of Psychiatry. Hysteria in 17th century case records and unpublished manuscripts.

Willis T (1684). An Essay of the Pathology of the Brain and Nervous Stock in which Convulsive Diseases are treated. Translated from Latin by Pordage S. T Dring, J Leigh and C Harper, London.

York GK, Steinberg DA (2009). Neurology in ancient Egypt. In: S Finger, F Boller, KI Tyler (Eds.), Handbook of Clinical Neurology, vol 95. Elsevier, Amsterdam, pp. 29–36. (Third Series). History of Neurology.

Handbook of Clinical Neurology, Vol. 139 (3rd series)
Functional Neurologic Disorders
M. Hallett, J. Stone, and A. Carson, Editors
http://dx.doi.org/10.1016/B978-0-12-801772-2.00002-3

Chapter 2

Charcot, hysteria, and simulated disorders

C.G. GOETZ*

Department of Neurology and Department of Pharmacology, Rush University Medical Center, Chicago, IL, USA

Abstract

Jean-Martin Charcot (1825–1893) was the 19th-century's premier international neurologist. One of his areas of focused interest was the neurologic disorder, hysteria, a condition with distinctive neurologic signs, but no established structural lesions identified at autopsy. Charcot considered hysteria as a physiologic disorder that affected specific neuroanatomic areas of the brain comparable to the same areas that were damaged by structural neurologic disorders provoking the same or similar signs. He considered hysteria primarily a hereditary disorder, but environmental factors including physical and emotional stress served as provoking factors. Charcot drew the strict distinction between hysteria and consciously simulated neurologic disorders, although he was keenly aware that the two disorders could occur in the same patients or be difficult to distinguish at times. He developed specific experimental techniques to separate hysteria from simulation. His studies of hysteria and simulation offer a basis for studies of functional neurologic disorders applicable to the 21st century.

INTRODUCTION

On his neurologic unit at the Salpêtrière Hospital in Paris, the 19th-century French neurologist, Jean-Martin Charcot, studied many patients who today would likely be considered to have functional neurologic disorders. Collectively diagnosed primarily under the designation hysteria, these patients had a variety of focal neurologic signs, sometimes static and sometimes fleeting. Tremors, dystonic postures, chorea, stereotypies, and complex, often bizarre contortions were among the phenomena Charcot documented.

Although Charcot's intense interest in hysteria has prompted some historians to label him incorrectly as a psychiatrist, his views remained strictly entrenched in neuroanatomy. As such, even if vague references can be identified to suggest that Charcot considered psychologic stress or trauma as having an influence on hysteria, these effects were not a primary cause. In his view, hysteria, like all primary neurologic disorders, was a hereditary condition. The signs themselves were induced by a dynamic or physiologic change in neural function that was strictly anchored in neuroanatomic patterns seen in structural disorders that shared similar, though not identical, neurologic signs. In the face of criticism that his hysteric patients were simulating disease, Charcot carefully outlined clinical strategies to separate the two disorders.

Though these studies have been largely forgotten, as the modern field of psychogenic neurology emerges as a new research arena, Charcot's work on hysteria requires review as a historic foundation for contemporary work. A reconsideration of primary source documents from his lectures, case histories, and hospital notes provides insight into Charcot's views on anatomic, hereditary, and physiologic issues that re-emerge in the modern study of neurologic functional disorders.

THE PROTAGONIST

Jean-Martin Charcot (1825–1893) was the premier clinical neurologist of the 19th century (Goetz et al., 1995). He spent his entire career at the Salpêtrière Hospital in Paris and raised the institution from a hospice for old

*Correspondence to: Christopher G. Goetz, MD, Professor of Neurological Sciences, Professor of Pharmacology, Rush University Medical Center, 1725 W. Harrison Street, Chicago IL 60612, USA. Tel: +1-312-942-8016, Fax: +1-312-563-2024, E-mail: cgoetz@rush.edu

women into a Mecca of neurologic study. His lectures drew students and colleagues from around the world and trained a generation of younger neurologists who would largely dominate the neurologic world in the generation after his death (Goetz, 1989). The Charcot service was organized as a very tight and authoritatively managed unit with a core team, termed the *circle intime* or inner circle. Around this halo, there was a large array of visitors and students (Goetz, 1987). In 1882, he was named as Professor of Diseases of the Nervous System, the first chaired professorship in neurology of international stature (Fig. 2.1).

Charcot contributed to many areas of neurology and medicine, but his most important areas of research focused on three issues: (1) the development of a nosology or classification system for neurology (Bouchara, 2014); (2) the practical application of the anatomoclinical method, whereby he correlated for the first time specific clinical neurologic signs with focal anatomic lesions (Charcot, 1887a); and (3) the study of the neurologic disorder, hysteria (Micale, 1989).

Modern readers may consider the topic of hysteria to be outside the realm of neurology and more suitable to the research career of a psychiatrist. In the 19th century, however, hysteria was a specific, and, largely due to Charcot's work, well-defined neurologic diagnosis. Within Charcot's cases of hysteria, modern neurologists will find numerous cases that fit well into the current classification of functional neurologic disorders. As only one example, the celebrated group portrait of Charcot and his students, *A Clinical Lesson at the Salpêtrière,* by Brouillet, shows Charcot conducting an experiment in hypnotism, involving a young hysteric with a focal dystonic hand contraction (Fig. 2.2). The term, functional neurologic disorder, today incorporates the focal, unconsciously generated neurologic syndromes that Charcot considered as hysteria, and, like the *Diagnostic and Statistical Manual of Mental Disorders*, 5th

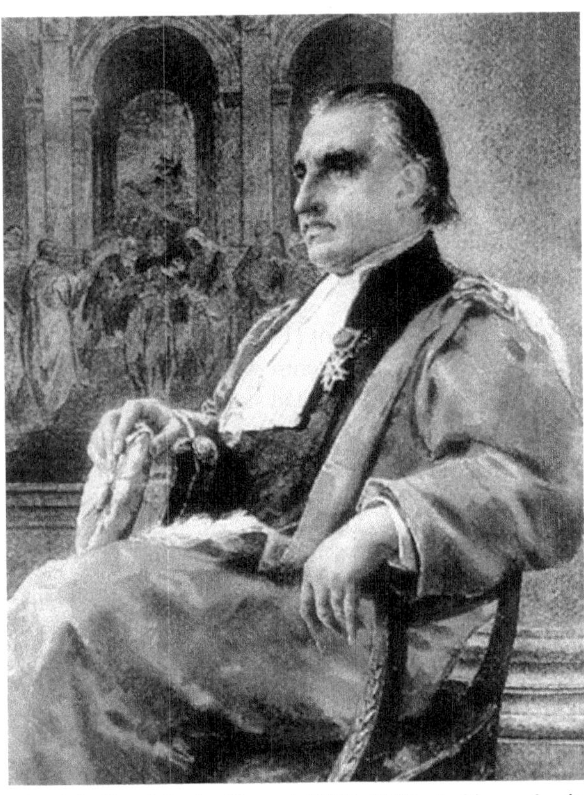

Fig. 2.1. Jean-Martin Charcot (1825–1893), in his academic robes, painted by E. Tofano in 1881. This portrait was commissioned and executed before Charcot was named as the newly created Chair of Diseases of the Nervous System in 1882. The picture is part of the personal collection of Christopher G. Goetz.

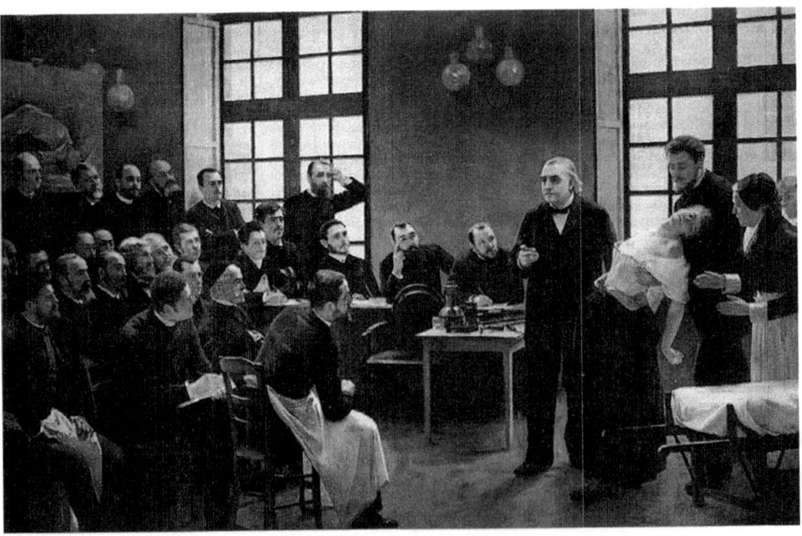

Fig. 2.2. *Une Leçon Clinique à la Salpêtrière* [*A Clinical Lesson at the Salpêtrière*] by Brouillet (1887), showing Charcot and a hysterical patient with a hand dystonia. The picture is of the personal collection of Christopher G. Goetz.

edition (DSM-5) (American Psychiatric Association, 2013), Charcot considered hysteria completely separate from malingering and conscious fabrication. Furthermore, psychogenic global symptoms of fatigue, headache, and malaise are encompassed in this modern term, though in the 19th century, they were considered under another diagnosis, neurasthenia, not specifically discussed in this presentation (Beard, 1869; Goetz, 2001).

To trace Charcot's neurologic contributions to psychogenic neurologic disorders, this study relies on primary source material written by Charcot and examines his views on the nosologic organization of neurologic disorders, his concept of disease etiology, and the diagnosis of hysteria as a primary neurologic disorder. A separate section discusses simulated neurologic illness and Charcot's methods for identifying such patients. With no attempt to obscure the theatric errors of Charcot's experiments on hysteria or his very likely misidentification of some subjects who were simulating their symptoms, this chapter offers modern neurologists a historic perspective of how the major 19th-century neurologist, whose training and fame were based on anatomic correlations with clinical signs, faced the reality that a group of patients with dramatic clinical signs had no evidence of structural anatomic lesions. His views offer a historic framework for current research efforts and emphasize that many seemingly modern concepts, physiologic, genetic, and environmental, were discussed and posited as research axes over a century ago.

CHARCOT'S NOSOLOGY: ORGANIC DISEASES AND THE *NÉVROSES*

Prior to Charcot, most neurologic disorders were described by large categories of symptoms and not by anatomic lesions. Motor disorders included weakness, spasms, and palsies. Multiple sclerosis and Parkinson's disease were not differentiated, and cases with either diagnosis were coalesced, because they both were marked by tremor. Charcot's clinical skills, discipline of a systematic methodology, and his large patient population allowed him to refine clinical categories, defining several disorders with both archetypal presentations as well as variants or *formes frustes*. With this clinical analysis, Charcot published the first major description of Parkinson's disease (Charcot, 1872a), supervised the seminal article by Gilles de la Tourette (1886) on tic disorders, and wrote on many forms of myelopathies (Charcot, 1877). These reports remain neurologic anchors of clinical description even in the 21st century.

The core of Charcot's approach was termed the "anatomoclinical method" or *méthode anatomoclinique*. Based on the model originally applied by Laennec, Charcot (1887a) sought to identify the anatomic basis of neurologic symptoms. In this two-part discipline, the first step involved the examination of thousands of patients and a careful description of their neurologic signs. Taking advantage of the vast population within the Salpêtrière wards, he culled the medical service to categorize patients by the signs they demonstrated, studying them in detail and documenting symptom evolution over time (Goetz, 2012).

The second phase of the anatomoclinic method involved autopsy examinations. Because the Salpêtrière patients were wards of the state, when they died, Charcot had ready access to nervous-system tissue. He developed a sophisticated neuropathology service and focused his postmortem studies on a systematic process that cross-referenced identified lesions to the clinical signs experienced during life. Charcot's crowning anatomoclinic research concerned the identification of amyotrophic lateral sclerosis, internationally still widely known as Charcot's disease. He demonstrated that spasticity and pseudobulbar affect related to upper motor neuron lesions of the lateral columns and corticobulbar tracts, whereas atrophy and fasciculations occurred in the body regions associated with anterior horn cell loss (Goetz, 2000a). Comparable anatomoclinic studies illuminated the pathologic basis of locomotor ataxia, stroke syndromes, and some of the early aphasias. As a group, these disorders, with a clear correlation between symptoms and structural anatomic lesions, formed the large category of "organic diseases," meaning diseases with a defined pathologic basis. In the naming of disease in this classification system, Charcot emphasized the structural, anatomic foundations of symptoms, choosing designations like neuropathy, myopathy, and myelopathy rather than clinical terms like weakness or spasms.

As dramatic as many of these discoveries were, the second phase of anatomoclinic method was not always revealing. Numerous entities, including several movement disorders, Parkinson's disease, choreas, tics, and dystonia, were not associated with anatomic lesions that Charcot could identify. Charcot established a new category of neurologic disorders, the *névroses* or neuroses, to classify the numerous neurologic conditions that were well characterized clinically, but still had no identifiable anatomic lesion (Goetz, 1989). Though neurosis today is a psychiatric term, it was strictly a neurologic terms in Charcot's era, and the newer usage dates to the 20th century. Because of the ambiguity of the English term, *névrose* will be used throughout this discussion. This category of *névroses* was intentionally tentative, as Charcot, an anatomist, anticipated that future studies would identify the responsible structural lesions directly allied to the typical clinical signs associated with most of these diagnoses.

Another group of disorders also were included under the designation of *névroses,* but for a different reason. In the cases of neurologic disorders with paroxysmal or sudden but transient signs, epilepsies, migraines, and hysteria, Charcot contended that the anatomic lesion underlying the disorder, though well defined, also was fluctuating, or, in his terms, "dynamic." Importantly, such physiologic dysfunction was not global throughout the brain, but confined within very specific neuroanatomic regions relating directly to the clinical signs manifested by the patient (Charcot, 1887b). Charcot was a strong advocate of localization theory, considering the brain a confederation of nuclei responsible for different functions, rather than a homogeneous organ controlling all functions (Goetz, 2000b). In patients with fluctuating signs, he deduced the involved brain regions by drawing parallels between focal signs seen during these episodes and anatomoclinic discoveries he had previously made with disorders showing similar, but static, signs and clear anatomic lesions at autopsy. The focal signs that occurred in the midst of focal epileptic spells, migraine attacks, or hysteric episodes therefore related to involvement of the same neuroanatomic regions affected in subjects with similar clinical signs due to strokes or abscesses. In this way, when he observed a focal seizure of the left hand with a temporary postictal paresis, Charcot concluded that the right motor cortex of the precentral gyrus was transiently affected, since he had seen this same area lesioned with tumors or strokes in cases of static left hand weakness. As a natural extension to any other similar *névrose,* including hysteria, he concluded, similarly, that the signs of transient paresis, blindness, contorted postures, and other focal signs had a specific neuroanatomic basis of physiologic or dynamic significance, but without an anticipated structural lesion at autopsy.

CHARCOT AND THE CAUSE OF NEUROLOGIC DISEASES

Charcot's observational skills and dispassionate evaluation of neurologic signs led him to see himself as "a photographer," and he was particularly conscious of the pitfalls of preconceived bias (Charcot, 1888a). Nonetheless, Charcot held to one primary preconception throughout his career, maintaining that the underlying cause of all primary neurologic disease was hereditary (Goetz et al., 1995). In his view, largely reflective of the 19th century as a whole, he adamantly held that patients with neurologic diseases inherited from prior generations a weakness or *tache* that predisposed them to neurologic disorders. Environmental factors, including cold, trauma, infections, and physical or emotional stress, influenced the underlying proclivity to disease and could provoke or exacerbate signs in hereditarily affected subjects. The same environmental factors, however, would have no impact on subjects without the familial *tache.* Conversely, within a family with neurologic disease, the avoidance of unhealthy influences could protect subjects, so that even with the hereditary condition, members who were careful in their lifestyle could remain asymptomatic or only mildly affected (Charcot, 1888b).

Charcot constructed extensive family trees in support of his premise and showed that most neurologically impaired patients had obvious or hidden family members with neurologic diseases. He emphasized, however, that the actual neurologic manifestations of disease varied among family members. In one genealogy (Fig. 2.3) (Charcot, 1888c), the parents were afflicted with aphasia, hemiplegia, and epilepsy, whereas the children revealed their neurologic disorder in the form of locomotor ataxia and general paresis (dissimilar inheritance). More rarely, the same manifestations of neurologic impairment passed between generations, as was the case in Huntington's disease (similar inheritance). Within Charcot's conceptual framework of the neuropathic family of diseases, disorders due to structural lesions and the *névroses* were equal in neurologic legitimacy, all being fundamentally hereditary and all intermingled within families.

Against this familial backdrop, the final clinical manifestations of the neurologic disorder depended largely on an array of environmental factors or *agents provocateurs.* For instance, in the case of tabes dorsalis, Charcot

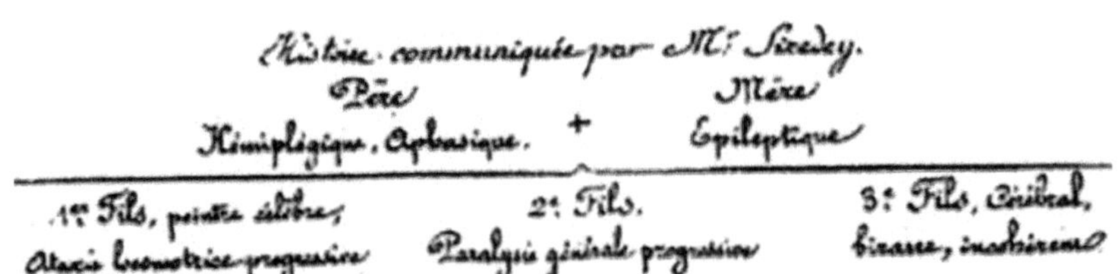

Fig. 2.3. Genealogic tree on a patient, showing Charcot's insistence on hereditary factors underlying neurologic disorders. A father with aphasia and hemiplegia and a mother with epilepsy had three children, one with locomotor ataxia, a second with general paresis, and a third with high intelligence but incoherent, bizarre behaviors. The picture is reproduced from Charcot (1888c), copied from the personal edition in the collection of Christopher G. Goetz.

held adamantly that syphilis was not the cause of the illness, but was frequently associated with the disorder because syphilis weakened the body:

> *There are conditions that relate to diseases as provocative agents. Trauma can unveil almost any illness to which a person is already predisposed. Syphilis too is undoubtedly important, and if we see many ataxics who were once syphilitic, we can reasonably ask whether ataxia would have ever developed without prior syphilis. Without syphilis, the tabes will not develop at all clinically, or, if it does, it will come later (Charcot, 1888b, French, no page number; English, p. 22).*

Given Charcot's unquestioned view of hereditary disease causation, the concept of primary psychogenic or functional neurologic disorders is a *non sequitur* in the strict sense. Nowhere in Charcot's writing will the reader find arguments that a healthy person without a hereditary proclivity to disease could develop a neurologic disorder from any psychologic influence, whether stress, trauma, excitement, or despair. On the other hand, as indicated previously, the roles of stress, emotional or minor physical trauma, and excitement were appreciated by Charcot as within the repertoire of *agents provocateurs*. These influences, though not restricted to one diagnosis, were particularly important when dealing with hysteria.

CHARCOT AND HYSTERIA

After 1870 and especially after 1880, Charcot devoted a particular effort to studying hysteria (Goetz et al., 1995). The clinical features of hysteria were varied but specific, including characteristic focal neurologic signs such as hemiparesis, hemianesthesia, contractures of the extremities, or bizarre involuntary movements. These findings could be statically present, but were often fleeting or intermittent. Males and females were affected, and within the hysteric's family tree, Charcot was consistently comfortable that he could establish the hereditary mark of neurologic disease.

Several specific features helped Charcot to identify hysterics. In comparing the distribution of weakness, sensory loss, or postures of these hysteric patients, Charcot acknowledged that the pattern of neurologic impairment closely resembled, but was usually not exactly the same as, the signs seen with classic structural lesions. Weakness was not necessarily accompanied by reflex changes and often involved only one extremity. Hemianesthesia tended to split the midline, and postures were more variable among hysteric subjects than the contractures he saw after strokes or other defined anatomic lesions (Charcot, 1872b). Furthermore, the degree of involvement was usually more intense and more disabling in hysteria than seen with a comparable lesion of structural origin. The most exotic of the movement disorders involved the celebrated *arc-en-cercle* opisthotonic posturing that occurred in the context of hysteroepileptic spells. Typically portrayed in images of women, the phenomenon occurred as well in men (Fig. 2.4). This neurologic sign was so characteristic of hysteria as encountered at the Salpêtrière that the patient displaying this behavior was usually diagnosed hysteric without further evaluations. Multiple hysteric signs often occurred simultaneously in a given patient or could be found in the past history; for example, a patient with hysteric monoplegia might have accompanying hemianesthesia or a past history of hysteroepilepsy.

Importantly, as well, hysteric signs were very often linked historically to a minor physical injury affecting the involved body part. This injury occurred in close juxtaposition to the neurologic signs that developed quickly

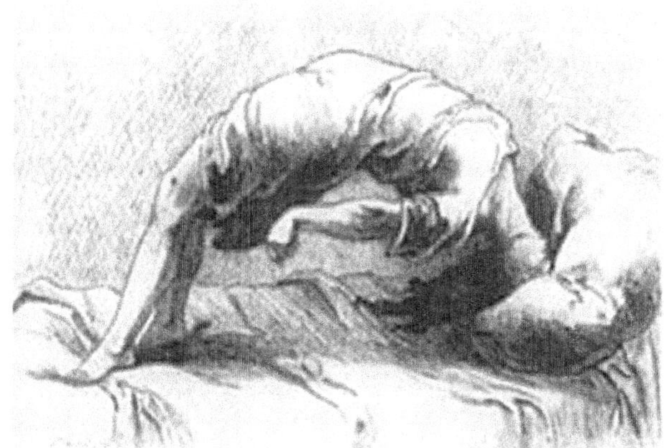

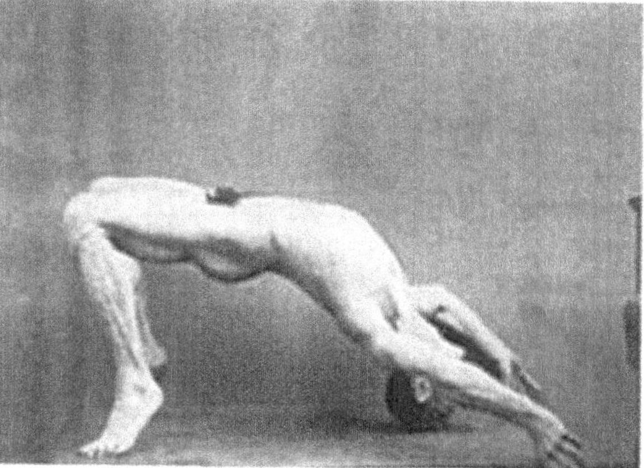

Fig. 2.4. The celebrated, exotic opisthotonic posturing (*arc-en-cercle*) seen as part of hysteria and specifically hysteroepilepsy. Whereas most patients with this behavior were women, the movement disorder syndrome also occurred in men. Both the lithograph (Richer, 1885) and the photograph, given to the author by Dr. J.J. Hauw, are from the personal collection of Christopher G. Goetz.

and fully, rather than showing a slow evolution. Finally, hysteric signs often resolved under the influence of hypnosis and could be treated with posthypnotic suggestion in some cases. Collectively, these features helped Charcot in classifying hysteria as a unified entity, and, because the presumed neurologic impairment was fundamentally dynamic or physiologic rather than structural, the observed patterns validated the relationship between the *névroses* and the organic disorders. Commenting specifically on the dynamic lesion site in a case of hysteric upper-extremity paralysis, Charcot drew his anatomic conclusions from parallels with structural lesions: "It is, I contend, in the gray matter of the cerebral hemisphere on the side opposite the paralysis and more precisely in the motor zone of the arm" (Charcot, 1887b, French, p. 318; English, p. 276).

As a group, the hysterics typically also showed an emotional affect of exotic elaboration, and though this feature aggravated the practical study of hysterics, it also helped to set them apart nosologically from subjects with other diagnoses. The issue of elaboration or exotic signs should not imply that Charcot considered hysteria as either neurasthenia or malingering. The focal neurologic presentation of hysteria distinguished the condition categorically from neurasthenia, where global fatigue and vague symptoms predominated the presentation. The transient nature of many hysteric spells and the patients' elaboration of signs always prompted Charcot's consideration of malingering or attempted deception on the part of the patient. In this context, Charcot was severe in his scrutiny, and he weeded out elements of conscious fabrication among hysterics through a number of physiological studies to demonstrate that the specific hysteric signs were involuntary and unconscious. Speaking of simulation as a comorbidity within the context of underlying hysteria, he warned of:

> *the slyness, cleverness and unexpected tenacity that women will show in trying to fool people in the midst of their hysteria, especially when the would-be victim is a doctor (Charcot, 1872c, French, p. 280; English, p. 230).*

Given the overlap association, Charcot devised very specific means to separate simulation from the *névroses* and specifically from hysteria (see later section).

HYSTERIA AND PSYCHOLOGIC INFLUENCES: THE ROLE OF SUGGESTION

To study hysteria in an experimental setting, Charcot invoked two previously highlighted observations: first, the close temporal link between hysteric signs and an event involving emotional stress or minor physical trauma; and, second, the facility by which physicians could hypnotize hysteric patients. Whereas the emotional stresses recounted by hysterics were of a wide variety and included fear, abandonment, and intense passion, cases involving minor trauma were more homogeneous and became a particularly rich resource for study. Charcot was a consulting physician for the national railroad company and hence evaluated a large number of patients who endured injuries in the context of their work. Though there were many serious injuries, Charcot was impressed with the number of neurologic cases seen after seemingly inconsequential physical trauma (Charcot, 1887c). The neurologic signs among these latter railway workers included weakness, anesthesia, or spasms that fit best into the category of hysteria (Micale, 1995). Charcot dispelled the historic bias that hysteria occurred only in women and effeminate young men. Discussing this point in his classroom of predominantly male doctors, he stated:

> *Male hysteria is not at all rare, and just among us, if I can judge from what I see each day, these cases are often unrecognized by even distinguished doctors. One can concede that a young and effeminate man might develop hysterical findings after experiencing significant stress, sorrow or deep emotions. But that a strong and vital workman, for instance, a railway engineer, fully integrated into the society and never prone to emotional instability before, should become hysteric – just as a woman might – this seems to be beyond imagination. And yet, it is a fact – one that we must get used to. Such was the case with so many other ideas today so universally accepted because they are founded on demonstrable evidence; but for so long, they met only skepticism and sarcasm – it is only a matter of time (Charcot, 1887d, French, p. 255; English, p. 222).*

Basing his diagnosis on the criteria for hysteria outlined above, Charcot considered the medical literature from England where railway accidents were of particular public and medical concern. He discovered the writings of the Englishman, J. Russell Reynolds (1826–1896), specifically his 1869 article, titled, "Certain forms of paralysis depending on idea" (Reynolds, 1869). With this foundation, Charcot considered whether emotional stress or a minor traumatic event could provoke focal neurophysiologic alterations in the brain of predisposed hysterics, with resultant neurologic impairments. Repeated thoughts of the original inducing event could somehow unleash the same physiologic dysfunction that, repetitively, in Charcot's words, "for want of a better term, we designate *dynamic or functional lesions* (Charcot, 1887b, French, p. 319; English, p. 278)." Charcot's terminology for this latter construct was autosuggestion. Charcot's perspective, however, remained always founded in neuroanatomy:

> *I have lightly struck the man's shoulder. In his case, as with any particularly predisposed neurologic subject, this minor trauma, this focal jolt, is sufficient to induce throughout his entire arm, a feeling of numbness and heaviness, the essence of paralysis; by the means of autosuggestion, this trace paralysis rapidly becomes complete. It is within the center controlling psychological processes, by that I mean within the cerebral hemispheres, that the phenomenon clearly is taking place (Charcot, 1888d, no page numbering).*

In parallel with these ideas of autosuggestion, Charcot had begun work on hypnotism at the Salpêtrière. He was impressed that hysterics were easily hypnotized and, during a trance, the physician could induce or dissipate hysteric signs by suggestion. This construct integrated well with the observations of autosuggestion and led Charcot to propose that suggestion, whether internally or externally generated, must play a pivotal role as an *agent provocateur* for the unleashing of the dynamic, physiologic lesions underlying typical hysteric symptoms. Whereas the original provoking forces may have been external in the form of stress or trauma, the physician-induced suggestion could rekindle the same neurologic events in the experimental setting of hypnosis. As such, autosuggestion accounted for the spontaneous and self-perpetuating spells that caused the patient's neurologic disability (Charcot, 1887e). In the view of the Salpêtrière school, hysteria and a proclivity to hypnosis thereby became interchangeable. The Charcot classroom and hospital ward served increasingly as an experimental human laboratory, where repeated hypnotic inductions allowed Charcot and his students to study the gamut of hysteric signs and their phases of development as well as resolution (Goetz et al., 1995).

Charcot's work with hypnotism brought him both fame and condemnation (Goetz, 2006). Many neurologists of the day dispelled these demonstrations as theatric maneuvers of no scientific value, and considered the exotic disorders seen at the Salpêtrière to be too frequent and too unusual to be independent of Charcot's own charisma. Disputes occurred over the requisite link between hysteria and hypnotism. Throughout this late period, covering the end of the 1880s up to his death in 1893, Charcot found his work on hysteria eroding on all fronts from the unquestioned acceptance of dynamic nervous system lesions to the categoric hereditary etiology of neurologic disorders, the role of autosuggestion to hysteria, and the pathognomonic hypnosis–hysteria link (Widlocher and Dantchev, 1994).

In the final years of Charcot's life, he produced very limited writing to clarify his final stand on hysteria as a neurologic entity, but the few documents that do exist suggest considerable self-questioning and the recognition of the need to reformulate his thinking (Goetz, 2003) After Charcot's death, his assistant Georges Guinon wrote a reflective essay, titled "Charcot intime," describing his last meeting with Charcot (Guinon, 1925). Guinon recounted that Charcot specifically discussed hysteria and considered his original concept obsolete and in need of full revision. Guinon provided no indication of the type of revamping needed, but his text clearly indicates that the topic of hysteria remained of intense interest to Charcot and that new work was envisioned. The only comment directly written by Charcot comes from a very brief preface written to introduce a monograph by his colleague, Janet (Charcot, 1892). Here, Charcot alludes to a pivotally new idea, but he presents it casually, as if readers could find extensive documentation elsewhere in his writings:

> *These works confirm a point of view that I have oftentimes expressed – which is that hysteria is for the most part a mental illness. This particular aspect of the disorder should not be neglected, if one wants to understand and treat hysteria (Charcot, 1892, p. iii).*

Within Charcot's extensive publications and formal texts on hysteria, no other statement ascribes a predominant role of mental or psychiatric causation to hysteria. Even though a number of Charcot's later lectures on hysteria approached topics that could be considered in the realm of mental disorders, double personalities, and very unusual forms of amnesias, he emphatically retained his neuroanatomic perspective (Gelfand, 1993). As a group, although the collective evidence suggests that Charcot may have been moving towards ideas that would today be considered closely linked to a true psychogenic cause of neurologic signs, his actual writings do not establish a solid argument for any fundamental change in Charcot's thinking on hysteria.

CHARCOT AND FREUD: THE MENTOR'S NEVER-SATED OBSESSION

Much has been written about the relationship between Sigmund Freud's seminal psychoanalytic works on the causes of diseases and his mentorship by Charcot (Goldstein, 1987; Gelfand, 1993; Widlocher and Dantchev, 1994). This relationship, however, should not be overinflated. Freud came to Paris for a short period in 1885 to study neuropathology with Charcot. During this sojourn, he witnessed Charcot's demonstrations of hysteria, participated in hypnosis sessions, and interacted with the circle of collaborators working on hysteria. Freud's diaries clearly confirm that this period of study with Charcot was a turning point in his own career and that the exposure was immeasurably important to his later development of psychoanalytic theory (Gelfand, 1993). Freud's pivotal theory that each patient's stress has symbolic importance and that this stress is actually at the origin of psychogenic neurologic or other signs may have indeed been inspired by these Salpêtrière experiences, but there is absolutely no indication that these conclusions originated with Charcot himself. Clearly, Charcot's neurologic emphasis precluded any particular concern over the type or nature of the provoking stimulus to hysteric spells. As such, because Freud's fundamental contributions are so related to symbolic importance of a given stress, it is historically inaccurate to ascribe to Charcot the role of Freud's pivotal predecessor in this domain (Gelfand, 1992; Goetz et al., 1995). As Gelfand points out:

> *it is simply anachronistic to assimilate Charcot to the genealogy of psychoanalysis constructed by Freud and dutifully repeated by generations of his followers where he tends to appear as a kind of John the Baptist figure announcing the coming of Freud (Goetz et al., 1995, p. 210).*

Freud's novel focus on the meaning behind stressful events related to hysteria launched him on an independent path, leaving Charcot still searching for neuroanatomic lesions. Charcot's student, Ballet, described his teacher as "haunted by the preoccupation" (Ballet, 1911, p. 379) to find the pathologic underpinnings of hysteric hemiplegia, as the professor continued to pose the question: "There is without doubt a lesion in the nervous centers, but where is it situated, and what is its nature?" (Charcot, 1887b, French, p 327; English, p. 286).

SIMULATION

As previously discussed, throughout his career, Charcot recognized that physicians needed to be constantly vigilant to identify patients who elaborated illness:

> *It is incontestable that in so many cases, patients have taken pleasure in distorting the principal elements of their disorder by exaggeration in order to make them appear extraordinary and more interesting or important (Charcot, 1872c, French, pp. 281–282; English, p. 230).*

Charcot's approach to dealing with conscious neurologic simulation, his medical attitudes toward malingering patients, and his diagnostic strategies to separate feigned illnesses from neurologic disorders were important contributions that would be amplified and expanded in the 20th century. Charcot discussed the overall challenges of dealing with difficult neurologic diagnoses in his introductory lecture that opens the third volume of the *Œuvres Complètes*. Part of this lecture alluded to the knotty problem of purposefully simulated illness, drawing a very clear distinction between feigned illness and the problems a clinician encounters when one disease mimics another because of overlapping signs.

> *While I am speaking to you of the difficulties that the physician encounters in the study of the* névroses *and of the means at his disposal for surmounting these obstacles, I wish to draw your attention to one point before finishing. I am speaking of* simulation: *not* imitation *of one disorder by another as we mentioned before, but of intentional and voluntary simulation, in which the patient exaggerates real symptoms or even creates an imaginary group of symptoms (Charcot, 1887a, French, p. 17; English, p. 14).*

The breadth of simulated symptoms was wide, but typical cases involved various forms of paresis (mono-, hemi-, quadra-), speech difficulties, and tongue weakness mimicking strokes. Contractures, blindness, and involuntary movements that ranged from tremor to wild gyrations and flamboyant behaviors were documented. Sudden attacks of vertigo or falls without clear explanation prompted investigation and the consideration of simulation. Charcot's suspicion of simulation increased when he identified neurologic signs that were inconsistent with objective disability and when findings occurred without the accompanying signs that typified recognized syndromes. He cautioned his students, however, on the expertise needed to detect simulation with authority:

> *But, to learn how to unveil simulation in such cases, at the very least, one must have completely studied the real condition in the greatest and most serious detail...and to know it in all its various forms (Charcot, 1887a, French, p. 18; English, p. 15).*

Charcot recognized the added problem that patients with clearly documented neurologic disease often confounded their own management by elaborating their symptoms. He was careful, however, to teach his students the necessity to extend their diagnostic skills beyond the superficial or cursory interview. Speaking of a case of a man who endured an accident several years ago and now complained of vertiginous attacks that would potentially allow him more workers' compensation, Charcot commented:

> *I have already shared with you my concern that this man has a tendency to amplify, to enhance*

the facts. He seems to want to simulate, *as we call it. On the other hand, amidst his exaggerations, is there a kernel of truth? It is for us to determine the answer to this question if we are to be equitable and truly fulfill our mission as doctors. It is insufficient to identify a tendency towards exaggeration or simulation as the grounds to condemn a subject in one quick assessment without further consideration. Such a judgment is both unjust and offensive. A more subtle evaluation of the details is required, and we must not forget that in certain real diseases, mental states, including the need to exaggerate or mislead, can be a marker of the primary disease. We need to know if these attacks that he says he is having resemble those that typify Ménière's syndrome, symptoms that are so characteristic, and yet so unexpected and little known that even many doctors do not recognize them (Charcot, 1888e, no page numbering).*

Of all neurologic diagnoses, Charcot found hysteria most frequently associated with simulation. Speaking to his students on this topic, he commented on the diagnostic overlap, but also provided a rare glimpse of his personal attitudes towards the creative spirit of simulators:

This leads me to say a word on simulation. *You will meet with it at every point when dealing with the history of hysteria. One sometimes catches oneself admiring the amazing craft, sagacity, and perseverance which women, under the influence of this great* névrose, *will mobilize for the purpose of deception – especially when a physician is to be the victim. (Charcot, 1872c, French, pp. 281–282; English, p. 230).*

The reader will note the gender-specific comment and might mistakenly interpret it as misogynous. The comment, however, related to the Salpêtrière inpatients, who were all women, the male counterpart in the French public health system being the Bicêtre Hospital outside of Paris. As already highlighted, one of Charcot's primary contributions to hysteria was his detailed descriptions of male hysterics, and these cases were derived from his outpatient and railway consultation experiences. His concern over simulation in men and women hysterics was entirely parallel (Goetz, 1999).

Charcot based most of his neurologic diagnoses on history, as the full neurologic examination was not codified until the next generation. However, he was well aware of typical gaits, tremors, movement disorders, and patterns of weakness that typified neurologic syndromes. He was keen on noting inconsistencies among his charges who lived within the confines of Salpêtrière and who could be monitored by his younger staff and his own watchful eye. Monoplegias were particularly suspicious, and simulated strokes were detected often by tongue deviation that did not parallel cortical or brainstem patterns in association with facial weakness. In his diagnostic quest, Charcot was not above slight trickery, and on one occasion when a reportedly deaf patient was presented, Charcot sat him in front of the audience and discussed his case, and then mumbled to his students with reference to the age-old ruses of street swindlers who play on sympathies: "These beggar schools seem to have produced a fine graduate," to which the patient spontaneously erupted: "I am no beggar."

Charcot's next words show his therapeutic, not punitive, intent:

Look here, you were so deaf a moment ago. See how you hear me now even though I am not speaking loudly at all ... I am not accusing you of being a beggar, but I claim with certainty that you exaggerate your situation which in fact hurts you in the long run. Tell me your story in simple detail, and tell me the truth and only the truth. Do not exaggerate, for I assure you that keeping to the truth will be much better for you (Charcot, 1888e, no page numbering).

The subject settled into an honest interview by which Charcot was able to elicit a history that allowed him to make a sound neurologic diagnosis aside from the reported simulated hearing loss.

Charcot prided himself on objective diagnostic measures and strove to develop actual criteria for the nosographic category of simulated neurologic disorders. To this end, when he considered a case of an unusual thumb contracture that he suspected was simulated, Charcot placed the patient's forearm on a table with the back of the hand secured. A sling containing the thumb was attached to a cord passing over two pulleys, and then a 1-kg weight was suspended to stretch the contracted thumb over 30 minutes (Fig. 2.5). In the case of a neurologically based contracture, during the stretching, the distance between the thumb and hand increased slowly and smoothly, and the patients showed no signs of effort or fatigue. After the stretching stopped, the thumb returned to its original position. In the patient simulating contractures, however, inconsistent distances between the finger and thumb developed with visible signs of fatigue. A pneumograph recording of breathing patterns during the test detected an increasingly irregular, deepening, and effortful inspiratory pattern in the simulator in contrast to the maintained, smooth, and regular pattern in the subject with an authentic contracture.

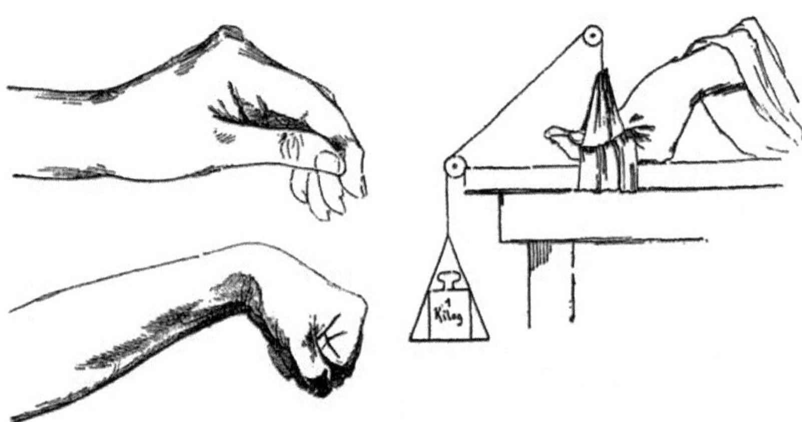

Fig. 2.5. Differentiating hysteric contractures from simulation. Charcot used this experimental apparatus that pulled on the thumb. By attaching a monitor to the chest, Charcot could measure respiratory movements during this stress. In hysteria, patients maintained their contractures in spite of a weighted stress without changing their respirations, whereas in simulating subjects fatigue developed, the thumb became jerky, and respirations became irregular. The pictures are reproduced from Charcot (1887c), copied from the personal edition in the collection of Christopher G. Goetz.

> *Thus you see, by an experiment of this kind, that fraud, if it existed, would have been easily recognized since we have in the study of the respiratory curve the means of unmasking it (Charcot, 1887c, French, p. 112; English, p. 97).*

A variation of this method was adapted for separating catalepsy from conscious simulation. As one of the more exotic signs typical of hysteria and a frequent finding among patients at the Salpêtrière, catalepsy was among the signs that critics considered simulated. Catalepsy is a behavior characterized by immobility and waxy flexibility of the limbs, so that patients can be moved into different postures and remain in those positions for prolonged period of time.

Charcot's scientific claims regarding hysteria were increasingly challenged in the later years of his career by allusions to his being duped by his own patients (Platel, 1883). In his own defense, he developed methods that he felt clearly identified the malingerer. When asked to extend the arms or legs, the true cataleptic extended the extremity unsupported for longer than the simulator, but eventually both fatigued, so that this test was deemed insufficient to ascertain a sure diagnosis. Charcot therefore developed a pressure drum with a recording pen fixed at the extremity of the outstretched limb to register the least oscillations of the arm, while the pneumograph again registered respiratory movements. In the cataleptic, the pen recorded regular extremity oscillations, whereas the tracing from the simulator was "crooked, very undulating, and marked in places by large oscillations arranged in series" (Charcot, 1887a, French, p. 20; English, p. 18). Simultaneously, the pneumographic recordings showed regular breathing that continued without variability in the cataleptic, whereas the simulator showed a pattern that quickly became highly irregular, with interspersed deep and rapid panting cycles occurring as fatigue and added effort developed. These same techniques were adopted by others and applied in cases of medical-legal controversy when simulation was considered (Goetz, 2004). Charcot felt these tests allowed the sophisticated diagnostician to deal effectively with simulation:

> *It is useless to insist further. A hundred other examples might be invoked which would only show that the simulation which is talked about so much when hysteria and allied affections are under consideration, is, in the current state of our knowledge only a perceived threat, before which only the insecure and inexperienced are stumped. In the future, it ought to be the province of the well-informed physician to dissipate chicanery wherever it occurs and to sort out the symptoms which form a fundamental part of the illness from those which are simulated and added to it by the artifice of the patient (Charcot, 1887a, French, pp. 20–21; English, p.18).*

In contrast to the underlying, though poorly defined, hereditary *tache* responsible for hysteria, with simulation, the underlying cause was more clearly identified. Charcot reflected on the potential benefits that patients might receive through deception, and though strict in front of malingerers, he also marveled at the highly developed ingenuity of some:

> *In fact, we all know that the desire to deceive, even without concrete benefit, but with a kind of disinterested worship of art for its own sake [*culte de l'art pour l'art*] or admittedly with the idea of*

provocation to excite pity or another emotion is a common enough occurrence (Charcot, 1887a, French, p. 17; English, p. 14).

In spite of these efforts, Charcot's scientific credibility was called into question by the issue of malingerers within his patient ranks. Accusations that Charcot wittingly or unwittingly fostered many of his patients' bizarre behaviors forced him into a turbulent and defensive close of his career (Goetz et al., 1995). Concerns that malingers had duped Charcot endured after his death, but the topic was specifically addressed by Blanche Wittman, one of Charcot's most celebrated hysterics and the patient depicted in the Brouillet painting, *A Clinical Lesson at the Salpêtrière* (Fig. 2.2) (Signoret, 1983). A. Boudouin, a physician of the generation after Charcot, interviewed Wittman:

"Listen Blanche, I know there are topics that you do not like to discuss. But as long as you have known me I have never been one to joke. I want you to tell me something about your episodes of the past." After a moment, she replied, "Alright, what do you want to know?" "It has been said that all these spells were simulated, that the patients just pretended to sleep and thereby made fun of the doctors. Is there any truth in that?" "None whatsoever; those are lies. We had those spells and were in those lethargic states because we could not do otherwise. Besides, there was nothing fun about it." And then she added: "Simulation! Do you think it would have been easy to fool Dr. Charcot? Oh yes, lots of fakes tried; he gave them one look and said "Be still" (Baudouin, 1935, p. 520).

These exact words cannot be specifically found in the direct patient interview transcriptions of Charcot's teaching lessons, but they are not far from the tenor of the cases already cited. Clearly, directness was a hallmark of Charcot, but, even in the context of his threatened credibility and even with his very modest trickery formerly cited, the existing primary documents reinforce his professionalism and the absence of the punitive postures. Perhaps the most salient contrast is with S. Weir Mitchell, Charcot's American colleague whose approach was more assertive and less nuanced. His student, B.R. Tucker, witnessed his teacher's treatment of a puzzling, bedridden woman with paralysis. After watching Mitchell's examination, the group left the patient's room to discuss the case in the hallway:

"Will she ever be able to walk?" asked one of the doctors. "Yes, in a moment," said Dr. Mitchell. Then the door of the room flew open and the paralyzed patient in her night gown rushed out and down the hall. Smoke exuded from the room. "What on earth is the matter?" asked someone. "I set the bedclothes on fires", said Dr. Mitchell. After this, the room was named the Weir Mitchell room (Tucker, 1936, p. 343).

CHARCOT IN A MODERN CONTEXT

Modern physicians dealing with functional neurologic disorders may rightly ask if we are any closer than Charcot in answering fundamental anatomic and physiologic questions. New functional imaging techniques, however, today provide researchers with direct tools to examine Charcot's putative dynamic lesions and to test his hypothesis that physiologically based focal central nervous system alterations in fact occur in psychogenic disorders. Functional magnetic resonance imaging techniques applied to study subjects with nondermatomal sensory loss, diagnosed as hysteric anesthesia, have documented anatomically specific changes (Mailis-Gagnon and Giannoylis, 2003), and regional cerebral blood flow studies in psychogenic visual loss detect perfusion alterations in the visual association cortex (Okuyama and Kawakatsu, 2002). The question of whether focal physiologic alterations should prompt neurodiagnosticians to revamp their diagnoses of psychogenic disorders or retain the diagnosis but broaden their concepts to embrace Charcot's original neuroanatomic constructs of hysteria is at the core of these new research efforts. In the therapeutic realm, neuroimaging studies demonstrating specific augmentation of dopaminergic function in subjects with Parkinson's disease who respond to placebo treatment reinforce the concept that psychologic mechanisms induce highly focal and disease-specific neuroanatomic effects (De la Fuente-Fernandez et al., 2001).

Charcot's emphasis on a hereditary basis of primary neurologic disorders, including hysteria, was largely discredited in the immediate generations after his death. New molecular biologic discoveries related to neurologic and psychiatric illness, however, rekindle Charcot's concepts of familial proclivity to disease. Psychogenic hand dystonia has been reported within a family with documented hereditary polyneuropathy and liability to pressure palsies (Strenge et al., 1996). Also, cases of psychogenic syncope occur in pedigrees of familial vasovagal syncope (Mathias et al., 2000). Familial psychogenic blindness and recurrent hysteric attacks within families have also occurred (Ziegler and Schlemmer, 1994; Matoo et al., 2002). The contributory issues of environment and heredity to these examples remain unexplored, but the increasing reliance on genetic markers of illness will likely provide more direct tests for Charcot's original hypotheses. Later sections of this volume of the *Handbook of Clinical Neurology* will address many of the issues discussed by Charcot as they relate to genetic predisposition, clinical manifestations, the prominent role of minor physical trauma, and physiologic changes associated with functional neurologic disorders. In this context, Charcot's words of advice to his students remain eminently modern in emphasizing the clinician's pre-eminent challenge when facing puzzling or poorly understood disorders:

> *Above all other things, clinical medicine is the study of the difficult aspects and complexities of diseases. When a patient calls on you, he is under no obligation to have a simple disease just to please you. He has every right to have a disease presenting as an extremely complex case (Charcot 1888b, French, no page numbering; English, p. 15).*

References

American Psychiatric Association (2013). Diagnostic and statistical manual of mental disorders. 5th edn. American Psychiatric Association, Washington, DC.

Ballet G (1911). La domaine de la psychiatrie. Presse Méd 377–380. May 10.

Baudouin A (1935). Quelques souvenirs de la Salpêtrière. Par Méd 26: 517–520.

Beard GM (1869). Neurasthenia or nervous exhaustion. Boston Med Surg J 80: 217–221.

Bouchara C (2014). Charcot: une vie avec l'image. Philippe Rey, Paris.

Charcot J-M (1872a). De la paralysie agitante. Œuvres Complètes, vol.1. Bureaux du Progrès Médical, Paris, pp. 155–188 [In English: Charcot J-M (1890). On paralysis agitans. Clinical Lectures on Diseases of the Nervous System, vol. 1. (transl. T. Savill). London: New Sydenham Society, pp. 129–156.].

Charcot J-M (1872b). De l'hystérie-épilepsie. Œuvres Complètes, vol.1. Bureaux du Progrès Médical, Paris, pp. 367–385 [In English: Charcot J-M (1890). Hystero-epilepsy (). Clinical Lectures on Diseases of the Nervous System, vol. 1. (transl. T. Savill). London: New Sydenham Society, pp. 300–316.].

Charcot J-M (1872c). De l'ischurie hystérique (). Œuvres Complètes, vol. 1. Bureaux du Progrès Médical, Paris, pp. 275–299 [In English: Charcot J-M (1890). Hysterical ischuria. Clinical Lectures on Diseases of the Nervous System, vol. 1. (transl. T. Savill). London: New Sydenham Society, pp. 225–245.].

Charcot J-M (1877). Prodromes anatomiques. Œuvres Complètes, vol. 2. Bureaux du Progrès Médical, Paris, pp. 1–19 [In English: Charcot J-M (1881). Anatomical Introduction. Lectures on Diseases of the Nervous System, vol. 2. (transl. G. Sigerson). London: New Sydenham Society, pp. 3–17.].

Charcot J-M (1887a). Sur deux cas de monoplégie brachiale hystérique de nature traumatique chez l'homme. Œuvres Complètes, vol. 3. Bureaux du Progrès Médical, Paris, pp. 315–343 [In English: Charcot J-M (1890). On two cases of hysterical brachial monoplegia in the male due to injury. Clinical Lectures on Diseases of the Nervous System, vol. 3. (transl. T. Savill). London: New Sydenham Society, pp. 274–295.].

Charcot J-M (1887b). Deux cas de contracture hystérique d'origine traumatique. Œuvres Complètes, vol. 3. Bureaux du Progrès Médical, Paris, pp. 97–124 [In English: Charcot J-M (1890), Two cases of hysterical contracture of traumatic origin. Clinical Lectures on Diseases of the Nervous System, vol. 3. (transl. T. Savill). London: New Sydenham Society, pp. 84–106.].

Charcot J-M (1887c). A propos de l'hystérie chez l'homme. Œuvres Complètes, vol. 3. Bureaux du Progrès Médical, Paris, pp. 253–280 [In English: Charcot J-M (1890). Concerning six cases of hysteria in the male. Clinical Lectures on Diseases of the Nervous System, vol. 3. (transl. T. Savill). London: New Sydenham Society, pp. 220–243.].

Charcot J-M (1887d). Deux nouveaux cas de paralysie hystéro-traumatique. Œuvres Complètes, vol. 3. Bureaux du Progrès Médical, Paris, pp. 441–463 [In English: Charcot J-M (1890). Two additional cases of hystero-traumatic paralysis in men. Clinical Lectures on Diseases of the Nervous System, vol. 3. (transl. T. Savill). London: New Sydenham Society, pp. 374–394.].

Charcot J-M (1887e). Leçon d'ouverture. Œuvres Complètes, vol. 3. Bureaux du Progrès Médical, Paris, pp. 1–22 [In English: Charcot J-M (1890). Introduction. Clinical Lectures on Diseases of the Nervous System, vol. 3. (transl. T. Savill). London: New Sydenham Society, pp. 1–19.].

Charcot J-M (1888a). In: Leçon du 28 février 1888. Leçons du Mardi à la Salpêtrière: 1887–1888, Bureaux du Progrès Médical, Paris. (no page numbering). [In English: Goetz CG (1987). Charcot's disease. Charcot, the Clinician: The Tuesday Lessons. New York: Raven Press, pp. 164–186.].

Charcot J-M (1888b). Leçon du 15 novembre 1888. Leçons du Mardi à la Salpêtrière: 1887–1888. Bureaux du Progrès Médical, Paris. (no page numbering). [In English: Goetz CG (1987). Syphilis, locomotor ataxia, facial paresis. Charcot, the Clinician: The Tuesday Lessons. New York: Raven Press, pp. 1–25.].

Charcot J-M (1888c). Leçon du 13 mars 1888. Leçons du Mardi à la Salpêtrière: 1887–1888. Bureaux du Progrès Médical, Paris. (no page numbering). [In English: Goetz CG (1987). Friedreich's disease: two young men with ataxia. Charcot, the Clinician: The Tuesday Lessons. New York: Raven Press, pp. 141–163.].

Charcot J-M (1888d). Leçon du 1 mai 1888. Leçons du Mardi à la Salpêtrière: 1887–1888. Bureaux du Progrès Médical, Paris. (no page numbering).

Charcot J-M (1888e). Leçon du 20 mars 1888. Leçons du Mardi à la Salpêtrière: 1887–1888. Bureaux du Progrès Médical, Paris. (no page numbering).

Charcot J-M (1892). Préface. In: P Janet (Ed.), Etat mental des hystériques: les stigmates mentaux. Rueff, Paris, p. iii.

De la Fuente-Fernandez R, Ruth TJ, Sossi V et al. (2001). Expectation and dopamine release: mechanism of the placebo effect in PD. Science 293: 1164–1166.

Gelfand T (1992). Sigmund-sur-Seine: Fathers and brothers in Charcot's Paris. In: T Gelfand, J Kerr (Eds.), Freud and the History of Psychoanalysis, Analytic Press, Hillsdale, NJ, pp. 29–57.

Gelfand T (1993). Becoming patrimony: when, how and why Charcot got into hysteria (). In: CG Goetz (Ed.), History of Neurology: Jean-Martin Charcot, American Academy of Neurology Publishing, Minneapolis, MN, pp. 53–68.

Gilles de la Tourette G (1886). Etude sur une affection nerveuse caractérisée par de l'incoordination motrice accompagnée d'écholalie et de copralalie. Arch Neurol (Paris) 9: 19–42. 158–200. [In English: Goetz, CG, Klawans, H (1982). Study of a neurologic condition characterized by motor incoordination accompanied by echolalia and coprolalia (jumping, latah, myriachit). Advances in Neurology 5: 12–43].

Goetz CG (1987). Charcot, the Clinician: The Tuesday Lessons, Raven Press, New York.

Goetz CG (1989). The father of us all – Jean-Martin Charcot: neurologist and teacher. In: FC Rose (Ed.), Neuroscience Across the Centuries, Smith-Gordon, London, pp. 139–149.

Goetz CG (1999). Charcot and the myth of misogyny. Neurology 52: 1678–1686.

Goetz CG (2000a). Amyotrophic lateral sclerosis: early contributions of Jean-Martin Charcot. Muscle and Nerve 23: 336–343.

Goetz CG (2000b). Battle of the titans: Charcot and Brown-Séquard on cerebral localization. Neurology 54: 1840–1847.

Goetz CG (2001). Poor Beard!! Charcot's internationalization of neurasthenia, the "American disease". Neurology 57: 510–514.

Goetz CG (2003). The prefaces of Charcot: Leitmotifs of an international career. Neurology 60: 1333–1340.

Goetz CG (2004). Medical-legal issues in Charcot's neurological career. Neurology 62: 1827–1883.

Goetz CG (2006). Charcot and psychogenic movement disorders. In: M Hallett, AE Lang, S Fahn et al. (Eds.), Psychogenic Movement Disorders, American Academy of Neurology Press, Minneapolis, MN, pp. 3–13.

Goetz CG (2012). Jean-Martin Charcot and the anatomo-clinical method of neurology. In: S Finger, F Boller, KL Tyler (Eds.), History of Neurology: Handbook of Clinical Neurology, vol. 95. Elsevier, Edinburgh, pp. 203–212.

Goetz CG, Bonduelle M, Gelfand T (1995). Charcot: Constructing Neurology. Oxford University Press, New York.

Goldstein J (1987). Console and Classify, Cambridge University Press, New York.

Guinon G (1925). Charcot intime. Paris Med 56: 511–516.

Mailis-Gagnon A, Giannoylis I (2003). Altered central somatosensory processing in chronic pain patients with "hysterical" anesthesia. Neurology 60: 1501–1507.

Mathias CJ, Deguchi K, Bleasdale-Barr K et al. (2000). Familial vasovagal syncope and pseudosyncope: observations in a case with both natural and adopted siblings. Clin Auton Res 10: 43–45.

Matoo SK, Gupta N, Lobana A et al. (2002). Mass family hysteria. Psychiatry Clin Neurosci 56: 643–646.

Micale MS (1989). Hysteria and its historiography: a review of past and present writings. Hist Sci 27 (223–261): 319–351.

Micale MS (1995). Charcot and les névroses traumatiques: scientific and historical reflections. J Hist Neurosci 4: 101–119.

Okuyama N, Kawakatsu S (2002). Occipital hypoperfusion in a patient with psychogenic visual disturbance. Psychiatry Res 114: 163–168.

Platel F (1883). Cabotinage. Le Figaro: 1. April 18.

Reynolds JR (1869). Certain forms of paralysis depending on idea. Oct 2, BMJ: 378–379. Nov 6::483–485.

Richer P (1885). Etudes cliniques sur la grande hystérie our l'hystéroépilepsie. Delahaye et Le Crosnier, Paris.

Signoret J-L (1983). Une leçon clinique à la Salpêtrière. Rev Neurol 139: 687–701.

Strenge H, Speidel H, Albert E (1996). Psychogenic hand dystonia and hereditary polyneuropathy with liability to pressure palsies. Fortschr Neurol Psychiatr 64: 20–25.

Tucker BR (1936). Speaking of Weir Mitchell. Am J Psychiatry 93: 341–346.

Widlocher D, Dantchev N (1994). Charcot et l'hystérie. Rev Neurol 150: 490–497.

Ziegler DK, Schlemmer RB (1994). Familial psychogenic blindness and headache. J Clin Psychiatry 55: 114–117.

Handbook of Clinical Neurology, Vol. 139 (3rd series)
Functional Neurologic Disorders
M. Hallett, J. Stone, and A. Carson, Editors
http://dx.doi.org/10.1016/B978-0-12-801772-2.00003-5

Chapter 3

Neurologic approaches to hysteria, psychogenic and functional disorders from the late 19th century onwards

J. STONE*

Department of Clinical Neurosciences, Centre for Clinical Brain Sciences, University of Edinburgh, Edinburgh, UK

Abstract

The history of functional neurologic disorders in the 20th century from the point of view of the neurologist is U-shaped. A flurry of interest between the 1880s and early 1920s gave way to lack of interest, skepticism, and concern about misdiagnosis. This was mirrored by increasing professional and geographic divisions between neurology and psychiatry after the First World War. In the 1990s the advent of imaging and other technology highlighted the positive nature of a functional diagnosis. Having been closer in the early 20th century but later more separate, these disorders are now once again the subject of academic and clinical interest, although arguably still very much on the fringes of neurology and neuropsychiatry. Revisiting older material provides a rich source of ideas and data for today's clinical researcher, but also offers cautionary tales of theories and treatments that led to stagnation rather than advancement of the field. Patterns of treatment do have a habit of repeating themselves, for example, the current enthusiasm for transcranial magnetic stimulation compared to the excitement about electrotherapy in the 19th century. For these reasons, an understanding of the history of functional disorders in neurology is arguably more important than it is for other areas of neurologic practice.

INTRODUCTION

This volume of *Handbook of Clinical Neurology* contains four chapters covering the history of hysteria and functional disorders. Michael Trimble and Ted Reynolds discussed hysteria from Babylon to Charcot (Chapter 1). Christopher Goetz described the contribution of Charcot and contemporaries (Chapter 2), and Richard Kanaan led us through 20th-century psychiatric thought, with a particular emphasis on Freud (Chapter 4). This chapter attempts to fill another piece in this history, and one that is relatively absent from many accounts of the topic, that of neurologic contributions and thought after Charcot. Although there was ongoing sustained interest in hysteria from neurologists and physicians of nervous disease, especially in France, Germany, and the USA until the First World War, it appeared to seriously wane after that. Researching this topic is largely a story of progressive lack of interest until the development of videotelemetry and magnetic resonance imaging in the 1990s. These new tools highlighted in more stark terms how commonplace functional disorders were in a neurology service and saw the rediscovery of functional clinical syndromes and signs, particularly in the fields of epilepsy and movement disorders. In this chapter I explore some of the themes in this story, not as a historian, but as a neurologist with an interest in the topic. Our intention is to provide a starting point for others wishing to explore the topic in more detail. We explore potential reasons for both the decline in interest and its more recent re-emergence within the specialty to whom patients with functional neurologic disorders usually present.

*Correspondence to: Jon Stone, Department of Clinical Neurosciences, Centre for Clinical Brain Sciences, University of Edinburgh, Crew Road, Edinburgh EH4 2 XU, UK. Tel: +44-131-537-1167, E-mail: jon.stone@ed.ac.uk

NEUROLOGIC APPROACHES TO HYSTERIA FROM CHARCOT TO WORLD WAR I

Babinski

After Charcot died in 1893, there was somewhat of a backlash against some of the more elaborate forms of hysteria that he had described. In particular, *la grande hystérie,* with its four phases, such as the *attitudes passionelles,* were derided as the product of coaching of patients in the Salpêtrière Hospital. Joseph Babinski (1857–1932), who stood behind Charcot waiting to catch Blanche Wittman in the famous painting by Brouillet (see Fig. 2.2 in Chapter 2), was especially keen on the idea that all hysteric symptoms were the result of suggestion. In his 1918 book he gave the disorder a new name, pithiatism, a compound of two Greek words, *peitha* ("I persuade") and *iatos* ("curable") (Babinski and Froment, 1918). He was keen to distance himself from some of Charcot's work on the subject, especially his views on the potential of a dynamic nervous system lesion as well as cases of hysteric fever, anuria, and circulatory disturbance. Perhaps most importantly, he did not think that hysteria could affect the deep tendon reflexes and plantar response which he had been so keen to promote. His view, in keeping in large part with Pierre Janet, was to move thinking towards a purely psychic disorder in which suggestion played a key role. He refers in his book several times to a 1908 meeting of the Paris Neurological Society during which this "modern conception of hysteria" was set out, to clear away the mistakes of the past. He noted that Charcot and others had placed a lot of weight on hysteric stigmata of hemianesthesia. Babinski, however, said he found no cases of hemianesthesia or narrowed visual field in over 100 cases when approached in a neutral way without suggestion.

He was particularly struck by a first-hand account of the wreck of a mail steamer by Clunet, a doctor who happened to be on board as the tragedy unfolded. He noted that in a life-threatening situation there were no "hysterical" symptoms, but these appeared as soon as people arrived at a place of safety, when Clunet had the clear-headedness to perform neurologic examinations on them, and then mostly disappeared within a week. He also mentions similar experience at the Battle of the Somme, where acute hysteria was not seen at the moment of the trauma but later on, away from the front. Babinski used this evidence to support his pithiatic notion that the symptoms arise out of autosuggestion at a time that is convenient for the patient and not from some innate conversion of emotion into physical symptom. Babinski acknowledges that Charcot had also noted this, calling it the "period of meditation." It would be simplistic to say that he was denying all his deceased boss had taught him. Charcot recognized the importance of suggestion and the "fixed idea" too, but Babinski clearly felt he was updating it to a more modern conception.

Janet

Pierre Janet (1859–1947) arguably became one of the first psychologists rather than a neurologist, although his thesis, later developed into the work *The Mental State of Hystericals* (Janet, 1901), was one of the last Charcot supervised. What is clear from reading his work are the very large numbers of patients he saw with functional disorders and the great thought and time that he spent in talking to them. His book *The Major Symptoms of Hysteria* reproduced a series of lectures he gave to Harvard Medical School in 1906 and remains one of the most perceptive books on the subject, with lucid and practical chapters on individual symptoms such as paralysis, visual disturbance, and seizures (Janet, 1907). Janet also promoted a "psychic" view of hysteria but introduced the concept of dissociation as an explanatory mechanism to understand how it was possible for someone to have a lack of integration of normal motor and sensory processing. The concept of dissociation has arguably had as much traction as conversion ever since and is discussed in more detail in Chapter 8 of this volume.

UK neurology before World War I

There were clearly many people working on hysteria, especially in France, Switzerland, and Germany at this time, including Sollier, Raymond, Binswanger, Oppenheim, Mills, Hellpach, Vogt, McDougall, Jules Dejerine, and Dubois. In 1911, Samuel Alexander Kinnier Wilson (1878–1937), who had trained with Babinski in Paris and later worked at Queen Square and Kings College in London, wrote a paper in *Brain* entitled "Some modern French conceptions of hysteria" (Kinnier Wilson, 1910) to discuss this material. Kinnier Wilson was an example of the neurologist at that time, like William Rivers, happy to cross over to psychiatry, at one stage being president of the psychiatry section of the Royal Society of Medicine. He commented that the "mere enumeration of these conflicting hypotheses may overwhelm the reader with a deep sense of despair at their hopeless dissimilarity, and he may reasonably fear that finality is as far off as ever." But in typical ironic style, he points out that they all have one thing in common, the earnestness with which their views are held based on their personally determined treatment. Wilson selected Babinski and Janet (and not Freud) for special and prolonged discussion. Wilson came back to hysteria on many further occasions in his career, providing excellent summaries of knowledge at the time (Wilson, 1931).

Oddly, his famous textbook, *Neurology* (Kinnier Wilson, 1940), did not include a chapter on the subject, probably due to his premature death (Reynolds, 2012b). He made several films of hysteria and other movement disorder in the mid-1920s supporting his interest in the topic (Reynolds et al., 2011; Sethi, 2011).

There had been some excellent work by British physicians. John Russell Reynolds' paper on the importance of idea (Reynolds, 1869), and Robert Todd's observations on paralysis had been seminal (Todd, 1854). Paget (1814–1899) did not write extensively about hysteria but his key observation, "She says, as all such patients do, 'I cannot'; it looks like 'I will not'; but it is 'I cannot will'," remains as popular as ever (Paget, 1873). William Gowers' (1845–1915) chapter on hysteria, from the heart of the National Hospital for Nervous Diseases in London, is especially rewarding and runs to 57 highly informative pages (Gowers, 1892). I discuss this chapter at some length here as an example of the sophistication of neurologic thinking at that time, reflected by many authors, which arguably became less rather than more over time.

Gowers' description of hysteria is one that is echoed by others in this period who viewed the mechanism as a disturbance of the function of the nervous system which could affect men as well as women.

> *The conditions of hemianaesthesia, paralysis and contracture must be regarded as the expression of a condition of restrained function (inhibition) or unrestrained activity, of certain cerebral centres, sensory and motor.*

Gowers went to a lot of effort to explain that he did not think the majority of his patients were simulating their symptoms.

> *It is now generally recognised that the malady is a real one, occasionally of great severity, and to a large extent beyond the direct influence of the patient's will.*

This appreciation of mechanism (the "how") was presented alongside a complex view of causation (the "why"). There was an appreciation of numerous potential predisposing, precipitating, and perpetuating factors, both mild and severe, which may be "either physical or mental influences." His thoughts on the interplay between ideas, fear, and desire are particularly interesting.

> *The nervous system is dominated by idea and by fear, as well as by desire; the definite conception of a symptom may lead to its occurrence; and when idea and emotion are conjoined, and a symptom is not only conceived but either dreaded or desired, its occurrence is still more easy.*

He also proposed a role for panic or depression in onset.

> *It may be a sudden alarm…it may be merely the depressing emotions from which no life is exempt, trifling in themselves, but potent because unresisted.*

He was especially forthright about the danger of iatrogenesis and unhelpful beliefs in relatives:

> *When the disease has once developed, it is often greatly increased by injudicious management. The near relatives of the hysterical are often conspicuously deficient in judgement, and the little common sense they may possess is often rendered useless by their affection for the sufferers.*

The importance of normal physiology was stressed in terms of how symptoms might develop.

> *Paraplegia is excited by emotion with especial frequency. Even in health a sensation of weakness in the legs may be caused by sudden alarm, and this, in hysteria, may be followed by a progressive loss of power. It is common for the onset of persistent weakness to be preceded by occasional momentary "giving way of the legs," at once recovered from – a very characteristic feature.*

He also appreciated the importance of pain in precipitating paralysis.

> *Spinal pain is very common in these cases, and being increased by standing, may distinctly excite the paralysis.*

In comparison to other countries there was, however, a dearth of original research and writing on the subject in the British literature. Kinnier Wilson suggested that, "Here in England hysteria has never been cultivated." He could only find 10 articles on it among the 350 in *Brain* published between its inception in 1877 and 1910, despite "seeing cases of functional disease in abundance." He suggested this was down to a lack of a *Maître* figurehead in the British establishment.

One exception to this was Henry Bastian (1837–1915), one of the senior staff at Queen Square who published a whole book about hysteric paralysis (Bastian, 1893). It is however, difficult to comprehend and I cannot help feeling that it shows the first signs of that particular author's journey to some peculiar ideas about life being able to appear from inanimate matter (Jellinek, 2000).

US neurology

In the USA the situation was slightly different. Silas Weir Mitchell (1829–1914), arguably the founder of US neurology, had taken a keen interest in neuroses and hysteria, including "soldier's heart" and "reflex paralysis", with and without nerve injury, the latter which later turned into reflex sympathetic dystrophy. One of his most well-known books, *Fat and Blood*, described a stringent treatment for hysteria based on a high-milk diet (to correct anemia) and enforced rest – the "rest cure" – both to isolate patients from a perceived toxic environment but also as a paradoxic intervention to make them desire activity. Contemporaries reflected that he mainly used the force of his personality to exact behavioral change. He became well known for other behavioral interventions for "hysteria," as this often-repeated anecdote testifies:

> *Dr Mitchell had run the gamut of argument and persuasion and finally announced: "If you are not out of bed in five minutes – I'll get in to it with you!" He thereupon started to remove his coat, the patient still obstinately prone – he removed his vest, but when he started to take off his trousers – she was out of bed in a fury (Burr, 1929).*

George Beard (1839–1883), one of the first doctors to call himself a neurologist, and the first elected member of the American Neurological Association, also devoted a lot of his energy to this area in the 1870s. He popularized the diagnosis of "neurasthenia," to describe a state of chronic fatigue, especially as an affliction of men and, like many physicians at the time, was impressed with the results of electric therapy. Just as World War I would spark interest in functional disorders in Europe, the American Civil War also brought this problem into sharper focus for the physicians of the day.

In the late 19th and early 20th century a group of American neurologists and psychiatrists in Boston promoted a unified approach to brain and mind. James Jackson Putnam (1846–1918) was the first neurologist at the Massachusetts General Hospital in 1872 and later president of the American Neurological Association in 1888. He had a keen interest in psychiatry throughout his career. He remained good friends with his neuropsychiatric colleague Adolf Meyer, who later, at Johns Hopkins, would be a keen Freudian instrumental in the spread of psychoanalysis in the USA. Putnam became the first president of the American Psychoanalysis Society in 1911 and wrote of his experiences as an analyst, something that is far removed from neurologic practice in the UK at the time and now (Goetz et al., 2003). Charles Franklin Hoover (1865–1927), a professor of medicine in Cleveland, Ohio, deserves special mention in this section on pre-war US neurology. His 1908 letter in *JAMA*, entitled "A new sign for the detection of malingering and functional paresis of the lower extremities," is notable for its brevity and the fact that he had only observed it in 4 patients (Hoover, 1908).

Oppenheim and traumatic neurosis

In Germany at the same time, Hermann Oppenheim (1858–1919), Professor in Berlin, was one of the preeminent neurologists of the time, also famous for a two-volume single-author textbook (Oppenheim and Mayer (transl.), 1900). Oppenheim fought powerfully from the late 1880s to World War I for the idea that "traumatic neurosis" was a condition separate and distinct from hysteria. He proposed that in patients with apparently "functional" symptoms after head or peripheral injury there was a different mechanism to those patients with what he admitted were identical symptoms as a part of hysteria. His clinical descriptions over 137 densely packed pages are excellent, but it is quite hard now to see why he thought traumatic neurosis was different, other than the obvious fact that men much more commonly fell into the "traumatic neuroses" category, just as they had also appeared disproportionately among cases of neurasthenia in the USA.

Oppenheim proposed that traumatic neurosis was due to molecular changes not present in hysteria, and whilst some of his work heads towards a progressive biopsychosocial model, it seems to do so only for patients with physical injury. He also included speculation on "fine organic changes" in the vessel walls and myelin of the brain which were different from the dynamic lesion of Charcot. Arguments ensued between Oppenheim and psychiatrists (Holdorff and Dening, 2011), with themes recurrent in older debates from the 1860s about "railway spine" and which continue to this day with whiplash injury, postconcussion syndrome, and complex regional pain syndrome (Trimble, 1981b; Malleson, 2002). Two books on malingering highlighted increasing concerns about the effects of workers' compensation legislation at this time and remain clinically relevant (Collie, 1913; Jones and Llewellyn, 1917).

WORLD WAR I

Shell shock, the term used for a variety of physical and psychologic consequences of trench warfare in the First World War, crystallized many issues between neurology and psychiatry, between the clinicopathologic method and Freudian theory. This debate spilled out to the general public, who often appeared to be more sympathetic to the soldiers than the neurologists looking after them. Around 80 000 soldiers had the diagnosis, which encompassed a wide variety of physical and psychologic presentations, including nightmares, anxiety, tremors, gait disorders, and panic attacks (Shephard, 2002; Wessely and Jones, 2005; Moscovich et al., 2013).

When soldiers started returning from war with physical complaints, the first line of enquiry was along the

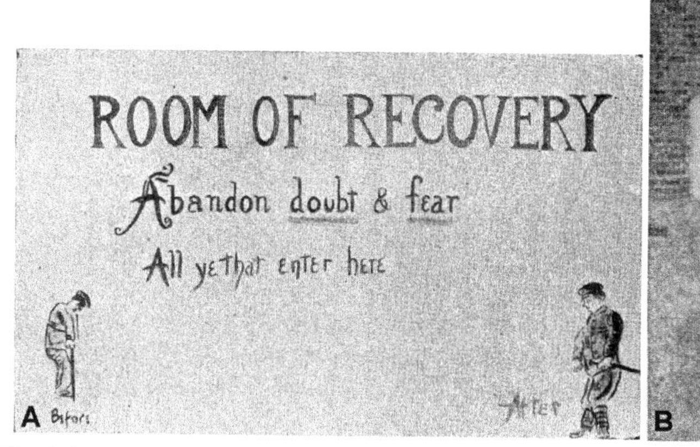

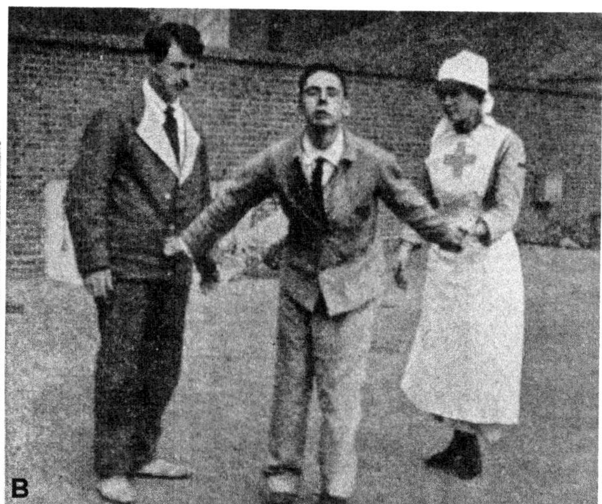

Fig. 3.1. (**A**) Notice made for Frederick Mott's door at the Maudsley Hospital, London, by a satisfied patient and (**B**) a case of astasia abasia. (Reproduced from Mott, 1919.)

lines of Oppenheim's molecular theory of traumatic neurosis. Frederick Mott (1853–1926) was a neurologist, pathologist, and psychiatrist, who with Henry Maudsley had founded the Maudsley Psychiatric Hospital in south London. He published some of the early pathologic studies of men who had been near an exploding shell, although his later work made it clear that he regarded most cases he was seeing as variants of a functional disorder (Mott, 1919) (Fig. 3.1).

Across the river in Queen Square, the much younger Lewis Yealland (1884–1954) began vigorously treating soldiers with hysteric symptoms such as mutism and paralysis with electricity. His book, *Hysterical Disorders of Warfare*, gives a very close narration of his techniques, which involved a great deal of persistence on his part, sometimes for hours on end (Yealland, 1918). Subsequent historians and novelists (Barker, 1991) have focused on the undoubtedly barbarous aspects of his method. Yealland treated 196 of the 323 cases of functional disorder at that hospital during the war. Review of this material highlights that he worked very hard for his patients, many of whom were tearfully grateful for his intervention in improving their symptoms (Linden et al., 2013). Yealland communicated, and apparently accepted, a functional model of the symptoms to his patients, something for which he was strongly criticized by Charles Myers, one of the chief figures during the war and in the UK at that time.

Charles Myers (1873–1946) had been appointed Specialist in Nerve Shock to the British Expeditionary Force in France at the beginning of the war by Gordon Holmes, neurologist, also at Queen Square. Myers had initially coined the term "shell shock," although as early as 1916 had realized that it was misleading, and suggested it be replaced by "concussion" and "nervous shock." By 1917 Myers had successfully lobbied for some of the treatment to occur on a psychologic basis near the front, whereas Holmes' view that shell shock was as a consequence of defective morale and character was very close to attributing the whole problem to malingering. Foster Kennedy, the US neurologist, in a private letter, explained how, after the war, Holmes had told him to "go back … to America … and see to it that the care of functional and organic cases there be put on the right basis – which basis is almost anything other than Freudian" (Casper, 2014).

In January 1917 Myers eventually had to accept a lesser position in the military set-up back in England, and it appears that Holmes maneuvered to remove responsibility for psychologic cases from him. Later Myers, clearly bitter at the experience, writing in his autobiography did not disguise his views on what had happened.

> *Colonel Holmes had previously told me that "functional" nervous disorders always formed a very large part of the civilian neurologist's practice. Naturally, therefore, he was little disposed to relinquish in army life what was so important a source of income in time of peace. Although he confessed that (like most "pure" neurologists) he took little interest in such cases (quoted in Shephard, 2014).*

The treatment of the psychologic and functional neurologic disorders that arose in the war formed the basis of several new institutions, notably Littlemore in Oxford and Maghull near Liverpool, where Grafton Elliott Smith (1871–1937) and William Rivers (1864–1922) were faced with large numbers of working-class soldiers requiring physical and psychologic rehabilitation. They were enthused by the "new psychology" of Freud, Janet, and Jung, but their experiences of trying to provide therapy to ordinary infantrymen through techniques such as the interpretation of dreams proved disappointing. Rivers, who had a background in both neurology and anthropology, only found these techniques more interesting when he moved to Craiglockhart in Edinburgh, where he was asked to treat the officer classes.

> *The dreams of uneducated persons are exceedingly simple and their meaning is often transparent ... it was only when I began to work in Scotland that my growing interest in the psychological problems suggested by war-neurosis began to compete and conflict with my interest in ethnology (quoted in Shephard, 2014).*

Arthur Hurst (1879–1944) had worked as a neurologist in Guys Hospital, London, before the war. He is best known for a series of films he made of patients with shell shock at Netley Hospital, a vast military hospital in Hampshire near Southampton and in Seale-Hayne, further west in Devon. His films, which show patients with movement disorders such as dystonia and gait disorder, have been pored over by interested neurologists and historians (Moscovich et al., 2013). Some of the purported cures after 30 minutes or 1 hour are remarkable, although Edgar Jones (2012) has pointed out that some of the "before" scenes were staged after recovery. Hurst's subsequent book on hysteria, *The Psychology of the Special Senses and their Functional Disorders,* is arguably more of a substantial contribution to the field and includes interesting clinical observations, especially on the role of suggestion (Hurst, 1920).

THE 1920S TO THE 1960S

After the war a committee investigated the phenomenon of shell shock. Both neurologists and psychiatrists made substantial contributions to this process (HMSO, 1922). There was widespread acceptance that the diagnostic label was not helpful and that it hid a number of separate issues that were difficult to disentangle, including genuine psychologic problems and brain injury, but also malingering and cowardice (Wessely, 2006). Ultimately, after a few years it appeared that the whole experience had left most clinicians sated and keen to move on to different topics.

Working through the table of contents of journals such as *Brain* and *Journal of Neurology and Psychopathology* (later *JNNP*) reveals very few articles on the topic.

One exception to this was an article in the *British Medical Journal* of 1922 by Henry Head (1861–1940), neurologist at Queen Square, one which clearly indicates his acceptance of the ideas of Freud and Janet but embeds them within a more recognizable pragmatic approach to both diagnosis, based on positive physical signs, and treatment (Head, 1922). His opening remarks provide some evidence of the state of play at that time, although the whole article can be thoroughly recommended to any reader of this chapter.

> *Our knowledge of the nature and causes of functional nervous disorders has been revolutionized during the last fifteen years, and more recently the prevalence of the war neuroses has aroused a widespread interest in morbid psychology. Rival theorists contend for the truth of dogmas they have elevated to the solemn position of a religious cult. Moreover, the treatment of functional neuroses has become a special branch of medical practice carried out by men who see comparatively little of organic disease (Head, 1922).*

Unfortunately, shortly after this Head developed Parkinson's disease and had to retire. From both a neurologic and psychiatric perspective, hysteria went in to a long period of neglect that lasted until the 1990s. The psychoanalytic view had been articulated as early as 1913 by Ernest Jones, a neurologist and evangelist for Freudian ideas in the UK, who wrote the following discussion of Charcot's ideas regarding a dynamic/functional lesion of the brain in hysteria.

> *The microscope obstinately refusing to reveal any changes in such centres, the conclusion was reached that the fault lay in the imperfections of the microscope, and that these changes were too minute to betray themselves except by disturbances in function. An interesting relic of this fiction is to be found in the now antiquated expression of "functional nervous disorder," which is still used in many medical and even in some neurological text-books (Jones, 1913).*

Stanley Fahn has reviewed in detail descriptions of psychogenic movement disorders in textbooks over the last century (Fahn, 2005). We carried out a survey of neurology textbooks over the 20th century to work out the proportion of each devoted to functional neurologic disorders. The data show how the topic was gradually squeezed out of the curriculum over that time (Stone et al., 2008) (Fig. 3.2).

Some authors have suggested that the reason for this lack of interest was because the disorders themselves became less common with time. This forms one of the central hypotheses in Ed Shorter's book, *From Paralysis to Fatigue*, in which he suggested that dramatic symptoms such as paralysis have been replaced over time with more vague and sophisticated symptoms such as pain and fatigue (Shorter, 1992). Harold Merskey, a

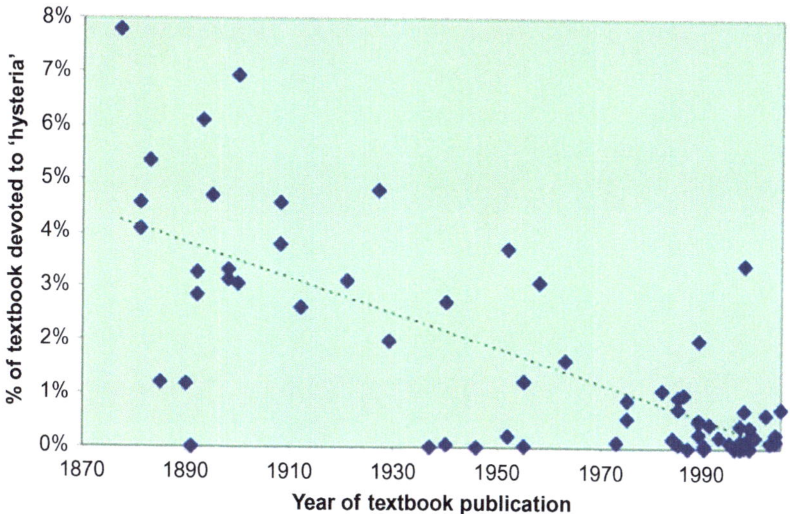

Fig. 3.2. Proportion of 68 textbooks devoted to hysteria from 1870 to 2005 (line is linear trend). (Modified from Stone et al., 2008.)

psychiatrist with an interest in hysteria, also commented in 1975 that "the classic anesthesisa, paralyses, amnesia, blindness and so forth, are now extremely rare except in certain clinical settings" (Merskey and Buhrich, 1975).

It is not easy collecting data on the topic but there is scattered evidence that in neurologic practices at least these patients remained common and had the same clinical presentation over time. This is the neurologist Georges Guillain (1876–1961) in Paris comparing his clinical practice in 1955 to that of Charcot from 1890:

> *In my recent outpatient consultations in the same hospital in the 20th century, I have the same number of sick patients but they are no longer given the name "hysteria," but instead* "psycho-nervose" *or* "troubles fonctionnels." *These illnesses have exactly the same symptoms as the illnesses which presented to Charcot. In reality, the illnesses have not changed since Charcot, it is the words we use to describe them that have changed (Guillain, 1955).*

The frequency of inpatient admission for hysteria between 1951 and 1971 at the National Hospital for Nervous Disease in Queen Square stayed fairly static at around 1% (Trimble, 1981a). It seems likely that several biases in the same direction make this an underestimate. Perkin, a London neurologist, found that 4% of his outpatients had a diagnosis of "conversion hysteria" (Perkin, 1990).

Between the 1930s and 1960s, Freudian ideas became more and more embedded in psychiatric practice and theory, especially in the USA. Hysteria, the prototypical disorder that started it all off, was in a privileged position during this time. Questioning the psychologic basis of that disorder would have been an attack on the whole of psychoanalysis. Books like Wilfred Abse's *Hysteria and Related Mental Disorders* from 1966 indicate the prevailing conversion hypothesis with pictures of symbolic symptoms (Fig. 3.3). Textbooks such as that of Purves-Stewart that did discus hysteria epitomized the predominantly diagnostically focused approach, with the patient's life story and background little discussed (Purves-Stewart and Worster-Drought, 1952). Neurologic asssociations such as the Association of British Neurologists, formed in the 1930s, had no members with an interest in functional disorders (Ted Reynolds, personal communication).

During World War II, cases of hysteria did not appear as frequent, or if they were present, perhaps were less well publicized. A remarkable 1946 US education film, *Let There be Light,* directed by John Huston and made to assist military health personnel, from that period contains sequences, filmed with real patients, of an abreaction with sedation for a patient with a functional gait disorder. The soldier is led in barely able to walk but after sedation and suggestion can stand and walk normally (Fig. 3.4). Another scene documented verbal abreaction for post-traumatic stress.

By the 1960s there was very little research on hysteria. Eliot Slater (1904–1983), a psychiatrist appointed to the National Hospital, took a particular interest carrying out one of the only genetic studies of the disorder in the late 1950s (Slater, 1961). By the mid-1960s however he was disillusioned. Data collected by his colleague Eric Glithero appeared to suggest a high rate of misdiagnoses. It is hard to summarize the data in Slater's follow-up study of 112 patients over a 9-year period because it is so poorly presented (Slater, 1965; Slater and Glithero, 1965). Authors trying to do so have come up with figures ranging from 20% to 60%. Slater mixed presumed misdiagnosis (hysteric weakness turning into "atypical myopathy") with diagnoses that were probably incidental (renal cancer)

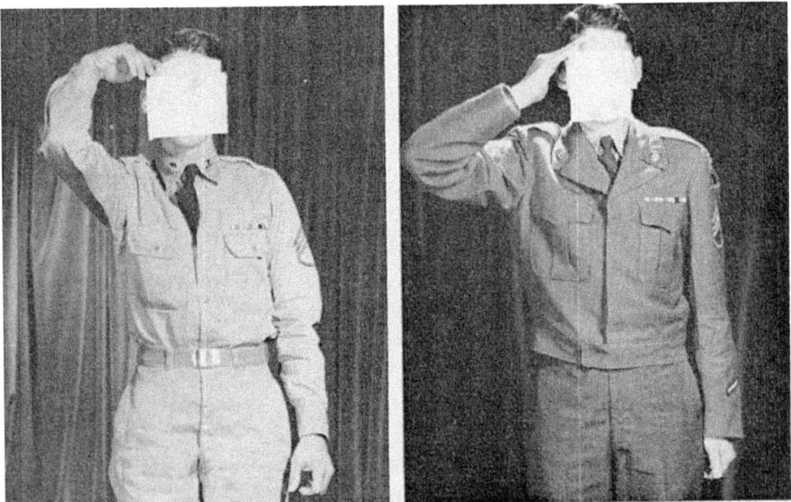

Fig. 3.3. A man with difficulty saluting (**A**) before treatment and (**B**) after treatment is a perfect example of Freudian symbolism in conversion disorder. (Reproduced from Abse, 1966.)

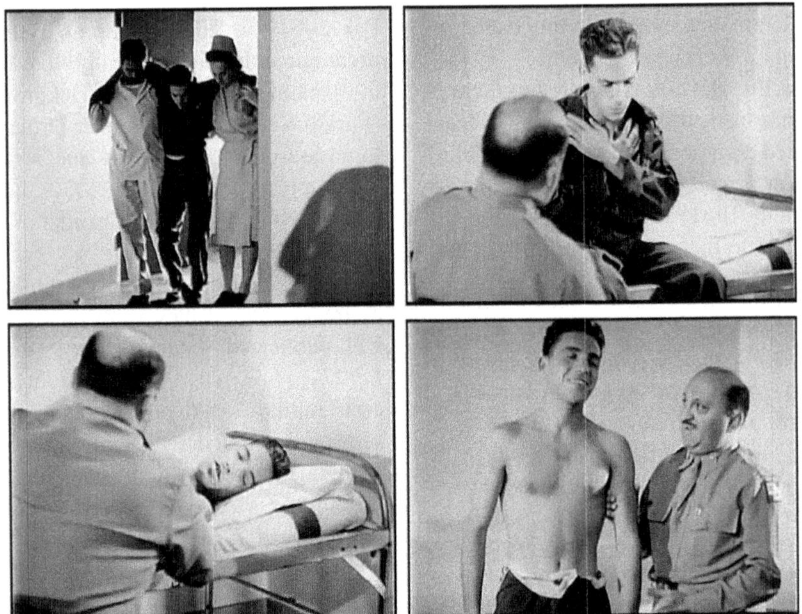

Fig. 3.4. Abreaction of a soldier with functional gait disorder, from *Let There be Light*, a US army film from 1946 directed by John Huston and featuring real patients. From top left clockwise: abnormal gait; explaining the onset with chest pain and back pain; abreaction with discussion of life stress; resolution of symptoms.

and later pathologic findings of dubious significance (cortical atrophy). Slater famously concluded that hysteria did not exist and that the diagnosis was a delusion. Sir Francis Walshe (1885–1973), a neurologist not known for his interest in the topic, nonetheless wrote a fierce reply suggesting Slater's stance was just a way of avoiding the patient.

> *Alas! We are not all cast in his mould, and, liable to frustration in the handling of the subject of hysteria as we are, it is only too easy to resent our dilemma; so that when presented with an essentially curable clinical state that we still cannot banish, we suggest to ourselves that there is no such illness (Walshe, 1965).*

St. Louis "hysteria" and the systematization of symptoms

In the 1950s and 1960s the St. Louis school, Eli Robins (1921–1994) and Samuel Guze (1923–2000), carried out a series of systematic studies of patients with hysteria, including a case-control study (Purtell et al., 1951), a retrospective and then prospective cohort study testing new criteria for the diagnosis (Guze, 1967). They suggested a new operationalized approach to the diagnosis of hysteria based on a history of 25 multiple physical symptoms over a long period and beginning before the age of 35. Their scientific approach was incorporated into the *Diagnostic and Statistical Manual of Mental Disorders* (3rd edn: DSM-III: American Psychiatric Association, 1980) definition of somatization disorder. Also in this period an outstanding Swedish retrospective cohort study of 381 patients and their relatives by Lennart Ljungberg, published as a 26-chapter supplement, deserves a mention (Ljungberg, 1957).

1970S TO 1990S

From a neurologic perspective, though, there was little sign of renewed interest until the late 1980s. Many books and articles in these decades promoted the view that patients with conversion disorders were often histrionic or seductive. *La belle indifférence* often featured prominently as a diagnostic sign, although subsequent controlled studies do not support its use (Stone et al., 2006) (Fig. 3.5).

Ted Reynolds, one of the first epileptologists in the UK, remembers that, training in the 1960s at Queen Square, "none of the neurologists were interested in hysteria and the patients were promptly shunted out or sometimes over to Eliot Slater."

C. David Marsden (1938–1998), neurologist at Kings College Hospital and later Queen Square, was instrumental in reclassifying the focal and task-specific dystonias as neurologic diseases and not as psychogenic phenomena (Quinn et al., 2012). One can see at the time that the existing psychiatric models for such symptoms, such as torticollis as a "turning away from responsibility," were especially unsatisfactory. Marsden reclaimed an earlier strand of thinking in which these dystonias had already been considered disease states, but set them on a much firmer footing (Munts and Koehler, 2010). Marsden's careful work arguably influenced a generation of movement disorders to be especially careful about labeling presentations as "psychogenic." His long-standing colleague at Kings College Hospital, Ted Reynolds, remembers him, however, as being prepared to diagnose functional or psychogenic disorder and doing it often (Ted Reynolds, personal communication).

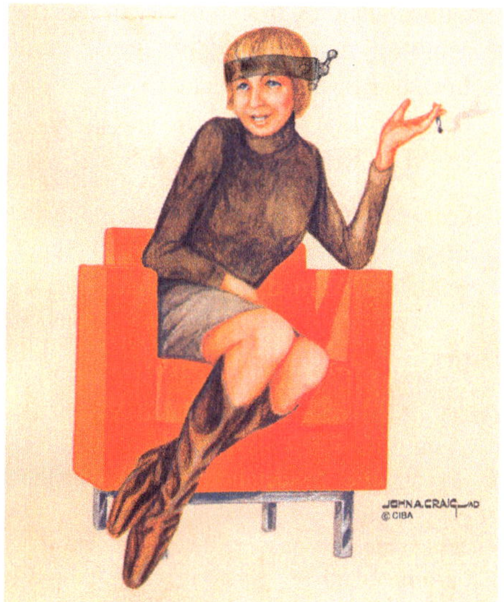

Fig. 3.5. 1970s Depiction of *la belle indifférence* in relation to headache betrays a sexualized and derogatory view. (Reproduced from Weintraub, 1977.)

Marsden and Reynolds were neurologists in the heart of the Institute of Psychiatry, part of Kings College London, and as such rekindled the older firmer relationships with psychiatry that had faded in the middle of the century. Ted Reynolds, for example, was one of the founding neurologists of the British Neuropsychiatry Association in 1987 and edited a volume called *The Bridge between Neurology and Psychiatry* in 1989 with Michael Trimble, based at the Institute of Neurology (Reynolds and Trimble, 1989). Marsden wrote an excellent review of hysteria in 1986 for *Psychological Medicine* and was a coauthor on the 1998 study, "Slater revisited," which demonstrated again how incorrect Slater had been about the stability of the diagnosis when made by neurologists (Crimlisk et al., 1998). Studies from the early 1970s had been turning up misdiagnosis rates of around 4% (Stone et al., 2005), but this was a particular turning point, partly because it was done in the same institution as Slater's original study.

From the mid-1980s, videotelemetry offered epilepsy specialists a whole new level of clinical certainty about seizure disorders. Series of patients with "pseudoseizures" began to appear in the literature, notably from Gates in the USA (Gates et al., 1985), Lempert and colleagues in Berlin (Lempert and Schmidt, 1990), and from a team in Queen Square led by Simon Shorvon (Meierkord et al., 1991).

Stan Fahn and Dan Williams in New York wrote one of the earliest case series of psychogenic movement disorders, a case series of psychogenic dystonia (Fahn and Williams, 1988), a condition for which they provided inpatient multidisciplinary treatment (see Chapter 51). Others followed on psychogenic tremor (Koller et al., 1989), gait (Lempert et al., 1991), myoclonus (Monday and Jankovic, 1993), and parkinsonism (Lang et al., 1995), focusing once again on the positive diagnostic signs that had been in the canon of the neurologist since the 1880s but had become somewhat lost along the way.

The first functional imaging study of a functional neurologic disorder was a single-case positron emission tomography study from Oxford and London (Marshall et al., 1997). The finding, abnormal activation of right orbitofrontal and anterior cingulate activity when attempting to move a paralyzed leg, reopened the debate started by Charcot when he had suggested a mechanism for hysteria could involve a "dynamic" lesion of the nervous system.

DEVELOPMENTS SINCE 2000 AND THE FUTURE

It is, of course, risky to write about the recent past from a historic perspective. It does seem likely, though, that the period from 1995 onwards will be seen as a renaissance of interest in the area of functional neurologic disorders, even if not quite an explosion.

Research groups across the world, especially in the UK, USA, Netherlands, and Switzerland, have increased in number and productivity. A survey suggested there were 180 articles on psychogenic nonepileptic seizures in the journal *Epilepsy and Behavior* alone over this period (Brigo and Igwe, 2014). Studies have covered semiology, etiology, mechanism, and treatment. Randomized trials, especially larger ones, are however still in short supply (Goldstein et al., 2010; Jordbru et al., 2014; LaFrance et al., 2014).

Several books have arisen from international meetings on functional/psychogenic disorders in Woodstock, Oxfordshire (2000) (Marshall et al., 2001), Atlanta (2003) (Hallett et al., 2005), and Washington (2009) (Hallett et al., 2011). Gates and Rowan's initial 1993 book on pseudoseizures is about to enter its fourth edition (Schacter and LaFrance, 2010). The book for which this chapter has been written, *Handbook of Clinical Neurology*, is in a series stretching back to 1968 which has never had a comparable volume. It appears that functional disorders are also beginning to make a comeback in textbook, neurologic curricula, and general neurology journals, although progress is slow and undoubtedly patchy.

Information for patients (e.g. www.neurosymptoms.org, currently receiving 60 000 hits a month) and patient organizations (e.g. www.fndhope.org) are also new in the history of functional neurologic disorders. They create new opportunities for treatment and also challenges for health professionals not used to transparency or working alongside patients whom they have often tended to keep at arm's length.

From a classification perspective, functional disorders have never figured in the *International Classification of Disesases* (ICD) "neurology" section, although they do appear as "dissociative (conversion) disorders" in the psychiatry section and other functional disorders, for example, irritable-bowel syndrome, appear in the "gastroenterology" section. From ICD-11 they will appear in both the neurology and psychiatry sections, perhaps marking an era in which they sit more comfortably at the interface between neurology and psychiatry rather than exclusively within psychiatry (Stone et al., 2014). Ultimately, a single section for neurologic and psychiatric disease would make more sense (Reynolds, 2012a).

CONCLUSIONS

The history of functional neurologic disorders in the 20th century from the point of view of the neurologist appears to be U-shaped. Between the 1880s and early 1920s professional structures and working practices allowed some neurologists to maintain an interest in psychiatry. This gave way in the 1930s to professional separation, lack of interest, and skepticism, and in the 1950s and 1960s concern from psychiatry about misdiagnosis. In the 1980s interest in collaboration between neurologists and psychiatrists led to a resurgence of these professional relationships and by the 1990s the advent of imaging and other technology highlighted the positive nature of a functional diagnosis. These disorders are now once again the subject of academic and clinical interest, although arguably still very much on the fringes of neurology and neuropsychiatry. Revisiting older material provides a rich source of ideas and data for today's clinical researcher but also offers cautionary tales of theories and treatments that led to stagnation rather than advancement of the field. Patterns of treatment do have a habit of repeating themselves, for example, the current enthusiasm for transcranial magnetic stimulation compared to the excitement about electrotherapy in the 19th century (McWhirter et al., 2015). For these reasons, an understanding of the history of functional disorders in neurology is arguably more important than it is for other areas of neurologic practice.

ACKNOWLEDGMENTS

I would like to thank Ted Reynolds, who made a valuable contribution to this chapter. Also thanks to Alan Carson, Mark Hallett, Bilal Ahmed, and Michael Okun.

References

Abse WD (1966). Hysteria and Related Mental Disorders, John Wright, Bristol.

American Psychiatric Association (1980). Diagnostic and Statistical Manual of Mental Disorders, 3rd edn. American Psychiatric Association, Washington, DC.

Babinski J, Froment J (1918). Hysteria or Pithiatism (transl. by JD Rolleston), University of London Press, London.

Barker P (1991). Regeneration, Viking, London.

Bastian HC (1893). Various Forms of Hysterical or Functional Paralysis, Lewis, London.

Brigo F, Igwe SC (2014). Psychogenic nonepileptic seizures are Cinderella seizures, and Epilepsy & Behavior is their Prince Charming. Epilepsy Behav: 7–8.

Burr AR (1929). Weir Mitchell, His Life and Letters, Duffield, New York.

Casper ST (2014). The Neurologists - a History of a Medical Specialty in Modern Britain c.1789–2000, Manchester University Press, Manchester.

Collie J (1913). Malingering, Arnold, London.

Crimlisk HL, Bhatia K, Cope H et al. (1998). Slater revisited: 6 year follow up study of patients with medically unexplained motor symptoms. BMJ 316: 582–586.

Fahn S (2005). The History of Psychogenic Movement Disorders. In: M Hallett, AE Lang, S Fahn et al. (Eds.), Psychogenic Movement Disorders, Lippincott Williams and Wilkins and the American Academy of Neurology, Philadelphia.

Fahn S, Williams DT (1988). Psychogenic dystonia. Adv Neurol 50: 431–455.

Gates JR, Ramani V, Whalen S et al. (1985). Ictal characteristics of pseudoseizures. Arch Neurol 42: 1183–1187.

Goetz CG, Chmura TA, Lanska D (2003). Part 1: the history of 19th century neurology and the American Neurological Association. Ann Neurol 53 (Suppl 4): S2–S26.

Goldstein LH, Chalder T, Chigwedere C et al. (2010). Cognitive-behavioral therapy for psychogenic nonepileptic seizures: a pilot RCT. Neurology 74: 1986–1994.

Gowers WR (1892). Hysteria. In: A Manual of diseases of the Nervous System, Churchill, London, pp. 903–960.

Guillain G (1955). Charcot: 1825–1893. Sa vie, son oeuvre, Masson, Paris.

Guze SB (1967). The diagnosis of hysteria: what are we trying to do? Am J Psychiatry 124: 491–498.

Hallett M, Cloninger CR, Fahn S et al. (2005). Psychogenic Movement Disorders. Lippincott Williams & Wilkins and the American Academy of Neurology, Philadelphia, PA.

Hallett M, Lang AE, Jankovic J et al. (2011). Psychogenic Movement Disorders and Other Conversion Disorders. Cambridge University Press, Cambridge.

Head H (1922). The diagnosis of hysteria. BMJ i: 827–829.

HMSO (1922). Report of the War Office Committee of Enquiry into "Shell Shock.", HMSO, HMSO. London.

Holdorff B, Dening DT (2011). The fight for "traumatic neurosis", 1889–1916: Hermann Oppenheim and his opponents in Berlin. Hist Psychiatry 22: 465–476.

Hoover CF (1908). A new sign for the detection of malingering and functional paresis of the lower extremities. JAMA 51: 746–747.

Hurst A (1920). The Psychology of the Special Senses and their Functional Disorders, Henry Frowde, Hodder & Stoughton, Oxford University Press, London.

Janet P (1901). The Mental State of Hystericals, Putnams, New York.

Janet P (1907). The Major Symptoms of Hysteria, Macmillan, London.

Jellinek EH (2000). Dr H C Bastian, scientific Jekyll and Hyde. Lancet 356: 2180–2183.

Jones E (1913). The treatment of the psychoneuroses. In: WA White, SE Jelliffe (Eds.), The Modern Treatment of Nervous and Mental Diseases (p. 350), Henry Kimpton, London, p. 350.

Jones E (2012). War neuroses and Arthur Hurst: a pioneering medical film about the treatment of psychiatric battle casualties. J Hist Med Allied Sci 67: 345–373.

Jones AB, Llewellyn LJ (1917). Malingering or the Simulation of Disease, William Heinemann, London.

Jordbru AA, Smedstad LM, Klungsøyr O et al. (2014). Psychogenic gait disorder: a randomized controlled trial of physical rehabilitation with one-year follow-up. J Rehabil Med 46: 181–187.

Kinnier Wilson SA (1910). Some modern French conceptions of hysteria. Brain 33: 293–338.

Kinnier Wilson SA (1940). Neurology, Edward Arnold, London.

Koller W, Lang A, Vetere-Overfield B et al. (1989). Psychogenic tremors. Neurology 39: 1094–1099.

LaFrance WC, Baird GL, Barry JJ et al. (2014). Multicenter pilot treatment trial for psychogenic nonepileptic seizures: a randomized clinical trial. JAMA Psychiatry 71: 997–1005.

Lang AE, Koller WC, Fahn S (1995). Psychogenic parkinsonism. Arch Neurol 52: 802–810.

Lempert T, Schmidt D (1990). Natural history and outcome of psychogenic seizures: a clinical study in 50 patients. J Neurol 237: 35–38.

Lempert T, Brandt T, Dieterich M et al. (1991). How to identify psychogenic disorders of stance and gait. A video study in 37 patients. J Neurol 238: 140–146.

Linden SC, Jones E, Lees AJ (2013). Shell shock at Queen Square: Lewis Yealland 100 years on. Brain 136: 1976–1988.

Ljungberg L (1957). Hysteria: a clinical, prognostic and genetic study. Acta Psychiatr Neurol Scand Suppl 112: 1–162.

Malleson A (2002). Whiplash and Other Useful Illnesses, McGill-Queen's University Press, Montreal.

Marsden CD (1986). Hysteria – a neurologist's view. Psychol Med 16: 277–288.

Marshall JC, Halligan PW, Fink GR et al. (1997). The functional anatomy of a hysterical paralysis. Cognition 64: 1–8.

Marshall JC, Halligan PW, Bass CM (2001). Contemporary Approaches to the Study of Hysteria. Oxford University Press, Oxford.

McWhirter L, Carson A, Stone J (2015). The body electric: a long view of electrical therapy for functional neurological disorders. Brain 138: 1113–1120.

Meierkord H, Will B, Fish D et al. (1991). The clinical features and prognosis of pseudoseizures diagnosed using video-EEG telemetry. Neurology 41: 1643–1646.

Merskey H, Buhrich NA (1975). Hysteria and organic brain disease. Br J Med Psychol 48: 359–366.

Mitchell SW (1877). Fat and Blood: And How to Make Them. J.B. Lippincott, Philadelphia.

Monday K, Jankovic J (1993). Psychogenic myoclonus. Neurology 43: 349–352.

Moscovich M, Estupinan D, Qureshi M et al. (2013). Shell shock: psychogenic gait and other movement disorders – a film review. Tremor and Other Hyperkinetic Movements 3: 1–7.

Mott FW (1919). War Neuroses and Shell Shock, Henry Frowde, Hodder & Stoughton, Oxford University Press, London.

Munts AG, Koehler PJ (2010). How psychogenic is dystonia? Views from past to present. Brain 133: 1552–1564.

Oppenheim H, Mayer (transl.) EE (1900). Diseases of the Nervous System: A Textbook for Student and Practitioner of Medicine, J.B. Lippincott, Philadelphia, PA.

Paget J (1873). Nervous mimicry. In: S Paget (Ed.), Selected Essays and Addresses by Sir James Paget, Longmans, Green, London.

Perkin GD (1990). Outpatient referrals. J Neurol Neurosurg Psychiatry 53: 535–536.

Purtell JJ, Robins E, Cohen ME (1951). Observations on clinical aspects of hysteria; a quantitative study of 50 hysteria patients and 156 control subjects. JAMA 146: 902–909.

Purves-Stewart J, Worster-Drought C (1952). The psychoneuroses and psychoses. In: Diagnosis of Nervous Diseases, Williams and Wilkins, Baltimore, MD, pp. 661–758.

Quinn N, Rothwell J, Jenner P (2012). Charles David Marsden. 15 April 1938–29 September 1998. Biographical Memoirs of Fellows of the Royal Society 58: 203–228.

Reynolds JR (1869). Paralysis and other disorders of motion and sensation dependent on idea. BMJ i: 483–485.

Reynolds EH (2012a). Hysteria, conversion and functional disorders: a neurological contribution to classification issues. Br J Psychiatry 201: 253–254.

Reynolds EH (2012b). Kinnier Wilson on hysteria: a missing chapter? J Neurol Neurosurg Psychiatry 83: 464–465.

Reynolds EH, Trimble M (Eds.), (1989). The Bridge Between Neurology and Psychiatry, Churchill Livingstone, Edinburgh.

Reynolds EH, Healy DG, Lees AJ (2011). A film of patients with movement disorders made in Queen Square, London in the Mid-1920s by Samuel Alexander Kinnier Wilson. Mov Disord 26: 2453–2459.

Schacter S, LaFrance Jr WC (2010). Gates and Rowan's Nonepileptic Seizures, 3rd edn. Cambridge University Press, Cambridge.

Sethi KD (2011). The Wilson films – psychogenic. Mov Disord 26: 2467–2468.

Shephard B (2002). War of Nerves: Soldiers and Psychiatrists, 1914–1994. Pimlico, London.

Shephard B (2014). Headhunters: The Search for a Science of the Mind, The Bodley Head, London.

Shorter E (1992). From Paralysis to Fatigue, The Free Press, New York.

Slater ET (1961). Hysteria 311. J Ment Sci 107: 359–381.

Slater ET (1965). Diagnosis of "Hysteria". Br Med J 1: 1395–1399.

Slater ET, Glithero E (1965). A follow up study of patients diagnosed with hysteria. J Psychosom Res 9: 9–13.

Stone J, Smyth R, Carson A et al. (2005). Systematic review of misdiagnosis of conversion symptoms and "hysteria". BMJ 331: 989.

Stone J, Smyth R, Carson A (2006). La belle indifférence in conversion symptoms and hysteria: systematic review. Br J Psychiatr 188: 204–209.

Stone J, Hewett R, Carson A et al. (2008). The "disappearance" of hysteria: historical mystery or illusion? J R Soc Med 101: 12–18.

Stone J, Hallett M, Carson A, Bergen D, Shakir R (2014). Functional disorders in the Neurology section of ICD-11: a landmark opportunity. Neurology 83: 2299–2301.

Todd RB (1854). Clinical Lectures on Paralyses, Diseases of the Brain, and Other Affections of the Nervous System, J. Churchill, London.

Trimble MR (1981a). Neuropsychiatry, John Wiley, Chichester.

Trimble MR (1981b). Post-Traumatic Neurosis: from Railway Spine to the Whiplash, John Wiley, Chichester.

Walshe F (1965). Diagnosis of hysteria. BMJ 2: 1451–1454.

Weintraub MI (1977). Hysteria. A clinical guide to diagnosis. Clin Symp 29: 1–31.

Wessely S (2006). The life and death of Private Harry Farr. J R Soc Med 99: 440–443.

Wessely S, Jones E (2005). Shell Shock to PTSD: Military Psychiatry from 1900 to the Gulf War, Psychology Press, London.

Wilson SAK (1931). The approach to the study of hysteria. J Neurol Psychopath 11: 193–206.

Yealland LR (1918). Hysterical Disorders of Warfare, Macmillan, London.

Handbook of Clinical Neurology, Vol. 139 (3rd series)
Functional Neurologic Disorders
M. Hallett, J. Stone, and A. Carson, Editors
http://dx.doi.org/10.1016/B978-0-12-801772-2.00004-7

Chapter 4

Freud's hysteria and its legacy

R.A.A. KANAAN*

Department of Psychiatry, University of Melbourne, Austin Hospital, Heidelberg, Australia

Abstract

Though Freud was himself interested in neurologic disorders, the model of hysteria he developed – of the repression of painful experiences, and their conversion into physical symptoms – made the disorder psychiatric, as the increasingly complex explanations came to rely on the "meaning" of events, which could not easily be understood neurologically. This evolved to become a prototype for psychiatric illness more broadly, a model which, though challenged by the First World War, enjoyed great success, notably in the USA, dominating psychiatric thinking for most of the 20th century. Concerns about the empiric basis for his ideas latterly led to a rapid decline in their importance, however, exemplified by 1980's "etiologically neutral" DSM-III. Hysteria, now renamed conversion disorder, retained its Freudian explanation for another 30 years, but as psychiatry lost its faith in Freud, so psychiatrists stopped seeing the disorder he had made theirs, and returned it once more to neurology.

INTRODUCTION

In the long history of hysteria, its brief time as a psychiatric illness begins, and in a sense ends, with Freud. Though he, and his work, inevitably had antecedents and collaborators, his contribution was unrivaled in its novelty, scope, and impact. He made hysteria a psychiatric illness with a model that dominated psychiatry's thinking for over half a century, and rendered it seemingly inescapably different from the rest of medicine. Such was the grip of that model on generations of psychiatrists that even when his ideas were finally rejected, wholesale, by the *Diagnostic and Statistical Manual of Mental Disorders* (3rd edition) (DSM-III) in 1980 (APA, 1980) a special case for a Freudian hysteria was made for 30 years more. I shall outline that model and how it fared in the 20th century, charting the rise and fall of a "golden age" for hysteria, when it stood as a paragon of illness, instead of as a reproach.

FREUDS HYSTERIA

At the time when he began working with hysteric patients, hysteria was effectively a neurological disorder, and Freud was a neurologist. It was a time of great interest in hysteria (Shorter, 1986), which had become a particular focus of the greatest neurologist of his time, Jean-Martin Charcot. Freud undertook a fellowship with him, and was clearly inspired (Freud, 1953c), though his own work in hysteria soon surpassed that of his teacher.

Those works were among Freud's earliest,[1] in a huge corpus that underwent considerable evolution. Hysteria was the first subject he explored with the methods that made his fame; his interest then seemed to wane as he

[1]In approximate chronological order (roman numerals refer to the volume of the standard edition): Charcot, 1893, III; On the Psychical Mechanism of Hysterical Phenomena: A lecture, 1893, III; Some Points for a Comparative Study of Organic and Hysterical Motor Paralyses, 1893, I; The Neuro-Psychoses of Defence, 1894, III; Studies on Hysteria, 1895, II; Further Remarks on the Neuro-Psychoses of Defence, 1896, III; The Aetiology of Hysteria, 1896, III; Fragment of an Analysis of a Case of Hysteria, 1905, VII; Some General Remarks on Hysterical Attacks, 1908, VIII; Hysterical Phantasies and their relation to Bisexuality, 1908, IX; Five Lectures on Psycho-Analysis, 1910, XI; The Psycho-Analytic View of Psychogenic Disturbance of vision, 1910, XI; Beyond the Pleasure Principle, 1922, XVIII.

*Correspondence to: Richard A.A. Kanaan, Department of Psychiatry, Lance Townsend Level 10, Austin Hospital, Heidelberg, VIC 3084, Australia. Tel: +61-9496-3351, E-mail: richard.kanaan@unimelb.edu.au

extended his psychology to neuroses in general, though he continued to refer to his early work with approval (describing his 1895 *Studies in Hysteria* as "valuable first approximations" in 1908 (Breuer and Freud, 1953, p. xxxi)). At its simplest, his model had two parts, the repression of a "traumatic" idea and its conversion into physical symptoms: "she repressed her erotic idea and transformed the amount of its affect into physical sensations of pain" (Breuer and Freud, 1953, p. 164). The repression involved doing something to an unwelcome idea that rendered it less conscious, or separate from our primary consciousness (latterly, the ego). The conversion cooperated in this, as the "excitation" of the traumatic idea was converted into a physical symptom, so discharging its affective energy and helping to keep the idea repressed. Both parts, the repression and the conversion, were present in some form from the start of Freud's work and retained throughout. The conversion concept was not developed much, but the repression aspect was greatly elaborated as his work progressed and is difficult to singly define.

REPRESSION

Repression is one of Freud's most enduring notions. He started from the principle that we normally know what it is that upsets us – what makes us cry, for example – so that if we accept that something has upset someone without them recognizing it, then we should accept that there are unconscious ideas (Breuer and Freud, 1953, p. 221; Freud, 1953c, p. 19). Of the many metaphors that were used to describe such unconscious ideas, the first was of a "foreign body" in flesh:

> *her love ... was present in her consciousness like a foreign body, without having entered into relationship with the rest of her ideational life ... We do not mean that their consciousness was of a lower quality or of a lesser degree, but that they were cut off from free associative connection of thought with the rest of the ideational content of her mind (Breuer and Freud, 1953, p. 165).*

This was possible even when an idea was traumatic because the affect – the emotional charge – had been converted. The idea remained, but its affect was stripped, allowing it to be easily overlooked: "the idea that gave rise to them is no longer coloured with affect and no longer marked out among other ideas and memories" (Breuer and Freud, 1953, p. 208). This was carried out deliberately, to avoid thinking of the painful experience:

> *The actual traumatic moment, then, is the one at which the incompatibility forces itself upon the ego and at which the latter decides on the repudiation of the incompatible idea. That idea is not annihilated by a repudiation of this kind, but merely repressed into the unconscious ... The splitting of the consciousness in these cases of acquired hysteria is accordingly a deliberate and intentional one. At least it is often introduced by an act of volition; for the actual outcome is something different from what the subject intended. What he wanted was to do away with an idea, as though it had never appeared, but all he succeeds in doing is to isolate it psychically (Breuer and Freud, 1953, p. 123).*

Though the repression may have been deliberate, the effects were unintended – "the formation of dangerous substitutes for the repressed" (Freud, 1953h, p. 215), which would include conversion when the conditions were right.

The intentional nature of this contributed to the sense of illness deception, as Freud was well aware. He appreciated that the functions that patients reported missing were "still there" (Freud, 1953h, p. 212), and would be available to them if the situation were critical (Freud, 1953e, p. 45). He saw that patients had a need to be ill (Breuer and Freud, 1953, p. 243), derived clear benefits from being ill (Freud, 1953e, p. 42), and showed resistance to a therapy designed to make them well (Breuer and Freud, 1953, p. 270). He knew that doctors seeing this concluded it was deliberate pretense (Freud, 1953c), and he was equally explicit that his own account was of a process initiated deliberately (Freud, 1953f, p. 47), willfully (Freud, 1953f, p. 46), intentionally (Freud, 1953e, p. 45): the reason he insisted the patient was the victim as much as the perpetrator in all this was, of course, the unconscious.

The nature of the unconscious and of repression famously underwent considerable development in the topographic and structural models – the conscious, subconscious, and preconscious; the ego, superego, and id. But these did not intrude much into Freud's discussion of hysteria. What did change was the complexity of the repressed material, its associations, and its accessibility. Though he remained wedded to the cathartic model – that articulating the repressed ideas would be curative – the ideas that must be articulated became increasingly diffuse: "no hysterical symptom can arise from a real experience alone, but that in every case the memory of earlier experiences awakened in association to it plays a part in causing the symptom" (Freud, 1953a, p. 197). In Freud's first studies, it was enough for the patient to recall the traumatic event, under hypnosis, or even under his "pressure technique" (which was little more than insisting his patients remember) for cure to be effected (Breuer and Freud, 1953, Part IV). But, as some articulations failed to cure, and he found it hard to get people to recall when directly challenged, Freud traced the symptoms through their associations (Freud, 1953e, p. 12), circuitously and further back in time, to childhood and even infancy (Freud, 1953f, p. 165). Equally, the associations became more complex, and the formulation "overdetermined," with multiple causal and associative chains leading to the same symptom (Breuer and Freud, 1953, p. 293). Associations were no longer simply temporal, but also symbolic, increasingly sexual, and highly elaborate:

> *No one, I believe, can have had any true conception of the complexity of the psychological events in a case of hysteria … The emphasis laid by Janet upon the* "idée fixe" *which becomes transformed into a symptom amounts to no more than an extremely meagre attempt at schematization (Freud, 1953e, p. 114).*

CONVERSION

Exploring the mechanics of conversion, we find a similar progression. Initially, the conversion – the transformation of the traumatic idea into symptoms – was little more than a behavioral description: problems lead to symptoms. Of course, there was that word "transformation" in addition, but neither "transformation" nor "conversion" told us much. Both suggested an almost alchemic process where substances were changed into one another, and at least initially this seems to have been Freud's view, in terms of the conversion of energies. He had ambitions to render this in neurological terms (Freud, 1953g), albeit with a more sophisticated, network model (Guenther, 2013), and initially employed physiological language, such as "cortical excitation" and "somatic innervation," though he was clear there was no specific evidence for these, and his use was thus both hypothetical and metaphorical. He postulated that all stimulation, whether sensory or ideational, would lead to increased excitation, and activity, such as motor acts or talking, would decrease excitation; and that "there exists in the organism a '*tendency to keep intracerebral excitation constant*'" (Breuer and Freud, 1953, p. 197), so that acts of revenge, for example, or even replying to insults, could be effective in decreasing the excitation in a nonpathologic way. Without these, a conversion (like a "short circuit") would be a risk (Breuer and Freud, 1953, p. 201).

> *I cannot, I must confess, give a hint of how a conversion of this kind is brought about … It is a process which occurs under the pressure of the motive of defence in someone whose organization … has a proclivity in that direction … If we venture a little further and try to represent the ideational mechanism in a kind of algebraical picture, we may attribute a certain quota of affect to the … feelings which remained unconscious, and say that this quantity (the quota of affect) is what was converted (Breuer and Freud, 1953, p. 166).*

In the *Studies*, it was argued that this affective energy was channeled to the brain regions responsible for the motor and sensory activity, giving rise to the symptoms directly: "Since hallucinations of pain arise so easily in hysteria, we must posit an abnormal excitability of the apparatus concerned with sensations of pain" (Breuer and Freud, 1953, p. 189). However Freud had earlier evinced a clear grasp of the ways in which hysterical symptoms did not fit with anatomy and physiology (Freud, 1953j), so that excitation of a motor area would be a very poor fit for hysterical motor phenomena: in his later works this simplistic model of conversion was dropped, replaced by something altogether more profound – and obscure.

As he dispensed with the conversion of a single, specific trauma, whether recent or of childhood (the "seduction theory") in favor of infantile sexuality, and then in favor of a response to a complex of incompatible ideas, it became clear there could be no simple alchemical conversion of a memory into a symptom, and after 1909 he no longer referred to a mechanism, so much as a syndrome. Employing his "topographical model" of the conscious, subconscious, and preconscious, Freud outlined this new process in the case of hysterical blindness. By then his view was that the repressed ideas were of sexual desire – sexual instincts, in fact – and that these conflicted with other psychological forces over their "use" of vision:

> *Let us suppose that the sexual component instinct which makes use of looking has drawn upon itself defensive action by the ego-instincts …so that the ideas in which its desires are expressed succumb to repression and are prevented from becoming conscious; in that case there will be a general disturbance of the relation of the eye and of the act of seeing to the ego and consciousness. The ego will have lost its dominance over the organ, which will now be wholly at the disposal of the repressed sexual instinct. It looks as though the repression had been carried too far by the ego, as though it had emptied the baby out with the bath-water: the ego refuses to see anything at all any more (Freud, 1953h, p. 216).*

Freud had dispensed with any notion that the disorder was of the effector system, in this case the visual system, and claimed it now lay in its "use." Whatever had wrested control of vision had imposed its "idea" of functioning on it, leaving intact vision sustained in the unconscious, but the hysteric unaware of it: "Excitation of the blind eye may have certain psychical consequences … even though they do not become conscious. Thus hysterically blind people are only blind as far as consciousness is concerned; in their unconscious they see" (Freud, 1953h, p. 212). It is difficult to translate this into the language of physiology, or even cognitive psychology, and Freud did not try: the mind was divided, and the symptoms then arose from the interplay of its parts rather than by any (specified) relationship with the nervous system.

Freed from the constraints of even a speculative neurophysiology, the relationships that Freud then described were not those of chemistry or electricity, but of meaning in all its forms – symbolic, associative, contradictory. The accessibility of these relationships has surely contributed much to Freud's enduring appeal. Though some of those associations are explicitly paradoxical (such as "reaction formation"), they are understandable by all, just like a novel.

> *I have not always been a psychotherapist … it still strikes me as strange that the case histories I write should read like short stories and that, as one might say, they lack the serious stamp of science. I must console myself with the reflection that the nature of the subject is evidently responsible for this … The fact is that … a detailed description of mental processes such as we are accustomed to find in the works of imaginative writers enables me, with the use of a few psychological formulas, to obtain at least some kind of insight into the course of that affection (Breuer and Freud, 1953, pp. 160–161).*

THE THIRD INGREDIENT

There was initially a third component whose nature varied over the course of Freud's work (Breuer and Freud, 1953, Part 3; Freud, 1953d, lectures 1 and 2) before it was eventually eliminated. This was the special state the patient needed to be in or conditions she needed to meet in order to develop the symptoms as she did; to answer the questions "why her, why then, why that symptom?" At first Freud used the idea of the "hysterical disposition," an idea adopted from the neurologist Paul Julius Moebius. He then adopted "dissociation" – a splitting of consciousness, a weakness in the ability to synthesize perceptions – from Pierre Janet. Freud's collaborator on the *Studies*, Josef Breuer, introduced the idea of "hypnoid states" based on Anna O.'s "auto-hypnosis": just as hysteria appeared to be inducible under hypnosis, so a similar state could operate at the time that symptoms were created, perhaps due to the fright that the traumatic experience generated. Freud later dropped this concept entirely and merged the third component with repression. To the extent that a prerequisite remained, it became a repressed traumatic history, typically of sexual abuse (Freud, 1953f); the only dissociation was of the unconscious, repressed material (Freud, 1953h, p. 213), though this material assumed an increasing degree of organization as his writing progressed. He later dropped the abuse requirement as well in favor of a relevant fantasy life, and generalized this to the extent that the sexual fantasies of children became schematized in the Oedipal complex. So in his later writings there did not appear to be any distinctive state required for hysteria (nor for neuroses in general: Freud, 1953d, p. 51), except for a "somatic compliance" – some tendency in that part of the body to permit the "discharge" of this excitation in that way. This might come from a previous injury or, in his later work, from a personal symbolic relation. It was what, he thought,

> *differentiates [hysteria] from other psychoneuroses. The mental events in all psychoneuroses proceed for a considerable distance along the same lines before any question rises of the "somatic compliance" which may afford the unconscious mental process a physical outlet. When this factor is not forthcoming, something other than a hysterical symptom will arise (Freud, 1953e, p. 51).*

It is unclear how these ideas developed, as Freud largely stopped writing about hysteria after his well-received Clark lectures in the USA (Freud, 1953d) in 1909 (Tomlinson, 2005; Guttman, 2006), and stopped aligning specific etiologies with specific neuroses. Conversion became a process that could occur in anyone, and hysteria a syndrome (Mace, 1992). Thereafter, the history of Freudian hysteria was largely determined by other writers, and by the Great War.

SHELL SHOCK AND PSYCHOSOMATICS

In the First World War (1914–1918) there was an epidemic of functional neurological symptoms. Of the huge number of casualties from that unimaginable slaughter – one million from the Battle of Somme alone – 40% were deemed psychiatric, mainly functional symptoms of one type or another (Young, 1995). The extraordinary explosion of what came to be called shell shock was unprecedented, and has never been repeated. In the field of hysteria it had several consequences: it confirmed that such symptoms were not inherently gynecological, and that sexual trauma or libidinal fixations alone could not be the cause of the problem (Mace, 1992); it renewed the quiescent debate over whether these symptoms were conscious (malingering) or subconscious (Wessely, 2003), and created immense pressure on doctors to differentiate the two (Kanaan and Wessely, 2010); and it created an enduring interest in psychosomatics (Brown, 2000).

Freud responded to this epidemic, and to the responses of other psychoanalytic writers, with 1922's "Beyond the Pleasure Principle." Though he did not equate shell shock with hysteria, he saw them as similar enough – as "fixations to the experience that started the illness" (Freud, 1953b, p. 13) – to necessitate an explanation, which he provided in the form of the death instinct. Debate over the role of this, and the relative importance of Oedipal or pre-Oedipal developmental stages, came to dominate the discussion of hysteria within psychoanalysis (Guttman, 2006), though Freud did not contribute further to the debate. He did give his blessing (Brown, 2000), however, to writers such as Groddeck and Ferenzci, who argued for a broadening of symbolic meanings beyond those of the Clark lectures to any physical condition, so that even a cancerous tumor, for example, could be understood analytically – in this case as a wish to be pregnant (Gottlieb, 2003). This attempt at a psychoanalytic explanation for all illness has been regarded as such obvious "over-reaching" (Tomlinson, 2005) that it seriously hampered broader acceptance of psychoanalysis within medicine (Brown, 2000).

Within psychiatry, however, psychoanalysis enjoyed some impressive success. While its success was perhaps to be expected in its European heartland, in the USA it was more of a surprise. It owed much to the financial backing it received from the Rockefeller Foundation, and to the influential support of Adolf Meyer, the first psychiatrist-in-chief at Johns Hopkins Hospital who, though not an analyst himself, introduced it to a wide audience as part of his "biopsychosocial" formulation (Brown, 2000). It was strengthened by émigré European analysts fleeing the rise of Nazism, and with the American Psychoanalytic Association's insistence that all analysts be medically trained, contrary to Freud's wishes (Freud, 1953i). Psychoanalysis became the *de facto* model for psychiatry in the USA, even as its "over-reaching" interpretations limited its integration with medicine more broadly.

Franz Alexander was one such émigré, who took the narrower, Clark lectures, view, and combined this with his interest in physiology, and the considerable backing of the Rockefeller Foundation, to develop the field, and journal, of psychosomatic medicine in 1939, to much optimism and great popularity throughout the 1950s; but this splintered and declined in the 1960s (Guttman, 2006), with the growth of experimental clinical psychologists, and their interest in neuroscience, and the observable (Brown, 2000).

SCIENTISTS AND PHILOSOPHERS

Psychoanalysis never had the same grip on psychiatry in the UK as it did in the USA, though it benefitted from émigré analysts too, notably Freud himself. Though his ideas were cautiously received before 1914 (Loughran, 2008), they were championed during the war by W.H.R. Rivers (Young, 1995), Charles Myers, and Ernest Jones (Forrester, 2008). But attempts to institutionalize an analytic model of medicine at Cambridge after the war foundered with Rivers' early death. Instead, the newly founded Maudsley Hospital and Institute of Psychiatry became the focus of British psychiatry, and under the empirical influence of Sir Aubrey Lewis, adopted a notably antipsychoanalytic approach. The Freudian model for hysteria was rejected as "false and absurd" (Lewis, 1975), and Freudian theory more generally rejected as unscientific (Eysenck, 2004).

This critique originated in British philosophy of science. Because interpretations were so multiply realizable and the decision about their correctness so unverifiable, it was argued, any interpretation could be sustained (Wittgenstein, 1982). This was most clearly so as Freud's work progressed, when the interpretations became increasingly metaphorical and complex: a single item in a dream might come to stand for itself, its opposite, and symbolically many other things, all at the same time (Freud, 1953d, p. 35) – indeed, he noted that an interpretation that was too straightforward could not be etiologically relevant (Freud, 1953e, p. 17f). This was used to argue that Freudian theory could not be scientific, since it could not be falsified (Popper, 1963). As the scientific development of psychiatry and its integration with medicine assumed greater importance in the 20th century, a Freudian model would therefore become problematic. Arguably his greatest contribution – the importance of meaning – would be a significant obstacle, as the impossibility of locating meanings "inside the head" seemed to render them essentially different from the neurological (Putnam, 1975). Researchers looking to reconcile neuroscience with the psychological in hysteria (Vuilleumier, 2005) would increasingly find a more sympathetic model in Pierre Janet (Gottlieb, 2003).

It was nevertheless against the tide of a robustly psychoanalytic American psychiatry (Young, 1995) that Robert Spitzer was appointed chair of the task force for the immensely influential DSM-III (APA, 1980). The second edition, like the first, had been almost exclusively psychoanalytic in its construction, but Spitzer's pursuit of observable criteria in the interests of a scientific understanding of psychiatry led to the expulsion of Freudian ideas from its pages – and, in relatively short order, from American psychiatry (Young, 1995): only in hysteria, now named conversion disorder, were they retained. But, though the Freudian criteria were weakened with each iteration (Martin, 1992), it was not until DSM-5 (APA, 2013), over 30 years later, that they were finally removed from its last corner. The criteria for conversion disorder that remain no longer show any trace of Freud's influence – but nor, indeed, do they now include any feature that is obviously psychiatric: by these criteria, conversion disorder once again seems to be a neurological disorder, albeit an unexplained one.

HYSTERIA IS DEAD; LONG LIVE FUNCTIONAL NEUROLOGIC SYMPTOMS

In the 1960s there appeared a number of psychiatric articles noting the disappearance of hysteria (Kanaan and Wessely, 2010). Outside of psychiatry, too, hysteria came to be treated as an historical entity, an odd cultural phenomenon ripened by, if not born from, particular Victorian medical and sexual mores (Micale, 1995). By way of illustration, a Hollywood romantic comedy was released in 2011 with the simple title *Hysteria*: one only has to contemplate the impossibility of a similar comedy with the title *Leukaemia*, for example, to appreciate how great the fall of hysteria has been, and how far from a serious concern it has become, from the exemplar of psychiatry to a laughing stock.

What is most striking about this, however, is that it isn't true – its disappearance, at least. Whatever has changed does not appear to be related to any change in the prevalence of the condition (Stone et al., 2008). Hysteria presents with undiminished frequency to neurologists today, but it is no longer at the core of psychiatry, either conceptually or clinically. So what happened?

No adequate explanation has been formulated for this, to my knowledge, and one will not be attempted here – though its relationship with the fall of Freud cannot be ignored. Of course, the change of name from "hysteria" to "conversion disorder" may have contributed to the sense of its disappearance, but changes of name are not uncommon in medicine, or psychiatry, without attendant mysteries. More important seems to have been the publication of Eliot Slater's study claiming that hysteria was, at least in a large minority of cases, simply neuropathology that had been missed by neurologists (Slater and Glithero, 1965). Though that particular paper has been justly criticized (Stone et al., 2005), its core finding of extensive neurological comorbidity found a sympathetic ear with more than one author (Marsden, 1986), and its impact is still readily apparent today. If once treated with derision (Freud, 1953c), conversion disorder came to be treated by neurologists with a concern approaching trepidation (Kanaan et al., 2009).

By contrast, apart from those working in liaison with neurology, psychiatrists no longer seemed to treat it at all, at least not in the West (Najim et al., 2011). This is a return to the situation pre-Freud, when hysteria sat, uncomfortably, within neurology. It was Freud who made it into a psychiatric condition, and as his ideas have been discredited, so has the very foundation for considering conversion disorder to be psychiatric. It is not merely that psychiatrists don't come across it any longer: it's that when they do, they don't see it as psychiatric. The regular lament of neurologists sending their "functional" cases to psychiatrists today is that they are simply sent back, with a note saying there is "nothing psychiatrically wrong with them" (Espay et al., 2009; Kanaan et al., 2011).

Alarming as that must sound, there is a sense in which those psychiatrists are right. Though there has been a resurgence of interest in the neuroscientific investigation of Freudian ideas (Panksepp and Solms, 2012), even in hysteria (Brown et al., 2013; Aybek et al., 2014), the battle was lost with DSM-III, and the slow death of psychoanalytic training (Damsa et al., 2010). Psychoanalysis was never about diagnosis (how could it be, when the analyst might not offer an interpretation for many months?) so much as formulation – understanding patients (Young, 1995). Though psychosocial formulation was retained to a degree in the criteria for conversion disorder, psychiatrists working in the field routinely ignored that criterion, and argued for its removal (Kanaan et al., 2010; Stone et al., 2011) – for pragmatic reasons, yes, but also because without employing a Freudian, or similar, model, there was really no way a psychiatrist could formulate a case of conversion disorder (Nicholson et al., 2011). That conversion disorder stayed Freudian for as long as it did afterwards is a testament, not only to the lingering influence of his ideas, therefore, but because it was only by defining it in such terms that it made sense for it to remain in a psychiatric classification at all. If there are no diagnostic interpretations to be made, no repressed traumas to be therapeutically revealed, no neurological symptoms which have been converted: without Freud, or someone like him, what is psychiatry to do with hysteria, after a hundred years, but send it back?

References

APA (1980). Diagnostic and statistical manual of mental disorders, 3rd edn. Washington, D.C., American Psychiatric Association.

APA (2013). Diagnostic and statistical manual of mental disorders: DSM-5, Washington, D.C., American Psychiatric Association.

Aybek S, Nicholson TR, Zelaya F et al. (2014). Neural correlates of recall of life events in conversion disorder. JAMA Psychiatry 71: 52–60.

Breuer J, Freud S (1953). Studies on Hysteria. In: S Freud, A Freud, A Strachey et al. (Eds.), The standard edition of the complete psychological works of Sigmund Freud, Hogarth Press, London.

Brown TM (2000). The Rise and Fall of American Psychosomatic Medicine, New York Academy of Medicine, New York.

Brown LB, Nicholson TR, Aybek S et al. (2013). Neuropsychological function and memory suppression in conversion disorder. J Neuropsychol 8: 171–185.

Damsa C, Bryois C, Morelli D et al. (2010). Are psychiatric residents still interested in psychoanalysis? A brief report. Am J Psychoanal 70: 386–391.

Espay AJ, Goldenhar LM, Voon V et al. (2009). Opinions and clinical practices related to diagnosing and managing patients with psychogenic movement disorders: An international survey of movement disorder society members. Mov Disord 24: 1366–1374.

Eysenck HJ (2004). Decline & fall of the Freudian empire, New Brunswick, N.J; Transaction.

Forrester J (2008). 1919: Psychology and Psychoanalysis, Cambridge and London - Myers, Jones and MacCurdy. Psychoanal Hist 10: 37–94.

Freud S (1953a). The Aetiology of Hysteria. In: S Freud, A Freud, A Strachey et al. (Eds.), The Standard Edition of the complete psychological works of Sigmund Freud, Hogarth Press, London.

Freud S (1953b). Beyond the Pleasure Principle. In: S Freud, A Freud, A Strachey et al. (Eds.), The Standard Edition of the complete psychological works of Sigmund Freud, Hogarth, London.

Freud S (1953c). Charcot. In: S Freud, A Freud, A Strachey et al. (Eds.), The Standard Edition of the complete psychological works of Sigmund Freud, Hogarth Press, London.

Freud S (1953d). Five Lectures on Psycho Analysis. In: S Freud, A Freud, A Strachey et al. (Eds.), The standard edition of the complete psychological works of Sigmund Freud, Hogarth Press, London.

Freud S (1953e). A Fragment of an Analysis of a Case of Hysteria. In: S Freud, A Freud, A Strachey et al. (Eds.), The Standard Edition of the complete psychological works of Sigmund Freud, Hogarth Press, London.

Freud S (1953f). Further remarks on the Neuro-Psychoses of Defence. In: S Freud, A Freud, A Strachey et al. (Eds.), The Standard Edition of the complete psychological works of Sigmund Freud, Hogarth Press, London.

Freud S (1953g). Project for a Scientific Psychology. In: S Freud, A Freud, A Strachey et al. (Eds.), The standard edition of the complete psychological works of Sigmund Freud, Hogarth Press, London.

Freud S (1953h). The Psycho-Analytic View of Psychogenic Disturbance of Vision. In: S Freud, A Freud, A Strachey et al. (Eds.), The Standard Edition of the complete psychological works of Sigmund Freud, Hogarth Press, London.

Freud S (1953i). The Question of Lay Analysis. In: S Freud, A Freud, A Strachey et al. (Eds.), The Standard Edition of the complete psychological works of Sigmund Freud, Hogarth, London.

Freud S (1953j). Some Points for a Comparative Study of Organic and Hysterical Motor Paralyses. In: S Freud, A Freud, A Strachey et al. (Eds.), The Standard Edition of the complete psychological works of Sigmund Freud, Hogarth Press, London.

Gottlieb RM (2003). Psychosomatic medicine: the divergent legacies of Freud and Janet. J Am Psychoanal Assoc 51: 857–881.

Guenther K (2013). The disappearing lesion: Sigmund Freud, sensory-motor physiology, and the beginnings of psychoanalysis. Mod Intellect Hist 10: 569–601.

Guttman S (2006). Hysteria as a Concept. Mod Psychoanal 31: 182–228.

Kanaan RA, Wessely SC (2010). The origins of factitious disorder. Hist Human Sci 23: 68–85.

Kanaan R, Armstrong D, Barnes P et al. (2009). In the psychiatrist's chair: how neurologists understand conversion disorder. Brain 132: 2889–2896.

Kanaan RA, Carson A, Wessely SC et al. (2010). What's so special about conversion disorder? A problem and a proposal for diagnostic classification. Br J Psychiatry 196: 427–428.

Kanaan RA, Armstrong D, Wessely SC (2011). Neurologists' understanding and management of conversion disorder. J Neurol Neurosurg Psychiatry 82: 961–966.

Lewis A (1975). The survival of hysteria. Psychol Med 5: 9–12.

Loughran T (2008). Hysteria and neurasthenia in pre-1914 British medical discourse and in histories of shell-shock. Hist Psychiatry 19: 25–46.

Mace CJ (1992). Hysterical conversion. I: A history. Br J Psychiatry 161: 369–377.

Marsden CD (1986). Hysteria – a neurologist's view. Psychol Med 16: 277–288.

Martin RL (1992). Diagnostic issues for conversion disorder. Hosp Community Psychiatry 43: 771–773.

Micale MS (1995). Approaching hysteria : disease and its interpretations, Princeton University Press, Princeton, N.J.

Najim H, Al-Habbo DJ, Sultan KO (2011). Trends of admissions of conversion disorder in Mosul Iraq. Psychiatr Danub 23 (Suppl 1): S29–S31.

Nicholson TR, Stone J, Kanaan RA (2011). Conversion disorder: a problematic diagnosis. J Neurol Neurosurg Psychiatry 82: 1267–1273.

Panksepp J, Solms M (2012). What is neuropsychoanalysis? Clinically relevant studies of the minded brain. Trends Cogn Sci 16: 6–8.

Popper KR (1963). Conjectures and Refutations. The growth of scientific knowledge. (Essays and lectures.), Routledge & Kegan Paul, London.

Putnam H (1975). The meaning of 'meaning'. Minnesota Studies in the Philosophy of Science 7: 131–193.

Shorter E (1986). Paralysis: the rise and fall of a "hysterical" symptom. J Soc Hist 19: 549–582.

Slater ET, Glithero E (1965). A follow-up of patients diagnosed as suffering from "hysteria". J Psychosom Res 9: 9–13.

Stone J, Warlow C, Carson A et al. (2005). Eliot Slater's myth of the non-existence of hysteria. J R Soc Med 98: 547–548.

Stone J, Hewett R, Carson A et al. (2008). The 'disappearance' of hysteria: historical mystery or illusion? J R Soc Med 101: 12–18.

Stone J, LaFrance Jr WC, Brown R et al. (2011). Conversion disorder: current problems and potential solutions for DSM-5. J Psychosom Res 71: 369–376.

Tomlinson WC (2005). Freud and Psychogenic Movement Disorders. In: M Hallett, CR Cloninger, S Fahn et al. (Eds.), Psychogenic Movement Disorders, Lippincott Williams & Wilkins.

Vuilleumier P (2005). Hysterical conversion and brain function. Prog Brain Res 150: 309–329.

Wessely S (2003). Malingering: Historical perspectives. In: PW Halligan, CM Bass, DA Oakley (Eds.), Malingering and illness deception, Oxford University Press, New York.

Wittgenstein L (1982). Conversations with Rush Rees. In: R Wollheim, J Hopkins (Eds.), Philosophical essays on Freud, Cambridge University Press, Cambridge.

Young A (1995). The harmony of illusions: inventing post-traumatic stress disorder, Chichester, Princeton University Press, Princeton, N.J.

Section 2

Epidemiology, etiology, and mechanism

Handbook of Clinical Neurology, Vol. 139 (3rd series)
Functional Neurologic Disorders
M. Hallett, J. Stone, and A. Carson, Editors
http://dx.doi.org/10.1016/B978-0-12-801772-2.00005-9

Chapter 5

Epidemiology

A. CARSON[1]* AND A. LEHN[2]

[1]*Departments of Clinical Neurosciences and of Rehabilitation Medicine, NHS Lothian and Centre for Clinical Brain Sciences, University of Edinburgh, Edinburgh, UK*

[2]*Department of Neurology, Princess Alexandra Hospital and School of Medicine, University of Queensland, Brisbane, Australia*

Abstract

The epidemiology of functional neurologic disorders (FND) is complex and has been hampered over the years by a lack of clear definition, with previous definitions struggling with an uneasy mix of both physical and psychologic components. The recent changes in DSM-5 to a definition based on positive identification of physical symptoms which are incongruent and inconsistent with neurologic disease and the lack of need for any associated psychopathology represent a significant step forward in clarifying the disorder. On this basis, FND account for approximately 6% of neurology outpatient contacts and putative community incidence rates of 4–12 per 100 000 per annum. Comorbid neurologic disease occurs in around 10% of cases. The diagnosis is reliable, with revision rates less than 5%. Of note, this revision rate was consistent prior to the widespread utilization of computed tomography and magnetic resonance imaging. FND symptoms are disabling and associated with significant distress. They are more common in women and have a peak incidence between the ages of 35 and 50; however the presentation is common in men and throughout the lifespan. The issues surrounding case definition, ascertainment, misdiagnosis, and risk factors are discussed in detail.

INTRODUCTION: WHICH DIAGNOSIS IN WHICH POPULATION?

One of the best definitions of epidemiology is given by Wikipedia – it is the study of the patterns, causes, and effects of health and disease conditions in defined populations. The definition is straightforward but alerts us to two central problems for the study of functional neurologic disorders (FND) – what actually is the disease condition and how are we defining our population? This is not mere pedantry but can have a substantial effect on rates and risks.

In terms of what the "disease" actually is, there has been a historic tension between competing views of how FND should be categorized. The 20th-century name "conversion disorder" carries an explicit assumption that the etiology of the condition is based on psychic trauma, the memories of which are repressed but the ensuing psychologic tension, caused by this repression, escapes in the form of physical symptoms. This definition stems directly from a Freudian model (see Chapter 10) and is held with an almost theologic degree of worship by some. The problem for epidemiology is: how do we measure something that is not apparent on the surface? If patients can report it freely and easily, then by definition they are not repressing it. *Diagnostic and Statistical Manual of Diseases,* fourth edition (DSM-IV: American Psychiatric Association, 2000) had an uneasy compromise, stating that "psychological factors are judged to be associated with the symptom or deficit because the initiation or exacerbation of the symptoms or deficit is preceded by conflicts or other stressors," but never really grappled with whose judgment, how this judgement would be made, or, critically, what the diagnosis was in patients who had similar physical symptom presentations but in whom such a stressor or conflict could not be found. There was no clue for the epidemiologist as how

*Correspondence to: Dr. Alan Carson, MD MPhil FRCPsych FRCP, Robert Fergusson Unit, Royal Edinburgh Hospital, Morningside Terrace, Edinburgh EH10 5HF, UK. Tel: +44-131-537-6896, E-mail: a.carson@ed.ac.uk

this might be standardized. Furthermore, conceptually it introduced a tautology by defining a disorder according to an, as yet, unproven hypothesis.

DSM-5 represents a significant improvement: the explicit psychologic factors were dropped from the definition on the grounds that they were untestable and of uncertain significance (American Psychiatric Association, 2013). The new definition is based around the presentation of neurologic symptoms that are internally inconsistent or incongruent with the patterns of pathophysiologic disease. This offers an overt and testable definition and forms the basis of a coherent approach that has been taken forward for specific subsets of functional disorders, e.g., functional dystonia and functional tremor, and has even allowed for associated laboratory criteria to be appended (Schwingenschuh et al., 2016). The important feature is that this is not simply based on the exclusion of neurologic disease, but on the basis of positive features showing inconsistency with neurologic disease.

This approach has been exemplified in the field of functional movement disorders, which saw a push in recent years towards new diagnostic criteria to increase diagnostic sensitivity and specificity and to improve case ascertainment. Where the past criteria relied heavily on psychiatric features and historic background (Fahn and Williams, 1988; Shill and Gerber, 2006), Espay and Lang (2015) recently published a new approach. They proposed a phenotypic-specific classification exclusively reliant on clinical examination without regard for historic and psychiatric features, having removed clinically probable and possible categories. The hope is that the use of these criteria minimizes diagnostic errors. While these criteria will likely be helpful in functional movement disorders, such an approach would need to be adapted for other functional neurologic motor disorders. A similar approach has been proposed in dissociative seizures (LaFrance et al., 2013; see Chapter 17).

What remains an epidemiologic issue is the definition of how severe a symptom must be before we classify it as a "disorder." Within DSM, there is a global approach which is slightly loose: "The symptom or deficit causes clinically significant distress or impairment in social, occupational, or other important areas of functioning or warrants medical evaluation." This is pragmatic, but where cutoffs should be set is not clear. At the milder end of the spectrum, FND starts to merge with normal function. If we think away from neurologic symptoms briefly: we have all stood outside an exam hall with our stomach tied in knots, a highly unpleasant experience, but few of us would think of this as a clinical disorder. What about a newly qualified doctor, anxious at her new responsibilities, who has diarrhea for 3 months and has some investigations? Should that be considered a disorder? Or do we wait for the most extreme case of a patient who has 15 episodes of diarrhea a day and cannot leave the house without planning a route around a public toilet? Does it matter which bodily system the symptom occurs in? It is difficult to think of a severe case of functional paralysis ever being considered normal, but what about mild collapsing weakness in someone with known neuropathic pain, or cases of odd, isolated tingling in an arm? It may be functional, or it may be pain inhibiting motor function, and do we really class it as a disorder? This remains unresolved. Whilst in clinical practice common sense renders this a nonissue, for epidemiologic purposes a more precise cutoff is required. Attempts have been made to solve it by counting the number of different symptoms suffered or by looking at the disability associated with an individual symptom or by combinations of the two, with no universally accepted solution emerging.

A TECHNICAL BARRIER TO EPIDEMIOLOGIC RESEARCH

The limitation on severity aside the DSM-5 and related criteria-based definitions offers a definite improvement in that they describe objective features that can be tested, including their own utility, but in doing so they raise a major technical barrier. Making the diagnosis requires considerable medical training for it to be reliable. Carson et al. (2000) compared primary care physician (general practitioner) diagnoses to those made in neurology clinics and found general practitioners did little better than chance on whether a symptom was functional. However, with diagnoses made in neurology clinics, the diagnosis remained stable at follow-up (Stone et al., 2009b). If our "defined population" is of neurology clinic attenders, this is unlikely to be a problem, but for any other population it may present a major barrier to case ascertainment. Healthcare utilization is known to be affected by a range of gender, psychologic, and social factors. If we are trying to study the potential etiologic role of any such factors in functional symptoms (and all are valid candidates as risk factors), conducting studies in secondary care or even tertiary care settings will inevitably bias the sample.

We are unaware of any study that has had proper neurologically diagnosed case ascertainment at a population or even primary care level of FND; the costs and time would be prohibitive. Researchers generally try to get round this problem in one of three ways.

The simplest approach is to conduct studies based in services which they hope have a good level of population coverage; so one might conduct a study in a service which is theoretically the only point of contact with a neurologist for that population (for example, see Stone et al. (2010b) or Duncan et al. (2011)). However, there are many means by which patients can slip through such an ascertainment net, by not reporting their symptoms, having them dealt with by a primary care doctor and not referred on, being seen in the emergency room or a general secondary care service and not being referred to neurologists, being referred to a neurologist not involved in the study who fails to notify the researcher of the case, and so on. These studies give a good minimum prevalence level but it can be safely assumed do not detect all cases. The unanswered question therefore is: is noninclusion a genuinely random chance or is there a systematic bias that explains why a patient does not get included? Experience dictates the latter is usually the case.

An alternate approach that has gained popularity in recent years has been to use proxy measures based on screening questionnaires. This is based on the principle that patients who have FND often report multiple somatic symptoms. This increased symptom reporting has been recommended as being a useful clue to making the diagnosis (Stone et al., 2005), leading to proposals that high scores on self-rating scales of somatic symptoms will identify patients likely to have FND. Such a methodology is highly desirable as it can be administered quickly and easily, and is suitable for household surveys. A widely used example of such a scale is the Patient Health Questionnaire (PHQ-15); higher numbers of somatic symptoms on this scale have been consistently found to correlate with FND, poorer outcomes, higher healthcare use, and higher rates of depression/anxiety (Carson et al., 2011). However, a correlation analysis is not the same as testing the diagnostic sensitivity and specificity. This is particularly the case when the method allows large numbers to be recruited. Highly significant (i.e., nonchance) correlations can be found, but they often have little explanatory power, since they explain only a small proportion of the variance. In a review of the use of the PHQ-15 (Carson et al., 2011), we found 18 studies on 43 360 patients where it had been used as a diagnostic measure for somatoform symptoms and a further seven studies in which it had been used as a quasidiagnostic measure on 17 016 patients. These were large-scale studies with significant impact and the measure was being recommended for use as a diagnostic tool in primary care despite a lack of validation against a gold standard of assessment by experienced clinicians. As above, when we examined the PHQ-15 in a prospective study, we too found highly significant correlations between increased scores on the PHQ and FND, but when we examined the actual diagnostic accuracy of any given cutoff score we found a performance little better than chance (Figs 5.1 and 5.2).

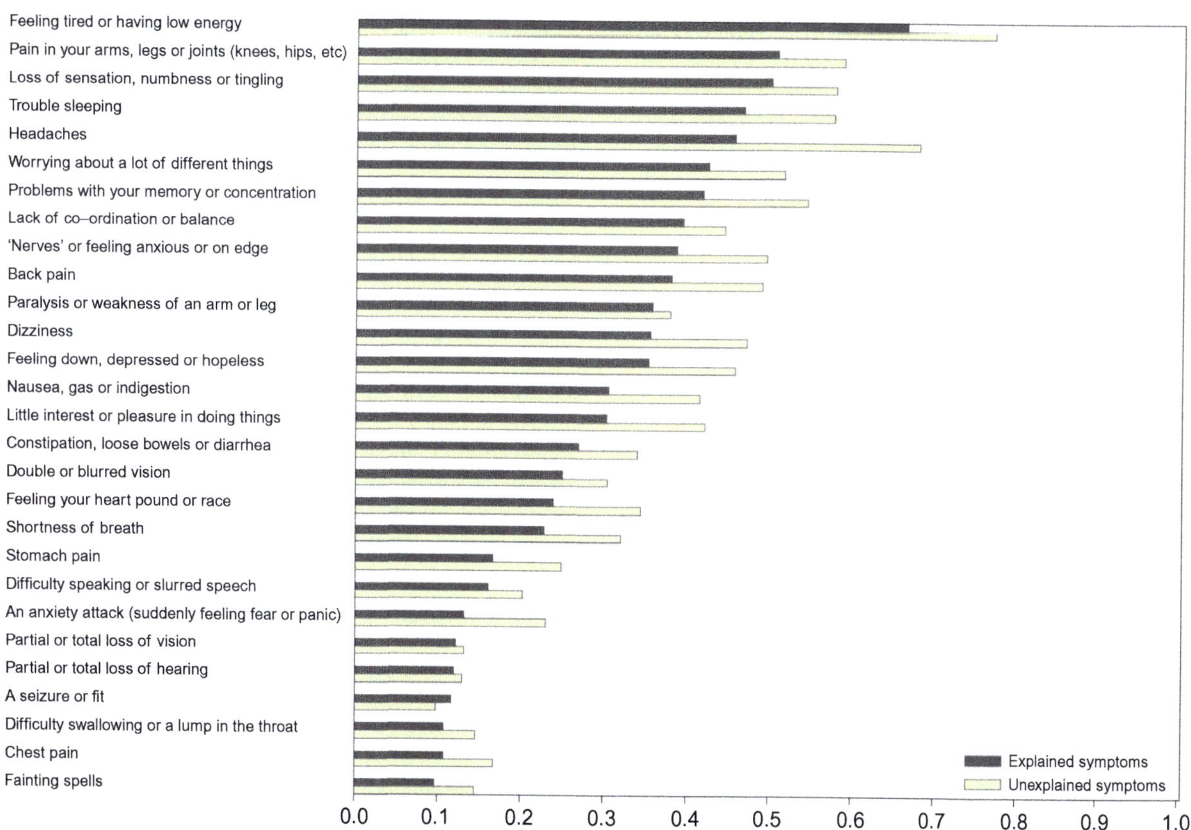

Fig. 5.1. Rates of endorsement of individual symptoms by new patients attending Scottish neurology clinics (shown as percentage with 1.0 = 100%: $n = 3781$). (Reproduced from Carson et al., 2014, with permission from BMJ Publications.)

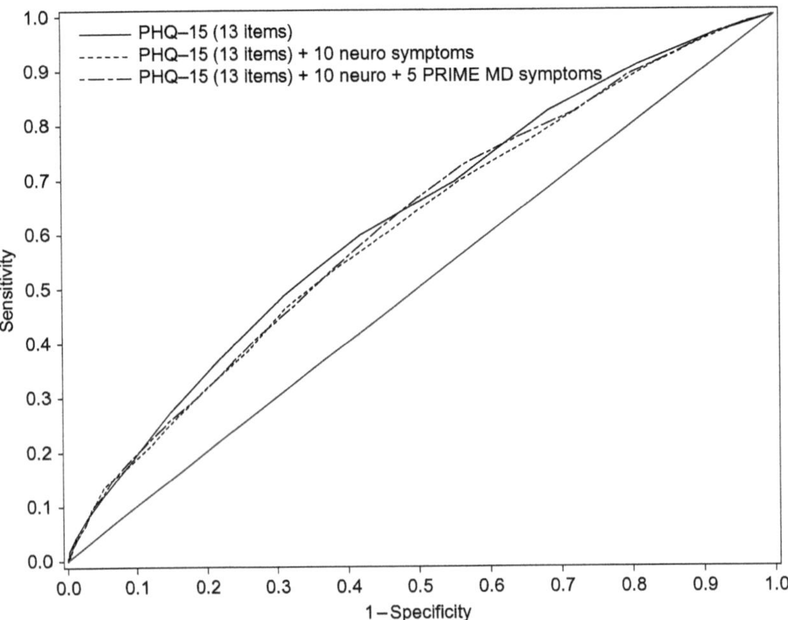

Fig. 5.2. Use of symptom counts as a diagnostic tool on the same population. PHQ-15, Patient Health Questionnaire; PRIME MD. (Reproduced from Carson et al., 2014, with permission from BMJ Publications.)

This raises concerns about the accuracy of a number seminal studies such as the Epidemiological Catchment Area study (Escobar et al., 1987), which used methodology based on related approaches.

A third approach is the use of case registries. Case registries, if based on normal practice, tend to be prone to underidentification of cases, even for a well-specified, neurologic disorder. When one starts to consider disorders such as FND, which can be classed under multiple names and which some clinicians still feel uncomfortable about diagnosing for fear of upsetting the patient, this problem will almost certainly be magnified.

INCIDENCE

For these reasons definitive, high-quality studies of the general population incidence of FND are lacking. Nonetheless, there is some consistency of results, despite different methodologies and geographic settings, with reported rates of "conversion disorder" of 4–12 per 100 000 population per year (Stefansson et al., 1976; Stevens, 1989; Binzer et al., 1997; Stone et al., 2010b). One of the better studies of functional weakness, based in Scotland (Stone et al., 2010b), and a similar study in Sweden (Binzer et al., 1997) both found an estimated minimum incidence of 4–5 per 100 000 per year for motor conversion symptoms. By way of comparison, these conservative estimates are broadly equivalent to the incidence of multiple sclerosis (Mackenzie et al., 2014).

Dissociative seizures studies have an estimated incidence of 1.5–4.9 per 100 000 population per year for video-electroencephalogram-confirmed cases (Sigurdardottir and Olafsson, 1998; Szaflarski et al., 2000; Duncan et al., 2011), but it is acknowledged that many more cases will not have been subject to this degree of scrutiny and this is likely to be an underestimate.

In children aged below 16, estimates of incidence of 1.3–4.3 per 100 000 per annum have been made (Kozlowska et al., 2007; Ani et al., 2013).

PREVALENCE

Accepting the limitations, the lower estimates of community prevalence of FND, extracted from population-based case registers, are around 50/100 000 population (Akagi and House, 2001). The prevalence of dissociative seizures has been estimated at 2–33/100 000 (Benbadis and Allen, 2000). The figure rises depending on the definition studied, in particular how the overlap with other somatoform symptoms is considered and the time frame of sampling with annual prevalence figures being roughly double that of point prevalence figures.

Frequency in neurology settings

There are more reports of prevalence figures from neurology clinic settings reflecting the ease of case ascertainment (Table 5.1). However, they are liable to a range of potential biases depending on clinic sampled.

In a national study in Scotland (Stone et al., 2009b), involving all but two neurologists, in a consecutive series of 3781 patients we found 1144 patients were found to have symptoms unexplained by neurologic disease

Table 5.1

Studies measuring the frequency of symptoms unexplained by disease in neurology outpatient clinics

Study	Location	*n*	% unexplained by disease
Carson et al. (2000)	Edinburgh, UK	300	30% (11% "not at all" and 19% "somewhat" explained by disease)
Bateman and Harrison (2000)	Bath, UK	356	26% no neurologic disorder
Nimnuan et al. (2001)	London, UK	103	62% had "medically unexplained" symptoms
Stone and Sharpe (2002)	Edinburgh, UK	89	36% (7% "not at all" and 29% "somewhat" explained by disease)
Stone et al. (2004)	Colchester, UK	100	45% had a "nonneurologic" diagnosis
Snijders et al. (2004)	Utrecht, Netherlands	208	35% considered to have "medically unexplained" symptoms
Fink et al. (2005)	Vejle, Denmark	198*	61% had "medically unexplained" symptoms, 39% had a somatoform disorder
Stone et al. (2010a)	Aberdeen, Dundee, Edinburgh, Glasgow, UK	3781	30% (12% "not at all" and 18% "somewhat" explained by disease)
Ahmad and Ahmad (2016)	Sydney, Australia	884	15% had functional neurologic disorder

*Mixture of inpatients and outpatients.

(Table 5.2). Twenty-five percent of these 1144 patients had a coexisting neurologic disorder (8% of all neurology cases) and another 25% had headache disorders. Typical FND cases comprised a smaller, but nonetheless significant, group of 18% (5.4% of all cases).

Age and sex

There is uniformity in cited studies that FND are more frequent in women, with estimates tending to be around 60–75% female (Monday and Jankovic, 1993; Lang, 1995; Williams et al., 1995; Kim et al., 1999; Feinstein et al., 2001; Thomas et al., 2006; plus studies cited above). It should be noted, however, that these are generally clinic-based samples and women are more likely to present to health services in general by a factor of 1.5:1. However, this is not always the case and, in some specific presentations – late-onset dissociative seizures (Duncan et al., 2006) and functional myoclonus – the frequency is the same in both genders.

There was similar consistency with regard to age, with onset tending to be 35–50 years old within the studies cited above, but clinicians should note that one message coming from reported cases series is that incident cases are reported in both sexes and all ages, from young children to the elderly.

Geographic and historic epidemiology

Most studies of FND have been conducted in industrialized countries. It has generally been accepted in academic textbooks that rates are higher in nonindustrialized countries and that the prevalence has dramatically decreased in the industrialized nations during the 20th century. A number of extravagant anthropologic explanations have been provided for this. However, the theories do seem to have run ahead of the data, which are notably absent (Stone et al., 2008). There have been a small number of high-quality international studies of general somatoform disorders and they have concluded very similar rates internationally (Simon et al., 1996). Also, a recent study from the Middle East showed a similar prevalence of dissociative seizures seen in the Western world (Farghaly et al., 2013).

Historic comparators are equally hard to achieve; however, where available, they are notably in keeping with modern figures. Sydenham (trans. Latham, 1848), suggested that a third of the patients he was seeing with neurologic symptoms had "the vapours" (the equivalent of functional symptoms), a figure strikingly close to modern data. Charcot's assistant, Guinon, reported a frequency of 8% for hysteria in 3168 consultations (Guinon, 1889), again, a figure very in keeping with current estimates. Interpretation of such historic data is fraught with complications, but does at least suggest that we should be highly sceptical of historically revisionist claims that hysteria was once frequent and is now rare.

ONSET

There is agreement that it is difficult and unreliable to use history alone to differentiate an FND from an "organic" neurologic disorder. Nonetheless, a sudden onset is often seen in functional movement disorders, with a frequency of 54–92% (Factor et al., 1995; Deuschl et al., 1998; Kim et al., 1999; Feinstein et al., 2001; Ertan et al., 2009). However, "sudden" generally means over the course of 10 minutes to 1 hour (Stone et al., 2013), and not the truly sudden onset of a vascular event. Physical injury or pain at onset is particularly typical in sudden-onset cases. The injury, as in patients with complex regional pain

Table 5.2

Diagnoses in 1144 patients with symptoms unexplained by neurological disease

Neurologist diagnosis	Number of patients (%)	Age (mean, years)	Female *n* (%)
Neurologic or medical disorder*	**297 (26%)**	**47**	**171 (58%)**
Headache	**285 (25%)**	**42**	**185 (65%)**
Chronic daily headache	112	42	61
Migraine	49	44	41
Other headache	124	42	83
Conversion symptoms	**209 (18%)**		
Functional blackouts/pseudoseizures	*85 (7.4%)*	*38*	*62 (73%)*
Functional sensory	*68 (5.9%)*	*44*	*36 (53%)*
Functional sensory	54	44	30
Hemisensory disturbance – NE or SE	12	44	5
Visual symptoms – NE or SE	2	46	1
Functional weakness/gait/movement	*56 (4.9%)*	*45*	*45 (80%)*
Functional gait	2	56	2
Functional mixed motor/sensory	10	50	10
Functional movement disorder	9	51	7
Functional weakness	35	41	26
Other			
Functional	*103 (9.0%)*	*43*	*72 (70%)*
? Nonorganic – NOS	15	43	8
Functional and organic	3	48	3
Hyperventilation	8	35	7
No diagnosis – NE or SE	22	45	13
Nonorganic – NOS	46	43	35
Physiologic	9	41	6
Psychiatric disorder	*77 (6.7%)*	*43*	*58 (75%)*
Alcohol excess	3	47	1
Anxiety and depression	68	44	53
Other psychiatric	5	38	3
Psychosis	1	28	1
Pain symptoms	*63 (5.5%)*	*46*	*48 (76%)*
Atypical facial/TMJ pain – NE or SE	9	50	7
Fibromyalgia	7	43	6
Pain symptoms – NE or SE	35	46	24
Spinal pain – NE or SE	12	41	11
Dizzy symptoms – NE or SE	*32 (2.8%)*	*45*	*24 (75%)*
Fatigue symptoms – NE or SE	*29 (2.5%)*	*43*	*25 (86%)*
Cognitive symptoms – NE or SE	*22 (1.9%)*	*44*	*9 (41%)*
Posttraumatic	*27 (2.4%)*	*36*	*12 (44%)*
Post head injury symptoms – NE or SE	19	34	10
Post traumatic headache	7	42	1
Repetitive strain injury	1	38	1
Total	1144		

(From Stone et al. 2010a, with permission.)

*Comprising: neurologic other (49), peripheral neuropathy (48), spinal disorders (36), demyelination/multiple sclerosis (32), epilepsy (31), general medical (25), syncope (25), parkinsonism/movement disorder (20), stroke (17), brain tumor (6), muscle/neuromuscular junction (3), dementia (1). NE or SE, not explained or somewhat explained by disease; NOS, not otherwise specified; TMJ, temporomandibular joint.

syndrome type 1 (discussed in Chapter 41), is often relatively trivial. In Schrag et al.'s (2004) series of patients with fixed dystonia, physical injury occurred in 63% of 103 patients. In a systematic review of 132 studies ($n = 869$) looking at physical injury in motor and sensory conversion disorder, we found that physical injury was reported in 34% of 357 cases of FND (the overall rate for all symptoms was 37%) (Stone et al., 2009a). The methodology of this analysis has limitations, but the frequency of physical injury is striking. A subsequent prospective study also noted the compelling association of a range of events causing unpleasant sensations at the time of symptom onset (Pareés et al., 2014).

A frequency of litigation of 15–30% in FND (Factor et al., 1995; Crimlisk et al., 1998; Kim et al., 1999; Feinstein et al., 2001; Schrag et al., 2004) has been commented on by several studies. Although this must raise suspicion of malingering in some cases, it could also simply reflect a close relationship between physical injury and FND.

PHYSICAL SYMPTOM AND DISEASE COMORBIDITY

FNDs do not usually present as an isolated physical symptom. Pain, fatigue, mixed patterns of weakness and sensory disturbance, and multiple functional symptoms are all very common (Koller et al., 1989; Kim et al., 1999; Carson et al., 2000). Neurologic disease is also more common than would be expected by chance (Stone et al., 2012) and occurred in approximately 1 in 10 cases.

DISABILITY

Descriptions of disability in FND are infrequent but fairly consistent in their findings. In general, and perhaps not surprisingly, physical measures of disability tend to describe a clinical impact of roughly similar severity to the equivalent "organic" neurologic disorder but substantially increased rates of total symptom burden and mental distress (Carson et al., 2000, 2011; Anderson et al., 2007). Even on long-term follow-up, FNDs have a significant impact on patient disability as well as functioning in regard to working life (Rask et al., 2015). Illness perception in early stages was shown to be a predictor for disability and work ability (Sharpe et al., 2010). This work reports self-rated disability. However, it seems unlikely that observer-derived disability scores would lead to different conclusions; if a patient with a substantive functional motor disorder in the form of the typical "dragging" leg rates himself as having difficulty climbing stairs on the physical function subscale of the Short Form health survey (SF-36), an observer-rated scale such as the Rankin or Barthel will come to the same conclusion if applied in the setting of a clinic or home visit. However, whilst one might reasonably assume some consistency in such a score following a stroke or other structural lesion, that same assumption cannot be made in association with functional motor disorder. Gaining evidence about the degree of fluctuation of disability in conversion disorder is a priority in this field.

One fascinating study comparing patient diaries of tremor frequency to actigraphic measurement showed that in both organic and functional tremor patients overestimate how often they are shaking. However, whilst organic-group patients reported 28% more tremor than actigraphy recordings, in the functional group the rates of perceived tremors were 65% higher than recorded. This discrepancy was so great that it suggested that attention was a major factor in symptom creation, somewhat akin to the refrigerator light: when the patient looked, the tremor was always on (Pareés et al., 2011).

PSYCHOLOGIC COMORBIDITY

Rates of psychologic comorbidity are also consistently higher than comparable neurologic disorders, with rates of depression between 20% and 40% (Crimlisk et al., 1998; Carson et al., 2000, 2011) and anxiety probably somewhat higher. In Feinstein et al.'s (2001) study the frequency of a current anxiety disorder was 38%. Our own experience, especially with tremor and other hyperkinetic movement disorders, is that anxiety is very common but that it may not present overtly. The interpretation of standard diagnostic structured interviews can be problematic, as the question "do you feel anxious?" will get a very different response from "do your symptoms make you feel anxious?" Overall, around two-thirds to three-quarters of patients with FND will have some kind of axis 1 emotional disorder. By contrast, patients with equivalent disability from neurologic disease tend to report rates of around half to two-thirds that of the corresponding conversion disorder (Carson et al., 2000, 2011; Stone et al., 2010b; Diprose et al., 2016).

These figures offer clear support for the notion that emotional factors are a significant risk factor for FND, but for those who cite such figures as proof of the "conversion" hypothesis there are two problems. First, what is the mechanism in the one-third of patients in whom there is no emotional distress? Second, if the mechanism is based on conversion of psychic trauma into a physical symptom as a form of ego defense, then why are such a substantive proportion of patients still distressed?

One potential explanation for the "third" without distress is that there are serious problems with using standardized methodologies for diagnosis of psychiatric disorder in this group of patients, especially questionnaires. Patients with FND may go to some effort to try to persuade the examining doctor (and sometimes themselves in the process) that they do not have any difficulties with anxiety or low mood (Stone et al., 2010b). The alternative explanation, and null hypothesis, however, is that psychologic distress is not an essential ingredient for the development of FND.

Studies of personality are difficult to interpret in FND as multiple definitions of personality are used and also there is a distinction to be made between personality type and personality disorder. Furthermore, although most clinicians believe there is some form of relationship between FND and personality, from an epidemiologic perspective the diagnosis of personality disorder is fraught with issues of validity and reliability. Early attempts were confused, as the term hysteria might apply to the physical symptom or a psychologic trait or a personality type (Chodoff and Lyons, 1958). The work of Robert Cloninger (1986) is highly cited and illustrates the attempt to link personality traits (using a three-trait model) to personality disorders, centering on histrionic and obsessive disorders, and suggesting these combinations of traits are particularly linked to conversion disorders, which are really viewed as somatic displays of anxiety. The literature on this topic is more developed in somatoform disorders in general and a good mainstream, if slightly dated, review can be found in Bass and Murphy (1995). Although high rates of personality disorder are reported (Binzer et al., 1997; Roelofs et al., 2005; Scévola et al., 2013), caution is warranted as these studies are on selected groups of patients and the diagnosis does not appear to have been made on the basis of lifelong informant information, making it difficult to know whether displayed personality is the cause or effect. In our experience (writing as a neurologist and psychiatrist), the patients referred to psychiatry from neurology often have increased rates of personality disorder. One would be hard-pushed to find an experienced clinician who didn't think that personality was important in the field of FND, but you would be even harder pushed to find a clinician who could accurately define personality in a reliable and valid manner.

To examine the question from the perspective of traditional classifications of personality may be an example of putting in screws with a hammer simply because we have one, rather than searching for a screwdriver. A more fruitful endeavor, albeit currently in its infancy in the field of FND, may be the examination of specific cognitive subtypes which can be tested using neuropsychologic paradigms. In an interesting study, Pareés et al. (2012) asked patients to decide whether a jar contained mainly blue balls or mainly red balls by serial extraction of one ball at a time. FND patients made a decision after drawing only one or two balls, suggesting a cognitive bias towards arriving at firm conclusions before adequate data were available. In another early example, Bakvis et al. (2009) used a masked emotional Stroop test to evaluate the association between increased threat vigilance, rates of dissociative seizures, and childhood sexual assault.

OUTCOME: MISDIAGNOSIS

Misdiagnosis is often a significant clinical fear. However, more recent evidence does not support the apparent degree of worry. In a systematic review of 27 studies of conversion symptoms ($n=1466$), we found the reported frequency of misdiagnosis has been consistently around 4% since 1970 (Stone et al., 2005; Fig. 5.3). This figure

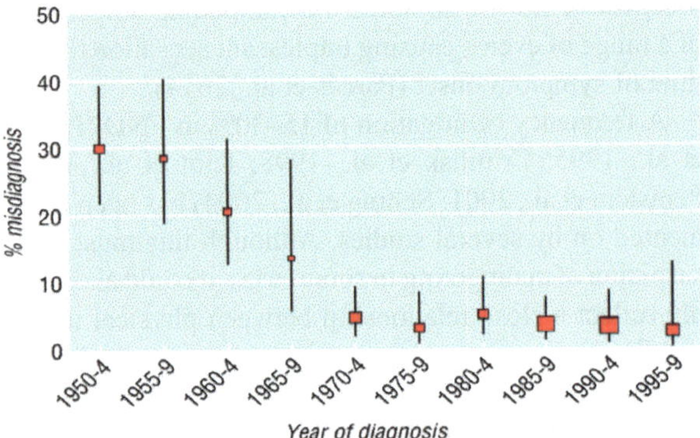

Fig. 5.3. Misdiagnosis of conversion symptoms and hysteria (mean %, 95% confidence intervals, random effects) plotted at midpoint of 5-year intervals according to when patients were diagnosed. Size of each point is proportional to number of subjects at each time point (total $n=1466$). (Reproduced from Stone et al., 2005, with permission from BMJ Publications.)

was unaffected by the widespread introduction of clinical imaging. We concluded that the higher rates of misdiagnosis reported in earlier studies largely reflected poor case definition and study methodology rather than recently enhanced diagnostic skills.

In the Scottish Neurological Symptoms Study (SNSS) (Stone et al., 2009b) we found, at baseline, that 1144/3781 patients had neurologic symptoms that were either "not at all" or only "somewhat" explained by neurologic disease. At 12-month follow-up we had diagnostic outcome data on 1030/1144 of these patients (90%) and 9 deaths. We realized that the analysis of misdiagnosis was not straightforward; in particular, clinical error leading to misdiagnosis was only one of a number of explanations for diagnostic revision in an outcome study. We operationalized criteria for describing diagnostic revision according to criteria described in Table 5.3.

We found 45 diagnostic revisions, but only four of the 45 were category 1 misdiagnoses; the others were differential diagnostic change ($n=12$), diagnostic refinement ($n=22$), *de novo* development of disease ($n=1$), and disagreement between doctors ($n=6$).

These data should not lead to complacency. Our personal experience is that nonneurologists can struggle to distinguish between psychogenic and "organic" neurologic diagnoses. Too often they are swayed by factors such as the presence of obvious psychiatric or personality factors or apparent "bizarreness" of symptoms, especially in gait or movement disorders. It is also important to remember that misdiagnosis of an organic disorder when FND was the true cause can be an equally damaging experience for the patient. There is little systematic study of this form of misdiagnosis, but in our personal experience the symptoms looking too "real" or the patient being too "normal" are common reasons (Stone et al., 2013). Studies of

Table 5.3

A new classification for diagnostic revision used in the Scottish Neurological Symptoms Study

Type of diagnostic revision	Example	Degree of clinician error
1 Diagnostic error	Patient presented with symptoms that were plausibly due to MS, but the diagnosis of MS was not considered and was unexpected at follow-up	Minor–major
2 Differential diagnostic change	Patient presented with symptoms that were plausibly related to a number of conditions. Doctor suggested chronic fatigue syndrome as most likely, but considered MS as a possible diagnosis. Appropriate investigations and follow-up confirmed MS	None–minor
3 Diagnostic refinement	Doctor diagnosed epilepsy but at follow-up the diagnosis is refined to juvenile myoclonic epilepsy	Minor
4 Comorbid diagnostic change	Doctor correctly identified the presence of both epilepsy and nonepileptic seizures in the same patient. At follow-up, one of the disorders has remitted	None
5 Prodromal diagnostic change	Patient presented with an anxiety state. At follow-up the patient has developed dementia. With hindsight, anxiety was a prodromal symptom of dementia, but the diagnosis could not have been made at the initial consultation, as the dementia symptoms (or findings on examination/ investigation) had not developed	None
6 *De novo* development of disease	Patient is correctly diagnosed with chronic fatigue syndrome. During the period of follow-up, the patient develops subarachnoid hemorrhage as a new condition	None
7 Disagreement between doctors – without new information at follow-up	Patient is diagnosed at baseline with chronic fatigue syndrome and at follow-up with chronic Lyme disease by a different doctor, even though there is no new information. However, if the two doctors had both met the patient at baseline, they would still have arrived at the same diagnosis. This would be reflected in similar divided opinion among their peers	None
8 Disagreement between doctors – with new information at follow-up	Patient is diagnosed at baseline with chronic fatigue syndrome and at follow-up with fatigue due to a Chiari malformation by a different doctor because of new information at follow-up (in this case, an MRI scan ordered at the time of the first appointment). However, the first doctor seeing the patient again at follow-up continues to diagnose chronic fatigue syndrome, believing the Chiari malformation to be an incidental finding, This would be reflected in divided opinion among their peers	None

MS, multiple sclerosis; MRI, magnetic resonance imaging.

misdiagnosis will need to continue, especially as the diagnosis is made more often. Recognizing that different kinds of diagnostic change occur will be useful for any such studies.

RISK FACTORS

Epidemiologic studies have highlighted a range of risk factors for the occurrence of FND. One particular issue with reporting is that results are often shown in terms of their significance as a p-value, an odds ratio, or within multiple regression analyses. However, because the population prevalence of the risk factor is seldom known, a relative risk is seldom possible. Studies also generally fail to report any analysis of the variance – in other words, how much of the overall risk the disorder explains.

The risk factors are similar to those described for disorders in the neurotic spectrum and include: predisposing factors; precipitating factors; and perpetuating factors.

Predisposing factors

As discussed above, female sex and younger age are associated with FND. Also emotional and personality disorders are predisposing factors. The coexistence of other health issues, difficulties in interpersonal relationships, and previous life events such as bereavement are other risk factors (Duncan et al., 2006; Reuber et al.,

2007; Creed et al., 2012). Evidence on educational background and IQ as risk factors is rather mixed, although it seems they have little effect on outcome (Ljungberg, 1957; Williams et al., 1995; Binzer and Kullgren, 1998; Gelauff et al., 2013).

The prevalence of adverse childhood experiences (including physical and sexual abuse) is often overestimated by clinicians and particularly the data for functional movement disorders are not clear. While some studies suggested early-life stressors as a risk factor for functional movement disorders (Kranick et al., 2011), others showed different results (Binzer and Kullgren, 1998). However, there is an association between adverse childhood experiences and dissociative attacks (Stone et al., 2004b). A meta-analysis of 34 studies found that 33% of patients with dissociative attacks had reported a history of sexual abuse (Sharpe and Faye, 2006). Exposure to functional or organic movement disorders among friends and family may be a risk factor for developing functional movement disorders (Stamelou et al., 2013; Pellicciari et al., 2014). Similar disease modeling can play a role in dissociative attacks (Asadi-Pooya and Emami, 2013).

Precipitating factors

Particular prominence has been given to the issue of life events as a precipitant to "conversion disorders" and this was supported within the DSM-IV definition. Despite the dominance of this hypothesis, the actual epidemiologic evidence in support of it is notable in its paucity and inconsistency. The issues are described in detail in Chapter 13.

Perpetuating factors

There are multiple factors that play a role in perpetuating FNDs (for a more detailed discussion, see Chapter 12). These include biologic factors such as central nervous system plasticity and deconditioning as well as psychologic factors like abnormal illness beliefs and the perception of symptoms as being irreversible (Moss-Morris and Chalder, 2003; Sharpe et al., 2010). Social factors such as secondary gain, diagnostic uncertainty, and receiving health benefits have been suggested as well (Reuber et al., 2007; Hingray et al., 2011). Despite the prominence given to illness beliefs, patients with functional weakness (Stone et al., 2010b) and nonepileptic attacks (Stone et al., 2004a) have been found to have similar illness beliefs to their corresponding disease counterparts, except that paradoxically they are slightly less likely to attribute their symptoms to stress than patients with disease (Sharpe et al., 2010). These findings do not mean that illness beliefs are unimportant; rather, they highlight a problem with attribution error, which can be on the part of patient or researcher. If a patient declares that she considers her condition to be genetic, this may be an attribution error on her part if she is considering a mechanism such as that of Huntington's disease. However, if as researchers we regard this belief as maladaptive, it could be that we are making the attribution error, as the patient may be endorsing a complex biopsychosocial model in which genetic risk does play a part (see Chapter 12). There have been some suggestions from qualitative research (Salmon et al., 1999) that patients are sometimes more comfortable with a genuine biopsychosocial model than we are as clinicians, where the phrase is trotted out, but actually what ensues is a form of psychologic reductionism and the "bio" is forgotten.

We have already discussed the role of physical injury in FND. Other research has found a high frequency of panic symptoms in patients with dissociative seizures (Goldstein and Mellers, 2006; Dimaro et al., 2014; Hendrickson et al., 2014). In line with 19th-century thinking on the topic, we think there is value in exploring more "proximal" events in the onset of FND. Our own experience is that an acute panic attack (a "shock," in 19th-century parlance), a dissociative episode, an episode of sleep paralysis, or general anesthetic may provide more of a window to understanding the onset of FND that a thorough exploration of life events and childhood factors may miss.

We do not wish to suggest that life events and other stressors are irrelevant or unimportant but simply we need more data and better understanding of their role before assumptions about the universality of their etiologic role can be made.

EPIDEMIOLOGY OF FUNCTIONAL NEUROLOGIC DISORDER SUBTYPES: LUMPING OR SPLITTING?

One issue that has to be addressed when discussing epidemiology of FNDs is the question of whether the various clinical phenotypes are all different manifestations of the same underlying pathology or if they are in fact different disorders. Dissociative attacks and functional movement disorders, for example, have always been grouped together in diagnostic criteria such as DSM, and this is still the case with the current DSM-5. Several studies compared these two subtypes: Patients with dissociative attacks are generally younger at symptom onset, more likely to report adverse childhood experiences, and more likely to be female than patients with functional movement disorders (Stone et al., 2004b; Driver-Dunckley et al., 2011; Hopp et al., 2012). However, the two disorders commonly coexist in patients (Lempert et al., 1990), and there is a significant overlap in clinical presentations: some patients might present with intermittent acute events that could well be diagnosed as dissociative attacks but are afterwards left with ongoing functional weakness. Also regarding the underlying (psycho) pathology, there are more similarities than differences: the two groups are both characterized by increased levels of chronic pain and fatigue (Driver-Dunckley et al., 2011) and both have similar psychologic profiles with high levels of emotional disorders and personality disorders (Stone et al., 2004a; Hopp et al., 2012).

The above-mentioned cross-sectional studies are helpful in order to assess baseline characteristics, but what is really needed is to look prospectively at the natural history of patients with functional symptoms. This would allow us, for example, to see if patients with dissociative attacks are prone to develop functional weakness at a later stage. Two systematic reviews were published in recent years summarizing currently available outcome data (of largely retrospective studies) for dissociative attacks (Durrant et al., 2011) and functional weakness (Gelauff et al., 2013). They confirm that symptom persistence is common but do not give us further information about symptom cross-over between dissociative attacks and functional weakness. In the absence of better evidence, this still leaves us with the question of whether we should lump or split the various types of functional symptoms.

PATIENT OUTCOMES AND MORTALITY

Patient outcomes and mortality are discussed in Chapter 43.

ECONOMICS

FND is associated with substantive increased healthcare utilization and consequently increased direct and indirect costs. The major supporting factor for high associated costs is simply that FND very commonly presents across all healthcare settings and therefore must have a substantive associated cost. In a study from the USA, Barsky et al. (2005) found that, compared with patients suffering from organic disorders, FND patients had more primary care visits, more specialty visits, more emergency department visits, more hospital admission, and higher inpatient as well as outpatient costs. They estimated that annual direct medical costs attributable to FNDs alone for the USA were $256 billion. A recently published study from Ireland evaluated the economic cost and the treatment costs of dissociative attacks (Magee et al., 2014). Based on a retrospective chart review, the author estimated that direct annual medical costs of dissociative attacks in Ireland are 5429.30 euros per patient. They also calculated the total annual costs (direct and indirect) of undiagnosed dissociative attacks as about 21 000 euros. The combined cost of diagnosis and treatment of dissociative attacks was calculated as 8728 euros per person. Based on a prevalence of 31 per 100 000, Magee estimated the national annual cost of dissociative attacks in Ireland (population about 4.5 million) as over 27 million euros.

As with every disorder, the distribution of healthcare utilization is highly skewed, with a small group of patients consuming a substantive proportion of the resources – such "fat file" FND patients are very familiar but are probably outliers. The extent of resource utilization in the majority of patients is less certain. In unpublished data from SNSS, we found a significant excess utilization of a variety of outpatient clinics in the 12 months after the initial neurology consultation. However, this was largely at lower-cost outpatient clinics rather than inpatient services, where there was also an excess, but much less marked.

From the data above the potential for planned interventions can be associated with cost savings, but the size of these effects is not always as dramatic as people think and depends to some extent on the cost model of the healthcare service involved. For example, Razvi et al. (2012) reported a substantive reduction in emergency room (ER) usage following the setting up of a dedicated one-stop diagnostic service for new-onset dissociative seizures and suggested this offset the costs of the clinic. This style of service undoubtedly has much to recommend it, but the assumption of associated cost savings was a fallacy. ER consults are very cheap, and in the context of the UK, where service is free at point of delivery, there was not in fact any real cost savings as the numbers of patients with dissociative seizures passing through each ER, compared to ER general activity, was minimal, so there was no evidence of downscaling of required staff in the department, so the only true savings were marginal and undoubtedly less than the new intervention of the dedicated clinic. The same improvements however in a health service where an insurer underwrites an individual patient's care may have differentially greater impact. This is not to say that such service should not be set up, but just to caution that one has to specify and target what the cost savings associated may actually be in terms of the healthcare system involved rather than simply adding up the cost per care episode.

In terms of "nonhealthcare" costs, rates of unemployment owing to sickness and capacity-related benefits are obvious areas of concern. Within the context of SNSS (Carson et al., 2011), we found a slight excess of FND patients permanently off work through sickness and of FND patients claiming capacity-related benefits, but this was proportionate to their increased disability rates. Looked at the other way, the rate of FND patients currently working was exactly the same as the rates of current work in neurology patients in general. Receipt of invalidity benefits was associated with a poorer outcome independently of baseline disability rates (see Chapter 43), but given the crudeness of measurement of disability, we should still be cautious about the direction of causality in this association.

A systematic review of 13 studies looking into the economics of FNDs found significant direct and indirect costs constituting the economic burden of these disorders. In cost-of-illness studies, excess costs ranged from \$432 to \$5353 (in 2006 prices) per patient and year compared to patients without functional symptoms (Konnopka et al., 2012). Depending on cost stratification used, the bulk of direct costs is due to inpatient care and/or diagnostic procedures. This suggests that early and appropriate management of FNDs could reduce direct costs by avoiding unnecessary diagnostic procedures and hospital admissions.

The systematic review identified nine economic evaluations in the management of FNDs. Some of the studies focused on interventions targeting the primary care-giver (evaluating the impact of consultation letters and educational training) whereas others focused on cognitive-behavioral therapy approaches for patients. Most studies were small and of limited quality and, while the majority of them found cost reductions due to the interventions, they often didn't reach statistical significance. Another problem with a large number of these studies was that they only compared costs but neglected to measure differences in health effects. Ignoring these potential changes is an issue, as an intervention might well result in cost savings, but also lead to adverse health effects.

In summary, while there are increasing data for the economic burden of FNDs and some emerging evidence for interventions leading to savings in the direct costs, clearly more research is needed assessing effects on indirect costs and cost-effectiveness.

CONCLUSION

Epidemiologic studies of FND pose many technical problems. Nonetheless, it is clear that FND can be diagnosed accurately and is much more common than many realize, accounting for between 1 in 20 and 1 in 10 neurologic presentations. It is associated with a substantive disease burden. Yet FND has received far less attention than many other disorders of significantly lower prevalence and lower burdens on society.

References

Ahmad O, Ahmad KE (2016). Functional neurological disorders in outpatient practice: an Australian cohort. J Clin Neurosci 28: 93–96.

Akagi H, House A (2001). The epidemiology of hysterical conversion. In: PW Halligan, C Bass, JC Marshall (Eds.), Contemporary approaches to the study of hysteria: clinical and theoretical perspectives, Oxford University Press, Oxford, pp. 73–87.

American Psychiatric Association (2000). Diagnostic and Statistical Manual of Diseases, 4th edn. American Psychiatric Association, Washington, DC. Text Revision.

American Psychiatric Association (2013). Diagnostic and Statistical Manual of Mental Disorders (5th edn.; DSM-5), American Psychiatric Association, Washington, DC.

Anderson KE, Gruber-Baldini AL, Vaughan CG et al. (2007). Impact of psychogenic movement disorders versus Parkinson's on disability, quality of life, and psychopathology. Mov Disord 22 (15): 2204–2209.

Ani C, Reading R, Lynn R et al. (2013). Incidence and 12-month outcome of non-transient childhood conversion disorder in the UK and Ireland. Br J Psychiatry 202 (6): 413–418.

Asadi-Pooya AA, Emami M (2013). Demographic and clinical manifestations of psychogenic non-epileptic seizures: the impact of co-existing epilepsy in patients or their family members. Epilepsy Behav 27 (1): 1–3.

Bakvis P, Roelofs K, Kuyk J et al. (2009). Trauma, stress, and preconscious threat processing in patients with psychogenic nonepileptic seizures. Epilepsia 50 (5): 1001–1011.

Barsky AJ, Orav EJ, Bates DW (2005). Somatization increases medical utilization and costs independent of psychiatric and medical comorbidity. Arch Gen Psychiatry 62 (8): 903–910.

Bass C, Murphy M (1995). Somatoform and personality disorders: syndromal comorbidity and overlapping developmental pathways. J Psychosom Res 39 (4): 403–427.

Bateman DE, Harrison FM (2000). Psychiatric disorder in neurology clinics. Association of British Neurologists (conference abstract) University of Exeter 2000: 44.

Benbadis SR, Allen HW (2000). An estimate of the prevalence of psychogenic non-epileptic seizures. Seizure 9 (4): 280–281.

Binzer M, Kullgren G (1998). Motor conversion disorder. A prospective 2- to 5-year follow-up study. Psychosomatics 39: 519–527.

Binzer M, Andersen PM, Kullgren G (1997). Clinical characteristics of patients with motor disability due to conversion disorder: a prospective control group study. J Neurol Neurosurg Psychiatry 63 (1): 83–88.

Carson AJ, Ringbauer B, Stone J et al. (2000). Do medically unexplained symptoms matter? A prospective cohort study of 300 new referrals to neurology outpatient clinics. J Neurol Neurosurg Psychiatry 68 (2): 207–210.

Carson A, Stone J, Hibberd C et al. (2011). Disability, distress and unexployment in neurology outpatients with symptoms 'unexplained by disease'. J Neurol Neurosurg Psychiatry 82: 810–813.

Carson AJ, Stone J, Holm Hansen C et al. (2014). Somatic symptom count scores do not identify patients with symptoms unexplained by disease: a prospective cohort study of neurology outpatients. J Neurol Neurosurg Psychiatry. jnnp-2014.

Chodoff P, Lyons H (1958). Hysteria, the hysterical personality and "hysterical" conversion. Am J Psychiatry 114 (8): 734–740.

Cloninger CR (1986). A unified biosocial theory of personality and its role in the development of anxiety states. Psychiatr Dev 3 (2): 167–226.

Creed FH, Davies I, Jackson J et al. (2012). The epidemiology of multiple somatic symptoms. J Psychosom Res 72 (4): 311–317.

Crimlisk HL, Bhatia K, Cope H et al. (1998). Slater revisited: 6 year follow up study of patients with medically unexplained motor symptoms. BMJ 316 (7131): 582–586.

Deuschl G, Koster B, Lucking CH et al. (1998). Diagnostic and pathophysiological aspects of psychogenic tremors. Mov Disord 13 (2): 294–302.

Dimaro LV, Dawson DL, Roberts NA et al. (2014). Anxiety and avoidance in psychogenic nonepileptic seizures: the role of implicit and explicit anxiety. Epilepsy Behav 33C: 77–86.

Diprose W, Sundram F, Menkes DB (2016). Psychiatric comorbidity in psychogenic nonepileptic seizures compared with epilepsy. Epilepsy Behav 56: 123–130.

Driver-Dunckley E, Stonnington CM, Locke DEC et al. (2011). Comparison of psychogenic movement disorders and psychogenic nonepileptic seizures: is phenotype clinically important? Psychosomatics 52 (4): 337–345.

Duncan R, Oto M, Martin E et al. (2006). Late onset psychogenic nonepileptic attacks. Neurology 66: 1644–1647.

Duncan R, Razvi S, Mulhern S (2011). Newly presenting psychogenic nonepileptic seizures: incidence, population characteristics, and early outcome from a prospective audit of a first seizure clinic. Epilepsy Behav 20 (2): 308–311.

Durrant J, Rickards H, Cavanna AE (2011). Prognosis and outcome predictors in psychogenic nonepileptic seizures. Epilepsy Res Treat 2011.

Ertan S, Uluduz D, Ozekmekci S et al. (2009). Clinical characteristics of 49 patients with psychogenic movement disorders in a tertiary clinic in Turkey. Mov Disord 24 (5): 759–762.

Escobar JI, Burnam MA, Karno M et al. (1987). Somatization in the community. Arch Gen Psychiatry 44: 713–718.

Espay AJ, Lang AE (2015). Phenotype-specific diagnosis of functional (psychogenic) movement disorders. Curr Neurol Neurosci Rep 15 (6): 1–9.

Factor SA, Podskalny GD, Molho ES (1995). Psychogenic movement disorders: frequency, clinical profile, and characteristics. J Neurol Neurosurg Psychiatry 59 (4): 406–412.

Fahn S, Williams DT (1988). Psychogenic dystonia. Adv Neurol 50: 431–455.

Farghaly WMA, El-Tallawy HN, Rageh TA et al. (2013). Epidemiology of uncontrolled epilepsy in the Al-Kharga District, New Valley, Egypt. Seizure 22 (8): 611–616.

Feinstein A, Stergiopoulos V, Fine J et al. (2001). Psychiatric outcome in patients with a psychogenic movement disorder: a prospective study. Neuropsychiatry Neuropsychol Behav Neurol 14 (3): 169–176.

Fink P, Steen HM, Sondergaard L (2005). Somatoform disorders among first-time referrals to a neurology service. Psychosomatics 46 (6): 540–548.

Gelauff J, Stone J, Edwards M et al. (2013). The prognosis of functional (psychogenic) motor symptoms: a systematic review. J Neurol Neurosurg Psychiatry. jnnp-2013.

Goldstein LH, Mellers JD (2006). Ictal symptoms of anxiety, avoidance behaviour, and dissociation in patients with dissociative seizures. J Neurol Neurosurg Psychiatry 77 (5): 616–621.

Guinon G (1889). Les agents provocateurs de l'hysterie. Delahaye & Lecrosnier, Paris.

Hendrickson R, Popescu A, Dixit R et al. (2014). Panic attack symptoms differentiate patients with epilepsy from those with psychogenic nonepileptic spells (PNES). Epilepsy Behav 37: 210–214.

Hingray C, Maillard L, Hubsch C et al. (2011). Psychogenic nonepileptic seizures: characterization of two distinct patient profiles on the basis of trauma history. Epilepsy Behav 22 (3): 532–536.

Hopp JL, Anderson KE, Krumholz A et al. (2012). Psychogenic seizures and psychogenic movement disorders: are they the same patients? Epilepsy Behav 25 (4): 666–669.

Kim YJ, Pakiam AS, Lang AE (1999). Historical and clinical features of psychogenic tremor: a review of 70 cases. Can J Neurol Sci 26 (3): 190–195.

Koller W, Lang A, Vetere-Overfield B et al. (1989). Psychogenic tremors. Neurology 39 (8): 1094–1099.

Konnopka A, Schaefert R, Heinrich S et al. (2012). Economics of medically unexplained symptoms: a systematic review of the literature. Psychotherapy and psychosomatics 81: 265–275.

Kozlowska K, Nunn KP, Rose D et al. (2007). Conversion disorder in Australian pediatric practice. J Am Acad Child Adolesc Psychiatry 46 (1): 68–75.

Kranick S, Ekanayake V, Martinez V et al. (2011). Psychopathology and psychogenic movement disorders. Mov Disord 26 (10): 1844–1850.

LaFrance WC, Baker GA, Duncan R et al. (2013). Minimum requirements for the diagnosis of psychogenic nonepileptic seizures: a staged approach: a report from the International League Against Epilepsy Nonepileptic Seizures Task Force. Epilepsia 54: 2005–2018.

Lang AE (1995). Psychogenic dystonia: a review of 18 cases. Can J Neurol Sci 22 (2): 136–143.

Lempert T, Dieterich M, Huppert D et al. (1990). Psychogenic disorders in neurology: frequency and clinical spectrum. Acta Neurol Scand 82 (5): 335–340.

Ljungberg L (1957). Hysteria: a clinical, prognostic and genetic study. Acta Psychiat Neurol Scand Suppl 112: 1–162.

Mackenzie IS, Morant SV, Bloomfield GA et al. (2014). Incidence and prevalence of multiple sclerosis in the UK 1990–2010: a descriptive study in the General Practice Research Database. J Neurol Neurosurg Psychiatry 85 (1): 76–84.

Magee JA, Burke T, Delanty N et al. (2014). The economic cost of nonepileptic attack disorder in Ireland. Epilepsy Behav 33: 45–48.

Monday K, Jankovic J (1993). Psychogenic myoclonus. Neurology 43 (2): 349–352.

Moss-Morris R, Chalder T (2003). Illness perceptions and levels of disability in patients with chronic fatigue syndrome and rheumatoid arthritis. J Psychosom Res 55 (4): 305–308.

Nimnuan C, Hotopf M, Wessely S (2001). Medically unexplained symptoms: an epidemiological study in seven specialities. J Psychosom Res 51: 361–367.

Pellicciari R, Superbo M, Gigante AF et al. (2014). Disease modeling in functional movement disorders. Parkinsonism Relat Disord 20: 1287–1289.

Pareés I, Kassavetis P, Saifee TA et al. (2012). 'Jumping to Conclusions' bias in functional movement disorders. J Neurol Neurosurg Psychiatry. jnnp-2011.

Pareés I, Kojovic M, Pires C et al. (2014). Physical precipitating factors in functional movement disorders. J Neurol Sci 338 (1–2): 174–177.

Pareés I, Saifee TA, Kassavetis P et al. (2011). Believing is perceiving: mismatch between self-report and actigraphy in psychogenic tremor. Brain. awr292.

Rask MT, Rosendal M, Fenger-Grøn M et al. (2015). Sick leave and work disability in primary care patients with recent-onset multiple medically unexplained symptoms and persistent somatoform disorders: a 10-year follow-up of the FIP study. Gen Hosp Psychiatry 37 (1): 53–59.

Razvi S, Mulhern S, Duncan R (2012). Newly diagnosed psychogenic nonepileptic seizures: health care demand prior to and following diagnosis at a first seizure clinic. Epilepsy Behav 23 (1): 7–9.

Reuber M, Howlett S, Khan A et al. (2007). Non-epileptic seizures and other functional neurological symptoms: predisposing, precipitating, and perpetuating factors. Psychosomatics 48 (3): 230–238.

Roelofs K, Spinhoven P, Sandijck P et al. (2005). The impact of early trauma and recent life-events on symptom severity in patients with conversion disorder. J Nerv Ment Dis 193 (8): 508–514.

Salmon P, Peters S, Stanley I (1999). Patients' perceptions of medical explanations for somatisation disorders: qualitative analysis. BMJ 318 (7180): 372–376.

Scévola L, Teitelbaum J, Oddo S et al. (2013). Psychiatric disorders in patients with psychogenic nonepileptic seizures and drug-resistant epilepsy: a study of an Argentine population. Epilepsy Behav 29 (1): 155–160.

Schrag A, Trimble M, Quinn N et al. (2004). The syndrome of fixed dystonia: an evaluation of 103 patients. Brain 127 (Pt 10): 2360–2372.

Schwingenschuh P, Saifee TA, Katschnig-Winter P et al. (2016). Validation of 'laboratory-supported' criteria for functional (psychogenic) tremor. Mov Disord 31: 555–562.

Sharpe D, Faye C (2006). Non-epileptic seizures and child sexual abuse: a critical review of the literature. Clin Psychol Rev 26: 1020–1040.

Sharpe M, Stone J, Hibberd C et al. (2010). Neurology outpatients with symptoms unexplained by disease: illness beliefs and financial benefits predict 1-year outcome. Psychol Med 40 (4): 689–698.

Shill H, Gerber P (2006). Evaluation of clinical diagnostic criteria for psychogenic movement disorders. Mov Disord 21 (8): 1163–1168.

Sigurdardottir KR, Olafsson E (1998). Incidence of psychogenic seizures in adults: a population-based study in Iceland. Epilepsia 39 (7): 749–752.

Simon G, Gater R, Kisely S et al. (1996). Somatic symptoms of distress: an international primary care study. Psychosom Med 58 (5): 481–488.

Snijders TJ, de Leeuw FE, Klumpers UM et al. (2004). Prevalence and predictors of unexplained neurological symptoms in an academic neurology outpatient clinic – an observational study. J Neurol 251 (1): 66–71.

Stamelou M, Cossu G, Edwards MJ et al. (2013). Familial psychogenic movement disorders. Mov Disord 28: 1295–1298.

Stefansson JG, Messina JA, Meyerowitz S (1976). Hysterical neurosis, conversion type: clinical and epidemiological considerations. Acta Psychiatr Scand 53 (2): 119–138.

Stevens DL (1989). Neurology in Gloucestershire: the clinical workload of an English neurologist. J Neurol Neurosurg Psychiatry 52 (4): 439–446.

Stone J, Sharpe M (2002). Amnesia for childhood in patients with unexplained neurological symptoms. J Neurol Neurosurg Psychiatry 72: 416–417.

Stone J, Sharpe M, Deary I et al. (2004). Functional paresis - paradoxes in illness beliefs and disability in 107 subjects. J Neurology, Neurosurg Psychiatry 75: 519.

Stone J, Binzer M, Sharpe M (2004a). Illness beliefs and locus of control: a comparison of patients with pseudoseizures and epilepsy. J Psychosom Res 57 (6): 541–547.

Stone J, Sharpe M, Binzer M (2004b). Motor conversion symptoms and pseudoseizures: a comparison of clinical characteristics. Psychosomatics 45 (6): 492–499.

Stone J, Carson A, Duncan R et al. (2012). Which neurological diseases are most likely to be associated with "symptoms unexplained by organic disease". J Neurol 259 (1): 33–38.

Stone J, Smyth R, Carson A et al. (2005). The misdiagnosis of conversion symptoms / hysteria - a systematic review. BMJ 331: 989–991.

Stone J, Hewett R, Carson A et al. (2008). The 'disappearance' of hysteria: historical mystery or illusion? J R Soc Med 101 (1): 12–18.

Stone J, Carson A, Aditya H et al. (2009a). The role of physical injury in motor and sensory conversion symptoms: a systematic and narrative review. J Psychosom Res 66 (5): 383–390.

Stone J, Carson A, Duncan R et al. (2009b). Symptoms 'unexplained by organic disease' in 1144 new neurology out-patients: how often does the diagnosis change at follow-up? Brain 132 (Pt 10): 2878–2888.

Stone J, Carson A, Duncan R et al. (2010a). Who is referred to neurology clinics? The diagnoses made in 3781 new patients. Clin Neurol Neurosurg 112: 747–751.

Stone J, Warlow C, Sharpe M (2010b). The symptom of functional weakness: a controlled study of 107 patients. Brain 133: 1537–1551.

Stone J, Reuber M, Carson A (2013). Functional symptoms in neurology: mimics and chameleons. Pract Neurol 13: 104–113.

Sydenham T (1848). In: WA Greenhill, RG Latham (Eds.), The works of Thomas Sydenham, vol. 1, Sydenham Society, London. English edition by.

Szaflarski JP, Ficker DM, Cahill WT et al. (2000). Four-year incidence of psychogenic nonepileptic seizures in adults in Hamilton County, OH. Neurology 55 (10): 1561–1563.

Thomas M, Vuong KD, Jankovic J (2006). Long-term prognosis of patients with psychogenic movement disorders. Parkinsonism Relat Disord 12 (6): 382–387.

Williams DT, Ford B, Fahn S (1995). Phenomenology and psychopathology related to psychogenic movement disorders. Adv Neurol 65: 231–257.

Handbook of Clinical Neurology, Vol. 139 (3rd series)
Functional Neurologic Disorders
M. Hallett, J. Stone, and A. Carson, Editors
http://dx.doi.org/10.1016/B978-0-12-801772-2.00006-0

Chapter 6

Neurophysiologic studies of functional neurologic disorders

M. HALLETT*
Human Motor Control Section, National Institute of Neurological Disorders and Stroke, Bethesda, MD, USA

Abstract

Functional neurologic disorders are largely genuine and represent conversion disorders, where the dysfunction is unconscious, but there are some that are factitious, where the abnormality is feigned and conscious. Malingering, which can have the same manifestations, is similarly feigned, but not considered a genuine disease. There are no good methods for differentiating these three entities at the present time. Physiologic studies of functional weakness and sensory loss reveal normal functioning of primary motor and sensory cortex, but abnormalities of premotor cortex and association cortices. This suggests a top-down influence creating the dysfunction. Studies of functional tremor and myoclonus show that these disorders utilize normal voluntary motor structures to produce the involuntary movements, again suggesting a higher-level abnormality. Agency is abnormal and studies shows that dysfunction of the temporoparietal junction may be a correlate. The limbic system is overactive and might initiate involuntary movements, but the mechanism for this is not known. The limbic system would then be the source of top-down dysfunction. It can be speculated that the involuntary movements are involuntary due to lack of proper feedforward signaling.

INTRODUCTION

Almost by definition, functional neurologic disorders (FNDs) have no identifiable, responsible pathology. Yet, something is wrong. As we often say to patients (and which may be at least partly true), "the hardware is all right, it's the software that is the problem." The prevailing etiologic theories are psychosocial and still strongly dominated by the Freudian concept of conversion. A psychologic symptom is converted into a somatic symptom as a way of dealing with the distress of the symptom. With the conversion, the distress is ameliorated, and in fact by this logic, if the conversion is successful, the psychologic symptom is gone. Even if this is in some sense what happens, there still needs to be a physiologic mechanism responsible. The software is the way the brain functions, and this is amenable to study. Physiologic studies are necessary to understand what is happening, and they are beginning to illuminate the pathophysiology. These studies also define methods to help with diagnosis of FNDs, and "laboratory-supported" criteria can make a diagnosis more secure (Lang and Voon, 2011; Schwingenschuh et al., 2011b). Functional neuroimaging is a method of neurophysiology, but since this topic will be the focus of the next chapter, this chapter will only touch on functional neuroimaging results briefly.

This chapter will focus on conversion, a type of somatic symptom disorder, which has a fundamental feature of being the product of an unconscious process. Two other entities may have a similar clinical presentation: factitious disorder and malingering. The critical feature of these two entities separating them from conversion is that the symptoms are feigned; they are voluntarily produced. Factitious disorder arises to satisfy a psychologic need for medical care and is a psychiatric disorder also categorized under somatic symptom disorder. Malingering is the feigning of symptoms for nonhealthcare reasons and without any psychiatric disorder. In both

*Correspondence to: Mark Hallett, MD, Human Motor Control Section, National Institute of Neurological Disorders and Stroke, National Institutes of Health, Building 10, Room 7D37, 10 Center Drive, Bethesda MD 20892-1428, USA. Tel: +1-301-496-9526, Fax: +1-301-480-2286, E-mail: hallettm@ninds.nih.gov

factitious and malingering disorders, although the symptoms may look the same as with conversion disorders, the patients are lying. Unfortunately, doctors (and everyone else) are not good at determining whether someone is lying (Levine and Bond, 2014).

Secret surveillance has been used to document these disorders, but generally physicians do not hire detectives. The lie detector test depends on autonomic responses, but has many false-positive and negative results (Grubin, 2010). Eye blink frequency declines with deception, but it also has false positives and negatives (Perelman, 2014). Electroencephalogram (EEG) methods, such as event-related potentials (Proverbio et al., 2013; Rosenfeld et al., 2013; Pfister et al., 2014), and functional magnetic resonance imaging (fMRI) methods (Rusconi and Mitchener-Nissen, 2013; Farah et al., 2014) have also been proposed to evaluate truth or lying, but these too are not definitive. As to the physiology, presumably in factitious and malingering disorders the findings would be the same as in normal persons, although there may be excessive autonomic activity. In conversion disorders, the abnormality is unconscious and the physiology should differ in some ways from normal processing. In conversion blindness, the patient does not see; in conversion movement disorders, the movement is involuntary. In this chapter, there are some reports of physiologic changes in conversion. In order to understand FNDs completely, it is really necessary to understand the physiology of consciousness. If it would be possible to read the content of consciousness, we could more easily differentiate conversion from factitious disorder and malingering.

We certainly do not understand consciousness at this time, but some generalities can be stated. The brain is likely doing many things at all times. Information of many types is being passed around brain networks. At any one moment, only one (or very few) of these processes is manifest in consciousness. It is possible that conscious awareness is associated with a greater prominence of activity within the specific network for that process (Baars et al., 2013; Barttfeld et al., 2015). Increased activity and higher probability of getting into consciousness may result from bottom-up or top-down mechanisms (Corradi-Dell'Acqua et al., 2015). Consider why a sensory stimulus might get into consciousness. Bottom-up would be a strong sensory stimulus, such as an acute pain. That will come into consciousness almost no matter what else is happening. Top-down likely implies a cortical process which can regulate which networks have prominence. It is as if there is a conscious decision to pay attention to sensory stimuli of a certain type, and then even a weak stimulus would be appreciated. In relation to the issues discussed here, top-down mechanisms could also prevent a process from coming into consciousness. It is likely, for example, that this is the reason that soldiers in the heat of battle often do not feel their injuries.

FUNCTIONAL WEAKNESS AND PARALYSIS

In the face of functional weakness, routine nerve conduction studies are normal. In the electromyogram (EMG) examination, there is no spontaneous activity and motor units are normal. The interference pattern, however, is reduced. There is no clear difference of a reduced interference pattern from decreased effort and from a central nervous system lesion. In both circumstances there is reduced central nervous system drive.

A method that can separate a central nervous system lesion and reduced effort is transcranial magnetic stimulation (TMS) of the motor cortex. TMS will produce a normal motor evoked potential (MEP) with normal latency in the setting of functional weakness, and routine studies of motor cortex excitability are normal (Liepert et al., 2008). Such studies are abnormal with lesions anywhere along the corticospinal tract from motor cortex to spinal cord (Hallett, 2007). With severe lesions, the MEP will be absent. With compressive lesions, such as cervical spondylosis, or demyelinating disorders, such as multiple sclerosis, the central motor conduction time may be prolonged. Not only can a normal MEP be diagnostic, it can also be therapeutic. Patients have been described who improve after normal motor responses are produced by stimulation (Chastan and Parain, 2010; Pollak et al., 2014).

From the early days of TMS studies, it has been appreciated that motor imagery of moving a body part will increase the MEP amplitude of muscles acting on that part. In patients with functional paresis, opposite to normal, motor imagery suppresses the MEP amplitude (Fig. 6.1) (Liepert et al., 2009, 2011). Normal subjects feigning weakness also show reduced MEP amplitude (Liepert et al., 2014). On the other hand, movement observation, which also increases MEP amplitude in normal subjects, similarly increases the MEP in functional patients (Liepert et al., 2011). Motor imagery of simple movements in normal subjects in fMRI produces activations in most of the same parts of the motor system as does actual movement, except for the motor cortex (Hanakawa et al., 2008). There have not been similar studies with fMRI in patients. However, there have been functional studies in patients attempting to make movements, which have not occurred. In these few studies, dysfunctional activation is seen in the frontal lobes (Nowak and Fink, 2009), and the frontal areas are particularly strongly connected to the "paretic" motor cortex (Cojan et al., 2009).

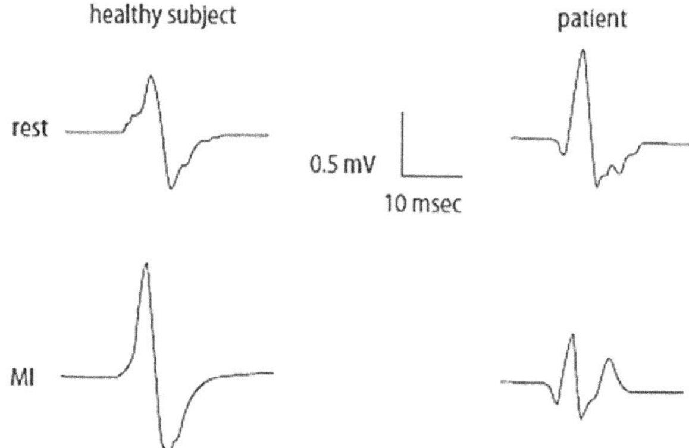

Fig. 6.1. Examples of motor evoked potentials during the resting condition and while performing motor imagery (MI). Electromyogram recording is from the right first dorsal interosseous muscle, and the subjects are asked to imagine a tonic adduction of the right index finger. (Reproduced from Liepert et al., 2009, with permission.)

The physiology of motor preparation in patients with conversion paresis has been studied with the contingent negative variation (CNV), a widespread cortical negativity measured with EEG in between a warning stimulus (S1) and the go stimulus (S2). Patients with unilateral conversion weakness were compared to normal subjects performing normally and normal subjects feigning weakness (Blakemore et al., 2015). A low-amplitude CNV was found only for the symptomatic hand of the conversion patients. In this study only partial information for the required movement was given with S1. In an earlier study by the same group (Blakemore et al., 2013), S1 conveyed full information about the upcoming movement and the emphasis of the study was on the response to S1 and less on the movement preparation. The authors interpreted this study as showing a larger than normal P3 (or P300), and that this positivity drove the EEG down so that the subsequent CNV was low for that reason, but the CNV could be interpreted similarly to their later experiment. In regard to the large P3, one possible interpretation offered by the authors was that it might have been due to increased emotional response to an instructed movement of the affected limb. It is certainly of interest that the findings in these two studies were restricted to the affected limb of conversion patients and were not seen in feigned weakness. The low-amplitude CNV could well be indicative of suppressed motor preparation.

Interpretation

The motor system from motor cortex to muscle is fully normal. With motor imagery of movement, the motor cortex is depressed rather than facilitated. There also appears to be reduced motor preparation. With "voluntary attempts" to move, there is activation of frontal areas that have been associated with "voluntary inhibition" of movement. Voluntary inhibition can be studied in a number of different tasks. One such task is the "stop signal task," where subjects get a second stimulus to inhibit a movement shortly after a first stimulus to make the movement. In one study, the right inferior frontal gyrus was particularly activated in stop trials (Sebastian et al., 2016). In another study, the inferior frontal cortex bilaterally was a critical node for other cortical areas and the subthalamic nucleus (Rae et al., 2015). These results would seem consistent with a top-down inhibition of the motor system causing the weakness or paralysis. As noted by Cojan and colleagues (2009), the areas of frontal cortex activated are related to emotional regulation. An additional conclusion appears to be that abnormalities are brought out with attention to the weak body part.

FUNCTIONAL SENSORY LOSS

Somatic sensation

Somatosensory evoked potentials (SEPs) are good probes for the large-fiber, dorsal-column, primary sensory cortex pathway. The presence of good potentials documents that this pathway is intact and is not compatible with total anesthesia. Such studies with normal potentials have been reported in the literature (Halliday, 1968; Kaplan et al., 1985), and although there are not many contemporary studies, this is the expected result. However, there was a case report of a patient with a functional sensory loss whose SEP was abnormally low in the anesthetic limb, but then became normal when the patient was put under light general anesthesia (Hernandez Peon et al., 1963). The authors postulated that a top-down control of sensory input might be responsible for the findings. In another case report of functional sensory loss, the SEP was absent with weak stimuli but normal with stronger stimuli, and again the authors postulated a top-down explanation (Levy and Behrman, 1970). It is important to be aware that there might well be false positives and false negatives (Howard and Dorfman, 1986). Using magnetoencephalography, it is possible to pick up a signal from the secondary somatosensory cortex, and, in a small case series of 3 patients, they all showed normal responses in both primary and secondary cortices (Hoechstetter et al., 2002).

Later SEP components are not often studied, but indicate further processing of the sensory stimuli. A P300 potential is seen in response to a rare stimulus in a series of stimuli with both common and rare stimuli. In 1 patient, the P300 component produced by stimulating the anesthetic limb was absent, whereas it was present on the normal limb and also present in a normal subject feigning sensory loss to mimic malingering (Lorenz et al., 1998).

If the symptom is restricted to loss of pain or small-fiber sensation, the ordinary SEP would not be a good test. To evaluate the spinothalamic tract, there are now methods coming into more routine use to look at sensory evoked potentials from heat stimuli. One method for doing this is laser stimulation, and at least in 1 patient with a functional sensory loss, the potential was normal (Lorenz et al., 1998). Another method is the "contact heat-evoked potentials." Test–retest reliability for this technique has been demonstrated (Kramer et al., 2012), but this has not been applied to the study of functional patients as yet.

Neuroimaging of sensory responses in functional sensory loss has only limited results. In one study of 4 patients (who had normal SEPs), there was actually a deactivation of primary and secondary somatosensory cortices, decreased activation of more upstream areas, but increased activation of the anterior cingulate cortex (Mailis-Gagnon et al., 2003). An older study using single-photon emission computed tomography in a single patient with functional sensory loss had similar findings of normal SEP, and decreased parietal perfusion and increased frontal perfusion with median nerve stimulation (Tiihonen et al., 1995). In 7 patients with functional sensorimotor symptoms, bilateral vibration led to asymmetric depressed response only in contralateral thalamus and basal ganglia (Vuilleumier et al., 2001). Three patients with unilateral sensory loss were studied with fMRI and vibrotactile stimulation (Ghaffar et al., 2006). With stimulation of the anesthetic limb, there was no activation of the primary sensory cortex. With bilateral stimulation, however, there was activation of the primary sensory cortex opposite the anesthetic limb, as well as the "normal" activation of the cortex opposite the normal limb. Hence, it appears that the primary sensory cortex can be activated, even if not by stimulation of the anesthetic limb by itself.

Vision

Visual evoked potentials (VEPs) can be done with full-field or hemifield stimulation of each eye and explored objectively for uniocular or hemifield abnormality. The stimulus is typically patterned, such as a checkerboard. The prominent potentials come from the primary visual cortex. If a subject does not look at the stimulus, then there might be a false-positive abnormality. It is also possible to do just a flash evoked response, which does not require attention. Retinal function can be examined with electroretinograms.

In nonorganic visual loss, VEPs can be normal (Kramer et al., 1979; Yoneda et al., 2013). When normal, that almost always indicates functioning of the early parts of the visual pathway, although there are some patients who do have abnormalities but still test normal. Decreased amplitude of the VEP is also reported (Schoenfeld et al., 2011). When abnormal, it is more difficult to interpret due to the possibility of false positives, as noted already. When abnormal in a patient with conversion, it might be possible to change the result to normal using distraction. This was noted in a case report (Manresa et al., 1996).

An interesting case report of a patient with multiple personalities was published in German (Waldvogel et al., 2007) and subsequently in English also (Strasburger and Waldvogel, 2015). In some personalities, the patient could see and VEPs were present, and in other personalities, the patient could not see and VEPs were absent. Whether this was a conversion patient or a factitious patient with "defocusing" is not clear.

Using pattern VEPs with different check size, it is possible to get an objective measure of acuity. Using this method in malingering patients, it was possible to show better acuity than claimed (Gundogan et al., 2007).

The P300 was evaluated in 2 patients with malingering and 1 patient with conversion, and it was present in all 3 (Towle et al., 1985). All 3 patients did have VEPs at least some of the time. While statistics were not possible in these few cases, the authors did comment that the P300 amplitude seemed small in the conversion patient.

Audition

Auditory evoked potentials, as ordinarily done, explore the brainstem pathway for auditory information. There is a potential as well from auditory cortex. Late potentials have been studied in this situation also, and the P300 was reduced unilaterally in a patient with functional hearing loss (Fukuda et al., 1996). Mismatch negativity is an electrographic component similar to the P300, seen with target stimuli in the midst of background stimuli. In a group of 10 patients with somatization disorder, the mismatch negativity was smaller than normal (James et al., 1989).

Interpretation

In all these sensory functional disorders, it is usually possible to demonstrate normal functioning of the early part of the afferent pathway, including the primary sensory cortices. Beyond the primary sensory cortices, the information is less clear since the understanding of later evoked potential waves is not well known and less studied. Perception certainly involves brain structures beyond the primary cortices. However, it does seem that the P300 can be abnormal in conversion and this has interesting implications. On the other hand, the P300 might be normal in malingering, and this may well have diagnostic value for differentiating it from conversion.

Sensory systems have top-down operations as well as bottom-up. Attention can certainly modulate sensation, and top-down mechanisms can shut down sensory activity (Nunez and Malmierca, 2007). The notion of increased inhibition of sensory function in conversion disorders by corticofugal tracts has been proposed (Ludwig, 1972).

FUNCTIONAL MOVEMENT DISORDERS

Functional myoclonus

The methods for analysis of myoclonus (Hallett and Shibasaki, 2008) and for functional myoclonus (Hallett, 2010) in particular have been described in detail, and will only be summarized here. There are three steps in the evaluation of myoclonus: (1) the analysis of the EMG underlying the movement, generally with at least the simultaneous recording of both muscles of an antagonist pair; (2) to record the EEG simultaneously with the EMG to look at their correlation; and (3) to analyze reflex myoclonus, if present, for EMG latencies and EEG evoked responses.

In myoclonus that is a fragment of epilepsy, the EMG burst length is generally 30–50 ms and antagonist muscles are always synchronous. In other forms of myoclonus, the EMG burst length is longer and antagonist muscle relationships are variable. Functional myoclonus falls into this latter category. Hence, epileptic myoclonus can be ruled out with this method, but nonepileptic myoclonus cannot be. Additionally, some forms of nonepileptic myoclonus have characteristic EMG patterns, and this would help identify them as such. For example, in startle, orbicularis oculi is the first and most consistent muscle, sometimes with apparent double burst. This is followed by activity in lower cranial nerve muscles and subsequently by upper cranial nerve muscles and limb muscles (Matsumoto and Hallett, 1994). Functional myoclonus may well show highly variable patterns.

The EEG correlate is obtained by backaveraging the EEG using the onset of EMG (or movement) as the fiducial point. Each type of epileptic myoclonus has a characteristic EEG correlate. The best known is the potential associated with cortical myoclonus, a brief negative–positive potential about 20 ms prior to the EMG. In nonepileptic myoclonus, generally a potential is not identified. In functional myoclonus, very frequently a normal-looking Bereitschaftspotential can be identified (Fig. 6.2) (Terada et al., 1995). This indicates activity in the premotor cortex (Shibasaki and Hallett, 2006). In a study of 29 patients with functional myoclonus, 25 had a Bereitschaftspotential (van der Salm et al., 2012). As an unexpected finding in the latter study, there was often an absent Bereitschaftspotential prior to a voluntary wrist flexion movement. The explanation for this is unclear, and the authors raised issues of attention and motivation.

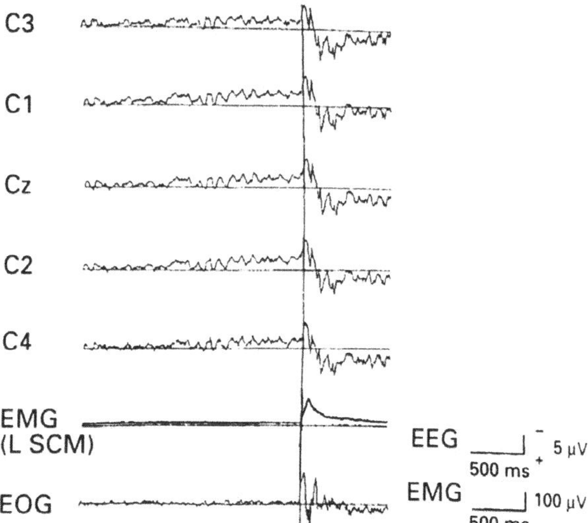

Fig. 6.2. Electroencephalogram (EEG) backaverage from functional myoclonus showing a normal-looking Bereitschaftspotential. L SCM, left sternocleidomastoid; EOG, electro-oculogram; EMG, electromyogram. (Reproduced from Terada et al., 1995, with permission.)

The physiologic correlate of reflex myoclonus is called the C-reflex. In organic myoclonus syndromes the C-reflex comes from hyperexcitability of one of several long-latency reflex pathways. All of these pathways produce shorter latencies than the fastest voluntary reaction times, about 40–50 ms. In functional reflex myoclonus, the latencies are variable and similar to, and never faster than, the fastest voluntary reaction time, 100 ms or longer depending on the type of sensory stimulus (Thompson et al., 1992).

Interpretation

Functional myoclonus has the EMG signature of voluntary movement and even the expected EEG correlate of a Bereitschaftspotential. Since functional myoclonus is involuntary, the presence of a Bereitschaftspotential in this situation is evidence that the Bereitschaftspotential is not indicative of voluntariness. What it does appear to indicate is movement preparation in the premotor cortex. Another feature of functional myoclonus similar to normal voluntary movement is reaction time latencies. Hence it appears that normal voluntary mechanisms are utilized to produce functional myoclonus and that these mechanisms are operating normally. It must be that some top-down process co-opts this mechanism to produce movement, but not the sense of willing the movement.

Functional tremor

As with functional myoclonus, the testing for functional tremor is very good, and should be able to support the diagnosis. Tremor can be measured with EMG and/or with accelerometry, or both. Functional tremor may show marked variation in frequency and amplitude (O'Suilleabhain and Matsumoto, 1998). Additionally, functional tremor is typically exactly the same frequency and in phase in different limbs; this virtually never happens in organic tremors. This can be formally assessed with coherence analysis (McAuley and Rothwell, 2004).

The most useful physiologic method is the entrainment test (Hallett, 2010). In this test, the patient is asked to tap voluntarily at various frequencies with a body part unaffected by the tremor. If all body parts show tremor, this still can be done, with voluntary tapping of one body part while monitoring the response of the "involuntary" tremor in another body part. The tremor is entrained if the tremor takes up the frequency of the voluntary tapping. Another clue of psychogenicity is that the patient might have considerable difficulty in doing the voluntary tapping at the requested rate (Zeuner et al., 2003). Most commonly the test is done by measuring tremor of one hand and performing voluntary tapping with the other hand at a series of different frequencies. The different frequencies can be demonstrated for the subject with a metronome. The tremor might stop completely, change its frequency, or will take up the frequency of the voluntary tapping. Coherence analysis can quantify this. While this is a very good test, there are some functional tremors that do not entrain (Raethjen et al., 2004). The ballistic movement test is a variation on entrainment (Kumru et al., 2004). Here, patients are asked to make a quick movement with one limb. In functional tremor, there might be a pause in the tremor during the movement.

In a small group of patients, their functional tremor has been compared to voluntarily mimicked tremor using fMRI (Voon et al., 2010b). The most prominent difference was in the activation of the temporoparietal junction (TPJ) region, including connectivity of this area to parts of the motor system. As the TPJ appears relevant to the sense of self-agency for movement (Nahab et al., 2011), the lack of activation was speculated to be a correlate for the tremor being involuntary. Abnormal activation of the TPJ was also seen in conversion disorder patients when recalling past stressful life events (Aybek et al., 2014).

Interpretation

Similar to functional myoclonus, functional tremor appears to use a normally functioning motor system for the manifestation of the movement disorder. A higher-level brain network controls the motor network to produce tremor without producing the sense of voluntariness or agency. The lack of TPJ activation could be due to a failure of feedforward signaling at the time of movement generation.

Further evidence for a failure of feedforward signaling comes from studies of sensory gating. Sensory gating is the reduction of sensation and SEPs from a limb at the onset of, and during, self-generated movement. Studied in a mix of functional movement disorder patients, sensory gating was decreased in the patients (Pareés et al., 2014; Macerollo et al., 2015b). In one study of force matching, patients did not overestimate the force required as the normal controls did, indicating that they did not have normal gating (Pareés et al., 2014). In an SEP study, the N20 and N30 potentials were not suppressed at all (Macerollo et al., 2015b). Gating must be due to feedforward signaling from the motor command to the sensory system, thus dampening the sensory feedback from the movement. This avoids the brain being "bothered" by expected sensory events. There are two important implications. First, this is evidence for abnormal top-down control of sensation in these patients. Second, a loss of the gating function would mean that the movement related to the sensation would be more likely to be interpreted as externally generated rather than internally generated; this would then lead to a loss of the sense of agency.

However, the ultimate source of the motor command remains unknown. Imaging studies do suggest that the limbic system is overactive in functional movement disorders in general (Voon et al., 2011). As the limbic system provides important drive to movement, this could be the primary source, but this remains speculative.

Functional dystonia

Functional dystonia is often difficult to diagnose even with physiologic testing. For some reason, not yet fully understood, functional dystonia and organic dystonia often show the same findings.

Dystonic movement is usually characterized by co-contraction of antagonist muscles, but this is not always the case (Malfait and Sanger, 2007). In a study of patients with fixed dystonia and acquired (secondary) dystonia, those with fixed dystonia had less co-contraction as a group, but there was significant overlap between the findings in the two groups (Macerollo et al., 2015a). Hence, while lack of (or less) co-contraction might suggest that the disorder is functional, this is not a definitive observation. A pathologic drive at 4–7 Hz to muscles in patients with cervical dystonia and DYT1 dystonia was not seen in normal subjects and patients with fixed dystonia (assumed to be mostly functional) (Grosse et al., 2004). However, such drive was not seen in patients with writer's cramp (Cordivari et al., 2002). Hence, this observation cannot be used as a definitive test either.

There are a large number of physiologic abnormalities in organic dystonia, most relating to loss of inhibition. These abnormalities can be seen at spinal level, such as reciprocal inhibition, and cortical level, such as short intracortical inhibition assessed with TMS. Most of these abnormalities are shared with functional dystonia (Espay et al., 2006; Avanzino et al., 2008). Temporal discrimination is also similarly abnormal in organic and functional dystonia (Morgante et al., 2011). One inhibitory mechanism not shared is the blink reflex recovery curve (Schwingenschuh et al., 2011a). In organic dystonia affecting cranial muscles, there is a loss of normal inhibition in blink reflex recovery. There is no such loss in functional blepharospasm. Eye blink conditioning is similarly normal in unmedicated patients with fixed dystonia (Janssen et al., 2014).

One important physiologic difference might be a measure of central nervous system plasticity called paired-associative stimulation. This method repetitively pairs a shock to the median nerve with a TMS to the motor cortex. Similar to long-term potentiation, this repetitive pairing leads to an increase in excitability of the motor cortex as assessed by the amplitude of the MEPs in muscles innervated by the median nerve and adjacent muscles. While organic dystonia shows an increased plasticity with this method, functional dystonia does not show this abnormality (Quartarone et al., 2009).

Interpretation

The physiologic overlap of organic and functional dystonia is not understood. One possibility is that the physiologic abnormalities indicate a propensity to dystonia that can be either organic or functional in the correct setting. Another possibility is that they are the result of dystonia rather than the cause. There are some tests that are different, including the blink reflex recovery curve and the paired-associative stimulation. However, how they illuminate the nature of functional dystonia is not clear.

OTHER FUNCTIONAL MOVEMENT DISORDERS

Functional gait disorders are common, but there are no physiologic studies. Most patients complain of poor balance, but it is clear from observing the gait that balance is very good. Quantitative balance testing has been undertaken. In one study, balance was assessed in conversion disorder patients and controls standing quietly, standing with eyes closed, and standing with an attention-demanding cognitive task (Stins et al., 2015). Sway increased more in patients in the eyes-closed condition, but it normalized in the attention task. Presumably, when the patients focused attention away from balance, it became normal. In another study, conversion disorder patients were compared with controls and patients with multiple sclerosis, in eight conditions, standing on solid floor or foam, eyes open or closed, and with and without distraction (Wolfsegger et al., 2013). Distraction here was recognizing numbers drawn on the back. Again, balance improved with distraction only in the conversion disorder patients.

Functional parkinsonism is not common, and again there have not been any physiologic investigations other than examination of tremor, as described above.

Functional seizures (psychogenic nonepileptic seizures: PNES)

Video-EEG is the standard technique for evaluating patients with suspected PNES (Gedzelman and LaRoche, 2014). A normal EEG in the face of an episode is strong evidence for its functional nature. There are some examples of false negatives, particularly frontal-lobe sources, which are sometimes missed with scalp recordings. Nocturnal dystonia was a subclass of paroxysmal dystonia until it was recognized that this was a form of epilepsy. It is also fair to say that an EEG is full of movement and muscle artifacts during any seizure, making the identification of subtle changes difficult to identify. Curiously, interictal epileptiform abnormalities are almost twice as common in PNES patients as in normal subjects, but it is not clear what that means (Reuber et al., 2002).

Resting EEG networks have been investigated in PNES patients. In general, these studies show a variety of weakened connections between parts of the brain (Knyazeva et al., 2011; Barzegaran et al., 2012, 2016). Perhaps most interesting is the finding of decreased prefrontal and parietal synchronization. Speculatively, that could underlie a weakness of possible feedforward connections in the brain.

Interpretation

While useful for diagnosis, a normal EEG does not inform us much about the pathophysiology of nonepileptic attacks. More work might be undertaken to study brain networks in these patients, including during the seizures themselves.

Synthesis

The physiology of conversion is not well understood, and motor and sensory disorders should be particularly helpful in studying this phenomenon since they can be objectively measured. The evidence seems clear that the

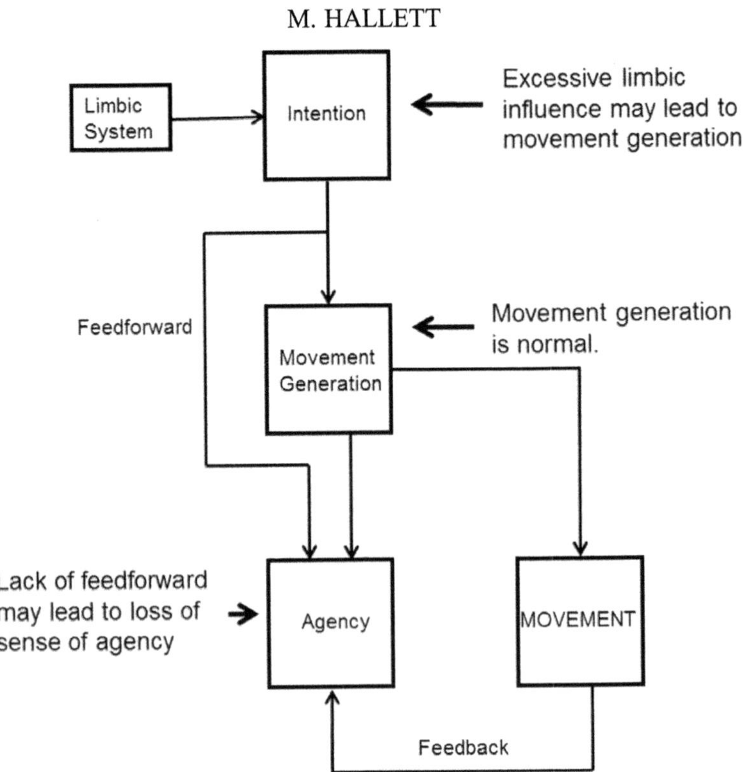

Fig. 6.3. Model of how involuntary movements might be generated and how they might not acquire a sense of agency. The model speculates that excessive limbic activity leads to movement generation, but does not produce a normal feedforward signal. Although movement is generated in a normal fashion and feedback occurs, there is a mismatch between feedforward and feedback and agency is not generated.

elementary motor efferent system beginning in motor cortex and the elementary sensory afferent systems extending to primary sensory cortices are functioning normally. The premotor systems and the sensory association areas are where the dysfunction is. fMRI, which is a major addition to clinical neurophysiology in assessing brain networks beyond primary cortices, is already shedding some light on these higher-level functions.

There is much evidence supporting an abnormality of top-down control with derangement of feedforward signaling. Attention to a disorder seems to aggravate or maintain it, while distraction might improve function. The failure of feedforward communication in the brain appears to give rise to sense of loss of control.

The primary site of the functional abnormalities, if there is one, is not clear. As noted earlier, some studies give evidence of increased influence of the limbic system in driving movement. Patients with functional movement disorders show an increased startle response to positive affective pictures as well as negative ones, indicating abnormal regulation of the startle response (Seignourel et al., 2007). In an fMRI study of faces showing different affects, patients with functional movement disorders showed increased activation of the right amygdala (Voon et al., 2010a). In a choice reaction time task, patients with functional movement disorders showed increased limbic activity and increased connectivity of the limbic system to the motor system (Voon et al., 2011). The limbic system can drive the motor system. Indeed, emotions are one of the major factors influencing movement choice. Limbic structures, such as the amygdala, can be influenced by genetic factors and/or early life stress. At this time, the idea is rather speculative, but it could be that abnormal functioning of the limbic system, both because of intrinsic "vulnerability" as well as traumatic life experiences, upsets brain networks and leads to functional disorders by deranged top-down control (Fig. 6.3). Freud might well have liked that idea.

ACKNOWLEDGMENT

This work is supported by the National Institute of Neurological Disorders and Stroke (NINDS) intramural program. I am grateful to Dr. Timothy Nicholson for thoughtful comments on an early draft of this chapter.

References

Avanzino L, Martino D, van de Warrenburg BP et al. (2008). Cortical excitability is abnormal in patients with the "fixed dystonia" syndrome. Mov Disord 23 (5): 646–652.

Aybek S, Nicholson TR, Zelaya F et al. (2014). Neural correlates of recall of life events in conversion disorder. JAMA Psychiatry 71 (1): 52–60.

Baars BJ, Franklin S, Ramsoy TZ (2013). Global workspace dynamics: cortical "binding and propagation" enables conscious contents. Front Psychol 4: 200.

Barttfeld P, Uhrig L, Sitt JD et al. (2015). Signature of consciousness in the dynamics of resting-state brain activity. Proc Natl Acad Sci U S A 112 (3): 887–892.

Barzegaran E, Joudaki A, Jalili M et al. (2012). Properties of functional brain networks correlate with frequency of psychogenic non-epileptic seizures. Front Hum Neurosci 6: 335.

Barzegaran E, Carmeli C, Rossetti AO et al. (2016). Weakened functional connectivity in patients with psychogenic non-epileptic seizures (PNES) converges on basal ganglia. J Neurol Neurosurg Psychiatry. 87 (3): 332–337.

Blakemore RL, Hyland BI, Hammond-Tooke GD et al. (2013). Distinct modulation of event-related potentials during motor preparation in patients with motor conversion disorder. PLoS One 8 (4): e62539.

Blakemore RL, Hyland BI, Hammond-Tooke GD et al. (2015). Deficit in late-stage contingent negative variation provides evidence for disrupted movement preparation in patients with conversion paresis. Biol Psychol 109: 73–85.

Chastan N, Parain D (2010). Psychogenic paralysis and recovery after motor cortex transcranial magnetic stimulation. Mov Disord 25 (10): 1501–1504.

Cojan Y, Waber L, Carruzzo A et al. (2009). Motor inhibition in hysterical conversion paralysis. Neuroimage 47 (3): 1026–1037.

Cordivari C, Lees AJ, Misra VP et al. (2002). EMG-EMG coherence in writer's cramp. Mov Disord 17 (5): 1011–1016.

Corradi-Dell'Acqua C, Fink GR, Weidner R (2015). Selecting category specific visual information: top-down and bottom-up control of object based attention. Conscious Cogn 35: 330–341.

Espay AJ, Morgante F, Purzner J et al. (2006). Cortical and spinal abnormalities in psychogenic dystonia. Ann Neurol 59 (5): 825–834.

Farah MJ, Hutchinson JB, Phelps EA et al. (2014). Functional MRI-based lie detection: scientific and societal challenges. Nat Rev Neurosci 15 (2): 123–131.

Fukuda M, Hata A, Niwa S et al. (1996). Event-related potential correlates of functional hearing loss: reduced P3 amplitude with preserved N1 and N2 components in a unilateral case. Psychiatry Clin Neurosci 50 (2): 85–87.

Gedzelman ER, LaRoche SM (2014). Long-term video EEG monitoring for diagnosis of psychogenic nonepileptic seizures. Neuropsychiatr Dis Treat 10: 1979–1986.

Ghaffar O, Staines WR, Feinstein A (2006). Unexplained neurologic symptoms: an fMRI study of sensory conversion disorder. Neurology 67 (11): 2036–2038.

Grosse P, Edwards M, Tijssen MA et al. (2004). Patterns of EMG-EMG coherence in limb dystonia. Mov Disord 19 (7): 758–769.

Grubin D (2010). The polygraph and forensic psychiatry. J Am Acad Psychiatry Law 38 (4): 446–451.

Gundogan FC, Sobaci G, Bayer A (2007). Pattern visual evoked potentials in the assessment of visual acuity in malingering. Ophthalmology 114 (12): 2332–2337.

Hallett M (2007). Transcranial magnetic stimulation: a primer. Neuron 55 (2): 187–199.

Hallett M (2010). Physiology of psychogenic movement disorders. J Clin Neurosci 17 (8): 959–965.

Hallett M, Shibasaki H (2008). Myoclonus and myoclonic syndromes. In: J Engel Jr, TA Pedley (Eds.), Epilepsy: A Comprehensive Textbook, Lippincott, Williams & Wilkins, Philadelphia, pp. 2765–2770.

Halliday AM (1968). Computing techniques in neurological diagnosis. Br Med Bull 24 (3): 253–259.

Hanakawa T, Dimyan MA, Hallett M (2008). Motor planning, imagery, and execution in the distributed motor network: a time-course study with functional MRI. Cereb Cortex 18 (12): 2775–2788.

Hernandez Peon R, Chavez Ibarra G, Aguilar Figueroa E (1963). Somatic evoked potentials in one case of hysterical anaesthesia. Electroencephalogr Clin Neurophysiol 15: 889–892.

Hoechstetter K, Meinck HM, Henningsen P et al. (2002). Psychogenic sensory loss: magnetic source imaging reveals normal tactile evoked activity of the human primary and secondary somatosensory cortex. Neurosci Lett 323 (2): 137–140.

Howard JE, Dorfman LJ (1986). Evoked potentials in hysteria and malingering. J Clin Neurophysiol 3 (1): 39–49.

James L, Gordon E, Kraiuhin C et al. (1989). Selective attention and auditory event-related potentials in somatization disorder. Compr Psychiatry 30 (1): 84–89.

Janssen S, Veugen LC, Hoffland BS et al. (2014). Normal eyeblink classical conditioning in patients with fixed dystonia. Exp Brain Res 232 (6): 1805–1809.

Kaplan BJ, Friedman WA, Gravenstein D (1985). Somatosensory evoked potentials in hysterical paraplegia. Surg Neurol 23 (5): 502–506.

Knyazeva MG, Jalili M, Frackowiak RS et al. (2011). Psychogenic seizures and frontal disconnection: EEG synchronisation study. J Neurol Neurosurg Psychiatry 82 (5): 505–511.

Kramer KK, La Piana FG, Appleton B (1979). Ocular malingering and hysteria: diagnosis and management. Surv Ophthalmol 24 (2): 89–96.

Kramer JL, Taylor P, Haefeli J et al. (2012). Test-retest reliability of contact heat-evoked potentials from cervical dermatomes. J Clin Neurophysiol 29 (1): 70–75.

Kumru H, Valls-Sole J, Valldeoriola F et al. (2004). Transient arrest of psychogenic tremor induced by contralateral ballistic movements. Neurosci Lett 370 (2–3): 135–139.

Lang AE, Voon V (2011). Psychogenic movement disorders: past developments, current status, and future directions. Mov Disord 26 (6): 1175–1186.

Levine TR, Bond Jr CF (2014). Direct and indirect measures of lie detection tell the same story: a reply to ten Brinke, Stimson, and Carney (2014). Psychol Sci 25 (10): 1960–1961.

Levy R, Behrman J (1970). Cortical evoked responses in hysterical hemianaesthesia. Electroencephalogr Clin Neurophysiol 29 (4): 400–402.

Liepert J, Hassa T, Tuscher O et al. (2008). Electrophysiological correlates of motor conversion disorder. Mov Disord 23 (15): 2171–2176.

Liepert J, Hassa T, Tuscher O et al. (2009). Abnormal motor excitability in patients with psychogenic paresis. A TMS study. J Neurol 256 (1): 121–126.

Liepert J, Hassa T, Tuscher O et al. (2011). Motor excitability during movement imagination and movement observation in psychogenic lower limb paresis. J Psychosom Res 70 (1): 59–65.

Liepert J, Shala J, Greiner J (2014). Electrophysiological correlates of disobedience and feigning-like behaviour in motor imagery. Clin Neurophysiol 125 (4): 763–767.

Lorenz J, Kunze K, Bromm B (1998). Differentiation of conversive sensory loss and malingering by P300 in a modified oddball task. Neuroreport 9 (2): 187–191.

Ludwig AM (1972). Hysteria. A neurobiological theory. Arch Gen Psychiatry 27 (6): 771–777.

Macerollo A, Batla A, Kassavetis P et al. (2015a). Using reaction time and co-contraction to differentiate acquired (secondary) from functional 'fixed' dystonia. J Neurol Neurosurg Psychiatry 86 (8): 933–934.

Macerollo A, Chen JC, Pareés I et al. (2015b). Sensory attenuation assessed by sensory evoked potentials in functional movement disorders. PLoS One 10 (6): e0129507.

Mailis-Gagnon A, Giannoylis I, Downar J et al. (2003). Altered central somatosensory processing in chronic pain patients with "hysterical" anesthesia. Neurology 60 (9): 1501–1507.

Malfait N, Sanger TD (2007). Does dystonia always include co-contraction? A study of unconstrained reaching in children with primary and secondary dystonia. Exp Brain Res 176 (2): 206–216.

Manresa MJ, Bonaventura I, Martinez I et al. (1996). Voluntary changes of visual evoked potentials in cases with hysteria and/or simulation. Rev Neurol 24 (127): 285–286.

Matsumoto J, Hallett M (1994). Startle syndromes. In: CD Marsden, S Fahn (Eds.), Movement Disorders 3, Butterworth-Heinemann, Oxford, pp. 418–433.

McAuley J, Rothwell J (2004). Identification of psychogenic, dystonic, and other organic tremors by a coherence entrainment test. Mov Disord 19 (3): 253–267.

Morgante F, Tinazzi M, Squintani G et al. (2011). Abnormal tactile temporal discrimination in psychogenic dystonia. Neurology 77 (12): 1191–1197.

Nahab FB, Kundu P, Gallea C et al. (2011). The neural processes underlying self-agency. Cereb Cortex 21 (1): 48–55.

Nowak DA, Fink GR (2009). Psychogenic movement disorders: Aetiology, phenomenology, neuroanatomical correlates and therapeutic approaches. Neuroimage 47 (3): 1015–1025.

Nunez A, Malmierca E (2007). Corticofugal modulation of sensory information. Adv Anat Embryol Cell Biol 187. 1 p following table of contents, -74.

O'Suilleabhain PE, Matsumoto JY (1998). Time-frequency analysis of tremors. Brain 121 (Pt 11): 2127–2134.

Pareés I, Brown H, Nuruki A et al. (2014). Loss of sensory attenuation in patients with functional (psychogenic) movement disorders. Brain 137 (Pt 11): 2916–2921.

Perelman BS (2014). Detecting deception via eyeblink frequency modulation. PeerJ 2. e260.

Pfister R, Foerster A, Kunde W (2014). Pants on fire: the electrophysiological signature of telling a lie. Soc Neurosci 9 (6): 562–572.

Pollak TA, Nicholson TR, Edwards MJ et al. (2014). A systematic review of transcranial magnetic stimulation in the treatment of functional (conversion) neurological symptoms. J Neurol Neurosurg Psychiatry 85 (2): 191–197.

Proverbio AM, Vanutelli ME, Adorni R (2013). Can you catch a liar? How negative emotions affect brain responses when lying or telling the truth. PLoS One 8 (3): e59383.

Quartarone A, Rizzo V, Terranova C et al. (2009). Abnormal sensorimotor plasticity in organic but not in psychogenic dystonia. Brain 132 (Pt 10): 2871–2877.

Rae CL, Hughes LE, Anderson MC et al. (2015). The prefrontal cortex achieves inhibitory control by facilitating subcortical motor pathway connectivity. J Neurosci 35 (2): 786–794.

Raethjen J, Kopper F, Govindan RB et al. (2004). Two different pathogenetic mechanisms in psychogenic tremor. Neurology 63 (5): 812–815.

Reuber M, Fernandez G, Bauer J et al. (2002). Interictal EEG abnormalities in patients with psychogenic nonepileptic seizures. Epilepsia 43 (9): 1013–1020.

Rosenfeld JP, Hu X, Labkovsky E et al. (2013). Review of recent studies and issues regarding the P300-based complex trial protocol for detection of concealed information. Int J Psychophysiol 90 (2): 118–134.

Rusconi E, Mitchener-Nissen T (2013). Prospects of functional magnetic resonance imaging as lie detector. Front Hum Neurosci 7: 594.

Schoenfeld MA, Hassa T, Hopf JM et al. (2011). Neural correlates of hysterical blindness. Cereb Cortex 21 (10): 2394–2398.

Schwingenschuh P, Katschnig P, Edwards MJ et al. (2011a). The blink reflex recovery cycle differs between essential and presumed psychogenic blepharospasm. Neurology 76 (7): 610–614.

Schwingenschuh P, Katschnig P, Seiler S et al. (2011b). Moving toward "laboratory-supported" criteria for psychogenic tremor. Mov Disord 26 (14): 2509–2515.

Sebastian A, Jung P, Neuhoff J et al. (2016). Dissociable attentional and inhibitory networks of dorsal and ventral areas of the right inferior frontal cortex: a combined task-specific and coordinate-based meta-analytic fMRI study. Brain Struct Funct 221 (3): 1635–1651.

Seignourel PJ, Miller K, Kellison I et al. (2007). Abnormal affective startle modulation in individuals with psychogenic [corrected] movement disorder. Mov Disord 22 (9): 1265–1271.

Shibasaki H, Hallett M (2006). What is the Bereitschaftspotential? Clin Neurophysiol 117 (11): 2341–2356.

Stins JF, Kempe CL, Hagenaars MA et al. (2015). Attention and postural control in patients with conversion paresis. J Psychosom Res 78 (3): 249–254.

Strasburger H, Waldvogel B (2015). Sight and blindness in the same person: gating in the visual system. Psych J 4 (4): 178–185.

Terada K, Ikeda A, Van Ness PC et al. (1995). Presence of Bereitschaftspotential preceding psychogenic myoclonus: clinical application of jerk-locked back averaging. J Neurol Neurosurg Psychiatry 58: 745–747.

Thompson PD, Colebatch JG, Brown P et al. (1992). Voluntary stimulus-sensitive jerks and jumps mimicking myoclonus or pathological startle syndromes. Mov Disord 7 (3): 257–262.

Tiihonen J, Kuikka J, Viinamaki H et al. (1995). Altered cerebral blood flow during hysterical paresthesia. Biol Psychiatry 37 (2): 134–135.

Towle VL, Sutcliffe E, Sokol S (1985). Diagnosing functional visual deficits with the P300 component of the visual evoked potential. Arch Ophthalmol 103 (1): 47–50.

van der Salm SM, Tijssen MA, Koelman JH et al. (2012). The bereitschaftspotential in jerky movement disorders. J Neurol Neurosurg Psychiatry 83 (12): 1162–1167.

Voon V, Brezing C, Gallea C et al. (2010a). Emotional stimuli and motor conversion disorder. Brain 133 (Pt 5): 1526–1536.

Voon V, Gallea C, Hattori N et al. (2010b). The involuntary nature of conversion disorder. Neurology 74: 223–228.

Voon V, Brezing C, Gallea C et al. (2011). Aberrant supplementary motor complex and limbic activity during motor preparation in motor conversion disorder. Mov Disord 26 (13): 2396–2403.

Vuilleumier P, Chicherio C, Assal F et al. (2001). Functional neuroanatomical correlates of hysterical sensorimotor loss. Brain 124 (Pt 6): 1077–1090.

Waldvogel B, Ullrich A, Strasburger H (2007). Sighted and blind in one person: a case report and conclusions on the psychoneurobiology of vision. Nervenarzt 78 (11): 1303–1309.

Wolfsegger T, Pischinger B, Topakian R (2013). Objectification of psychogenic postural instability by trunk sway analysis. J Neurol Sci 334 (1–2): 14–17.

Yoneda T, Fukuda K, Nishimura M et al. (2013). A case of functional (psychogenic) monocular hemianopia analyzed by measurement of hemifield visual evoked potentials. Case Rep Ophthalmol 4 (3): 283–286.

Zeuner KE, Shoge RO, Goldstein SR et al. (2003). Accelerometry to distinguish psychogenic from essential or parkinsonian tremor. Neurology 61 (4): 548–550.

Handbook of Clinical Neurology, Vol. 139 (3rd series)
Functional Neurologic Disorders
M. Hallett, J. Stone, and A. Carson, Editors
http://dx.doi.org/10.1016/B978-0-12-801772-2.00007-2

Chapter 7

Imaging studies of functional neurologic disorders

S. AYBEK[1,2]* AND P. VUILLEUMIER[2]

[1]*Neurology Service, Geneva University Hospitals, Geneva, Switzerland*

[2]*Laboratory for Behavioural Neurology and Imaging of Cognition, Department of Neuroscience, University of Geneva-Campus Biotech, Geneva, Switzerland*

Abstract

Brain imaging techniques provide unprecedented opportunities to study the neural mechanisms underlying functional neurologic disorder (FND, or conversion disorder), which have long remained a mystery and clinical challenge for physicians, as they arise with no apparent underlying organic disease. One of the first questions addressed by imaging studies concerned whether motor conversion deficits (e.g., hysteric paralysis) represent a form of (perhaps unconscious) simulation, a mere absence of voluntary movement, or more specific disturbances in motor control (such as abnormal inhibition). Converging evidence from several studies using different techniques and paradigms has now demonstrated distinctive brain activation patterns associated with functional deficits, unlike those seen in actors simulating similar deficits. Thus, patients with motor FND show consistent hypoactivation of both cortical and subcortical motor pathways, with frequent increases in other brain areas within the limbic system, but no recruitment of prefrontal regions usually associated with voluntary motor inhibition. Other studies point to a dysfunction in sensorimotor integration and agency – related to parietal dysfunction – and abnormal motor planning related to supplementary motor area and prefrontal areas. These findings not only suggest that functional symptoms reflect a genuine brain dysfunction, but also give new insights into how they are produced. However, fewer studies attempted to understand why these symptoms are produced and linked to potential psychologic or emotional risk/triggering factors. Results from such studies point towards abnormal limbic regulation with heightened emotional arousal and amygdalar activity, potentially related to engagement of defense systems and stereotyped motor behaviors, mediated by medial prefrontal cortex and subcortical structures, including the periaqueductal gray area and basal ganglia. In addition, across different symptom domains, several studies reported abnormal recruitment of ventromedial prefrontal cortex (vmPFC), a region known to regulate emotion appraisal, memory retrieval, and self-reflective representations. The vmPFC might provide important modulatory signals to both cortical and subcortical sensorimotor, visual, and even memory circuits, promoting maladaptive self-protective behaviors based on personal affective appraisals of particular events. A better understanding of such a role of vmPFC in FND may help link how and why these symptoms are produced. Further research is also needed to determine brain activation patterns associated with FND across different types of deficits and different evolution stages (e.g., acute vs. chronic vs. recovered).

BACKGROUND

Functional neurologic disorders (FND), formerly called hysteria, and also called conversion disorder, have represented an enormous challenge over the centuries in terms of comprehension of the psychologic and biologic mechanisms responsible for various deficits which mimic neurologic diseases without organic damage (Vuilleumier, 2009). After the ancient explanatory model involving

*Correspondence to: Dr. Selma Aybek, Cheffe de Clinique Scientifique, FNS Ambizione, Service de Neurologie, Hôpitaux Universitaires Genevois, Rue Gabrielle Perret-Gentil 4, 1205 Geneva, Switzerland. Tel: +41-795533819, E-mail: Selma.aybek@unige.ch

an unstable wandering uterus, leading to the term of hysteria, these symptoms were long recognized as a dysfunction of a normally structured brain. Doubts, however, have always haunted both clinicians and theorists as to whether this was a medical disorder after all or simply a fabricated simulation from the sufferers.

When functional neuroimaging was developed in the 1990s, a new opportunity was offered to finally address this question: are FNDs really about dysfunction of the brain or do patients just not activate the corresponding brain regions on purpose? The very first imaging studies thus addressed this issue by probing for the neural correlates of these symptoms (Tiihonen et al., 1995; Marshall et al., 1997; Vuilleumier et al., 2001) and comparing them to those of fake symptoms that are voluntarily produced by simulators/feigners (Spence et al., 2000; Stone et al., 2007; Cojan et al., 2009b). The findings converged to suggest distinctive changes in brain activation patterns in patients, and thus triggered a novel line of research trying to understand how (Stone et al., 2010b; Vuilleumier, 2014) these symptoms are produced, i.e., which brain circuits are functionally altered during conversion symptoms.

Accordingly, in the last decade, several imaging studies were conducted which employed different tasks tailored to the clinical presentation (e.g., motor preparation/execution for symptoms of weakness or movement disorder; visual stimuli for functional visual loss; tactile stimulation for somatosensory disorders). Only a handful of more recent studies have focussed on trying to understand why these symptoms are produced and proposed to revisit psychodynamic (e.g., Freudian) theories that have highlighted psychologic trauma and abnormal emotional regulation as causal factors. Together, these approaches set the stage for modern theories of conversion that aim to reconcile both lines of research, linking the how of symptoms to the why, and paving the way to new paradigms to be tested in the future.

This chapter will first review the functional neuroimaging literature on conversion, exploring both "how" and "why" symptoms are produced, and then also cover other related areas of neuroimaging based on structural and resting-state techniques.

Are functional symptoms simulated?

This question was first addressed in a positron emission tomography (PET) study (Spence et al., 2000), comparing 3 patients with a diagnosis of conversion upper-limb motor loss relative to 4 actors instructed to fake an arm paralysis. Patients attempting to move their weak hand (relative to rest), unlike both healthy controls moving normally and actors feigning weakness, showed reduced activation of the left dorsolateral prefrontal cortex (DLPFC). This was interpreted as suggesting some genuine anomalies in conscious action control mechanisms in conversion disorder mediated by DLPFC, a key region for volition. The fact that feigning weakness did not show the same pattern was taken to support distinct mechanisms between conversion and voluntary simulation, because only feigners exhibited right anterior prefrontal hypoactivation, not conversion patients.

Another functional magnetic resonance imaging (fMRI) study (Stone et al., 2007) also compared attempted movements with affected or normal leg in 4 patients with motor conversion, as well as 4 controls who feigned leg weakness. Conversion patients, but not feigners, showed activations in the basal ganglia, insula, lingual gyri, and inferior frontal cortex in association with movement of the weak limb. On the contrary, controls feigning weakness, but not patients, activated the contralateral supplementary motor area (SMA) moving the weak ankle compared with moving the normal ankle. These data suggest some impairment in motor control in patients, possibly reflecting effortful and uncoordinated movements with the affected limb, which is different from feigners.

Another fMRI study (Cojan et al., 2009a) used a go-nogo paradigm in order to test two alternative hypotheses concerning the motor paralysis: whether this results from deficient intention or from active inhibition of motor action. Thirty healthy participants were cued to prepare a movement with either the right or left hand based on a corresponding hand picture presented on the screen, which would then either turn green to instruct the subject to press a button (go), or red to instruct the subject to inhibit the prepared movement (no go). A subset of 24 healthy participants were asked to perform the task normally, whereas 6 others were asked to behave "as if" they were suffering from left-hand weakness. The no-go condition (voluntary inhibition) activated the right inferior frontal gyrus in healthy controls, as expected given the role of this region in inhibitory control (Robbins, 2007; Xue et al., 2008). The right inferior frontal gyrus was also activated in the go condition, when subjects were instructed to feign a paralysis, but this was not the case in one 36-year-old female patient suffering from motor conversion disorder in the upper limb. This result suggests that conversion paralysis does not result from voluntary movement inhibition, although further studies in larger groups and different symptoms are still needed to confirm these results.

Another study examined both motor execution and motor imagery in a group of 12 patients with conversion motor symptoms and 13 healthy controls feigning weakness, as well as 21 healthy controls moving normally (van Beilen et al., 2011). Both conversion patients and feigners showed abnormal movement preparation but in different ways: patients showed increased activation of dorsolateral premotor areas – possibly reflecting a greater preparatory effort, while feigners showed increased pre-SMA activity – presumably reflecting a modulation of voluntary movement planning. Also, a distinctive pattern of contralateral (opposite to the side of limb weakness) parietal hypoactivation was specifically observed in patients when compared to normal movement and feigned weakness, during both motor execution and motor imagery in flipped data. In addition, in unflipped data, a consistent right-sided supramarginal gyrus (in the temporoparietal junction (TPJ)) hypoactivation was found, suggesting a consistent role for this region in the disorder, independently of the side of limb weakness. The authors proposed that this may reflect an abnormal interaction of bodily scheme information (see also discussion below on self-agency) and environmental cues, resulting in ineffective movement initiation in patients

The notion of voluntary versus involuntary control in conversion patients was also tested in a study (Voon et al., 2010b) that investigated brain activity when patients were spontaneously experiencing/exhibiting their involuntary conversion tremor, as compared to a condition where they were asked to "mimic" their own tremor on purpose. Right TPJ hypoactivation was found during the involuntary abnormal movement, attributed to impairment in the sense of agency and self-monitoring (see below for more discussion on this finding).

To sum up, when compared to subjects consciously producing similar symptoms, motor conversion patients consistently demonstrated abnormal patterns of brain activity that seem different from changes observed in feigners, suggesting that their symptoms cannot be reduced to conscious feigning. There is some evidence suggesting a more "effortful" involvement of motor circuits, possibly subsequent to the sensorimotor deficit itself, and a frequent involvement of abnormal parietal and prefrontal activity, possibly responsible for altered sensorimotor integration and reflecting the genuine sense reported by these patients that they cannot control their movements or do not experience them as "normally" controlled. However, it remains possible that these differences between patients and feigners reflect at least partly other factors related to their medical history, comorbidity, and emotional state during fMRI scanning. Further work comparing patients with different symptoms and different evolution course will be necessary to disentangle these issues.

How are functional neurologic symptoms produced?

How then are the symptoms and signs produced, if they are not feigned? In the 1990s, the hypothesis of "central inhibition" (Ludwig, 1972) was endorsed by a single-photon emission computed tomography (SPECT) study (Tiihonen et al., 1995) in a woman with left sensorimotor hemisyndrome, who presented with hypoperfusion in the contralateral parietal region and increased perfusion in the frontal region during symptoms. These changes recovered when symptoms disappeared. This pattern was supported by a PET study of a patient with hemiparesis (Marshall et al., 1997), where again increased activity was found in frontal regions including the anterior cingulate and orbitofrontal cortex. The authors proposed that frontal regions could inhibit the motor and premotor areas when patients tried to move their affected limb, as if their "center of volition" or "motivation" was malfunctioning.

However, another fMRI task (Burgmer et al., 2006) did not show evidence of active inhibition during attempted movements (such as increased activity of right inferior frontal gyrus; see also Cojan et al., 2009a) but revealed abnormal motor activation contralateral to the affected hand during movement observation. These results suggest not only a dysfunction in movement initiation but also in movement conceptualization.

Other data on motor functioning with both negative motor symptoms (weakness) (Vuilleumier et al., 2001) and positive motor symptoms (dystonia) (Schrag et al., 2013) suggest abnormal basal ganglia activation in functional disorders. Decreased putamen, caudate, and thalamus activation was found during symptoms in 7 patients with sensorimotor deficits (Vuilleumier et al., 2001), which recovered when symptoms disappeared in a subgroup of patients (Fig. 7.1). The longitudinal aspect of this study not only offered the opportunity to underscore the functional nature of the disorder, since it revealed a reversible hypoactivation that was linked to the presence of symptoms; but also this longitudinal design allowed the researchers to control for possibly confounding effects of comorbidity (depression, anxiety) and medical history of patients that cannot be achieved by cross-sectional comparisons of patients vs. healthy controls.

Interestingly, in contrast, another study reported increased activity in the caudate and thalamus in psychogenic dystonia patients compared to controls across three different conditions (rest, fixed posturing, and movement). This opposite pattern is interesting as it might suggest a link with the nature of the motor symptom (hyperkinetic versus hypokinetic). Moreover, functional connectivity analyses suggested that the changes in caudate and thalamus during symptoms were associated with differential coupling with activity in inferior and ventral prefrontal regions, which are known to provide affective and motivational inputs to the basal ganglia (Vuilleumier et al., 2001).

Other studies investigating motor function revealed abnormal frontal activations in regions close to the

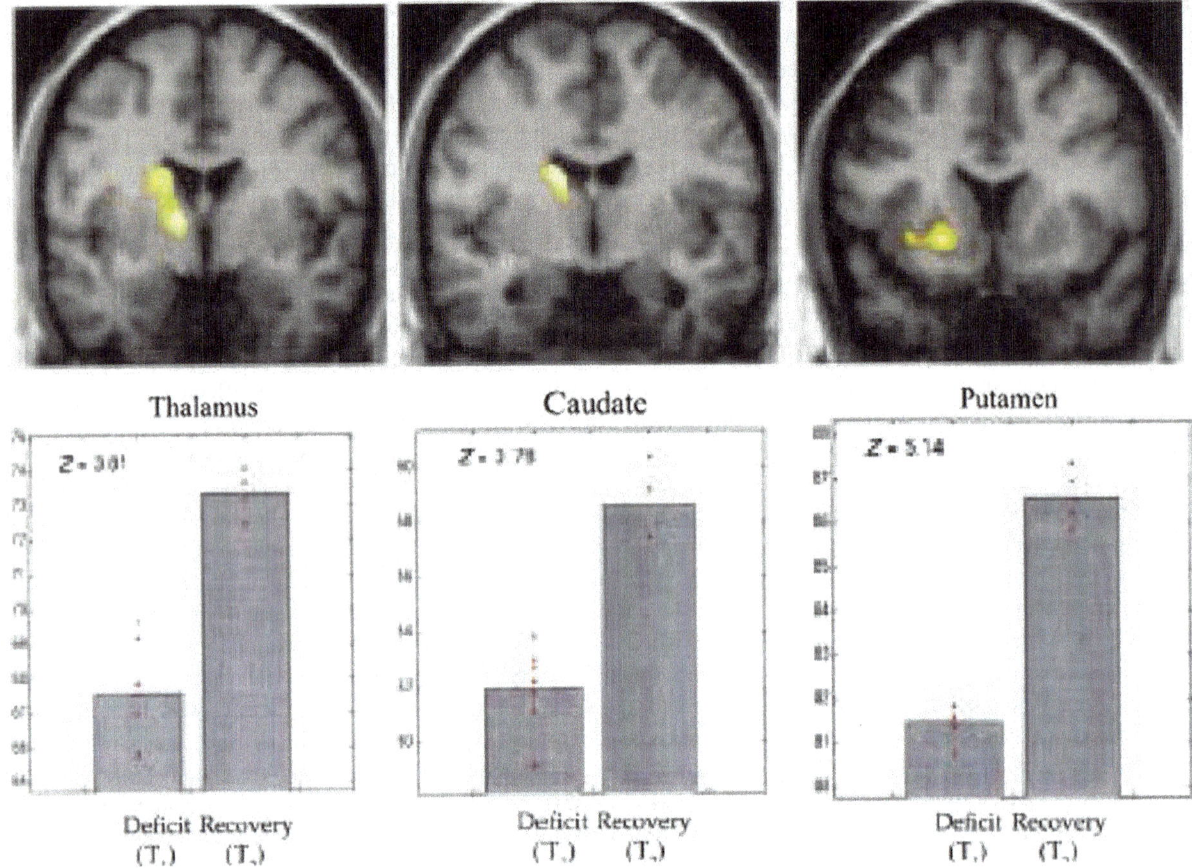

Fig. 7.1. Transitory hypoactivation in the basal ganglia during motor functional neurologic disorder. Decreased cerebral blood flow (single-photon emission computed tomography) in thalamus, caudate, and putamen while symptomatic (T^1), as compared to after symptom recovery (T^2). (Reproduced from Vuilleumier et al., 2001.)

orbitofrontal cortex and anterior cingulate cortex (ACC) areas described by Marshall et al. (1997). An increased medial prefrontal cortex activation was found in a group of 8 patients (de Lange et al., 2007) compared to healthy controls during a motor imagery task. The authors suggested that this corresponds to a failure to deactivate these regions while performing a motor task, which could be interpreted as a heightened/abnormal self-monitoring of movements.

The same group of researchers (de Lange et al., 2008) further investigated the role of implicit versus explicit movement control. They found longer reaction times during the explicit motor paradigm (voluntary motor imagery of own hands) versus the implicit condition (mental rotation of seen hands), in accordance with greater task demand in explicit motor actions. When comparing the healthy to the affected hand sides, they found that only during implicit movements the affected hand showed increased ventromedial prefrontal cortex (vmPFC) activity (just as in their previous study). During the explicit task, no differences were found in vmPFC. This suggests that implicit and explicit movements induce different self-monitoring demands. This may echo clinical observations that patients vary in their motor performance depending on which movement they initiate. For example, some patients display severe leg paresis while examined in bed and asked to move their limb against resistance, but are then able to stand up and put their trousers back on while standing – a clinical sign described as "motor inconsistency." One might argue that trying to lift a leg from the examination bed implies an explicit movement whereas getting dressed induces an implicit motor program.

These data converge to support the concept that what is observed clinically in the form of discordance, inconsistency, and variability in motor performances may not necessarily reflect a conscious defect in subjects' effort and willed action, but it could relate to abnormalities in different underlying motor programs, a concept already very well summarized by Paget, who remarked that conversion patients appeared to suffer from what he called "nervous mimicry of organic diseases": i.e., when the patient says "I cannot," it looks like "I will not,“ but it is "I cannot will" (Paget, 1873).

This voluntary / involuntary dichotomy in the perception of movement and its control, together with the fact that functional patients do not have a reliable judgment of their actual movement production (Stone et al., 2010c), might be imputed to an abnormal sense of self-agency. Agency refers to the experience that we are the cause of our own actions. This subjective sense has been related to recent models of motor control proposing that generation of a motor program in the brain also involves the generation of an efferent copy which is then compared to proprioceptive feedback resulting from the executed action; if a mismatch is detected between the feedback and the efferent copy of the intended movement, the movement can be corrected online. The comparison of feedforward (also linked to prior expectation) and feedback (sensory information) signals will lead to the perception that the movement was made according to plan and is voluntary. In the case of functional disorders, it has been hypothesized that a modification of the feedforward or prior expectation/beliefs might play a role in the emergence of motor deficits, leading the subjects to perceive their movements (which look voluntary) as involuntary or not "normally" under their control (Edwards et al., 2012).

An fMRI study (Voon et al., 2010b) directly addressed this issue by comparing brain activity during a voluntary motor action (intentionally produced tremor) and an involuntary one (functional tremor) and revealed hypoactivity in the right TPJ during the spontaneous (involuntary) functional tremor (Fig. 7.2). The right TPJ is known to play a key role in the computational comparison of internal predictions with actual external events (Spengler et al., 2009), leading the authors to interpret their findings of reduced TPJ activity during functional tremor as either the cause or the consequence of abnormal sense of agency in these patients.

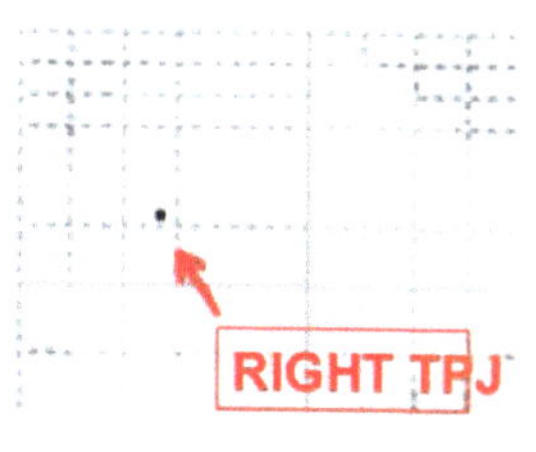

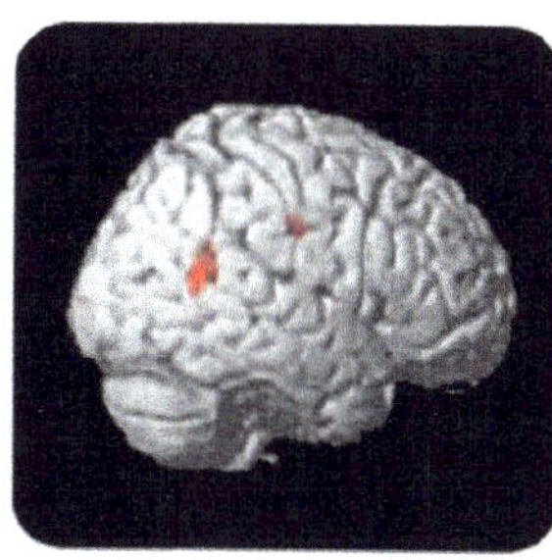

Fig. 7.2. Involvement of the right temporoparietal junction (TPJ) in motor functional neurologic disorder. Right TPJ hypoactivation when patients experience their functional involuntary tremor (compared to a condition where a voluntary similar abnormal movement is actively produced). This region is interpreted as being linked to the sense of self-agency (feeling in control of one's own movement). (Adapted from Voon et al., 2010b, with permission from Wolters Kluwer Publishing.)

Further work is needed to better understand these potential changes in self-agency and abnormal movement control (including the role of prior beliefs) in functional patients. Promising pilot works have opened new hypotheses. For example, patients might exhibit particular cognitive processing traits (Pareés et al., 2012), leading them to "jump to conclusions," which could also underlie abnormal inferences about their bodily afferent sensory inputs. This might contribute to partly explain why functional symptoms often follow a mild physical injury (Stone et al., 2009; Pareés et al., 2014), as abnormal beliefs and sense of agency might emerge from altered or unusual sensory inputs. Remarkably, similar dysfunction in feedforward motor control models, belief formations, and meta-awareness of action were proposed to account for the syndrome of anosognosia (Berti et al., 1996, Vocat et al., 2013; Saj et al., 2014), which is characterized by a mirror dissociation, where patients with true paralysis after brain damage deny any conscious experience of paralysis.

Why are functional neurologic symptoms produced?

For more than a century, the causal factors for conversion disorder have been rooted in psychologic grounds; the term "conversion" itself refers to the transformation of psychologic stressor into physical symptoms. This concept has been recently challenged; however (Stone and Edwards, 2011), as stressors can be linked to many medical conditions (Sibai and Armenian, 2000; Cohen et al., 2007; Sorenson et al., 2013), its specificity to conversion disorder can be disputed. Also, should the diagnosis of conversion disorder be excluded in a patient who shows the typical clinical presentation but does not disclose any obvious psychologic stressor (as is often the case)? This question has been addressed by experts (Nicholson et al., 2011; Stone et al., 2010a, 2011), when reframing the new Diagnostic and Statistical Manual of Mental Disorders, 5th edition (DSM-5) criteria (American Psychiatric Association, 2013). It has been estimated that an explicit criterion requiring "a psychological factor with a temporal link to the symptoms" should be eliminated, as it is often impossible to ascertain the presence of a psychologic factor in many patients, and even harder to verify its causal link with symptoms. This is a major issue for clinicians, because it implies that the diagnosis now mostly relies on the neurologic examination, and thus signifies a shift from a purely psychiatric condition to a condition essentially diagnosed by neurologists. In order to avoid further separation between neurology and psychiatry, however, conversion disorder should be seen as a true "neuropsychiatric" condition (Carson, 2014), much in keeping with the tradition of the late 19th century.

Indeed, although the role of psychologic factors is no longer understood as a unique causal factor, it is still of high importance. It has been shown that adverse life events often – even if not always – precede the symptoms (Roelofs et al., 2005; Aybek et al., 2010), and psychologic dimensions may have some explanatory meaning in relation to the nature of the symptoms (e.g., motor, visual), as notoriously postulated by Freud and others. Moreover, traumatic childhood experience (Roelofs et al., 2002) have been reported to be of longer duration and more frequently located in the close familial circle in conversion patients, as compared with other affective disorder patients, suggesting that exposure to early trauma combined with a lack of familial protection might constitute a specific risk factor for the development of conversion disorder.

Moreover, documented childhood abuse and neglect have been linked to abnormal emotion regulation in adulthood, including in particular changes in amygdalar activity (Woon and Hedges, 2008; van Harmelen et al., 2010; Grant et al., 2011). A recent neuroimaging study of implicit emotion perception in patients with motor functional disorder (Voon et al., 2010a) revealed a lack of differential valence responses, unlike healthy controls, who normally displayed greater activation of the right amygdala to negative vs. positive emotion. Thus, amygdalar activity in FND was sensitive to emotional arousal irrespective of valence.

This study also highlighted an abnormal functional connectivity between the amygdala and the SMA, a key region for motor planning. This suggests an abnormal interaction between limbic structures and motor programming. Further work in this direction demonstrated similar abnormal SMA activity in FND patients in response to more specific emotional stimuli, when subjects had to recall a relevant traumatic life event (Aybek et al., 2014b). These effects in SMA, alongside abnormal right TPJ activity (Fig. 7.3), were found only in FND subjects, but not in healthy controls undergoing the same task (i.e., also recalling a recent traumatic event). This again provides evidence to support a role for traumatic psychologic stressors, and brings new light to the classic concept of conversion being caused by past trauma, as recognized by early clinicians (and further elaborated by Freud in relation to unconscious repression). Additionally, these new data provide new hints for the possible neural pathways mediating the emergence of these symptoms.

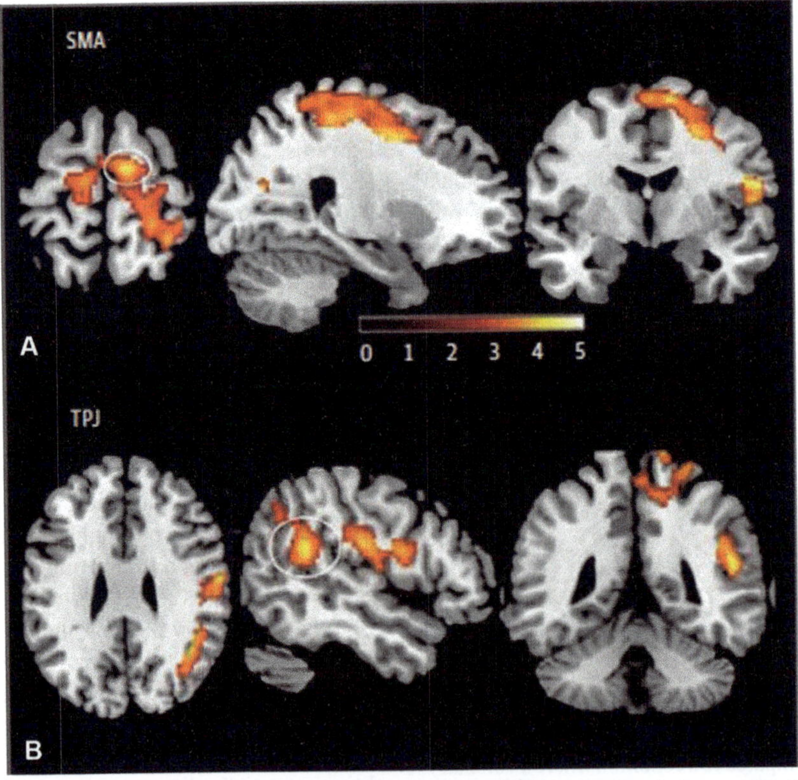

Fig. 7.3. Supplementary motor area (SMA) and temporoparietal junction (TPJ) activation during recall of traumatic event, suggesting a link between aversive memories and sensorimotor circuits compatible with a psychodynamic influence on motor processes. Statistical parametric maps showing significant clusters of activation ($p < 0.05$ familywise error and cluster corrected). Red indicates a significant group–condition interaction for the contrast-relevant traumatic event > control event in patients > healthy controls, with peak activations in the right SMA and right TPJ. (Reproduced with permission from Aybek et al., 2014b. Copyright © (2014) American Medical Association. All rights reserved.)

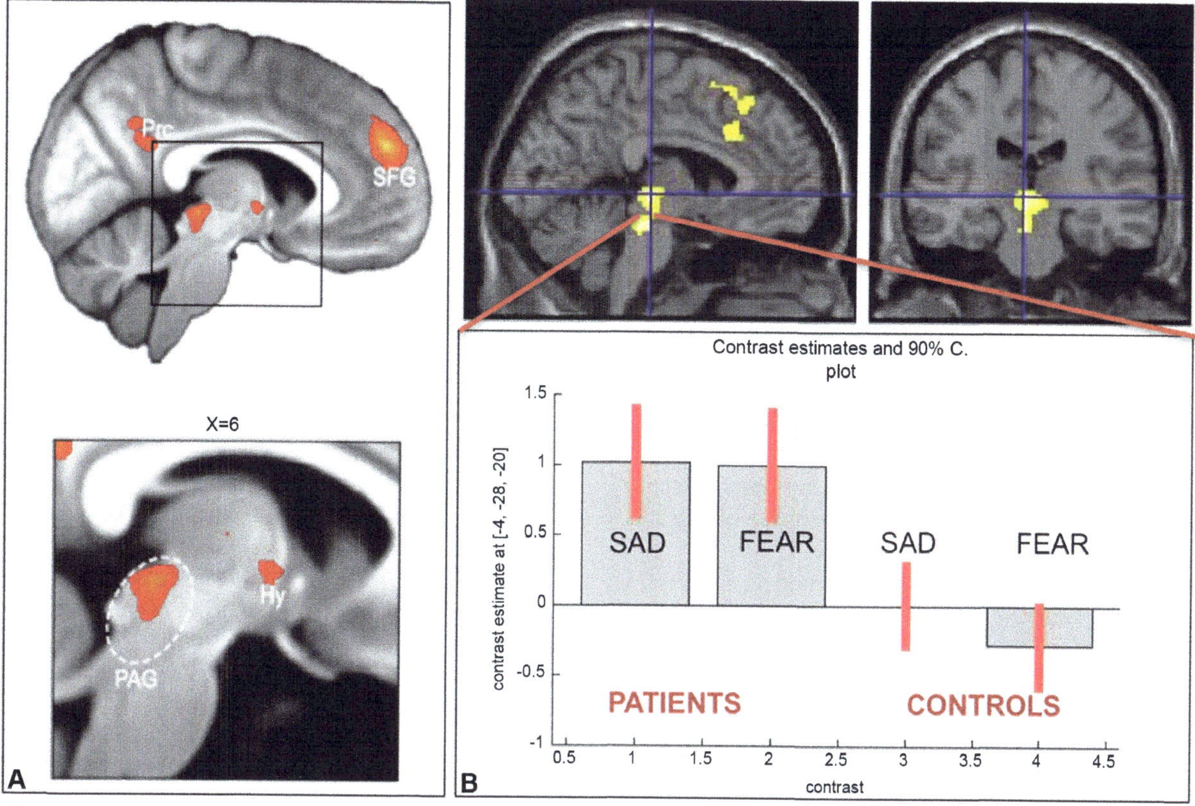

Fig. 7.4. Involvement of periaqueductal gray (PAG) area in functional neurologic disorder (FND). (**A**) PAG activation during physiologic freeze response in humans. (Adapted from Hermans et al., 2013.) (**B**) Increased PAG activation for negative emotions (sad and fearful faces) in patients with FND compared to healthy controls. (Adapted from Aybek et al., 2015.)

Other evidence suggesting abnormal emotional regulation in FND comes from an fMRI study using incidental negative emotion (Aybek et al., 2015) (sad and fearful faces) in 11 patients compared to 14 healthy controls. Results showed increased amygdalar activity in patients for both emotions, confirming a general hyperarousal state evoked by negative stimuli. This was accompanied by a lack of sensitization over time, selective for fearful faces, suggesting more prolonged hyperarousal in a threatening context. Also, this study showed increased periaqueductal grey (PAG) area activity across both emotions (Fig. 7.4), suggesting that patients may be more prone than healthy controls to automatic motor defense behavior, such as freeze response, as the PAG has been consistently implicated in the freeze response in animal (Koutsikou et al., 2015) and human studies (Hermans et al., 2013; Blakemore et al., 2016).

Linking the how and why: a role for medial prefrontal areas?

A promising hypothesis has recently emerged based on repeated observation of dysfunction in the medial prefrontal areas (particularly vmPFC) in functional patients (see above), suggesting that these patients might have an abnormal affective representation of self-relevant information encoded in this region (see below), and that the latter might induce particular patterns of behavior through interaction with sensorimotor circuits (Vuilleumier, 2014). The vmPFC is a major part of the default-mode network (Greicius et al., 2003), known to be implicated in the access to self-relevant affective representations and memories (D'Argembeau et al., 2008). Thus, this is a key limbic structure that may play an important role as a relay between emotion regulation and complex bodily function control.

In an early PET study (Marshall et al., 1997), increased vmPFC activity was observed during attempted movements with the affected limb in a patient with conversion paralysis. In a subsequent SPECT study performed in a larger sample of 7 patients (Vuilleumier et al., 2001), during a passive vibrotactile stimuli (sensorimotor stimuli), functional network analyses showed that activity decreases in striatothalamic circuits were correlated with concomitant changes in the coupling between these regions and inferior and ventromedial prefrontal areas of the same hemisphere, contralateral to the motor symptoms. This increased coupling suggests an important role for the vmPFC in modulating motor activity.

A more recent study (Cojan et al., 2009a) compared motor preparation, execution, and inhibition for both the affected and intact hand in a single patient with a unilateral functional paralysis. A selective increase in the connectivity between vmPFC and primary motor cortex contralateral to paralysis was observed in the patient (Fig. 7.5B), not seen when paralysis was induced by hypnosis or simulated in healthy volunteers, while reduction between the primary cortex and premotor cortex was observed in all groups (Cojan et al., 2009b, 2015). Similarly, increased activity was observed in vmPFC during motor imagery in patients with motor conversion deficits (Fig. 7.5A), specifically for conditions involving the affected hand (de Lange et al., 2007).

Another fMRI study (Mailis-Gagnon et al., 2003) reported a complex pattern of changes in 4 patients with chronic sensory loss and pain in one or more limbs. Non-noxious or noxious tactile stimulation was applied to both the affected and unaffected limbs. Noxious and non-noxious stimulations on the affected limb (which were not perceived) did not activate the thalamus, insula, inferior frontal, and posterior cingulate regions, as compared to stimulation on the normal side. Moreover, ACC and vmPFC showed significant increased activity during unperceived stimulation on the affected limb than during perceived stimulation on the normal side (Fig. 7.5C). These changes were interpreted as the result of attentional and emotional processes triggered by stressful or painful conditions, perhaps exacerbated by individual predispositions or developmental factors.

Other evidence supporting the role of medial prefrontal cortex comes from two studies of functional visual loss. In a first study (Werring et al., 2004), occipital cortical areas showed reduced responses to visual stimulation by whole-field color flickers, accompanied by decreased activation in ACC. In another study (Becker et al., 2013), occipital cortex showed normal responses to simple geometric stimulation but decreased responses to faces, together with selective increases in vmPFC. Functional connectivity analysis also revealed increased coupling between vmPFC and occipital areas during blindness episodes.

Finally, an fMRI study exploring the neural correlates of internally and externally generated movements found decreased SMA activity together with abnormal increased activity in the amygdala, anterior insula, and posterior cingulate (limbic structures) in conversion patients (Voon et al., 2011). Moreover, lower coupling between the SMA and the DLPFC during internally generated action suggested an impaired prefrontal top-down regulation during action control. The authors suggested that previously mapped conversion motor representation

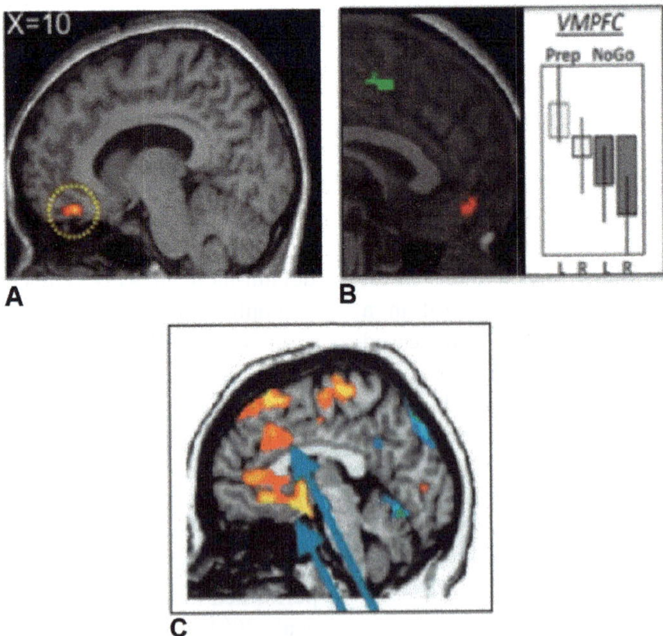

Fig. 7.5. Activation of the vmPFC in a motor imagery task (panel **A**, adapted from DeLange et al., 2007), a go-nogo task (panel **B**, adapted from Cojan et al., 2009a), a sensory task (panel **C**, adapted from Mailis-Gagnon et al., 2003). See text for details of the paradigms.

may, in arousing context, hijack the voluntary action selection system, favoring a theory of abnormal emotion–motor interaction in FND.

Taken together, these findings converge to indicate that FND might be associated with abnormal recruitment of medial limbic areas (posterior cingulate and vmPFC) whose exact role remains to be determined. However, vmPFC is well known to operate at the interface of processes regulating emotion appraisal and memory retrieval, mediate the access to self-reflective representations, and provide important modulatory signals to both cortical and subcortical sensorimotor circuits, which could thus modulate behavior based on personally relevant affective information.

STRUCTURAL IMAGING

As shown above, a fair amount of literature has emerged on functional brain imaging of FND over the last decades, but very few focused on structural imaging, probably due to the fact that clinical brain scans are typically expected to be normal in functional patients. This fits with Charcot's view that no "organic" lesion can be found in FND, but maybe a "dynamic" functional lesion. Some studies, however, recently reported structural abnormalities in groups of patients with functional disorders.

The first controlled study used a region of interest to study 12 motor FND patients and 12 age- and gender-matched healthy controls. Individual manual tracing measured subcortical MRI structures (Atmaca et al., 2006) and demonstrated significant reductions in volume for bilateral basal ganglia structures (caudate and lentiform nuclei) and right thalamus in patients as compared to controls. All patients were right-handed and had unilateral motor symptoms, although data on the proportions of left- and right-sided symptoms were not given.

A more recent MRI study (Nicholson et al., 2014) also explored anatomic differences in basal ganglia in an a priori region-of-interest analysis for 14 motor FND patients compared to 31 healthy controls. Significant reduced left thalamic volume was found in patients, but no correlation with symptom duration was observed. Another controlled study analyzed 20 patients with positive motor symptoms (psychogenic nonepileptic seizures: PNES) compared to 40 age- and sex-matched healthy controls by using a whole-brain voxel-based morphometry analysis, as well as cortical thickness analysis (Labate et al., 2012). This study showed significantly decreased cortical thickness in both motor and premotor regions in the right hemisphere and bilaterally in the cerebellum in patients compared to controls. In contrast, another voxel-based morphometry study (Aybek et al., 2014a) found increased cortical thickness in bilateral premotor cortex of 15 conversion patients suffering from negative motor symptoms (weakness) compared to 25 matched controls. The apparently contradictory results of these two studies may again relate to the type of symptoms, where motor weakness represents a lack of movement (hypokinesia), whereas PNES represents an excess of paroxysmal movements (hyperkinesia). These differences in motor cortex would accord with the previous observation of opposite findings of increased/decreased activity of the basal ganglia in two different types of motor symptoms (Vuilleumier et al., 2001; Schrag et al., 2013), as discussed above.

These structural changes need, however, further confirmation in larger samples in order to verify if these abnormalities are specific to FND (and not related to-confounding factors such as depression, for example), and whether they are trait- or state-dependent, meaning that they should be considered as a cause (e.g., subsequent to history or trauma), a risk factor (e.g. developmental or genetically determined predisposition), or a mere consequence (through a plasticity phenomenon, for instance) of the physical symptom. It will therefore be important to examine the reversibility of these anomalies in longitudinal studies.

Resting-state imaging

Finally, brain function can also be explored using resting-state imaging (Raichle et al., 2001; Leonardi et al., 2013) without asking patients to perform specific tasks. Some valuable information has been gathered from a few studies in the field.

An early SPECT study (Yazici and Kostakoglu, 1998) looked at brain perfusion at rest in 5 motor conversion patients suffering from psychogenic gait disorders. In 4 patients, left temporal hypoperfusion was found, whereas a fifth patient had left parietal hypoperfusion.

A group analysis using PET data in 16 PNES patients compared to 16 healthy controls reported right inferior parietal and ACC hypometabolism. These findings may relate to abnormal sensorimotor integration and agency mediated by parietal areas, while ACC changes may relate to abnormal emotion regulation, as discussed above in task-specific imaging findings.

Another recent fMRI study (van der Kruijs et al., 2014) used resting state to probe intrinsic functional brain networks using independent component analysis (particularly the executive, frontoparietal, sensorimotor, and default-mode networks) in 21 PNES patients compared to 27 healthy controls. Significantly increased activity was observed in patients for several nodes of these networks, including within the executive network (ACC and insula), within the frontoparietal network (orbitofrontal cortex, insula), within the sensorimotor network (ACC, parietal, motor, and premotor), as well as within the default-mode network (precuneus). Also, the connectivity strength correlated with clinical scores of dissociation obtained from three questionnaires (Dissociative Experience Scale (DES), Dissociation Questionnaire (DIS-Q), and Somatoform Dissociation Questionnaire (SDQ-20)). The authors suggested that these areas represent the neural correlates of the dissociative phenomenon that occurs in PNES.

Notably, a similar independent component analysis approach to fMRI activity was applied to brain network activity during a motor task (Cojan, 2012), rather than resting state. Results revealed selective changes for two intrinsic networks: the sensorimotor network, to which primary motor cortex and basal ganglia were less connected in patients with hand paralysis due to either conversion or simulation, whereas the SMA was less connected to this network during simulation only; and the default-mode network, to which the vmPFC was less connected in conversion patients only, relative to both normal controls and simulators. This again points to a differential recruitment of the vmPFC, abnormally connected to motor pathways in these patients, rather than the default-mode network observed at rest (Cojan et al., 2009a).

SUMMARY

To sum up, many brain imaging studies have been conducted in the past decade aiming to better understand the mechanisms underlying FND. As reviewed, many different tasks and various clinical samples were used, rendering difficult any attempt to do a meta-analysis and draw definite conclusions.

Many valuable clues, however, point to an important role for frontal dysfunction (DLPFC) in the top-down regulation of lower-order areas in emotional contexts, with an implication of affective and perhaps mnemonic representations in medial regions (vmPCF, precuneus), as well as a role for parietal areas (especially right TPJ) in the abnormal sense of agency implied by motor conversion symptoms. Also, abnormal limbic function can be postulated given observations of heightened amygdalar activity and increased amygdala–SMA coupling, suggesting abnormal limbic–motor or limbic–sensory interaction. Further, most imaging studies focused on motor symptoms, but the brain substrates associated with other manifestations remain to be clarified (Vuilleumier, 2005; Aybek, 2016).

One emerging hypothesis postulates that functional patients may have abnormal affective representation and/or emotion regulation mechanisms – possibly due to prior experience or partly genetically determined or both – which interact with lower-order functions mediating motor, visual, sensory, or even memory processes, leading to the production of the conversion symptoms. However, much further empiric research is needed to better understand this fascinating and debilitating condition, as well as to derive new perspectives for more efficient therapeutic interventions in these patients.

ACKNOWLEDGMENTS

The authors' work is supported by LEENAARDS and FNS.

REFERENCES

American Psychiatric Association (2013). Diagnostic and statistical manual of mental disorders, 5th ed. American Psychiatric Association, Washington, DC.

Atmaca M, Aydin A, Tezcan E et al. (2006). Volumetric investigation of brain regions in patients with conversion disorder. Prog Neuropsychopharmacol Biol Psychiatry 30: 708–713.

Aybek SVP (2016). Self-awareness disorders in conversion hysteria. In: S Laureys, O Gosseries, G Tononi (Eds.), The Neurology of Consciousness, 2nd edn. Elsevier, San Diego.

Aybek S, Nicholson T, Craig T et al. (2010). Life events in conversion disorder: Role of timing and nature of events. In: Journal of Psychosomatic Research, 605–679.

Aybek S, Nicholson TR, Draganski B et al. (2014a). Grey matter changes in motor conversion disorder. J Neurol Neurosurg Psychiatry 85: 236–238.

Aybek S, Nicholson TR, Zelaya F et al. (2014b). Neural correlates of recall of life events in conversion disorder. JAMA Psychiatry 71: 52–60.

Aybek S, Nicholson TR, O'daly O et al. (2015). Emotion–motion interactions in conversion disorder: an FMRI study. PLoS One 10: e0123273.

Becker B, Scheele D, Moessner R et al. (2013). Deciphering the neural signature of conversion blindness. Am J Psychiatry 170: 121–122.

Berti A, Ladavas E, Della Corte M (1996). Anosognosia for hemiplegia, neglect dyslexia, and drawing neglect: clinical findings and theoretical considerations. J Int Neuropsychol Soc 2: 426–440.

Blakemore RL, Rieger SW, Vuilleumier P (2016). Negative emotions facilitate isometric force through activation of prefrontal cortex and periaqueductal gray. Neuroimage 124: 627–640.

Burgmer M, Konrad C, Jansen A et al. (2006). Abnormal brain activation during movement observation in patients with conversion paralysis. Neuroimage 29: 1336–1343.

Carson AJ (2014). Introducing a 'neuropsychiatry' special issue: but what does that mean? J Neurol Neurosurg Psychiatry 85: 121–122.

Cohen S, Janicki-Deverts D, Miller GE (2007). Psychological stress and disease. JAMA 298: 1685–1687.

Cojan YVP (2012). Functional brain inaging of psychogenic paralysis during conversion and hypnosis. In: M Hallett (Ed.), Psychogenic Movement Disorders and Other Conversion Disorders, Cambridge University Press, Cambridge.

Cojan Y, Waber L, Carruzzo A et al. (2009a). Motor inhibition in hysterical conversion paralysis. Neuroimage 47: 1026–1037.

Cojan Y, Waber L, Schwartz S et al. (2009b). The brain under self-control: modulation of inhibitory and monitoring cortical networks during hypnotic paralysis. Neuron 62: 862–875.

Cojan Y, Piguet C, Vuilleumier P (2015). What makes your brain suggestible? Hypnotizability is associated with differential brain activity during attention outside hypnosis. Neuroimage 117: 367–374.

D'Argembeau A, Feyers D, Majerus S et al. (2008). Self-reflection across time: cortical midline structures differentiate between present and past selves. Soc Cogn Affect Neurosci 3: 244–252.

De Lange FP, Roelofs K, Toni I (2007). Increased self-monitoring during imagined movements in conversion paralysis. Neuropsychologia 45: 2051–2058.

De Lange FP, Roelofs K, Toni I (2008). Motor imagery: a window into the mechanisms and alterations of the motor system. Cortex 44: 494–506.

Edwards MJ, Adams RA, Brown H et al. (2012). A Bayesian account of 'hysteria'. Brain 135: 3495–3512.

Grant MM, Cannistraci C, Hollon SD et al. (2011). Childhood trauma history differentiates amygdala response to sad faces within MDD. J Psychiatr Res 45: 886–895.

Greicius MD, Krasnow B, Reiss AL et al. (2003). Functional connectivity in the resting brain: a network analysis of the default mode hypothesis. Proc Natl Acad Sci U S A 100: 253–258.

Hermans EJ, Henckens MJ, Roelofs K et al. (2013). Fear, bradycardia and activation of the human periaqueductal grey. Neuroimage 66: 278–287.

Koutsikou S, Watson TC, Crook JJ et al. (2015). The periaqueductal gray orchestrates sensory and motor circuits at multiple levels of the neuraxis. J Neurosci 35: 14132–14147.

Labate A, Cerasa A, Mula M et al. (2012). Neuroanatomic correlates of psychogenic nonepileptic seizures: a cortical thickness and VBM study. Epilepsia 53: 377–385.

Leonardi N, Richiardi J, Gschwind M et al. (2013). Principal components of functional connectivity: a new approach to study dynamic brain connectivity during rest. Neuroimage 83: 937–950.

Ludwig AM (1972). Hysteria. A neurobiological theory. Arch Gen Psychiatry 27: 771–777.

Mailis-Gagnon A, Giannoylis I, Downar J et al. (2003). Altered central somatosensory processing in chronic pain patients with "hysterical" anesthesia. Neurology 60: 1501–1507.

Marshall JC, Halligan PW, Fink GR et al. (1997). The functional anatomy of a hysterical paralysis. Cognition 64: B1–B8.

Nicholson TR, Stone J, Kanaan RA (2011). Conversion disorder: a problematic diagnosis. J Neurol Neurosurg Psychiatry 82: 1267–1273.

Nicholson TR, Aybek S, Kempton MJ et al. (2014). A structural MRI study of motor conversion disorder: evidence of reduction in thalamic volume. J Neurol Neurosurg Psychiatry 85: 227–229.

Paget J (1873). Clinical lectures on the nervous mimicry of organic diseases. Lancet .

Pareés I, Kassavetis P, Saifee TA et al. (2012). Jumping to conclusions' bias in functional movement disorders. J Neurol Neurosurg Psychiatry 83: 460–463.

Pareés I, Kojovic M, Pires C et al. (2014). Physical precipitating factors in functional movement disorders. J Neurol Sci 338: 174–177.

Raichle ME, Macleod AM, Snyder AZ et al. (2001). A default mode of brain function. Proc Natl Acad Sci U S A 98: 676–682.

Robbins TW (2007). Shifting and stopping: fronto-striatal substrates, neurochemical modulation and clinical implications. Philos Trans R Soc Lond B Biol Sci 362: 917–932.

Roelofs K, Keijsers GP, Hoogduin KA et al. (2002). Childhood abuse in patients with conversion disorder. Am J Psychiatry 159: 1908–1913.

Roelofs K, Spinhoven P, Sandijck P et al. (2005). The impact of early trauma and recent life-events on symptom severity in patients with conversion disorder. J Nerv Ment Dis 193: 508–514.

Saj A, Vocat R, Vuilleumier P (2014). Action-monitoring impairment in anosognosia for hemiplegia. Cortex 61: 93–106.

Schrag AE, Mehta AR, Bhatia KP et al. (2013). The functional neuroimaging correlates of psychogenic versus organic dystonia. Brain 136: 770–781.

Sibai AM, Armenian HK (2000). Long-term psychological stress and heart disease. Int J Epidemiol 29: 948.

Sorenson M, Janusek L, Mathews H (2013). Psychological stress and cytokine production in multiple sclerosis: correlation with disease symptomatology. Biol Res Nurs 15: 226–233.

Spence SA, Crimlisk HL, Cope H et al. (2000). Discrete neurophysiological correlates in prefrontal cortex during hysterical and feigned disorder of movement. Lancet 355: 1243–1244.

Spengler S, Von Cramon DY, Brass M (2009). Was it me or was it you? How the sense of agency originates from ideomotor learning revealed by fMRI. Neuroimage 46: 290–298.

Stone J, Edwards MJ (2011). How "psychogenic" are psychogenic movement disorders? Mov Disord 26: 1787–1788.

Stone J, Zeman A, Simonotto E et al. (2007). FMRI in patients with motor conversion symptoms and controls with simulated weakness. Psychosom Med 69: 961–969.

Stone J, Carson A, Aditya H et al. (2009). The role of physical injury in motor and sensory conversion symptoms: a systematic and narrative review. J Psychosom Res 66: 383–390.

Stone J, Lafrance Jr WC, Levenson JL et al. (2010a). Issues for DSM-5: Conversion disorder. Am J Psychiatry 167: 626–627.

Stone J, Vuilleumier P, Friedman JH (2010b). Conversion disorder: separating "how" from "why". Neurology 74: 190–191.

Stone J, Warlow C, Sharpe M (2010c). The symptom of functional weakness: a controlled study of 107 patients. Brain 133: 1537–1551.

Stone J, Lafrance Jr WC, Brown R et al. (2011). Conversion disorder: current problems and potential solutions for DSM-5. J Psychosom Res 71: 369–376.

Tiihonen J, Kuikka J, Viinamaki H et al. (1995). Altered cerebral blood flow during hysterical paresthesia. Biol Psychiatry 37: 134–135.

Van Beilen M, De Jong BM, Gieteling EW et al. (2011). Abnormal parietal function in conversion paresis. PLoS One 6: e25918.

Van Der Kruijs SJM, Jagannathan SR, Bodde NMG et al. (2014). Resting-state networks and dissociation in psychogenic non-epileptic seizures. J Psychiatr Res 54: 126–133.

Van Harmelen AL, Van Tol MJ, Van Der Wee NJ et al. (2010). Reduced medial prefrontal cortex volume in adults reporting childhood emotional maltreatment. Biol Psychiatry 68: 832–838.

Vocat R, Saj A, Vuilleumier P (2013). The riddle of anosognosia: does unawareness of hemiplegia involve a failure to update beliefs? Cortex 49: 1771–1781.

Voon V, Brezing C, Gallea C et al. (2010a). Emotional stimuli and motor conversion disorder. Brain 133: 1526–1536.

Voon V, Gallea C, Hattori N et al. (2010b). The involuntary nature of conversion disorder. Neurology 74: 223–228.

Voon V, Brezing C, Gallea C et al. (2011). Aberrant supplementary motor complex and limbic activity during motor preparation in motor conversion disorder. Mov Disord 26: 2396–2403.

Vuilleumier P (2005). Hysterical conversion and brain function. Prog Brain Res 150: 309–329.

Vuilleumier P (2009). The neurophysiology of self-awareness disorders in conversion hysteria. In: S Laureys, G Tononi (Eds.), The neurology of consciousness, Elsevier, Amsterdam, pp. 282–302.

Vuilleumier P (2014). Brain circuits implicated in psychogenic paralysis in conversion disorders and hypnosis. Neurophysiol Clin Clin Neurophysiol 44: 323–337.

Vuilleumier P, Chicherio C, Assal F et al. (2001). Functional neuroanatomical correlates of hysterical sensorimotor loss. Brain 124: 1077–1090.

Werring DJ, Weston L, Bullmore ET et al. (2004). Functional magnetic resonance imaging of the cerebral response to visual stimulation in medically unexplained visual loss. Psychol Med 34: 583–589.

Woon FL, Hedges DW (2008). Hippocampal and amygdala volumes in children and adults with childhood maltreatment-related posttraumatic stress disorder: a meta-analysis. Hippocampus 18: 729–736.

Xue G, Aron AR, Poldrack RA (2008). Common neural substrates for inhibition of spoken and manual responses. Cereb Cortex 18: 1923–1932.

Yazici KM, Kostakoglu L (1998). Cerebral blood flow changes in patients with conversion disorder. Psychiatry Res 83: 163–168.

Handbook of Clinical Neurology, Vol. 139 (3rd series)
Functional Neurologic Disorders
M. Hallett, J. Stone, and A. Carson, Editors
http://dx.doi.org/10.1016/B978-0-12-801772-2.00008-4

Chapter 8

Dissociation and functional neurologic disorders

R.J. BROWN*
Division of Psychology and Mental Health, University of Manchester, Manchester, UK

Abstract

Dissociation has been cited as a possible psychologic mechanism underpinning functional neurologic disorders (FND) since the 19th century. Since that time, changes in psychiatric classification have created confusion about what the term dissociation actually means. The available evidence suggests that it now refers to at least two qualitatively distinct types of phenomena: detachment (an altered state of consciousness characterized by a sense of separation from the self or world) and compartmentalization (a reversible loss of voluntary control over apparently intact processes and functions), as well as their underlying mechanisms. This chapter considers some of the problems with conflating these phenomena under a single heading as well as the relationship between detachment, compartmentalization, and FND. It is argued that FNDs are fundamentally compartmentalization disorders, but that detachment is often part of the clinical picture and may contribute to the development and maintenance of functional symptoms in many cases. By this view, understanding compartmentalization requires an appreciation of the mechanisms involved in controlling and accessing mental processes and contents. Two possible mechanisms in this regard are described and the evidence for these is considered, followed by a discussion of clinical and empiric implications.

INTRODUCTION

Clinical use of the term dissociation originated in the 19th-century work of Pierre Janet, who used it (or its French translation, *desagrégation*) to refer to a psychologic process whereby the mind fragments into separate compartments in response to extreme stress or trauma. This process of "compartmentalization" (Holmes et al., 2005) was said to be responsible for a range of symptoms, including amnesia, multiple personality states, automatisms, and other phenomena said to be characteristic of hysteria, such as the somatic symptoms that we now recognize as functional neurologic disorders (FND). For most contemporary clinicians, however, "dissociation" refers to something quite different, namely a subjective state of unreality in which individuals feel detached from themselves (so-called depersonalization) or the world (derealization; see, e.g., Stone et al., 2012). This experience may be chronic and disabling, as seen in depersonalization disorder and some cases of posttraumatic stress disorder (PTSD), or an acute state triggered by fatigue, intoxication, intense emotion, and/or potentially traumatizing events (so-called peritraumatic dissociation). From this perspective, someone who is experiencing such a state of detachment is said to be "dissociating." Detached states of this sort were never part of Janet's model of dissociation, and recent evidence suggests that detachment and compartmentalization are qualitatively distinct phenomena (Holmes et al., 2005; Brown, 2006a). In this chapter we will consider the evidence pertaining to detachment and compartmentalization in FND and the relevance of these concepts for understanding and working with functional symptoms.

PSYCHIATRIC CLASSIFICATION AND THE DISSOCIATIVE EXPERIENCES SCALE

Consistent with the distinction between detachment and compartmentalization, the first two editions of the

*Correspondence to: Richard J. Brown, 2nd Floor Zochonis Building, Brunswick Street, Division of Psychology and Mental Health, University of Manchester, Manchester M13 9PL, UK. Tel: +44-161-306-0400, E-mail: richard.j.brown@manchester.ac.uk

Diagnostic and Statistical Manual of Mental Disorders (DSM: American Psychiatric Association, 1952, 1968) classified depersonalization separately from hysteric phenomena. DSM-III, in contrast, adopted a descriptive approach to classification, which saw depersonalization classified as a dissociative disorder alongside psychogenic amnesia, fugue states, and multiple personality disorder, on the grounds that to feel unreal is to lose an important aspect of one's identity (American Psychiatric Association, 1980). In contrast, functional neurologic symptoms (FNS) were separated from their hysteric counterparts and classified alongside other "unexplained" physical symptoms in the somatoform disorders. Although DSM-III was meant to be atheoretic, this new approach to classification had a profound effect on how "dissociation" was studied and understood. In particular, it led to the development of the Dissociative Experiences Scale (DES: Bernstein and Putnam, 1987), which sought to quantify dissociation as defined in the DSM. Following that scheme, the DES was comprised of items pertaining to experiences of amnesia, identity disturbance, depersonalization, derealization, and absorption; being classified elsewhere, FNS were not included in the measure. A central assumption of the DES is that a "tendency to dissociate" manifests in a greater range of more intense dissociative symptoms and therefore a higher score on the measure. Intrinsic to this concept of "trait" dissociation is the idea of an underlying dissociative process (i.e., a loss of mental integration) that can give rise to different symptoms, with the number and severity of symptoms reflecting the extent of this disintegration; this is sometimes referred to as the "continuum" of dissociation.

Since then, hundreds of studies have used the DES (as well as other measures based on similar concepts, e.g., the Dissociation Questionnaire, DIS-Q: Vanderlinden et al., 1993) in different populations, with results seeming to confirm the underlying model. Thus, patients with dissociative identity disorder (DID; formerly multiple personality disorder) have, on average, the highest DES scores, followed by patients with dissociative disorder not otherwise specified (DDNOS; a less severe form of DID) and those with PTSD, with these groups scoring substantially higher than psychiatric controls (e.g., Van Izjendoorn and Schuengl, 1996). As a result, these measures have increasingly influenced what people regard as dissociation and how they understand it as a concept. In particular, the symptoms on the DES have come to be regarded as paradigmatic instances of dissociation rather than the FNS that originally exemplified the concept.

Numerous commentators have since criticized the separation of FNS from the dissociative disorders, reprising the notion that they constitute a physical (i.e., "somatoform") manifestation of dissociation that involves a similar process to "psychoform" symptoms like identity disturbance, amnesia, and depersonalization (e.g., Kuyk et al., 1996; Nijenhuis et al., 1996; Bowman, 2006; Brown et al., 2007). Indeed, the *International Classification of Diseases* (ICD-10: World Health Organization, 1992) still classifies the two alongside one another; even DSM-5 (American Psychiatric Association, 2013) now makes explicit reference to their potential overlap, despite categorizing them separately.

"TRAIT DISSOCIATION" AND FUNCTIONAL NEUROLOGIC SYMPTOMS

The argument that FNS involve dissociative mechanisms is partly based on the claim that somatoform and psychoform dissociation are commonly comorbid, typically informed by studies using scales like the DES in patients with FND, or measures of functional symptoms in patients with DSM-defined dissociative disorders.

Physical symptoms in patients with dissociative disorders

Brown et al. (2007) reviewed 11 studies investigating physical symptom reports in patients with dissociative disorders (mostly DID or DDNOS rather than depersonalization disorder), of which seven were controlled studies with mixed psychiatric comparison groups. Of these, five used the Somatoform Dissociation Questionnaire (SDQ-20: Nijenhuis et al., 1996), which has several items pertaining to functional neurologic complaints (e.g., "I am paralyzed for a while"; "I have an attack that resembles an epileptic seizure"). In all seven studies, scores were significantly higher in the dissociative disorder group than in the controls. Whether this reflects a greater prevalence of functional symptoms in the dissociative disorder groups is unclear, however, since none of the participants was subject to formal medical evaluation and many of the items on the SDQ-20 do not pertain to FNS.

More recently, Simeon et al. (2008) found that patients with depersonalization disorder scored significantly higher on the SDQ-20 than healthy controls, but that the patients' mean score (28.2) was lower than the cut-off of 30 normally recommended as indicating a possible dissociative disorder; moreover, the items that differentiated the groups were mainly those pertaining to depersonalization-like experiences (e.g., "I see things around me differently than usual"; "I hear sounds from nearby as if they were coming from far away") rather than neurologic symptoms as such. Further studies addressing whether FNS are more common in depersonalization disorder are clearly required.

"Psychoform" dissociative symptoms in patients with nonepileptic seizures

Numerous studies have compared trait dissociation in patients with psychogenic nonepileptic seizures (PNES) and controls with epilepsy, with both significant and nonsignificant between-group differences on the DES and DIS-Q being found (Alper et al., 1997; Wood et al., 1998; Kuyk et al., 1999b; Litwin and Cardena, 2000; Fleisher et al., 2002; Dikel et al., 2003; Reuber et al., 2003; Akyuz et al., 2004; Van Merode et al., 2004; Goldstein and Mellers, 2006; Lawton et al., 2008; Ito et al., 2009; Mazza et al., 2009). Combining data across all of these studies, there is a difference between the two groups of about 9 points on the DES, which amounts to a moderate effect size. The average DES score in the PNES group is just over 20, which is only slightly higher than that seen in patients with depression or schizophrenia (Van Izjendoorn and Schuengl, 1996; Moene et al., 2001); it is also substantially below those for patients with PTSD, DDNOS, or DID, as well as the score of 30 thought to indicate a possible dissociative disorder. It is noteworthy that the largest DES study in this area ($n = 137$) found a much lower mean DES score of 15 (Alper et al., 1997), which may be attributable to their exclusion of patients with "nonconversion" PNES, whose attacks are attributable to a diagnosable condition like panic disorder or psychosis.

"Psychoform" dissociative symptoms in patients with functional motor symptoms

Comparatively few studies have measured comorbid dissociation in patients with FND other than PNES. Of these, one found a significant difference between patients with motor FND and mixed psychiatric controls (Spitzer et al., 1999), whereas two others did not (Moene et al., 2001; Roelofs et al., 2002a). Similarly, one study found significantly lower dissociation scores in a group with motor FNS compared to patients with PNES (Guz et al., 2003), whilst another study found very similar scores in the two groups (Spinhoven et al., 2004). In all cases, average dissociation scores were relatively low in the FND group.

Is comorbidity evidence for a dissociative mechanism in FND?

Taken together, the available studies present a rather inconsistent picture regarding the comorbidity between psychoform dissociative symptoms and FND, raising more questions than they answer. It is apparent, for example, that patients presenting with FND typically have fewer, less severe psychoform dissociative symptoms than patients presenting with conditions like PTSD, DID, and DDNOS. Does this mean that FNDs, when occurring in isolation, involve less extensive dissociation than these conditions? Whilst this may be possible, what are we to make of the many FND patients whose dissociation scores are in the normal range? Is dissociation not relevant for understanding these conditions? Are there dissociative and nondissociative subtypes of FND? Even when comorbidity is apparent, does it in itself constitute evidence for FND being dissociative phenomena? A similar argument could just as easily be applied to depression, which is also commonly comorbid with FND, but few claim that similar psychologic processes are involved in each case.

The problem seems to stem from the assumption that scales like the DES measure a process (i.e., "dissociation") rather than just a set of symptoms, with the same process being responsible for all of the scale items. This ignores the fact that many items are nonspecific, such as those pertaining to memory disturbance. It is also inconsistent with research and theory suggesting that detachment and compartmentalization phenomena involve fundamentally different mechanisms (Holmes et al., 2005; Brown, 2006a). As such, two people with high scores on the DES may have very different problems. The distinction between psychoform and somatoform dissociation is problematic for the same reason, since the former is a heterogeneous category that encompasses both detachment (e.g., depersonalization) and compartmentalization symptoms (e.g., identity alteration), as well as those that could be attributable to either (e.g., amnesia). A recent model of compartmentalization suggests that somatoform dissociative phenomena like FND belong in that category, separately from detachment (e.g., Brown, 2002a, b, 2006b, 2013a, b).

It is also a mistake to suggest that a low score on a measure like the DES necessarily implies the absence of dissociation. A single dissociative symptom can be extremely debilitating, for example, but would attract a much lower score on the DES regardless of whether it involves the same mechanisms as those responsible for multiple symptoms. As such, it is impossible to conclude from these studies whether FNDs involve a dissociative process or not.

"STATE" DISSOCIATION AND FUNCTIONAL NEUROLOGIC SYMPTOMS

If the presence (or absence) of comorbid dissociative symptoms (i.e., "trait" dissociation) does not constitute evidence for (or against) FNS being dissociative phenomena in their own right, then what might? One possibility is dissociative experiences that arise immediately before or during the functional neurologic complaints themselves (i.e., an association between FNS and "state" dissociation). Stone et al. (2012), for example, found that 39% of their patients with sudden-onset functional weakness reported depersonalization or derealization in the 24 hours prior to developing the symptom; this was much less common in patients with waking (19%) or gradual-onset (12%) weakness. Stone et al. (2012) interpret these findings as indicating that functional weakness may involve a dissociative mechanism; by this logic, however, such a mechanism is either only operating in a minority of patients, or it only manifests as depersonalization-derealization in some cases.

With regard to other FNS, Goldstein and Mellers (2006) found that patients with PNES reported an average of three detachment symptoms (mainly depersonalization-derealization) during their attacks; a comparable rate was also seen in a control group with epilepsy, however. More recently, Hendrickson et al. (2014) found that just over 60% of a large sample of patients with PNES "always" or "sometimes" experienced depersonalization or derealization immediately before, during, or after their attacks, more than twice as often as a control group with epilepsy. In both studies, the detachment symptoms occurred alongside several other panic attack symptoms, including shortness of breath, dizziness, sweating, paresthesias, heart palpitations, and so on, many of which were also more common in the patients with PNES (see also Vein et al., 1994; Galimberti et al., 2003; Reinsberger et al., 2012).

These studies seem to suggest that detachment symptoms are part of the phenomenology of PNES for many patients, which may explain the moderate elevations seen on the DES in some studies. It is apparent that the experience is not one of a prototypic panic attack, however. In particular, the symptoms of autonomic arousal that occur in PNES tend to arise without the subjective anxiety said to define panic (so-called "panic without panic"). One interpretation of this is that PNES constitute a dissociative response to autonomic arousal that serves to reduce intense anxiety (Goldstein and Mellers, 2006); in other words, PNES detach or "dissociate" the individual from a threatening emotional experience. A similar phenomenon is said to occur in depersonalization disorder, which also has emotional numbing as a central feature. According to Sierra and Berrios (1998), depersonalization results from a hard-wired neurobiologic process in which prefrontal brain systems inhibit emotional processing in the anterior cingulate and amydalae, creating a state of vigilant attention and hypoemotionality that is adaptive in threatening situations. Future research should consider whether a related process is also operating in many PNES.

COMPARTMENTALIZATION AND FND

Whilst detachment might be a common experience for patients with PNES at the time of their attacks, there remains the issue of how to explain the seizure-like motor/behavioral (e.g., limb thrashing) and experiential features (e.g., alteration of consciousness) that distinguish PNES from phenomena like pure depersonalization, as well as other cases of nonfearful panic (the latter actually constitute nearly a third of all panic attacks and are much less likely to be characterized by depersonalization than fearful panic; Chen et al., 2009). It also seems unlikely that episodic detachment and emotional numbing could account for the signs and symptoms of other FND, such as paralysis, gait disturbance, blindness, and so on.

I have argued previously that the concept of compartmentalization may be particularly useful for understanding these phenomena (e.g., Brown, 2002a, b, 2006a, 2013a, b). Holmes et al. (2005) define compartmentalization phenomena as those in which individuals lose the ability to control processes or actions that they would normally have volitional control over. In each case, the affected functions are otherwise operating normally and can influence processing more generally; in this sense, the affected functions are said to be "compartmentalized," that is, separated from normal executive control. The deficit is reversible in principle, but this cannot be achieved through a deliberate act of will. By this view, the experiential and motor/behavioral features of PNES and other FNS would reflect a loss of control over the cognitive and behavioral control structures responsible for managing the functions in question.

A particularly compelling example of compartmentalization is provided by Kuyk et al. (1999a), who compared patients reporting profound postictal amnesia following generalized PNES or epileptic seizures. Both groups were hypnotized and given the suggestion that they could retrieve information about events occurring during the ictus. Under hypnosis, 85% of the PNES group recalled material pertaining to ictal events that they had previously been amnesic for, and which was corroborated by independent observers. If one takes the initial amnesia of the patients with PNES at face value, these findings suggest that the relevant material was always available in the cognitive system but inaccessible (i.e., compartmentalized) due to a retrieval deficit, which was subsequently reversed by the hypnotic intervention. In contrast, none of the patients with epilepsy were able to recall additional information during hypnosis, indicating a lack of encoding and therefore irreversible amnesia. Another striking example is the below-chance performance on perceptual discrimination tasks exhibited by some patients with functional sensory deficits (Kihlstrom, 1992). More prosaic examples include the simple bedside phenomena that are used to diagnose FND by demonstrating intact functioning alongside the subjective deficit (e.g., Hoover's sign; see Stone et al., 2011). Transient sensorimotor deficits induced using suggestion also fall in this category, suggesting a continuum of compartmentalization severity ranging from nonpathologic to massively disabling (Holmes et al., 2005).

According to this purely descriptive account, FNDs involve dissociation by definition, that is, dissociation between the individual's subjective experience of functioning and objective evidence pertaining to it. By this view, there is no need to look for additional symptoms or experiences in order to posit that FNS are dissociative phenomena: the symptom is the dissociation. This definition is theory-neutral, although it does imply that a successful account of these phenomena will appeal to the mechanisms responsible for controlling and accessing mental processes and contents. Although theories vary, two basic mechanisms have been identified in this regard: (1) compartmentalization due to a monitoring problem; and (2) compartmentalization due to a control problem.

Compartmentalization due to a monitoring problem

In Janet's original dissociation model of hysteria, fragmentation of the personality into separate compartments was regarded as an abnormal process triggered by extreme stress or emotion in the constitutionally weak mind of the hysteric individual. Subsequent developments of the model, in contrast, suggest that compartmentalization is inherent to mental processing in general. Hilgard's (1977) neodissociation theory, for example, suggests that the vast majority of processing is managed outside of awareness by low-level control systems with awareness, attention, and volition (functions of a so-called executive ego or "self") only being needed for the initial selection of those systems. By this view, most routine functions are "dissociated" from executive control, in the same way that most operations of a company are performed without direct involvement from its chief executive, who simply makes the initial decisions to perform them. This mental organization leaves the executive free to engage in other, more attention-demanding and strategic operations without interference from routine activity. A common example of this is driving a car whilst holding a conversation. When we are first learning to drive, the activity is novel and requires considerable attention while we develop the necessary processing routines; at this stage, our ability to perform concurrent actions, like holding a conversation, is extremely limited. Over time, however, our processing routines become sufficiently developed for the behavior to be managed with only minimal attention and awareness, freeing up executive resources to engage in other activities, such as conversation.

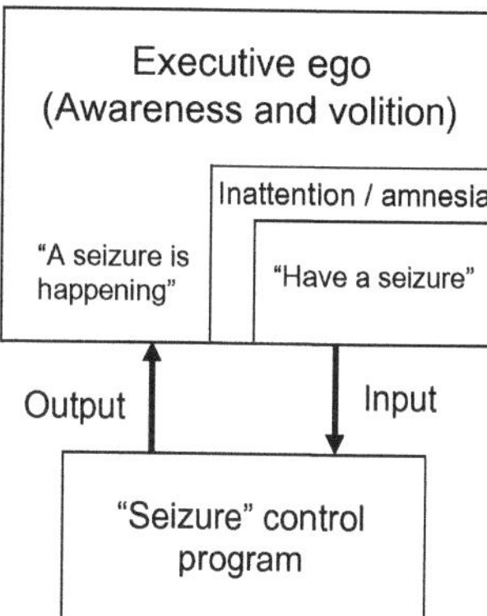

Fig. 8.1. Control structures involved in functional neurologic symptoms according to dissociated experience concept. (Adapted with permission from Kirsch and Lynn, 1995.)

Although the neodissociation model posits that any activity performed without ongoing executive input is technically dissociated, in the majority of cases the activity remains accessible to the executive, which can intervene should the need arise. If an unexpected event occurs whilst driving, for example, conversation will typically cease while executive attention and decision making are applied to the task in hand. In this sense, such activities are not true compartmentalization phenomena. That term mainly applies to situations where executive access to, or control over, lower-level processing is compromised for some reason, and which are much more relevant from a clinical perspective.

Consider the scenario where we (or, more specifically, the executive) instigate (i.e., "on purpose") a behavior that we subsequently realize is inconsistent with our goals. In this case, the experience will be one of having made a mistake (i.e., "I did that, but I shouldn't have"). This only applies, however, if we know that the behavior was performed on purpose. If we don't know this, perhaps because we forgot, we weren't paying attention, or we didn't represent it in this way to ourselves, then we will experience the behavior as happening by itself (i.e., to us, not by us). In this way, unwanted and seemingly involuntary actions can arise, such as those that characterize FND (note here that we are defining action broadly as referring to both overt behaviors and covert cognitive processes, including those that inhibit action or processing). By this view, therefore, FNDs arise when we trigger a behavior or process but are not aware that we triggered it due to a monitoring problem; as a result, we experience it as involuntary (Fig. 8.1).

Compartmentalization due to a control problem

In the monitoring explanation of compartmentalization symptoms it is the experience of control that is

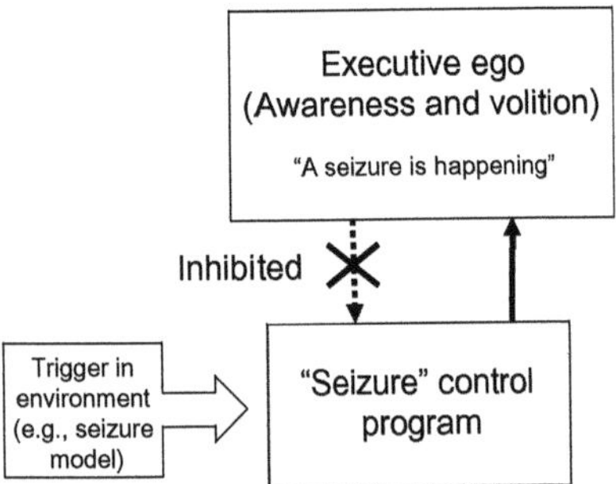

Fig. 8.2. Control structures involved in functional neurologic symptoms according to dissociated control concept. (Adapted with permission from Kirsch and Lynn, 1995.)

dissociated from awareness. A variation on the neodissociation model suggests that compartmentalization phenomena could also reflect an actual loss of executive control over lower-level systems. This "dissociated control" account suggests that much lower-level processing is automatically triggered by cues in the environment, without direct input from the executive itself (Fig. 8.2). By this view, the executive only serves to influence the likelihood of particular processes being triggered, or to inhibit them once they are running (Norman and Shallice, 1986; Woody and Bowers, 1994). If the executive is inhibited for some reason, then the ability to influence or inhibit the activity of lower-level systems is reduced, making the system vulnerable to stimulus-driven activation of unintended behaviors/processes, such as those seen in FND. In this account, the symptoms are experienced as involuntary because they bypass the systems responsible for initiating intentional action. By this view, functional symptoms are similar to the everyday action slips that occur in moments of inattention (e.g., dialing a familiar but out-of-date telephone number; Reason, 1979), as well as the utilization behavior seen in some patients with frontal-lobe damage. This echoes Janet's original dissociation model, which posits that attentional dysfunction and heightened suggestibility confer vulnerability to the development of hysteric symptoms.

The Integrative Cognitive Model

In my previous work, I have incorporated the concepts of dissociated experience and dissociated control within a broader biopsychosocial model of medically unexplained symptoms and FND (Brown, 2002a, 2004, 2006a, 2013a, b). According to the Integrative Cognitive Model, phenomena such as FND reflect the overactivation of ideas about illness in memory (i.e., "rogue representations"), distorting consciousness and cognitive control accordingly. This process may be moderated by various factors that contribute to the activation levels of these rogue representations, and/or compromise the individual's ability to inhibit them. Dissociated control is a central concept in this model, which assumes that FNS result from the automatic activation of lower-level structures, without requiring any input from executive systems at all. Indeed, this process would be facilitated by a deficit in executive functioning, which would cede further control of processing to the lower level. However, executive processes may play a more direct role in triggering symptoms in cases where attentional processes such as looking out for, focusing on, or actively trying to control or inhibit symptoms increases the activation of the underlying rogue representations. Symptoms generated in this way are experienced as involuntary, however, because the individual's intention is to prevent rather than initiate them. This aspect of the Integrative Cognitive Model is consistent with the concept of dissociated experience.

According to the Integrative Cognitive Model, many different factors influence the activation of rogue representations and thereby contribute to symptom experience. Particularly important in this regard are factors that encourage chronic symptom-focused attention, such as worry, rumination, and hypervigilance (Brown, 2013a). This may include the individual's context, mood, and illness beliefs and behaviors, as well as the motivational value of particular states and experiences. With regard to the latter, focusing attention on physical symptoms may be an effective way of avoiding thinking about other, more threatening material (e.g., aversive memories or situations), whilst expressing distress and soliciting care from others. In this way, the model offers a contemporary spin on the psychodynamic concepts of conversion and somatization, without insisting that these defense mechanisms are either necessary or sufficient for FND to develop (see Brown, 2013a, for case examples illustrating how such factors can be, but are not always, clinically relevant).

EVIDENCE FOR COMPARTMENTALIZATION IN FUNCTIONAL NEUROLOGIC DISORDERS

On a purely descriptive level, the idea that FND is characterized by compartmentalization seems uncontroversial in many cases: it is evident in the disabling nature of these conditions coupled with the preservation of function often observed during bedside testing. This is less obvious for some symptoms (e.g., PNES), but can be studied using appropriate methods such as the implicit perception and memory paradigms described above.

With regard to the processes underpinning compartmentalization, there is some evidence that motor FND patients have difficulties when actions (including imagined actions) are explicitly initiated, but not when they are evoked implicitly, which is consistent with the dissociated control account (Roelofs et al., 2001, 2002b; Cojan et al., 2009; Liepert et al., 2011; Pareés et al., 2013). Similarly, a number of studies have identified attentional disturbances in patients with PNES (Pouretemad et al., 1998; Bakvis et al., 2010; Strutt et al., 2011; Almis et al., 2013; cf. Bakvis et al., 2009) and motor FND (Roelofs et al., 2003, 2006; de Lange et al., 2007; van Poppelen et al., 2011). These include problems with inhibiting irrelevant stimuli, potentially implicating the executive deficit cited by dissociated control, and heightened self-monitoring, which fits with the concept of dissociated experience. There is also some evidence of increased hypnotic suggestibility in patients with FND (Kuyk et al., 1999a; Barry et al., 2000; Roelofs et al., 2002a), which is predicted by Janet's dissociation model of hysteria and further implicates altered attentional processing in this group (Brown and Oakley, 2004).

More recently, Edwards et al. (2011) found evidence for a delayed sense of volition accompanying the voluntary actions of patients with psychogenic tremor, which is consistent with the dissociated experience idea that there is a misrepresentation of intentionality in FND. More direct evidence for executive attention contributing to symptoms is provided by Stins et al. (2015), who found that patients with functional paresis exhibited a greater decrease in postural control when attending to their movements than age-matched controls, an effect that was normalized when the patients performed an attention-demanding cognitive task. Across the groups, the decrease in postural control when attending to movements correlated with self-reported state dissociation on the Clinician Administered Dissociative States Scale (Bremner et al., 1998), which mainly consists of items pertaining to detachment phenomena. This suggests that the experience of detachment might modulate the occurrence of compartmentalization, which could account for the apparent overlap between the two phenomena.

Taken together, the available evidence supports predictions from both the dissociated experience and dissociated control accounts of FND. The studies are small in most cases, however, and the evidence is often indirect (e.g., for attentional dysfunction rather than automatic activation of a behavior). It is a challenge for future researchers to develop paradigms that allow these predictions to be assessed more directly.

TRAUMA AND FUNCTIONAL NEUROLOGIC DISORDERS

Given the focus of this chapter, it is noteworthy that there has been little mention so far of the concept of trauma, which is often seen as inextricably linked with dissociation (see, e.g., Dalenberg et al., 2012). Indeed, there are studies indicating that exposure to potentially traumatizing events, such as childhood sexual, physical, and emotional abuse, is more common in patients with FND than controls (see, e.g., Fiszman et al., 2004; Brown, 2005; Sharpe and Faye, 2006; Roelofs and Spinhoven, 2007), which is often cited as evidence in favor of a dissociative interpretation of these complaints (Kuyk et al., 1996; Bowman, 2006; Brown et al., 2007). Notwithstanding the numerous methodologic problems with research in this area (see, e.g., Sharpe and Faye, 2006), it is apparent that not all patients with FND have been exposed to events of this sort (Brown, 2005). Whilst some might regard this as a challenge to the dissociation model of FND, there is no necessary link between dissociation and traumatic experiences in Janet's original model (Dorahy and Van der Hart, 2007) or in contemporary models based on this concept (e.g., Oakley, 1999; Brown, 2002a, 2004, 2006a, 2013a). Whilst outright trauma may play a role in the development of FND in some cases, in others the emotional antecedents are more subtle (Brown et al., 2005; Brown, 2013a, b). Nevertheless, exposure to potentially traumatizing events constitutes a vulnerability factor for both detachment and compartmentalization, through a number of different pathways. For example, attempts to suppress or avoid memories of adverse events could result in compartmentalization of the associated material, consistent with the idea that dissociation serves a defensive purpose. This may be particularly likely where peritraumatic detachment has compromised the encoding of trauma memories, giving rise to flashbacks and other distressing intrusions that motivate avoidance behavior (Brewin et al., 2010). Intense traumatic affect could also trigger depersonalization via its effect on frontal inhibitory systems (Sierra and Berrios, 1998). In terms of more indirect effects, early adversity could influence emotion regulation abilities via its impact on prefrontal functioning and the hypothalamic–pituitary–adrenal axis, compromising cognitive control at times of stress and intense emotion (Roelofs and Spinhoven, 2007). As such, exposure to traumatic events may be an important moderator of the tendency to experience FND, even if it does not mediate the development of these conditions.

SUMMARY, IMPLICATIONS, AND FUTURE DEVELOPMENTS

The term "dissociation" means different things to different people, with the available evidence suggesting that it refers to at least two qualitatively distinct types of phenomena: detachment and compartmentalization. Failing to distinguish between these phenomena leads to theoretic confusion, as well as the use of heterogeneous groups and inappropriate measures in research. Also problematic is the tendency to conflate processes with symptoms, which is apparent when people describe dissociation as a defense mechanism or cite the presence of comorbid detachment as evidence that a dissociative mechanism is responsible for FND. It is mainly for these reasons that it is impossible to draw firm conclusions about mechanisms from studies that have used measures like the DES to quantify "trait" dissociation in patients with FND. Ultimately, we need to be much more precise about the phenomena and processes that we are (and are not) referring to when we use the term.

Despite these caveats, there is good reason to believe that detachment and compartmentalization are relevant for understanding both the mechanisms of FND and the management of patients with these conditions. To begin with, it is apparent that a substantial proportion of patients with PNES experience detachment immediately before, during, and/or after their attacks. There is also some evidence that detachment is associated with the onset of functional weakness in some cases, although further studies on this and other FNS are required. This suggests that assessing and treating detachment may be an important aspect of managing FNS, which may include reducing autonomic arousal, providing education about depersonalization to help challenge catastrophic appraisals (e.g., "I'm going crazy"), and targeting other cognitive, behavioral, and psychodynamic maintenance factors (e.g., Simeon and Abugel, 2006; Stone, 2006; Baker et al., 2007). It is also important to consider the potential for misdiagnosing episodic depersonalization and nonfearful panic attacks as FND. This is true both clinically and when conducting research on symptoms such as PNES.

It is nevertheless noteworthy that many patients, particularly those with FND other than PNES, do not report detachment. What I have tried to demonstrate in this chapter is that FND may still involve "dissociation" (i.e., compartmentalization) even if detachment is absent. Conversely, the mere presence of detachment does not mean that it is the mechanism underlying FNS. On a purely descriptive level, all FNS involve dissociation by definition, that is, dissociation between objective data and subjective experience. The various examples that illustrate this phenomenon are useful both in terms of diagnosis and explaining this to patients. Whilst some might argue that the concept of dissociation (or, more specifically in this case, compartmentalization) is not necessary for these purposes, such phenomena illustrate that disturbances in consciousness, cognitive control, and the experience of agency are central to FNS. Models implicating these processes in the development of compartmentalization symptoms help explain FNS in a non-blaming way and are growing in empiric support. According to these models, acute experiences of detachment may trigger compartmentalization phenomena or moderate their occurrence, but are not the source of the FNS themselves. There is now a pressing need for studies investigating these hypotheses in larger groups with a range of different FNS, using both cognitive and neurobiological methods.

References

Akyuz G, Kugu N, Akyuz A et al. (2004). Dissociation and childhood abuse history in epileptic and pseudoseizure patients. Epileptic Disord 6: 187–192.

Almis BH, Cumurcu BE, Unal S et al. (2013). The neuropsychological and neurophysiological profile of women with pseudoseizure. Compr Psychiatry 54: 649–657.

Alper K, Devinsky O, Perrine K et al. (1997). Dissociation in epilepsy and conversion nonepileptic seizures. Epilepsia 38: 991–997.

American Psychiatric Association (1952). Diagnostic and Statistical Manual of Mental Disorders (DSM), American Psychiatric Press, Washington, DC.

American Psychiatric Association (1968). Diagnostic and Statistical Manual of Mental Disorders, 2nd Edition (DSM-II), American Psychiatric Press, Washington, DC.

American Psychiatric Association (1980). Diagnostic and Statistical Manual of Mental Disorders, 3rd Edition (DSM-III), American Psychiatric Press, Washington, DC.

American Psychiatric Association (2013). Diagnostic and statistical manual of mental disorders, 5th ed. American Psychiatric Association, Washington, DC.

Baker D, Hunter E, Lawrence E et al. (2007). Overcoming depersonalization and feelings of unreality. A self-help guide using CBT techniques, Robinson, London.

Bakvis P, Roelofs K, Kuyk J et al. (2009). Trauma, stress, and preconscious threat processing in patients with psychogenic non-epileptic seizures. Epilepsia 50: 1001–1011.

Bakvis P, Spinhoven P, Putman P et al. (2010). The effect of stress induction on working memory in patients with psychogenic nonepileptic seizures. Epilepsy Behav 19: 448–454.

Barry J, Atzman O, Morrell M (2000). Discriminating between epileptic and nonepileptic events: the utility of hypnotic seizure induction. Epilepsia 41: 81–84.

Bernstein E, Putnam FW (1987). Development, reliability, and validity of a dissociation scale. J Nerv Ment Dis 174: 727–735.

Bowman E (2006). Why conversion seizures should be classified as a dissociative disorder. Psychiatr Clin North Am 29: 185–211.

Bremner JD, Krystal JH, Putnam FW et al. (1998). Measurement of dissociative states with the clinician-administered dissociative states scale (CADSS). J Trauma Stress 11: 125–136.

Brewin CR, Gregory JD, Lipton M et al. (2010). Intrusive images in psychological disorders: characteristics, neural mechanisms, and treatment implications. Psychol Rev 117: 210–232.

Brown RJ (2002a). The cognitive psychology of dissociative states. Cogn Neuropsychiatry 7: 221–235.

Brown RJ (2002b). Epilepsy, dissociation and nonepileptic seizures. In: MR Trimble, B Schmitz (Eds.), The Neuropsychiatry of Epilepsy, Cambridge University Press, Cambridge, UK.

Brown RJ (2004). Psychological mechanisms of medically unexplained symptoms: an integrative conceptual model. Psychol Bull 130: 793–812.

Brown RJ (2005). Dissociation and conversion in psychogenic illness. In: M Hallett, S Fahn, J Jankovic et al. (Eds.), Psychogenic movement disorders: Psychobiology and treatment of a functional disorder, Lippincott, Williams & Wilkins, Philadelphia.

Brown RJ (2006a). Different types of "dissociation" have different psychological mechanisms. J Trauma Dissociation 7: 7–28.

Brown RJ (2006b). Medically unexplained symptoms. In: N Tarrier (Ed.), Case Formulation in Cognitive Behaviour Therapy: The Treatment of Challenging and Complex Cases, Brunner-Routledge, London.

Brown RJ (2013a). Dissociation and somatoform disorders. In: F Kennedy, H Kennerley, D Pearson (Eds.), Cognitive Behavioural Approaches to the Understanding and Treatment of Dissociation. Routledge, London.

Brown RJ (2013b). Explaining the unexplained. Psychologist 26: 868–872.

Brown RJ, Oakley DA (2004). An integrative cognitive theory of hypnosis and high hypnotizability. In: M Heap, RJ Brown, DA Oakley (Eds.), The Highly Hypnotizable Person: Theoretical, Experimental and Clinical Issues. Brunner-Routledge, London.

Brown RJ, Schrag A, Trimble MR (2005). Dissociation, childhood interpersonal trauma and family functioning in somatisation disorder. Am J Psychiatry 162: 899–905.

Brown RJ, Cardena E, Nijenhuis E et al. (2007). Should conversion disorder be reclassified as a dissociative disorder in DSM-V? Psychosomatics 48: 369–378.

Chen J, Tsuchiya M, Kawakami N et al. (2009). Non-fearful vs. fearful panic attacks: a general population study from the National Comorbidity Survey. J Affect Disord 112: 273–278.

Cojan Y, Waber L, Carruzzo A et al. (2009). Motor inhibition in hysterical conversion paralysis. Neuroimage 47: 1026–1037.

Dalenberg CJ, Brand BL, Gleaves DH et al. (2012). Evaluation of the evidence for the trauma and fantasy models of dissociation. Psychol Bull 138: 550–588.

De Lange FP, Roelofs K, Toni I (2007). Increased self-monitoring during imagined movements in conversion paralysis. Neuropsychologia 45: 2051–2058.

Dikel TN, Fennell EB, GIlmore RL (2003). Posttraumatic stress disorder, dissociation and sexual abuse history in epileptic and nonepileptic seizure patients. Epilepsy Behav 4: 644–650.

Dorahy MJ, Van der Hart O (2007). Relationship between trauma and dissociation: A historical analysis. In: E Vermetten, MJ Dorahy, D Spiegel (Eds.), Traumatic Dissociation: Neurobiology and treatment, American Psychiatric Publishing, Arlington, VA.

Edwards MJ, Moretto G, Schwingenschuh P et al. (2011). Abnormal sense of intention preceding voluntary movement in patients with psychogenic tremor. Neuropsychologia 49: 2791–2793.

Fiszman A, Alves-Leon SV, Nunes RG et al. (2004). Traumatic events and posttraumatic stress disorder in patients with psychogenic nonepileptic seizures: a critical review. Epilepsy Behav 5: 818–825.

Fleisher W, Staley D, Krawetz P et al. (2002). Comparative study of trauma-related phenomena in subjects with pseudoseizures and subjects with epilepsy. Am J Psychiatry 159: 660–663.

Galimberti C, Teresa Ratti M, Murelli R et al. (2003). Patients with psychogenic nonepileptic seizures, alone or epilepsy-associated, share a psychological profile distinct from that of epilepsy patients. J Neurol 250: 338–346.

Goldstein L, Mellers J (2006). Ictal symptoms of anxiety, avoidance behaviour, and dissociation in patients with dissociative seizures. J Neurol Neurosurg Psychiatry 77: 616–621.

Guz H, Doganay Z, Ozkan A et al. (2003). Conversion disorder and its subtypes: a need for a reclassification. Nord J Psychiatry 57: 377–381.

Hendrickson R, Popescu A, Dixit R et al. (2014). Panic attack symptoms differentiate patients with epilepsy from those with psychogenic nonepileptic spells (PNES). Epilepsy Behav 37: 210–214.

Hilgard ER (1977). Divided consciousness: Multiple controls in human thought and action, Wiley, New York.

Holmes EA, Brown RJ, Mansell W et al. (2005). Are there two qualitatively distinct forms of dissociation? A review and some clinical implications. Clin Psychol Rev 25: 1–23.

Ito M, Adachi N, Okazaki M et al. (2009). Evaluation of dissociative experiences and the clinical utility of the Dissociative Experience Scale in patients with coexisting epilepsy and psychogenic nonepileptic seizures. Epilepsy Behav 16: 491–494.

Kihlstrom JF (1992). Dissociative and conversion disorders. In: DJ Stein, J Young (Eds.), Cognitive science and clinical disorders, Academic Press, San Diego, CA.

Kirsch I, Lynn SJ (1995). The altered state of hypnosis: changes in the theoretical landscape. Am Psychol 50: 846–858.

Kuyk J, Van Dyck R, Spinhoven P (1996). The case for a dissociative interpretation of pseudoepileptic seizures. J Nerv Ment Dis 184: 468–474.

Kuyk J, Spinhoven P, Van Dyck R (1999a). Hypnotic recall: a positive criterion in the differential diagnosis of epileptic and pseudoepileptic seizures. Epilepsia 40: 485–491.

Kuyk J, Spinhoven P, Van Emde Boas W et al. (1999b). Dissociation in temporal lobe epilepsy and pseudo-epileptic seizure patients. J Nerv Ment Dis 187: 713–720.

Lawton G, Baker G, Brown RJ (2008). Comparison of two types of dissociation in epileptic and non-epileptic seizures. Epilepsy Behav 13: 333–336.

Liepert J, Hassa T, Tüscher O et al. (2011). Motor excitability during movement imagination and movement observation in psychogenic lower limb paresis. J Psychosom Res 70: 59–65.

Litwin R, Cardena E (2000). Demographic and seizure variables, but not hypnotizability or dissociation, differentiated psychogenic from organic seizures. J Trauma Dissociation 1: 99–122.

Mazza M, Della Marca G, Martini A et al. (2009). Non-epileptic seizures (NES) are predicted by depressive and dissociative symptoms. Epilepsy Res 84: 91–96.

Moene FC, Spinhoven P, Hoogduin K et al. (2001). Hypnotizability, dissociation and trauma in patients with a conversion disorder: an exploratory study. Clin Psychol Psychother 8: 400–410.

Nijenhuis ER, Spinhoven P, Van Dyck R et al. (1996). The development and psychometric characteristics of the Somatoform Dissociation Questionnaire (SDQ-20). J Nerv Ment Dis 184: 688–694.

Norman DA, Shallice T (1986). Attention to action: Willed and automatic control of behavior. In: RJ Davidson, GE Schwartz, D Shapiro (Eds.), Consciousness and self-regulation. Advances in research and theory, Volume 4. Plenum Press, New York.

Oakley DA (1999). Hypnosis and conversion hysteria: A unifying model. Cogn Neuropsychiatry 4 (3): 243–265.

Pareés I, Kassavetis P, Saifee TA et al. (2013). Failure of explicit movement control in patients with functional motor symptoms. Mov Disord 28: 517–523.

Pouretemad HR, Thompson PJ, Fenwick PB (1998). Impaired sensorimotor gating in patients with non-epileptic seizures. Epilepsy Res 31: 1–12.

Reason JT (1979). Actions not as planned. In: G Underwood, R Stevens (Eds.), Aspects of Consciousness, Volume 1: Psychological Issues, Academic Press, London.

Reinsberger C, Perez DL, Murphy MM et al. (2012). Pre- and postictal, not ictal, heart rate distinguishes complex partial and psychogenic nonepileptic seizures. Epilepsy Behav 23: 68–70.

Reuber M, House A, Pukrop R et al. (2003). Somatization, dissociation and general psychopathology in patients with psychogenic non-epileptic seizures. Epilepsy Res 57: 159–167.

Roelofs K, Spinhoven P (2007). Trauma and medically unexplained symptoms: towards an integration of cognitive and neuro-biological accounts. Clin Psychol Rev 27: 798–820.

Roelofs K, Näring GWB, Keijsers GPJ et al. (2001). Motor imagery in conversion paralysis. Cogn Neuropsychiatry 6: 21–40.

Roelofs K, Hoogduin KA, Keijsers GP et al. (2002a). Hypnotic susceptibility in patients with conversion disorder. J Abnorm Psychol 111 (2): 390–395.

Roelofs K, van Galen GP, Keijsers GP et al. (2002b). Motor initiation and execution in patients with conversion paralysis. Acta Psychol (Amst) 110: 21–34.

Roelofs K, van Galen GP, Eling P et al. (2003). Endogenous and exogenous attention in patients with conversion paresis. Cogn Neuropsychol 20: 733–745.

Roelofs K, de Bruijn ER, Van Galen GP (2006). Hyperactive action monitoring during motor-initiation in conversion paralysis: an event-related potential study. Biol Psychol: 71.

Sharpe D, Faye C (2006). Non-epileptic seizures and child sexual abuse: a critical review of the literature. Clin Psychol Rev 26: 1020–1040.

Sierra M, Berrios GE (1998). Depersonalization: neurobiological perspectives. Biol Psychiatry 44: 898–908.

Simeon D, Abugel J (2006). Feeling unreal: Depersonalization disorder and the loss of the self. Oxford University Press, New York.

Simeon D, Smith RJ, Knutelska M et al. (2008). Somatoform dissociation in depersonalization disorder. J Trauma Dissociation 9: 335–348.

Spinhoven P, Roelofs K, Moene F et al. (2004). Trauma and dissociation in conversion disorder and chronic pelvic pain. Int J Psychiatry Med 34: 305–318.

Spitzer C, Spelsberg B, Grabe H-J et al. (1999). Dissociative experiences and psychopathology in conversion disorders. J Psychosom Res 46 (3): 291–294.

Stins JF, Kempe CA, Hagenaars MA et al. (2015). Attention and postural control in patients with conversion paresis. J Psychosom Res 78: 249–254.

Stone J (2006). Dissociation: what is it and why is it important? Pract Neurol 6: 308–313.

Stone J, LaFrance WC, Brown RJ et al. (2011). Conversion disorder: current problems and potential solutions for DSM-5. J Psychosom Res 71: 369–376.

Stone J, Warlow C, Sharpe M (2012). Functional weakness: clues to mechanism from the nature of onset. J Neurol Neurosurg Psychiatry 83: 67–69.

Strutt A, Hill S, Scott B et al. (2011). A comprehensive neuropsychological profile of women with psychogenic nonepileptic seizures. Epilepsy Behav 20: 24–28.

Van Izjendoorn MH, Schuengl C (1996). The measurement of dissociation in normal and clinical populations: meta-analytic validation of the Dissociative Experiences Scale. Clin Psychol Rev 16: 365–383.

Van Merode T, Twellaar M, Kotsopoulos I et al. (2004). Psychological characteristics of patients with newly developed psychogenic seizures. J Neurol Neurosurg Psychiatry 75: 1175–1177.

Van Poppelen D, Saifee TA, Schwingenschuh P et al. (2011). Attention to self in psychogenic tremor. Mov Disord 26: 2575–2576.

Vanderlinden J, Dyck RV, Vandereyken H et al. (1993). The Dissociation Questionnaire: development and characteristics of a new self-reporting questionnaire. Clin Psychol Psychother 1: 21–27.

Vein AM, Djukova GM, Vorobieva OV (1994). Is panic attack a mask of psychogenic seizures? A comparative analysis of phenomenology of psychogenic seizures and panic attacks. Funct Neurol: 153–159.

Wood B, McDaniel S, Burchfiel K et al. (1998). Factors distinguishing families of patients with psychogenic seizures from families of patients with epilepsy. Epilepsia 39: 432–437.

Woody EZ, Bowers KS (1994). A frontal assault on dissociated control. In: SJ Lynn, JW Rhue (Eds.), Dissociation: Clinical and Theoretical Perspectives, Guilford Press, New York.

World Health Organization (1992). The ICD-10 Classification of Mental and Behavioural Disorders: Clinical Descriptions and Diagnostic Guidelines, World Health Organization, Geneva, Switzerland.

Handbook of Clinical Neurology, Vol. 139 (3rd series)
Functional Neurologic Disorders
M. Hallett, J. Stone, and A. Carson, Editors
http://dx.doi.org/10.1016/B978-0-12-801772-2.00009-6

Chapter 9

Hypnosis as a model of functional neurologic disorders

Q. DEELEY*

Department of Forensic and Neurodevelopmental Sciences, Institute of Psychiatry, Kings College, London, UK

Abstract

In the 19th century it was recognized that neurologic symptoms could be caused by "morbid ideation" as well as organic lesions. The subsequent observation that hysteric (now called "functional") symptoms could be produced and removed by hypnotic suggestion led Charcot to hypothesize that suggestion mediated the effects of ideas on hysteric symptoms through as yet unknown effects on brain activity. The advent of neuroimaging 100 years later revealed strikingly similar neural correlates in experiments matching functional symptoms with clinical analogs created by suggestion. Integrative models of suggested and functional symptoms regard these alterations in brain function as the endpoint of a broader set of changes in information processing due to suggestion. These accounts consider that suggestions alter experience by mobilizing representations from memory systems, and altering causal attributions, during preconscious processing which alters the content of what is provided to our highly edited subjective version of the world. Hypnosis as a model for functional symptoms draws attention to how radical alterations in experience and behavior can conform to the content of mental representations through effects on cognition and brain function. Experimental study of functional symptoms and their suggested counterparts in hypnosis reveals the distinct and shared processes through which this can occur.

HYPNOSIS AS A MODEL

Introduction

Apparent similarities between hysteria and hypnosis have been noted from the 19th century onwards. In particular, the process of suggestion has been viewed as a potential explanation of hysteric symptoms, operating via effects on brain function (e.g., Charcot and Marie, 1892; Oakley, 1999a). This chapter considers the relationship between hypnosis and hysteria, now described as "functional neurologic symptoms." Characteristics of hypnosis are outlined before considering ways in which hypnosis might act as a model for functional symptoms. This provides a basis for evaluating past and current attempts to explain functional symptoms by analogy with hypnosis.

HYPNOSIS AND SUGGESTIBILITY

In a report on hypnosis for the British Psychological Society, hypnosis was defined as:

an interaction between one person, the "hypnotist", and another person or other people, the "subject" or "subjects". In this interaction the hypnotist attempts to influence the subjects' perceptions, feelings, thinking and behaviour by asking them to concentrate on ideas and images that may evoke the intended effects. The verbal communications that the hypnotist uses to achieve these effects are termed "suggestions" (Heap et al., 2001).

Autosuggestions refer to suggestions that are self-administered, while the "classic suggestion effect" entails that responses elicited by suggestions that are experienced as "involuntary and effortless" (Weitzenhoffer, 1980). Although suggestion is employed in hypnosis, it has a broader definition as "a form or type of communicable belief capable of producing and modifying experiences, thoughts and actions. Suggestions can be (a) intentional/nonintentional, (b) verbal/nonverbal, or (c) hypnotic/nonhypnotic" (Halligan and Oakley, 2014).

*Correspondence to: Dr. Quinton Deeley, Department of Forensic and Neurodevelopmental Sciences, Institute of Psychiatry, De Crespigny Park, London SE5 8AZ, UK. E-mail: peter.q.deeley@kcl.ac.uk

Suggestive processes have formed part of cultural practices since recorded history, but the explicit recognition of suggestion as a psychologic process that can be deliberately used to produce specific effects dates from the 19th century (Ellenberger, 1994). In the case of hypnosis, verbal suggestions to relax and focus attention, generally administered in a standardized way as a "formal induction procedure," are used to establish a hypnotic state or "trance." In keeping with the content of typical suggestions in the induction procedure, the hypnotic state is characterized by attentional absorption, disattention to extraneous stimuli, and relaxation. Induction of the hypnotic state increases responses to further suggestions (e.g., of limb paralysis), although some individuals respond to the same suggestions without a formal induction procedure (Braffmann and Kirsch, 1999).

A variety of scales have been developed to measure individual responsiveness to suggestions, such as the Harvard Group Scale of Hypnotic Susceptibility (Shor and Orne, 1962). These scales generally include a hypnotic induction followed by test suggestions and an assessment of the subject's response to each. "Hypnotizability" or "hypnotic suggestibility" is typically defined as the number of suggestions that an individual responds to on a standard scale of this type. A resemblance between hypnosis and functional neurologic symptoms has been noted at this basic level of how hypnotic responsiveness is determined; as Kirsch (1990) put it, "Hypnotized subjects are asked to experience paralysis, amnesia, anaesthesia, involuntary movements and hallucinations. In fact, hypnotizability is measured as the number of conversion and dissociation symptoms that the person is able to display." This resemblance is central to the claim that hypnosis can act as a model for functional symptoms. Before examining the evidence for this claim in more detail, we will first consider how hypnosis might act as a model for functional symptoms based on recent accounts of models in scientific explanation.

EXPLANATORY MODELS IN SCIENTIFIC EXPLANATION

An explanatory model allows "the construction of hypotheses about unobservable processes and structures that can be used to explain observable phenomena" (Harré, 2002, p. 54). Explanatory models rest on a particular use of analogy, in which, first, patterns of similarity and difference between the source model and subject are identified, and second, the source model and subject are recognized as subtypes of an overarching category or "supertype" which defines the characteristics they share in common. The source model of hypnosis allows the construction of an overarching category which also includes functional neurologic symptoms – specifically, a category of phenomena characterized by subjectively realistic, involuntary alterations in experience and behavior that conform to ideas, beliefs, and expectations. Hypnotic phenomena and functional neurologic symptoms "inherit" this shared characteristic as members of the category (Harré, 2002).

In some cases the success of an explanatory model can be demonstrated through experiments in which features of the subject are represented and investigated by controlled manipulation of the source which would be impossible or difficult in the subject itself. Hypnosis has been extensively used to model functional symptoms in this way (Bell et al., 2011) – for example, by using suggestion to reproduce and then remove specific functional symptoms in healthy participants whilst measuring brain activity. This allows much more precise comparison of hypnotic phenomena and functional symptoms than would otherwise be the case.

If hypnosis is a good explanatory model for functional neurologic symptoms then it should display certain characteristics. It should be ontologically plausible (involve the same kind of processes); the processes should clearly relate to general theories of cognition and brain function and apply to both hypnosis and functional symptoms; and the model should allow prediction of features of functional symptoms (such as brain mechanisms), and vice versa.

Features of what would count as a successful use of hypnosis as a model for functional neurologic symptoms can be tested against successive versions of this model since the 19th century.

THE INITIAL CONSTRUCTION OF HYPNOSIS AS A MODEL FOR HYSTERIA

Many psychiatrists, neurologists and psychologists explored the relationship between hypnosis, suggestion, and hysteria in the 19th and early 20th centuries (Ellenberger, 1994). Here we focus on the work of the pioneering neurologist Jean-Martin Charcot (1825–1893) and the philosopher, psychiatrist, and experimental psychologist Pierre Janet (1859–1947). This is not only because of their central influence in their own time, but also because their proposals continue to inform contemporary research.

Charcot proposed that motor symptoms of hysteria derived from unconscious "fixed" ideas based on suggestions or autosuggestions "remaining isolated from the rest of the mind and expressing themselves outwardly through corresponding motor phenomena" (Ellenberger, 1994). Charcot used the recently discovered technique of hypnosis to produce and remove hysteric symptoms. He proposed that the effects of fixed ideas in both hysteria and hypnosis operated via as yet unexplained "dynamic or functional lesions" in the cortical motor area opposite the paralysis (Charcot, 1889). These dynamic lesions produced a temporary version of the more permanent loss of function due to structural damage caused by conditions such as stroke, which had been well described in the 19th century. In Charcot's words, it was "one of those lesions which escape our present means of anatomical investigation" (Charcot, 1889).

Charcot's proposal that brain function could be reorganized by ideas to produce involuntary symptoms radically differed from the dominant clinicoanatomic method in medicine and neurology that viewed symptoms as solely arising from discrete brain lesions. Charcot's views had been influenced by the English neurologist John Russell Reynolds, who in 1869 had introduced the concept of "psychic paralysis." Reynolds wrote:

> *some of the most serious disorders of the nervous system, such as paralysis, spasm, pain, and otherwise altered sensations, may depend upon a morbid condition of emotion, or idea and emotion, or of idea alone ... they sometimes associate themselves with distinct and definite diseases of the nervous centers, so that it becomes very important to know how much a given case is due to an organic lesion, and how much to morbid ideation (Reynolds, 1869).*

Reynolds gave an example of a young woman whose father had become paralyzed after a reversal of fortune. She had to support the household by giving lessons, which involved long walks around the town. As Binet and Féré summarized the case in their book *Animal Magnetism*:

> *influenced by the fatigue caused by so much walking, it occurred to her that she might become paralysed and that their situation then would be terrible. Haunted by this idea, she felt a growing weakness in her limbs, and after a while was quite unable to walk. The pathology of the affection was understood by Reynolds who prescribed moral treatment. He finally convinced the patient that she was able to walk, and in fact she resumed the practice (Binet and Féré, 1891, p. 323f).*

As Charcot put it, hysteric paralysis arose when "the idea comes to the patient's mind that he might become paralysed; in one word through autosuggestion, the rudimentary paralysis becomes real" (Charcot and Marie, 1892).

The influence of ideas on the symptoms of hysteria and their hypnotic counterparts was also emphasized by Charcot's younger colleague Pierre Janet. Janet, like Charcot, considered both hysteria and hypnosis to operate through the suggestive effects of ideas. Indeed, Janet felt that suggestion based on ideas was so central to both hysteric and hypnotic phenomena that, without exposure to relevant ideas, the respective effects would not occur (Ellenberger, 1994). Janet originated the modern notion of dissociation as a "narrowing of the field of consciousness," resulting in an abnormal splitting off or compartmentalization of mental functions that are normally closely associated (Janet, 1907). Janet viewed dissociation as influenced by the suggestive effect of "fixed ideas" based on unresolved traumatic memories. Suggestibility was defined as the tendency for a simple idea to develop into chains of association which then influence mental function and behavior (Halligan and Oakley, 2014). Janet's masterly case studies showed how the involuntary behavior of hysterics, performed without awareness of recollection, reproduced and indirectly expressed earlier traumatic experiences (Janet, 1907). While Janet's approach was similar to Charcot's in many respects, he did not accept Charcot's thesis that hysteric symptoms were caused by temporary "dynamic" lesions by analogy with "structural" lesions causing more permanent deficits. The question of the brain basis of dissociation and suggested effects could not be addressed until the invention of neuroimaging about 100 years after the death of Charcot.

CONTEMPORARY VERSIONS OF HYPNOSIS AS A MODEL FOR FUNCTIONAL SYMPTOMS

Developments in cognitive neuropsychology and neuroimaging have led to a re-examination of earlier proposals about hypnosis as model for hysteria (see in particular the influential paper of Oakley, 1999a). Here we consider these recent developments.

Neuroimaging studies

Hypnotic suggestion has been used to create experimental models of a range of functional or dissociative symptoms, in some cases allowing comparison of brain correlates of symptoms and their suggested analogues.

Limb paralysis

In a positron emission tomography study, Halligan and colleagues used suggestion to produce a left-leg paralysis in a single hypnotized participant that reproduced the functional paralysis of the patient in their prior study (Marshall et al., 1997; Halligan et al., 2000). Attempted movement of the paralyzed limb was associated with increased right anterior cingulate cortex (ACC) and orbitofrontal cortex, resembling activation changes of the clinical study. It was concluded that similar processes of executive inhibition might underpin hypnotically suggested and functional paralysis. A follow-up study with 12 highly hypnotizable participants addressed the criticism that the hypnotized subject might have feigned the paralysis (Ward et al., 2003). While independent clinically trained observers were not able to distinguish suggested and feigned paralysis, brain activity to suggested paralysis largely replicated the previous single case study (although ACC activation was not found) and markedly differed from the feigned condition (Ward et al., 2003).

Functional magnetic resonance imaging (fMRI) studies of suggested limb paralysis have also been conducted, noting that the fMRI environment does not interfere with response to suggestions (Oakley et al., 2007). Cojan and colleagues (2009a, b) used hypnotically suggested paralysis to replicate their earlier study that used the Go NoGo task in functional paralysis patients. Suggested paralysis was also associated with normal motor cortex activation during the preparation phase, supporting the view that paralysis was not working through suppression of motor intention. They also found that anterior prefrontal and ACC activity was increased in all hypnosis conditions, not just suggested paralysis, which they took as evidence of state-related hypnosis changes rather than a mechanism to inhibit movement. As with their study of functional paralysis, they reported increased functional connectivity between the motor cortex and precuneus, proposing that in both cases motor inhibition (paralysis) may be mediated through mental imagery and self-reflective processing rather than executive inhibition. Also, functional paralysis but not suggested paralysis was associated with modulation of ventromedial prefrontal cortex (VMPFC) (Cojan et al., 2009b). This was interpreted as evidence of involvement of affectively laden self-representations and memories in modulating motor function in functional but not suggested paralysis.

The question of whether functional and suggested motor inhibition (paralysis) is mediated through executive inhibition, or modulation by emotion, memory, and self-related processing, or some combination of these processes appears unresolved at present. For example, a study of hypnotically induced left-hand paralysis using resting-state fMRI showed changes in resting-state networks that could be associated with both altered self-related processing and engagement of executive inhibition (Pyka et al., 2011), while a recent fMRI study of suggested left upper-limb paralysis was consistent with a selective role for ACC in movement inhibition (Deeley et al., 2013a). Inconsistent findings may be partly attributable to differences in experimental design. Nevertheless, similar patterns of brain activity have been found when studies with functional paralysis patients have been closely reproduced with suggested paralysis – except for activation of VMPC in functional paralysis, but not suggested paralysis in Cojan and colleagues' studies. This draws attention to the important issue of potential differences in the role of emotion and memory processing between functional and suggested symptoms, which we discuss further below.

Functional amnesia

Mendelsohn and colleagues (2008) used suggestion in hypnosis to selectively block memory-specific aspects of a cue when a posthypnotic cue was given. Only the highly hypnotically responsive group showed impaired recall compared to low responders and a control group instructed to feign high hypnotizability. Reduced recall was associated with reduced activity in left extrastriate occipital lobe and the left temporal pole, as well as increased activity in the left rostrolateral PFC. These effects were reversed when the posthypnotic amnesia suggested was removed. These findings are consistent with studies of functional amnesia which show increased activity of prefrontal inhibitory regions and decreased activity of medial temporal-lobe memory systems during attempted recall (reviewed in Bell et al., 2011).

Loss of agency and awareness

Functional neurologic symptoms include loss of the sense of agency or perceived self-initiation and control of movements. For example, involuntary movements present as convulsions in nonepileptic seizures, or complex automatisms in fugues or other dissociative episodes. Reductions of agency in functional disorders can also be accompanied by loss or narrowing of awareness – as occurs, for example, in about half of patients with nonepileptic seizures (Brown et al., 2011). Alterations of agency and awareness also form part of other pathologic conditions such as schizophrenia, in which loss of agency is illustrated by passivity phenomena such as alien control of movement. In this syndrome movements are interpreted and experienced as under the control of an external agent. Disruptions of agency involve not only movements but also the sense of control and ownership of mental contents such as thought, emotion, and personal identity – as in dissociative identity disorder, in which speech and actions occur as if under the control of an alternate indwelling personality; and thought insertion in schizophrenia, in which thoughts are experienced as introduced into the mind by an external agent. Alien control of thought or movement – sometimes associated with loss of awareness – is also described in culturally influenced dissociative phenomena such as spirit possession, mediumship, and shamanism (Oesterreich, 1974; Rouget, 1985). These closely related alterations in experience across pathologic conditions and cultural settings raise the question of whether they involve changes in shared cognitive and brain systems involved in the usual sense of agency and awareness. Suggestion has been used to address this question because it allows the creation of experimental analogs of closely related alterations in experience.

Nonepileptic seizures, involuntary movement, and loss of awareness

While suggested convulsions cannot be safely or informatively produced in an fMRI scanner, it is possible to model nonepileptic seizures by suggesting involuntary movements with and without loss of awareness. Suggested simple involuntary actions (joystick movement) were associated with altered functional connectivity between motor-planning brain regions (supplementary motor area, SMA) and regions involved in movement execution (e.g., premotor areas, M1, S1) (Deeley et al., 2013b). Reduced awareness of hand movement was associated with decreased activity in brain areas involved in bodily awareness (BA 7) and sensation (insula), suggesting a mechanism for the loss or narrowing of awareness reported in about half of patients with nonepileptic seizures (Brown et al., 2011), as well as other forms of dissociation.

Dissociative identity changes

In some forms of dissociative identity disorder and the similar phenomenon of "lucid possession" (Oesterreich, 1974), the subject is aware of the mental contents of an alternate personality or possessing agent but otherwise unable to control his or her speech or actions (Deeley et al., 2014). An experimental model of these experiences and attributions of control by another agent involved a suggestion of an engineer conducting research into limb movement. The engineer had found a way to enter the subject and control movement from within. The subject was aware of the thoughts and motives of this possessing agent but unable to control the hand movements produced by it. Suggested control by the external agent was associated with an increase in functional connectivity between M1 (a key movement implementation region) and BA 10, demonstrating functional coupling with brain regions involved in the representation of agency in experiences of loss of motor control to another agent (Deeley et al., 2014).

Complex automatisms and loss of awareness

Brain mechanisms for complex automatisms have been investigated in experiments employing suggestions for automatic writing, in which control of movement (hand writing) and thought (thinking of a sentence ending) is attributed to an engineer (Walsh et al., 2014, 2015b). An additional experimental condition involved loss of awareness for automatic writing. At a phenomenologic level the suggestions for external control were associated with a sense of reduced ownership as well as control for movement and thought (Walsh et al., 2014, 2015b). The experiments therefore modeled loss of control, ownership, and awareness of complex movement and thought. These experiential changes can occur in pathologic and culturally normative dissociative states, as well as alien control of movement and thought insertion occurring in schizophrenia. Loss of perceived control of movement and thought were associated with largely nonoverlapping changes in brain activity and connectivity. In the case of movement, involuntary hand writing was associated with increased activity of a left-lateralized cerebellar-parietal network. This is consistent with a "forward model" account, that increased activity in this network during involuntary movement reflects loss of the suppression of sensory processing of self-generated movement that accompanies voluntary actions (Blakemore et al., 2003; Frith, 2005). Thought insertion, by contrast, was associated with reduced activity in networks supporting language and self-related processing. However, in addition to these modality-specific changes in brain activity, both experiences involved a reduction in activity of left SMA and altered functional connectivity between SMA and brain regions involved in movement implementation and language processing respectively. Similar changes did not occur during a simulation condition.

Taken together, these results suggest that reduced SMA activity may represent a general mechanism for the experience of loss of control and ownership of thought and action, acting with distinct changes in brain function and connectivity that underpin specific features of each phenomenon. On this account the earlier experiment showing reduced connectivity between SMA and M1 during involuntary simple movement of a joystick was powered to detect changes in SMA connectivity but not activity (Deeley et al., 2013b). Reduction of SMA activity during involuntary simple movement can be tested in a follow-up study with a larger sample size.

A prediction arising from these symptom-modeling studies is that loss of perceived control for movement and thought in dissociative psychopathology and schizophrenia involves disruption of SMA activity and connectivity, even if the factors modulating this disruption are specific to each condition (Deeley et al., 2013b).

These findings illustrate the importance of a transdiagnostic approach when attempting to understand basic mechanisms involved in disruptions of agency. Also, loss of awareness for involuntary writing was associated with reduced activity of left-sided posterior cortical network including BA 7 (superior parietal lobule and precuneus), and posterior cingulate cortex, demonstrating overlapping brain processes in loss of awareness of both simple and complex movement (Deeley et al., 2013b; Walsh et al., under review).

Integrative models of functional and suggested phenomena

These brain imaging studies identify the immediate changes in brain activity underpinning specific changes in experience and behavior, but raise the question of how we should conceptualize the wider processes leading to these changes. In other words, how do ideas, or – in the language of cognitive neuroscience – mental representations such as concepts, images, memories, beliefs, and expectancies, alter brain function to produce functional symptoms or suggested alterations in experience?

Mesulam (1998) observed how "our highly edited subjective version of the world" is the product of extensive associative elaboration and modulation of sensory information across the processing hierarchy of the brain. Integrative theories of functional and suggested phenomena identify cognitive and brain processes which affect this "editing" of information before its presentation to conscious awareness as a late stage of processing (Brown and Oakley, 2004; Brown, 2006; Oakley, 1999a,b, 2009a,b; Bell et al., 2011; Brown et al., 2011). While these theories have undergone extensive development in response to refinement of general accounts of cognitive architecture and brain function, they share features in common. The contents of consciousness are viewed as a working model of the environment produced by the interpretation and organization of sensory data by information in memory (Oakley, 1999b; Brown et al., 2011). The working model guides behavioral responses to the environment. Routine behavior is controlled by learned cognition and action programs selected automatically with minimal conscious effort or awareness. Novel actions, by contrast, engage attention and a sense of effort and self-awareness. In both cases there is generally little or no introspective access to the selection of representations from memory that inform consciousness and behavior. This means that consciousness and behavior can be "distorted by disproportionately active material in memory, leaving us prone to both misperceptions and behaviors that conflict with goals in self-awareness" (Brown et al., 2011). In this view the content of "rogue representations" mobilized from memory informs functional symptoms and suggested effects, respectively. In the case of symptoms or suggested effects that involve disruptions of agency (such as paralysis or involuntary movements), the representations may not only establish an expectancy that a type of experience or behavior will occur, but critically that it is not self-caused – the difference between "your arm is rising" rather than "you are raising your arm" (Spanos and Gorassini, 1984; Brown and Oakley, 2004).

The content of "rogue" representations can have many sources. In the case of functional illness their content may be based on experiences of illness in oneself or others, cultural learning, or expectancies established by the verbal communications of healthcare providers. They may also assume different forms – imagery-based schemata, verbal representations, episodic memories, or cue-driven action programs based on associative learning. In the case of hypnosis, the representational content of suggestions is typically verbally encoded. However, posthypnotic suggestion can establish automatic response tendencies to internal or external cues which operate outside awareness. In many cases this may be closer to the cognitive processes generating functional symptoms.

The "rogue representations" underpinning functional symptoms may be cued by many psychologic processes – such as anxious anticipation of symptoms (as in the case of the young woman described by Reynolds (1869)); attention to and misinterpretation of bodily sensations; as well as social reinforcement in settings such as work, health, and social care, and personal relationships. The emphasis of integrative approaches on the influence of diverse mental representations and causal attributions on functional symptom formation is consistent with a recently proposed hierarchic Bayesian model of functional symptoms derived from computational neuroscience (Edwards et al., 2012). This model provides a detailed account of how prior beliefs interact with sensory processing across different levels of neural organization to generate functional motor and sensory symptoms (Edwards et al., 2012).

Emotional arousal or specific types of emotion are not present in hypnotic models of functional symptoms, which employ induction procedures that establish a state of relaxation. This recalls the finding that functional paralysis, but not suggested paralysis, is associated with modulation of VMPFC, interpreted as indicating affectively laden cognitive processing in functional but not suggested paralysis (Cojan et al., 2009b). However, it is only by convention that hypnotic induction procedures establish a state of emotional calm and relaxation. Suggestions reproducing affective and self-representational aspects of functional paralysis would be predicted to enlist VMPC (assuming these cognitive processes explain its engagement). In other words, to paraphrase Reynolds (1869), there is no inherent reason why suggestions should not only produce the ideas but also the ideas coupled with emotions that can elicit functional symptoms. The greatest challenge here may be to elicit verbal descriptions of the subjective experience of symptom onset in patients with functional symptoms that could then be modeled with hypnotic suggestions. This difficulty reflects the tendency of patents with functional disorders not to acknowledge psychologic factors in symptom onset, or indeed because the relevant psychologic processes may be hard to describe or largely operate outside conscious awareness.

RELATIONSHIPS BETWEEN FUNCTIONAL SYMPTOMS, SUGGESTIVE PROCESSES, AND HYPNOSIS

A prediction arising from hypnosis as a model for functional symptoms is that highly hypnotically responsive individuals should be more likely to develop functional symptoms. Some studies have shown an association between hypnotizability and a tendency to develop sensorimotor functional symptoms (Bliss, 1984; Moene et al., 2001; Roelofs et al., 2002a, b). Also, a recent study shows that hypnotizability is associated with susceptibility to the rubber-hand illusion (Walsh et al., 2015a). In this illusion the perceived location of a hand being stroked out of sight is mislocalized to the position of a rubber hand being stroked in view. The rubber hand acts as a nonverbal, visually based implicit suggestion. Greater susceptibility to the illusion in more hypnotically responsive individuals may indicate a more general responsiveness to nonverbal, implicit suggestive processes that contribute to functional symptoms – such as a symptom observed in another. Despite this, high hypnotic responsiveness (or, indeed, susceptibility to the rubber-hand illusion) may not be necessary for functional symptoms to arise (Popkirov et al., 2015; Ricciardi et al., 2016). This is not only because most people respond to at least some suggestions, but also because, irrespective of hypnotizability, individuals may be more responsive to the suggestive effects of a relevant illness representation under conditions of stress, trauma, social conflict, preoccupation, or other factors motivating symptom formation and the adoption of an illness role.

While the subjective experience of symptom formation in functional patients is difficult to access, there may be scope for eliciting patient descriptions based on psychologic treatment where trust with a therapist and self-reflection are established. Case histories of this kind could help determine whether there are "styles" of functional symptom formation, by analogy with "styles" of hypnotic responding that are associated with differing degrees of automaticity. Hypnotic subjects with a "concentrative" response style focus their attention of the content of the suggestion and tend to experience the suggested effects as "happening by themselves." By contrast, those with a "constructive" response style who engage in mental imagery have a greater awareness of actively contributing to the suggested effects – although once established, they are nevertheless experienced as involuntary and realistic (Brown and Oakley, 2004).

Cultural and historic variation in functional symptoms, as well as hypnosis, draws attention to how radical alterations in experience and behavior can conform to the content of mental representations (Deeley, 2003, 2013). For example, the widespread category of spirit possession is constituted by dissociative identity change, often accompanied by phenomena such as collapse, convulsions, paralysis, and aphonia (Rouget, 1985; Deeley, 1999). Research on "harmful" spirit possession following political violence shows cultural influences on dissociative responses to trauma (Igreja et al., 2010). Alternatively, some societies enlist powerfully suggestive ritual practices to induce and reverse forms of dissociation, such as spirit possession as part of healing or other socially valued experiences (Seligman and Kirmayer, 2008). Cross-cultural research is important because it extends understanding of the full range of functional and dissociative phenomena. It also reveals the suggestive effects of explicitly directive speech and actions and implicit social modeling outside hypnotic procedures, as well as the social and psychologic values attached to some forms of dissociation (Deeley, 2016). In terms of the explanatory model we are considering in this chapter, functional neurologic symptoms, other cultural forms of dissociation, and hypnosis all belong to an overarching category of "suggestive-dissociative phenomena." As such, research into one subtype should provide insights into the others.

One of the more obvious dissimilarities between functional symptoms and suggested effects relates to time scale. Functional symptoms presenting to health services usually (but not always) persist for much longer than hypnotically suggested effects – days to years, rather than minutes to hours. The persistence of functional symptoms may be due to psychologically relevant needs, but may also relate to secondary social, neurocognitive, and bodily adaptation that influence how the symptoms are maintained. Physical changes such as atrophy or contracture of a chronically underused limb are unlikely to be well modeled with suggestion.

From a neurocognitive perspective, chronicity of symptoms may be associated with changes in underlying mechanism. For example, in some cases there may be a transition from symptom maintenance based on representations derived from explicit memory (such as mental imagery of symptoms) to engagement of implicit associative learning (such as conditioned inhibition of limb movement countermanding an intention to move). Hypnotic suggestion could potentially be employed to model this kind of neurocognitive adaptation to symptom maintenance over extended time periods. Studies of this kind could help understand not only the range of neurocognitive mechanisms that can mediate functional symptoms, but also their potential temporal relationships.

CONCLUSION

In the 19th century it was recognized that neurologic symptoms could be caused by "morbid ideation" as well as organic lesions (Reynolds, 1869). The subsequent observation that hysteric symptoms could be produced and removed by hypnotic suggestion led Charcot to hypothesize that suggestion mediated the effects of ideas on functional symptoms through as yet unknown effects on brain activity. The advent of neuroimaging 100 years later revealed strikingly similar neural correlates in experiments matching functional symptoms with clinical analogs created by suggestion. Integrative models of suggested and functional symptoms regard these alterations in brain function as the endpoint of a broader set of changes in information processing due to suggestion. These accounts consider that suggestions alter experience by mobilizing internal representations from memory systems, and altering causal attributions, during preconscious processing which alters the content of what is provided to our highly edited subjective version of the world. "Suggestion" in this sense is a broad term which recognizes that representations underlying symptom formation can be embedded in a variety of cognitive processes (explicit or implicit memory, verbal or nonverbal) and be linked to a range of internal or external cues.

Future studies with closer symptom matching can test whether all brain correlates of functional symptoms can be reproduced in suggested analogs. This will require a more refined understanding of the phenomenology of functional symptom formation to guide symptom modeling with suggestion. Suggestion and fMRI have also been used to model functional symptoms such as involuntary movements, loss of awareness, identity change, and complex automatisms. While these functional symptoms have been little studied with neuroimaging – not least because of the problem of capturing symptoms in the scanner – the hypnotic models identify potential brain mechanisms for their functional counterparts and may inform their experimental study.

Perhaps the deeper significance of hypnosis as a model for functional symptoms is that hypnosis, as well as cultural and historic variation in functional symptoms, draws attention to how radical alterations in experience and behavior can conform to the content of prior mental representations through effects on cognition and brain function. Experimental study of functional symptoms and their suggested counterparts in hypnosis reveals the distinct and shared processes through which this can occur.

References

Bell V, Oakley DA, Halligan PW et al. (2011). Dissociation in hysteria and hypnosis: evidence from cognitive neuroscience. J Neurol Neurosurg Psychiatry 82 (3): 332–339.

Binet A, Féré C (1891). Animal magnetism, Kegan Paul, Trench, Trübner, London.

Blakemore SJ, Oakley DA, Frith CD (2003). Delusions of alien control in the normal brain. Neuropsychologia 41 (8): 1058–1067.

Bliss EL (1984). Hysteria and hypnosis. J Nerv Ment Dis 172 (4): 203–206.

Braffman W, Kirsch I (1999). Imaginative suggestibility and hypnotizability: an empirical analysis. J Pers Soc Psychol 77 (3): 578.

Brown RJ (2006). Different types of "dissociation" have different psychological mechanisms. J Trauma Dissociation 7 (4): 7–28.

Brown RJ, Oakley DA (2004). An integrative cognitive theory of hypnosis and high hypnotizability. In: High hypnotizability: Theoretical, experimental and clinical perspectives, pp. 152–186.

Brown RJ, Syed TU, Benbadis S et al. (2011). Psychogenic nonepileptic seizures. Epilepsy Behav 22 (1): 85–93.

Charcot JM (1889). Lectures on the Diseases of the Nervous System (Vol. 3), New Sydenham Society, London.

Charcot JM, Marie P (1892). Hysteria. In: DH Tuke (Ed.), Dictionary of psychological medicine, Churchill, London, UK.

Cojan Y, Waber L, Carruzzo A et al. (2009a). Motor inhibition in hysterical conversion paralysis. Neuroimage 47 (3): 1026–1037.

Cojan Y, Waber L, Schwartz S et al. (2009b). The brain under self-control: modulation of inhibitory and monitoring cortical networks during hypnotic paralysis. Neuron 62 (6): 862–875.

Deeley Q (1999). Ecological understandings of mental and physical illness. Philos Psychiatr Psychol 6 (2): 109–124.

Deeley Q (2003). Social, cognitive, and neural constraints on subjectivity and agency: implications for dissociative identity disorder. Philos Psychiatr Psychol 10 (2): 161–167.

Deeley Q (2013). Hypnosis. In: Encyclopedia of Sciences and Religions, Springer, Netherlands, pp. 1031–1036.

Deeley Q (2016). Transforming experience through the meditation and ritual of chod: insights from hypnosis research. In: A Raz, M Lifshiz (Eds.), Hypnosis and Meditation: towards an integrative science of conscious planes, Oxford University Press, Oxford.

Deeley Q, Oakley DA, Toone B et al. (2013a). The functional anatomy of suggested limb paralysis. Cortex 49 (2): 411–422.

Deeley Q, Walsh E, Oakley DA et al. (2013b). Using hypnotic suggestion to model loss of control and awareness of movements: an exploratory fMRI study. PLoS One 8 (10): e78324.

Deeley Q, Oakley DA, Walsh E et al. (2014). Modelling psychiatric and cultural possession phenomena with suggestion and fMRI. Cortex 53: 107–119.

Edwards MJ, Adams RA, Brown H et al. (2012). A Bayesian account of 'hysteria'. Brain 135 (11): 3495–3512.

Ellenberger HF (1994). The discovery of the unconscious: the history and evolution of dynamic psychiatry, Fontana Press, London.

Frith C (2005). The self in action: lessons from delusions of control. Conscious Cogn 14 (4): 752–770.

Halligan PW, Oakley DA (2014). Hypnosis and beyond: Exploring the broader domain of suggestion. Psychology of Consciousness: Theory, Research, and Practice 1 (2): 105.

Halligan PW, Athwal BS, Oakley DA et al. (2000). Imaging hypnotic paralysis: implications for conversion hysteria. Lancet 355 (9208): 986–987.

Harré R (2002). Cognitive science: a philosophical introduction, Sage, London.

Heap M, Alden P, Brown RJ et al. (2001). The nature of hypnosis: Report prepared by a working party at the request of the Professional Affairs Board of the British Psychological Society, British Psychological Society, Leicester.

Igreja V, Dias-Lambranca B, Hershey DA et al. (2010). The epidemiology of spirit possession in the aftermath of mass political violence in Mozambique. Soc Sci Med 71 (3): 592–599.

Janet P (1907). The major symptoms of hysteria. Classics of Psychiatry & Behavioral Sciences Library, Division of Gryphon Editions, New York.

Kirsch I (1990). Changing expectations: a key to effective psychotherapy, Brooks, Pacific Grove, CA.

Marshall JC, Halligan PW, Fink GR et al. (1997). The functional anatomy of a hysterical paralysis. Cognition 64 (1): B1–B8.

Mendelsohn A, Chalamish Y, Solomonovich A et al. (2008). Mesmerizing memories: brain substrates of episodic memory suppression in posthypnotic amnesia. Neuron 57 (1): 159–170.

Mesulam MM (1998). From sensation to cognition. Brain 121 (6): 1013–1052.

Moene FC, Spinhoven P, Hoogduin K et al. (2001). Hypnotizability, dissociation and trauma in patients with a conversion disorder: an exploratory study. Clin Psychol Psychother 8: 400–410.

Oakley DA (1999a). Hypnosis and conversion hysteria: a unifying model. Cogn Neuropsychiatry 4 (3): 243–265.

Oakley DA (1999b). Hypnosis and consciousness: a structural model. Contemp Hypn 16 (4): 215–223.

Oakley DA, Deeley Q, Halligan PW (2007). Hypnotic depth and response to suggestion under standardized conditions and during fMRI scanning. Int J Clin Exp Hypn 55 (1): 32–58.

Oesterreich TK (1974). Possession and exorcism, Causeway Books, New York. (first published 1921).

Popkirov S, Grönheit W, Wellmer J (2015). A systematic review of suggestive seizure induction for the diagnosis of psychogenic nonepileptic seizures. Seizure 31: 124–132.

Pyka M, Burgmer M, Lenzen T et al. (2011). Brain correlates of hypnotic paralysis – a resting-state fMRI study. Neuroimage 56 (4): 2173–2182.

Reynolds JR (1869). Remarks on paralysis, and other disorders of motion and sensation, dependent on idea. Br Med J 2 (462): 483.

Ricciardi L, Demartini B, Crucianelli L et al. (2016). Interoceptive awareness in patients with functional neurological symptoms. Biol Psychol 113 (2016): 68–74.

Roelofs K, Hoogduin KA, Keijsers GP et al. (2002a). Hypnotic susceptibility in patients with conversion disorder. J Abnorm Psychol 111: 390–395.

Roelofs K, Keijsers GP, Hoogduin KA et al. (2002b). Childhood abuse in patients with conversion disorder. Am J Psychiatry 159: 1908–1913.

Rouget G (1985). Music and trance: A theory of the relations between music and possession, University of Chicago Press, Chicago, IL.

Seligman R, Kirmayer LJ (2008). Dissociative experience and cultural neuroscience: Narrative, metaphor and mechanism. Cult Med Psychiatry 32 (1): 31–64.

Shor RE, Orne EC (1962). Harvard Group Scale of Hypnotic Susceptibility, Form A, Consulting Psychologists Press, Palo Alto, CA.

Spanos NP, Gorassini DR (1984). Structure of hypnotic test suggestions and attributions of responding involuntarily. J Pers Soc Psychol 46 (3): 688.

Walsh E, Mehta MA, Oakley DA et al. (2014). Using suggestion to model different types of automatic writing. Conscious Cogn 26: 24–36.

Walsh E, Guilmette DN, Longo MR et al. (2015a). Are you suggesting that's my hand? The relation between hypnotic suggestibility and the rubber hand illusion. Perception 44 (6): 709–723.

Walsh E, Oakley DA, Halligan PW et al. (2015b). The functional anatomy and connectivity of thought insertion and alien control of movement. Cortex 64: 380–393. Mar.

Walsh E, Oakley DA, Halligan PW et al. (under review). Brain mechanisms for loss of awareness of thought and movement.

Ward NS, Oakley DA, Frackowiak RSJ et al. (2003). Differential brain activations during intentionally simulated and subjectively experienced paralysis. Cogn Neuropsychiatry 8 (4): 295–312.

Weitzenhoffer AM (1980). Hypnotic susceptibility revisited. Am J Clin Hypn 22: 130–146.

Handbook of Clinical Neurology, Vol. 139 (3rd series)
Functional Neurologic Disorders
M. Hallett, J. Stone, and A. Carson, Editors
http://dx.doi.org/10.1016/B978-0-12-801772-2.00010-2

Chapter 10

Psychologic theories in functional neurologic disorders

A. CARSON*, L. LUDWIG, AND K. WELCH

Departments of Clinical Neurosciences and of Rehabilitation Medicine, NHS Lothian and Centre for Clinical Brain Sciences, University of Edinburgh, Edinburgh, UK

Abstract

In this chapter we review key psychologic theories that have been mooted as possible explanations for the etiology of functional neurologic symptoms, conversion disorder, and hysteria. We cover Freudian psychoanalysis and later object relations and attachment theories, social theories, illness behavior, classic and operant conditioning, social learning theory, self-regulation theory, cognitive-behavioral theories, and mindfulness. Dissociation and modern cognitive neuroscience theories are covered in other chapters in this series and, although of central importance, are omitted from this chapter. Our aim is an overview with the emphasis on breadth of coverage rather than depth.

INTRODUCTION

In this chapter we aim to provide a brief synopsis of the main psychologic and social theories that are described in the context of the study of functional neurologic disorder. This chapter is primarily aimed at clinicians with an interest in functional symptoms but without expert knowledge of these fields. We cover psychodynamic theories, learning theories, cognitive-behavioral theory, the sick role, illness behavior, and diagnostic operationalization. The descriptions are unashamedly a crib for the uncertain: the expert will find nothing new and perhaps only gain a sense of frustration that he or she could have described the terms better. Dissociation (including the work of Janet) and modern cognitive neuroscience theories are dealt with elsewhere in the book and are omitted.

PSYCHODYNAMIC THEORIES

Early psychodynamic theories were led by the ideas and writings of Sigmund Freud. He had a dominant personality and it may be no coincidence that his biographer Stafford-Clark (1967) describes Freud's early ambition as being a great general, like Hannibal. From the beginning there was a quasi-religious atmosphere to the development of his theories and early followers were invited to his Wednesday Club, where his was "the first and last word" (Freud, in a letter to Fleiss: quoted by Stafford-Clark, 1967).

The key tenet of Freudian therapy was that humans had a range of distressing or guilt-inducing thoughts and memories that were repressed and inaccessible to normal conscious thought but the associated emotions could still exert a psychic influence. In essence, what was being said was, that which cannot be remembered cannot be emotionally forgotten. The role of therapy was to bring both the thought and, critically, the feeling into the patient's conscious awareness. The notion, although in some ways originally expressed, was not dissimilar from previous theories of some form of driving forces present in the brain, often described as the passions, which in turn borrowed heavily on ideas of Galenic spirits and Newtonian mechanics.

Freud initially used hypnosis to try to release these repressed thoughts, but his breakthrough moment, described along with Joesph Breuer in *Studies on Hysteria*, was when he realized that talking alone could produce the same results. Initially he pressed his hand heavily on the patient's forehead but that too was soon forgotten – talking alone was enough. The classic vision

*Correspondence to: Dr. Alan Carson, MD MPhil FRCPsych FRCP, Robert Fergusson Unit, Royal Edinburgh Hospital, Morningside Terrace, Edinburgh EH10 5HF, UK. E-mail: a.carson@ed.ac.uk

is the patient lying on the couch staring into space with little to interfere with her flow of thought, but early psychoanalytic sessions were just as likely to happen on a long walk through the Viennese woods. The very airing of the thoughts and the experiencing of the emotions were held to have a cathartic effect. As Freud developed his theories, the discussion and interpretation of dreams, then free association, in which patients let their mind wander, reporting all thoughts regardless of triviality or sense of guilt or shame, became key techniques. With specific regard to hysteria:

> *the causal relation between the determining psychical trauma [trauma is taken from the Greek for wound] and the hysterical phenomenon is not of a kind implying that the trauma merely acts as an agent provocateur in releasing the symptom, which thereafter leads an independent existence. We must presume rather that the psychical trauma – or more precisely the memory of the trauma – acts like a foreign body which long after its entry must continue to be regarded as an agent that is still at work; and we find the evidence for this in a highly remarkable phenomenon which at the same time lends an important practical interest to our findings.*
>
> *For we found, to our great surprise at first, that each individual hysterical symptom immediately and permanently disappeared when we had succeeded in bringing clearly to light the memory of the event by which it was provoked and in arousing its accompanying affect, and when the patient had described that event in the greatest possible detail and had put the affect into words. Recollection without affect almost invariably produces no result (Breuer and Freud, preliminary communication, 1955).*

Central to this theory was the notion of the twin concepts of repression and resistance: "that the hysterical patient's 'not knowing' was in fact 'a not wanting to know' – a not wanting which might be to a greater or lesser extent conscious" (Breuer and Freud, 1955).

The role of therapy was: "by means of my psychical work I had to overcome a psychical force in patients which was opposed to the pathogenic ideas becoming conscious (being remembered)" (Breuer and Freud, 1955).

Freud acknowledged that at this stage "I cannot, I must confess, give any hint of how a conversion of this kind is brought about." However, in the preface to the second edition 10 years later, he commented that the "attentive reader will be able to detect in the present book the germs of all that has since been added to the theory of catharsis: for instance, the part played by psychosexual factors and infantilism, the importance of dreams and of unconscious symbolism" (Breuer and Freud, 1955).

However, Freud himself recognized the limitations of the treatment, if not the theory:

> *I do not maintain that I have actually got rid of all the hysterical symptoms that I have undertaken to influence by the cathartic method. But it is my opinion that the obstacles have lain in the personal circumstances of the patients and have not been due to any question of the theory (Breuer and Freud, 1955).*
>
> *I am justified in leaving these unsuccessful cases out of account in arriving at judgment, just as a surgeon disregards cases of death which occur under anaesthesia, owing to post-operational haemorrhage, accidental sepsis, etc. (Breuer and Freud, 1955).*

The further caution is added that treatment is for the actual functional symptom only and not the underlying predisposition. Furthermore, Freud felt that on a personal level he would be unable to treat anyone "who struck me as low-minded and repellent" and "the treatment not applicable at all below a certain level of intelligence." It should be highlighted that all the modern psychodynamic therapists known to the authors would completely reject these latter statements and find them offensive. However, both comments highlight ongoing debates that are current. Advocates of dynamic psychotherapy often differ from Freud himself and claim that intrinsically the treatment treats the underlying cause of the problem, not "just the symptoms." Critics would claim, on the basis of empiric evidence, that there is a bias in access to therapy towards the young, well educated, and Caucasian (Mind Report, 2013).

Although Freud always acknowledged that there would be neurobiologic underpinnings for his theories, he did not regard it, quite reasonably, as his role to uncover them. He concentrated instead on describing psychologic models. Although viewed as a criticism by some, it is worth noting this is no different from the approach of modern cognitive neuroscience, and if Freud had had access to functional magnetic resonance imaging and magnetoencephalography, his own approach to testing theories, at least in the early stages of his work, may well have been quite different. Among his core theories were:

- The topographic model: Freud's original psychologic model divided our psychologic structure into three areas: the unconscious, preconscious, and conscious. Although not actually articulated in the original *Studies on Hysteria* one can see it is based on this conceptual approach and remains the one most readily recognizable to clinicians today (Freud, 1953–1957, vol. XV).

- The structural model: on top of the topographic model was placed the structural model of id, ego, and superego. Freud himself did not use these terms but wrote of the "das Es," "das Ich," and "das Über-Ich": "the It," "the I," and "I above." The subsequent change to Latin was by his translator James Strachey. The "it" was the original drive state seen in the new infant and ungoverned by any awareness other than its own needs. From Freud's perspective it worked on the "pleasure principle," or the immediate gratification of its own needs and desire without concern for the consequences. Critically, in this state contrary impulses can exist side by side. The "I" brings with it socialization and the "reality principle." It works to delay the immediate impulse for gratification of needs in favor of a view of long-term benefit. The "I" allows the human to live and function in the real world where giving way solely to the "it" would lead to grief; the "it" contains the passions whereas the "I" judgment and common sense (Freud, 1953–1957, vol. XIV).
- The "I above" represents a more idealized, self-policing version of rules and cultural norms, viewed as an internalization of parental guidance. The "I" in Freud's model had to serve three masters – the passions of the "it," the rules of the "I above," and the real world – and still keep the person free from distress or anxiety. To assist it in this thankless task it employed a range of subterfuge and tricks to distort reality, known as defense mechanisms: denial, displacement, intellectualization, fantasy, compensation, projection, rationalization, reaction formation, regression, repression, and sublimation.

These structures were not mutually exclusive and compartmentalized but rather ran seamlessly into each other. Similarly, in the overlap with the topographic model, although the "it" was predominantly unconscious and the "I" conscious, the components of the structural model may exist in the conscious or the unconscious mind.

Transference and countertransference

The concept of transference was initially viewed by Freud as an impediment to the therapeutic process but was subsequently seen as a key tool in gaining an understanding of unconscious processes. Transference occurred when patients imbued in their doctor or therapist ideas, traits, or characteristics that were not based on the doctor's behavior but rather were unconscious representations of previous experiences or expectations, in turn often based on their relationships with their parents. Countertransference is the reverse, when the doctor/therapist imbues in the patient ideas, thoughts, or behaviors that relate to his or her own needs and desires. Arguably, these two concepts are ones that all doctors practicing in this area need to be most aware of. One can make sense of many failed doctor–patient relationships and the opposite, many heroic yet doomed attempts at, particularly surgical, treatment, through such a lens (Rycroft, 1995; Gay, 2006).

Primary and secondary gain

The primary gain was the development of the hysterical physic symptom which acted as a psychologic defense against these internal psychologic conflicts. The physical symptom in some way assisted in keeping the repressed thoughts or emotions repressed by allowing the dissipation of psychic energy. This was seen as the primary gain and is the origin of the term conversion. Of note, this does not mean that the patient cannot be externally distressed, anxious, or depressed, but refers solely to control of unconscious conflicts. Secondary gain, which can be either conscious or unconscious, refers to the external or material advantages of being ill, such as avoidance of some unwanted task or financial gain, and can apply across any illness (Rycroft, 1995; Gay, 2006).

Sexual theories

Freud initially postulated the seduction theory – that infantile sexual molestation caused such traumatic repressed memories that this was the main cause of adult hysterical neurosis (McCullough, 2001). Initially he presented no data to support the notion; it has been suggested that he felt, perhaps not unreasonably, that the notion may be too repellent for people to believe, although why he thought a lack of data would assist is unclear. In fact, the idea was not new and Paul Briquet, in his landmark monograph on hysteria, arguably the first case-control study in psychiatry, had conclusively demonstrated some 10 years earlier an association between sexual abuse and the development of hysteric symptoms (Carson and Stone, 2015). Freud however quickly became increasingly concerned by the theory. He viewed hysteric symptoms as increasingly common and held that such widespread perversions against children were unlikely. He replaced the original theory with one of infantile sexuality and phantasy (note in psychoanalytic speak that phantasies refer to infants' view of the world and fantasies normal daydreams). In this he felt that the repressed ideas of sexual molestation had their origins in fantasies, not reality. This led on to the idea of normal infant development passing through stages of oral, anal, phallic, latent, and genital stages, where the "it's" source of pleasure was derived primarily from stimulation of these regions, usually via normal processes such as eating and learning to defecate. Development could be arrested or corrupted.

From this model arose the now famous notion of the Oedipal complex (Rycroft, 1995). This occurs during the phallic stage of development, where the child develops a competitive relationship for one parent with the opposite-sex parent. It is resolved when the child identifies with the same-sex parent, incorporating that parent's image and values into his/her "I above." Within this lies the idea of choice: that the child has chosen to learn and accepts the benefit of abiding by values for both him/herself and the common good. By contrast, a failure to do so results in a pseudocompliance driven solely from a fear of punishment that results in an internal sense of distress and anguish.

The abandonment of the seduction theory has led to considerable, and justifiable, criticism and left a difficult legacy of many victims of molestation having the reality of the ordeal being denied (Masson, 1984). This is a difficult area and even today many of Freud's devoted followers struggle to acknowledge its consequences. At the time Freud was moving from a theory of hysteria as a synonym for a functional neurologic symptom to theory of general psychic distress, and to suggest that all psychic distress was secondary to child sexual abuse would be as ludicrous now as it seemed then. The lesson was, and it remains a valuable one today, that there may be more than one etiology behind common and varied phenomena; but Freud too needed to remember that (McCullough, 2001).

It is also unclear to what extent Freud's immediate colleagues genuinely believed these theories. Freud himself expressed his frustrations at this.

> *Not long ago Breuer made a big speech about me at the Doktorenkollegium, in which he announced his conversion to belief in the sexual aetiology. When I took him on one side to thank him for it, he destroyed my pleasure by saying: 'All the same I don't believe it.' Can you understand that? I can't (Freud in a letter to Fleiss, quoted in Stafford-Clark, 1967).*

It can be difficult to gauge whether these ideas had much of an impact on contemporary mainstream neurologic practice, even though the experience of treatment of shellshock in World War I was associated with universal acceptance and sophisticated understanding of the role of psychologic factors in the creation and maintenance of hysteric symptoms.

Symbolism

Symbolism, of all the Freudian theories, is perhaps the most widely recognized by the general public but unfortunately the hardest to nail down as to what was actually said or meant. It did not feature in his early work in the *Studies on Hysteria* but began to be articulated in the context of the interpretation of dreams. Dreams were viewed by Freud as a means of unlocking the closed world of the unconscious and in that context symbols were seen as a means of decoding the content of the dreams. As Freud developed his ideas over the course of his career, he became more interested in the use of symbols as a form of phylogentic inheritance, a universal language shared by all humans, as evidenced by a universal understanding and similarity of art and folk wisdom.

Whilst there is little doubt that there is a shared semiotic that is transcultural, it is difficult to know whether at the phantasy level Freud's ideas of a universal symbolism are true – does fear of beheading really represent fear of castration or is having one's head cut off scary in its own right? Part of the problem is that Freud's ideas are now so universal that the semiotic of a cigar as a phallus is generally held: but was it always thus?

With regard to hysteric symptoms, Freud's use of hysteria from a state of a conversion disorder as we would currently understand the condition to a more generalized neurotic state without the need for a physical symptom makes it hard to know exactly where symbolism fitted into his views on the formation of what we would now call a functional neurologic symptom. His immediate followers, most infamously Ferenczi, would relate it to a mix of sexual phantasies and fantasies; thus the woman with globus had a secret fear of fellatio – an idea widely and justly ridiculed. In the modern era therapists will often enthusiastically quote symbolism in a fairly direct way as involving a symbolic representation of the underlying psychologic fear in the display of the physical symptom as part of an illness "narrative." Thus the abused woman harboring repressed fantasies of stabbing her husband may develop a paralysis of her dominant arm. There is no scientific support for these notions but they are largely untestable owing to the very nature of symbolism as a symbol.

Object relations theory and attachment theory

After Freud's death, whilst the Second World War raged in Europe, a different war was raging in West London. A protracted and acrimonious series of scientific meetings were taking place at the British Psychoanalytical Society, the "controversial discussions," between the Viennese school led by Freud's daughter Anna, the supporters of Melanie Klein, and the Middle Group, later to be known as the Independent Group; at stake was the future direction of psychoanalysis. An uncomfortable tripartite approach was the outcome, the legacy of which was Anna Freud's theories holding particular influence in the USA, Klein in South America, and the Independents in the UK. For mainstream current medical practice it is perhaps the ideas arising from this Independent Group that survive to the current day, with Klein and both Freuds largely historic figures. The ideologic stance of the Independents was to not be constrained by ideology, but rather to use what worked.

Arguably, the key figure for modern psychodynamic theory was the relatively unknown Edinburgh analyst Ronald Fairbairn. Fairbairn was the first to wholly and publicly break with Freud's notion that the primary drive or libido of humans was the pleasure principle; in Fairbairn's view it was to form relationships to other humans. He gave the original description and coined the phrase object relations theory. The process started in infancy with the infant's attachment to his/her parents. The quality of the attachment formed to the parents was so strong and fundamental that it would shape the quality of future relationships throughout the lifespan. These relationships were internalized and formed a prototype for future relationships. This internalization was what Fairbairn referred to as "internal objects" – i.e., a relationship that existed in the person's thoughts. For the early infant it was not possible to initially tell who was doing what or to have a fully integrated view and the infant would relate to part objects – i.e., was the mother that fed the child the same mother who withheld food when it was desired in these early days? However, this realization that the part objects were one and the same person came with early maturation.

For those who had a healthy relationship with parents this would lead to a normal pattern of looking outwards and forming healthy relationships with real people or external objects that could fulfill a person's needs. By contrast, when the parental experience was poor and the parents unavailable to provide appropriate nurture and support, the child struggled to deal with this. He or she would solve it by simply accepting the responsive part of the parents as being real and a good object and internalize the unresponsive "unsatisfying object" as part of him- or herself. This was known as "splitting," where at a fantasy level the good and bad parts of the parental figures were kept separate and thus controlled, rather than dealing with the distressing problem of ambivalent feelings and recognition of good and bad points in the one person. At its worst, this process can be seen in abuse victims who carry the blame themselves for all that happened – what Fairbairn described as a "moral defence"; the idea being that this allowed them to perpetuate the inner fantasy that they had loving, nurturing parents.

From this came the acceptance that parents did not have to be infallible but simply "goodenough" – the oft-quoted phrase of Donald Winnicott, the unofficial leader of the Independent Group. Winnicott held that "the foundations of health are laid down by the ordinary mother in her ordinary loving care of her own baby." Often described as theoretically elusive, Winnicott spoke of a "true self" and a "false self"; the idea of sense of self being complex or, as Winnicott said, "a word like self…knows more than we do." The true self is a free-feeling, internal state, creative and alive. The false self is a public face made for acceptance. In an ordinarily healthy person the two will still coexist but their goals and values will be closely enough aligned that they will have no adverse effects. By contrast with poor early experience, the need to adopt an ever greater false self as a protection will be such that it dominates and smothers the true self, leaving a person feeling dead inside or "phoney" (Rodman, 2003).

Another member of this group, John Bowlby, emphasized the central role of attachment to this process (Bowlby, 1951). Attachment took place between infants and adults who were able to be sensitive to their need for social interaction and comfort. The infant, when dealing with any difficult, novel, or stressful situation, was viewed seeking a reduction in distress by being close to the adult. This was referred to as "proximity seeking" for the "attachment figure." It was considered to be an evolutionary protective mechanism. The key period for developing such attachment was between 6 months and 2 years. The adult's responses would be processed by the infant and developed into "internal working models" that would form the basis of attachment and emotions for future relationships. Infants would develop internal models to guide both their own behavior but also their expectation of the behavior of others. Unlike Freudian ideas, these theories have been subject to empiric and rigorous scientific research, both in humans and animal models, and whilst not all aspects of the theories can be tested, the basic tenet of the central and core need for attachment for human emotional development has been undeniably confirmed.

What has not been tested empirically, and remains a hypothesis, is how much, if at all, this maps on to functional symptoms. Fairbairn (1944) viewed the concepts of hysteria as being discovered by Janet with his description of dissociation. Fairbairn modified Janet's theories in line with his own theories of object relations psychology. In all of these theories, hysteric or conversion symptoms arose as a means of coping with the distress caused by interpersonal problems. As Fairbairn put it:

> *Hysterical conversion is of course a defensive technique – one designed to prevent the conscious emergence of emotional conflicts involving object-relationships. Its essential and distinctive feature is the substitution of a bodily state for a personal problem; and this substitution enables the personal problem as such to be ignored. All personal problems are basically problems involving personal relationships with significant objects; and the objects involved in the conflicts of the hysteric are essentially internal objects – and more specifically the exciting and frustrating objects (Fairbairn, 1954).*

Although a generalization, in the second half of the 20th century the psychoanalytic movement did not really appear to think of hysteria or functional neurologic symptoms from the perspective that we use in this book of a physical symptom to be explained, but rather as a psychologic mindset which may or may not be associated with a physical symptom. The result can often be a sense of comparing apples and oranges.

The social model

The 20th century was not solely about psychoanalysis. The discipline of sociology was also postulating important theoretic inroads. Foremost among them was Talcott Parsons' *The Social System* (1951). Parsons was an unapologetic theorist who conducted little empiric research, although he did not dismiss it. He was clearly influenced by the contemporary zeitgeist of psychoanalysis, but he thought that individual dynamic insights were of little value if viewed without the context of the wider social structures in which they were made. Parsons' primary consideration was what it meant to be sick. It should be noted he was not thinking specifically of functional disorders but of all ill health in general. He considered it inappropriate to be thinking of sickness in terms of "a condition" described by (psycho)pathophysiology; rather, it was a "prescribed role" that had a range of cultural rules and expectations and could not be considered without reference to this wider context. He argued that the test was "the existence of a set of institutionalized expectations and the corresponding sentiments and sanctions" (Parsons, 1951).

There were four aspects to the institutionalized expectation system relative to the sick role. First, the sick individual was exempt from his or her normal social responsibilities to a nature and extent relative to the degree of illness severity. This required legitimization and that came from a physician, who was thus placed in the role of arbiter. This was clearly a protection against "malingering" at a societal level. Second, the sick person could not be expected to get better simply by "pulling himself together", it was critical that the illness was due to "a condition," not an "attitude." Third, the sick person had to want to get better, and fourth, s/he had an obligation to seek "technically competent" help (Parsons, 1951). Parsons argued that, defined in this way, the sick role became the object of significant secondary gain, which the patient could be unconsciously motivated to secure. The problem for functional neurologic disorders was one of legitimization – symptoms could not be defined, nor accurately separated from malingering, except on a basis of trust. The sick role offered an explanation of the subjective overwhelming need in patients for a legitimizing diagnosis, as well as explaining a punitive attitude held by some doctors and society at large.

It also offers an interesting insight into doctors' responses to those who don't fit into the pre-prescribed roles. In discussing unnecessary surgery, Parsons quotes the ideas of Malinowski:

> *a pseudo-scientific element in the technical competence of the medical profession which is more than simply an expression of the relative lack of scientific development of the field; it is positively motivated...cluster about situations where there is an important uncertainty factor and where there are strong emotional interests in the success of the action...[such as]...gardening and deep sea fishing...[this form of] pseudo-science is the functional equivalent of magic in the modern medical field...it is to bolster the self-confidence of actors [surgeons] in situations where energy and skill do make a difference but because of uncertainty factors, outcome cannot be guaranteed. This suits both participants, i.e. doctor and patient (Parsons, 1951).*

ILLNESS BEHAVIOR

Further sociologic understanding of illness came from the work of David Mechanic. Mechanic had been stimulated by the work of Koos (1954), *The Health of Regionville*. Koos described the views on health of 500 families in a small American town. He made the striking discovery that people experienced many more symptoms than they presented to doctors with. That may seem rather obvious, but at the time it represented a radical challenge to the pathoanatomic medicine of the 19th and early 20th century (Armstrong, 1986). Mechanic attempted to explain this phenomenon in terms of illness behavior, which he defined as "the way in which given symptoms may be differentially perceived, evaluated and acted upon (or not acted upon) by different kinds of person" (Mechanic, 1962). Illness behavior could therefore be influenced by cultural, social, or sex-role expectations or may be subject to variation as a result of previous illness experiences, situational factors, or adaptive needs. The key factor was that different people would react differently to the same pathology, as a result of a diverse array of psychologic and social variables (Mechanic, 1977). It also offered a patient-centered view, and as such one that was directly applicable, rather than the societal-level view of the sick role which necessitated the reactions of others. Although the theory was predominantly centered around pathologic disease processes, it still influenced a significant shift from analytic thinking as it allowed, and validated, the patient's thoughts and previous experience rather than consigning them to unconscious sources of trauma.

ABNORMAL ILLNESS BEHAVIOR

Pilowsky (1969) recognized that, although Mechanic's theory was intended to be universal, the main concern was, in reality, the underreporting of symptoms. Pilowsky, through his interest in functional symptoms, was by contrast more concerned with those who overreported symptoms. Borrowing from Mechanic, he felt such patients may be best described as having abnormal illness behavior. Implicit within this definition lies the idea that functional symptoms could have a heterogeneous etiology. Pilowsky, himself, recommended physicians inquire into the nature of the somatic component of patients' symptoms, but also their ideation and affect, their attitude to others, their motivations, and any relevant cultural factors in order to understand the presentation. One potentially useful, but scientifically difficult, aspect of this concept was that it allowed for coexistence of both somatoform symptoms and pathologic disease.

Some have criticized this model as paternalistic and making a social judgment. This is articulated by Armstrong (1986), who criticizes these models for assuming that the doctor is at the rational center, and it is with the patient that the "problem" lies; rather than the limitations of medical theory and practice.

> *Put simply it is not the illness which brings the patient to see the doctor but the theory...Abnormal illness behaviour was invented to cope with a problem, namely symptoms without disease, which was medically incomprehensible. But is it patient behaviour which is "abnormal", "maladaptive", or just plain wrong, or is it medical theory itself which cannot adequately account for the phenomena it observes? Why is it that doctors react with such strong emotion, "hostility", or feeling hunted, to patients with symptoms but without an organic lesion? Is it not the doctor's response which is abnormal? (Armstrong, 1986).*

DIAGNOSTIC OPERATIONALIZATION

The psychodynamic school of thinking held influence over psychiatry through the first half of the 20th century. The idea of diagnoses drifted, judgments were made on patients on the basis of an individual analysis of the psychologic processes, which effectively allowed clinicians to describe someone as having a disease if they thought the person showed evidence of such thought processes. This mode of assessment became so extreme at one stage that one could have functional symptoms without actually having any physical complaints but just by thinking in the manner of someone who might.

To Samuel Guze, a psychiatrist in St. Louis, however, this was nonsensical and, one suspects, intolerable. He practiced psychiatry from the perspective of his background medical training looking for features of commonality between individual clinical presentations. In his seminal paper (Guze, 1967), he outlined his view that psychiatric diagnosis could be described by operationalized criteria according to the following underlying principles. He thought that a reliable and valid classification was the essential foundation for communication, teaching, comparison, and evaluation. He set out to describe this approach using hysteria as a model (Carson and Stone, 2015).

> *The diagnosis of a functional psychiatric illness may be considered if the patients do not develop features of a different illness, if they have a similar course, and if an increased prevalence of the same disorder is encountered among their relatives (Guze, 1967).*

This seemingly obvious approach was considered heretic when the dominant view of psychiatric disorder was of a highly idiosyncratic reaction to the particular circumstances of an individual's life. His group proposed a definition based solely on observed clinical features of multiple unexplained symptomatology: a minimum of 25 symptoms, including at least one neurologic symptom, distributed across a range of body systems with onset before age 35 without imposing any etiologic framework. They demonstrated that such diagnoses could be made accurately between clinicians and were stable over time. They found a familial aggregation and noted an association with antisocial personality disorder in familial clusters. They paid homage to Briquet's influential work and named the disorder after him.

The classification proposed by Guze has remained reliable but it is now recognized that "Briquet's syndrome" is a relatively rare and severe form of presentation of somatoform symptoms occurring in only 0.1–0.2% of the population, compared to a general-population prevalence of somatoform symptoms of 5–15%, depending on what definition is used.

The importance of Guze's contribution to the field was less his actual definition of Briquet's syndrome but more the underlying principle of his approach that patients could be objectively measured in terms of the presenting symptoms and clustered into groups in a meaningful way to allow quantitative measurement: a head-on collision with the psychodynamic zeitgeist of the era.

The influence of Guze's work extended far beyond functional symptoms and has come to dominate psychiatric practice. The methods he laid out for an operationalized approach to psychiatric diagnosis changed the landscape, and along with similar work he subsequently conducted on schizophrenia, and the UK–US diagnostic study on schizophrenia based on the same methods, led directly to *Diagnostic and Statistical Manual of Mental Disorders,* 3rd edition (DSM-III: American Psychiatric Association, 1980) and a whole new, and improved, era of psychiatric diagnosis.

Guze's influence on operationalized diagnosis for functional symptoms remains into the current revisions of DSM-5 (American Psychiatric Association, 2000).

LEARNING THEORIES

The mechanisms of how learning occurs are not only key to the understanding of human behavior in general, but also give insight into the ways in which maladaptive behaviors are established and with that an essential starting point for psychotherapy. The basic learning theories are briefly presented here. Their implications for cognitive-behavioral therapy (CBT), particularly in patients with functional neurologic symptoms, are discussed further below. A more detailed discussion can be found in Lieberman (2012).

Despite the ongoing debate on the extent of determinism versus free will, one of the basic assumptions in learning theory is that behavior is predictable and governed by biologic laws. In the 17th century, Descartes provided one of the first detailed physiologic explanations for human behavior, when proposing that reflexes are the basis for all automatic, involuntary reactions. His assumption that these reflexes were based on animal spirits flowing through the nerves was quickly falsified. However, he shaped the research that followed with his concept of the explicability of human behavior in a mechanistic way. The British Associationists, including John Locke, David Hume, and others, expanded on Descartes' ideas of movement based on association, but transferred this concept to mental processes. According to them, ideas are formed through the principle of association. When two sensations occurred together, they became associated and the strength of their association was assumed to depend on: (1) contiguity (how close in time are the events occurring together?); (2) frequency (how often are they occurring together?); and (3) intensity (how intense are the feelings that accompany these events?). These laws of association, postulated initially by Aristotle (≈300 BC), still provide the basis for modern learning theories. However, back then, these assumptions were solely based on introspection, and lacked an objective method for verification (Lieberman, 2012).

Classic conditioning

Almost two centuries later, Ivan Pavlov discovered, during his research on the physiology of the digestive system of dogs, an important objectifiable mechanism of learning, namely classic conditioning. He observed that dogs not only salivated when food was presented to them, but also in other specific and related situations, such as when the regular feeder entered the room. Salivation was found by Pavlov to be an automatic, reflexive response that is normally elicited by contact of the mouth with food. That this response could apparently be evoked also by other stimuli, and the notion that there must be an underlying law to predict this behavior, was fascinating to him and led to a number of experimental investigations, using physiologic methods in a highly controlled laboratory environment in order to understand this psychologic phenomenon. In the typical experiment a dog learns to salivate solely by the sound of a bell which was previously presented together with food. Before this association has been formed, salivation is the only reflexive response towards the presentation of food. Therefore, the presentation of food acts as an unconditioned stimulus (US) causing salivation as its innate unconditioned response (UR). The sound of the bell, on the contrary, is initially a neutral stimulus (conditioned stimulus, CS) to the extent that it does not elicit salivation on its own and also does not suppress it either. The conditioning takes place when the tone is paired with the food in the course of the experiment. Gradually, the dog learns to respond to the CS with salivation. This response is the result of the conditioning that took place over a number of paired presentations of US and CS, and is called conditioned response (CR).

Such conditioning can occur over multiple exposures or during a single event if the experience is sufficiently aversive. Many of us will have experienced single-event aversive conditioning during a bout of food poisoning. When we are re-exposed to the food we associate with our episode of sickness, we will often feel nauseated and unable to eat it. Of note, it does not have to be the food that actually caused the problem, but simply the food that the subject associates mentally with the problem, often the most recent meal rather than necessarily the true culprit. Panic can be a potent cause/response of single-event conditioning.

In the maintenance/manifestation of dissociative (functional) seizures classic conditioning, mediated via panic as the CR, is suspected to yield a possible explanation in some patients. This hypothesis is supported by the two clinical experiences. One, the first seizure experienced is often more typical of a simple faint, but occurring in a situation that may have been paired with agoraphobic anxieties, i.e., a busy bar or similar. The second observation is that many subsequent seizures occur without an identifiable warning or an obvious trigger. In those cases the seizures are assumed to be triggered by slight emotional fluctuations or neutral stimuli through conditioning mediated by panic (Roberts and Reuber, 2014). This would be in accordance with a finding by Reuber et al. (2011), who reported that more patients experience their seizures as always coming "out of the blue" than occurring due to emotional stress. In some patients with functional movement disorders a link to physical triggers is suggested. Pareés et al. (2014) found that 38% of those patients with a physical triggering event such as mild physical trauma also fulfilled the criteria for a panic attack at the time of the event. Given the role of the amygdala in fear conditioning (Hitchcock and Davis, 1986), the authors concluded that panic may be a potent conditioning factor in the development of the symptoms.

Operant conditioning

While Pavlov combined two stimuli in order to build an association, Thorndike postulated in his *Law of Effect* (1898, 1911) a mechanism of learning based on the contingency between a response and a stimulus. He basically showed how a specific response is learned/likely to recur if it produces a favorable outcome or satisfaction. This is termed reinforcement and was investigated within a number of experiments. Skinner, who was a learning theorist and very influential in animal learning research, developed the so-called Skinner box, in which the animal under testing could be presented with stimuli and then make choices and gain rewards. For example, when a red light shines if a lever is pressed, a food pellet is gained, but not if the lever is pressed in response to a green light (Schacter et al., 2011). Hence, once conditioned, the animal will manifest behavior (lever press) to the red light, but not to the green light. Operant conditioning in the case of functional symptoms will often concern steps taken to avoid the physical manifestations of anxiety. The subsequent avoidance paradoxically serves to promote and reinforce anxiety. Typical operant conditioning includes a fear of falls, leading to mobilizing only when holding on to furniture or walls, or agoraphobic-like symptoms where all physical symptoms come on shortly after leaving the house.

Conditioning, whether classic or operant, might in some cases contribute to the development and maintenance of functional symptoms, and should then be shared as one part of an explanatory model with the patient. Clearly, this does not yield a full etiologic explanation. Behavioral conceptualizations with a too-narrow view may potentially be even harmful or offending when emphasis is placed on reinforcement of sick-role behavior. However, knowledge and use of these learning concepts as part of a broader treatment are likely to be beneficial in the treatment of functional symptoms, such as the extinction of maladaptive behaviors promoting alternative responses to warning signals and also changing behavior and cognitions that perpetuate the symptoms (such as agoraphobic avoidance (Goldstein and Mellers, 2006) and negative thoughts (Goldstein et al., 2015)).

The role of operant conditioning factors in the development, maintenance, but also in the treatment of functional neurologic symptoms has been discussed by several authors. Viewed purely as operational conditioning it is quite rare but it is more common as an integrated part of CBT, described below. A "controlled" single-subject design study was presented by Mizes back in 1985, describing the use of contingent reinforcement in the treatment of a young patient with functional weakness. Behavioral changes, such as gradually lifting the weak leg, were dependent on how powerful the rewards were. Facing the fact that gains were made initially but were not maintained, the author discusses potential harmful countereffects of social reinforcement of a sick role. Klonoff and Moore (1986) used monitored electromyogram signals as biofeedback in 2 functional motor patients in order to cause symptom change so that this could then be systematically reinforced. As well as the direct reinforcement of success on the biofeedback, further operant conditioning took place in that conversations which did not discuss symptoms were positively reinforced by praise and attention from the nursing staff and in a second phase by the parents as well. Both patients seem to have benefitted. These two studies demonstrate how operant conditioning has been used in this patient group; however, reviewing the literature indicates a lack of randomized controlled trials that would support this approach as an isolated treatment.

The concept of reinforcement has also been used as a treatment principle in physiotherapy in functional motor symptoms by a couple of studies, summarized in a systematic review on physiotherapy by Nielsen et al. (2013). The minimization of reinforcement of abnormal movement and maladaptive behaviors was eventually incorporated by Nielsen et al. (2015) in their consensus recommendation for physiotherapy in functional symptoms. One can view reinforcement in this context as both the positive reinforcement of being ill, i.e., medical attendants or relatives paying more attention to someone who is more unwell and less attention as the person improves, and negative reinforcement, which is the removal of an unpleasant stimulus encouraging a maladaptive behavior, i.e., if the patient tries to mobilize he/she gets an increase in pain and anxiety, whereas by staying in bed this is avoided.

Social learning theory

While psychodynamic theories depicted behavior as a result of inner drives, behaviorists focused on the other extreme, eschewing inner causes and postulating that behavior is solely environmentally determined, denying any sort of power of self-direction. The social learning theory by Albert Bandura expands on these behaviorist concepts, but emphasizes cognition as the foundation of learning (Bandura, 1971). The internal processes which happen in a social context are considered crucial. According to the theory, learning therefore occurs not only through direct reinforcement but through observational learning when behavior is simply observed, and indirectly through observation of rewards and punishments (vicarious reinforcement). One of Bandura's most famous experiments investigated how children's behavior changes after they have watched an adult model acting aggressively towards a doll, depending on whether the adult model got punished, rewarded, or experienced no consequence for beating the doll.

Within the social learning theory and its emphasis on self-regulatory processes, Bandura also coined the term self-efficacy – a psychologic construct defined as belief in the ability to succeed in specific tasks or situations based on one's own competencies, even if facing obstacles. The locus of control is defined by the extent to which a person ascribes events and actions to internal factors (e.g., own behavior, characteristics) or to external factors (e.g., chance, other people). Great importance is attached to these concepts in health psychology as a determinant of health behavior and the strengthening of self-efficacy and an appropriate internal locus of control are often key elements of psychotherapy.

Cohen et al. (2014) found that distress and also the locus of control predicted higher levels of dissociative symptoms in patients with nonepileptic seizures with stronger perceived external control by others and a weaker perceived control by doctors being associated with higher levels of dissociation. Self-efficacy, despite being frequently discussed, had no predictive power in this particular study and has – to the knowledge of the authors – not been extensively researched in the context of functional symptoms. Stone et al. (2004) found that patients with nonepileptic seizures have a more external locus of control, experiencing seizures as unpredictable and out of their control, than those with epilepsy. Targeting beliefs about locus of control may therefore yield fruitful possibilities for psychotherapy in these patients. To a certain extent this is an essential component of any behavior change, whether or not one labels it formally as a locus of control.

Self-regulation theory

Following the belief that cognitions underlie human behavior, Leventhal and colleagues provided an influential theoretic framework which suggests that it is individuals' illness beliefs, in other words, their cognitive representation of the illness, that will influence the coping strategies applied and the appraisal of their efficacy (Cameron and Leventhal, 2003). Based on this theory the Illness Perception Questionnaire (IPQ) was developed, in which illness representations are assumed to be based on five distinct elements: identity (associated symptoms), cause, consequences (effects on life), timeline, and cure/control (Weinman et al., 1996). Discrepancy between the patient's health belief and the given health advice are likely to influence adherence to treatment and may present potential illness-perpetuating factors. Thus a patient may have a strong belief that he has a demyelinating illness as an explanation for functional paralysis and may have researched information on this on the internet; when a doctor says there is no neurologic disease, this fails to match with the patient's internal model and is rejected and the patient seeks further opinions or tests. However, if a doctor understands the components of why the patient has come to this conclusion based on asking about these five factors (Table 10.1) and can tailor her explanation of the complaint around the patient's constructs, but modifying them in the process, this may lead to a much more successful consultation, modification of the patient's underlying beliefs to accommodate this new information, and subsequent treatment adherence.

In patients with functional neurologic symptoms, illness beliefs are considered to play an important role (Sharpe et al., 2010; Edwards et al., 2012). Application of Leventhal's self-regulation theory to functional neurologic symptoms has been scarce but increased over the last years. One striking finding was that functional patients compared with equally disabling neurologic diseases (such as epilepsy or multiple sclerosis) often share quite similar beliefs about the impact of their illness, whereas functional patients are more likely to reject

Table 10.1

The common-sense model of illness regulation (after the work of Leventhal and Weinman)

Element	Cognition	Distortions
Identity	What are these symptoms?	Symptoms cause labels But labels also lead to the self-generation of symptoms
Cause	What caused these symptoms?	
Consequences	What effects will the symptoms have on my life?	Cog representations guide subsequent behaviour; i.e., if patients believe symptoms brought on by overactivity, they may engage in excessive rest which will exacerbate fatigue
Timeline	How long will the symptoms last?	
Cure and control	What will help make the symptoms better?	Change in symptoms provides feedback on coping strategies and may result in reappraisal of symptoms or adoption of maladaptive strategies, i.e., pain on activity leading to increased down time

psychologic factors as relevant to their illness (Stone et al., 2004, 2010; Ludwig et al., 2015). Further discrepancies in illness beliefs were found between nonepileptic seizure patients and their neurologists (Whitehead et al., 2013). The findings suggested a mismatch between the assumed cause of the illness as well as in regard to beliefs about the personal control.

Cognitive-behavioral therapy

CBT is a combination of concepts and techniques taken from cognitive and behavioral therapies. Behavioral therapy, developed originally from learning theory, suggests that how we behave depends on previous learned experiences and the processes of classic and operant conditioning. Therapy aims to relieve symptoms by changing behavior and the environmental factors that control behavior. By contrast, cognitive therapy aims to identify and modify patterns of negative automatic thinking. These approaches were combined into CBT in the 1960s and 1970s by Aaron T. Beck, who promoted the treatment and demonstrated efficacy for depression (Rush et al., 1977). The underlying idea was not, however, new: Stoic philosopher Epictetus recognized the link between events, thoughts, and emotions long before then, reportedly stating in the second century: "People are disturbed not by things, but by the view which they take of them."

The central idea of a person's percepts as a unique subjective experience was emphasized by Kant: "certain internal sensations which are not the expression of real disease cause nonetheless great anxiety about having one."

Kant went on to explain that humans have the characteristic of magnifying a sensation by concentrating upon it (Kant, 1800). This was formalized into a form of therapy based on rational persuasion developed by Swiss family physician Paul Dubois.

These central observations, expanded to emphasize that physiology and behavior are also interlinked with thoughts, emotions, and life circumstances, are the foundation upon which CBT is built. An example of how these intertwined experiences can interact to produce progressively worsening symptoms is illustrated by the cross-sectional CBT formulation in Figure 10.1. An important implication is that (though inadvertent), patients' solutions to their difficulties are actually the problem, maintaining symptoms, distress, and handicap.

CBT is a structured, problem-focused intervention. The therapist uses Socratic questioning to support patients to develop their own hypotheses regarding problems, explore assumptions and contradictions, and try to generate potential solutions. Most of the actual process of treatment takes place without therapy sessions, this being facilitated by planning and reviewing homework. In contrast to psychodynamic therapy, the therapist is open and explicit about the approaches being used.

Reflecting its intermingling of cognitive and behavioral theories, a CBT model of functional neurologic symptoms posits that the processes of classic and operant conditioning and emotional arousal interact with an individual's pre-existing conceptualization of illness to give rise to symptoms. In some individuals vulnerabilities such as early maladaptive experiences influencing unconscious processing of health-related information may be relevant, but this is not universal. Dissociation (discussed further in Chapter 8) is thought to be an important process in how symptom representations in memory can be expressed as physical symptoms (Brown, 2013). Once manifest, symptoms are perpetuated by unhelpful illness beliefs and counterproductive coping behaviors (safety behaviors, avoidance, symptom vigilance, and monitoring), which interact with the participant's emotional and physiologic state and interpersonal situation to form self-perpetuating vicious cycles of symptoms and disability. A proposed model is outlined in Figure 10.2.

Therapy aims to bring about improvement by addressing maintaining factors. This generally includes

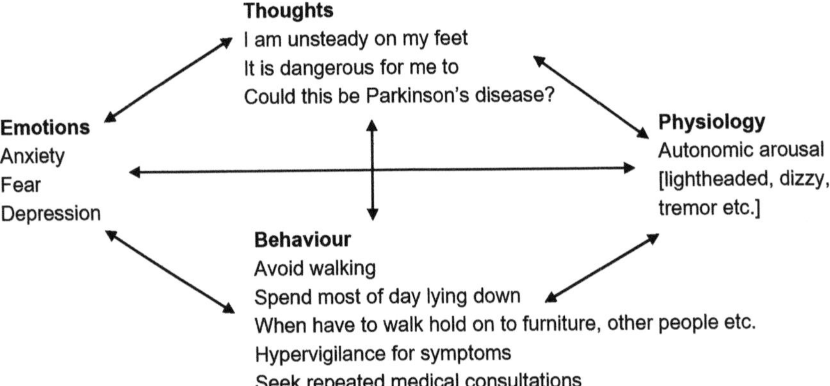

Fig. 10.1. Model formulation for maintaining processes in a patient with functional balance problems.

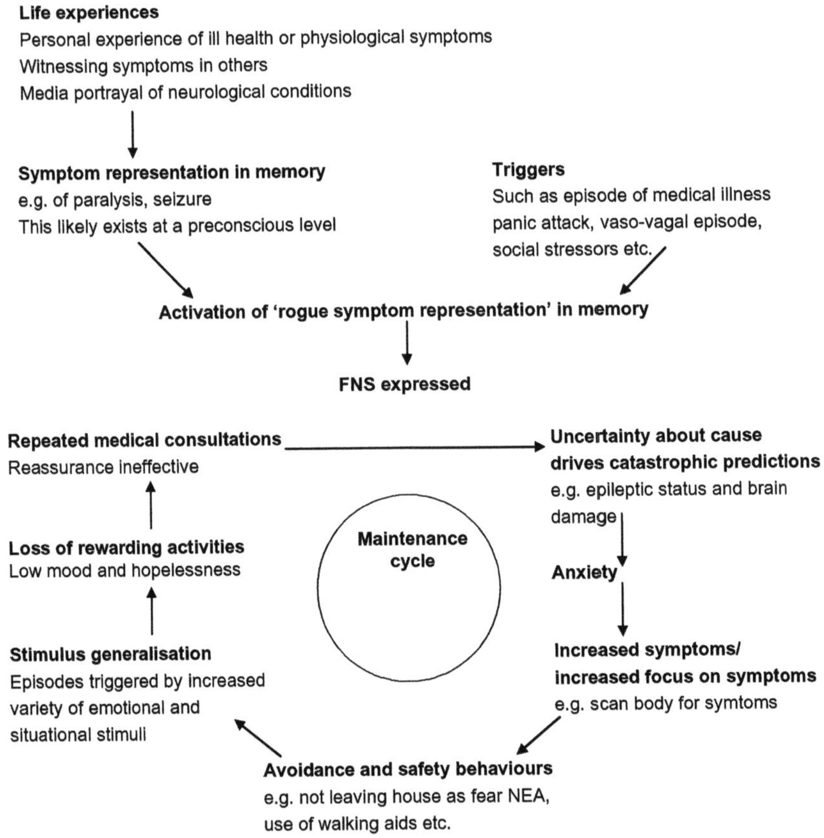

Fig. 10.2. Potential CBT formulation for how FNS come about and are maintained. (Influenced by Brown, 2013.)

changing unhelpful beliefs, teaching the patient relaxation techniques to manage anxiety, and replacing behaviors maintaining symptoms with ones fostering recovery.

Treatment begins with eliciting patients' own model of illness to establish what erroneous or otherwise unhelpful health beliefs they hold, and how they appraise and cope with their situation. Ideally, a neurologist has already provided an alternative, plausible, and hopefully acceptable explanation for symptoms. Research is limited here, but an explanation based on mechanism rather than cause, emphasizing "functional" disruption, for example, using the analogy of a computer in which the hardware is fine but the software crashes, is often adequate initially (Stone et al., 2005). An emphasis on the positive findings supportive of a diagnosis of functional symptoms makes such an explanation credible, and these can be referred to (and even re-elicited) in subsequent discussions. If done effectively, this explanation undermines the common and frightening conviction that symptoms reflect unidentified underlying pathology. These beliefs both directly cause distress (with its associated emotional arousal and physiologic symptoms) and promote the process of aberrant attentional focus on the body believed so important in producing and maintaining functional neurologic symptoms. The explanation also provides a rationale for CBT as an appropriate treatment and logically leads to identifying and attempting to address maintaining factors. On this basis, a shared multifactorial understanding of their illness, focusing on the "here and now," but exploring if previous life events can explain the origins of beliefs and behaviors can be formulated. Of course, despite these efforts, patients often remain convinced they have a pathophysiologically based rather than functional condition. This should not preclude treatment, and these patients may still benefit from CBT.

It is important that the initial assessment details current level of functioning. As well as providing a baseline from which to build activity levels, a focus on what the patient is doing to cope with symptoms and what changes in activities have occurred since symptom onset can reveal the extent of avoidance and associated maintaining factors. These often include well-meaning but damaging facilitation of avoidance by family members or even formal carers, and unhelpful use of the healthcare system and medications. Following their identification, treatment aims to collaboratively address maintaining factors. Given they have prevented feared exposures (to situations, thoughts, or emotions), avoidance and safety behaviors have been intensely reinforced and are daunting for the patient to address. This is openly acknowledged, and patients are provided with attentional refocusing and/or relaxation techniques to support them in taking this step. The patient is warned that, as exposure begins, symptoms may transiently worsen, but this is a crucial step to improving function. A program to address avoided exposures is then agreed, the nature of this program varying depending on the specific symptoms being addressed. In patients with functional balance problems the target may be addressing the safety behavior of touching walls or holding on to furniture as they walk; in the patient with nonepileptic attacks it may be not leaving the house alone for fear of having a seizure; in the patient with functional tremor it may be actively using the affected hand in day-to-day activities.

Often a graded exposure program must be devised, specific behaviors being rated by how challenging/anxiety provoking they seem and the program beginning with activities which, though daunting, are not completely overwhelming. Each exposure must be repeated regularly until the anxiety/symptom experience associated with it has diminished by at least 50%; the patient can then progress to the next step in the hierarchy. Fundamental to the success of this treatment is that the activity is engaged in long enough for anxiety to diminish. If the duration of exposure is insufficient for this to occur, it will simply further sensitize the patient and potentially worsen symptoms.

While some patients will respond to an explanation of the model and a simple program of activity scheduling, many require unhelpful health beliefs to be explicitly addressed before improvement is seen. Various approaches such as behavioral experiments and symptom-monitoring charts (thought records) can facilitate this process (Table 10.2). The latter technique is useful for eliciting negative automatic thoughts; these are automatic appraisals of events which influence moment-to-moment symptom experience and reflect pervasive health (or more general) beliefs. In some patients addressing avoidance will itself result in reappraisal of negative automatic thoughts. For example, the fact they were not robbed despite having a nonepileptic attack in the supermarket undermines the conviction they can't leave the house in case this occurs. In other patients, however, the thoughts maintaining avoidance will need direct work before progress can be made. This will necessitate eliciting the automatic thoughts as accurately as possible, examining the evidence for and against them, and constructing more balanced thoughts that incorporate all the evidence available. The original thoughts have generally been greatly influenced by thinking errors (such as catastrophizing, generalizations, or perfectionism) whereas the balanced thoughts are not; consequently they are not associated with the same negative affect, and are less of a barrier to the proposed exposure.

As avoidance reduces and engagement in activities increases, a virtuous self-reinforcing cycle can quickly lead to considerable improvement in function. A major strength of CBT, deriving from the open and explicit manner in which techniques are introduced, is that treatment will ideally result in participants becoming expert in managing their problems. Consequently, by the end of treatment they are able to maintain and build on their progress.

It may that during the course of treatment other psychologic symptoms such as panic, depression, posttraumatic stress disorder, or personality disorder become evident. Alternatively the patient may have specific skills deficits, such as in assertiveness or sleep hygiene. CBT can help with these difficulties, and, if present, treatment of

Table 10.2

Commonly encountered CBT techniques

Guided discovery (or Socratic questioning)	Constructing questions in a manner which helps patients clarify their thoughts and beliefs. The aim is to help clients to work out alternative ways of looking at things and to test out the usefulness of new perspectives for themselves.
Behavioural assessment	Collation of information about activities engaged in currently and in the past. Want to establish both activities patient is currently engaging in and what they are avoiding.
Activity record	Prospective record compiled by the patient of activities. The patient is often asked to record intensity of symptom experience during each activity. This can help to identify activities associated with improvement or worsening of symptom experience.
Activity scheduling	A basic technique often used early in CBT to programme pleasant or satisfying activities and improve mood. It is however a fundamental part of the treatment of FNS, in which avoided activities must be identified and specifically programmed. The consequent increase in positive interactions with the world will itself improve feelings of wellbeing and sense of productivity. In essence pathogenic contingencies of reinforcement are replaced with salutary ones. If fatigue is prominent activities should be planned to gradually increase as stamina improves to prevent precipitating aversive post-exertional fatigue.
Exposure plus response prevention	Exposure to feared/triggering stimuli without escape or avoidance. Through habituation and extinction the exposure loses ability to trigger symptoms.
Graded exposure	Increasing exposure to avoided, anxiety-inducing stimulus in a planned, gradually increasing way. For therapeutic benefit the discomfort associated with a planned level of exposure must be tolerable, or it will simply result in escape/avoidance. Increases in intensity of exposure only occur when the patient has sufficiently de-sensitised to the current level of exposure such that it leads only to modest levels of anxiety.
Behavioural experiment	Planned intervention to gather information about consequences of changing a particular behaviour. They are used to test and modify dysfunctional beliefs. An example of how a behavioural experiment may be used could be to test the consequences of not sitting down as soon as they feel dizzy, but instead keep walking for five minutes to see what happens. They note what happens and then reflect on the implications of this for thinking and behaviour.
Problem solving	Structured process to identify the problems to be solved and the steps a person might take to try to solve them. It includes outlining the pros and cons of each potential option to help decide on and plan a specific course of action. Most people do not lack problem-solving skills, but they may be avoiding their problems.
Functional analysis	A process for clarifying what is maintaining behaviours which involves looking at their triggers and consequences.
Relaxation training	Approaches which aim to lower physiological arousal. Diaphragmatic breathing and progressive muscle relaxation (sequentially tensing and then relaxing all the muscle groups of the body) are most commonly used.
Symptom monitoring form (or thought record)	Form on which symptoms are monitored together with the situation the patient is in and associated emotions and thoughts. They gather information on potential triggers for symptoms as well as gathering information about (often catastrophic) thoughts and provide the patient with practice in recognising the emotions they experience.

conditions such as panic attacks or low mood will likely be important for improvement in functional neurologic symptoms to occur. More enduring problems (such as severe posttraumatic stress disorder or the sequelae of childhood sexual abuse) may require referral to practitioners with particular expertise in treating these conditions.

MINDFULNESS

In the late 1980s a new group of therapies based on acceptance rose to prominence. Mindfulness, derived from traditional Buddhist practice and based around the regular practice of meditation, was prominent amongst these. A core goal of mindfulness is to develop metacognitive awareness, which is the ability to experience cognitions and emotions as mental events that pass through the mind and may or may not be related to external reality. The focus is not to change "dysfunctional" thoughts, but to learn to experience them as internal events separated from the self (Segal et al., 2012). As a key aim of treatment of functional neurologic symptoms is for patients to develop the ability to tolerate symptoms whilst not letting them dictate behavior, it has been suggested that these approaches may have particular utility for this patient group (Baslet et al., 2015; Detert, 2015). Whilst currently very popular, the efficacy of mindfulness remains to be properly tested. A note of caution should be sounded, as in other fields of anxiety and depression, randomized trials, as opposed to case series, of mindfulness-based CBT are not showing improved outcomes compared to traditional CBT practice, although the quality of studies is in general low, preventing a definitive statement of mindfulness's utility being made (Hofmann et al., 2010; Hunot et al., 2013).

CONCLUSIONS

A range of psychologic theories have been proffered over the years to attempt to explain functional symptoms. No comprehensive explanatory framework exists and most have significant limitations. One can see helpful elements within the majority of theories, but one is equally reminded that anyone who thinks s/he holds all the answers psychologically or that a single theory is explanatory is probably woefully naive.

References

American Psychiatric Association (1980). Diagnostic and statistical manual of mental disorders (3rd ed., text rev.), American Psychiatric Association, Washington, DC.

American Psychiatric Association (2000). Diagnostic and statistical manual of mental disorders (4th ed., text rev.), American Psychiatric Association, Washington, DC.

Armstrong D (1986). Illness behaviour revisited. In: Proceedings of the 15th European Conference on Psychosomatic Research, Libbey, London.

Bandura A (1971). Social learning theory, General Learning Press, New York.

Baslet G, Dworetzky B, Perez DL et al. (2015). Treatment of psychogenic nonepileptic seizures: updated review and findings from a mindfulness-based intervention case series. Clin EEG Neurosci 46: 54–64.

Bowlby J (1951). Maternal care and mental health. Bull WHO 3: 355–534.

Breuer J, Freud S (1955). Studies on Hysteria. Translated from the German, In: J Strachey (Ed.), The Standard Edition of the Complete Psychological Works of Sigmund Freud, Vol. II. Hogarth Press, London.

Brown RJ (2013). Dissociation and somatoform disorders. In: F Kennedy, H Kennerley, D Pearson (Eds.), Cognitive Behavioural Approaches to the Understanding and Treatment of Dissociation, Routledge, Abingdon, UK, pp. 133–138.

Cameron LD, Leventhal H (2003). The Self-regulation of Health and Illness Behaviour, Routledge, London.

Carson A, Stone J (2015). Functional symptoms. In: M Turner, M Kiernan (Eds.), Landmark papers in Neurology, Oxford University Press, Oxford.

Cohen ML, Testa SM, Pritchard JM et al. (2014). Overlap between dissociation and other psychological characteristics in patients with psychogenic nonepileptic seizures. Epilepsy Behav 34: 47–49.

Detert NB (2015). Mindfulness for neurologists. Pract Neurol 15 (5): 369–374.

Edwards MJ, Adams RA, Brown H et al. (2012). A Bayesian account of 'hysteria'. Brain 135: 3495–3512.

Fairbairn WRD (1944). Endopsychic structure considered in terms of object-relationships. Int J Psychoanal 25: 70–92.

Fairbairn WRD (1954). Observations on the nature of hysterical states. Br J Med Psychol 27: 105–125.

Freud S (1953–1957) (edited and transl. Strachey J), The Standard Edition of the Complete Psychological Works of Sigmund Freud. London: Hogarth Press and the Institute of Psycho-Analysis.

Gay P (2006). Freud: A Life for Our Time, W. W. Norton, London.

Goldstein LH, Mellers JDC (2006). Ictal symptoms of anxiety, avoidance behaviour, and dissociation in patients with dissociative seizures. J Neurol Neurosurg Psychiatry 77: 616–621.

Goldstein LH, Mellers JDC, Landau S et al. (2015). Cognitive behavioural therapy vs standardised medical care for adults with dissociative non-epileptic seizures (CODES): a multicentre randomised controlled trial protocol. BMC Neurol 15: 98.

Guze SB (1967). The diagnosis of hysteria: what are we trying to do? Am J Psychiatry 124: 491–498.

Hitchcock J, Davis M (1986). Lesions of the amygdala, but not of the cerebellum or red nucleus, block conditioned fear as measured with the potentiated startle paradigm. Behav Neurosci 100 (1): 11.

Hofmann SG, Sawyer AT, Witt AA et al. (2010). The effect of mindfulness-based therapy on anxiety and depression: a meta-analytic review. J Consult Clin Psychol 78 (2): 169–183.

Hunot V, Moore THM, Caldwell DM et al. (2013). 'Third wave' cognitive and behavioural therapies versus other psychological therapies for depression. Cochrane Database Syst Rev (10): Art. No.: CD008704.

Kant I (1800). Lectures on Logic (The Cambridge Edition of the Works of Immanuel Kant). Cambridge University Press, Cambridge, 2000. 2nd Print edition (17 April 2009).

Klonoff EA, Moore DJ (1986). 'Conversion reactions' in adolescents: a biofeedback-based operant approach. J Behav Ther Exp Psychiatry 17: 179–184.

Koos EL (1954). The health of Regionville: what people thought and did about it. Columbia University Press, New York.

Lieberman DA (2012). Human learning and memory, Cambridge University Press, Cambridge.

Ludwig L, Whitehead K, Sharpe M et al. (2015). Differences in illness perceptions between patients with non-epileptic seizures and functional limb weakness. J Psychosom Res 79: 246–249.

Masson JM (1984). The assault on truth, Freud's suppression of the seduction theory. Farrar, Straus and Giroux, New York.

McCullough ML (2001). Freud's seduction theory and its rehabilitation: a saga of one mistake after another. Rev Gen Psychol 5: 3–22.

Mechanic D (1962). The concept of illness behaviour. J Chron Dis 15: 189–194.

Mechanic D (1977). Illness behaviour, social adaptation, and the management of illness. J Nerv Ment Dis 165: 79–87.

Mind Report (2013). We still need to talk: a report on access to talking therapies. Mind, London.

Mizes JS (1985). The use of contingent reinforcement in the treatment of a conversion disorder: a multiple baseline study. J Behav Ther Exp Psychiatry 16: 341–345.

Nielsen G, Stone J, Edwards MJ (2013). Physiotherapy for functional (psychogenic) motor symptoms: a systematic review. J Psychosom Res 75: 93–102.

Nielsen G, Stone J, Matthews A et al. (2015). Physiotherapy for functional motor disorders: a consensus recommendation. J Neurol Neurosurg Psychiatry 86: 1113–1119.

Pareés I, Kojovic M, Pires C et al. (2014). Physical precipitating factors in functional movement disorders. J Neurol Sci 338: 174–177.

Parsons T (1951). The Social System, The Free Press of Glencoe, New York.

Pilowsky I (1969). Abnormal illness behaviour. Br J Med Psychol 42: 347–351.

Reuber M, Jamnadas-Khoda J, Broadhurst M et al. (2011). Psychogenic nonepileptic seizure manifestations reported by patients and witnesses. Epilepsia 52: 2028–2035.

Roberts NA, Reuber M (2014). Alterations of consciousness in psychogenic nonepileptic seizures: emotion, emotion regulation and dissociation. Epilepsy Behav 30: 43–49.

Rodman FR (2003). Winnicott: Life and work, Perseus, Cambridge, MA.

Rush AJ, Beck AT, Kovacs M et al. (1977). Comparative efficacy of cognitive therapy and pharmacotherapy in the treatment of depressed outpatients. Cognit Ther Res 1: 17–37.

Rycroft C (1995). A Critical Dictionary of Psychoanalysis. Penguin Books, London. p. 59.

Schacter DL, Gilbert DT, Wegner DM (2011). B. F. Skinner: The Role of Reinforcement and Punishment Psychology. 2nd Edition, Worth, New York.

Segal ZV, Williams JMG, Teasdale JD (2012). Mindfulness-based cognitive therapy for depression. Guilford Press, New York.

Sharpe M, Stone J, Hibberd C et al. (2010). Neurology outpatients with symptoms unexplained by disease: illness beliefs and financial benefits predict 1-year outcome. Psychol Med 40: 689–698.

Stafford-Clark D (1967). What Freud really said. MacDonald, London.

Stone J, Binzer M, Sharpe M (2004). Illness beliefs and locus of control: a comparison of patients with pseudoseizures and epilepsy. J Psychosom Res 57: 541–547.

Stone J, Carson A, Sharpe M (2005). Functional symptoms and signs in neurology: assessment and diagnosis. J Neurol Neurosurg Psychiatry 76 (Suppl 1): i2–i12.

Stone J, Warlow C, Sharpe M (2010). The symptom of functional weakness: a controlled study of 107 patients. Brain 133: 1537–1551.

Thorndike, E. L. (1898, 1911) Animal intelligence: an experimental study of the associative processes in animals. Psychological Monographs #8.

Weinman J, Petrie KJ, Moss-Morris R et al. (1996). The illness perception questionnaire: a new method for assessing the cognitive representations of illness. Psychol Health 11: 431–445.

Whitehead K, Kandler R, Reuber M (2013). Patients' and neurologists' perception of epilepsy and psychogenic nonepileptic seizures. Epilepsia 54: 708–717.

Handbook of Clinical Neurology, Vol. 139 (3rd series)
Functional Neurologic Disorders
M. Hallett, J. Stone, and A. Carson, Editors
http://dx.doi.org/10.1016/B978-0-12-801772-2.00011-4

Chapter 11

Voluntary or involuntary? A neurophysiologic approach to functional movement disorders

M.-P. STENNER[1,2] AND P. HAGGARD[3]*
[1]*Wellcome Trust Centre for Neuroimaging, Institute of Neurology, London, UK*
[2]*Department of Neurology, Otto-von-Guericke-University Magdeburg, Magdeburg, Germany*
[3]*Institute of Cognitive Neuroscience, London, UK*

Abstract

Patients with functional movement disorders (FMD) experience movements as involuntary that share fundamental characteristics with voluntary actions. This apparent paradox raises questions regarding the possible sources of a subjective experience of action. In addition, it poses a yet unresolved diagnostic challenge, namely how to describe or even quantify this experience in a scientifically and clinically useful way. Here, we describe recent experimental approaches that have shed light on the phenomenology of action in FMD. We first outline the sources and content of a subjective experience of action in healthy humans and discuss how this experience may be created in the brain. Turning to FMD, we describe implicit, behavioral measures that have revealed specific abnormalities in the awareness of action in FMD. Based on these abnormalities, we propose a potential, new solution to the paradox of volition in FMD.

was ist das, was übrigbleibt, wenn ich von der Tatsache, dass ich meinen Arm hebe, die abziehe, dass mein Arm sich hebt?

[what is left over if I subtract the fact that my arm goes up from the fact that I raise my arm?] Ludwig Wittgenstein, *Philosophische Untersuchungen* (1953)

wehe der verhängnisvollen Neubegier, die durch eine Spalte einmal aus dem Bewußtseinszimmer heraus und hinabzusehen vermöchte [...] der Mensch ruht in der Gleichgültigkeit seines Nichtwissens und gleichsam auf dem Rücken eines Tigers in Träumen hängend.

[woe betide him, who, out of ominous curiosity, dares to look down through a crack in his chamber of consciousness [...] man rests in indifference to his own ignorance, caught in dreams, as it were, on the back of a tiger.] Friedrich Nietzsche (1973), *Über Wahrheit und Lüge im außermoralischen Sinn* (1870–1873)

INTRODUCTION

Motor symptoms in functional neurologic disorders, specifically in functional movement disorders (FMD), have characteristics that imply voluntary control. They are typically enhanced by attention and alleviated by distraction (e.g., Kenney et al., 2007), suggesting that their generation requires allocation of attention. In addition, these movements may entrain to the frequency of concurrent voluntary actions such as voluntary finger tapping (e.g., Schwingenschuh et al., 2011), may occur at latencies after sensory triggers that resemble voluntary reaction times, and may be preceded by cortical potentials characteristic of self-paced voluntary actions (Edwards and Bhatia, 2012). Consequently, neurologists frequently regard aberrant movement generation in FMD as voluntary (but see, e.g., Edwards et al., 2012). Yet a hallmark of FMD is that patients experience these movements as involuntary. How can movements that display fundamental features of voluntary control be experienced as involuntary?

*Correspondence to: Patrick Haggard, Institute of Cognitive Neuroscience, 17 Queen Square, London WC1N 3AR, UK. Tel: +44-20-7679-1153, E-mail: p.haggard@ucl.ac.uk

It is difficult to establish objective criteria that uniquely classify human movements as voluntary or involuntary. One possible approach comes from considering the linkage between an action and its current sensory context. Voluntary actions are often considered "free from immediacy" (Shadlen and Gold, 2004), i.e., internally motivated rather than stimulus-driven (Haggard, 2008). However, this definition raises further questions, e.g., how free from external preconditions an action must be to be considered voluntary, or indeed how free it can be, and how volition and external preconditions are precisely related. Most would agree that movements driven purely by spinal reflexes are involuntary. But other actions seem finely balanced between voluntary actions and stereotyped responses to an external stimulus. Is someone who waits for the green man to appear, and then crosses the road, really less voluntary than another individual who walks across the road deep in thought without attending to the lights? We suggest that the former action, although stimulus-dependent, is arguably as voluntary as, or even more voluntary than, the same action performed endogenously but without particular thought. Thus, even in healthy humans, there is no sharp and unique divide between actions that appear voluntary vs. involuntary. Indeed, most actions are a mixture of more reflexive and less reflexive elements: some features of an action may seem like reflexive responses to current stimulation, while others may seem purely endogenous. Perceptual discrimination of these different contributions is surprisingly poor (Ghosh and Haggard, 2014). Thus, dichotomously classifying any particular action as either voluntary or involuntary is unrealistic (Schüür and Haggard, 2011).

An alternative approach to volition in general, and the paradox of volition in FMD in particular, is based on accepting subjective descriptions of an action as voluntary or involuntary, and then investigating the specific causes and consequences of these descriptions. Following this approach, we first outline the bases of a subjective experience of volition in healthy humans (in the section entitled 'What are we aware of when we act?') and review how this experience may be created in the human brain (in the section 'Neurophysiology of action awareness'). We then turn to the phenomenology of action in FMD. FMD patients experience motor symptoms as involuntary, and this contributes essentially to patients' beliefs about illness and, consequently, their suffering. Understanding how and why movements are perceived differently in FMD may thus inform positive diagnostic criteria and, ultimately, improve treatment.

However, this approach to FMD via the subjective experience of volition poses an unresolved diagnostic problem, namely how to describe, and even quantify, first-person, "private" experiences, such as feelings of voluntariness or involuntariness in a way that is scientifically and clinically useful, without reverting to naïve reliance on subjective reports. The second part of this chapter therefore outlines several behavioral methods that aim to qualify and quantify aspects of the phenomenology of action and reviews how these methods have recently revealed specific alterations in action awareness in FMD (see section 'Action awareness and agency in functional movement disorders').

In the third part, we propose a potential new solution to the paradox of volition in FMD (section 'Expected and experienced control'). Specifically, we suggest that FMD patients may expect conscious access to, and explicit control over, a full and detailed range of motor parameters. Since, in fact, the lower levels of the motor hierarchy produce actions involuntarily, following a principle of delegated control (Bernstein, 1967), this expectation is not fulfilled. That is, FMD patients may experience a need or desire for conscious control over their own actions that their motor system is physiologically unable to provide. We discuss how this may contribute to the observed alterations in action awareness and agency, as well as to the generation of aberrant movements in FMD (section 'Generation of "involuntary" movements in FMD'). Finally, we suggest a possible research agenda that could test predictions of our model.

WHAT ARE WE AWARE OF WHEN WE ACT?

Awareness of the motoric details of what we do is surprisingly limited and does not provide a veridic readout of motor action. As a result, humans may think they move when they do not, or they may be unaware of movements that they in fact control. Patients with anosognosia for hemiplegia, for example, may obstinately claim to actively and successfully move a plegic and therefore immobile limb (e.g., Berti et al., 2005). Conversely, patients with visual agnosia may be unable to consciously access information about object features while readily integrating this information into actions that involve these objects. For example, patients may rotate their hand before inserting it into an elongated slot whose orientation they cannot consciously discriminate (Milner et al., 1991). These patients are thus described as performing functional goal-directed actions, but without conscious awareness. In some cases, limited insight into motoric details may lead to confusion whether one even performed a particular action or not, creating a deficit in action recognition tasks. For example, patients with left parietal lesions and apraxia may misinterpret visual feedback from someone else's (correct) movements as feedback from their own (incorrect) movements despite discrepant movement execution (Sirigu et al., 1999).

In a seminal study, Desmurget et al. (2009) showed that intraoperative electric stimulation of parietal cortex in awake subjects could induce unprompted reports of a "will," "desire," or "wanting" to move certain body parts, without producing overt movement or electromyogram activity. With higher amplitudes of parietal stimulation, subjects were convinced that they had actually moved. Stimulation of frontal cortex, on the other hand, produced movements of which patients claimed to be unaware. This strongly suggests that, at least in the protocol employed in this study, certain aspects of action awareness can dissociate from actual motor output. While the frontal cortex may trigger physical movement, their data suggest it does not underlie movement awareness. In contrast, parietal cortex activity appears to be sufficient for movement awareness.

A similar dissociation of physical and perceived movement may also occur in healthy humans and in more natural settings. Fourneret and Jeannerod (1998) observed that subjects accurately adjust the trajectory of a reaching movement to counter a visuomotor rotation, but they either underestimate this adjustment or even misjudge its direction. Similarly, Marcel (2003) reported that an illusory displacement of the position of one hand (induced by tendon vibration) led a majority of subjects to misjudge the direction of an active hand movement, in some cases despite explicit knowledge of this error. Implicit motor adjustments, e.g., during learning of a visuomotor rotation, are not only elusive to the agent, but may even impede explicit, conscious task strategies at the expense of task performance (Mazzoni and Krakauer, 2006).

Many of the above phenomena have been interpreted as evidence that a conscious experience of action does not depend on actual motor execution as much as on prior goals, intentions, or predictions (e.g., Desmurget and Sirigu, 2009). The idea of prospective components of action awareness is now widely accepted. Prospective action awareness has been theoretically related to forward modeling in motor control (Blakemore and Frith, 2003) and integrated in models of neuropsychiatric disorders to explain, for example, delusions of control in schizophrenia (Voss et al., 2010; Moore et al., 2013).

On the other hand, there is evidence that postdictive, reconstructive mechanisms contribute to aspects of action awareness. Following Wegner (2003), experiencing oneself as an agent depends on a *post hoc* comparison between sensory input and pre-movement thoughts, together with an assessment of potential alternative causes. In agreement with a retrospective contribution to action awareness in addition to prospection, Lau et al. (2007) demonstrated that transcranial magnetic stimulation after action execution, targeting the presupplementary motor area, advances the perceived onset of an intention to act. The authors argued that their manipulation added noise to peri- and postaction components of action awareness, leading to stronger reliance on earlier, prospective components. A similar combination of pre- and postdiction is thought to contribute to the "sense of agency," i.e., the subjective experience of control over external consequences of an action (Moore and Haggard, 2008). Taken together, different aspects of the conscious awareness of action are influenced by a combination of prospective and retrospective processes. Conscious access to motoric details of an action, on the other hand, is limited and readily overridden by prediction and reconstruction.

NEUROPHYSIOLOGY OF ACTION AWARENESS

Several lines of research have investigated the neurophysiology of action awareness. One line of experimental work is based on the "Libet experiment." Libet et al. (1983) studied the temporal relationship between electroencephalographic brain potentials that signal preparation of an upcoming motor action and the perceived time of an associated intention to act. In the Libet experiment, subjects watch a clock hand rotating at ~0.4 Hz, press a button at a time of their choice, and then report which clock hand position they perceived either at the time when they pressed the button or at the time when they first felt the "urge" to press the button. Typically, both events are perceived to occur before action execution, but the "urge" to move is judged to be significantly earlier, around 200 ms before the button press. Crucially, this urge to move is reported significantly later than the onset of the readiness potential – a gradual, ramp-like increase in neural activity generated by medial frontal cortex, among other areas. The method has been criticized for several reasons (e.g., Guggisberg et al., 2011; Schurger et al., 2012). Notwithstanding these criticisms, the main result has been replicated, and the method has been an important driver of neurophysiologic studies of the processes that may underlie an experience of intention and action (e.g., Haggard and Eimer, 1999; Lau et al., 2004; Sirigu et al., 2004; Hallett, 2007; Fried et al., 2011). The classic interpretation of this experiment draws two conclusions: first, initiation of voluntary action is based on increasing neuronal activity in medial frontal areas that generate the readiness potential; and second, the conscious experience of controlling a voluntary action is a consequence, rather than a cause, of this preparatory neural activity.

Several studies have followed along the same broad line of research. Sirigu et al. (2004) found that patients with focal parietal lesions showed a delayed awareness of intention relative to controls, suggesting a role of parietal cortex in the experience of voluntary action, in addition to the established role of medial frontal cortex. However, Lafargue and Duffau (2008) did not find the same effect in a small group of patients with neurosurgical resections of parietal cortex. Haggard and Eimer (1999) asked participants to choose freely between moving either their left or their right hand. They found that the experience of intention was associated with the late lateralization of the readiness potential to the hemisphere contralateral to the moving hand, rather than the earlier onset of the midline readiness potential.

However, other studies did not find this association (Schlegel et al., 2013). Lau et al. (2004) repeated the core conditions of the Libet experiment in functional magnetic resonance imaging. They found a stronger blood oxygen level-dependent signal in presupplementary motor area, dorsolateral prefrontal cortex, and the intraparietal area when subjects judged the time of their intention to act, as opposed to the time of their action. Soon et al. (2008) combined a modified version of the Libet task with a multivoxel pattern-decoding approach. They were able to predict which of two actions people would freely choose to make several seconds before the movement itself, and prior to participants' reports of when they decided on their action. The frontopolar cortex contained the earliest information about the movement choice.

A second important strand of information comes from stimulation studies in awake human patients undergoing mapping prior to neurosurgery. Stimulation of a number of areas was reported to produce an experience of an "urge" or "intention" to move. These areas were located in the medial frontal cortex (Fried et al., 1991) and also in the parietal cortex (Desmurget et al., 2009). Based on the precise phrasing of subjective reports during stimulation, it has been suggested that the parietal cortex and medial frontal cortex are associated with distinct phenomenologic components, namely "conscious intentions" vs. an experience of "imminence" of a movement, respectively (Desmurget and Sirigu, 2009).

The above experiments ignore one important feature of voluntary actions, namely that they aim at an external goal. Healthy adults have the experience of determining a particular course of action because of a goal they wish to achieve, and then achieving their goal through the corresponding action. This produces a distinctive "sense of agency" with respect to one's own actions, and also with respect to the external consequences of such actions. Thus, an important feature of the perception of voluntary action is the perception of its goal-directedness. This has been measured both using explicit agency ratings and also using implicit measures, such as the compression of perceived time between an action and its outcome, a phenomenon called temporal (or intentional) binding. For example, the perceived time of a tone is bound backward towards a voluntary action that causes it, but not towards an involuntary movement of the same muscles (Haggard et al., 2002). Thus, whether or not a movement "feels voluntary" might potentially be tested by asking participants to judge the perceived time of a subsequent sensory consequence of this movement. One merit of measures like temporal binding is that they are essentially implicit. The interest in such measures for disorders such as FMD is evident (e.g., Kranick et al., 2013; see next section). The neural correlates of the intentional binding effect are not fully understood, but stimulation, pharmacologic and neuroimaging evidence point towards an involvement of medial frontal cortex Moore et al., 2010a,b; Kühn et al., 2013), as well as parietal cortex (Khalighinejad and Haggard, 2015).

ACTION AWARENESS AND AGENCY IN FUNCTIONAL MOVEMENT DISORDERS

A positive diagnosis of FMDs implies criteria that are not solely based on exclusion of "organic" disorders. To date, a positive diagnosis relies to a large extent on clinical signs that reveal characteristics of voluntary control, e.g., symptom exacerbation by attention, or presence of a pre-movement readiness potential (Edwards and Bhatia, 2012). In principle, however, it would appear desirable to take into account cardinal symptoms as positive diagnostic criteria. In the case of FMD, this would mean including the patients' experience that their motor symptoms are produced involuntarily. Importantly, implicit measures would be required to capture this experience without reverting to patients' self-reports. This would be the only way to avoid an influence of patient expectation or feigning. In this section, we outline three behavioral methods that aim to objectify aspects of action awareness, two of which provide clearly implicit measures. We then review recent studies that have employed these methods to examine the phenomenology of action in FMD.

The first approach to FMD is based on the Libet experiment, described above. Edwards et al. (2011) showed that patients with functional tremor perceive both the time of their first intention and the time of action execution later than age-matched healthy controls. Interestingly, the perceived time of intention was more delayed, relative to controls, than the perceived time of action. These effects were similar for tremulous and unaffected limbs and were therefore interpreted as a manifestation of a trait instead of an effector-specific abnormality. The direction of the effect – i.e., a delay in the perception of intention – would be expected for movements experienced as involuntary. However, because perceived intentions of voluntary movements were delayed, Edwards et al.'s (2011) finding may represent a more general predisposition to experience movements as involuntary. A general, trait-like change in action awareness across effectors could, in principle, explain why motor manifestations in individual FMD patients are variable over time, e.g., why new functional symptoms can be provoked by directing the patient's attention to them. While Edwards et al. (2011) interpreted the observed shift in the perceived time of action execution as a general impairment of time perception in FMD, it could also reflect a shift in perception towards motoric details of an action, away from intentional signals. We will discuss this possibility in the next section.

The second method considered here also relies on time judgments, specifically on the perceived times of an action and of a delayed sensory consequence. Haggard et al. (2002) observed an attraction between the perceived time of an action and a tone presented a few hundred milliseconds later, relative to baseline conditions in which the two events occurred in isolation. This phenomenon, called temporal or intentional binding, is often considered an index of an implicit sense of agency, i.e., an experience of control, via one's actions, over events in the world (Moore and Obhi, 2012).

A recent study reported reduced temporal binding in a group of FMD patients with various motor symptoms, including patients with functional tremor, functional myoclonus, functional dystonia, and gait disturbance (Kranick et al., 2013). This effect appeared to be largely driven by a reduced attraction of the outcome towards the action that caused it. The effector-specificity of this effect was not examined. The authors proposed that reduced temporal binding in FMD reflects an altered sense of control across patients with distinct motor manifestations. In particular, one might conjecture that the voluntary actions of FMD patients are less prone than those of healthy controls to structure the perception of an outcome event, consistent with a reduced perception of volition. Alternatively, reduced binding could be interpreted as the result of more accurate time perception of an action and its consequence, a point we come back to in the following section.

Similar to the temporal binding paradigm, the third method also aims at a perceptual effect that occurs when an action has a predictable sensory consequence. This effect, called sensory attenuation, is a reduction in the perceived intensity of touch or force generated by one's own movement compared to physically identical, but externally generated, touch or force. Sensory attenuation has been explained by a cancellation of predicted reafferent sensory input (e.g., Cullen, 2004) or, alternatively, as a decrease in the precision of sensory input during movement (Brown et al., 2013). Like temporal binding (Moore et al., 2010a), sensory attenuation has been associated with medial frontal cortex function (Haggard and Whitford, 2004) and, rather speculatively, with perceptual discrimination of self-caused vs. externally generated sensory input (Shergill et al., 2005).

Following this interpretation and, at the same time, testing a prediction from their neurobiologic model (Edwards et al., 2012; see Chapter 12), Pareés et al. (2014) tested sensory attenuation in FMD patients (primarily functional fixed dystonia), and healthy controls. They employed a well-established paradigm in which subjects have to match different test forces applied to one hand, either by pressing on that hand with their other hand or by operating a robot via a joystick. Typically, healthy subjects overestimate required forces when pressing on their hand directly, relative to the joystick condition, indicating that they attenuate perceived force that is an immediate consequence of their own movement. Pareés et al. (2014) demonstrated that FMD patients in their study did not show sensory attenuation. Instead, they perceived force similarly in both conditions, and were consequently more accurate than healthy subjects in perceiving force that was immediately caused by their own movement. The authors correctly concluded that this speaks strongly against feigning.

Indeed, sensory attenuation is arguably the "most implicit" of the three measures considered here, since it reflects behavioral inaccuracy of which subjects are not (explicitly) aware and which they probably do not expect, given that the task probes an apparently simple, fundamental ability. Similarly to the delayed awareness of intention and action in Edwards et al. (2011) and the reduced temporal binding in Kranick et al. (2013), this loss of sensory attenuation in FMD was evident for body parts that showed no functional symptoms. From this, Pareés et al. (2014) concluded that a loss of sensory attenuation in FMD may result from an increase in body-focused attention. The authors interpreted a loss of sensory attenuation in FMD as evidence for an essential role of attentional gain or precision in the generation of functional (motor) symptoms (Edwards et al., 2012), within the context of a recent neurobiologic account of motor control (active inference; e.g., Brown et al., 2013). However, Pareés et al.'s (2014) data show an increase in accuracy, not a change in precision, as predicted by the model. We will discuss a different interpretation of this loss of sensory attenuation in the next section.

In all three studies (Edwards et al., 2011; Kranick et al., 2013; Pareés et al., 2014), FMD patients were compared to healthy controls, but not to patients with organic movement disorders and similar involuntary movements. We acknowledge the difficulty of conducting studies with two matched control groups, and the difficulties involved in matching clinical symptom severity. However, as a result, the reported abnormalities in action awareness could, in principle, reflect more general, epiphenomenal changes that occur as a result of the presence of involuntary movements *per se*. Similar to patients with FMD (Edwards et al., 2011), adolescents with Tourette syndrome and strong premonitory urges also display a delayed awareness of intention (but no delay in the perceived time of action; Ganos et al., 2014). Some of the reported abnormalities in FMD could therefore reflect more general consequences of frequent experience of involuntary movements, rather than a marker for any specific pathology.

EXPECTED AND EXPERIENCED CONTROL

FMD patients display more accurate awareness of movement onset (Edwards et al., 2011) and more accurate perception of the sensory consequences of movement (Kranick et al., 2013; Pareés et al., 2014) compared to healthy subjects, and they perceive their first intention to move closer to their actual motor execution (Edwards et al., 2011). In agreement with a role of attention for symptom manifestation (e.g., Kenney et al., 2007), this pattern is consistent with an enhanced focus of action awareness on motoric details in FMD, i.e., enhanced attention to parameters of motor execution. What could explain such a shift in attention?

In their recently proposed pathophysiologic model of FMD, Edwards et al. (2012) emphasize the role of precipitating physical events in functional neurologic disorders, including, for example, physical injury or panic attacks. They propose that these events instantiate false prior beliefs and endow them with high certainty by directing undue attention towards them. Crucially, these prior beliefs are assumed to reside at an intermediate level in a cortical hierarchy, below levels at which intentions are conscious (2012). Under the assumption that prior beliefs with high certainty can generate movements via spinal reflex arcs (active inference; Adams et al., 2013; Brown et al., 2013), Edwards et al. (2012) explained the perceived involuntariness in FMD as a misinterpretation of these movements, which are in some real sense attended and expected, as being neurologic symptoms. In the model, this misinterpretation arises because higher cortical levels, at which conscious awareness of intention emerges, have no access to the content of these false prior beliefs at intermediate levels. It is unclear, however, why precipitating events would trigger false beliefs specifically at these intermediate levels. Furthermore, a strong prior of a specific sensation or movement seems at odds with the common clinical observation that symptoms in individual FMD patients may vary strongly over time (Edwards and Bhatia, 2012).

Instead of interpreting a perceived loss of control as a "secondary failure" (Edwards et al., 2012), we propose that it may actually constitute the primary factor in a pathophysiologic chain. On this view, the precipitating events, such as physical injury or panic attacks, are interpreted subjectively as the consequence of a loss or insufficiency of control. This interpretation might lead to increased monitoring of voluntary control, and thus to an expectation of a strong, conscious, and vivid experience in controlling actions. As outlined in the first section of this chapter, humans have relatively limited conscious access to motoric details of their own actions. Stripped of their immediate goals, abstract reasons, and a nonobservational knowledge of being "immersed" in action (e.g., Marcel, 2003), movements provide only a "thin" (Pacherie, 2008) momentary experience of control. Patients who go on to develop functional symptoms may in fact have the same, limited conscious access to their intentional actions as other people. Like other people, they may also have only a limited, background feeling of control over the movements that they make. However, unlike other people, they interpret this "thin" phenomenology of action as pathologic.

Why are physical injuries or other somatic events followed by a manifestation of functional symptoms in some individuals, but not in others? One plausible explanation draws on an intriguing finding by Pareés et al. (2012). In this study, patients with FMD drew as many beads from a jar as they considered necessary to reach a decision whether the jar contained predominantly blue or red beads. In this probabilistic decision-making task, patients showed a "jumping to conclusions" style of reasoning, i.e., they tended to base decisions on relatively little sensory evidence. Furthermore, they were biased towards new evidence even when it conflicted with previously accumulated, stronger evidence. Individuals who develop FMD may thus have a predisposition to weight recent experience more strongly than prior beliefs (which seems at odds with the assumption of a strong prior expectation that overwhelms sensory evidence in Edwards et al.'s (2012) model). Individuals who go on to develop FMD would be more likely to conclude a loss of voluntary control when faced with an unexpectedly "thin" experience of control over motoric details of their action, especially if this experience persists upon further monitoring.

Unlike false prior beliefs about specific sensations or movements assumed in Edwards et al.'s (2012) model, an aberrant expectation of a strong phenomenology of control over motoric details of an action does not assume a specific sensory or motor content. This interpretation is therefore more consistent with a high variability of FMD movements over time. Furthermore, it does not assume any resemblance between precipitating events and subsequent functional symptoms that persists over time.

GENERATION OF "INVOLUNTARY" MOVEMENTS IN FMD

If a perceived loss of control due to an excessive expectation of control is a "primary" failure in FMD, the question arises whether and how this may generate motor symptoms. Edwards et al.'s (2012) model explains aberrant movement generation in FMD by mechanisms of active inference, a neurobiologic theory that translates principles of Bayesian inference in perception to motor action (Adams et al., 2013; Brown et al., 2013). Alternatively, one could speculate that patients with FMD develop first motor symptoms through an interaction of incidental, overt motor noise, detected by excessive conscious monitoring, and a predisposition to "jump to conclusions" (Pareés et al., 2012), e.g., to misinterpret noise according to lay beliefs about neurologic disorders (Edwards et al., 2012). Strong expectations, together with excessive monitoring, i.e., attention, may in turn bias motor output towards movements that comply with these lay beliefs through a recently proposed accumulator mechanism.

Schurger et al. (2012) argued that a commitment to move is characterized by a threshold crossing of an accumulator that takes stochastic fluctuations into account. They have provided evidence that the onset of a self-initiated movement and the preceding readiness potential may depend on ongoing, random fluctuations of neuronal activity in motor cortical areas. Following the idea of an accumulator in the motor system, enhanced attention towards details of motor execution, specifically of movements that are strongly expected, could, in principle, increase the gain of a biased accumulator. Consequently, execution of specific motor plans that are compatible with patients' strong expectations would become more susceptible to noise, leading to overt, stereotyped movements that would otherwise be inhibited.

Voon et al. (2013) have recently shown that patients with FMD display an inhibition deficit relative to healthy controls, with an increase in commission errors in a NoGo task. This could reflect an increased level of motor noise and a consequent, premature commitment to (voluntary) movement.

CONCLUSIONS AND RESEARCH AGENDA

The idea that patients with FMD have abnormal expectations of control over motoric details of their actions makes several testable predictions. First, in agency tasks, patients should be strongly "retrospectivist," i.e., their awareness of action should be strongly influenced by actual outcomes. In a variant of the temporal binding paradigm described above (see section, Action awareness and agency in functional movement disorders), Moore and Haggard (2008) manipulated the contingency between an action and a consequent tone, such that the action caused a tone only in some trials. In a low-contingency (50%) condition, they observed that healthy subjects showed a later awareness of an action when it was followed by a tone, as compared to when it was not. Because the occurrence of the tone was unpredictable in this condition, this shift was interpreted as a retrospective component of action awareness, i.e., one that occurred at the time of outcome presentation. When the action/tone contingency was high (75%), on the other hand, the action was perceived later even in trials in which it was not followed by a tone. This was interpreted as a prospective contribution to action awareness. If, as we propose, patients with FMD attempt to access and control details of motor execution, instead of deriving their awareness of action from goals and predictions, they should show strong retrospective and weak prospective binding. In addition, patients should perform better than healthy subjects in detecting their own adjustment of a reaching movement to a visuomotor rotation (Fourneret and Jeannerod, 1998), and their perception of movement direction should be less susceptible to illusory limb displacement (Marcel, 2003).

Furthermore, as a result of a strongly retrospective awareness of action, patients with FMD should not show an "intentional capture" of involuntary movements (Jensen et al., 2014): When voluntary and involuntary, e.g., transcranial magnetic stimulation-induced, movements occur at the same time, but in different hands, healthy subjects tend to (falsely) remember that the involuntary movement involved the hand which in fact executed the voluntary movement. Jensen et al. (2014) interpreted this effect as evidence of a voluntary capture of involuntary movements, supporting intentional agency theories. A strong reliance on retrospective awareness of action, as proposed for patients with FMD, would predict that this effect is absent in these patients.

Enhanced attention to motoric details of action execution in patients with FMD would also predict a specific change in pre-movement electrophysiologic potentials. Schurger et al. (2012) tested a variant of the classic Libet experiment that involved infrequent, unpredictable Go signals. When comparing pre-movement potentials in trials in which subjects responded slowly vs. quickly to this Go signal, they observed an amplitude difference that occurred well before the Go signal. This was interpreted as evidence that the time at which a voluntary movement is executed is influenced by spontaneous random fluctuations of neural activity in motor cortex that are integrated by an accumulator. If patients with FMD overattend to motor execution and, thereby, increase the gain of this accumulator, they should show an even bigger amplitude difference between trials with fast vs. slow responses before the Go signal. This would also predict a larger standard deviation of reaction times to unpredictable, infrequent Go signals in patients with FMD.

Taken together, the pathophysiology of FMD is likely to involve abnormalities in the way that attention and expectation shape action execution and action awareness. Well-characterized, implicit behavioral tests are available to examine the precise nature of this interaction in FMD. Conversely, the paradox of volition in FMD offers a unique view on mechanisms of action awareness in humans that has the potential to inform research on human volition in general.

References

Adams RA, Shipp S, Friston KJ (2013). Predictions not commands: active inference in the motor system. Brain Struct Funct 218 (3): 611–643.

Bernstein N (1967). The control and regulation of movements, Pergamon Press, London.

Berti A, Bottini G, Gandola M et al. (2005). Shared cortical anatomy for motor awareness and motor control. Science 309 (5733): 488–491.

Blakemore S-J, Frith C (2003). Self-awareness and action. Curr Opin Neurobiol 13 (2): 219–224.

Brown H, Adams RA, Parees I et al. (2013). Active inference, sensory attenuation and illusions. Cogn Process 14 (4): 411–427.

Cullen KE (2004). Sensory signals during active versus passive movement. Curr Opin Neurobiol 14 (6): 698–706.

Desmurget M, Sirigu A (2009). A parietal-premotor network for movement intention and motor awareness. Trends Cogn Sci 13 (10): 411–419.

Desmurget M, Reilly KT, Richard N et al. (2009). Movement intention after parietal cortex stimulation in humans. Science 324 (5928): 811–813.

Edwards MJ, Bhatia KP (2012). Functional (psychogenic) movement disorders: merging mind and brain. Lancet Neurol 11 (3): 250–260.

Edwards MJ, Moretto G, Schwingenschuh P et al. (2011). Abnormal sense of intention preceding voluntary movement in patients with psychogenic tremor. Neuropsychologia 49 (9): 2791–2793.

Edwards MJ, Adams RA, Brown H et al. (2012). A Bayesian account of "hysteria". Brain 135: 3495–3512.

Fourneret P, Jeannerod M (1998). Limited conscious monitoring of motor performance in normal subjects. Neuropsychologia 36 (11): 1133–1140.

Fried I, Katz A, McCarthy G et al. (1991). Functional organization of human supplementary motor cortex studied by electrical stimulation. J Neurosci 11: 3656–3666.

Fried I, Mukamel R, Kreiman G (2011). Internally generated preactivation of single neurons in human medial frontal cortex predicts volition. Neuron 69 (3): 548–562.

Ganos C, Asmuss L, Bongert J et al. (2014). Volitional action as perceptual detection: predictors of conscious intention in adolescents with tic disorders. Cortex 64C: 47–54.

Ghosh A, Haggard P (2014). The spinal reflex cannot be perceptually separated from voluntary movements. J Physiol 592: 141–152.

Guggisberg AG, Dalal SS, Schnider A et al. (2011). The neural basis of event-time introspection. Conscious Cogn 20 (4): 1899–1915.

Haggard P (2008). Human volition: towards a neuroscience of will. Nature reviews. Neuroscience 9 (12): 934–946.

Haggard P, Eimer M (1999). On the relation between brain potentials and the awareness of voluntary movements. Exp Brain Res 126 (1): 128–133.

Haggard P, Whitford B (2004). Supplementary motor area provides an efferent signal for sensory suppression. Brain research. Cogn Brain Res 19 (1): 52–58.

Haggard P, Clark S, Kalogeras J (2002). Voluntary action and conscious awareness. Nat Neurosci 5 (4): 382–385.

Hallett M (2007). Volitional control of movement: the physiology of free will. Clin Neurophysiol 118: 1179–1192.

Jensen M, Vagnoni E, Overgaard M et al. (2014). Experience of action depends on intention, not body movement: An experiment on memory for mens rea. Neuropsychologia 55: 122–127.

Kenney C, Diamond A, Mejia N et al. (2007). Distinguishing psychogenic and essential tremor. J Neurol Sci 263: 94–99.

Khalighinejad N, Haggard P (2015). Modulating human sense of agency with non-invasive brain stimulation. Cortex 69: 93–103.

Kranick SM, Moore JW, Yusuf N et al. (2013). Action-effect binding is decreased in motor conversion disorder: implications for sense of agency. Mov Disord 28 (8): 1110–1116.

Kühn S, Brass M, Haggard P (2013). Feeling in control: Neural correlates of experience of agency. Cortex 49: 1935–1942.

Lafargue G, Duffau H (2008). Awareness of intending to act following parietal cortex resection. Neuropsychologia 46: 2662–2667.

Lau HC, Rogers RD, Haggard P et al. (2004). Attention to intention. Science 303 (5661): 1208–1210.

Lau HC, Rogers RD, Passingham RE (2007). Manipulating the experienced onset of intention after action execution. J Cogn Neurosci 19 (1): 81–90.

Libet B, Gleason CA, Wright EW et al. (1983). Time of conscious intention to act in relation to onset of cerebral activity (readiness-potential). Brain 106 (3): 623–642.

Marcel A (2003). The sense of agency: awareness and ownership of action. In: J Roessler, N Eilan (Eds.), Agency and self-awareness: Issues in Philosophy and Psychology, Oxford University Press, New York.

Mazzoni P, Krakauer JW (2006). An implicit plan overrides an explicit strategy during visuomotor adaptation. J Neurosci 26 (14): 3642–3645.

Milner AD, Perrett DI, Johnston RS et al. (1991). Perception and action in "visual form agnosia." Brain 114: 405–428.

Moore J, Haggard P (2008). Awareness of action: Inference and prediction. Conscious Cogn 17 (1): 136–144.

Moore JW, Obhi SS (2012). Intentional binding and the sense of agency: a review. Conscious Cogn 21 (1): 546–561.

Moore JW, Ruge D, Wenke D et al. (2010a). Disrupting the experience of control in the human brain: pre-supplementary motor area contributes to the sense of agency. Proc Biol Sci 277 (1693): 2503–2509.

Moore JW, Schneider SA, Schwingenschuh P et al. (2010b). Dopaminergic medication boosts action-effect binding in Parkinson's disease. Neuropsychologia 48 (4): 1125–1132.

Moore JW, Cambridge VC, Morgan H et al. (2013). Time, action and psychosis: using subjective time to investigate the effects of ketamine on sense of agency. Neuropsychologia 51 (2): 377–384.

Nietzsche F (1973). (1870–1873) Über Wahrheit und Lüge im außermoralischen Sinn [On Truth and Lies in a Nonmoral Sense.] Colli G, Montinari M (eds) Nietzsche Werke, Kritische Gesamtausgabe, 3. Abteilung, 2. Band, Nachgelassene Schriften 1870-1873, Walter de Gruyter, Berli.

Pacherie E (2008). The phenomenology of action: a conceptual framework. Cognition 107 (1): 179–217.

Pareés I, Kassavetis P, Saifee TA et al. (2012). "Jumping to conclusions" bias in functional movement disorders. J Neurol Neurosurg Psychiatry 83 (4): 460–463.

Pareés I, Brown H, Nuruki A et al. (2014). Loss of sensory attenuation in patients with functional (psychogenic) movement disorders. Brain 137: 2916–2921.

Schlegel A, Sinnott-Armstrong W, Parker Wheatley T et al. (2013). Barking up the wrong free: readiness potentials reflect processes independent of conscious will. Exp Brain Res 229: 329–335.

Schurger A, Sitt JD, Dehaene S (2012). An accumulator model for spontaneous neural activity prior to self-initiated movement. Proc Natl Acad Sci U S A 109 (42): E2904–E2913.

Schüür F, Haggard P (2011). What are self-generated actions? Conscious Cogn 20: 1697–1704.

Schwingenschuh P, Katschnig P, Seiler S et al. (2011). Moving toward "laboratory-supported" criteria for psychogenic tremor. Mov Disord 26 (14): 2509–2515.

Shadlen M, Gold J (2004). The neurophysiology of decision-making as a window on cognition. In: M Gazzaniga (Ed.), The Cognitive Neurosciences, MIT Press, Cambridge, MA.

Shergill SS, Samson GG, Bays PM et al. (2005). Evidence for sensory prediction deficits in schizophrenia. Am J Psychiatry 162 (12): 2384–2386.

Sirigu A, Daprati E, Pradat-Diehl P et al. (1999). Perception of self-generated movement following left parietal lesion. Brain 122: 1867–1874.

Sirigu A, Daprati E, Ciancia S et al. (2004). Altered awareness of voluntary action after damage to the parietal cortex. Nat Neurosci 7 (1): 80–84.

Soon CS, Brass M, Heinze HJ et al. (2008). Unconscious determinants of free decisions in the human brain. Nat Neurosci 11 (5): 543–545.

Voon V, Ekanayake V, Wiggs E et al. (2013). Response inhibition in motor conversion disorder. Mov Disord 28 (5): 612–618.

Voss M, Moore J, Hauser M et al. (2010). Altered awareness of action in schizophrenia: a specific deficit in predicting action consequences. Brain 133 (10): 3104–3112.

Wegner D (2003). The mind's best trick: How we experience conscious will. Trends Cogn Sci 7 (2): 65–69.

Wittgenstein L (1953). Philosophische Untersuchungen. [Philosophical Investigations.], Basil Blackwell, Oxford.

Handbook of Clinical Neurology, Vol. 139 (3rd series)
Functional Neurologic Disorders
M. Hallett, J. Stone, and A. Carson, Editors
http://dx.doi.org/10.1016/B978-0-12-801772-2.00012-6

Chapter 12

Neurobiologic theories of functional neurologic disorders

M.J. EDWARDS*

Department of Molecular and Clinical Sciences, St George's University of London and Atkinson Morley Regional Neuroscience Centre, St George's University Hospitals NHS Foundation Trust, London, UK

Abstract

Although neurobiologic theories to explain functional neurologic symptoms have a long history, a relative lack of interest in the 20th century left them far behind neurobiologic understanding of other illness. Here we review the proposals for neurobiologic mechanisms of functional neurologic symptoms that have been made over time and consider how they might inform our diagnostic and treatment methods, and how they integrate with psychologic formulations of functional symptoms. Modern approaches map on to recent developments in theoretic models of brain function, and suggest a key role for processes affecting attention, beliefs/expectations, and a resultant impairment of sense of agency.

INTRODUCTION

This chapter aims to address the question: How is it proposed that functional neurologic symptoms (FNS) are implemented within the anatomy and physiology of the brain? This question is certainly an interesting one, and is one where answers will help us move forward in our search for improved diagnosis and treatment of patients with FNS. However, it is also a question that has little meaning when considered in isolation. Neurobiologic understanding of FNS only makes an impact on health when it is coupled with an understanding of the psychologic and social dimensions of the illness. The importance of a biopsychosocial approach to human health and ill health is often highlighted but rarely practiced. It is perhaps for people with FNS where this approach is most acutely required, and why therefore care for people with FNS is often so acutely lacking. A one-dimensional approach to FNS, for example, a purely psychologic interpretation of symptoms and mode of treatment, or one that highlights neurobiologic mechanisms while ignoring the level of cognitive and psychologic experience, is doomed to failure. In particular situations, focusing on a specific level of "processing" (biologic, psychologic, social, and the myriad gradations of these broad concepts) can be appropriate and very useful. However, if we lose sight of the whole picture then we will never be able to meet our goal of improving the health of those with FNS.

I would like to provide one further caveat to this chapter: a warning regarding the allure of neurobiologic research methods. Our ability to "see into" the brain with functional imaging and, to a slightly less alluring extent with neurophysiologic techniques such as electroencephalography, can result in some dangerous patterns of thinking. If we are studying a particular illness and an area of the brain "lights up" in a functional imaging study in our patients and not in controls, it is easy to start thinking that we have found the bit of the brain that is causing the illness. It is a short step from there to saying that illness *x* is damage/dysfunction of brain area *y*. This naïve reductionism is attractive but very flawed. Any alteration of perception/movement will have a neural correlate, so the mere finding of differences between patients with FNS and healthy controls is entirely expected and is not in itself that useful. It is the interpretation of these findings which is key, and how they can inform testable theories for the neurobiology of FNS.

HISTORIC NEUROBIOLOGIC THEORIES

Much has been made of the scientific ignorance (and latent misogyny) expressed by the term "hysteria" to

*Correspondence to: Professor Mark J. Edwards, Department of Cell Sciences, St. George's University, Cranmer Terrace, London SW17 0RE, UK. E-mail: medwards@sgul.ac.uk

describe patients with FNS. While not seeking to defend use of this term, it is worthwhile pointing out that the (biologic) idea of uterine dysfunction as the cause of functional symptoms was not particularly out of step with pathophysiologic thinking on many other medical conditions at the time this hypothesis was advanced and then over most of the next 2500 years of medical progress. But progress in neurobiologic understanding was made over time. Thomas Willis, for example, suggested that the brain was the source of hysteria. Then, in a flurry of activity in the latter part of the 19th and early 20th centuries there was considerable interest and development of neurobiologic theories (see below). Perhaps part of the problem is that there was then relative lack of interest and even an active disregard for neurobiologic theories in relation to FNS from the 1920s until recent times (with a few notable exceptions). In this way, "hysteria" missed out on the revolution in biologic understanding of many illnesses that took place in the 20th century, and thus appears as rather an anomaly amongst the biologic reassessment of the pathophysiology of illness that occurred in so many other areas of neurology and psychiatry.

Briquet, Janet, Charcot, and Freud all made contributions towards neurobiologic theories of FNS, and though the attempts may seem at first sight rather limited in scope and detail, by the standards of the time and with the knowledge of brain anatomy and physiology available to them, they are impressive. Key observations which were made included the role for attention in manifestation of symptoms, the difference of functional symptoms from feigning, the role for physical and affective triggers to symptoms and the role of physical and psychologic treatment. Charcot proposed that hysteria was a disorder that could be understood with reference to knowledge regarding brain function and dysfunction that occurred in other disorders of the nervous system: "[hysterical symptoms] do not form, in pathology, a class apart, governed by other physiological laws other than the common one" (Charcot, 1889). As an example of this approach he related a biologic understanding of limb postures seen in spasticity to those seen in hysteria, and specifically how hysteric fixed postures often resulted from minor physical trauma:

> *there exists in cases of paralysis due to material lesion a hyper-excitability of the grey substance, and particularly of the motor cells of the anterior horns, a special state. Then, a cutaneous irritation, irritations of the centripetal nerves in general, augments the already excited conditions of the motor cells. ... Now to return to hysteria, in many hysterical patients ... exists an exaggerated reflex excitability. Hence, it is not astonishing to find that an excitation of the centripetal nerves ... produces the same effects as in cases where there exists a lesion of the nervous system (Charcot, 1889).*

His subsequent interest in hypnotism as a treatment indicated a willingness to accept that psychologic factors also played a role in the pathophysiology of hysteria.

Janet (1859–1947) drove a careful middle line between the "clinical period" of Charcot and his followers who emphasized the biologic nature of hysteria and the "psychological period" following on from Freud and Breuer. He criticized both for being overly simplistic: Charcot for being "carried along by habits as a clinician" and Freud and others for being

> *seduced by the psychological explanation ... It seemed to them that the mere words "moral" and "thought" were enough to explain everything, and as people generally like simple explanations, physicians are too disposed nowadays to be content with a vaguely mental explanation.*

Janet's major neurobiologic contribution was in the development of the theory of dissociation as an explanation for how hysteric symptoms might arise. He proposed a key role for attention in the pathophysiology of hysteria, and specifically that a "retraction of the field of consciousness" drove the development of symptoms (Janet, 1907). Janet held that functional sensory loss was a key manifestation of hysteria, and proposed that there was excessive activity of the normal mechanism that filters out extraneous sensory input. A retraction of the field of consciousness occurred, and with it a loss of normal awareness of sensory input. He proposed that the retraction in the field of consciousness often affected a part of the body that was already "weak," for example, a limb that was previously injured (Janet, 1907). This theory accounts well for losses of function such as loss of sensation, but fares less well when considering functional tremor, for example, where Janet himself acknowledged that distraction of attention, for example on to another task, could improve the tremor.

Breuer and Freud, in *Studies on Hysteria* (1893–1895), proposed explicitly not to directly discuss biology in their book: "in what follows, little mention will be made of the brain and none whatever of molecules. Physical processes will be dealt with in the language of psychology; and indeed it cannot possibly be otherwise" (Breuer and Freud, 1974). However, they do on some level attempt to provide a theory for how symptoms might develop in terms which are biologic. They proposed that in health a normal level of "intracerebral tonic excitation" exists in the brain, and excess excitation can be released via motor discharge or secretions, such as jumping for joy or crying. They proposed that a system of "resistance" existed in health, preventing the general distribution of excitation to the vital organs of the body. In hysteria, Freud and Breuer suggested that there was a natural excess of excitation which increased during and after puberty coupled with a lack of innate resistance to the spread of this excitation. Thus, the excess excitation triggered by emotional events is "converted" into somatic phenomena, a process that "follows the principle of least resistance and takes place along paths whose resistances have already been weakened by concurrent circumstances." This theory provided the rationale behind trying to access, via psychotherapy and/or hypnosis, the traumatic event, to allow the release of associated excitation via normal affective responses, hence abolishing the associated somatic symptoms.

20TH-CENTURY NEUROBIOLOGIC THEORIES

Kretschmer (1926) made links between two broad patterns of hysterical symptoms and two instinctive behavioral responses seen in animals. By doing this, he was echoing Janet (1907), who proposed that: "Action, by becoming unconscious in hysterics, by separating from consciousness, loses something of its dignity ... and assumes an appearance that recalls the action of visceral muscles, the action of the lower animals." Kretschmer highlighted two common behavioral responses to threat seen in animals: the "violent motor response," for example, seen when a bird is cornered, and the "sham-death" response, characterized by a lack of movement accompanied by atonia or rigidity. Kretschmer related these instinctive patterns to patterns of symptoms seen in hysteria, for example, convulsive dissociative seizures and violent tremors and conversely paralysis and "fall down and lie still" dissociative seizures. Kretschmer proposed that an initial triggering of this behavior, by a chance (traumatic) event or even done deliberately to escape from a difficult situation, could via repetition become more and more habitual and automatic, a conditioned response no longer requiring the presence of the inciting event.

Whitlock (1967) proposed a biologic basis for hysteria, relating it to corticofugal inhibition of afferent input at the level of the reticular formation which caused a "selective depression of awareness of a bodily function." In this way, attentional diversion away from the symptomatic area caused an inhibition of afferent input from the area, leading to loss of function. This clearly relates closely to Janet's "retraction of the field of consciousness." However in the case of Whitlock, and later, Ludwig (1972), the motivation for the corticofugal inhibition theory seems to have come from the presence of "*la belle indifférence*," a (supposed) lack of attention or concern exhibited by those with hysteria regarding their symptoms.

Both Whitlock and Ludwig link the concept of corticofugal inhibition to the normal phenomenon of lack of awareness of somatic sensation when attention is diverted, for example, on the battlefield or playing field, with Ludwig also pointing to evidence from some studies using evoked potentials in patients with hysteric sensory loss showing a reduction in evoked potential amplitude on the affected side. Ludwig makes a distinction between hysteria and hypochondriasis, proposing that they are "two sides of the same coin." He proposes that patients with hysteria have a "dissociation of attention" from their symptoms, while hypochondriacs have their attention "locked to their symptoms." Ludwig proposes that in hypochondriasis:

> *excessive attention becomes directed and locked to a source of afferent stimulation ... corticofugal inhibition of afferent stimulation (both corticocortical and corticoreticular) becomes reduced or "hypotonic" thereby permitting the greater intrusion of afferent stimulation into conscious awareness. A closed feedback loop then becomes established, whereby unchecked afferent stimulation produces a greater conscious awareness of it; this then produces reduced corticofugal inhibition which, in turn, allows greater afferent activity, and so on.*

Ludwig uses his proposal of increased corticofugal inhibition in hysteria to account for the "propensity toward 'exaggerated absentmindedness' and a continuous amnesia for immediate events" seen in hysteria, a clinical observation that he ascribes to Janet. He suggested that the presence of excessive corticofugal inhibition is in keeping with resolution of symptoms that was reported with sedation and "psychological maneuvers (e.g. hypnosis, relaxation procedures) having disinhibitory effects." He also proposed that suggestibility in hysteria would be predicted from the weakness of their attentional focus due to corticofugal inhibition and hence that attention (and belief, one assumes) could be easily captured by an external stimulus/suggestion and cause a "suspension of critical faculties and enhanced credulity."

Basing a neurobiologic theory on the phenomenon of "*la belle indifférence*" is likely to be a dangerous thing to do. The use of the term as Whitlock and Ludwig propose it – a lack of concern and attention towards symptoms – is probably not its original use, and is certainly not a clinical sign with any useful discriminating value between patients with FNS and those with organic neurologic disease (Stone et al., 2006). It also fails to account for why attention is required for many FNS to manifest (e.g., paralysis, tremor) and why such symptoms improve when attention is distracted away. Indeed, the description

Ludwig gives of the neurobiology of hypochondriasis seems to provide a better model for explaining such clinical phenomena.

21ST-CENTURY NEUROBIOLOGIC MODELS

The very end of the 20th and the early 21st century brought a renewed clinical interest in FNS, and also the use of modern investigative techniques, in particular functional imaging. Limited patient numbers in these studies (including many with single subjects) makes interpretation difficult and, not surprisingly, conflicting results have emerged. Also, with one exception, studies tend to occur at a single time point and do not look at patients before and after treatment. This latter approach is a powerful way in which to minimize the impact of comorbidities that are present in many patients with functional symptoms and to be able to see more clearly what imaging features are related to the presence of the functional symptoms themselves.

The study of a single patient with unilateral functional leg weakness by Marshall et al. (1997) marked a watershed in approach to study of FNS. They employed new technology (functional imaging) and made an interpretation of the data (orbitofrontal and anterior cingulate activation during attempted movement of the weak leg inhibiting prefrontal cortex activation) that was relatively free from speculation about psychologic underpinnings of the disorder. Studies by Spence et al. (2000) and Maruff and Velakoulis (2000) found what appeared to be normal preparatory activity for upcoming movement in single patients with functional paralysis, but then differences from healthy controls and those feigning paralysis with respect to prefrontal cortex activation. This was interpreted as the presence of abnormal prefrontally driven inhibition of a normally functioning motor system, echoing previous theories such as those of Ludwig (1972) and Whitlock (1967). Vuilleumier et al. (2001) took subjects with unilateral sensory loss and examined activations using single-positron emission computed tomography (SPECT) occurring during vibration of the healthy and affected sides. A reduction in blood flow was seen in the thalamus, caudate, and putamen contralateral to the affected side, and this resolved in those patients who experienced resolution of symptoms when they were rescanned some months later. This was interpreted as showing the presence of a more "basic," low-level dysfunction in patients with functional symptoms that could not so easily be explained by the presence of excessive higher-level inhibition.

In a clear step beyond the existing rather broad suggestions of "excess inhibition" present in neurobiologic theories to date, Voon and Hallett proposed a new theory for how functional movement disorders (FMD) might arise, developed against the background of a number of important functional imaging and behavioral studies in FMD (Voon et al., 2010a, b, 2011, 2013). These studies proposed the concept of a "previously mapped conversion motor representation," a (conditioned) pattern of movement established by a previous triggering event.

Functional imaging studies provided evidence for hypoactivity in areas usually associated with action selection (e.g., supplementary motor area: SMA), as well as abnormally strong connectivity between limbic structures (e.g., amygdala) and SMA (Voon et al., 2010b, 2011), enhanced by emotional stimuli. The hypoactivity of the SMA provides a substrate for an impairment in the ability to inhibit or stop an action. In an arousing context, the previously mapped conversion motor representation is activated in part because of the abnormal functional connectivity between limbic structures and SMA, and cannot be inhibited because there is a disconnection between SMA and areas (prefrontal cortex, for example) that could usually inhibit unwanted action. The result is a movement that arises without a normal prediction of its sensory consequences (in the language of motor control theory, without an efference copy) and is therefore experienced by patients as arising spontaneously and without will or control (Voon et al., 2011).

This theory is supported by imaging studies from within the group and others – for example, it fits well with findings of prefrontal cortex hypoactivity in studies by Spence et al. (2000). It also provides a mechanism for the "involuntariness" of symptoms as reported by patients. The "previously mapped conversion representation" fits with previous proposals regarding the conditioning of responses from inciting events proposed by Kretschmer, and others before him, including Freud and Janet.

In my own work, developed with a number of other researchers, including Isabel Pareés, Rick Adams, and Karl Friston, I have been interested in building a neurobiologic model of functional symptoms from "the ground up" – in other words, starting with basic clinical observations, and devising a set of principles that must be accounted for by any neurobiologic theory. The resulting principles (which are certainly not new nor complete, but perhaps bring together previous observations in a novel way) can be summarized as follows.

Co-occurrence of symptoms

While the phenomenology of FNS is clearly very diverse, such symptoms commonly co-occur. It is therefore most likely that there is a unifying underlying pathophysiology for functional symptoms that cuts across different physical manifestations.

Attention

Attention towards motor symptoms (both "positive" ones such as tremor and "negative" ones such as paralysis) can clearly be seen as necessary for the symptom to be present, and when it is absent, the symptom resolves. If principle 1 (co-occurrence of symptoms) is correct, then an abnormal switch of attention towards the body/symptom must be a key pathophysiologic feature of all functional symptoms.

Beliefs/expectations

Symptoms are clearly influenced by beliefs about how the brain and body work and how they may go wrong, producing symptoms which are incongruent with basic anatomic and physiologic (and even physical) principles. Examples of this include tubular visual fields and patterns of psychogenic amnesia. Therefore, a mechanism by which belief/expectations about symptoms can affect function must be incorporated in any pathophysiologic theory.

Agency

Movements that require attention to manifest and which stop on distraction are characteristically experienced as voluntary. Therefore disruption of a sense of agency for movement (and perception) must be accounted for by any pathophysiologic theory.

We used a modern biologic theory of brain function called active inference as a foundation for our neurobiologic theory of FNS (Edwards et al., 2012). Active inference is based on a statistical theory advanced by Bayes (1702–1761) and proposals from Helmholtz (1821–1894). The brain is considered as a hierarchic structure with a flow of information in two directions, from sense organs (e.g., proprioception, visual input) upwards ("bottom-up") and from the cortex down ("top-down"). At each level in the hierarchy, bottom-up data meet top-down predictions (called "priors") about the content of that data. Bottom-up data and top-down priors are "compared" in a statistical fashion that takes into account different weightings given to the data/predictions. Thus, in certain circumstances (for example, when priors are down-weighted and bottom-up data are weighted more strongly), the resulting perception or movement is more strongly influenced by the nature of the bottom-up data than the prior. In a real-world example, if you are navigating round an unfamiliar hotel bedroom in the dark, the weighting or "precision" of your priors about where the bathroom door is located is low. You therefore move very slowly, feeling your way along the wall, sensitive to any bottom-up sensory data that you encounter. This increased sensitivity or precision on the bottom-up data might even lead you to misperceive things, for example, the faint glow of the television standby light might be misperceived as light coming from the door to the bedroom, and you may go off in the wrong direction. In contrast, if you are in your own bedroom, the precision/weighting of your priors about the layout of the room is high, and you may stride out confidently across the room. This may lead to lack of sensitivity to salient "bottom-up" data, for example, that the pattern of light in the room indicates that the door is half-closed, something you do not perceive until you stub your toe on it. Though this example is a little trivial, it highlights a crucial point, that our perception and control of movement are not fixed, but can be influenced by both our predictions and data we receive from the world. Attention plays a key role in changing the precision or weighting of both bottom-up data and priors.

Our proposal (Edwards et al., 2012) with regard to FNS is that an event induces the formation of an abnormally strong (precise) prior. These events may be normal physiologic experiences (e.g., sleep paralysis, hypnic jerks, fasciculations), pathophysiologic experiences (e.g., migraine, pain following injury, symptoms of neurologic disease such as multiple sclerosis or epilepsy), or psychophysiologic experiences (e.g., symptoms associated with panic). Obviously these may co-occur in the same person (e.g., symptoms from migraine causing additional symptoms caused by panic). Crucially for a universal theory for the generation of FNS, it is the nature of the prior that determines the symptoms the patient experiences. It does not matter if the symptom is a "positive" one such as pain or tremor, or a "negative" one such as anesthesia or paralysis: the mechanism is the same. This overcomes the problematic issue with previous theories since the time of Janet, where it is difficult to reconcile within the same theory the presence of positive and negative functional symptoms (which can coexist in the same patient). It is the case that the nature of the prior for some positive symptoms (tremor, choreiform movements, bizarre gait abnormalities) appears complex and more difficult to define compared to a symptom such as unilateral sensory loss. However, priors relating to complex movement are proposed to exist in health, permitting the generation of complex voluntary movements.

The movements that occur in patients with FMDs are within the bounds of those that can be produced voluntarily, and so the existence of priors that could define very complex movement patterns that could be triggered without will is feasible. The theory proposes that "misdirected" attention towards the body and specifically towards the symptom itself (and beliefs/expectations around it) increases the precision of the abnormal prior, overwhelming any "bottom-up" data that are out of keeping with it. This is consistent with the lack of awareness of many patients with functional symptoms of their own inconsistencies where, for example, they say that they cannot move their arm, but then it can be clearly seen to move when they are distracted.

The lack of sense of agency over functional movement symptoms can also be explained within this theory. The (voluntary) action that triggers the functional symptom is the turning of attention towards the body, though, as explained here (Edwards et al., 2012), this turning of attention towards the body may happen by a much more involuntary "capture" of attention. However, this is where the voluntariness stops, as the resulting percept or movement that is triggered by the turning of attention towards the body does not occur in a normal manner. It happens without the normal series of events that would lead to a normal sensation of voluntariness, a sense that "I willed that."

This theory leads to some testable predictions about, for example, abnormalities in the behavioral and electrophysiologic phenomenon of sensory attenuation that accompanies normal voluntary movement, and the effect of attention towards the limb on somatosensory evoked potentials in patients with functional sensory loss. So far, these predictions have been borne out by experimental work (Pareés et al., 2014; Macerollo et al., 2015; Brown et al., 2016), though much more needs to be done.

CONCLUDING REMARKS

The main components of neurobiologic theories of FNS have been present for a century or more. Russell Reynolds' insights on the influence of "idea" (i.e., belief/expectation) on motor and sensory function (Reynolds, 1869) deserve a special mention, as does Richard Brown's highly influential cognitive model for "medically unexplained symptoms" (Brown, 2004). Modern neuroscience provides the tools for closer examination of theoretic predictions, and should lead to refinement of neurobiologic theories in due course.

However, the biggest step forward in this field of study has come not from the theories themselves, but from developments in clinical practice. Though many neurologists, almost in secret, had an interested and enlightened view of patients with FNS in their personal practice, published data and doctrine from most of the 20th century paint a fairly uninspiring, enormously simplistic, and ultimately nihilistic picture of the role of biologic understanding in FNS. Pioneering work on the epidemiology of FNS (Stone et al., 2009, 2010), work that challenged accepted doctrine on issues such as misdiagnosis (Crimlisk et al., 1998), and work that advocated a broad nonjudgmental approach to considering etiology, was all crucial in providing fertile ground for neurobiologic studies to emerge. Providing this broad consensus can continue, avoiding splitting into biologic and psychologic "camps," the future for a neurobiologic understanding of functional symptoms is very bright indeed.

References

Breuer J, Freud S (1974). Studies on Hysteria. The Pelican Freud Library. Penguin Books, Harmondsworth.

Brown RJ (2004). Psychological mechanisms of medically unexplained symptoms: an integrative conceptual model. Psychol Bull 130: 793–812.

Brown H, Adams RA, Stone J, et al. (2016). Attentional processing in functional anaesthesia. Am J Psychiatry (in press).

Charcot JM (1889). Clinical Lectures on Diseases of the Nervous System. The New Sydenham Society, London.

Crimlisk HL, Bhatia K, Cope H et al. (1998). Slater revisited: 6-year follow-up study of patients with medically unexplained motor symptoms. BMJ 316: 582–586.

Edwards MJ, Adams RA, Brown H et al. (2012). A Bayesian account of 'hysteria'. Brain 135: 3495–3512.

Janet P (1907). The Major Symptoms of Hysteria, Macmillan, London.

Kretschmer E (1926). Hysteria, Nervous and Mental Disease Publishing, New York.

Ludwig AM (1972). Hysteria: a neurobiological theory. Arch Gen Psychiatr 27: 771–777.

Macerollo A, Chen JC, Pareés I et al. (2015). Sensory attenuation assessed by sensory evoked potentials in functional movement disorders. PLoS One 10 (6): e0129507.

Marshall JC, Halligan PW, Fink GR et al. (1997). The functional anatomy of a hysterical paralysis. Cognition 64 (1): B1–B8.

Maruff P, Velakoulis D (2000). The voluntary control of motor imagery. Imagined movements in individuals with feigned motor impairment and conversion disorder. Neuropsychologia 38: 1251–1260.

Pareés I, Brown H, Nuruki A et al. (2014). Loss of sensory attenuation in patients with functional (psychogenic) movement disorders. Brain 137: 2916–2921.

Reynolds JR (1869). Paralysis and other disorders of motion and sensation dependent on idea. BMJ. i: 483–485.

Spence SA, Crimlisk HL, Cope H et al. (2000). Discrete neurophysiological correlates in prefrontal cortex during hysterical and feigned disorder of movement [letter]. Lancet 355: 1243–1244.

Stone J, Smyth R, Carson A et al. (2006). La belle indifférence in conversion symptoms and hysteria: systematic review. Br J Psychiatry 188: 204–209.

Stone J, Carson A, Duncan R et al. (2009). Symptoms 'unexplained by organic disease' in 1144 new neurology outpatients: how often does the diagnosis change at follow-up? Brain 132: 2878–2888.

Stone J, Carson A, Duncan R et al. (2010). Who is referred to neurology clinics? The diagnoses made in 3781 new patients. Clin Neurol Neurosurg 112: 747–751.

Voon V, Gallea C, Hattori N et al. (2010a). The involuntary nature of conversion disorder. Neurology 74: 223–228.

Voon V, Brezing C, Gallea C et al. (2010b). Emotional stimuli and motor conversion disorder. Brain 133: 1526–1536.

Voon V, Brezing C, Gallea C et al. (2011). Aberrant supplementary motor complex and limbic activity during motor preparation in motor conversion disorder. Mov Disord 26: 2396–2403.

Voon V, Ekanayake V, Wiggs E et al. (2013). Response inhibition in motor conversion disorder. Mov Disord 28: 612–618.

Vuilleumier P, Chicherio C, Assal F et al. (2001). Functional neuroanatomical correlates of hysterical sensorimotor loss. Brain 124: 1077–1090.

Whitlock FA (1967). The aetiology of hysteria. Acta Psychiatr Scand 43: 144–162.

Handbook of Clinical Neurology, Vol. 139 (3rd series)
Functional Neurologic Disorders
M. Hallett, J. Stone, and A. Carson, Editors
http://dx.doi.org/10.1016/B978-0-12-801772-2.00013-8

Chapter 13

Stress, childhood trauma, and cognitive functions in functional neurologic disorders

K. ROELOFS[1,2]* AND J. PASMAN[1]
[1]*Behavioural Science Institute, Radboud University Nijmegen, Nijmegen, The Netherlands*
[2]*Donders Institute for Brain Cognition and Behaviour, Nijmegen, The Netherlands*

Abstract

Conversion disorder (CD) has traditionally been ascribed to psychologic factors such as trauma, stress, or emotional conflict. Although reference to the psychologic origin of CD has been removed from the criteria list in DSM-5, many theories still incorporate CD as originating from adverse events.

This chapter provides a critical review of the literature on stressful life events in CD and discusses current cognitive and neurobiologic models linking psychologic stressors with conversion symptomatology. In addition, we propose a neurobiologic stress model integrating those cognitive models with neuroendocrine stress research and propose that stress and stress-induced changes in hypothalamus–pituitary–adrenal (HPA) axis function may result in cognitive alterations, that in turn contribute to experiencing conversion symptoms. Experimental studies indeed suggest that basal as well as stress-induced changes in HPA axis responding lead to alterations in attentional processing in CD. Although those changes are stronger in traumatized patients, similar patterns have been observed in patients who do not report a history of traumatic events.

We conclude that, whereas adverse events may play an important role in many cases of CD, a substantial proportion of patients do not report a history of traumatization or recent stressful events. Studies integrating effects of stress on cognitive functioning in CD are scarce. We propose that, instead of focusing research on defining etiologic events in terms of symptom-eliciting events, future research should work towards an integrated mechanistic account, assessing alterations in cognitive and biologic stress systems in an integrated manner in patients with CD. Such an account may not only serve early symptom detection, it might also provide a starting point for better-targeted interventions.

INTRODUCTION

Medically unexplained neurologic symptoms have been observed in over 30% of patients presenting in specialized neurologic clinics (Carson et al., 2000). The official rates for conversion disorder (CD) are lower: only 5% of referrals to neurology clinics are diagnosed with CD, and the incidence in the general population is estimated to be 2–5 per 100 000 per year (American Psychiatric Association, 2013). This discrepancy is in part due to scarce psychiatric evaluation and underreporting in nonpsychiatric settings (Akagi and House, 2002; Nicholson et al., 2011). Given the prevalence and because conversion symptoms are associated with individual suffering and excessive public health costs, it is highly relevant to gain more insight into the underlying etiologic mechanisms (Konnopka et al., 2012).

CD has traditionally been ascribed to psychologic stress factors such as trauma, adverse life events, or emotional conflicts. Until the introduction of the fifth edition of the *Diagnostic and Statistical Manual of Mental Disorders* (DSM-5: American Psychiatric Association,

*Correspondence to: Prof. Dr. K. Roelofs, Donders Institute for Brain, Cognition and Behaviour, Kapittelweg 29, 6525 EN Nijmegen, The Netherlands. E-mail: k.roelofs@donders.ru.nl

2013) this etiologic factor even belonged to the main criteria for the diagnostic entity of CD, stating that the symptom initiation or exacerbation should be preceded by conflicts or other stressors (fourth edition, text revision: American Psychiatric Association, 2000). Because the DSM is a descriptive manual and because it is extremely difficult, if not impossible, to prove that a psychologic event has a causal relationship with the onset or exacerbation of a symptom, this criterion has now been removed from the current DSM-5. The presence of psychologic stressors is now handled as a specifier that can be added to the diagnosis. Note that in the revised 10th version of the *International Classification of Diseases* (ICD-10: World Health Organization, 2010), CD is still assumed to be "associated closely in time with traumatic events, insoluble and intolerable problems, or disturbed relationships" (article F44).

Not only diagnostic manuals but also traditional theories on CD have been dominated by the view that the symptoms would be caused by a psychologic stressor or an emotional conflict. Throughout history, philosophers like Plato, physicians such as Breuer, neurologists such as Freud, and pioneer psychiatrists such as Janet have tried to explain how conversion symptoms could arise from such stress factors. Before describing current theories on conversion symptoms, we will first present an overview of the literature on comparative studies that reported on the occurrence of stressful life events or trauma in the history of patients diagnosed with CD. Thereafter, we will present explanatory models, mostly of cognitive nature. Finally, those models will be integrated with recent neurobiologic findings in CD and we will end with setting an agenda for research needed to advance this emerging and interesting field of medically unexplained somatic symptoms.

TRAUMA AND LIFE EVENTS IN CONVERSION DISORDER: A LITERATURE REVIEW

Literature on life adversities generally distinguishes between trauma and recent stressful events (e.g., Roelofs et al., 2005; Reuber et al., 2007; Bakvis et al., 2009b). For trauma it is common to further distinguish between emotional, physical, and sexual abuse (e.g., Alper et al., 1993; Bakvis et al., 2009b, 2010a; Baslet, 2011; Almis et al., 2013; Baker et al., 2013). In the present literature review we will follow these distinctions, resulting in four subcategories of life adversities (physical abuse, sexual abuse, emotional abuse/neglect, and life events). Some studies report specifically on childhood trauma; if this was the case, it will be reported in the review. Because the literature only reports on retrospective studies on life adversities in CD and because the reliability of various retrospective assessment methods may vary, we decided to indicate the assessment method (interview, questionnaire, or both) in our literature review. In addition, we excluded studies with fewer than 10 subjects in the experimental group and studies that did not have a control group. Following these criteria, we conducted a literature review in online databases (PsycINFO and Medline 1990–September 2014), using a range of keywords describing variants of CD (conversion, hysteria, hysterical, functional, pseudoneurologic, pseudoepileptic, psychogenic or medically unexplained symptoms or disorders) combined with variants of traumatic experiences (trauma, life event, adverse event, abuse, neglect, assault). In addition, the reference lists of the found studies were explored to detect other relevant citations. Please note that we did not include a systematic quality assessment and do not claim that this review is complete. The results of the literature review are presented in Table 13.1. Articles that report on stressful life events without specifically referring to trauma are not included in the table, but are discussed below in the section on Life events. Depending on the availability of data and results, trauma rates (in percentages) and/or the significance of differences between subsamples (in *p*-value) have been reported.

Trauma rates in conversion disorder

A total of 32 studies was selected. Most studies distinguished between various subtypes of trauma; physical and sexual abuse were common categories. Trauma was measured using a structured interview, questionnaire, or a clinical (unstructured) interview. The outcome of the present literature overview gives no indication of systematic variance related to use of assessment instrument.

In 22 studies, total trauma rates for CD patients were compared to those in a control sample. Fifteen of those studies reported total trauma percentages, ranging from 14% to 100% for CD samples (and 9–66% for controls; organic, psychiatric, or healthy). At first sight, the trauma rates for CD seem higher than those in the normal population, where estimates of trauma exposure vary between 14.2% and 56% (Breslau et al., 1991; Kessler et al., 1995; Perkonigg et al., 2000). In 18 of the 22 studies the group differences in trauma rates were statistically tested (using occurrence rates or questionnaire scores). In 17 of these 18, total trauma experience was significantly higher in the CD sample than in the control sample. One study found no significant difference (no. 18). In the remaining four studies, that provided no formal statistical testing of group differences, the pattern was in the same direction. Below we detail findings for separate trauma categories: physical, sexual, and emotional abuse.

Table 13.1

Review of the literature on the occurrence rates of (childhood) trauma and recent stressful events in different conversion disorder samples

	Article	Measurement instrument	L/C*	Sample characteristics	Physical abuse		Sexual abuse	Emotional abuse/ neglect		Total trauma[†]	Recent life events[‡]
1	Almis et al. (2013)	Structured Clinical Interview for DSM-IV	C	22 PNES, 100% female, age 25	5%		9%			14%	
				22 healthy controls, 100% female, age 25	5%		5% $p = 0.550$			9% (abuse)	
2	Alper et al. (1993)	Structured Clinical Interview for DSM-IV	C	71 PNES, 73% female, age 32	16%		24%			32%	
				140 epilepsy, 51% female, age 32	3%		7%			9% (abuse)	
3	Arnold and Privitera (1996)	Own instrument	L	14 PNES, 64% female, age 33	43%		0%			86%	
				27 ES, 48% female, age 35	0%		11% (incl. physical)			33% (any trauma) $p = 0.004$	
4	Akyuz et al. (2004)	Childhood Abuse and Neglect Questionnaire	C	33 PNES, 100% female, age 28	79%		33%	61%	42%		
				30 ES, 100% female, age 28	17% $p < 0.001$		7% $p = 0.009$	13% (abuse) $p < 0.001$	27% (neglect) $p = 0.190$	(abuse and neglect) $p < 0.001$	
5	Baker et al. (2013)	Life Events and Difficulties Schedule	L	73 functional voice disorder, 100% female, age 47	41%	14%	32%			49%	74%
				55 organic voice disorder, age 48	29%	7%	18%			33%	22%
				66 nonrandom control group, age 47	14% (violence) $p = 0.002$	2% (strangulation) $p = 0.025$	11% $p = 0.008$			21% (abuse) $p = 0.002$	14% (severe events) $p < 0.001$
6[§]	Bakvis et al. (2009b)	Traumatic Experiences Checklist	L	19 PNES, 79% female, age 28	63%		74%	74%		89%	
				20 healthy controls, 90% female, age 22	5% $p < 0.001$		5% $p < 0.001$	11% $p < 0.001$		11% (interpersonal) $p < 0.001$	
7[§]	Bakvis et al. (2010a)	Traumatic Experiences Checklist	L	18 PNES patients, 61% female, age 32	33%		39%	44%		61%	
				19 healthy controls, 47% female, age 35	16% $p = 0.021$		11% $p = 0.044$	21% (abuse) $p = 0.129$		26% (interpersonal) $p = 0.033$	

Continued

Table 13.1

Continued

	Article	Measurement instrument	L/C*	Sample characteristics	Physical abuse	Sexual abuse	Emotional abuse/ neglect	Total trauma[†]	Recent life events[‡]
8	Berkhoff et al. (1998)	Own interview	C	10 PNES, 50% female, age 44	10%	20%			
				10 ES, 50% female, age 43	0% $p = 0.317$	0% $p = 0.179$			
9	Betts and Boden (1992)	Case history	C	96 PNES, 85% female, age ?		54%			
				132 ES, 61% female, age ?		25%			
				87 psychiatric control, 67% female, age ?		32%			
10	Binzer and Eisemann (1998)	Own memories of childrearing experiences	C	30 PMD, 60% female, age 39		3.3%			
				30 neurological motor disorder, 70% female, age 34		0% $p > 0.05$			
11	Binzer et al. (2004)	Own memories of childrearing experiences	C	20 PNES, 75% female, age 27		30%			(year prior to onset) $p < 0.001$
				20 ES, 60% female, age 27		5% (incest) $p = 0.090$			
12	Bowman and Markand, (1996)	Own trauma experience checklist	C	45 PNES, 78% female, age 38	67%	69%		84% (any trauma) $p < 0.001$	
				Unspecified comparable sample		38% (females) $p < 0.010$			
13	Dikel et al. (2003)	Life Events Checklist	L	17 PNES, 76% female, age 39		71%		100%	
				34 ES, 50% female, age 35		32% (childhood) $p = 0.010$		67.6% (any assault) $p = 0.008$	
14	Jawad et al. (1995)	Own interview	C	46 PNES, 100% female, age 29		9%			
				50 psychiatric control, age 32		8% $p = 0.900$			

15	Kaplan et al. (2013)	Childhood Trauma Questionnaire	C	91 PNES, 90% female, age 42	35%	38%	44%	30%		
				81 ES, 68% female, age 40	20% $p = 0.030$	25% $p = 0.050$	30% (abuse) $p = 0.054$	17% (neglect) $p = 0.005$		
16	Kozlowska et al. (2011)	Linguistic analysis of interview	C	76 conversion, 70% female, age 13	15%	7%	13% (neglect)		75%,	27% (bereavement)
				76 healthy controls, matched for age and sex					12% (unresolved loss/trauma) $p < 0.001$	
17	Kranick et al. (2011)	Childhood Trauma Questionnaire	C	64 PMD, 72% female, age 45	$p = 0.090$	$p = 0.700$	$p < 0.050$		(abuse and neglect) $p < 0.001$	
				39 focal hand dystonia, 74% female, age 4939 healthy controls, 74% female, age 49						
18	Kuyk et al. (1999)	Trauma Questionnaire	L	27 PNES, 77% female, age 29	26%	33%	37%		44%	
				47 temporal-lobe epilepsy (TLE), 36% female, age 39	6%	4%	23%		26%	
				25 non-TLE , 38% female, age 35	16% PNES vs. other: $p = 0.053$	0% PNES vs. other $p < 0.001$	16% PNES vs. other: $p > 0.05$		24% (abuse) PNES vs. other: $p > 0.05$	
19	Litwin and Cardeña (2000)	Dissociative Disorders Interview Schedule	L	10 PNES, 100% female, age 31	50%	60%				
				31 ES, 45% female, age 35	29% $p > 0.050$	13% $p < 0.005$				
20	McDade and Brown (1992)	Own interview	C	18 PNES, 38% female, age 34		17%				
				18 ES, 44% female, age 32		5%				
21	Mökleby et al. (2002)	MINI International Neuropsychiatric Interview	L	23 PNES, 83% female, age 32					30%	
				23 other somatoform disorder, 83% female, age 32					17%	
				23 healthy controls, 83% female, age 30					0% (abuse)	

Continued

Table 13.1

Continued

	Article	Measurement instrument	L/C*	Sample characteristics	Physical abuse	Sexual abuse	Emotional abuse/ neglect	Total trauma†	Recent life events‡
22	Ozcetin et al. (2009)	Childhood Trauma Questionnaire	C	56 PNES, 100% female, age 34 59 healthy controls, 100% female, age 34	$p < 0.001$	$p < 0.001$	$p < 0.001$	(abuse and neglect) $p < 0.001$	
23	Plioplys et al. (2014)	Children's Hassles Scale	C	55, 71% female, age 15 35 healthy siblings, 51% female, age 14	13% 6% $p = 0.300$	15% 3% $p = 0.200$	42% 17% (abuse) $p = 0.010$	(adversities) $p = 0.020$	
24	Proença et al. (2011)	Childhood Trauma Questionnaire	C	20 PNES 20 ES No significant differences in age or gender	$p = 0.144$	$p = 0.123$	$p > 0.05$ for every subcategory	(abuse) $p = 0.014$	
25	Reilly et al. (1999)	Medical History Questionnaire	L	40 PNES, 73% female, age 34	53% 18%	53% 18%	60% 45%		
				40 ES, 60% female, age 34	40% 23%	40% 23%	45% 33%		
				40 medically unexplained gastrointestinal symptoms, 75% female, age 41	13% (childhood) 0% (adulthood) PNES vs. other $p < 0.001$	13% (childhood) 0% (adulthood) PNES vs. other $p < 0.010$	23% (childhood) 13% (adulthood) PNES vs. other $p < 0.001$		
26	Roelofs et al. (2002a)	Structured Trauma Interview	C	54 conversion, 83% female, age 38	28%	24%		44%	
				50 affective disorder, 82% female, age 36	20% $p = 0.280$	14% $p = 0.85$		24% (abuse) $p < 0.050$	
27	Salmon et al. (2003)	Medical History Questionnaire Parental Bonding Instrument	L	81 PNES, 69% female, age 35	36% 14%	31% 32%	53% 31%		
				81 ES, 69% female, age 35	21% (childhood) $p < 0.050$ 4% (adulthood) $p < 0.050$	16% (childhood) $p < 0.050$ 15% (adulthood) $p < 0.001$	32% (childhood) $p < 0.010$ 26% (adulthood) $p > 0.050$		

28	Şar et al. (2009)	Own interview (A-criterion DSM-IV)	C	274 conversion symptoms 32 somatization with conversion 322 no conversion total sample: 100% female, age 35	12% 19% 5% $p = 0.001$	3% 9% 1% $p = 0.019$	37% 63% 15% $p < 0.001$	43% 66% 32% (abuse and neglect) $p < 0.001$	
29	Scévola et al. (2013)	Structured Clinical Interview for DSM-IV	L	35 PNES, 77% female, age 38 49 ES, 59% female, age 35	14% 12% (incl. other violence) $p = 0.410$	26% 4% $p = 0.007$		49% 25% (any trauma) $p = 0.020$	
30	Steffen et al. (2015)	Early Trauma Inventory Life Events Questionnaire	L	45 FND (excl. PNES), 71% female, age 40 45 healthy controls, 69% female, age 45	$p > 0.050$	$p > 0.050$	$p < 0.001$	(general trauma) $p < 0.010$	(in past year) $p < 0.001$
31	Tojek et al. (2000)	Life Events Checklist	L	25 PNES, 88% female, age 44 33 ES, 91% female, age 40	(adulthood) $p = 0.030$	(childhood) (adulthood) $p = 0.350$ $p = 0.100$		44% 33%	$p < 0.050$
32	Van Merode et al. (2015)	Childhood Trauma Questionnaire	C	40 PNES, 65% female, age 49 138 ES, 50% female, age 35				(abuse) (abuse and neglect) $p = 0.030$	

DSM-IV: *Diagnostic and Statistical Manual of Mental Disorders*, 4th edn (American Psychiatric Association, 2000); PNES, psychogenic nonepileptic seizures; ES, epileptic seizures; PMD, psychogenic motor disorder; FND, functional neurological disorder.

Empty cells: type of trauma was not assessed or figure was not reported. Red marking: group difference was significant; blue marking: group difference was non-significant; white: group difference was not statistically tested.

[*] L/C: specifies the investigated period of trauma occurrence, with L standing for "at any point in lifetime" and C standing for "anywhere during childhood" (before age 18).

[†] The "total trauma" category follows the definition as cited in the respective paper.

[‡] The "stressful events" category includes bereavement and other loss, accidents, change in health or employment status, and interpersonal conflict.

[§] Please note that some overlap in the patient samples of these two articles could not be ruled out.

Physical abuse

In 22 studies, physical abuse rates for CD patients were compared to those in a control sample. Absolute physical abuse rates (based on 19 of those studies) ranged from 5% to 79% for CD samples and rates from 0% to 40% for control samples. Ten out of 19 studies that statistically tested for group differences in physical abuse rates found significantly higher rates or scores in the CD group. In the other nine studies, there were no significant differences. In two out of the three final studies (nos. 1–3) that did not test for significant differences, physical abuse rates followed the pattern of being higher in CD samples than in controls. In 11 of the 22 studies that reported on physical abuse, specific rates were provided for childhood abuse (before age 18). In six out of those 11 studies, a significantly higher rate was found in CD compared to controls. In three of the remaining five, the difference did not reach significance (nos. 9, 17, and 24). In the final two no formal statistical testing was provided, but the physical abuse rates showed the pattern of being higher in CD than in control samples (nos. 1 and 2).

Sexual abuse

Thirty studies reported on sexual abuse. The rates of sexual abuse ranged between 0% and 74% in CD samples and between 0% and 40% in controls (based on 25 studies). In 13 out of the 26 studies that statistically tested for group differences, rates of sexual abuse were significantly higher in CD compared to at least one control group. When specifically looking at childhood sexual abuse, seven out of 18 studies that statistically tested for group differences found a significant difference, with higher rates of childhood sexual abuse in CD patients than in at least one control group. In the other 11, no significant differences were found. Three studies (nos. 2, 8, and 20) did not test for significance, but did report childhood sexual abuse rates, and those followed the pattern of being higher in the CD samples than in controls.

Emotional abuse or neglect

A total of 14 studies looked into emotional abuse and/or neglect. Rates for the total category or of abuse or neglect only were 30–74% for CD samples and 11–63% for control samples (based on nine studies). Thirteen of the 14 studies statistically tested the difference in rates between CD and control samples, with 10 finding a significant effect for the total category or at least one subcategory of emotional abuse and neglect. One study (no. 18) found a significant difference in the opposite direction, with rates being higher in the psychiatric control group than in CD. Six studies found no significant differences in the total category or in a subcategory. In 10 of the 14 studies, the occurrence of neglect/emotional abuse in childhood (under age 18) was under investigation. Of those studies, nine tested for group differences in this category. Eight of those found significantly higher rates in CD samples compared to controls, although in two the rates were only significantly higher in CD for some subtype of emotional abuse or neglect (nos. 4 and 15). One study (no. 24) showed no significant difference and the final study only reported an occurrence rate for their CD sample (no. 16).

In conclusion, the reported trauma rates are generally found to be higher for CD compared to healthy and organic disorder control groups. Studies specifically targeting childhood experiences reported comparable findings to those investigating adverse events during adulthood or any time in life. Note that only three studies included a psychiatric control group. Two of those studies reported slightly higher childhood trauma rates in CD (nos. 14 and 26), but the third failed to find this (no. 9). Only two studies compared CD directly to other somatoform disorders and found trauma rates to be higher in the former samples. Finally, it is important to realize that if 14–100% of CD patients have experienced trauma, the remaining 0–86% have not. Concluding, in general trauma rates (childhood or adult) appear to be higher in CD than in healthy or organic disorder control groups, but this is not universally so, and more research is needed to determine whether trauma rates in CD are elevated in comparison to other psychiatric disorders, too.

Life events

Of all studies focused on traumatic events reviewed in Table 13.1, only five studies reported separately on life events (adverse events, not necessarily traumatic, that have typically preceded the onset of symptoms: nos. 5, 11, 16, 30, and 31). Four of those studies reported significantly higher life event rates/scores for CD compared to a control group. The last one did not report comparison rates and did not test for statistical differences. Apart from the articles reviewed above, other studies have specifically focused on stressful life events. These studies are not reported in Table 13.1 as it reviews studies on trauma, but they will be briefly discussed below. In these studies life events are typically defined as "change" events that have occurred within a year prior to symptom onset or assessment time. They include changes in health, relationships, housing, or employment status. It is often found that CD patients have experienced more of such events than controls (Grattan-Smith et al., 1988; Binzer et al., 1997; Roelofs et al., 2005; Bodde et al., 2013). However, other studies failed to find this (e.g., Voon et al., 2010; Czarnecki and Hallett, 2012; Testa et al., 2012).

The relation between life events and CD seems to be not so clearcut. For example, one study (Binzer et al., 2004) found no group differences between psychogenic nonepileptic seizures (PNES) and epileptic seizures (ES) patients in the number of events in the 3 months prior to symptom onset, but did so when accounting for events during the whole year prior to symptom onset. One older study (House and Andrews, 1988) found that women with functional dysphonia had not experienced more stressful events in general, but did experience more "conflicts over speaking out." In another study, among 40 subjects with PNES compared to 60 without, Testa et al. (2012) found that PNES patients did not experience higher frequency or severity of stressful life events, although they did rate them as more distressing. Testing 54 patients with CD, Roelofs et al. (2005) did find a link between severity of life events and conversion symptoms. In addition and most critically, they showed that the relationship between childhood trauma and the severity of conversion symptoms was mediated by the occurrence of recent stressful events (Roelofs et al., 2005).

To conclude, a large percentage (14–100%) of CD patients report having experienced some traumatic event in their history. In addition, they also report relatively more recent stressful life events, that may mediate the link between trauma and CD. Although adverse life events may have occurred in a large number of CD patients, it is important to note that many other patients do not report trauma (0–86%) or stressful life events. Also, note that all studies relied on retrospective reports for measuring life adversities. Underreporting and overreporting may have biased the results.

OTHER VULNERABILITY FACTORS

Life adversity will not result in psychopathology in everyone: multiple factors will determine vulnerability (e.g., Belsky and Pluess, 2009). As risk factors for psychopathology, gender, socioeconomic status (SES), social support, personality and genetic factors have been identified (for an overview, see Rolf and Garmezy, 1992). In CD, some of these factors have been confirmed to play a role. In particular, female gender (Bodde et al., 2009) and low SES (Stefánsson et al., 1976) have been identified as predisposing risk factors. In addition, avoidant and borderline personality have been reported as risk factors (e.g., Reuber et al., 2004; Bodde et al., 2009), though only once (to our knowledge) in a prospective study (Binzer et al., 2004). Genetic factors are still unknown, although scarce evidence in mixed samples of somatoform disorders seems to indicate a role for serotonergic pathway genes (Hennings et al., 2009; Koh et al., 2011). As for precipitating factors, context variables as social support are relevant to take into account when considering the effects of adverse events (e.g., Mehnert et al., 2010). Unfortunately, in only one of the above-reported studies (Table 13.1) was social support taken into account (no. 4). Importantly, this study found social support to be lower in the CD sample.

In sum, besides life adversities, other predisposing and precipitating factors (such as gender, SES, genetics, social context) as well as their interactions should be considered. There is a lack of studies that have tested these factors and their interactions in CD. Nevertheless it is relevant to consider how adversities could lead to CD. The next section describes relevant cognitive and neurobiologic models of conversion symptoms and explores whether and how adverse life events can be linked to conversion symptomatology.

EXPLANATORY MODELS

Historic models of conversion and dissociation

Freud and Breuer) were the first to propose that hysteric symptoms could arise when affect related to psychologic stress factors or conflicts was "converted" into somatic symptoms (Breuer and Freud, 2009). Those stress factors or conflicts could be subconscious and were assumed to be often sexual or aggressive in nature. Although very influential, this theory and later modifications of it have been criticized for circular reasoning and for being untestable (e.g., Miller, 1999; Brown, 2004). Also, evaluation of the original conversion hypothesis does not suggest that psychologic distress symptoms are successfully converted into somatic symptoms: CD patients still experience a lot of psychologic discomfort (e.g., Lader and Sartorius, 1968; Brown, 2004).

Instead of "direct" conversion as described by Freud, Janet proposed dissociation as a mechanism that could explain conversion symptoms (Janet, 1907). According to dissociation theories, sensory processing that occurs via different sensory channels can be modified via attentional mechanisms that may block processing of some channels, but not the processing of other sensory channels. Later modifications of dissociation theory by Kihlstrom (1992) and Oakley (1999) integrated these attentional accounts with current hierarchic cognitive models (Norman and Shallice, 1986) and suggested that CD is an autosuggestive disorder that may lead to dissociative symptoms that are characteristic of conversion but also of hypnotic states (e.g., Oakley, 1999; Bell et al., 2010). Original conversion and dissociation accounts have been largely abandoned, but dissociation as a descriptive cognitive phenomenon referring to state, characterized by a dissociation between implicit and explicit information processing, still plays an important role in many modern explanatory models of CD.

Cognitive hierarchic models

One of the first cognitive hierarchic models of CD was described by Brown (2004). Like Oakley (1999), Brown based his model on the hierarchic attention model of Norman and Shallice (Norman and Shallice, 1986; Shallice, 1988), adopting the view that there is a supervisory attentional system and a more automated "contention-scheduling" system that generates reflex-like actions based on learned schemata. Schemata or representations on motor and/or sensory functions would be altered in CD. This would lead to altered allocation of attentional function to certain sensory states, resulting in activation of dysfunctional hypotheses about sensory and motor outcome (e.g., "I will not be able to move my leg"; "I'll experience pain in that leg") and eventually feeding back into dysfunctional mental representations. Brown called these altered mental representations mental "rogue" representations. He proposed that these "rogue" representations could be formed through various routes, including autosuggestion (see Oakley, 1999), the presence of examples or "models" in the environment, but also via earlier experiences (e.g., by re-experiencing physical symptoms initially experienced during trauma exposure). There is indeed accumulating evidence suggesting that attention can alter actual sensory processing, and that participants reporting medically unexplained somatic symptoms pay more attention to hypotheses they have about sensorimotor processes and are less responsive to actual sensory input (Bogaerts et al., 2008; Brown et al., 2010; Miles et al., 2011; Pareés et al., 2012; Schaefer et al., 2012).

Building on this line of reasoning, Edwards et al. (2012) further specified the role of attentional processes on sensory gating in CD by applying a Bayesian computational view based on the free-energy theory of Friston et al. (2006). In this predictive coding model, neuronal prediction units predict the outcome of a particular sensory (perception) or motor system (action). Lower-order units feed back a prediction error if the expectation did not come true. According to the free-energy principle, the brain will always try to minimize prediction error. Therefore, the subject will alter his or her prediction ("prior"). The prediction error feeds back into the prediction system of the subject. In some situations, however, it makes more sense to change the motor action or the perception itself instead of the prior prediction. Now the prediction error feeds forward into motor action.

According to Edwards, these feedback and feedforward processes, that play a role in many situations, are disturbed in CD patients. A problem in feedback processes may, for example, arise when an individual experiences a "real" somatic symptom, for example, is not able to lift his or her hand for a moment. The person may start to belief that he or she will never be able to lift the hand and, instead of feeding forward the prediction error and changing the outcome (lifting the hand), it is fed back and the prior is changed (paralysis belief). Feedforward problems in CD may arise when priors about outcome of behavior or sensation are given too much attention. To prevent prediction error, motor action or perception is adapted to what was expected. This, in turn, will reinforce the prior and result in a self-sustaining circle. Although this Bayesian predictive coding theory is particularly valuable in specifying how attention beliefs may eventually lead to actual symptoms in CD, it does not specify how stress may amplify this system.

Neurobiologic stress models

Neurobiologic stress models (Vuilleumier, 2005; Roelofs and Spinhoven, 2007; Kozlowska, 2013) of CD propose a link between major biologic stress/emotion systems and somatic symptoms. For example, Kozlowska (2005) applied the somatic marker theory of Damasio (1994) to explain conversion symptoms. According to this hypothesis, some emotional stimulus activates neural emotion-processing systems, which leads directly to a "body map," a representation of body state. Such a body map becomes part of an "as-if" loop, in which the body state associated with some emotion is directly produced, without real evaluation of the body. This system could be distorted in CD patients in such a way that false associations between emotional and bodily states arise in the as-if loop. For example, it may be that there is some innate or learned link between an emotion and a motor response (e.g., trembling or freezing), and an automatically processed emotion may involuntarily give rise to that same response or body map, immediately resulting in, for example, trembling or freezing. Accordingly, increased emotional reactivity (Roberts and Reuber, 2014) could give rise to a high motor readiness to respond with tremors or spasms to emotional stimuli (Kozlowska, 2013).

Vuilleumier et al. (2001) indeed found altered function of striatothalamocortical brain circuits during sensory stimulation in patients with CD. These circuits are known to be implicated in intentional movement and sensory processing and receive input from the limbic (emotional) structures in the brain (Vuilleumier, 2005). The authors proposed that affective and stress-related factors can result in conversion symptoms through reflexive alertness processes and interactions between limbic and sensorimotor networks. Although these neural circuits may provide a mechanism through which emotions may affect sensory and/or motor representations in CD, few studies have attempted to integrate these findings with findings on neurobiologic stress systems such as the hypothalamic–pituitary–adrenal (HPA) axis or on cognitive processes in CD. The next sections will describe cognitive dysfunctions in CD and the way these may interact with stress factors and alterations in major neurobiologic stress systems such as the HPA axis.

Cognitive dysfunction in CD: empiric support

Studies on general neuropsychologic function in CD have not resulted in a clear explanatory model of CD. Many studies have reported neuropsychologic impairments in CD patients (e.g., Kalogjera-Sackellares and Sackellares, 1999; Drane et al., 2006; Binder and Salinsky, 2007; Almis et al., 2013; Bodde et al., 2013; Demir et al., 2013). Some studies find intelligence to be somewhat lower, too (Kalogjera-Sackellares and Sackellares, 1999; Van Beilen et al., 2010). However, these impairments are not worse in psychogenic neurologic disorders than in organic neurologic disorders (Binder et al., 1998; Van Beilen et al., 2010; Heintz et al., 2013).

Evidence for abnormalities in voluntary attention is more unequivocal. Impairment in higher-order, voluntarily controlled attention came, for example, from a study using exogenous and endogenous cueing tasks, showing that patients with CD have reduced attentional guiding by endogenous cues, indicative of impaired voluntary attention, but show no problem in automatic exogenous cueing of attention (Roelofs et al., 2003; Pareés et al., 2013).

Self-focused attention, in particular, may be enhanced in patients with motor CD. Several event-related potential and functional magnetic resonance studies have shown increased action monitoring and heightened prefrontal cortex activity (mainly stemming from the anterior cingulate and medial prefrontal cortices) during voluntary motor processes, consistent with amplified self-directed attention to affected limbs in CD (Roelofs et al., 2006; De Lange et al., 2008, 2010; Cojan et al., 2009; Van Beilen et al., 2010). CD patients also show reduced motor excitability during explicit motor performance compared to implicit motor tasks (Liepert et al., 2011). This may explain why several studies have indicated that, whereas mental movements can be elicited implicitly (by task requirements), there are problems when (mental) movements are under explicit control (Roelofs et al., 2002b; Roelofs et al., 2003; Pareés et al., 2013). Interestingly, and in line with the role of self-focused attention in CD, attentional distraction can reduce motor conversion symptoms (e.g., Monday and Jankovic, 1993; Lang et al., 1995; McAuley and Rothwell, 2004; Kumru et al., 2007; Wolfsegger et al., 2013; Stins et al., 2015). A next question to address is whether and how stress and neurobiologic stress reactions can alter cognitive processes in patients with CD.

Stress and cognitive function in CD

There is increasing evidence that patients with CD show increased attentional and memory processing of emotional stimuli. In a study assessing attention to subliminally presented negative, positive, and neutral face stimuli, patients with PNES displayed a clear attentional bias specific for negative (angry-looking) faces. In addition, the magnitude of this bias was positively correlated to trauma rates (Bakvis et al., 2009a). There are also indications for increased startle responses (Seignourel et al., 2007) and increased amygdalar activity in reaction to emotional faces in CD (Voon et al., 2010). Moreover, processing threat stimuli was associated with altered connectivity between the amygdala and motor areas in the brain (Voon et al., 2010; Aybek et al., 2014). Aybek et al. tested CD patients during reactivation of adverse memories, from which patients were or were not able to escape through developing physical symptoms (as judged by independent raters). During reactivation of escape memories versus nonescape memories, CD patients showed increased activity in the left dorsolateral prefrontal cortex and decreased activity in the left hippocampus, accompanied by increased activity in right supplementary motor area and temporoparietal junction. These findings were taken to suggest that abnormal emotion and memory control are associated with alterations in symptom-related motor planning in CD.

Another line of evidence suggests altered stress sensitivity in major neuroendocrine and arousal systems in CD. For example, PNES patients were found to have lower heart rate variability, which is taken as an indication of hyperarousal (Bakvis et al., 2009b). In addition, PNES patients were found to show higher baseline cortisol levels (Mehta et al., 1994; Tunca et al., 2000; Bakvis et al., 2010a), which may be related to the experience of trauma (Bakvis et al., 2009b, 2010a). Based on these and other findings, several literature reviews have suggested that CD is associated with a general state of hyperarousal (Lang and Voon, 2011; Van der Kruijs et al., 2011; Reuber and Mayor, 2012; Kozlowska, 2013). The question arises whether these stress mechanisms function independently of cognitive mechanisms in the production of CD, or whether a more integrative account should be proposed.

TOWARDS AN INTEGRATION

To our knowledge, only few studies have actually tested the premise that alterations in cognitive functions relate to heightened stress sensitivity in the case of CD.

Bendefeldt et al. (1976) were among the first to explore whether neuropsychologic functioning of CD patients altered after stress induction. In both stress and nonstress conditions, CD patients (compared to clinical controls) scored worse on measures of controlled attention, but performance was even worse in the stress condition. This first finding thus suggested that there may be an amplifying effect of stress on attentional processes relevant for CD. Recent findings confirmed this hypothesis. Bakvis et al. (2010b) found that PNES patients, compared to healthy controls, showed more working-memory interference when exposed to emotional stimuli and this working-memory deficit was stronger after stress induction. Also, heightened cortisol stress reactivity predicted the magnitude of this deficit in CD patients. Another study on attentional function showed that basal cortisol levels predict attentional bias to angry-face cues in CD patients, type PNES (Bakvis et al., 2009a). Thus, there is emerging evidence for a link between neurobiologic stress sensitivity and altered attentional function in CD.

How can we integrate those findings? Based on our earlier model of medically unexplained somatic symptoms (Roelofs and Spinhoven, 2007), as well as the current review, we suggest that life adversities may affect medically unexplained somatic symptoms via at least two routes: via associative learning and via their effect on relevant neurobiologic stress systems. Below we detail these routes.

Associative learning leads to altered mental representations

As for the first, somatosensory experiences during traumatic events may directly be linked to affective states and later activation of those affective states may reactivate the somatosensory experience (or "body maps": Kozlowska, 2005, or mental symptom representations: Brown, 2004) that in turn leads to symptom expectations (or priors, Edwards et al., 2012; see Fig. 13.1, route a).

Life events lead to alterations in neurobiologic stress systems

As for the second, life adversities may lead to alterations in the responsiveness of major stress system like the HPA axis (e.g., Sapolsky, 1996; Anisman et al., 1998; McEwen, 1998; Elzinga et al., 2003). Scarce studies in CD show a similar relation between early trauma and HPA axis hyperresponsiveness (Bakvis et al., 2010a, b; Fig. 13.1, route b). Note that HPA axis hyperresponding may also arise from different factors, such as temperament or genetic predisposition.

Stress and stress-induced cortisol increases may in turn affect attentional processes in CD (Fig. 13.1, route b), in particular by increasing attention to emotional stimuli (Bakvis et al., 2009a, b, 2010a; Grisham et al., 2014). These findings can be combined with findings on higher arousal, as described above; it was found that individuals who frequently report physical symptoms experience more symptoms in reaction to negative stimuli only when their arousal is high (Constantinou et al., 2013). Stress has also been shown to increase action monitoring and self-focused attention, while impairing voluntary attention (Wegner and Giuliano, 1980; Vedhara et al., 2000; Braunstein-Bercovitz, 2003; Hsu et al., 2003; Liston et al., 2006, 2009; Roelofs et al., 2006), which may in turn worsen (motor) performance (Baumeister and Steinhilber, 1984; Schücker et al., 2013). Such mechanisms may be relevant because CD has consistently been associated with increased self-focused attention (Roelofs et al., 2006; De Lange et al., 2007, 2008, 2010; Cojan et al., 2009) and because self-focused attention may lead to increased symptom perception (Brown, 2004). The Bayesian predictive coding model by Edwards et al. (2012) offers a valuable explanatory framework detailing how such an increase in symptom perception occurs through enhancement of the precision of the predicted sensory or motor outcome (Fig. 13.1 route c), that in turn leads to perception of sensory and motor symptoms (Fig. 13.1 route d).

Concluding, we extend cognitive models where life adversities lead to abnormal priors (through representations and beliefs, route a) with the notion that life events may also lead to changes in neurobiologic stress systems, such as the HPA axis, that in turn amplify the attention processes that are at the core of the symptoms (route b). When given too much attention, priors may become

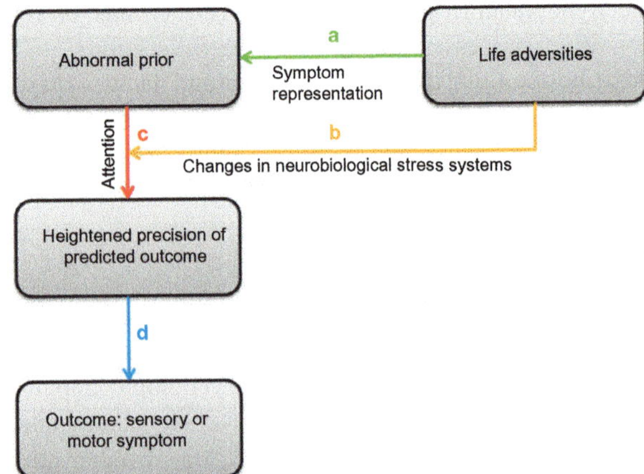

Fig. 13.1. Schematic illustration of the proposed mechanisms by which life adversities may affect conversion disorder symptoms. The tentative model is based on the integration of neurobiological stress models, associative learning models, and predictive coding models of medically unexplained somatic symptoms.

overly precise (route c) and act in a self-fulfilling manner, leading to sensory or motor symptoms (route d).

SUMMARY AND RESEARCH AGENDA

In sum, from the literature review on life adversities in CD, we can conclude that CD is associated with slightly increased trauma reports. A substantial proportion of CD patients (ranging from 0% to 86%) do not report having experienced traumatic events in their history. However, in those studies where trauma reports were linked to symptom severity in CD, it was consistently found that the presence and severity of life adversities were related to greater symptom severity in CD.

Therefore, we propose that explanatory models of CD should account for mechanisms that may explain symptoms without a role of trauma history as well as for mechanisms that may be amplified by trauma and alterations in stress-responsiveness. The present chapter provides such integration, by reviewing current major cognitive models and by integrating the most relevant Bayesian predictive coding model by Edwards et al. (2012) on the role of attention and beliefs in CD with emerging evidence on the relation between stress and attention functioning in CD. We propose that stress and stress-related factors may affect symptom beliefs (via learning mechanisms) and may affect attentional mechanisms (partly via its effect on neurobiologic stress systems).

Future research should directly test premises of Bayesian feedforward and feedback mechanisms proposed for CD and should test whether stress can amplify both these processes. There is a great need for large-cohort longitudinal studies on the development and maintenance of medically unexplained somatic symptoms, including CD. Such studies are needed to determine predisposing, precipitating, and consequential factors that affect the development and maintenance of the disorder. As regards predisposing factors, not only trauma history but also demographic, personality, genetic, neurobiologic, and context variables should be taken into account. As regards precipitating factors, cognitive processes (attention, memory, and belief biases) should be directly tested and monitored over time. The present chapter did not cover consequential factors, such as change of context due to having CD, although it acknowledges that those factors should be monitored as well to get a complete picture.

Finally, in the presented model attention processes are considered to be central to CD. The role of attention in interaction with stress factors may not only be of mechanistic value. The clinical relevance of each of the processes could be investigated in intervention studies where the proposed underlying components of CD are treated in isolation. For example, initial evidence shows that attention distraction can reduce conversion symptoms momentarily. It would be important for future studies to integrate attentional, belief, and stress physiology assessments before and after treatment and to investigate whether these factors should be directly targeted in effective treatments for CD.

ACKNOWLEDGMENTS

K. Roelofs was funded by a VICI grant (#453-12-001) from the Netherlands Organization for Scientific Research (NWO) and a starting grant from the European Research Council (ERC_StG2012_313749).

References

Akagi H, House H (2002). The clinical epidemiology of hysteria: Vanishingly rare, or just vanishing? Psychol Med 32: 191–194.

Akyuz G, Kugu N, Akyuz A et al. (2004). Dissociation and childhood abuse history in epileptic and pseudoseizure patients. Epileptic Disord 6: 187–192.

Almis BH, Cumurcu BE, Unal S et al. (2013). The neuropsychological and neurophysiological profile of women with pseudoseizure. J Comp Psych 54: 649–657.

Alper K, Devinsky O, Perrine K et al. (1993). Nonepileptic seizures and childhood sexual and physical abuse. Neurology 43: 1950–1953.

American Psychiatric Association (2000). Diagnostic and statistical manual of mental disorders (4th ed., text rev.), American Psychiatric Association, Washington, DC.

American Psychiatric Association (2013). Diagnostic and statistical manual of mental disorders, 5th edn. American Psychiatric Association, Washington, DC.

Anisman H, Zaharia MD, Meany MJ et al. (1998). Do early-life events permanently alter behavioral and hormonal responses to stressors? Int J Dev Neurosci 16: 149–164.

Arnold LM, Privitera MD (1996). Psychopathology and trauma in epileptic and psychogenic seizure patients. Psychosomatics 37: 438–443.

Aybek S, Nicholson TR, Zelaya F et al. (2014). Neural correlates of recall of life events in conversion disorder. JAMA Psychiatry 71: 52–60.

Baker J, Ben-Tovim D, Butcher A et al. (2013). Psychosocial risk factors which may differentiate between women with functional voice disorder, organic voice disorder and a control group. Inter J Speech Lang Pathol 15: 547–563.

Bakvis P, Spinhoven P, Roelofs K (2009a). Basal cortisol is positively correlated to threat vigilance in patients with psychogenic nonepileptic seizures. Epilepsy Behav 16: 558–560.

Bakvis P, Roelofs K, Kuyk J et al. (2009b). Trauma, stress, and preconscious threat processing in patients with psychogenic nonepileptic seizures. Epilepsia 50: 1001–1011.

Bakvis P, Spinhoven P, Giltay EJ et al. (2010a). Basal hypercortisolism and trauma in patients with psychogenic nonepileptic seizures. Epilepsia 51: 752–759.

Bakvis P, Spinhoven P, Putman P et al. (2010b). The effect of stress induction on working memory in patients with psychogenic nonepileptic seizures. Epilepsy Behav 19: 448–454.

Baslet G (2011). Psychogenic non-epileptic seizures: a model of their pathogenic mechanism. Seizure 20: 1–13.

Baumeister RF, Steinhilber A (1984). Paradoxical effects of supportive audiences on performance under pressure: the home field disadvantage in sports championships. J Pers Soc Psychol 47: 85–93.

Bell V, Oakley DA, Halligan PW et al. (2010). Dissociation in hysteria and hypnosis: evidence from cognitive neuroscience. J Neurol Neurosurg Psychiatry 82: 332–339.

Belsky J, Pluess M (2009). Beyond diathesis stress: differential susceptibility to environmental influences. Psychol Bull 135: 885–908.

Bendefeldt F, Miller LL, Ludwig AM (1976). Cognitive performance in conversion hysteria. Arch Gen Pscyhiatry 33: 1250–1254.

Berkhoff M, Briellmann RS, Radanov BP et al. (1998). Developmental background and outcome in patients with nonepileptic versus epileptic seizures: a controlled study. Epilepsia 39: 463–469.

Betts T, Boden S (1992). Diagnosis, management and prognosis of a group of 128 patients with non-epileptic attack disorder. Part II. Previous childhood sexual abuse in the aetiology of these disorders. Seizure 1: 27–32.

Binder LM, Salinsky MC (2007). Psychogenic nonepileptic seizures. Neuropsychol Rev 17: 405–412.

Binder LM, Kindermann SS, Heaton RK et al. (1998). Neuropsychologic impairment in patients with nonepileptic seizures. Arch Clin Neuropsychol 13: 513–522.

Binzer M, Eisemann M (1998). Childhood experiences and personality traits in patients with motor conversion symptoms. Acta Psychiatr Scand 98: 288–295.

Binzer M, Andersen PM, Kullgren G (1997). Clinical characteristics of patients with motor disability due to conversion disorder: a prospective control group study. J Neurol Neurosurg Psychiatry 63: 83–88.

Binzer M, Stone J, Sharpe M (2004). Recent onset pseudoseizures: Clues to aetiology. Seizure 13: 146–155.

Bodde NMG, Brooks JL, Baker GA et al. (2009). Psychogenic non-epileptic seizures – Definition, etiology, treatment and prognostic issues: a critical review. Seizure 18: 543–553.

Bodde NMG, Van der Kruijs SJM, Ijff DM et al. (2013). Subgroup classification in patients with psychogenic non-epileptic seizures. Epilepsy Behav 26: 279–289.

Bogaerts K, Millen A, Li W et al. (2008). High symptom reporters are less interoceptively accurate in a symptom-related context. J Psychosom Res 65: 417–424.

Bowman ES, Markand ON (1996). Psychodynamics and psychiatric diagnoses of pseudoseizure subjects. Am J Psychiatry 153: 57–63.

Braunstein-Bercovitz H (2003). Does stress enhance or impair selective attention? The effects of stress and perceptual load on negative priming. Anxiety Stress Coping 16: 345–357.

Breslau N, Davis GC, Adreski P et al. (1991). Traumatic events and posttraumatic stress disorder in an urban population of young adults. Arch Gen Psychiatry 48: 216–222.

Breuer J, Freud S (2009). Studies on hysteria, Basic Books Classics, New York.

Brown RJ (2004). Psychological mechanisms of medically unexplained symptoms: an integrative conceptual model. Psychol Bull 130: 793–812.

Brown RJ, Danquah AN, Miles E et al. (2010). Attention to the body in nonclinical somatoform dissociation depends on emotional state. J Psychosom Res 69: 249–257.

Carson AJ, Ringbauer B, MacKenzie L et al. (2000). Neurological disease, emotional disorder, and disability: They are related: A study of 300 consecutive new referrals to a neurology outpatient department. J Neurol Neurosurg Psychiatry 68: 202–206.

Cojan Y, Waber L, Carruzzo A et al. (2009). Motor inhibition in hysterical conversion paralysis. Neuroimage 47: 1026–1037.

Constantinou E, Bogaerts K, Van Diest I et al. (2013). Inducing symptoms in high symptom reporters via emotional pictures: the interactive effects of valence and arousal. J Psychosom Res 74: 191–196.

Czarnecki K, Hallett M (2012). Functional (psychogenic) movement disorders. Curr Opin Neurol 25: 507–512.

Damasio A (1994). Descartes' error: Emotion, reason and the human brain, Putnam, New York.

De Lange FP, Roelofs K, Toni I (2007). Increased self-monitoring during imagined movements in conversion paralysis. Neuropsychologia 45: 2051–2058.

De Lange FP, Roelofs K, Toni I (2008). Motor imagery: a window into the mechanisms and alterations of the motor system. Cortex 44: 494–506.

De Lange FP, Toni I, Roelofs K (2010). Altered connectivity between prefrontal and sensorimotor cortex in conversion paralysis. Neuropsychologia 48: 1782–1788.

Demir S, Çelikel FÇ, Taycan SE et al. (2013). Neuropsychological assessment in conversion disorder. Turk Psikiyatri Derg 24: 75–83.

Dikel TN, Fennell EB, Gilmore RL (2003). Posttraumatic stress disorder, dissociation, and sexual abuse history in epileptic and nonepileptic seizure patients. Epilepsy Behav 4: 644–650.

Drane DL, Williamson DJ, Stroup E et al. (2006). Cognitive impairment is not equal in patients with epileptic and psychogenic nonepileptic seizures. Epilepsia 47: 1879–1886.

Edwards MJ, Adams RA, Brown H et al. (2012). A Bayesian account of "hysteria". Brain 135: 3495–3512.

Elzinga BM, Schmahl CG, Vermetten E et al. (2003). Higher cortisol levels following exposure to traumatic reminders in abuse-related PTSD. Neuropsychopharmacology 28: 1656–1665.

Friston K, Kilner J, Harrison L (2006). A free energy principle for the brain. J Physiol Paris 100: 70–87.

Grattan-Smith P, Fairley M, Procopis P (1988). Clinical features of conversion disorder. Arch Dis Child 63: 408–414.

Grisham JR, King BJ, Makkar SR et al. (2014). The contributions of arousal and self-focused attention to avoidance in social anxiety. Anxiety Stress Coping 28: 303–320.

Heintz CEJ, Van Tricht MJ, Van der Salm SMA et al. (2013). Neuropsychological profile of psychogenic jerky movement disorders: importance of evaluating non-credible cognitive performance and psychopathology. J Neurol Neurosurg Psychiatry 84: 862–867.

Hennings A, Zill P, Rief W (2009). Serotonin transporter gene promotor polymorphism and somatoform symptoms. J Clin Psychiatry: 1536–1539.

House AO, Andrews HB (1988). Life events and difficulties preceding the onset of functional dysphonia. J Psychosom Res 32: 311–319.

Hsu FC, Garside MJ, Massey AE et al. (2003). Effects of a single dose of cortisol on the neural correlates of episodic memory and error processing in healthy volunteers, Psychopharmacology (Berl) 167: 431–442.

Janet P (1907). The major symptoms of hysteria: fifteen lectures given in the medical school of Harvard university. Macmillan, New York.

Jawad SSM, Jamil N, Clarke EJ et al. (1995). Psychiatric morbidity and psychodynamics of patients with convulsive pseudoseizures. Seizure 4: 201–206.

Kalogjera-Sackellares D, Sackellares JC (1999). Intellectual and neuropsychological features of patients with psychogenic pseudoseizures. Psychiatry Res 86: 73–84.

Kaplan MJ, Dwivedi AK, Privitera MD et al. (2013). Comparisons of childhood trauma, alexithymia, and defensive styles in patients with psychogenic non-epileptic seizure vs. epilepsy: implications for the etiology of conversion disorder. J Psychosom Res 75: 142–146.

Kessler RC, Sonnega A, Bromet E et al. (1995). Posttraumatic stress disorder in the National Comorbidity Survey. Arch Gen Psychiatry 52: 1048–1060.

Kihlstrom JF (1992). Dissociative and conversion disorders. In: DJ Stein, J Young (Eds.), Cognitive science and clinical disorders, Academic Press, San Diego, CA, pp. 247–270.

Koh KB, Choi EH, Lee Y et al. (2011). Serotonin-related gene pathways associated with undifferentiated somatoform disorder. Psychiatry Res 189: 246–250.

Konnopka A, Schaefert R, Heinrich S et al. (2012). Economics of medically unexplained symptoms: a systematic review of the literature. Psychother Psychosom 81: 265–275.

Kozlowska K (2005). Healing the disembodied mind: contemporary models of conversion disorder. Harv Rev Psychiatry 13: 1–13.

Kozlowska K (2013). Functional somatic symptoms in childhood and adolescence. Curr Opin Psychiatry 26: 485–492.

Kozlowska K, Schier S, Williams LM (2011). Patterns of emotional-cognitive functioning in pediatric conversion patients: Implications for the conceptualization of conversion disorders. Psychosom Med 73: 775–788.

Kranick S, Ekanayake V, Martinez V et al. (2011). Psychopathology and psychogenic movement disorders. Mov Disord 26: 1844–1850.

Kumru H, Begeman M, Tolosa E et al. (2007). Dual task interference in psychogenic tremor. Mov Disord 22: 2077–2082.

Kuyk J, Spinhoven P, Van Emde B et al. (1999). Dissociation in temporal lobe epilepsy and pseudo-epileptic seizure patients. J Nerv Ment Dis 187: 713–720.

Lader M, Sartorius N (1968). Anxiety in patients with hysterical conversion symptoms. J Neurol Neurosurg Psychiatry 31: 490–495.

Lang AE, Voon V (2011). Psychogenic movement disorders: past developments, current status, and future directions. Mov Disord 26: 1175–1186.

Lang AE, Koller WC, Fahn S (1995). Psychogenic parkinsonism. Arch Neurol 52: 802–810.

Liepert J, Hassa T, Tüscher O et al. (2011). Motor excitability during movement imagination and movement observation in psychogenic lower limb paresis. J Psychosom Res 70: 59–65.

Liston C, Miller MM, Goldwater DS et al. (2006). Stress-induced alterations in prefrontal cortical dendritic morphology predict selective impairments in perceptual attentional set-shifting. J Neurosci 26: 7870–7874.

Liston C, McEwen BS, Casey BJ (2009). Psychosocial stress reversibly disrupts prefrontal processing and attentional control. Proc Natl Acad Sci U S A 106: 912–917.

Litwin R, Cardeña E (2000). Demographic and seizure variables, but not hypnotizability or dissociation, differentiated psychogenic from organic seizures. J Trauma Dissociation 1: 99–121.

McAuley J, Rothwell J (2004). Identification of psychogenic, dystonic, and other organic tremors by a coherence entrainment test. Mov Disord 19: 253–267.

McDade G, Brown SW (1992). Non-epileptic seizures: Management and predictive factors of outcome. Seizure 1: 7–10.

McEwen BS (1998). Protective and damaging effects of stress mediators. N Engl J Med 338: 171–179.

Mehnert A, Lehmann C, Graefen M et al. (2010). Depression, anxiety, post-traumatic stress disorder and health-related quality of life and its association with social support in ambulatory prostate cancer patients. Eur J Cancer Care 19: 736–745.

Mehta SR, Dham SK, Lazar AI et al. (1994). Prolactin and cortisol levels in seizure disorders. J Assoc Physicians India 42: 709–712.

Miles E, Poliakoff E, Brown RJ (2011). Medically unexplained symptom reports are associated with a decreased response to the rubber hand illusion. J Psychosom Res 71: 240–244.

Miller E (1999). Conversion hysteria: Is it a viable concept? Cogn Neuropsychiatry 4: 181–191.

Mökleby K, Blomhoff S, Malt UF et al. (2002). Psychiatric comorbidity and hostility in patients with psychogenic nonepileptic seizures comopared with somatoform disorders and healthy controls. Epilepsia 43: 193–198.

Monday K, Jankovic J (1993). Psychogenic myoclonus. Neurology 43: 349–352.

Nicholson TR, Stone J, Kanaan RA (2011). Conversion disorder: a problematic diagnosis. J Neurol Neurosurg Psychiatry 82: 1267–1273.

Norman DA, Shallice T (1986). Attention to action: willed and automatic control of behavior. In: RJ Davidson, GE Schwartz, DE Shapiro (Eds.), Consciousness and self-regulation: advances in research and theory, Plenum, New York, pp. 1–18.

Oakley DA (1999). Hypnosis and conversion hysteria: a unifying model. Cognit Neuropsychiatry 4: 243–265.

Ozcetin A, Belli H, Ertem U et al. (2009). Childhood trauma and dissociation in women with pseudoseizure-type conversion disorder. Nord J Psychiatry 63: 462–468.

Pareés I, Saifee TA, Kassavetis P et al. (2012). Believing is perceiving: mismatch between self-report and actigraphy in psychogenic tremor. Brain 135: 117–123.

Pareés I, Kassavetis P, Saifee TA et al. (2013). Failure of explicit movement control in patients with functional motor symptoms. Mov Disord 28: 517–523.

Perkonigg A, Kessler RC, Storz S et al. (2000). Traumatic events and post-traumatic stress disorder in the community: prevalence, risk factors and comorbidity. Acta Psychiatr Scand 101: 46–59.

Plioplys S, Doss J, Siddarth P et al. (2014). A multisite controlled study of risk factors in pediatric psychogenic nonepileptic seizures. Epilepsia 55: 1739–1747.

Proença ICGF, Castro LHM, Jorge CL et al. (2011). Emotional trauma and abuse in patients with psychogenic nonepileptic seizures. Epilepsy Behav 20: 331–333.

Reilly J, Baker GA, Rhodes J et al. (1999). The association of sexual and physical abuse with somatization: characteristics of patients representing with irritable bowel syndrome and non-epileptic attack disorder. Psychol Med 29: 399–406.

Reuber M, Mayor R (2012). Recent progress in the understanding and treatment of nonepileptic seizures. Curr Opin Psychiatry 25: 244–250.

Reuber M, Pukrop R, Bauer J et al. (2004). Multidimensional assessment of personality in patients with psychogenic non-epileptic seizures. J Neurol Neurosurg Pychiatr 75: 743–748.

Reuber M, Howlett S, Khan A et al. (2007). Non-epileptic seizures and other functional neurological symptoms: predisposing, precipitating, and perpetuating factors. Psychosomatics 48: 230–238.

Roberts NA, Reuber M (2014). Alterations of consciousness in psychogenic nonepileptic seizures: emotion, emotion regulation and dissociation. Epilepsy Behav 30: 43–49.

Roelofs K, Spinhoven P (2007). Trauma and medically unexplained symptoms: towards an integration of cognitive and neuro-biological accounts. Clin Psychol Rev 27: 798–820.

Roelofs K, Keijsers GPJ, Hoogduin KAL et al. (2002a). Childhood abuse in patients with conversion disorder. Am J Psychiatry 159: 1908–1913.

Roelofs K, Van Galen GP, Keijsers GPJ et al. (2002b). Motor initiation and execution in patients with conversion paralysis. Acta Psychol 110: 21–34.

Roelofs K, Van Galen GP, Eling P et al. (2003). Endogenous and exogenous attention in patients with conversion paresis. Cognitive Neuropsych 20: 733–745.

Roelofs K, Spinhoven P, Sandijck P et al. (2005). The impact of early trauma and recent life events on symptom severity in patients with conversion disorder. J Nerv Ment Dis 193: 508–514.

Roelofs K, De Bruijn ERA, Van Galen GP (2006). Hyperactive action monitoring during motor-initiation in conversion paralysis: an event-related potential study. Biol Psychol 71: 316–325.

Rolf J, Garmezy N (1992). Risk and protective factors in the development of psychopathology, Cambridge University Press, Cambridge.

Salmon P, Al-Marzooqi SM, Baker G et al. (2003). Childhood family dysfunction and associated abuse in patients with nonepileptic seizures: towards a causal model. Psychosom Med 65: 695–700.

Sapolsky RM (1996). Why stress is bad for your brain. Science 273: 749–750.

Şar V, Akyüz G, Dogan O et al. (2009). The prevalence of conversion symptoms in women from a general Turkish population. Psychosomatics 50: 50–58.

Scévola L, Teitelbaum J, Oddo S et al. (2013). Psychiatri disorders in patients with psychogenic nonepileptic seizures and drug-resistant epilepsy: a study of an Argentine population. Epilepsy Behav 29: 155–160.

Schaefer M, Egloff B, Witthöft M (2012). Is interoceptive awareness really altered in somatoform disorders? Testing competing theories with two paradigms of heartbeat perception. J Abnorm Psychol 121: 719–724.

Schücker L, Hagemann N, Strauss B (2013). Attentional processes and choking under pressure. Percept Mot Skills 116: 671–689.

Seignourel PJ, Miller K, Kellison I et al. (2007). Abnormal affective startle modulation in individuals with psychogenic (corrected) movement disorder. Mov Disord 22: 1265–1271.

Shallice T (1988). From neuropsychology to mental structure, Cambridge University Press, New York.

Stefánsson JG, Messina JA, Meyerowitz S (1976). Hysterical neurosis, conversion type: clinical and epidemiological considerations. Acta Psychiatr Scand 53: 119–138.

Steffen A, Fiess J, Schmidt R et al. (2015). "That pulled the rug out from under my feet!" Adverse experiences and altered emotion processing in patients with functional neurological symptoms compared to healthy comparison subjects. BMC Psychiatry 15: 133–142.

Stins JF, Kempe CLA, Hagenaars MA et al. (2015). Attention and postural control in patients with conversion paresis. J Psychosom Res 78: 249–254.

Testa SM, Krauss GL, Lesser RP et al. (2012). Stressful life event appraisal and coping in patients with psychogenic seizures and those with epilepsy. Seizure 21: 282–287.

Tojek TM, Lumley M, Barkley G et al. (2000). Stress and other psychosocial characteristics of patients with psychogenic nonepileptic seizures. Psychosomatics 41: 221–226.

Tunca Z, Ergene U, Fidaner H et al. (2000). Reevaluation of serum cortisol in conversion disorder with seizure (pseudoseizure). Psychosomatics 41: 152–153.

Van Beilen M, Vogt BA, Leenders KL (2010). Increased activation in cingulate cortex in conversion disorder: what does it mean? J Neurol Sci 289: 155–158.

Van der Kruijs SJM, Bodde NMG, Adenkamp APA (2011). Psychophysiological biomarkers of dissociation in psychogenic non-epileptic seizures. Acta Neurol Belg 111: 99–103.

Van Merode T, Twellaar M, Kotsopoulos IAW et al. (2015). Psychological characteristics of patients with newly developed psychogenic seizures. J Neurol Neurosurg Psychiatry 75: 1175–1177.

Vedhara K, Hyde J, Gilchrist ID et al. (2000). Acute stress, memory, attention and cortisol. Psychoneuroendocrinology 25: 535–549.

Voon V, Brezing C, Gallea C et al. (2010). Emotional stimuli and motor conversion disorder. Brain 133: 1526–1536.

Vuilleumier P (2005). Hysterical conversion and brain function. Prog Brain Res 150: 309–329.

Vuilleumier P, Chicherio C, Assal F (2001). Functional neuroanatomical correlates of hysterical sensorimotor loss. Brain 124: 1077–1090.

Wegner DM, Giuliano T (1980). Arousal-induced attention to self. J Pers Soc Psychol 38: 719–726.

Wolfsegger T, Pischinger B, Topakian R (2013). Objectification of psychogenic postural instability by trunk sway analysis. J Neurol Sci 334: 14–17.

World Health Organization (2010). The ICD-10 classification of mental and behavioural disorders: clinical descriptions and diagnostic guidelines, World Health Organization, Geneva.

Handbook of Clinical Neurology, Vol. 139 (3rd series)
Functional Neurologic Disorders
M. Hallett, J. Stone, and A. Carson, Editors
http://dx.doi.org/10.1016/B978-0-12-801772-2.00014-X

Chapter 14

Do (epi)genetics impact the brain in functional neurologic disorders?

T. FRODL*

Department of Psychiatry and Psychotherapy, Otto von Guericke University of Magdeburg, Germany and Department of Psychiatry, Trinity College, Dublin, Ireland

Abstract

Advances in neuropsychiatric research are supposed to lead to significant improvements in understanding functional neurologic disorders and their diagnosis. However, epigenetic and genetic research on conversion disorders and somatoform disorders is only at its start. This review demonstrates the current state within this field and tries to bridge a gap from what is known on gene–stress interactions in other psychiatric disorders like depression. The etiology of conversion disorders is hypothesized to be multifactorial. These considerations also suggest that potential etiologic factors lead to alterations in brain function, either episodically or chronically, eventually leading to structural brain changes. In particular, the knowledge of how the environment influences brain structure and function, e.g., via epigenetic regulation, may be interesting for future research in functional neurologic disorders. Reviewing the literature results in evidence that childhood adversities play a role in the development of functional neurologic disorders, whereby at present no reports exist about the interactive effect between childhood adversity and genetic factors or about the impact of epigenetics.

INTRODUCTION

Conversion disorder is a functional neurologic symptom disorder, as defined by the *Diagnostic and Statistical Manual of Mental Disorders*, 5th edition (DSM-5: American Psychiatric Assocation, 2013) – or, as defined in the *International Classification of Diseases* (ICD-10: World Health Organization, 2010), is a dissociative disorder – marked by the presence of pseudoneurologic symptoms. Criteria in DSM-5 now emphasize the importance of the neurologic examination, and recognize that relevant psychologic factors may not be demonstrable at the time of diagnosis. Despite research in this area, the etiology is largely unknown. It is hypothesized to be multifactorial, with stress–environmental factors and potentially some mediating genetic factors influencing the development of psychopathology (Krem, 2004).

ENVIRONMENTAL EFFECTS

First, environmental factors are hypothesized to play a major role in the development of psychiatric disorders. This is true also for conversion disorders. A few studies investigated the association between childhood trauma or adversity and conversion disorders. Within a literature review, nine out of nine studies showed that increased physical and sexual abuse was found in patients with conversion or somatization disorders compared to healthy, organic, or psychiatric controls. Psychologic abuse also was found to be more pronounced in conversion/somatization disorders compared to controls. The review also included other medically unexplained conditions.

The impact of childhood adversity is not unique to conversion disorders, since it can also be seen in irritable-bowel syndrome and chronic pelvic pain (Roelofs and Spinhoven, 2007). In one more recent study, 56 female

*Correspondence to: Thomas Frodl, Department of Psychiatry and Psychotherapy, Otto von Guericke University of Magdeburg, Germany. Tel: +49-391-67-15029, E-mail: Thomas.Frodl@med.ovgu.de

patients with conversion disorder, who had psychogenic nonepileptic seizures, were investigated using clinical interviews about dissociation and childhood trauma. The total score of the childhood trauma questionnaire as well as its subscales – emotional abuse, emotional neglect, physical abuse, and sexual abuse – was significantly higher in the conversion group compared to control subjects. Moreover, the amount of dissociation was statistically higher in the conversion group in line with a traumatic background (Ozcetin et al., 2009).

Furthermore, in an earlier study, 54 patients with conversion disorder reported a higher incidence of physical or sexual abuse, a larger number of different types of physical abuse, sexual abuse of longer duration, and incestuous experiences more often than 50 comparison patients with affective disorders (Roelofs et al., 2002). Moreover, a series of patients with conversion disorder presenting as epilepsy showed a significantly higher frequency of a history of sexual or physical abuse than 140 patients with complex partial epilepsy. Also severity of sexual but not physical abuse was significantly greater in the nonepileptic seizure group relative to controls (Alper et al., 1993).

Furthermore, a diagnosis of psychogenic nonepileptic seizures was associated with significantly higher rates of childhood trauma in addition to female sex in a sample of 82 subjects with epileptic seizures and 96 subjects with psychogenic nonepileptic seizures (Kaplan et al., 2013). There are many more studies in this area, already summarized in a review and meta-analysis that comes to the conclusion that there is growing evidence of an association between childhood sexual abuse and psychogenic nonepileptic seizures (Sharpe and Faye, 2006).

To summarize, these studies all show significant higher severity and rates of childhood adversity in functional neurologic disorders compared to healthy controls or patients with affective disorders. In particular, the comparison between functional neurologic disorders and affective disorders that already show higher rates of childhood adversities compared to controls suggests that childhood adversity might play a prominent role for later developing a functional neurologic disorder. However, to date these studies also have to be taken with caution because of methodologic difficulties, e.g., that there is no common definition of childhood abuse, childhood abuse is usually reported retrospectively, and case and comparison groups were recruited, often not in a way that was representative of the population.

LINK BETWEEN ENVIRONMENTAL FACTORS LIKE STRESS AND THE BRAIN SYSTEMS

Previous studies have suggested that a relationship exists between childhood maltreatment and an increased risk of developing a number of mental disorders in adulthood (Heim and Nemeroff, 2001; Taylor et al., 2006), including major depressive disorder (MDD) (Kessler, 1997), posttraumatic stress disorder (Bonne et al., 2008), anxiety disorders (Heim and Nemeroff, 2001), and substance abuse (Dube et al., 2003).

The association between social early-life stressors and development of psychiatric disorders has also been explored experimentally and there is evidence suggesting an impact of early-life adversity on brain function and structure. Until only a few years ago, the adult brain was considered to be an organ with a fixed structure, unable to remodel or repair itself. However, recent research shows that both structural and physiologic changes occur in the adult nervous system, some arising as a result of the individual's interaction with the surrounding environment and some from internal adaptation, also interacting with genetic factors.

Chronic social stress has been shown to induce glucocorticoid-mediated pyramidal dendrite retraction in the hippocampus and changes in dendrite arborization in the prefrontal cortex (Woolley et al., 1990; Magarinos et al., 1996; Wellman, 2001; Kole et al., 2004), which might be associated with the behavioral manifestations of stress-related disorders like MDD (Macqueen and Frodl, 2011). There is mounting evidence that specific neuronal circuits, particularly in the developing brain, are damaged by environmental stress-inducing changes in the hypothalamic–pituitary–adrenal (HPA) axis and inflammatory pathways (Krishnan and Nestler, 2008). Experimental studies have shown that stress or cortisol administration may lead to depressive-like states and atrophy of neurons in the hippocampus (Duman, 2002) and that therapy with antidepressants reverses these changes (Santarelli et al., 2003). Moreover, chronic hypercortisolism has been shown to enhance tryptophan breakdown in the brain and induce neurodegenerative changes (Capuron and Miller, 2011). Other research has shown that both physiologic and psychologic stress can induce increased production of proinflammatory mediators that can stimulate tryptophan catabolism in the brain (Myint et al., 2012), with consequences on neurotransmitter metabolism, neuroendocrine function, synaptic transmission, and neurocircuits that regulate mood, motor activity, motivation, anxiety, and alarm reactions (Capuron and Miller, 2011).

Neuroimaging studies provide growing evidence that childhood maltreatment, defined as maltreatment or trauma in the form of emotional, physical, or sexual abuse, or emotional or physical neglect, could have detrimental effects on brain structure. Vythilingam et al. (2002) compared 32 women with recurrent unipolar depression and prepubertal physical or sexual abuse to 11 women with depression without prepubertal abuse and to 14 healthy controls. They found that the left hippocampus was 18% smaller in women with depression and prepubertal abuse than those without abuse and 15% smaller than healthy controls.

Emotional neglect has also been found to be associated with smaller hippocampal volumes. Smaller left hippocampal white-matter volumes were reported in MDD patients who had experienced emotional childhood neglect compared to those without neglect. Both emotional neglect and brain structural abnormalities predicted cumulative illness duration (Frodl et al., 2010b). Eighty-four healthy controls and patients with MDD who reported a history of emotional maltreatment during childhood had smaller left dorsomedial prefrontal cortex volumes compared to 96 comparison subjects without maltreatment (van Harmelen et al., 2010).

Recent studies in healthy participants and community samples have added to the evidence indicating that childhood maltreatment is associated with morphologic brain changes. In a large study ($n = 193$) of young adults with and without childhood maltreatment, a reduction in left hippocampal subfields CA2–CA3 and CA4–DG, CA1 and subiculum was revealed. This population was not characterized by histories of MDD or posttraumatic stress disorder (Teicher et al., 2012). In 148 healthy participants, reduced gray-matter volumes in the hippocampus, insula, orbitofrontal cortex, anterior cingulate gyrus, and caudate were found to be associated with high scores of childhood maltreatment. This association was not influenced by trait anxiety, depression level, age, intelligence, education, or more recent stressful life events (Dannlowski et al., 2012).

In a single-voxel magnetic resonance spectroscopy study, the ratio of *n*-acetylaspartate to creatine was significantly lower in the anterior cingulate cortex in 11 maltreated subjects with posttraumatic stress disorder than in the comparison 11 subjects without maltreatment (De Bellis et al., 2000).

A study of 18 maltreated children, compared to 20 children who were not maltreated, showed reduced gray matter in the medial orbitofrontal cortex and the left middle temporal gyrus in those with maltreatment (De Brito et al., 2013).

To date, most studies have been conducted cross-sectionally in adults. A longitudinal magnetic resonance imaging study involving 15 children aged 7–13 years with childhood adversity and posttraumatic stress disorder symptoms reported that the presence of childhood maltreatment was related to a decrease in hippocampal volumes over a 12- and 18-month interval. However, this study did not have a comparison group of individuals who were not maltreated, hence no definite conclusion can be drawn about whether children with childhood maltreatment are more vulnerable for hippocampal changes over time (Carrion et al., 2007).

In contrast, maltreatment leading to childhood posttraumatic stress disorder has been reported to result in larger hippocampal volumes in comparison to matched healthy children who were not maltreated (Tupler and De Bellis, 2006). Recently, we demonstrated that gray-matter volume was significantly decreased in the hippocampus and significantly increased in the dorsomedial prefrontal cortex and the orbitofrontal cortex in subjects who had experienced childhood maltreatment in comparison to those who had not (Chaney et al., 2014).

Research in functional neurologic disorders is rare and no significant effects of childhood adversity on brain structure have been investigated in these disorders. Interestingly, significantly smaller left thalamic volumes were found in 14 patients with conversion disorder compared with 31 controls when corrected for intracranial volume (Nicholson et al., 2014). Another voxel-based morphometry and cortical thickness study in patients with psychogenic nonepileptic seizures revealed abnormal cortical atrophy of the motor and premotor regions in the right hemisphere and the cerebellum bilaterally (Labate et al., 2012). These differences may reflect a disease process, or could be a secondary consequence of having a symptom for a while, or even a consequence of comorbidities such as depression. Therefore, larger and longitudinal studies are required in the future to explore these effects in more detail.

Childhood adversity, inflammation, brain structure, and neurotrophic factors are not standalone measurements. They seem to be related to each other. A history of childhood trauma and high levels of recent stressors predicted lower brain-derived neurotrophic factor (BDNF) expression through an inflammation-mediated pathway and, in turn, lower BDNF expression, increased interleukin-6 expression, and increased cortisol levels significantly and independently predicted a smaller left hippocampal volume (Mondelli et al., 2011).

There is one study investigating BDNF blood levels in patients with conversion disorders. Interestingly, serum BDNF levels were found to be significantly smaller in 15 patients with conversion disorders compared to 26 healthy controls. Moreover, there was no difference between BDNF levels between patients with conversion disorders and patients with MDD. This suggests that BDNF level may be altered in a similar way in MDD and conversion disorders (Deveci et al., 2007). However, the impact of childhood adversity, other environmental stressors and genetics on inflammation, neurotrophic factors, and brain structure and function has not yet been explored in conversion disorders. There may be some systems like the stress hormone, neurotrophic and inflammation system that may be most interesting to look at with regard to genetic and epigenetic research.

GENETICS

The role of heritability in conversion and somatization disorders is far from being clear, and twin studies were not conclusive (Torgersen, 1986; Guze, 1993).

Studies in conversion disorders

A PubMed search with the words "conversion disorder" in the title/abstract and "genetics" only results in six literature hits. For a search on "conversion disorder" in title/abstracts and "epigenetics," there were no hits.

There is only one study that investigated the effect of a single-nucleotide polymorphism (SNP) (catechol-*O*-methyltransferase (COMT) polymorphism) on the occurrence of conversion disorders in 48 patients with conversion disorder and 48 control patients. Alterations in COMT activity are involved in various types of neurologic disorders. There was no significant difference between the groups (Armagan et al., 2013). Based on the sample size, it has to be argued that this study was underpowered to detect any significant effects.

Studies in somatoform disorders

Another study investigated whether there is an association between somatoform disorder symptoms with genetic variants that were found in previous studies to be associated with pain. Pain is a major symptom of somatoform disorders, including functional neurologic symptom disorders. A total of 148 somatoform patients with pain as the leading clinical symptom and 149 age- and gender-matched healthy controls participated in this study. Interestingly, the common G-allele of rs1800629 (tumor necrosis factor-α) occurred significantly more often in the control group than in the group of patients with somatoform disorder and thus seems to have protective effects. Being carrier of the A-allele on the other hand might be a risk factor for somatoform disorder (Gil et al., 2011).

Polymorphisms in the COMT gene are associated with COMT enzymatic activity and pain sensitivity; the effect of COMT polymorphisms was investigated in the same sample. None of the six SNPs investigated, including the functionally relevant common SNP in codon 158 (Val158Met), showed a statistically significant allelic, genotypic, or haplotypic association with multisomatoform disorder (Jakobi et al., 2010).

Another study investigated 102 patients with undifferentiated somatoform disorder, 106 patients with MDD, and 133 healthy subjects for differences in the genotype frequency of tryptophan hydroxylase gene polymorphism and associations between this polymorphism and aggression. No significant differences were found in TPH1 C-allele and CC homozygote frequencies between the undifferentiated somatoform disorder patients and the healthy subjects. The group of patients with MDD, however, had significantly higher frequencies of TPH1 C-allele ($p=0.0002$) and CC homozygosity ($p=0.0003$) than healthy subjects, with the same genotypes, regardless of sex and age. Moreover, TPH1 CC homozygotes in the MDD group scored significantly higher in terms of verbal aggression and total aggression questionnaire score than A-carrier genotypes, regardless of sex and age. While there was an association between frequency of this polymorphism and MDD and the polymorphism was associated with aggression within the group of patients with MDD, this was not found for somatoform disorder (Koh et al., 2012).

It has been suggested that serotonergic hypofunction and serotonergic pathway genes underlie the somatic symptoms of somatoform disorders. This hypothesis was investigated using a variety of serotonin-related gene polymorphisms to determine whether undifferentiated somatoform disorder is associated with specific serotonin-related gene pathways. A total of 102 patients with undifferentiated somatoform disorder and 133 healthy subjects were enrolled. Patients with undifferentiated somatoform disorder had higher frequencies of the TPH1 (A218C) C-allele than healthy controls, but the difference was not significant after Bonferroni correction. The frequency of TPH1 genotype in addition to TPH2 rs1386494, 5-HTR 2A-T102C, 5-HTR 2A-G1438A, and 5HTTLPR allele and genotype frequencies did not differ significantly between the two groups. These findings suggest that a variety of serotonin-related gene pathways are unlikely to be genetic risk factors for undifferentiated somatoform disorder. The authors thus concluded that the pathogenesis of the disorder may be related to epigenetic factors, including psychosocial and cultural factors (Koh et al., 2011).

In conclusion, so far there is only one study that reports an association between the SNP rs1800629 of the tumor necrosis factor-α gene in a rather moderate sample size. Thus, larger samples are needed to investigate the effects of rare copy number variants or for looking with a genomewide approach. Thus, no major significant effect of genetic polymorphisms has to date been observed for functional neurologic disorders.

ENVIRONMENT–GENE INTERACTIONS AND EPIGENETICS

A number of research groups have suggested that gene–environmental interactions may be important to consider. To date there are no studies available on the effects of epigenetics on conversion disorders, so we need to discuss this aspect more theoretically.

Studies show that patients with conversion disorders show an excess number of childhood adversity events compared to comparison subjects, so childhood adversity is one factor that should be taken into account. It is known that childhood adversity interacts with genetic predisposition to even influence brain development and brain structure. For example, previously, we found that childhood maltreatment interacts with the s allele of the 5-HTTLPR and is associated with smaller hippocampal volumes in patients with MDD (Frodl et al., 2010a).

Since there are no studies in conversion disorders, it is relevant to look at other studies that examined the association of other disorders, such as dissociation, with early-life adversity and genetics.

Dissociation is a failure of perceptual, memory, and emotional integration that is associated with a variety of psychiatric disorders and usually dissociative processes are related to childhood trauma. One study investigated whether there was a potential gene–childhood abuse interaction for dissociation in bipolar disorder subjects and their affected and unaffected relatives. A sample of 178 affected and unaffected family members from patients with bipolar disorder was investigated for this purpose. Interestingly, the low-activity Met allele of the Val66Met polymorphism of the BDNF gene was associated with lower levels of self-reported dissociation. The COMT Val158Met polymorphism interacted significantly with total abuse scores obtained from the childhood trauma questionnaire to impact on dissociation. Here the Val/Val genotype was associated with increasing levels of dissociation in participants exposed to higher levels of childhood trauma, whereby those with the Met/Met genotypes seemed to display decreased dissociation with increasing self-reported childhood trauma (Savitz et al., 2008). These findings increase the likelihood that conversion disorders may also be related to childhood adversity by gene–environment interactions.

The physiologic mechanisms accounting for such gene–environment interactions are not known. One of the potential mechanisms by which gene–environment interacts and affects brain development is via environmentally induced stable changes in genetic expression (Szyf, 2009; Booij et al., 2013; Nestler, 2014). These changes in stable expression are most probably caused by epigenetic mechanisms (Szyf, 2009; Booij et al., 2013; Nestler, 2014). Following the observation of tissue-specific DNA methylation changes in the hippocampal glucocorticoid receptor (GR) gene in postmortem brains of victims of childhood abuse (McGowan et al., 2009), a number of studies have analyzed DNA methylation processes in peripheral tissues. With regard to the 5-hydroxytryptamine (5-HT) system, an increasing number of studies have found associations between peripheral methylation in the SLC6A4 gene and early-life adversity (Booij et al., 2013), or depression (Nestler, 2014). Specifically, studies demonstrated that early stress, including a history of childhood abuse, was associated with altered levels of peripheral methylation in SLC6A4 promoter regions later in life (Beach et al., 2010, 2011; Devlin et al., 2010; van Ijzendoorn et al., 2010; Kang et al., 2013).

In addition, it was recently found in a healthy sample that DNA methylation at the SLC6A4 promoter in white blood cells of adults was associated with lower *in vivo* measures of brain 5-HT synthesis in the orbitofrontal cortex, irrespective of 5-HTTLPR genotype.

The functional relevance of DNA methylation in SLC6A4 promotor regulation was further demonstrated by an *in vitro* experiment, showing that DNA methylation of the SLC6A4 promoter in a luciferase reporter construct suppressed its transcriptional activity (Wang et al., 2012). These findings, taken together, suggest that DNA methylation in the SLC6A4 promoter may be one of the physiologic mechanisms of how early stress could translate into altered brain development. Hippocampal changes might be particularly relevant here, since this brain region is densely innervated with 5-HT, and highly involved in stress regulation (Lupien et al., 2009; Frodl and O'Keane, 2013). However, other candidate genes and the whole epigenome need to be investigated first to understand how specific these associations might be and also how many other methylation regions might be affected.

Recently we found that methylation of 5-HT transporter polymorphism was significantly associated with higher amount of childhood adversity and smaller hippocampal volumes (Booij et al., 2015). Moreover, methylation of 5-HT transporter polymorphism also was functionally relevant for brain activation during emotional attention-processing tasks, as measured using functional magnetic resonance imaging (Frodl et al., 2015).

We need to consider that multiple factors are interacting over time to explain the associations between early-childhood maltreatment, hippocampus, and HPA axis functioning. Other influences, like genetic and temperamental factors, probably also play a significant role. Key personality traits that have been demonstrated to predict HPA axis stress responses are self-esteem and an internal locus of control. In healthy subjects of all ages these traits are significantly correlated with hippocampal volume (Pruessner et al., 2005). Environmental factors like stress and genetic variation are linked together via epigenetic processes. Animal models tracking the trajectory from early-life stress to adult depression indicate that sustained stress during development leads to hypermethylation of the GR promoter gene, leading to reduced function of the GR and inability to shut down stress responses (McGowan et al., 2011). An impact of parental care on epigenetic regulation of hippocampal GR was demonstrated in a study observing that suicide victims with a history of early-life adversity display decreased GR mRNA expression and increased cytosine methylation of a neuron-specific GR (NR3C1) promoter in postmortem hippocampus compared to either suicide victims with no early-life adversity or controls (McGowan et al., 2009).

Epigenetic influences on the HPA system may also be transgenerational. One study has shown that maternal childhood abuse is associated with lower cortisol responses in their infants (Brand et al., 2010). Interestingly, HPA axis development commences *in utero*. For most of the duration of pregnancy, the baby and mother share a common corticotropin-releasing hormone (CRH)–adrenocorticotropic hormone (ACTH)–cortisol axis, because the placenta produces CRH (McLean et al., 1995). CRH production by the placenta is positively controlled by maternal and fetal cortisol, so that if mother or baby is stressed, CRH production will increase (Smith and Nicholson, 2007). Increased production of placental CRH will result in increased cortisol levels in baby and mother and, because of a positive feedforward loop between cortisol and placental CRH, there will be increased CRH production (McLean et al., 1995). Babies born to women who were psychologically stressed during pregnancy tend to have disorganized sleep, to be less responsive emotionally (Field, 2011), and to have higher cortisol responses to stressors (Davis et al., 2011). The HPA axis seems to be "programmed" *in utero*, via GR mechanisms, so that the developing brain is primed to respond to a fixed "set point" in postuterine life (Glover et al., 2010).

Thus, developmental factors may play a role in some cases of medically unexplained (or "functional") symptoms like conversion disorder (Buffington, 2009). Experimental data suggest that, when a pregnant mother perceives a threatening environment, this situation may be transmitted to the fetus when hormones cross the placenta and affect the course of fetal development (Meaney et al., 2007). These changes also appear to increase vulnerability to life stressors, putting these individuals at greater risk of developing disorders characterized by pain and discomfort (Bateson et al., 2004). Medically unexplained symptoms need to be considered from the perspective of underlying developmental influences involving epigenetic modulation of gene expression that affect function of a variety of organs based on familial (genetic and environmental) predispositions (Fig. 14.1).

These observations may also indicate that good maternal care could protect against excessive stress responses and result in larger brain structural volumes. Indeed, mothers who reported higher maternal care in childhood

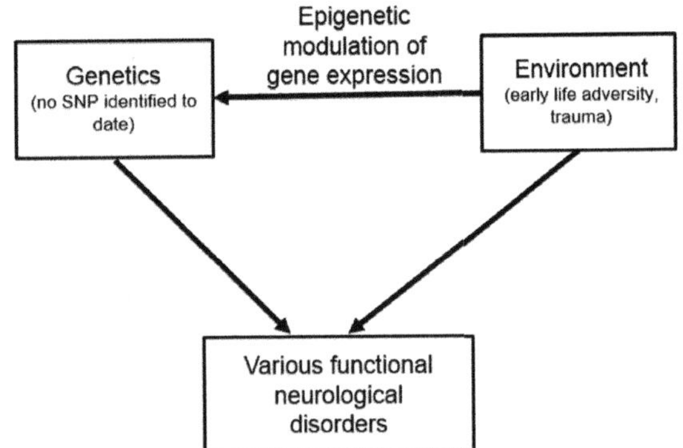

Fig. 14.1. There is some evidence that early-life adversity is associated with the development of functional neurologic disorders. While there is the assumption that stress–gene interaction plays a significant role, to date there is no study available showing that a genetic variation or single-nucleotide polymorphism (SNP) is clearly associated with functional neurologic disorders. However, samples investigated to date are clearly too small. Experimental data and observations about the stress–gene interactions suggest that epigenetic modulation of gene expression might play a central role. This idea needs further investigation.

showed larger gray-matter volumes in the superior and middle frontal gyri, orbital gyrus, superior temporal gyrus, and fusiform gyrus (Kim et al., 2010). Birth weight significantly positively predicted hippocampal volume in adulthood in female subjects reporting low maternal care, suggesting a complex picture with some protective factors (Buss et al., 2007). Thus, events postbirth may also reverse the damaging effects of a harsh intrauterine environment, and the greater plasticity within the HPA system during childhood can provide greater resilience for the developing adult (Fisher et al., 2006).

CONCLUSIONS

To date there is a significant lack of data about gene–environment interactions in functional neurologic disorders. Also to date there is no major evidence that genetics alone play a crucial role, although this research is limited by relatively small samples under investigation. Another limitation is that comorbidity with other psychiatric disorders is high in functional neurologic disorders and somatoform disorders, e.g., with affective disorders, substance use disorders, and personality disorders. Evidence already exists that childhood adversity is a factor influencing the vulnerability for functional neurologic disorders; however, again, the mechanism for how this is provided is unknown, in part because research on epigenetics in this area is just at its start.

References

Alper K, Devinsky O, Perrine K et al. (1993). Nonepileptic seizures and childhood sexual and physical abuse. Neurology 43: 1950–1953.

American Psychiatric Association (2013). Diagnostic and statistical manual of mental disorders, 5th edn. American Psychiatric Association, Washington, DC.

Armagan E, Almacioglu ML, Yakut T et al. (2013). Catechol-O-methyl transferase Val158Met genotype is not a risk factor for conversion disorder. Genet Mol Res 12: 852–858.

Bateson P, Barker D, Clutton-Brock T et al. (2004). Developmental plasticity and human health. Nature 430: 419–421.

Beach SRH, Brody GH, Todorov AA et al. (2010). Methylation at SLC6A4 is linked to family history of child abuse: An examination of the Iowa Adoptee sample. Am J Med Genet B Neuropsychiatr Genet 153B: 710–713.

Beach SRH, Brody GH, Todorov AA et al. (2011). Methylation at 5HTT mediates the impact of child sex abuse on women's antisocial behavior: an examination of the Iowa Adoptee Sample. Psychosom Med 73: 83–87.

Bonne O, Vythilingam M, Inagaki M et al. (2008). Reduced posterior hippocampal volume in posttraumatic stress disorder. J Clin Psychiatry 69: 1087.

Booij L, Wang D, Levesque ML et al. (2013). Looking beyond the DNA sequence: the relevance of DNA methylation processes for the stress-diathesis model of depression. Philos Trans R Soc Lond B Biol Sci 368: 20120251.

Booij L, Szyf M, Carballedo A et al. (2015). The role of SLC6A4 DNA methylation in stress-related changes in hippocampal volume: a study in depressed patients and healthy controls. Plos One 10: e0119061.

Brand SR, Brennan PA, Newport DJ et al. (2010). The impact of maternal childhood abuse on maternal and infant HPA axis function in the postpartum period. Psychoneuroendocrinology 35: 686–693.

Buffington CA (2009). Developmental influences on medically unexplained symptoms. Psychother Psychosom 78: 139–144.

Buss C, Lord C, Wadiwalla M et al. (2007). Maternal care modulates the relationship between prenatal risk and hippocampal volume in women but not in men. J Neurosci 27: 2592–2595.

Capuron L, Miller AH (2011). Immune system to brain signaling: neuropsychopharmacological implications. Pharmacol Ther 130: 226–238.

Carrion VG, Weems CF, Reiss AL (2007). Stress predicts brain changes in children: a pilot longitudinal study on youth stress, posttraumatic stress disorder, and the hippocampus. Pediatrics 119: 509–516.

Chaney A, Carballedo A, Amico F et al. (2014). Effect of childhood maltreatment on brain structure in adult patients with major depressive disorder and healthy participants. J Psychiatry Neurosci 39: 50–59.

Dannlowski U, Stuhrmann A, Beutelmann V et al. (2012). Limbic scars: long-term consequences of childhood maltreatment revealed by functional and structural magnetic resonance imaging. Biol Psychiatry 71: 286–293.

Davis EP, Glynn LM, Waffarn F et al. (2011). Prenatal maternal stress programs infant stress regulation. J Child Psychol Psychiatry 52: 119–129.

De Bellis MD, Keshavan MS, Spencer S et al. (2000). *N*-Acetylaspartate concentration in the anterior cingulate of maltreated children and adolescents with PTSD. Am J Psychiatry 157: 1175–1177.

De Brito SA, Viding E, Sebastian CL et al. (2013). Reduced orbitofrontal and temporal grey matter in a community sample of maltreated children. J Child Psychol Psychiatry 54: 105–112.

Deveci A, Aydemir O, Taskin O et al. (2007). Serum brain-derived neurotrophic factor levels in conversion disorder: Comparative study with depression. Psychiatry Clin Neurosci 61: 571–573.

Devlin AM, Brain U, Austin J et al. (2010). Prenatal exposure to maternal depressed mood and the *MTHFR C677T* variant affect *SLC6A4* methylation in infants at birth. PLoS One 5. e12201.

Dube SR, Felitti VJ, Dong M et al. (2003). Childhood abuse, neglect, and household dysfunction and the risk of illicit drug use: the adverse childhood experiences study. Pediatrics 111: 564.

Duman RS (2002). Pathophysiology of depression: the concept of synaptic plasticity. Eur Psychiatry 17 (Suppl 3): 306–310.

Field T (2011). Prenatal depression effects on early development: a review. Infant Behav Dev 34: 1–14.

Fisher PA, Gunnar MR, Dozier M et al. (2006). Effects of therapeutic interventions for foster children on behavioral problems, caregiver attachment, and stress regulatory neural systems. Ann N Y Acad Sci 1094: 215–225.

Frodl T, O'Keane V (2013). How does the brain deal with cumulative stress? A review with focus on developmental stress, HPA axis function and hippocampal structure in humans. Neurobiol Dis 52: 24–37.

Frodl T, Reinhold E, Koutsouleris N et al. (2010a). Childhood stress, serotonin transporter gene and brain structures in major depression. Neuropsychopharmacology 35: 1383–1390.

Frodl T, Reinhold E, Koutsouleris N et al. (2010b). Interaction of childhood stress with hippocampus and prefrontal cortex volume reduction in major depression. J Psychiatr Res 44: 799–807.

Frodl T, Szyf M, Carballedo A et al. (2015). DNA methylation of serotonin transporter gene (SLC6A4) associates with brain function involved in processing of emotional stimuli. J Psychiatr Neurosci 40: 296–305.

Gil FP, Giegling I, Reisch N et al. (2011). Association of somatoform disorder symptoms with genetic variants potentially involved in the modulation of nociception. Psychiatr Genet 21: 50.

Glover V, O'Connor TG, O'Donnell K (2010). Prenatal stress and the programming of the HPA axis. Neurosci Biobehav Rev 35: 17–22.

Guze SB (1993). Genetics of Briquet's syndrome and somatization disorder. A review of family, adoption, and twin studies. Ann Clin Psychiatry 5: 225–230.

Heim C, Nemeroff CB (2001). The role of childhood trauma in the neurobiology of mood and anxiety disorders: preclinical and clinical studies. Biol Psychiatry 49: 1023–1039.

Jakobi J, Bernateck M, Tran AT et al. (2010). Catechol-O-methyltransferase gene polymorphisms are not associated with multisomatoform disorder in a group of German multisomatoform disorder patients and healthy controls. Genet Test Mol Biomarkers 14: 293–297.

Kang HJ, Kim JM, Stewart R et al. (2013). Association of SLC6A4 methylation with early adversity, characteristics and outcomes in depression. Prog Neuropsychopharmacol Biol Psychiatry 44: 23–28.

Kaplan MJ, Dwivedi AK, Privitera MD et al. (2013). Comparisons of childhood trauma, alexithymia, and defensive styles in patients with psychogenic non-epileptic seizures vs. epilepsy: implications for the etiology of conversion disorder. J Psychosom Res 75: 142–146.

Kessler RC (1997). The effects of stressful life events on depression. Annu Rev Psychol 48: 191–214.

Kim P, Leckman JF, Mayes LC et al. (2010). Perceived quality of maternal care in childhood and structure and function of mothers' brain. Dev Sci 13: 662–673.

Koh KB, Choi EH, Lee YJ et al. (2011). Serotonin-related gene pathways associated with undifferentiated somatoform disorder. Psychiatry Res 189: 246–250.

Koh KB, Kim CH, Choi EH et al. (2012). Effect of tryptophan hydroxylase gene polymorphism on aggression in major depressive disorder and undifferentiated somatoform disorder. J Clin Psychiatry 73: e574–e579.

Kole MH, Czeh B, Fuchs E (2004). Homeostatic maintenance in excitability of tree shrew hippocampal CA3 pyramidal neurons after chronic stress. Hippocampus 14: 742–751.

Krem MM (2004). Motor conversion disorders reviewed from a neuropsychiatric perspective. J Clin Psychiatry 65: 783–790.

Krishnan V, Nestler EJ (2008). The molecular neurobiology of depression. Nature 455: 894–902.

Labate A, Cerasa A, Mula M et al. (2012). Neuroanatomic correlates of psychogenic nonepileptic seizures: a cortical thickness and VBM study. Epilepsia 53: 377–385.

Lupien SJ, Mcewen BS, Gunnar MR et al. (2009). Effects of stress throughout the lifespan on the brain, behaviour and cognition. Nat Rev Neurosci 10: 434–445.

Macqueen G, Frodl T (2011). The hippocampus in major depression: evidence for the convergence of the bench and bedside in psychiatric research? Mol Psychiatry 16: 252–264.

Magarinos AM, Mcewen BS, Flugge G et al. (1996). Chronic psychosocial stress causes apical dendritic atrophy of hippocampal CA3 pyramidal neurons in subordinate tree shrews. J Neurosci 16: 3534–3540.

Mcgowan PO, Sasaki A, D'Alessio AC et al. (2009). Epigenetic regulation of the glucocorticoid receptor in human brain associates with childhood abuse. Nat Neurosci 12: 342–348.

Mcgowan PO, Suderman M, Sasaki A et al. (2011). Broad epigenetic signature of maternal care in the brain of adult rats. PLoS One 6. e14739.

Mclean M, Bisits A, Davies J et al. (1995). A placental clock controlling the length of human pregnancy. Nat Med 1: 460–463.

Meaney MJ, Szyf M, Seckl JR (2007). Epigenetic mechanisms of perinatal programming of hypothalamic–pituitary–adrenal function and health. Trends Mol Med 13: 269–277.

Mondelli V, Cattaneo A, Belvederi Murri M et al. (2011). Stress and inflammation reduce brain-derived neurotrophic factor expression in first-episode psychosis: a pathway to smaller hippocampal volume. J Clin Psychiatry 72: 1677–1684.

Myint AM, Schwarz MJ, Muller N (2012). The role of the kynurenine metabolism in major depression. J Neural Transm 119: 245–251.

Nestler EJ (2014). Epigenetic mechanisms of depression. JAMA Psychiatry 71: 454–456.

Nicholson TR, Aybek S, Kempton MJ et al. (2014). A structural MRI study of motor conversion disorder: evidence of reduction in thalamic volume. J Neurol Neurosurg Psychiatry 85: 227–229.

Ozcetin A, Belli H, Ertem U et al. (2009). Childhood trauma and dissociation in women with pseudoseizure-type conversion disorder. Nord J Psychiatry 63: 462–468.

Pruessner JC, Baldwin MW, Dedovic K et al. (2005). Self-esteem, locus of control, hippocampal volume, and cortisol regulation in young and old adulthood. Neuroimage 28: 815–826.

Roelofs K, Spinhoven P (2007). Trauma and medically unexplained symptoms towards an integration of cognitive and neuro-biological accounts. Clin Psychol Rev 27: 798–820.

Roelofs K, Keijsers GP, Hoogduin KA et al. (2002). Childhood abuse in patients with conversion disorder. Am J Psychiatry 159: 1908–1913.

Santarelli L, Saxe M, Gross C et al. (2003). Requirement of hippocampal neurogenesis for the behavioral effects of antidepressants. Science 301: 805–809.

Savitz JB, Van der Merwe L, Newman TK et al. (2008). The relationship between childhood abuse and dissociation. Is it influenced by catechol-O-methyltransferase (COMT) activity? Int J Neuropsychopharmacol 11: 149–161.

Sharpe D, Faye C (2006). Non-epileptic seizures and child sexual abuse: a critical review of the literature. Clin Psychol Rev 26: 1020–1040.

Smith R, Nicholson RC (2007). Corticotrophin releasing hormone and the timing of birth. Front Biosci 12: 912–918.

Szyf M (2009). The early life environment and the epigenome. Biochim Biophys Acta 1790: 878–885.

Taylor SE, Eisenberger NI, Saxbe D et al. (2006). Neural responses to emotional stimuli are associated with childhood family stress. Biol Psychiatry 60: 296–301.

Teicher MH, Anderson CM, Polcari A (2012). Childhood maltreatment is associated with reduced volume in the hippocampal subfields CA3, dentate gyrus, and subiculum. Proc Natl Acad Sci U S A 109: E563–E572.

Torgersen S (1986). Genetics of somatoform disorders. Arch Gen Psychiatry 43: 502–505.

Tupler LA, De Bellis MD (2006). Segmented hippocampal volume in children and adolescents with posttraumatic stress disorder. Biol Psychiatry 59: 523–529.

Van Harmelen AL, Van Tol MJ, Van der Wee NJ et al. (2010). Reduced medial prefrontal cortex volume in adults reporting childhood emotional maltreatment. Biol Psychiatry 68: 832–838.

Van ijzendoorn MH, Caspers K, Bakermans-Kranenburg MJ et al. (2010). Methylation matters: interaction between methylation density and serotonin transporter genotype predicts unresolved loss or trauma. Biol Psychiatry 68: 405–407.

Vythilingam M, Heim C, Newport J et al. (2002). Childhood trauma associated with smaller hippocampal volume in women with major depression. Am J Psychiatry 159: 2072–2080.

Wang D, Szyf M, Benkelfat C et al. (2012). Peripheral SLC6A4 DNA methylation is associated with in vivo measures of human brain serotonin synthesis and childhood physical aggression. PLoS One 7. e39501.

Wellman CL (2001). Dendritic reorganization in pyramidal neurons in medial prefrontal cortex after chronic corticosterone administration. J Neurobiol 49: 245–253.

Woolley CS, Gould E, Frankfurt M et al. (1990). Naturally occurring fluctuation in dendritic spine density on adult hippocampal pyramidal neurons. J Neurosci 10: 4035–4039.

World Health Organization (2010). The ICD-10 classification of mental and behavioural disorders: clinical descriptions and diagnostic guidelines, World Health Organization, Geneva.

Section 3

Symptoms (including signs and investigations)

Handbook of Clinical Neurology, Vol. 139 (3rd series)
Functional Neurologic Disorders
M. Hallett, J. Stone, and A. Carson, Editors
http://dx.doi.org/10.1016/B978-0-12-801772-2.00015-1

Chapter 15

Assessment of patients with functional neurologic disorders

A. CARSON[1]*, M. HALLETT[2], AND J. STONE[3]

[1]*Departments of Clinical Neurosciences and of Rehabilitation Medicine, NHS Lothian and Centre for Clinical Brain Sciences, University of Edinburgh, Edinburgh, UK*

[2]*Human Motor Control Section, National Institute of Neurological Disorders and Stroke, Bethesda, MD, USA*

[3]*Department of Clinical Neurosciences, Centre for Clinical Brain Sciences, University of Edinburgh, Edinburgh, UK*

Abstract

We describe an overall approach and structure to the clinical assessment of the patient with a functional neurologic disorder. Whilst the primary purpose of the assessment is to make a diagnosis and develop a treatment plan, we believe the assessment also plays a key role in treatment in its own right, as it sets a tone and context for future clinical interactions. We aim to set up an atmosphere of collaboration based on taking the patient's problems seriously, and emphasizing that all facets of the patient's presentation – physical, psychologic, and social – are of importance. Patients with functional disorders can be perceived as difficult to help and yet with the correct approaches we believe the consultation can be much more satisfying for both patient and doctor. Finally, we discuss and list some of the common diagnostic pitfalls in the assessment of functional neurologic disorders, looking at features that lead to erroneous diagnosis of neurologic disease (such as old age, *la belle indifférence*, and lack of psychiatric comorbidity) and an erroneous diagnosis of a functional disorder (such as "bizarre" gait in stiff-person syndrome).

INTRODUCTION

In this chapter we describe our general approach to clinical assessment; individual symptoms and signs in specific functional presentations are described in other chapters. Here we shall concentrate on an overall approach and structure to the assessment. This is a topic we have written on at length in other review papers and the material presented here synthesizes many of these thoughts; in particular it either duplicates or draws heavily on material described in previous papers (Stone, 2009; Carson and Stone, 2013; Stone et al., 2013), and is reproduced with permission.

Whilst the primary purpose of the assessment is to make a diagnosis and develop a treatment plan, we believe the assessment also plays a key role in treatment in its own right as it sets a tone and context for future clinical interactions (Stone, 2014). In this regard we aim to set up an atmosphere of collaboration based on taking the patient's problems seriously, and emphasizing that all facets of the patient's presentation – physical, psychologic, and social – are of importance. Patients with functional disorders can be perceived as difficult to help (Carson et al., 2004), and yet with the correct approaches we believe the consultation can be much more satisfying for both patient and doctor, leading more productively to explanation (see Chapter 44) and further treatment.

PREPARATION AND START OF THE CONSULTATION

Setting

The initial contacts with healthcare services should take place in a medical setting where adequate examination facilities are available. Obviously this is the norm where the first contact is with a neurologist, but it is not uncommon in psychiatric facilities for there to be a lack of basic equipment such as examination couches and the standard tools of physical examination. Such facilities are seldom

*Correspondence to: Alan Carson, Robert Fergusson Unit, Royal Edinburgh Hospital, Tipperlin Road, Edinburgh EH10 5HF, UK. E-mail: a.carson@ed.ac.uk

available in psychotherapeutic settings. Even in situations where the primary purpose of the examination is to assess potential psychopathology, we believe that the willingness of clinicians to engage with physical examination is not just for diagnostic information but sends a clear signal that the physical element of the presentation is being taken seriously. It is sometimes suggested that patients might be referred directly from primary care to specialist psychotherapy. We think this approach is mistaken and that proper medical assessment is essential, partly because primary care diagnoses of functional neurologic disorder are often erroneous (Carson et al., 2000), and also because we think that the physical assessment and diagnosis are the key first steps in multidisciplinary treatment (Healthcare Improvement Scotland, 2012).

One core component of the examination is to allow enough time. Such consultations are always more satisfactory when there is enough time to deal with the patient's problems properly without either patient or doctor feeling rushed. Whilst consultations have to fit into the time available we generally find that 25 minutes or less is a false economy and an hour is preferable. In the UK 30 minutes is a squeeze but most of the key components can be addressed. Indeed, for complex patients longer may be advisable. It is far better to have time to attend to all aspects of the consultation and draw a meaningful conclusion than to have multiple return visits.

Table 15.1

Functional syndromes presenting to different medical specialties

Medical specialty	Functional symptom
Rheumatology	Fibromyalgia
Orthopedics	Chronic back pain
Neurology	Functional movement disorder
	Dissociative (nonepileptic) seizure
Ear, nose, and throat	Atypical facial pain
	Chronic unexplained dizziness
	Functional dysphonia
	Globus pharyngis
Infectious diseases	Chronic fatigue syndrome
Cardiology	Noncardiac chest pain
	Palpitations with normal investigations
Gastroenterology	Functional dyspepsia
	Irritable-bowel syndrome

Preparation

Where possible review the patient's past medical history from medical records. Patients tend to have inaccurate recall of their own medical records and the information provided by them during history taking can be misleading, possibly especially so in patients with functional disorders (Schrag et al., 2004a,b). A previous diagnosis of a functional disorder might have been made, but the patient may not mention it. A thick pile of records has been considered a possible sign indicating a functional disorder since these patients may well have multiple consultations and a large number of tests. A major predictor of a likely functional disorder is a previous history of functional disorder (Hotopf et al., 2000); this may be present but be given alternate, disease-based labels, by patients in their own report.

In our experience functional motor disorders, such as paralysis, are unusual first presentations of functional disorders. Although this does happen, we would look for evidence of prior problems with functional symptoms that are more on a spectrum with normal experience, such as irritable-bowel syndrome, heavy painful menstrual bleeding, a history of unexplained abdominal pain, or a history of chronic back pain. It should be noted that these disorders are common in the general population anyway and their presence should be viewed only as indicative of an increased risk (Table 15.1).

By contrast, a prior history of psychiatric disorder is often unhelpful or misleading. Whilst a previous history of anxiety disorders or depression increases the risk of having functional disorders (Katon et al., 2001), such disorders are also common in neurologic disease and indeed can increase the risk of many neurologic diseases. In an approximate summary an emotional disorder will be present in two out of three functional cases and one out of three neurologic cases, so as diagnostic markers they should be treated with caution. Interestingly, in our experience the presence of psychotic illnesses such as bipolar illness or schizophrenia is seldom associated with functional disorder. We are unaware of any high-quality epidemiology to support this assertion, but the lack of comorbidity has been notable in some case series (Kranick et al., 2011) and in clinic. We would certainly recommend caution around making the diagnosis of functional disorder in a patient with a psychotic illness; and it should be noted that history taking in this group of patients can on occasions be difficult and the range of tardive movement disorders secondary to antipsychotics is wide and can be bizarre (Owens et al., 1982).

The referral letter itself can provide clues and patients with functional disorder are more likely to have multiple symptoms and sometimes a less clearly identified primary complaint.

There is also an association between previous operative procedures in particular, appendicectomy (with normal appendix), hysterectomy and surgical sterilization, and functional disorders for reasons which are poorly understood but have been replicated in a number of studies.

Some clinicians like to use preclinic assessment questionnaires. These can be helpful but the risk is that they end up as a lesser substitute for the process of listening and recording the patient's difficulties in person. In particular, symptom count measures, despite their recent hype, have little predictive validity (Carson et al., 2014; see Chapter 5 in this volume).

Beginning a consultation

It is often helpful to begin the consultation by simply allowing patients to speak freely about the problem that has brought them to clinic without interrupting. The mean duration of spontaneous talking time without interruption was 92 seconds in a primary care study. By contrast, most doctors interrupt within 20 seconds, following which patients can be inhibited in introducing new issues (Gask and Usherwood, 2002; Langewitz et al., 2002). Patients, however, frequently do not begin with the symptom that is most important to them and therefore this brief period of free-flowing dialogue can often allow the doctor to get a far better idea of what the key issue is more quickly than otherwise might be the case.

Everyone has their own style of assessment but it is noticeable how often patients with functional disorders want to "start from the beginning" of the story. To ensure the consultation and treatment focus on current issues, disability, and obstacles to recovery, it is often helpful to indicate to the patient that you wish to focus initially on how things are now and that you will come back to the story of how it happened later.

THE ASSESSMENT OF PHYSICAL SYMPTOMS IN THE HISTORY

Make a list of physical symptoms

After this initial opening we think it is most helpful to get a list of all the symptoms currently being suffered. During this phase the patient can be discouraged from going into minute detail and this can be further signposted by leaving space on clinic notes which will obviously be annotated later. Again, we find this tends to save time, and by getting all the symptoms out into the open, one often realizes that a number of symptoms are actually more or less facets of the same issue but described in different ways. In this context it is important to ask about pain, memory, fatigue, dizziness, and sleep disturbance. It is also worth enquiring briefly about other bodily systems and generally encouraging disclosure: "Is there anything else? I want to make sure I know everything bothering you."

The sense that everything has been asked about and the assessment is complete will often do more than any other strategy to secure a good collaborative nature to the consult. When a core complaint is widespread bodily pain, the use of pain maps is often particularly helpful in allowing the patient to describe the symptomatology

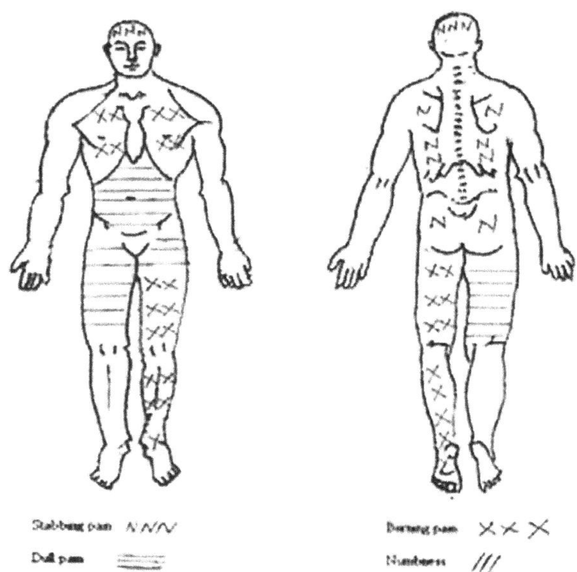

Fig. 15.1. The use of pain maps can help clearly transmit a lot of information about widespread pain quickly.

(Fig. 15.1). On completion of the list, do also ask: "What bothers you the most?"

Typical day and disability

It is often more informative to ask about what the patient can (rather than can't) do. Patients with functional symptoms have a tendency to report what they can no longer do rather than what they can. Whilst it is helpful to hear about previous function, ask them what they are able to do – do they enjoy it?

Taking a patient through a typical day provides information about levels of activity and social contacts and can give important supplementary information about mood and cognition. For example, if they enjoy a regular drama on TV then their mood may not be too bad and their cognition sufficient to follow the program.

Onset and course

The onset in patients with weakness and movement disorders is sudden in around 50% of cases. It is helpful to explore whether there was a trigger. Studies have found that patients with functional neurologic symptoms often report a physical injury, or some pathophysiologic disease or physiologic event at the time of onset. This event may well have a role in shaping the future functional symptoms. Thus, a painful injury to a leg may lead to functional paralysis, shaking from rigors may lead to functional tremor, traveler's diarrhea to irritable-bowel syndrome, or a simple faint to future dissociative seizures (Table 15.2 and Fig. 15.2).

Table 15.2

The etiology of functional symptoms (functional neurologic disorder: FND)

Precipitating	
FND is a disorder of sensorimotor processing in which erroneous health beliefs or expectations distort an, often noxious, somatosensory experience. This process is facilitated by misdirected and overly precise attention, anxiety, and dissociation. The symptom formation helps "make sense" of the amorphous somatic experience. The patient can be either consciously or preconsciously complicit in it	
Perpetuating	
Once present, FND can be perpetuated by maladaptive behavioral responses, both operant and classic learning, mood disorder, and central nervous system plasticity	
Predisposing	
Patients who have pre-existent mood/anxiety problems, excessive threat vigilance, or certain obsessive or rigid cognitive styles are more vulnerable; some of these risks may relate to the experience of abusive or aversive events currently, the recent past, or childhood. There is also a mild genetic risk and almost certainly other risk factors as yet unknown	

In this model the initially noxious somatic experience, whilst quite benign, is modified by a range of cognitive processes (see Chapter 10 and below) to create the functional symptom but it is that physical experience that dictates the timing of onset and possibly shapes the nature of symptom.

Such physical triggers may also include symptoms experienced as part of psychiatric or emotional states, in particular panic. Dissociation (see below) is also commonly experienced at onset. More gradual-onset symptoms are often associated with fatigue.

By contrast, the typical description of psychologically traumatic life event is less frequently reported (Stone et al., 2009a), although Nicholson et al. (2016) found that, with very detailed examination via the Life Events and Difficulties Scale interview schedule taken over several hours, such events occur more commonly than they are typically reported in clinic. Whatever the correct answer to this controversial topic, we believe that detailed exploration of the question of recent life events can usually be left to one side at first contact unless the patient is obviously keen to explore it.

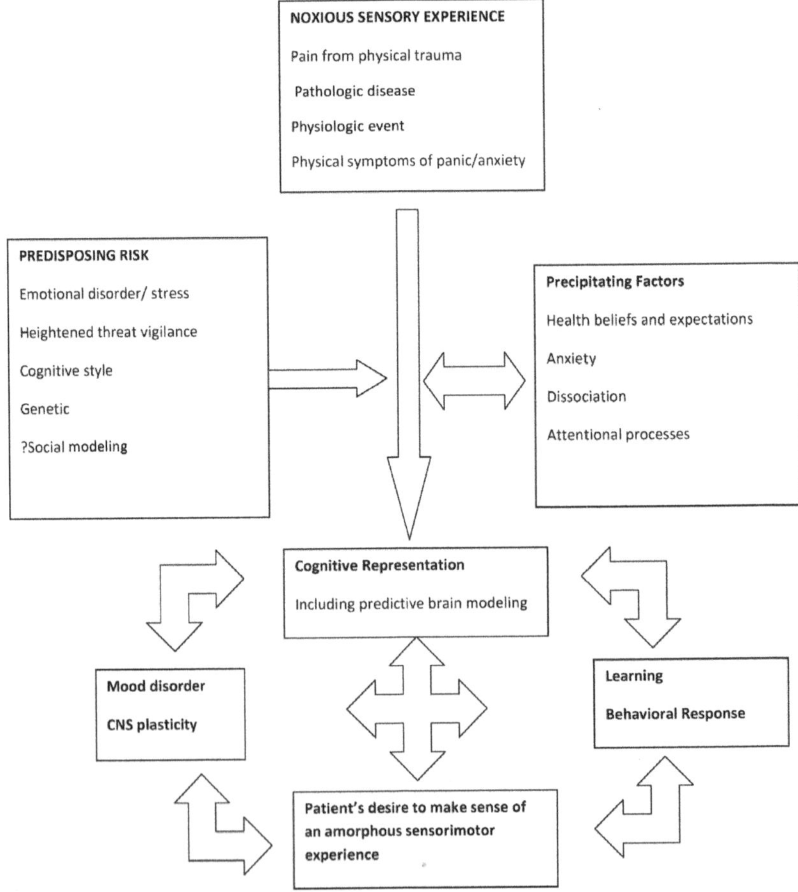

Fig. 15.2. Physical triggers to functional symptoms. CNS, central nervous system.

Trying to make sense of a long and complex history in a short consultation can be a challenge. The question, "When were you last really well, without any of these problems?" can be helpful, as can assessing the impact on work.

Mapping out the severity of the symptoms crudely on a graph of time vs. severity can help to understand the course and the relationship of symptoms to other medical interventions, illnesses, accidents, or life events.

Dissociative symptoms

We always ask specifically about symptoms of dissociation at time of onset. Dissociation is "a somewhat ambiguous collective term describing a range of psychopathological processes altering a person's level of awareness and/or the integration of sensorimotor function, emotions, thoughts, memories and identity which may be subjectively perceived as a sense of disconnection" (Carson et al., 2012). It can be conceptualized in a range of different ways (Holmes et al., 2005), but at this stage we ask in particular about symptoms of depersonalization and derealization (Stone, 2006; see Chapter 8).

Depersonalization, a sense of disconnection from the body, is commonly described as *I felt strange/weird, I felt as if I was floating away, I felt disembodied/disconnected/detached/far away from myself, apart from everything, in a place of my own/alone, like I was there but not there, I could see and hear everything but couldn't respond, like I was there but not there, I could see and hear everything but couldn't respond.* Or less commonly, as "puppet-like," "robot-like," "acting a part," *I couldn't feel any pain, like I was made of cardboard, I felt like I was just a head stuck on a body, like a spectator looking at myself on TV, an out-of-body experience, my hands or feet felt smaller/bigger, when I touched things it didn't feel like me touching them.* Sometimes with autoscopic experiences it can be that the patient's perceived actual movements and the false perception of movement are engaged in different tasks.

Derealization, a sense of disconnection from the environment, may be described as *My surroundings seemed unreal/far away, I felt spaced out, it was like looking at the world through a veil or glass, I felt cut off or distant from the immediate surroundings, objects appeared diminished in size/flat/dream-like/cartoon-like/artificial/unsolid.*

Patients may also describe other dissociative symptoms involving memory: *I drove the car home/got dressed/had dinner but can't remember anything about it, I don't know who I am or how I got here* (fugue state), *I remember things but it doesn't feel like it was me that was there.* They may describe their identity: *I feel like I'm two separate people/someone else* or distortions in time: *I felt like time was passing incredibly slowly/quickly*, or personal boundaries: *I get so absorbed in fantasy/a TV program that it seems real*, or a loss of "sense of being," *I felt an emptiness in my head as if I was not having any thoughts at all.*

We generally ask directly about a few such symptoms as we find patients are seldom willing to freely volunteer them as they seem so odd and they do not want to be considered as "going mad." After a patient discloses such symptoms it is helpful to offer a few words of reassurance that, despite the odd nature of the experience, such symptoms are commonplace, do not indicate "madness," are not sinister and in fact may help us to understand the nature of the complaints.

EXPLORING THE PATIENTS BELIEFS

It is vital to understand the patient's perspective on the cause of the symptoms. It is known that the patient's beliefs have a significant effect on outcome (Sharpe et al., 2010) and erroneous beliefs, and the sensory and motor distortions they produce in the nervous system, are increasingly believed to play a significant part in the etiology and mechanism of functional neurologic disorders (Edwards et al., 2012).

The assessment of a patient's views on the illness is best conducted in line with Leventhal's common-sense model of illness (Cameron and Leventhal, 2003). This is described in more detail in Chapter 10, but is outlined in brief in Table 15.3. The key in assessment is not just to ask about the five elements of illness belief but to be alert to areas of distortions of illness beliefs where the patient has followed a line of reasoning that at one level makes sense but that is ultimately maladaptive. A basic example of this might be a patient who hurts his back digging the garden. Rest helps the pain and when he returns to mobilization it is sore again, so he concludes that he must rest for longer rather than mobilize gradually until the pain eases. Although in the short term this might be reasonable behavior, if it continues day after day layers of avoidance and related anticipatory anxiety will lead to an escalation in pain and disability (Fig. 15.3).

One tip in the exploration of illness beliefs is to remember the effect of conditioning, in particular single-event aversive conditioning, in creating a link between two factors that should otherwise be physiologically unrelated, e.g., *whenever I drink tea I get severe paresthesia in my feet.* This type of linkage should be explored whenever patients report a clear association in their mind between two pathophysiologically implausible factors.

Some people require quite a lot of encouragement to admit their thoughts about what's wrong and may need encouragement to voice disagreement with previous medical opinion. It is possible and often helpful to allow

Table 15.3

The common-sense model of illness regulation

Element	Cognition	Distortions	Example in functional disorders
Identity	What are these symptoms?	Symptoms cause labels But labels also lead to the self-generation of symptoms	*I have limb weakness; I think it is a stroke*
Cause	What caused these symptoms?	Beliefs that symptoms are due to damage and therefore irreversible	*A stroke is a clot in the brain; I think it happened because I was overdoing it*
Consequences	What effects will the symptoms have on my life?	Cog representations guide subsequent behavior	*I am scared I could end up in a wheelchair or even die*
Time line	How long will the symptoms last?	Behaving and adjusting life in the belief something will go on for ever, i.e., quitting job, can become a self-fulfilling prophecy	*I don't think my leg will ever get better. What if I get more disabled?*
Cure and control	What will help make the symptoms better?	Change in symptoms provides feedback on coping strategies and may result in reappraisal of symptoms or adoption of maladaptive strategies, i.e., pain on activity leading to increased downtime	*I think I need to rest more to make sure this doesn't happen again. It is important I don't do anything to provoke it or cause it to recur*

From Stone et al. (2009b), by courtesy of the Guarantors of Brain.

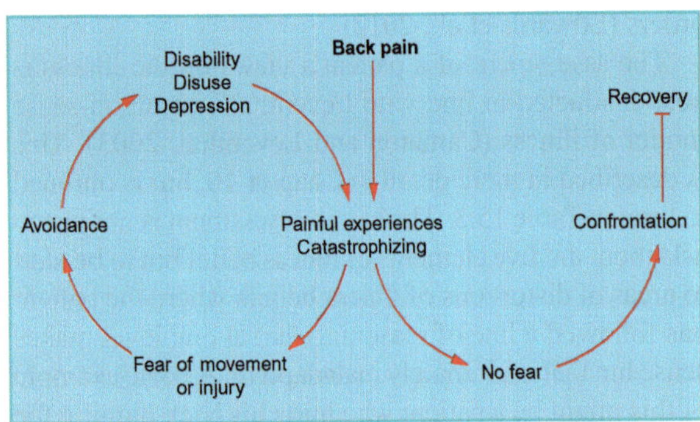

Fig. 15.3. The role of illness beliefs in the development of chronic back pain in the absence of structural disease. (From Main and Williams, 2002 with permission from BMJ Press.)

patients to vent feelings about prior diagnostic opinions without having to take sides. Some patients will "parrot" an explanation they have been given without necessarily believing it. Asking the patient what level of confidence they have in that diagnosis on a scale of one to 10 can be revealing:

"*Doctor: What do you think is the cause of your weak leg?*

Patient: They said it was some kind of dysfunction of the brain. They said it was like software, not hardware.

Doctor: Yes, but do you think that's correct?

Patient: Well, you're the doctor.

Doctor: I am, but it's important for me to know what you really think, or even if you just have a hunch about something, so that I can try to help. How confident are you that the diagnosis of functional disorder is correct? 20% confident? 80% confident?

Patient: About 50%.

Doctor: Are there any other conditions you were still wondering about or had niggling doubt about?

Patient: Well, I was wondering whether they could have missed multiple sclerosis."

Using some of the basic techniques of cognitive-behavioral therapy assessment can also be useful here. Asking patients not just what they think but what the personal significance of those thoughts are can be helpful. One can then ask them what they actually do when they have these thoughts or concerns and whether viewed objectively they make sense:

"*Patient: I am really frightened of the attacks in case they damage me [dissociative seizures].*

Doctor: Are you worried about any specific way they might damage you?

Patient: Yes, when I have had the attacks and have fallen and hurt myself, I've had quite a few injuries and had to go to casualty.

Doctor: Do you do anything to try to prevent that happening?

Patient: Yes, whenever I get any sense an attack is coming I run to the bathroom and lock myself in and sit on the toilet.

Doctor: If you fall in the bathroom is there much you can hit? (pause) How will people help if the door is locked?

Patient: Oh, it just sort of felt safe."

Finally, this part of the consultation is a useful point to establish what the patient was hoping that health professionals in general ought to do to help, and what, in particular s/he was hoping for from the assessment on the day.

Time spent on illness beliefs pays dividends later when helping the patient to understand the diagnosis. For example, if you haven't established that the patient is actually really concerned about a throwaway remark a junior doctor made about a scan showing some "high signal lesions," then progress with treatment may be slow. Alternatively, if you realize that the patient is only in the clinic because she had a new young general practitioner, she had accepted her disability years ago, and she wasn't really looking to engage in rehabilitation, then you could be talking at cross-purposes.

THE PSYCHOLOGIC ASSESSMENT OF PATIENTS WITH FUNCTIONAL DISORDERS

The basic assessment of depression, anxiety, and other psychologic disorders such as posttraumatic disorder or obsessive compulsive disorder can take place during a neurologic assessment and should be part of a psychiatric assessment. It is however not always essential to spend a lot of time on this. If you have discussed a typical day, fatigue, sleep, and concentration you will already have most of the relevant information. In addition, paying attention to some of the basic features of a mental state examination, such as eye contact, reactivity of mood, or agitation, can be revealing.

Asking about depression, anxiety, and other common psychologic symptoms

At the first assessment, overly blunt questioning in the domain of depression and anxiety can be counterproductive to a therapeutic relationship. The question of how detailed to make this should be led by cues from the patient, who is usually expecting an assessment of his weak leg or blackouts, not his mental state.

The typical patient with depression feels down, tearful, and lethargic. This is accompanied by a cognitive triad of distorted thoughts with a sense of hopelessness and futility about the future, a sense of worthlessness about the present, and a sense of guilt about the past. The symptom of anhedonia, the inability to experience pleasure, is central. There is usually a range of somatic symptoms, including disturbed sleep with early-morning wakening and lack of refreshment, loss of appetite, poor concentration, loss of libido, and a sense of general malaise.

Rarely, patients may be frankly suicidal and this represents a medical emergency to be dealt with immediately.

In many patients with functional symptoms detection is less straightforward. Patients may emphasize the somatic element of the presentation and view mood symptoms as a rational response to intolerable physical symptoms rather than an illness in their own right. The presence of low mood may be denied in response to direct questions, partly because the patient is aware that the doctor is "angling" for a psychiatric diagnosis. Exploring mood in this situation requires considerable tact. When suspicion is raised due to the presence of typical somatic symptoms (Fig. 15.3), sympathetic, leading questions can be more fruitful:

> *"It must be difficult living with all that pain … Have you cut down on your range of activities? … Do you find you stopped enjoying things that you can still manage to do physically? What about watching your favorite program on TV? Do you still enjoy it?"*

When assessing inpatients a critical question is often: *When friends or relatives come to visit do you look forward to their company as a break from the monotony? or do you just want to hide away and wish they would go?*

In patients who report mood symptoms a further diagnostic challenge is to separate out those with new symptoms from those who have dysthymic personalities by asking, *When did this first start? Have you always been like this since you were a teenager? Is this a change from your normal self?*

The core of an anxiety disorder is disproportionate, persistent, and unwelcome worry. Anxiety disorders present with a range of somatic symptoms such as muscle tension/pain, fatigue, tingling, nausea, and poor concentration, and symptoms associated with excessive, shallow, or disordered breathing. Abdominal bloating and borborygmi, from aerophagy are common. Peripheral paresthesiae affecting fingertips, toes, and perioral regions is common but tetany is rare. Patients will often report sensory symptoms as unilateral, but on questioning will usually disclose very mild symptoms on the opposite side. Patients often complain of fluid sensations under their scalp or tightly localized, transient headaches which they "can put a finger on." Commonly, anxiety tends to exacerbate existing primary headache disorders such as migraine.

Where anxiety disorders are suspected the key distinction is to separate generalized anxiety, which presents with ruminative worry about a wide range of topics with no consistency or theme, from phobic anxiety, in which anxiety presents in response to a given stimulus.

In patients with functional disorders a phobic component of anxiety may be obscured by misattribution to physical disease. This can follow an agoraphobic pattern.

For example, "attacks" attributed to effort occur on leaving the house: *My heart beats like crazy, my legs turn to jelly, I feel I am going to collapse, I just have to sit down, I can only manage to walk 200 yards before it happens*. Alternatively, the fear may be of a symptom – "bringing on pain" or "falling" both being common. This leads to cycles of decreased activity which can in turn lead to physiologic complications through disuse (see Chapter 10).

As with depression, be careful asking questions about anxiety and panic in patients with functional symptoms – there is a risk they will see you as criticizing them personally or labeling them a hypochondriac. Useful questions include:

> *"Do you often find yourself feeling worried about your symptoms? Do you often feel on edge or tense about things? Do you ever feel like you can't keep a lid on that worry? Do you ever get lots of physical symptoms all at once? Is it frightening when that happens?"*

Occasionally the unexpected *You're getting all these severe leg pains, you've been off work for 6 weeks and yet you are not worried – I would be!* pays dividends.

Many psychologic symptoms require specific questioning to elicit, sometimes because patients are embarrassed by them, sometimes because patients just don't realize they may be relevant or even pathologic, and sometimes because patients fear that a discussion of their psychologic state will detract from a proper physical assessment. The core of a posttraumatic stress state includes intrusive symptoms (such as nightmares and episodes where patients 'relive' traumatic experiences – so-called flashbacks), avoidance (e.g., avoiding driving after a car accident), negative feelings (e.g., feeling empty or having difficulty thinking about the future), and alterations in arousal (e.g., being hypervigilant or excessively "jumpy").

Obsessive compulsive symptoms are also not uncommon in patients with functional disorders but underreported by embarrassed patients. Obsessions are repetitive and intrusive thoughts or images that cause distress which the person tries to suppress. Compulsions are repetitive and excessive behaviors sometimes performed in response to obsessional thoughts which the person recognizes are excessive and which cause distress, take more than an hour a day or interfere with normal functioning, and tend to be underreported by patients who may be embarrassed by them. Full-blown obsessive compulsive disorder does not appear to be particularly common in patients with functional symptoms but by contrast obsessive traits do seem to be common. One can often spot circumlocution whilst taking the history, with a need to fill in every back clause in detail, including lots of extraneous material, without ever really coming to the point.

"Doctor: If I was looking at your cupboards at home, would I find everything was kept neatly in order, each thing with its own place?

Patient: Yes, my wife is always teasing me about it.

Doctor: What if I moved something – could you just leave it or would you be unable to relax until it was back in the proper place?"

It is conceptually helpful to think of pain communication behavior (Waddell et al., 1984) as part of the mental state examination. Pain itself is conceptually difficult (Perl, 2013), but one aspect of the consideration of pain, pain communication behavior, is best considered within the context of consideration of emotions. It is the interactive process between the patient and the clinician that surrounds the communication of pain. In essence the more the pain is communicated via sighing, grimacing, groaning, inappropriate response during examination, and so on, the higher the likelihood of a significant psychogenic component. This is separate from the simple hyperreactivity of pain response that can occur in a pure allodynia which should not be associated with the communicative element of pain but simply a reported response to soft or blunt touch on examination.

Family history, childhood, and recent stress

Functional symptoms are multifactorial in etiology. Genes may play a part (see Chapter 14), so remember to consider a family history from that perspective. Of course, one must be careful in ascribing familial clustering to a genetic cause and in some reports this has been explained by intrafamilial suggestibility and mimicry (Stamelou et al., 2013).

Childhood adverse experiences predispose to functional disorders in adult life. It is however important to remember that, whilst such aversive experiences increase the risk of a functional symptom, a significant proportion of patients, 30–60%, will have had no such experiences, with events such as sexual abuse being rarer still. Additionally, such experiences are unfortunately far from rare in the general population so, whilst they may be one of many relevant etiologic factors, when present they are not diagnostically helpful. Enquiry should be tactful and may be best left for a subsequent occasion if there are signs that it is a "difficult" first encounter. Even treatment of functional symptoms does not need patients to disclose every traumatic and abusive experience – indeed, in many circumstances that may be actively unhelpful.

What a psychiatrist, and sometimes the neurologist, may wish to gain is some general overview of childhood. If the patient discloses, or hints strongly at, significant physical or sexually abusive experiences it is often more helpful to let the patient set the pace of any disclosure rather than to push the issue: *Is that something you would be able to tell me a bit more about or is it something you would prefer to pass over for now?*

More commonly, however, the aversive experiences are milder; questions such as the following will help build a picture.

> *"Did you feel secure and cared for as a child? Did you feel a burden to your parents? Did you get bullied at school? What was the atmosphere like at home? Did your parents argue a lot? Did they ever hit each other? Did either of your parents drink too much?"*

Recent life events and stressors may also be important in some patients but, again, it's important to avoid assumptions. Studies of patients presenting to primary care with functional disorder show that they may volunteer explanations based around stress for their physical symptoms but doctors close down such enquiries too early in a rush to exclude biomedical causes of disease (Ring et al., 2005).

"*Patient: The pain is just kind of all over.*

Doctor And when does it come on?

Patient: It started shortly after my divorce.

Doctor: And are you OK generally, weight steady, no night sweats?"

In patients with functional neurologic disorders presenting to secondary care, however, there is some evidence that they are often less forthcoming. For example, patients with functional disorders are often less likely to attribute their symptoms to stress than patients with disease (Crimlisk et al., 1998; Stone et al., 2010) and will flatly deny any problems in their life even though you sense that they may be distressed by their personal circumstances. This can be difficult to deal with; challenging them usually just makes the patient defensive. Patience is usually the key, so keep a mental note that it is a subject to return to. Conversely, there are patients in whom stress and life events are really not a factor in the development of their symptoms. A recent study that evaluated a series of patients with functional movement disorders with diurnal cortisol levels did not find any difference from controls (Maurer et al., 2015). The take-home message is that it is important not to insist that the patient must be stressed.

Dealing with anger and excessive praise

Dealing with anger can be a problem when assessing patients with functional problems, but if the steps outlined in this chapter are followed, we hope it will be an unusual occurrence. However, no matter how well a consultation is conducted one will be faced with an angry patient on occasions. The first rule in dealing with this is not to get angry yourself. The patient's anger is often a sense of frustration secondary to a feeling that he or she is not being understood. It is important to remember that this may not be the result of your consultation but a legacy of previous contacts or other factors within the patient. Depending on the level of anger shown, acknowledging this either indirectly or, if required, directly is usually a helpful starting point.

> *"It can be very frustrating living with these symptoms every day – do you feel that we as doctors really understand how difficult it is?*
>
> *I am sorry, I am obviously frustrating you, I didn't mean to. What is it that you really want me to understand most?"*

The problems however may not be secondary to the patient's symptoms but secondary to some other problem. It may not be something you are able to help with but simply feeling you have understood the difficulty can often diffuse matters for the patient.

Try to understand what the patient thinks you are doing or thinking. This can often be done by summarizing the symptoms so far, and emphasizing the associated disability as you go – some of the technical information we wish to gather as clinicians to make a diagnosis can seem rather irrelevant to the patient – and asking, *Am I getting it right so far?*

Patients' anger can often relate to erroneous beliefs or fears. This may be about things you have never thought of or considered; try to understand what they are.

A proportion of patients who have had functional symptoms have suffered highly aversive and abusive experiences throughout their lives and have as a result distorted styles of attachment. Attachment style describes the way in which someone habitually approaches interpersonal relationships. Try to remember that experience has taught the patient that even if a person is nice today s/he may well horrendously assault the patient tomorrow. Trust is a commodity in scant supply – don't take it personally. Equally, remember the same processes can lead to overly idolizing attachments after minimal contact. It may be that you are *the best doctor ever* and *the only one who cares and understands*, but whilst such comments are always pleasing for the ego, they may relate more to an abnormal attachment style on the patient's part rather than your own brilliance. That doesn't mean one cannot politely accept a compliment but equally be careful if the consultation becomes overly familiar of if you are invited into conspiratorial conversations about the skills of a colleague, for example.

Sometimes patients become angry because they detect hostility, boredom, or anger in the clinician. There are several reasons why clinicians find patients with functional disorders difficult to help. These include the complex mixture of multiple problems, lack of training, lack of time, concerns about exaggeration (see below) and negative attitudes that clinicians often bring to the consultation (see Chapter 44). There are probably others, though, which are more on the patient's side of the equation. These include the presentation of distress and apparent request to help correct not just a neurologic symptom, but a whole set of symptoms and life circumstances. In addition some patients, most definitely the minority, appear to have a reduced sense of awareness of the time constraints of the clinic, reduced ability to take turns during conversations, and such a compulsive need to describe their problems at great length that they unwittingly reduce the time available to receive the help they crave. The clinician making the assessment should not be critical of the patient in this situation. The reasons for this behavior may relate again to attachment styles discussed earlier. The clinician can however strive to help direct the consultation so that the patient does feel listened to but still keep time to explain the diagnosis and move forward with treatment. And, as a final rule, don't get angry!

Exaggeration

During assessment, especially during the examination, the clinician may become aware of behavior that appears exaggerated. It is worth considering the various explanations for this, only one of which is that the patient is deliberately exaggerating.

An example of verbal exaggeration may be that the patient may report pain as 11 out of 10 in severity, even when you suggest that 10 out of 10 would be the worst pain imaginable, but is able to converse normally during the assessment. Putting a numeric value on an abstract sensation like pain is hard for anyone, but especially when measured against someone else's experience. The phrase "11 out of 10" should usually just be interpreted as meaning "it's really bad," although, paradoxically, these apparent verbal exaggerations often lead to clinicians devaluing the patient's complaints.

For some patients the more dismissive the clinician appears, the more likely they are to have pain communication behavior in a misguided, and usually nonwillful response to convince the clinician that there really is a problem. Again, paradoxically, this may make the clinician even more dismissive and the outcome is poor for both parties. One helpful question to ask yourself when you see something that any layperson would regard as exaggeration is 'is it "exaggeration to convince" or "exaggeration to deceive."?' Something similar has been described in functional gait disorder as the "huffing and puffing sign," where a gait is associated with signs of effort (Laub et al., 2015). A blinded study of video material concluded that 44% of 131 patients had at least mild signs of this whereas none of the 37 neurologic controls did.

The diagnosis of functional motor disorders is usually made on the basis of internal inconsistency. Most of the diagnostic maneuvers, for example, Hoover's sign or tremor entrainment, rely on the principle that the more the patient thinks about the movement, the worse it gets. Therefore, if a patient's gait is much worse during formal examination than it was when he walked in to the room, this is really just in keeping with a functional disorder relating to an abnormal attentional state and is not clearcut evidence of willful exaggeration, however much it may look like it. Clinicians should not be naïve either, but exaggeration can only be recorded with more confidence if there is a marked discrepancy between recorded and observed function. Even this can be problematic. A study of actigraphy in functional tremor showed that even patients who know they are being monitored are hopeless at guessing how bad their symptoms are. In this study, the 10 patients with functional tremor thought, on average, that their symptoms were present 83% of the time when in fact they were only present 4% of the time (compared to 58% reported vs. 24% observed in organic tremor) (Pareés et al., 2012). Factitious disorders and malingering are discussed in more depth in Chapter 42.

Mental state examination

The mental state examination in patients with functional symptoms is often relatively uninformative compared to gaining an understanding of the patient's illness beliefs and behaviors. Only in a minority of patients does the traditional picture of anxiety or depression presenting with physical symptoms apply. A significant proportion of patients will have relatively normal mental states on examination. Perhaps the single most important feature to be aware of is that this is perfectly compatible with a diagnosis of a functional disorder.

The most commonly encountered abnormal mental state is of a largely anxiety-driven hyperarousal accompanied by a slightly obsessive speech structure, anxiously driven, unfocused, and so full of subclauses that it is difficult to control the interview and "separate the wood from the trees." The patient is often in an egocentric state and relatively oblivious to normal social cues from the doctor (Stone and Carson, 2015a). There is a hypervigilance, often directed to perceived verbal slights surrounding the reality of the symptoms. This is often accompanied by an attentional bias towards the affected body area that shows itself by repeated checking and monitoring behavior, as well as eye gaze deviation. This can often change quite dramatically into a friendly and appreciative state if the consultation has gone well and, on occasion, anger if it has not.

The true anhedonic state of significant depressive illness, which is of emptiness rather than emotional upset, is, by contrast, relatively rare but is occasionally encountered in cases of depression presenting predominantly with physical symptoms. Here there is a monotonous, monosyllabic speech with little in the way of elaboration of answers. Eyes are cast downward, and the whole interview feels slow and lugubrious.

Pure "somatized" anxiety as opposed to anxiety comorbid to a functional disorder usually shows itself as a general health anxiety or a nonlocalized physical symptom but also tends to be accompanied by a lack of selective attentional bias to a specific body area.

Pseudohallucinations in which the patient recognizes the false sensory experience comes from her own mind are occasionally encountered along with occasional pareidolic phenomena (the seeing of clear illusory image when gazing at an ill-defined stimulus which intensifies with attention, e.g., seeing a face in a cloud), especially in patients with borderline/emotionally unstable personality types, but true hallucinosis with associated searching behavior, such as seeking the source of the voice or vision, are very rare indeed and should be a red flag for misdiagnosis.

Patients with functional symptoms often show high levels of selective attention, albeit towards their own bodies. A display of poor selective attention such as being distracted by every extraneous noise should suggest some alternate diagnosis.

Patients will often describe disruption of concentration and memory. The features of this are described in detail in Chapter 35 on functional cognitive disorders.

La belle indifférence

La belle indifférence (smiling indifference to disability) has appeared as a key diagnostic feature of conversion disorder for over a century and originated in the works of Freud and Janet. It epitomizes the "hydraulic" theory of conversion in which intrapsychic distress from a conflict is converted into a physical symptom, thus reducing distress, so-called primary gain. It is a difficult clinical sign to quantify and therefore study. However, data from 11 studies found that *la belle indifférence* occurs in a similar frequency in patients with functional disorders as those with neurologic disease (21% vs. 29%) (Fig. 15.4). There is also a differential diagnosis of indifference which the clinician should consider. The patient may just happen to have a stoic attitude to disability, whether caused by disease or not. Others are good at putting a "brave face" on for a clinician. Sometimes, perhaps especially in patients with functional disorders, this tendency is amplified by an awareness that the clinician is angling to find a psychiatric disorder. This perhaps is the commonest scenario in functional disorders in our experience. When the patient has a factitious disorder, this may be associated with indifference for obvious reasons. Neurologic diseases affecting frontal/executive function are particularly likely to lead to apathetic or indifferent states. One patient referred to us (JS) thought to have typical *la belle indifférence* turned out to have Wilson's disease. Finally, there are some patients who even on further assessment may be said to have true "indifference," but our own experience is that this is rare (Stone et al., 2006).

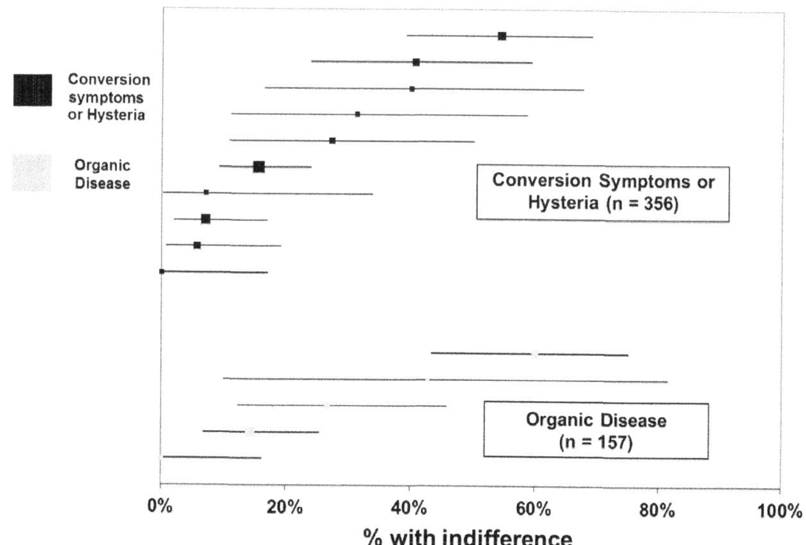

Fig. 15.4. Frequency of *la belle indifférence*. Each point represents an individual study, the size of the point represents the number of patients in the study, and the associated lines are 95% binomial confidence intervals. (From Stone et al., 2006 with permission from the Royal College of Psychiatrists.)

PHYSICAL EXAMINATION

The use of the physical examination, so essential to making a diagnosis of functional neurologic disorder, is discussed in each individual chapter in this book. Some common diagnostic pitfalls in relation to dissociative (nonepileptic) seizures and functional motor disorders are discussed below. Articles summarizing these physical signs are also available (Stone, 2009; Stone and Carson, 2015b). One aspect we would highlight here though is that we recommend explaining the features of particular positive signs during or at the end of the examination rather than keeping them as secrets (see Chapter 44).

PRINCIPLES OF DIAGNOSIS AND DIAGNOSTIC PITFALLS

Reaching a diagnosis

The guiding principle of diagnosis of most functional symptoms is that there should be inconsistency during the physical examination (so-called internal inconsistency) or incongruity with recognized neurologic disease. That is, there should be positive signs. Like much of neurology, there are gray areas, and patients for whom there is considerable diagnostic uncertainty. Clinicians perhaps tend to have a feeling that the important thing is not to diagnose a functional disorder and have it later transpire that there was an underlying disease explanation. However, if the consultation has been conducted in a collaborative fashion we generally find that patients are accepting of this. By contrast, clinicians seem to seldom worry about mislabeling functional symptoms as a neurologic disease, although in our experience this can often be more damaging and can lead to very difficult consultations when one tries to correct it (Coebergh et al., 2014).

Eight shades of diagnostic change

Even when the diagnosis does appear to change over time, it is rarely as simple as *I thought it was functional, but actually it is multiple sclerosis*. There are different kinds of diagnostic change with different degrees of error. As well as the best-known type of misdiagnosis – when you look back and think, *I got that wrong* – there are other types of change that could be construed as error when in fact they aren't (Table 15.4).

For example, someone presenting with functional hemiparesis who later goes on to develop motor neurone disease, may genuinely have had a functional hemiparesis; it's just that you didn't detect (and weren't able to detect) the comorbid neurologic disease predisposing to it at the time. Alternatively, a patient presenting with a functional movement disorder may 1 year later have a stroke, but it still doesn't account for the functional movement disorder. Diagnostic disagreements and patients where the diagnosis of functional symptoms is initially in the differential but then drops out also form part of the list of ways in which diagnoses may change over time without there necessarily being a "howler."

Diagnostic pitfalls – general considerations

Table 15.5 lists some factors that we often come across in patients who have been erroneously labeled as having a disease when they actually have a functional disorder, and vice versa.

"This patient is anxious/recently stressed/has a personality disorder," so must have functional symptoms

Probably the commonest source of diagnostic error is when the clinician pays too much attention to the patient's psychosocial history and not enough to the presenting symptom. A generation and more of doctors have been taught via psychiatric diagnostic criteria that functional neurologic symptoms are a form of conversion disorder and as such represent the conversion of recent stress into a physical symptom. As discussed earlier, recent and remote adverse experience as well as comorbid psychiatric disorder (such as anxiety, panic, and depression) and maladaptive personality traits (such as avoidant or borderline personality traits) are more common in patients with functional neurologic disorders in most studies. However, many patients with functional symptoms are psychiatrically normal and around a third of patients with defined neurologic disease have comorbid psychiatric symptoms.

The upshot of this is that it's dangerous to base your diagnosis on the psychosocial history, however tempting the narrative may appear. Just as you wouldn't make a diagnosis of stroke because someone smokes and has high blood pressure, these features should be regarded as supporting risk factors but not diagnostic in their own right. Be particularly careful of the patient who thinks the symptoms are stress-related, as patients with disease are more likely to present with psychosocial attributions than patients with functional symptoms (Stone et al., 2010).

"The patient is too normal/nice/stoic/male/young/old/intelligent/muchlike me," so must have a neurologic disease

The converse and quite common pitfall we have observed is the patient with functional symptoms who has the misfortune to share the same social and demographic features of the doctor attempting to make the

Table 15.4

Change in diagnosis doesn't necessarily mean you got it wrong first time round

Type of diagnostic revision	Example	Degree of clinician error
Diagnostic error	Patient presented with symptoms that were plausibly all due to multiple sclerosis but was diagnosed with functional symptoms. The diagnosis of multiple sclerosis had not been considered and was unexpected at follow-up	Major
Differential diagnostic change	Patient presented with multiple symptoms. Doctor suggested chronic fatigue syndrome as most likely but considered multiple sclerosis as a possible diagnosis. Appropriate investigations and follow-up confirmed multiple sclerosis	None to minor
Diagnostic refinement	Doctor diagnosed epilepsy but at follow-up the diagnosis is refined to juvenile myoclonic epilepsy	Minor
Comorbid diagnostic change	Doctor correctly identified the presence of both epilepsy and nonepileptic seizures in the same patient. At follow-up, one of the disorders has remitted	None
Prodromal diagnostic change	Patient presented with an anxiety state. At 1-year follow-up the patient has developed Alzheimer's disease. With hindsight, anxiety was a prodromal symptom of dementia but the diagnosis could not have been made at the initial assessment as the dementia symptoms (or findings on examination or investigation) had not developed sufficiently	None
De novo development of organic disease	Patient is correctly diagnosed with chronic fatigue syndrome. During the period of follow-up, the patient develops subarachnoid hemorrhage as a completely new and unrelated condition	None
Disagreement between doctors, without new information at follow-up	Patient is diagnosed at baseline with chronic fatigue syndrome and at follow-up with chronic Lyme disease by a different doctor even though there is no new information. However, if the two doctors had both met the patient at follow-up, they would still have arrived at the different diagnoses. This would be reflected in similar divided opinion among their peers	None
Disagreement between doctors, with new information at follow-up	Patient is diagnosed at baseline with chronic fatigue syndrome and at follow-up with fatigue due to a Chiari malformation by a different doctor because of new information at follow-up (in this case a magnetic resonance imaging scan ordered at the time of the first appointment). However, the first doctor seeing the patient again at follow-up continues to diagnose chronic fatigue syndrome, believing the Chiari malformation to be an incidental finding. This would be reflected in divided opinion among their peers	None

Adapted from Stone et al. (2009b) with permission from the Guarantors of Brain.

diagnosis. In line with the discussion above, middle-aged males, people who are "normal," "nice," or "seem genuine enough" can all develop functional symptoms, even dramatic ones (Carson et al., 2011). Studies on older patients with dissociative (nonepileptic) attacks show that they have an equal gender ratio and often suffer from potentially life-threatening disease (such as ischemic heart disease or severe asthma), triggering health anxiety which links to the attacks themselves (Duncan et al., 2006).

"I've made a diagnosis; there is no need for another one": the problem of comorbidity

The presence of any disease, however small, tends to "trump" the presence of functional symptoms. But the reality is that the experience of bodily dysfunction caused by neurologic disease is one of the most powerful risk factors for developing functional symptoms. Many patients have two diagnoses, for example: epilepsy and dissociative (nonepileptic) attacks; multiple sclerosis and functional limb weakness; idiopathic intracranial

Table 15.5

Functional disorders in neurology; general factors relevant to diagnostic error

Features of neurologic disease presentations that can lead erroneously to a diagnosis of a functional disorder	Diagnostic clues/how to avoid error
The presence of psychiatric disorder, especially personality disorder	Detecting psychiatric comorbidity may be useful in treating the patient but should be ignored in making the diagnosis. Focus on the nature of the attack / the physical examination. Are the physical features typical of functional symptoms?
Presence of schizophrenia or other psychotic illness	Such patients seldom have functional symptoms
The patient's presenting complaint is of new-onset mood or behavioral disturbance.	Patients with functional symptoms rarely complain of significant psychiatric or behavioral symptoms, e.g., panic, as their primary subjective complaint, even if it is clearly present
The presence of an obvious life event or stressor	Ignore the presence of recent stress in making the diagnosis even if this may be relevant for treatment
Failure to consider that the patient may have a functional disorder and a neurologic disease	Remember that neurologic disease is one of the most powerful risk factors for developing a functional disorder (e.g., epilepsy/dissociative (nonepileptic) attacks, MS/functional limb weakness)
Failure to consider that the patient may have functional disorder and a progressive neurologic disease which may be too early for you to diagnose (yet)	As above, but in some cases, especially where neuroimaging doesn't help, the disease may only become apparent on follow-up (e.g. motor neurone disease, Wilson's disease, Alzheimer's, myopathy)
La belle indifférence – apparent indifference to disability	This concept is wedded to conversion disorder and is of no diagnostic value, apparently occurring as frequently in neurologic disease, especially with frontal-lobe involvement (Stone et al., 2006)
Normal neuroimaging	Many neurologic diseases, e.g., epilepsy, amyotrophic lateral sclerosis, myopathy, spinocerebellar ataxia, have normal CNS imaging. Don't rely on it alone to exclude disease
Features of patients with functional symptoms that can wrongly put you off the diagnosis	
The patient is normal/nice/stoic/like me	Normal people get functional disorders too
The patient has no "form," i.e., previous functional symptoms	Patients can present with dramatic neurologic functional symptoms with no prior history
The patient has not been stressed	Between 1 in 3 and 1 in 4 patients have no evidence of recent stress
The patient is not tired/only has one symptom	Lack of fatigue or other symptoms should make you think twice about a diagnosis of functional symptoms but monosymptomatic presentations do occur
The symptoms came on after injury, minor pathologic disease	Commonplace in functional symptoms (Stone et al., 2012).
The patient suggests a psychologic causation	Around 1 in 4 patients with functional symptoms do think that psychologic factors are relevant
The patient has an established diagnosis of "known epilepsy, "known MS"	Always question other people's diagnoses (and your own!)
The patient is too old	Older patients with functional symptoms often have heath anxiety and comorbid disease (Duncan et al., 2006)
Incidental abnormalities on MRI (e.g. enlarged perivascular space, Chiari malformation, disc protrusion), EEG, serology, or other tests	Don't assume that all structural abnormalities are relevant

MS, multiple sclerosis; CNS, central nervous system; MRI, magnetic resonance imaging; EEG, electroencephalogram.

hypertension and functional visual symptoms. It is easy for the presence of disease to obscure the presence of functional symptoms. Conversely, recognizing the functional symptom diagnosis can assist in the patient's treatment as it will often have more potential for reversibility than the underlying disease. In our own Scottish study of 2467 outpatients with neurologic disease, around 12% also had a diagnosis of a functional symptom. In these 12% of patients, no one disease category was more common than another. In other words, patients with, for example, multiple sclerosis or Parkinson's disease do not appear to be more prone to functional symptoms than people with epilepsy or muscle disease (Stone et al., 2012).

Comorbidity can present concurrently; for example, a patient who presents acutely with a mild episode of demyelination in which the clinical features of the weakness are predominantly functional. Or functional symptoms can develop as a later complication of neurologic disease, with health anxiety often having a key etiologic role.

More problematically, some patients, especially those with degenerative and slowly progressive conditions, may present with functional symptoms years before the clear onset of their neurologic disease. In some cases, a definite functional diagnosis such as functional paralysis can present as part of the commonly encountered "psychiatric prodrome" in dementias. In others, it appears as if the experience of having a very mild ataxia, for example, in the very early stages of spinocerebellar ataxia, is enough to trigger the functional symptom. This has also been demonstrated for Parkinson's disease (Onofrj et al., 2010).

So always look for comorbid disease, even if the diagnosis of functional symptoms is clearcut, and make two diagnoses if necessary. If there is no disease consider whether there are features that deserve longer-term follow-up that might indicate the patient is in the early stage of a slowly progressive disease. Finally, accept that you will sometimes get it wrong or fail to anticipate the development of a disease, however careful you are. Studies of functional symptoms from the 1970s onwards coalesce around frequencies of misdiagnosis of about 5% after 5 years (Stone et al., 2005). This is the same rate of misdiagnosis for most neurologic and psychiatric disorders, and probably at least as common as misdiagnosis of functional symptoms as disease.

Overreliance on and poor interpretation of neuroimaging

There is a tendency among many physicians to forget that normal neuroimaging does not exclude neurologic disease. That list is very long indeed and includes amyotrophic lateral sclerosis, Parkinson's disease, epilepsy, and migraine.

Conversely, imaging frequently throws up incidental abnormalities which are of no relevance to the presentation. Many patients with functional disorders suffer iatrogenic damage from the failure of health professionals to place the results of spinal or brain imaging in the correct context.

As a general rule of thumb, your chance of seeing an incidental structural abnormality like a cavernoma or arachnoid cyst on neuroimaging is around 1 in 37 – the same as a roulette wheel. The chance of seeing any kind of "abnormality" such as white dot is around 1 in 6 for a 40-year-old – this time, Russian roulette (Morris et al., 2009).

For spinal magnetic resonance imaging, the frequency of disc degeneration, signal loss, and bulge is around 10% greater than numeric age in years. The frequency of disc protrusion is 30% by age 20 and climbs to 45% by age 80 (Brinjikji et al., 2014).

Diagnostic pitfalls in dissociative (nonepileptic) attacks

Several features can lead to confusion, both in terms of mistakenly calling attacks nonepileptic when they aren't (Smith, 2012), or missing the diagnosis of dissociative (nonepileptic) attacks (Table 15.6).

The diagnosis of dissociative attacks should be made on the basis of objective signs, such as eyes closed, resistance to eye opening, ictal or postictal weeping, and prolonged attacks (Avbersek and Sisodiya, 2010). The problem is that the evidence for many of these signs comes from videotelemetry studies and, in the real world, witnesses, including medical ones, can be very unreliable. For example, reports of eye closure from witnesses may be close to useless when compared with video-electroencephalogram evidence (Syed et al., 2008). Therefore the patient's subjective seizure experience is also important in giving additional clues. Simple questions such as whether the patient "remembers the shaking" can be helpful (Avbersek and Sisodiya, 2010) but there is also evidence that there are conversational features of seizure description typical of dissociative attacks, including reluctance to describe symptoms or giving a poorly detailed description (Plug and Reuber, 2009).

Frontal-lobe seizures can be associated with retained awareness or pelvic movements that can lead to assumptions that the patient may be "acting out" abuse (Geyer et al., 2000). It is particularly important to remember that in temporal-lobe epilepsy there can be quite a long prodrome lasting minutes in which the patient may have fear and dissociative symptoms similar to a patient having a dissociative (nonepileptic) attack (Goldstein and

Table 15.6

Dissociative (nonepileptic) attacks: mimics and chameleons

Feature of epilepsy and other neurologic disorders that can look like dissociative (nonepileptic) attacks	Diagnostic clues/how to avoid error
Generalized tonic-clonic seizure	Include: ictal guttural cry (not weeping) typically at onset, stertorous breathing, eyes open
Frontal-lobe seizures	Short duration (less than 30 seconds) Retained awareness during seizures Shouting, truncal, or cycling leg movements Onset often/mostly from sleep
Temporal-lobe seizures with ictal fear	Progression to generalized seizure. Structural cause. Many temporal-lobe features (e.g., olfactory hallucinations, macropsia) can appear in a dissociative nonepileptic attack
Self-induced epilepsy	Some patients with epilepsy can induce their own seizures, or may manipulate their medication to do so
Autoimmune limbic encephalitis (e.g., NMDA, anti-VGKC)	Patient may present with psychiatric symptoms, unusual behavior, and focal seizures
Stress-induced seizures or syncope	Some epileptic seizures and cardiac syncope (e.g., long QT-related) can be triggered by emotional stress
Features of dissociative (nonepileptic) attacks that can wrongly put you off the diagnosis	
Olfactory hallucinations	Reports of "burning rubber"/"feces"/"chemical smell" appear quite commonly in dissociative attacks
Dissociative experiences	Depersonalization, visual and perceptual changes in dissociative attacks can sound like temporal-lobe epilepsy
Eyes open	Although "eyes closed" is a good clue, some patients with dissociative attacks do open their eyes (with rolling) during attacks
Cyanosis/breath holding	Including low oxygen saturations
Injury	Bitten tongue (sometimes visibly), broken teeth, (recurrent) shoulder dislocation, and falls on stairs all occur in dissociative attacks. Reports of injury may be more common than actual injury
Incontinence	Urinary incontinence is common and fecal incontinence does happen in dissociative attacks
Seizures arising from sleep/when alone	Occurs in dissociative attacks
Response to trial of anticonvulsants/relapse of attacks when anticonvulsants withdrawn	Patients with dissociative attacks may experience both strong placebo effect when anticonvulsants are started and nocebo effect when they are stopped
The patient in ITU who several nonneurologist physicians and anesthetists are convinced is in status	Prolonged events are a risk factor for dissociative (nonepileptic) attacks. Up to 50% of patients attending hospital in apparent status have this diagnosis

NMDA, *N*-methyl-D-aspartate; VGKC, voltage-gated potassium channel; ITU, intensive therapy unit.

Mellers, 2006). Although ictal fear is usually distinguishable from a panic attack by the shorter duration, associated temporal-lobe features, and impaired awareness (Beyenburg et al., 2005), this is not such an easy distinction to make with dissociative nonepileptic attacks, which may have all of these features.

Features of dissociative attacks can easily put clinicians off the diagnosis, such as injury (Peguero et al., 1995) (and especially report of injury), olfactory hallucinations, and going blue.

In clinical practice it is not always possible to be sure what a patient's attack disorder is due to, even with all this information. For this reason, the careful neurologist strikes a balance between making confident diagnoses where possible, but saying "not sure" where appropriate. In any patient it is important not to completely close the book on the diagnosis, checking seizure descriptions each visit and watching out for the combination of both epilepsy and dissociative (nonepileptic) attacks.

Diagnostic pitfalls in functional motor disorders

The diagnosis of functional motor disorder should always be based on positive evidence on the examination of internal inconsistency (e.g., Hoover's sign for paralysis or a tremor that stops or entrains during contralateral cued rhythmic movement) (Stone, 2009). However, there can be difficulties in overinterpretation of these positive signs and it would be unreasonable to expect them to always perform, especially in isolation. The presence of pain in a limb, inattention or neglect, or simple failure to understand the examiner's instructions are all reasons why these signs may be false positive.

As with epilepsy, things that look bizarre, like stiff-person syndrome or generalized dystonia, particularly if they are inherently somewhat variable, can fool the unwary into a diagnosis of functional symptoms. The list in Table 15.7 is obviously not comprehensive. Orthostatic tremor (a movement disorder only present on standing), alien-limb phenomena in corticobasal degeneration, and the aura of paroxysmal kinesogenic dyskinesia are just some of the reasons why the diagnosis of functional neurologic disorders should usually be made by a neurologist familiar with the breadth of unusual presentation neurologic disease has to offer.

Conversely, in patients who do have functional disorder there can be surprising findings in some patients. Just as reflexes can be brisk in patients who are anxious, we have seen patients with unilaterally increased reflexes as a transient phenomenon. Such reflex asymmetry was well reported in the older literature (Allen, 1935). Occasionally patients with unilateral motor symptoms also develop something that looks very similar to ankle

Table 15.7

Diagnostic pitfalls in functional motor disorders

Neurologic diseases that can look like functional motor disorders	Diagnostic clues/how to avoid error
Higher cortical gait disturbance/bizarre gait	Don't rely on an odd gait to make the diagnosis
Acute parietal stroke/pathology	May have Hoover's sign/MRI brain
Stiff-person syndrome	Anti-GAD antibodies
Dystonia (*geste antagoniste*, better walking backwards or running)	Familiarity with clinical presentation of organic movement disorders
Myasthenia (variability, give-way weakness)	Avoid diagnostic weight on Tensilon tests, which can be false positive (even when blinded) in patients with chronic fatigue syndrome. Strong placebo response to steroids may also occur in patients with functional symptoms
Pain with weakness in limbs	Place less reliability on positive signs of functional weakness in presence of pain. Ask patient if s/he thinks pain is the reason the limb is weak
Paroxysmal dyskinesia, especially with aura and urge to move	Familiarity with clinical presentation of organic movement disorders
Tics/Tourette's	Ability to suppress with rebound movements (may be distractible)
Features of functional motor disorders that can wrongly put you off the diagnosis	
Variable ankle clonus	Happens
Facial symptoms	Common
Slightly asymmetric reflexes/mute plantar	Happens
Contractures in fixed dystonia	Happens
Migraine at onset	Separate trigger from current cause
Tremor unaffected by distraction	In chronic functional tremor motor distraction tasks sometimes no longer visibly affect the tremor. Tremor analysis or video recording may be helpful
Urinary retention	Appears to be quite common in patients with acute back pain and leg weakness in the absence of structural changes. Also occurs with opiate use (Hoeritzauer et al., 2015)
Axial propriospinal myoclonus	Usually functional (van der Salm et al., 2014)
Convergent spasm leading to apparent sixth-nerve palsy	Look for variability over the assessment or resolution with a more distant target

MRI, magnetic resonance imaging; GAD, glutamic acid decarboxylase.

clonus but is variable between assessments. It is not unusual for plantar responses to be mute on the same side as functional hemisensory loss.

Facial symptoms, typically with contraction of orbicularis oculis, oris, and platysma, and sometimes with jaw deviation are clinically quite common. They were well described in the older literature and have recently been described again in more detail (Fasano et al., 2012). Since these facial symptoms lead to an appearance of weakness (even though they are due to muscle overactivity), this can result in erroneous diagnosis of stroke if the presentation is acute.

Slightly better known, although still missed commonly, is the phenomenon of convergence spasm which is relatively common in patients with functional motor symptoms (Fekete et al., 2012). You can usually bring this out by asking the patient to converge on a near target for 10 seconds. In convergent spasm the convergence persists long enough to produce the appearance of impaired abduction, which can be mistaken for a sixth-nerve palsy. One way round this is to go back and test eye movements without convergence and using a more distant target at a different point in the assessment or just observe eye movement during the consultation to show the inconsistency.

Contractures can cause concern about a diagnosis of functional or fixed dystonia, but these do occur in patients who have been immobile for a long time, albeit they are rare and should at least prompt some reconsideration of the diagnosis. They can be demonstrated under anesthesia.

CONCLUSION

The assessment of patients with functional symptoms can be viewed as difficult, but we believe that, with an appropriate structure and technique, such consultations can be conducted in a much more collaborative fashion that is much more satisfactory for both doctor and patient.

Attention paid to all the physical symptoms in the presentation, exploration of illness beliefs, and a potential mechanism of onset can all pay dividends at the time of explanation (discussed separately in Chapter 44). The assessment of comorbid psychologic symptoms is not essential for diagnosis at the first assessment and is often best done at the patient's own pace. Psychologic comorbidity can lead to diagnostic pitfalls both when present and absent, leading to overdiagnosis and underdiagnosis of functional disorders respectively. The assessment of the neurologic symptoms themselves has many pitfalls, notably in the interpretation of investigations and in remembering that functional disorders and neurologic disease may coexist or the former may precede the latter.

References

Allen IM (1935). Observations on the motor phenomena of hysteria. J Neurol Psychopathol 16: 1–25.

Avbersek A, Sisodiya S (2010). Does the primary literature provide support for clinical signs used to distinguish psychogenic nonepileptic seizures from epileptic seizures? J Neurol Neurosurg Psychiatry 81: 719–725.

Beyenburg S, Mitchell AJ, Schmidt D (2005). Anxiety in patients with epilepsy: systematic review and suggestions for clinical management. Epilepsy Behav 7: 161–171.

Brinjikji W, Luetmer PH, Comstock B et al. (2014). Systematic literature review of imaging features of spinal degeneration in asymptomatic populations. Spine (Phila Pa 1976) 36: 811–816.

Cameron LD, Leventhal H (2003). The Self-Regulation of Health and Illness Behaviour, Routledge, London.

Carson A, Stone J (2013). Considering depression and anxiety. In: C Burton (Ed.), The ABC of Medically Unexplained Symptoms, BMJ Books/John Wiley, Chichester.

Carson AJ, Ringbauer B, Stone J et al. (2000). Do medically unexplained symptoms matter? A study of 300 consecutive new referrals to neurology outpatient clinics. J Neurol Neurosurg Psychiatry 68: 207–210.

Carson AJ, Stone J, Warlow C et al. (2004). What makes a neurologist find a patient difficult to help? J Neurol Neurosurg Psychiatry 75: 1776–1778.

Carson A, Stone J, Hibberd C et al. (2011). Disability, distress and unemployment in neurology outpatients with symptoms 'unexplained by organic disease'. J Neurol Neurosurg Psychiatry 82: 810–813.

Carson AJ, Brown R, David AS et al. (2012). Functional (conversion) neurological symptoms: research since the millennium. J Neurol Neurosurg Psychiatry 83: 842–850.

Carson AJ, Stone J, Hansen CH et al. (2014). Somatic symptom count scores do not identify patients with symptoms unexplained by disease: a prospective cohort study of neurology outpatients. J Neurol Neurosurg Psychiatry 86: 295–301.

Coebergh JA, Wren DR, Mumford CJ (2014). 'Undiagnosing' neurological disease: how to do it, and when not to. Pract Neurol 14: 436–439.

Crimlisk HL, Bhatia K, Cope H et al. (1998). Slater revisited: 6 year follow up study of patients with medically unexplained motor symptoms. BMJ 316 (7131): 582–586.

Duncan R, Oto M, Martin E et al. (2006). Late onset psychogenic nonepileptic attacks. Neurology 66: 1644–1647.

Edwards MJ, Adams RA, Brown H et al. (2012). A Bayesian account of 'hysteria'. Brain 135: 3495–3512.

Fasano A, Valadas A, Bhatia KP et al. (2012). Psychogenic facial movement disorders: clinical features and associated conditions. Mov Disord 27: 1544–1551.

Fekete R, Baizabal-Carvallo JF, Ha AD et al. (2012). Convergence spasm in conversion disorders: prevalence in psychogenic and other movement disorders compared with controls. J Neurol Neurosurg Psychiatry 83: 202–204.

Gask L, Usherwood T (2002). ABC of psychological medicine. The consultation. BMJ (Clinical research ed.) 324: 1567–1569.

Geyer JD, Payne TA, Drury I (2000). The value of pelvic thrusting in the diagnosis of seizures and pseudoseizures. Neurology 54: 227–229.

Goldstein LH, Mellers JD (2006). Ictal symptoms of anxiety, avoidance behaviour, and dissociation in patients with dissociative seizures. J Neurol Neurosurg Psychiatry 77: 616–621.

Healthcare Improvement Scotland (2012) Stepped care for functional neurological symptoms: a new approach to improving outcomes for a common neurological problem in Scotland, QIS Scotland.

Hoeritzauer I, Doherty CM, Thomson S et al. (2015). 'Scan-negative' cauda equina syndrome: evidence of functional disorder from a prospective case series. Br J Neurosurg 29: 178–180.

Holmes EA, Brown RJ, Mansell W et al. (2005). Are there two qualitatively distinct forms of dissociation? A review and some clinical implications. Clin Psychol Rev 25: 1–23.

Hotopf M, Wilson-Jones C, Mayou R et al. (2000). Childhood predictors of adult medically unexplained hospitalisations. Br J Psychiatr 176: 273–280.

Katon W, Sullivan M, Walker E (2001). Medical symptoms without identified pathology: relationship to psychiatric disorders, childhood and adult trauma, and personality traits. Ann Intern Med 134: 917–925.

Kranick S, Ekanayake V, Martinez V et al. (2011). Psychopathology and psychogenic movement disorders. Mov Disord 26: 1844–1850.

Langewitz W, Denz M, Keller A et al. (2002). Spontaneous talking time at start of consultation in outpatient clinic: cohort study. BMJ 325 (7366): 682–683.

Laub HN, Dwivedi AK, Revilla FJ et al. (2015). Diagnostic performance of the 'huffing and puffing' sign in functional (psychogenic) movement disorders. Mov Disord Clin Pract 2: 29–32.

Main CJ, Williams AC de C (2002). Musculoskeletal pain. BMJ : Br Med J 325: 534–537.

Maurer CW, LaFaver K, Ameli R et al. (2015). A biological measure of stress levels in patients with functional movement disorders. Parkinsonism Relat Disord 21: 1072–1075.

Morris Z, Whiteley WN, Longstreth WT et al. (2009). Incidental findings on brain magnetic resonance imaging: systematic review and meta-analysis. BMJ 339: b3016.

Nicholson TR, Aybek S, Craig T et al. (2016). Life events and escape in conversion disorder. Psychol Med 46: 2617–2626.

Onofrj M, Bonanni L, Manzoli L et al. (2010). Cohort study on somatoform disorders in Parkinson disease and dementia with Lewy bodies. Neurology 74: 1598–1606.

Owens DG, Cunningham E, Johnstone C et al. (1982). Spontaneous involuntary disorders of movement: their prevalence, severity, and distribution in chronic schizophrenics with and without treatment with neuroleptics. Arch Gen Psychiatry 39: 452–461.

Pareés I, Saifee TA, Kassavetis P et al. (2012). Believing is perceiving: mismatch between self-report and actigraphy in psychogenic tremor. Brain 135: 117–123.

Peguero E, bou-Khalil B, Fakhoury T et al. (1995). Self-injury and incontinence in psychogenic seizures. Epilepsia 36 (6): 586–591.

Perl ER (2013). Is pain a specific sensation? Principles, Practices, and Positions in Neuropsychiatric Research: Proceedings of a Conference Held in June 1970 at the Walter Reed Army Institute of Research, Washington, DC, in Tribute to Dr. David Mckenzie Rioch upon His Retirement as Director of the Neuropsychiatry Division of That Institute (p. 273), Elsevier.

Plug L, Reuber M (2009). Making the diagnosis in patients with blackouts – it's all in the history. Pract Neurol 9: 4–15.

Ring A, Dowrick CF, Humphris GM et al. (2005). The somatising effect of clinical consultation: what patients and doctors say and do not say when patients present medically unexplained physical symptoms. Soc Sci Med 61: 1505–1515.

Schrag A, Brown RJ, Trimble MR (2004a). Reliability of self-reported diagnoses in patients with neurologically unexplained symptoms. J Neurol Neurosurg Psychiatry 75: 608–611.

Schrag A, Trimble M, Quinn N et al. (2004b). The syndrome of fixed dystonia: an evaluation of 103 patients. Brain 127: 2360–2372.

Sharpe M, Stone J, Hibberd C et al. (2010). Neurology out-patients with symptoms unexplained by 'organic' disease in neurology outpatients: illness beliefs and financial benefits predict outcome. Psychol Med 40: 689–698.

Smith PE (2012). Epilepsy: mimics, borderland and chameleons. Pract Neurol 12: 299–307.

Stamelou M, Cossu G, Edwards MJ et al. (2013). Familial psychogenic movement disorders: Mov Disord 9. 1295–1298.

Stone J (2006). Dissociation: what is it and why is it important? Pract Neurol 6: 308–313.

Stone J (2009). The bare essentials: Functional symptoms in neurology. Pract Neurol 9: 179–189.

Stone J (2014). Functional neurological disorders: the neurological assessment as treatment. Neurophysiologie Clinique/Clinical Neurophysiology 44 (4): 363–373.

Stone J, Carson A (2015a). The 'cup of tea' sign in severe functional disorders. Cortex 64: 425.

Stone J, Carson A (2015b). Functional neurologic disorders. Continuum (N Y) 21: 818–837.

Stone J, Reuber M, Carson A (2013). Functional symptoms in neurology: mimics and chameleons. Pract Neurol 13 (2): 104–113.

Stone J, Smyth R, Carson A et al. (2005). Systematic review of misdiagnosis of conversion symptoms and "hysteria". BMJ 331 (7523): 989.

Stone J, Smyth R, Carson A et al. (2006). *La belle indifférence* in conversion symptoms and hysteria: systematic review. Br J Psychiatry 188: 204–209.

Stone J, Carson A, Aditya H et al. (2009a). The role of physical injury in motor and sensory conversion symptoms: a systematic and narrative review. J Psychosom Res 66: 383–390.

Stone J, Carson A, Duncan R et al. (2009b). Symptoms 'unexplained by organic disease' in 1144 new neurology out-patients: how often does the diagnosis change at follow-up? Brain 132: 2878–2888.

Stone J, Warlow C, Sharpe M (2010). The symptom of functional weakness: a controlled study of 107 patients. Brain 133: 1537–1551.

Stone J, Carson A, Duncan R et al. (2012). Which neurological diseases are most likely to be associated with "symptoms unexplained by organic disease"? J Neurol 259: 33–38.

Syed TU, Arozullah AM, Suciu GP et al. (2008). Do observer and self-reports of ictal eye closure predict psychogenic nonepileptic seizures? Epilepsia 49: 898–904.

van der Salm SM, Erro R, Cordivari C et al. (2014). Propriospinal myoclonus: clinical reappraisal and review of literature. Neurology 83: 1862–1870.

Waddell G, Main CJ, Morris EW et al. (1984). Chronic low-back pain, psychologic distress, and illness behavior. Spine 9 (2): 209–213.

Handbook of Clinical Neurology, Vol. 139 (3rd series)
Functional Neurologic Disorders
M. Hallett, J. Stone, and A. Carson, Editors
http://dx.doi.org/10.1016/B978-0-12-801772-2.00016-3

Chapter 16

The classification of conversion disorder (functional neurologic symptom disorder) in ICD and DSM

J.L. LEVENSON[1]* AND M. SHARPE[2]

[1]*Department of Psychiatry, Virginia Commonwealth University School of Medicine, Richmond, VA, USA*

[2]*Department of Psychiatry, University of Oxford, Oxford, UK*

Abstract

The name given to functional neurologic symptoms has evolved over time in the different editions of the *International Classification of Diseases* (ICD) and the *Diagnostic and Statistical Manual of Mental Disorders* (DSM), reflecting a gradual move away from an etiologic conception rooted in hysterical conversion to an empiric phenomenologic one, emphasizing the central role of the neurologic examination and testing in demonstrating that the symptoms are incompatible with recognized neurologic disease pathophysiology, or are internally inconsistent.

INTRODUCTION

Psychogenic neurologic symptoms were initially considered a form of hysteria, carrying forward a term from the ancient Greek concept that the symptoms were due to a wandering uterus. The term conversion itself expressed Sigmund Freud's theory that unconscious conflicts became converted into neurologic symptoms. Such symptoms were also conceptualized as one form of dissociation, reflecting Pierre Janet's theory. The name given to this disorder, and how it is classified, has evolved over the different editions of the *International Classification of Diseases* (ICD) and the *Diagnostic and Statistical Manual of Mental Disorders* (DSM), reflecting the move away from an etiologic conception of conversion to an empiric phenomenologic one. In formal diagnostic classifications, "conversion disorder" was first known by that exact term in DSM-III (published in 1980: American Psychiatric Association, 1980) and in a later versions of ICD-9 (ICD-9-CM: World Health Organization, 1979).

CONVERSION DISORDER IN THE *INTERNATIONAL CLASSIFICATION OF DISEASES* (ICD)

The *International Classification of Diseases* started out as the *International List of Causes of Death*. It was not until the sixth edition that it became a classification of diseases and injuries. ICD-6 (World Health Organization, 1948) divided psychoneuroses into those "without mention of somatic symptoms" and those "without mention of anxiety reaction." Within the latter category, listed under "hysteria" were a number of hysterical neurologic symptoms, including amnesia, anesthesia, anosmia, aphonia, blindness, convulsions, dyskinesia, mutism, paralysis, postures, tic, and tremor. Also on this list were "conversion" and "hysteroepilepsy," without explanation as to how these related to the other neurologic symptoms. ICD-7 (World Health Organization, 1957) changed terminology to "psychoneurosis with somatic symptoms affecting other systems." The systems designated included respiratory, genitourinary, cutaneous, and musculoskeletal

*Correspondence to: James L. Levenson, M.D., Virginia Commonwealth University School of Medicine, Box 980268, Richmond VA 23298-0268, USA. Tel: +1-804-828-0763, Fax: +1-804-828-7675, E-mail: jlevenson@mcvh-vcu.edu

(which included paralysis). This seems to have been a blurring of the boundary between psychophysiologic disorders and hysterical conversion. The other specific hysterical neurologic symptoms listed in ICD-6 no longer appeared in the classification.

The term "conversion" first appeared in ICD-8 (World Health Organization, 1968) as "conversion hysteria," a subtype of hysterical neurosis. Similarly, ICD-9 (World Health Organization, 1975) listed "conversion hysteria" as a subtype of hysteria. "Conversion disorder" first appeared in a later version, ICD-9-CM (World Health Organization, 1979). Conversion disorder was listed under the category titled "dissociative, conversion and factitious disorders," with subtypes of hysterical astasia-abasia, blindness, deafness, paralysis, and conversion hysteria or reaction. ICD-10 (World Health Organization, 1992) grouped dissociative and conversion disorders together, listing the diagnosis as "dissociative (conversion) disorder." In the current edition of ICD-10 (World Health Organization, 2016), conversion disorder is listed under dissociative and conversion disorders, with subtypes of motor symptom or deficit, seizures or convulsions, and sensory symptom or deficit.

One recent proposal for ICD-11 is to bring conversion back within the primary domain of neurology as functional neurologic disorders within the neurologic section of ICD (Stone et al., 2014). Like other conditions shared between neurologists and psychiatrists (e.g., Tourette syndrome and dementia), psychiatry would retain a code for functional neurologic disorders, ideally matching the one in neurology. The proposal aims to encourage neurologists to take clinical responsibility for these patients, making positive diagnoses rather than by exclusion; incorporate functional disorders into neurologic education; encourage neurologists to engage in related research; and promote collaboration between neurologists and psychiatrists.

CONVERSION DISORDER IN THE DSM, 1952–2000

In 1952, the American Psychiatric Association Committee on Nomenclature and Statistics published a variation of the mental disorder section of ICD-6 as the first edition of DSM (DSM-I) (American Psychiatric Association, 1952). "Conversion reaction" was listed alongside "dissociative reaction" among the "psychoneurotic disorders," which were defined as "disorders of psychogenic origin or without clearly defined tangible cause or structural change." The frequent use of the term "reaction" in DSM-I was a sign of the influence of Adolph Meyer's psychobiology in American psychiatry, with its emphasis on understanding mental illness as a reaction to life stress. Thus, conversion was considered a defense mechanism to cope with overwhelming anxiety generated by internal or external stressors.

In DSM-II (American Psychiatric Association, 1968), conversion was classified as "hysterical neurosis, conversion type," with the other hysterical neurosis being dissociative type. Hysterical neuroses were characterized by an involuntary psychogenic loss or disorder of function typically occurring in emotionally charged situations, and symbolic of the (presumed) underlying conflicts. Examples given of sensory or voluntary nervous system symptoms included blindness, deafness, anosmia, anesthesias, paresthesias, paralyses, ataxias, akinesias, and dyskinesias. The frequent presence of *la belle indifférence* and secondary gain was emphasized in the accompanying text. Differential diagnosis included psychophysiologic disorders (thought to be mediated by the autonomic nervous system), malingering (distinguished by being conscious behavior), and neurologic disease.

DSM-III (American Psychiatric Association, 1980) abandoned classification based on presumed etiology for an empiric approach classifying disorders by phenomenology. Conversion disorder was separated from the dissociative disorders and categorized under the somatoform disorders, a new section of DSM, along with hypochondriasis and somatization disorder. However, for historic continuity, conversion disorder was given a parenthetic optional name "hysterical neurosis, conversion type." The separation between conversion disorder and the dissociative disorders was maintained in all subsequent editions of DSM. The criteria for conversion disorder in DSM-III included loss or alteration in physical function, the clinician's judgment that psychologic factors were etiologically involved, determination that the symptoms were not under voluntary control, and after appropriate investigation not explained by known neuropathophysiology. Exclusions included symptoms limited to pain or sexual dysfunction, or when the symptoms were due to somatization disorder or schizophrenia.

DSM-III-R (American Psychiatric Association, 1987) retained the conversion disorder name, including the parenthetic option of calling it hysterical neurosis. The criteria were similar, though with some wording changes, and an additional exclusion when the symptom is "culturally sanctioned."

DSM-IV (American Psychiatric Association, 1994) extended DSM-III's move away from defining disorders by presumed etiology by dropping the reference to conversion disorder as a hysterical neurosis. In fact, the terms "hysteria," "hysterical," and "neurosis" do not appear in the DSM-IV index. The criteria were similar to DSM-III and DSM-III-R, but worded a bit differently, with the addition of the generic requirement applied to many other mental disorders that the symptom must cause significant distress or impairment. Subtypes were defined, including motor symptom or deficit, sensory symptom or deficit, seizures or convulsions, and mixed presentation. The text continued to mention *la belle indifférence* and secondary gain as common features, but also noted the inconsistency between the conversion symptom and known neuropathophysiology, demonstrated on the physical examination or testing. DSM-IV-TR (American Psychiatric Association, 2000) did not change any of the DSM diagnostic criteria, and there were no major changes in the text for conversion disorder.

CONVERSION DISORDER IN DSM-5

Whilst DSM-5 (American Psychiatric Association, 2013) retained elements of the prior criteria, i.e., altered voluntary motor or sensory function, causing significant distress or impairment (with the new addition of "or warrants medical evaluation"), and not better explained by another disorder, other components of the diagnosis were changed to address criticisms (Stone et al., 2010, 2011).

Name

The first problem was the name. "Conversion" refers to a psychoanalytic hypothesis, with little supportive empiric evidence. While some cases of conversion disorder seem to clinically fit the hypothesis, many others do not. Even the idea that the etiology of conversion symptoms is always psychogenic may not be correct. Furthermore, the name "conversion disorder" has not been widely accepted by neurologists or patients (Espay et al., 2009; Friedman and LaFrance, 2010). To be consistent with the movement, begun by DSM-III to avoid basing diagnoses on unproven etiology, the DSM-5 Work Group on the Somatic Symptom Disorders advocated for renaming the diagnosis to one commonly used in neurologic practice: "functional neurological disorder." This term was seen as relatively agnostic about etiology, to avoid mind–body dualism, and also to be more useful both for clinical practice and for stimulating research (Stone, 2009). However, others objected to the word "functional" as excessively vague and argued for retaining "conversion" for historic continuity, noting that we still use the term schizophrenia even though that disorder is not thought to be due to a "split mind." The solution was to retain the term conversion, with "functional neurological symptom disorder" in parentheses.

Feigning

While each was worded differently, DSM-III, DSM-III-R, and DSM-IV criteria all required the exclusion of feigning before one could diagnose conversion disorder. Proving feigning is difficult enough; proving the absence of feigning is arguably impossible. This requirement also seemed to be arbitrarily applied to conversion disorder; no other psychiatric diagnosis had this requirement, and there was no evidence to indicate that the feigning of neurologic symptoms was more common than the feigning of other physical (e.g., pain) or psychologic (e.g., anxiety) symptoms. This requirement was therefore dropped in the DSM-5 criteria, whilst retained as a differential for all DSM diagnoses.

Stressors

Previous DSM criteria also required the positive identification of associated psychologic factors preceding symptom onset or exacerbation before the diagnosis could be made. However, a number of problems were identified with this requirement. First, patients with conversion symptoms typically present to general medical settings, not mental health providers. Neurologists are less skilled at eliciting psychologic factors, especially sensitive histories of trauma or abuse. Second, the patient may not wish to reveal an underlying stressor, or be unable to, if not consciously aware of it. Indeed, if the psychoanalytic concept of conversion is correct, the recollection of related traumatic memory or anxiety-provoking conflict may only emerge within psychotherapy. Finally, empiric research has shown the requirement to identify an antecedent associated psychologic factor to be neither diagnostically reliable nor predictive of outcome (Roelofs et al., 2005). Even if one elicits a history of, for example, sexual abuse in childhood at the time of initial neurologic symptom presentation, it is unclear how to establish if it is etiologically relevant. Consequently, the requirement to identify an associated psychologic factor was removed from the criteria in DSM-5, but the importance of exploring psychologic stressors continued to be emphasized in the accompanying text (American Psychiatric Association, 2013).

Incompatibility with organic disease

In practice, conversion disorder is usually diagnosed only after a neurologist has identified a symptom as "nonorganic" because of findings on the physical examination or testing that are incompatible with recognized neurologic disease pathophysiology, or internally inconsistent (Stone, 2009). While previous DSM criteria required excluding symptoms due to neurologic disease, no guidance was provided in how to positively determine incompatibility with neurologic disease. The text in DSM-5 now provides examples of how this should be done; it requires the use of neurologic tests such as Hoover's sign, the tremor entrainment test, tubular visual fields, and simultaneous video and electroencephalogram monitoring of seizures (American Psychiatric Association, 2013). As a consequence, and perhaps controversially, conversion disorder is the only diagnosis in DSM that requires a neurologic examination and/or testing. It was the DSM-5 Work Group's hope that making incompatibility the defining criterion would improve psychiatric understanding and confidence in the diagnosis, and foster more cooperation between neurologists and psychiatrists.

Making the demonstration of incompatibility with organic disease the key criterion for the diagnosis of conversion disorder paradoxically was a move in the opposite direction from the DSM-5 Work Group's move away for other disorders, requiring that somatic symptoms be "medically unexplained." This was a major change from the conception of somatization disorder in DSM-III through DSM-IV-TR, to DSM-5's somatic symptom disorder. The essential criteria for somatic symptom disorder are that the patient's cognitive, affective, and behavioral responses to his or her somatic symptoms are grossly disproportionate. There is no requirement for the absence of a medical disorder causing the somatic symptoms. Reliance on medically unexplained symptoms as a key factor was considered very problematic because it fosters mind–body dualism; is based on a false assumption that lack of medical explanation is synonymous with psychogenicity; is unreliable; and leaves out those patients who have an organic disease "explanation" but still are somatizing. The reason criteria for CD were taken in the other direction is that neurologic symptoms in many cases can, with reasonable validity, be demonstrated to be incompatible with neuropathophysiology, and/or inconsistent in their presence, whereas that cannot be demonstrated for pain, nausea, sexual dysfunction, and other symptoms of medical diseases.

Specifiers

Finally, new optional specifiers were added, including symptom type (with weakness or paralysis, abnormal movement, attacks or seizures, special sensory symptom, speech symptoms, swallowing symptoms, or mixed symptoms), whether acute or chronic, and whether a psychologic stressor is present.

References

American Psychiatric Association (1952). Diagnostic and statistical manual: Mental disorders: DSM-I, American Psychiatric Association, Mental Hospital Service, Washington, DC.

American Psychiatric Association (1968). Diagnostic and statistical manual of mental disorders: DSM-II, American Psychiatric Association, Washington, DC.

American Psychiatric Association (1980). Diagnostic and statistical manual of mental disorders, 3rd edn. American Psychiatric Association, Washington, DC.

American Psychiatric Association (1987). Diagnostic and statistical manual of mental disorders (3rd ed., text rev), American Psychiatric Association, Washington, DC.

American Psychiatric Association (1994). Diagnostic and statistical manual of mental disorders, 4th edn. American Psychiatric Association, Washington, DC.

American Psychiatric Association (2000). Diagnostic and statistical manual of mental disorders (4th ed., text revision), American Psychiatric Association, Washington, DC.

American Psychiatric Association (2013). Diagnostic and statistical manual of mental disorders, 5th edn. American Psychiatric Association, Washington, DC.

Espay AJ, Goldenhar LM, Voon V et al. (2009). Opinions and clinical practices related to diagnosing and managing patients with psychogenic movement disorders: An international survey of movement disorder society members. Mov Disord 24 (9): 1366–1374.

Friedman JH, LaFrance Jr WC (2010). Psychogenic disorders: the need to speak plainly. Arch Neurol 67: 753–755.

Roelofs K, Spinhoven P, Sandijck P et al. (2005). The impact of early trauma and recent life-events on symptom severity in patients with conversion disorder. J Nerv Ment Dis 193: 508–514.

Stone J (2009). The bare essentials: functional symptoms in neurology. Pract Neurol 9: 179–189.

Stone J, LaFrance Jr WC, Levenson JL et al. (2010). Issues for DSM-5: conversion disorder. Am J Psychiatry 167: 626–627.

Stone J, LaFrance Jr WC, Brown R et al. (2011). Conversion disorder: current problems and potential solutions for DSM-5. J Psychosom Res 71: 369–376.

Stone J, Hallett M, Carson A et al. (2014). Functional Disorders in the Neurology section of ICD-11: a landmark opportunity. Neurology 83: 2299–2301.

World Health Organization (1948). Manual of the international statistical classification of diseases, injuries, and causes of death: Sixth revision of the international lists of diseases and causes of death, adopted 1948 (6th revision ed.), World Health Organization, Geneva, Switzerland.

World Health Organization (1957). Manual of the international statistical classification of diseases, injuries, and causes of death: Seventh revision of the international lists of diseases and causes of death, adopted 1957 (7th revision ed.), World Health Organization, Geneva, Switzerland.

World Health Organization (1968). Manual of the international statistical classification of diseases, injuries, and causes of death: Eighth revision of the international lists of diseases and causes of death, adopted 1968 (8th revision ed.), World Health Organization, Geneva, Switzerland.

World Health Organization (1975). International Classification of Diseases, 9th edn. Centers for Disease Control and Prevention, Atlanta, GA.

World Health Organization (1979). International Classification of Diseases. clinical modification, 9th edn. Centers for Disease Control and Prevention, Atlanta, GA.

World Health Organization (1992). International Statistical Classification of Diseases and Related Health Problems, 10th Revision (ICD-10), WHO, Geneva.

World Health Organization (2016). International Statistical Classification of Diseases and Related Health Problems, 10th Revision (ICD-10), Available online at: http://apps.who.int/classifications/icd10/browse/2016/en#/F44 (accessed March 21, 2016).

Handbook of Clinical Neurology, Vol. 139 (3rd series)
Functional Neurologic Disorders
M. Hallett, J. Stone, and A. Carson, Editors
http://dx.doi.org/10.1016/B978-0-12-801772-2.00017-5

Chapter 17

Neurologic diagnostic criteria for functional neurologic disorders

C. GASCA-SALAS[1,2] AND A.E. LANG[1]*

[1]*Morton and Gloria Shulman Movement Disorders Clinic and the Edmond J. Safra Program in Parkinson's Disease, University Health Network, Toronto Western Hospital, Toronto, Ontario, Canada*

[2]*HM CINAC-Hospital Universitario HM Puerta del Sur, Móstoles, Universidad CEU San Pablo, Madrid, Spain*

Abstract

The diagnosis of functional neurologic disorders can be challenging. In this chapter we review the diagnostic criteria and rating scales reported for functional/psychogenic sensorimotor disturbances, psychogenic nonepileptic seizures (PNES) and functional movement disorders (FMD). A recently published scale for sensorimotor signs has some limitations, but may help in the diagnosis, and four motor and two sensory signs have been reported as highly reliable. There is good evidence using eight specific signs for the differentiation of PNES from seizures. Recently, diagnostic criteria were developed for PNES; their sensitivity and specificity need to be evaluated. The definitive diagnosis of PNES can be made by recording typical positive features during the spells, and in a low proportion of cases, where the distinction with an organic etiology cannot easily be done, a normal electroencephalogram suggests the diagnosis. FMD diagnosis relies on diagnostic criteria, which have been refined over time and may be supplemented by laboratory tests in some phenotypes. Rating scales for PNES and FMD could be useful for severity measures, but several limitations remain to be addressed.

INTRODUCTION

Functional disorders are common in neurology; their diagnosis is not always easy and is commonly based on the neurologist's experience. Diagnosis should rely on the presence of positive signs and there must not be a better explanation for the symptoms, as emphasized in the recent published fifth edition of the *Diagnostic and Statistical Manual of Mental Disorders* (DSM-5: Stone et al., 2011; American Psychiatric Association, 2013; Daum et al., 2015). For that purpose, we need signs that are both sufficiently reliable in the detection of functional disorders and reproducible by different examiners. Moreover, DSM-5 does not require the presence of psychologic stressors as criteria for a diagnosis.

It is also important to take into account that patients may have a combination of an organic disease with a functional overlay (Stone et al., 2012, 2013).

In this chapter we will describe the validity and reliability of clinical signs as well as the diagnostic criteria and rating scales reported for different functional/psychogenic neurologic disorders, emphasizing sensory/motor disturbances, movement disorders, and nonepileptic events. Other symptoms, such as disturbances in level of consciousness, cognitive dysfunction, visual loss, and speech, eye movement, and auditory abnormalities, are dealt with in other chapters.

FUNCTIONAL MOTOR, SENSORY, AND GAIT DISORDERS

Reliable clinical signs and diagnostic criteria

Diagnostic criteria for functional disorders in neurology have been proposed in the fields of movement disorders and epilepsy. However, no criteria exist for other neurologic presentations, namely weakness, sensory or gait disorders (Daum et al., 2014). Therefore, we need valid positive signs suggestive of functional disorders to support the diagnosis, as negative signs of neurologic disease do not exclude an organic etiology. More than 50 positive signs have been identified for weakness,

*Correspondence to: Anthony E. Lang, MD, Movement Disorders Clinic, Toronto Western Hospital, 399 Bathurst St, 7 McL, Toronto, Ontario M5T 2S8, Canada. Tel: +1-416-603-5112, Fax: +1-416-603-5004, E-mail: lang@uhnres.utoronto.ca

sensory or gait disorders; however, not all have been properly assessed and there is no gold standard against which to compare these tests. Because of this, many studies have used the sign of interest in the diagnostic process, leading to an overestimated reported specificity (e.g., Tinazzi et al., 2008). This "diagnostic suspicion bias" and the lack of blinding in most of these studies reduce their validity generally, along with a number of generic limitations in studies of physical signs in this area (Table 17.1). Keeping these issues in mind, we will describe the most common and assessed signs, since some of them can still be regarded as helpful despite the absence of good validation.

In this regard, Daum et al. (2014) have recently reported 14 clinically validated positive signs in a systematic review; yet, none of these signs has been subject to really rigorous blind testing. Overall, these signs had good specificity but low sensitivity. The authors included studies with a minimum class III evidence level, and a controlled design.

Table 17.1

Limitations of the methodology of studies assessing the validity of clinical signs for the diagnosis of functional motor, sensory and gait disorders*

1. No gold standard against which to compare these tests
2. Diagnostic suspicion bias: many studies have used the studied sign in the diagnostic process, leading to an overestimated reported specificity
3. Most studies have based their validation on a single evaluation
4. Very few studies have been blinded (e.g., only Daum et al., 2015)
5. Possibility for some signs to be found in organic patients (e.g., give-way weakness: Gould et al., 1986, midline splitting and splitting of vibration: Rolak, 1988; Stone et al., 2010)
6. Potential for false positives: due the inability to understand the instructions, the presence of pain compromising patient compliance or even patients' eagerness to convince the doctor of their limitations. In all of these circumstances, patients with organic symptoms can demonstrate false-positive functional features (e.g., Hoover's sign, yes/no test)
7. Some studies did not specifically look at the reported deficit. For instance, in midline splitting sign for sensory disorders, only Rolak (1988) looked specifically at sensory deficit, whereas in Stone et al. (2010) and Chabrol et al. (1995) sensory deficits were not the main focus
8. Precise description of the clinical signs and interpretation of the findings is not always provided (e.g., Bowlus–Currier test, nonanatomic sensory loss)
9. Rating by videos instead of clinicians examining the same patients: limits the validity of inter-rater reliability assessment

*All these limitations could have introduced errors in the estimated sensitivity and specificity.

Subsequently, the authors further attempted to validate 10 signs previously suggested as valid and 28 previously unvalidated positive signs (13 motor/sensory, 14 gait, and one general sign) in a pilot study. The pilot study included 20 functional patients and 20 patients with an organic neurologic disorder as controls. For the first time, they calculated the inter-rater agreement of the positive signs in a controlled blind design (Daum et al., 2015). Twenty-three out of 38 signs had an acceptable inter-rater agreement. The "sternocleidomastoid" test (see Table 17.2 for explanation) and the presence of "falls that are always towards support" showed the highest inter-rater agreement (κ Cohen's$=0.83$). Six bedside positive signs that showed high specificity and good or excellent inter-rater agreement (κ Cohen's>0.6) in their study were proposed as "highly reliable," whereas 13 signs with high specificity and moderate to excellent inter-rater agreement (κ Cohen's>0.4) were considered as "reliable signs" (Tables 17.2–17.4). However, even though this study was blinded, it is a single study with a low sample size. Furthermore, the raters used videos instead of different clinicians examining the same patients, limiting the validity of inter-rater agreement assessment. Therefore, conclusions from this study should be interpreted with caution.

Positive signs for functional weakness, sensory and gait disorders

Suggested signs and their reliability

Weakness (Table 17.2)

Fifteen motor signs have been reported as valid; however, for many of them the data have been reported from only one study. Hoover's test has been considered the most useful test for nonorganic weakness (Stone et al., 2002). In addition, in certain case-control studies describing this test the main aim was not to evaluate Hoover's sign (Sonoo, 2004; Tinazzi et al., 2008; McWhirter et al., 2011). Other signs, such as the abductor sign, the abductor finger test, drift without pronation, and the spinal injury test, have shown high sensitivity and specificity, but the evidence comes from only one study each. Given their high specificity and "good or excellent" inter-rater agreement, Daum and coworkers (2015) proposed that give-way weakness, drift without pronation, and co-contraction are "highly reliable signs." Hoover's sign was also highly reliable; no inter-rater agreement was assessed, but it has a strong validation in several studies.

Sensory disorders (Table 17.3)

Despite many claims and attempts to demonstrate validity, sensory signs generally have poor specificity.

Table 17.2

Suggested positive signs for functional motor disorders

Sign	Description/assumption	Sensitivity	Specificity	Inter-rater agreement (κ Cohen's)* (Daum et al., 2015)	Reliability (Daum et al., 2015)	Comments (see Table 17.1 for generic methodologic issues)	References
Hoover's sign	Weakness of hip extension that resolves during contralateral hip flexion against resistance	63–100%	86–100%	–	Highly reliable	–	Ziv et al., 1998; Sonoo, 2004; Tinazzi et al., 2008; Stone et al., 2010; McWhirter et al., 2011; Daum et al., 2015
Abductor sign	Weakness of hip abduction that resolves with contralateral hip abduction against resistance	100%	100%	–	–	No inter-rater agreement provided information	Sonoo, 2004
Spinal injury center test	In patients unable to lift up their knees, legs are passively lifted up in a flexed posture. The paretic leg will not fall in nonorganic weakness	100%	13–98%	Moderate (0.52)	Reliable	Test limitations: only suitable for patients with bilateral leg paralysis	Yugue et al., 2004; Daum et al., 2015
Abduction finger test	In healthy subjects, abduction finger movements of one hand against resistance for 2 minutes will display a synkinetic abduction of the fifth finger of the contralateral (nonorganic paretic) hand	100%	100%	–	–	Test limitations: it can only be applied to patients with severe hand paresis	Tinazzi et al., 2008
Drift without pronation	Arms stretched out and palms in supinated position. Downward drift without pronation was described as a sign of functional paresis	61–100%	93–95%	Good (0.78)	Highly reliable	Only examined in one study of 26 patients	Babinski, 1907; Daum and Aybek, 2013; Daum et al., 2015
Collapsing weakness	In nonorganic weakness a limb collapses from a normal position with a light touch	44–70%	98–100%	Moderate (0.45)	Reliable	–	Stone et al., 2010; Daum et al., 2015
Give-way weakness	In functional paresis strength initially is normal during testing and then suddenly collapses	20–85%	95–100%	Good (0.61)	Highly reliable (Daum et al., 2015); highly unreliable (Gould et al., 1986)		Gould et al., 1986; Rolak, 1988; Daum et al., 2015

Continued

Table 17.2

Continued

Sign	Description/assumption	Sensitivity	Specificity	Inter-rater agreement (κ Cohen's)* (Daum et al., 2015)	Reliability (Daum et al., 2015)	Comments (see Table 17.1 for generic methodologic issues)	References
Co-contraction sign	Simultaneous contraction of the antagonist muscle (i.e., triceps) when the agonist muscle is being tested (biceps)	17–30%	100%	Good (0.77)	Highly reliable	False positive in spastic patients (excessive antagonist activation)	Knutsson and Martensson, 1985; Baker and Silver, 1987; Daum et al., 2015
Motor inconsistency	The impossibility to do a movement while another movement using the same muscle is possible	13%	98%	–	–	–	Chabrol et al., 1995
Sternocleidomastoid test	Weakness of head turning to the affected side in a patient with functional hemiparesis. (Sternomastoid has bilateral innervation)	31–80%	89–100%	Excellent (0.83)	Reliable	–	Diukova, 2001; Daum et al., 2015
Irregular drift	Same maneuver as "drift without pronation." In a nonorganic paresis the arm drifts irregularly	11%	95%	Good (0.72)	Suggestive	–	Daum et al., 2015
Nonconcavity of the palm of hand	Same maneuver as "drift without pronation." No concave/flexed position is observed in functional paresis	89%	65%	Good (0.65)	Reliable	–	Daum et al., 2015
Inconsistence of direction	Same maneuver as "drift without pronation." An oscillation of the arm is seen in functional paresis (downward, upward, downward…)	39%	95%	Moderate (0.42)	Reliable	–	Daum et al., 2015
Non digiti quinti sign	Same maneuver as "drift without pronation." In nonorganic paresis no abduction of the fifth finger is seen	0%	95%	Moderate (0.48)	Suggestive	–	Daum et al., 2015
Mingazzini: irregular drift	Mingazzini maneuver: patient in supine position, legs are bent 90° in the knees, and hips and eyes are closed for 5 seconds. In an organic paresis the leg drifts regularly whereas it drifts irregularly in a functional paresis	47%	95%	Moderate (0.60)	Reliable	–	Daum et al., 2015

Data from Daum et al. (2014, 2015).

*Inter-rater agreement: poor (<0.20), fair (0.21–0.40), moderate (0.41–0.60), good (0.61–0.80), excellent (0.81–1).

Table 17.3

Suggested positive signs for functional sensory disorders

Sign	Description/assumption	Sensitivity	Specificity	Inter-rater agreement (κ Cohen's)* (Daum et al., 2015)	Reliability in Daum et al. (2015) study	Comments (see Table 17.1 for generic methodologic issues)	References
Midline splitting	Exact splitting of sensory loss of half of the body cannot occur in organic disease, except thalamic lesions	18–42%	85–100%	Good (0.63)	Highly reliable	This sign can exist with thalamic lesions	Rolak, 1988; Chabrol et al., 1995; Stone et al., 2010; Daum et al., 2015
Splitting of vibration sense	There should not be differences in the sensation of a turning fork placed over the left or right side of the sternum or frontal bone as the same bone is involved	50–95%	14–88%	Good (0.66)	Highly reliable	–	Gould et al., 1986; Rolak, 1988; Stone et al., 2010; Daum et al., 2015
Nonanatomic sensory loss	Sensory deficits with nonanatomical distribution	74–80%	90–100%	Fair (0.23)	Reliable	–	Gould et al., 1986; Baker and Silver, 1987
Inconsistency	Findings are not consistent and not reproducible on repeated sensory testing	70%	100%	–	–	Sensory inconsistency not well defined in this small study. Parietal lesions can produce inconsistences in sensory testing (Magee, 1962; Critchley 1964)	Baker and Silver, 1987
Changing pattern of sensory loss	Changing boundaries of sensory loss	46%	20–52.5%	–	–	–	Gould et al., 1986; Chabrol et al., 1995
Systematic failure	The test is considered positive when the subject fails 100% of the time on a discrimination task (i.e., upgoing or downgoing joint)	8.7–15%	100%	Poor (0.16)	Reliable	Reported as "general sign"	Baker and Silver, 1987; Daum et al., 2015

*Inter-rater agreement: poor (<0.20), fair (0.21–0.40), moderate (0.41–0.60), good (0.61–0.80), excellent (0.81–1).

Table 17.4

Suggested positive signs for functional gait disorders and general sign

Sign	Description/assumption	Sensitivity	Specificity	Inter-rater agreement (κ Cohen's)* (Daum et al., 2015)	Reliability (Daum et al., 2015)	Comments (see Table 17.1 for generic methodologic issues)	References
Dragging monoplegic leg	In functional gait the leg is dragged after the patient "as it was inanimate matter" without circumduction seen in pyramidal weakness and typically with the forefoot in contact with the ground at all times (Todd, 1856)	8–11%	100%	Moderate (0.44)	Reliable	–	Ehrbar and Waespe, 1992; Stone et al., 2010; Daum et al., 2015
Chair test	Based on Blocq's (Blocq, 1888) description. Patients with nonorganic astasia-abasia despite apparently normal power can propel a swivel chair while sitting	89%	100%	–	–	No inter-rater reliability study	Okun et al., 2007
Falls always towards support	The patient falls in the direction of the examiner or another support	19%	93%	Excellent (0.83)	Suggestive	–	Daum et al., 2015
Psychogenic Romberg	Constant falls towards or away from the observer, large-amplitude body sway after a latency of a few seconds and improvement with distraction	39%	100%	Moderate (0.54)	Reliable	In the study of Lempert et al. (1991), this sign was present in 12 out of 25 patients and none of 13 healthy drama students simulators	Lempert et al., 1991; Daum et al., 2015
Noneconomic posture	A walking pattern that requires waste of muscle energy in order to maintain balance (for instance, standing and walking with flexion of hips and knees)	21%	100%	Moderate (0.53)	Suggestive	–	Lempert et al., 1991; Okun et al., 2007; Daum et al., 2015
Sudden knee buckling	Sudden knee buckling, usually with no falls	21%	95%	Moderate (0.52)	Suggestive	Infrequent sign. It can be found in chorea (Daum et al., 2015)	Keane, 1989; Lempert et al., 1991; Baik and Lang, 2007; Okun et al., 2007; Daum et al., 2015

Hesitation	The beginning of the movement is delayed or not possible	37%	100%	Good (0.66)	Reliable	Organic freezing of gait or start hesitation could be confused with this	Lempert et al., 1991; Daum et al., 2015
Tremulousness	Body tremor with up-and-down shaking of the body (flexion/extension of the knees), not compatible with an orthostatic tremor	16%	100%	Good (0.64)	Suggestive	–	Lempert et al., 1991; Daum et al., 2015
Bizarre excursion of the trunk	Bizarre excursions of the trunk, often building up over a few seconds; legs often unaffected	21%	100%	Moderate (0.48)	Reliable	–	Lempert et al., 1991; Daum et al., 2015
Excessive slowness	The slow motion is not consistent with an organic neurologic disorder	94%	32%	Moderate (0.47)		Common in functional gait disorders. moderate inter-rater agreement and high specificity (Daum et al., 2015)	Lempert et al., 1991; Baik and Lang, 2007; Okun et al., 2007; Daum et al., 2015
Expressive behavior (general sign)	Suffering or strained facial expression, moaning, mannered posture of hands, hyperventilation or grasping of the leg	55%	95%	Good (0.62)	Reliable	–	Lempert et al., 1991; Daum et al., 2015

*Inter-rater agreement: poor (<0.20), fair (0.21–0.40), moderate (0.41–0.60), good (0.61–0.80), excellent (0.81–1).

Although six sensory signs have been reported as valid, other studies have found high rates in controls with organic disease. For example, midline splitting and splitting of vibration showed a high inter-rater reliability in one study (Daum et al., 2015). However, this was based on a small sample size and other studies demonstrated these features in fairly high numbers of controls with neurologic disease (Rolak, 1988; Stone et al., 2010). Only two of the signs, the nonanatomic pattern sign and inconsistency, have demonstrated high sensitivity and specificity (Daum et al., 2014).

Gait disorders (Table 17.4)

In 1989, Keane assessed 60 patients with "hysterical gait disorders" and found that patterns rarely duplicated those of neurologic disability and were promptly suspected as functional by an experienced physician. Moreover, a dramatic cure was the best diagnostic evidence. Jordbru and colleagues (2012) provided a valuable categorization of psychogenic gait into three patterns – limping of one leg, limping of two legs, and truncal imbalance – and the reliability between independent raters was high. Baik and Lang (2007) found that 118 out of 279 (42.3%) patients with functional movement disorder (FMD) had an abnormal gait. Here they differentiated two groups of patients: those with psychogenic movement symptoms unrelated to walking but combined with an abnormal gait, where slowness of gait was the most common feature, and a second group with pure psychogenic gait, where buckling of the knee was the most common pattern, followed by astasia-abasia.

Eleven gait signs have been more carefully evaluated; most have low sensitivity and high specificity. The chair test presented the highest sensitivity and specificity (89% and 100% respectively), but was only evaluated in a single study (Okun et al., 2007). Daum and colleagues (2015) recently validated eight of these signs; however, none was considered as highly reliable and the chair test was not assessed. Lempert et al. (1991) identified six positive signs related to functional gait disorders (most were studied by Daum and colleagues but only in small numbers: momentary fluctuations of stance and gait, excessive slowness or hesitation, psychogenic Romberg test, uneconomic postures, "walking on ice," and sudden buckling of the knees), that were present alone or in combination in 97% of functional patients.

Less investigated signs (Table 17.5)

Ten motor, two sensory, and ten gait signs have been reported but not yet been evaluated in detail. Daum and coworkers (2015) aimed to validate some of these but, unfortunately, it was determined that further validation was required due to the poor to fair inter-rater agreement or because they are uncommon signs in functional patients.

Table 17.5

Less investigated positive signs for functional weakness, sensory and gait disorders

	Description/assumption	Comments	References
Weakness			
Nonpyramidal distribution of paresis	In organic lesions the weakness is greater distal > proximal and in flexor > extensor muscles. In functional paresis weakness is approximately equally distributed in all muscle groups	Not helpful to differentiate a peripheral lesion. Attempted validation by Daum et al. (2015). Fair inter-rater agreement (0.21)	Freud, 1895; Koehler, 2003; Daum et al., 2015
Arm drop test/hand strike	Patient lying supine, the limb is held over the patient's face and dropped by the examiner. In an organic paresis, the arm hits the patient's face. In functional paresis the arm regularly falls to the side, avoiding the face	Attempted validation by Daum et al. (2015); further validation required because it is a rare sign. It can only be applied in cases of complete upper-limb paralysis	Reeves and Bullen, 1994; Greer et al., 2005; Marcus et al., 2010; Stone et al., 2010; Daum et al., 2015
Barré test	Patient in prone position and legs bent at 90° in the knees. In pyramidal weakness, leg falls accompanied by contraction of hamstring muscle. In functional paresis, leg falls without contraction of the hamstrings or is maintained in the flexed position	Daum et al. (2015). Poor inter-rater agreement (0.03)	Barré, 1919; Daum et al., 2015

Table 17.5

Continued

	Description/assumption	Comments	References
Wrong-way tongue deviation	In organic hemiparesis a slight tongue deviation towards the paresis can be seen. A strong deviation away from the hemiparesis supports a functional paresis	–	Keane, 1986
Platysma sign	In organic paresis there is an asymmetry of platysma contraction when opening the mouth wide or when flexing the chin towards the chest against the examiner's pressure. This asymmetry is absent in functional cases	Expert opinion	Babinski, 1900
Babinski trunk-thigh test	The patient in supine position and arms across chest, is asked to sit up. In organic paresis, the weak limb raises above the bed and the contralateral shoulder makes a forward movement. In functional cases, the patient cannot sit or will sit but no asymmetry is seen	Expert opinion. Daum et al. (2015) attempted to validate; a poor inter-rater agreement (0.18)	Babinski, 1900; Daum et al. (2015)
Supine catch sign	Patient with a wrist drop is asked to put the hand in supination. In organic cases, the hand is maintained in neutral position with fingers flexed. In functional paresis, the wrist hyperextends with fingers extended	Reported in a case report of functional wrist drop	Sethi et al., 2010
Mingazzini: drift without extension	Mingazzini maneuver (see Table 17.1). In organic paresis there is a hip and knee extension with the downward drift. In functional paresis only the knee bends and drifts without an extension movement of the hip	Attempted validation by Daum et al. (2015). Fair inter-rater agreement (0.27)	Daum et al., 2015
Drift against gravity	Patient in supine position, arm held at 45° from the horizontal. In organic paresis arm drifts with the gravity. In functional cases arm raises against gravity	Attempted validation by Daum et al. (2015). Fair inter-rater agreement (0.36)	Daum et al. (2015)
"Elbow flex-ex"	Patient with unilateral arm weakness keeps elbows flexed at 30° and the examiner holds both forearms near the wrists. First part: Patient flexes or extends the normal arm at the elbow; in patients with nonorganic paresis the examiner simultaneously feels flexion or extension of the contralateral (paretic) arm. In organic paresis this contralateral movement is not significantly detectable. Second part: Patient flexes or extends the paretic arm at the elbow. In nonorganic weakness there is a simultaneous poor strength of extension of the normal limb. In organic weakness patient displays normal effort of the contralateral arm	–	Lombardi et al., 2014

Continued

Table 17.5

Continued

	Description/assumption	Comments	References
Sensory			
Bowlus–Currier test	Palms together, wrist crossed with thumbs down, interlock fingers (thumbs uncrossed), rotate hands, and keep them in front of the chest. The examiner starts touching on the fifth finger up to the thumb (which is uncrossed). In functional numbness, the patient will report anesthesia to all the fingers on that line, including the thumb, even though it belongs to the nonaffected side	Single study of 36 patients that did not provide a precise interpretation of the findings and whether it was independently tested	Bowlus and Currier, 1963
Yes/no test	Patient, with eyes closed, is asked to state "yes" when appreciating a touch stimulus and "no" when the stimulus is not appreciated. A "no" response in an anesthetic limb strongly suggests a functional deficit, because some degree of touch perception is preserved	Implies trickery on the part of the physician. The patient may think "no" means "no, I don't feel it as much," so it can be confusing – use with caution, is recommended. Attempted validation by Daum et al. (2015); further validation required because it is a rare sign	Magee, 1962; Stone et al., 2010; Daum et al., 2015
Gait			
Fluctuation	Gait disturbance with periods of normal gait. Often in response to suggestion	May occur in neurologic disease, for instance, myasthenia gravis	Lempert et al., 1991; Okun et al., 2007
"Walking on ice"	Patient walking pattern mimics ice skating or as if on slippery grounds	Attempted validation by Daum et al. (2015); further validation required because it is a rare sign	Lempert et al., 1991; Daum et al., 2015
Staggering long distance	Patient appears very unstable but doesn't fall, and will eventually find support, even if far out of reach	Attempted validation by Daum et al. (2015); further validation required because it is a rare sign	Keane, 1989; Daum et al., 2015
Exaggerated swaying without falling	Similar to the psychogenic Romberg sign (Table 17.3)	–	Keane, 1989
Astasia-abasia	Inability to stand and walk despite normal leg function in bed	In thalamic astasia the patient is also unable to stand	Knapp, 1891; Blocq, 1888; Lempert et al., 1991; Baik and Lang, 2007
Opposite of astasia-abasia	Inability to move legs in bed despite preserved capacity of stance and gait	–	Ehrbar and Waespe, 1992
Sudden side steps	Patient with functional gait will display a big displacement in his trajectory with sudden side steps, without falling	Attempted validation by Daum et al. (2015). Fair inter-rater agreement (0.37)	Diukova and Stoliarova, 2001; Daum et al., 2015
Cross legs	Functional patient will walk with crossed legs or scissoring pattern	–	Keane, 1989; Diukova and Stoliarova, 2001
Flailing arms	Exaggerated large-amplitude movements of the arms during walking apparently to maintain stability	Attempted validation by Daum et al. (2015). Poor inter-rater agreement (0.03)	Lempert et al., 1991; Daum et al., 2015
Robot walk	Robotic, stiff-legged, and square-cut walk	–	Southard, 1919; Keane, 1989; Daum et al., 2014

Inter-rater agreement: poor (< 0.20), fair (0.21–0.40), moderate (0.41–0.60), good (0.61–0.80), excellent (0.81–1).

Rating scales and their reliability

A sensorimotor scale for functional disorders was suggested by Daum and colleagues (2015) on the basis of their study. This scale was developed to help with the diagnosis and not as a severity scale. It combines six motor and four sensory validated "positive signs." This scale has a maximum score of 14 points. Two points are attributed to signs with a robust validation (Hoover's sign, the give-way weakness sign, the "drift without pronation" sign, and "splitting the midline" sign) and the remaining signs are given a score of 1 each (collapsing weakness, co-contraction, spinal injury test, splitting of vibration sense, nonanatomic sensory loss, and "systematic failure" – always choosing a wrong answer during sensory testing). A score of ≥ 4 showed 100% specificity and 95% sensitivity, suggesting that this scale can help in differentiating between organic and functional sensorimotor disorders. However, these results need to be interpreted with caution given the small study sample size and the use of a video for rater evaluation, which limits the assessment of inter-rater agreement (Daum et al., 2015).

PSYCHOGENIC NONEPILEPTIC SEIZURES

The most reliable diagnosis of psychogenic nonepileptic seizures (PNES) is provided by the clinical picture with the presence of clinical features consistent with a psychogenic/dissociative nonepileptic event (described below). In some cases where this distinction cannot be made easily (e.g., because the attack has not been witnessed), a video-electroencephalogram (EEG) recording of typical events will confirm the lack of electrographic changes and allow clinical features to be recorded (Syed et al., 2011). When trying to reach the diagnosis of PNES, it is important to consider that 10% of patients with PNES also have seizures (Benbadis et al., 2001) and, in these cases, clinical and laboratory criteria should be applied (Drazkowski and Chung, 2010).

Reliable clinical signs

Clinical signs that reliably distinguish between PNES and seizures have been extensively evaluated (Avbersek and Sisodiya, 2010) (Table 17.6). Selected motor signs have been reported in at least two controlled studies where a video-EEG was used to diagnose the events. Long duration, fluctuating course, asynchronous movements, pelvic thrusting, side-to-side head or body movement, closed eyes, ictal crying, and memory recall are signs with good evidence from literature that differentiate PNES from seizures. An occurrence from EEG-confirmed sleep and postictal confusion support an epileptic seizure. There is also good evidence from primary studies that postictal stertorous breathing supports epileptic seizure, but only in the case of convulsive events. Around 20% of "nonepileptic" events actually resemble syncope more than epilepsy. Here, a sudden collapse to the ground with eyes closed for more than 2 minutes is highly characteristic of a psychogenic nonepileptic event.

In addition, there are other potentially useful clinical signs that have been described. For example, ictal stuttering (Vossler et al., 2004) and the bringing of an age-inappropriate toy animal to the video-EEG monitoring ("teddy bear sign") (Burneo et al., 2003) were found in single studies to have a specificity of 100%, but they are not frequent, leading to a low sensitivity (9% and 5.2%, respectively).

The presence of somatic symptoms of anxiety during attacks seems to be more frequent in PNES compared to epileptic seizures, and could help in the diagnosis (Goldstein and Mellers, 2006). Hendrickson et al. (2014) recently reported that the presence, whether before, during, or after an attack, of at least four of the 13 panic attack symptoms of anxiety of the *Diagnostic and Statistical Manual* IV Text Revision (DSM-IV-TR: American Psychiatric Association, 2000) has a sensitivity of 83% and specificity of 65%. By increasing the number of these symptoms to five and six, the sensitivity reduces, but the specificity improves. These symptoms include: (1) palpitations, pounding heart, or accelerated heart rate; (2) sweating; (3) trembling or shaking; (4) sensations of shortness of breath; (5) feeling of choking; (6) chest pain or discomfort; (7) nausea or abdominal distress; (8) feeling dizzy, unsteady, lightheaded, or faint; (9) derealization or depersonalization; (10) fear of losing control or going crazy; (11) fear of dying; (12) paresthesias; and (13) chills or hot flushes.

Finally, there are six relatively common signs with insufficient evidence to support their usefulness: gradual onset, nonstereotyped movements, flailing or thrashing movements, opisthotonus, tongue biting, and urinary incontinence (Avbersek and Sisodiya, 2010).

The final diagnosis of PNES will require all available data and should not be led by only one clinical sign (Avbersek and Sisodiya, 2010). As mentioned above, all these signs are useful in the diagnosis of PNES, but the gold standard for the diagnosis is video-EEG monitoring and recording of typical positive features during the episodes.

Table 17.6

Clinical signs differentiating between epileptic seizure (ES) and nonepileptic events (NEE)/psychogenic nonepileptic seizures (PNES)

	Sensitivity per event	Sensitivity per patient	Specificity per event	Specificity per patient	Comments	References from controlled studies
Signs supporting NEE/PNES						
Fluctuating course	69%	47–88%	96%	96–100%	–	Vinton et al., 2004; Chen et al., 2008
Asynchronous movements	44–96%	9–56%	93–96%	93–100%	Limitation: frontal-lobe partial seizures are excluded	Gates et al., 1985; Azar et al., 2008; Chen et al., 2008
Pelvic trusting	1–31%	7.4–44%	96–100%	92–100%	Limitation: frontal-lobe partial seizures are excluded	Gates et al., 1985; Saygi et al., 1992; Devinsky et al., 1996; Geyer et al., 2000; Azar et al., 2008; Chen et al., 2008
Side-to-side head or body movement	25–63%	15–36%	96–100%	92–100%	Only applied for generalized tonic clonic seizures	Gates et al., 1985; Saygi et al., 1992; Pierelli et al., 1989; Azar et al., 2008; Chen et al., 2008
Closed eyes	34–88%	52–96%	74–100%	97%	–	DeToledo and Ramsay, 1996; Chung et al., 2006; Azar et al., 2008; Chen et al., 2008; Syed et al., 2008
Ictal crying	13–14%	3.7–37%	100%	37%	–	Slater et al., 1995; Devinsky et al., 1996; Walczak and Bogolioubov, 1996; Chen et al., 2008
Memory recall	63%	77–88%	96%	90%	–	Bell et al., 1998; Devinsky et al., 1996
Long duration	–	–	–	–	Events longer than 2 minutes are highly suggestive of NEE/PNES. However, partial ES may also last more than 2 minutes	Gates et al., 1985; Pierelli et al., 1989; Brown et al., 1991; Saygi et al., 1992; Henry and Drury, 1998; Jedrzejczak et al., 1999; Azar et al., 2008
Signs supporting ES						
Occurrence from sleep	31–59%	–	100%	–	Electroencephalogram is required to verify wakefulness	Pierelli et al., 1989; Saygi et al., 1992; Azar et al., 2008
Postictal confusion	61–100%	67%	88%	84%	–	Azar et al., 2008; Slater et al., 1995
Postictal stertorous breathing	61–91%	–	100%	–	Partial seizures are excluded	Sen et al., 2007; Azar et al., 2008; Chen et al., 2008

Modified from Avbersek and Sisodiya (2010), with permission from BMJ Publishing Group Ltd.

Diagnostic criteria

For the diagnosis of PNES, video-EEG monitoring has demonstrated a moderate inter-rater agreement ($\kappa = 0.57$) (Benbadis et al., 2009). In the absence of video-EEG recording, the diagnosis of PNES can be unreliable, with resulting false-positive diagnoses (Ramani et al., 1980; King et al., 1982; Gates et al., 1985; Parra et al., 1999). Specifically, a prospective study showed that epileptic seizures were misdiagnosed as PNES more frequently than the reverse (57% vs. 12%) (Parra et al., 1999). Moreover, epileptic seizures of frontomesial origin are often misdiagnosed as PNES, since they can semiologically mimic them and often fail to display an identifiable electrographic ictal pattern (Saygi et al., 1992).

Table 17.7

Proposed diagnostic levels of certainty for non-epileptic events (NEE)/ psychogenic nonepileptic seizures (PNES)

Diagnostic level	Witnessed event	EEG findings	Comments
Possible NEE/PNES	Self-reported and/or witness description of the events	No epileptiform activity (routine EEG or sleep-deprived interictal EEG)	–
Probable NEE/PNES	Physician witnessed the event or reviewed a video showing semiologic findings of PNES	No epileptiform activity (routine EEG or sleep-deprived interictal EEG)	Home video recording does not usually include the beginning of the event
Clinically established NEE/PNES	Clinician experienced in epilepsy reviewed the video or witnessed the event, typical of PNES	No epileptiform activity (routine EEG or ambulatory ictal EEG) during a typical event in which the semiology would expect epileptiform EEG activity during equivalent epileptic seizures	–
Documented NEE/ PNES	Clinician experienced in epilepsy reviewed the video or witnessed the event, typical of PNES	No epileptiform activity immediately before, during, and after the event captured on ictal video EEG	The recorded event on the EEG has to be typical of the patient's habitual ones

Reproduced from LaFrance et al. (2013), with permission from John Wiley.
EEG, electroencephalogram.

Recently, using different combinations of patient history, witness description, clinician observation, and EEG findings, diagnostic criteria have been developed for PNES. These four categories of certainty have been reported: "possible," "probable," "clinically established," and "documented PNES" (LaFrance et al., 2013). All levels need history characteristics consistent with PNES (Table 17.7). However, these are proposed criteria and their sensitivity and specificity have not yet been evaluated.

Rating scales and their reliability

Inspired by the Psychogenic Movement Disorders Scale (Hinson et al., 2005), Cianci et al. (2011) aimed to develop a rating scale for PNES (Table 17.8). For this purpose, 60 PNES patients were included; they had no epileptiform activity (ictal or interictal) and no postictal slowing. The diagnosis of PNES was confirmed by suggestion, which has shown a high sensitivity and specificity (Popkirov et al., 2015). This scale showed a good inter-rater reliability (measured by AC1 statistic, this ranged from 0.69 to 1 for the presence or absence of the motor phenomena and associated features). There was a moderate inter-rater agreement for the three scores of this scale (Kendall's concordance coefficients (KCC) 0.53–0.71 and intraclass correlation coefficient (ICC) 0.51–0.56). The results from this scale were compared to the Clinical Global Impression (CGI) scale, a nonspecific scale, to test the validity. There was a strong correlation (Spearman correlation score = 0.69) between the mean CGI and the mean total PNES score. Although this scale may be a valid assessment of PNES, it has several limitations, such as how the severity or the time of the episode should be judged or the evaluation of only one event per patient that prevents the assessment of the consistency or stereotyped nature of the events. In addition, some of the "associated features" support a diagnosis (but are nonspecific for PNES, i.e., crying), while others such as sphincteric incontinence are not specific for epilepsy. Finally, this test evaluated responsiveness during atonic/akinetic fits only, and not when other motor phenomena (i.e., tremor/oscillation, hypermotor/agitation, automatisms) were present, and so consciousness was not properly assessed.

FUNCTIONAL MOVEMENT DISORDERS

Diagnostic criteria and their degree of certainty

When dealing with FMDs or psychogenic movement disorders, the clinical picture should guide the diagnosis. Although no absolutely pathognomonic findings exist, there are important unequivocal clinical features, discussed in the following chapters (e.g., inconsistency and/or incongruity in the exam), that serve as critical cues to the diagnosis and are applicable to all types of movement disorders. (Table 17.9 provides a list of the historic and general examination clues to the diagnosis.) In addition to these features, there is a new sign that could be helpful in the diagnosis of any kind of hyperkinetic FMD, the "whack-a-mole" sign. This sign is characterized by the development of an abnormal movement in

Table 17.8

Rating scale for psychogenic nonepileptic seizures

Motor phenomena	Scale factors		
Tremor/oscillation	*Presence of motor phenomena*	*Severity*	*Duration*
Tonic Clonic/jerking Hypermotor/agitation Atonic/akinetic Automatisms	0 = absent 1 = present	0 = none 1 = minimal 2 = mild 3 = moderate 4 = severe	0 = none 1 = < 25% of the time 2 = 25–50% of the time 3 = 50–75% of the time 4 = > 75% of the time

Body parts considered: upper face, lips/perioral, jaw, neck, head, left shoulder, right shoulder, left upper extremity, right upper extremity, left lower extremity, right lower extremity, pelvis, trunk.

Associated features	Presence of associated features
Incontinence Tongue biting Drooling Eye closure Hyperventilation Lament/crying	0 = absent 1 = present

Modified from Cianci et al. (2011).

There are three scores for this scale: (1) the total scores for phenomena, calculated as the sum of the severity and duration rating of all phenomena considering all body regions affected; (2) the total scores for associated phenomena, calculated as the sum of the scores for the presence of the different signs; and (3) the total psychogenic nonepileptic seizure score, calculated as the addition of the total phenomenology score and the total associated phenomena score.

Table 17.9

Clues suggesting a functional/psychogenic cause of a movement disorder

Historic	General examination
Abrupt onset (symptoms often maximal at that time) Static course Spontaneous remissions/cures Paroxysmal symptoms (generally nonkinesigenic)* Psychiatric comorbidities† Secondary gain (often not apparent) Risk factors for conversion disorder (sexual and physical abuse, trauma) Psychological stressors Multiple somatizations/undiagnosed conditions Employed in allied health professions (infrequent)	Movement inconsistent • Variability over time (frequency, amplitude, direction/distribution of movement) • Distractibility reduces or resolves, attention increases movement • Selective disability • Entrainment (especially with tremor) Movement incongruous with organic movement disorders • Mixed (often bizarre) movement disorders • Paroxysmal attacks (including pseudoseizures) • Precipitated paroxysms (often suggestible/startle) Suggestibility Effortful production or deliberate slowness (without fatiguing) of movement Self-inflicted injury (caution: tic disorders) Delayed and excessive startle response to a stimulus Burst of verbal gibberish or stuttering speech False (give-away) weakness Nonanatomic sensory loss or spread of movement Certain types of abnormal movements common in individuals with functional movement disorders‡ Functional disability out of proportion to examination findings

Data from Gupta and Lang (2009).

*Separation from organic paroxysmal dyskinesias can be challenging, particularly if they occur infrequently with prolonged symptom-free periods.

†Psychiatric diseases can also coincide with organic illness or present as part of the organic movement disorder.

‡Such movements include dystonia that begins as a fixed posture (particularly if abrupt onset, painful, and early contractures are seen); bizarre gait; twisting facial movements that move mouth to one side or the other (organic dystonia of the facial muscles usually does not pull the mouth sidewise).

another limb when the affected limb's movement is restricted by the examiner holding it (Park et al., 2015). Unlike the field of epilepsy, where a normal EEG can be useful in the diagnosis of PNES in specific cases, in FMD the laboratory is only of help in providing positive diagnostic information in cases of tremor and myoclonus.

The diagnosis of FMD should not be considered a diagnosis of exclusion. Instead, it should rely on positive signs and other features for which laboratory findings may help (Espay et al., 2009; Gupta and Lang, 2009).

In 1988, Fahn and Williams first proposed criteria for the diagnosis of psychogenic dystonia, that can be applied to all movement disorders. They categorized patients into four levels of certainty: "documented," "clinically established," "probable," and "possible" (Table 17.10). Later, Williams et al. (1994) proposed the combination of "documented" and "clinically established" degrees as "clinically definite," since both may imply a definite diagnosis.

Shill and Gerber proposed criteria in 2006. They defined the following levels of certainty: clinically proven FMD when it remits with psychotherapy, while unobserved, or if there is premovement Bereitschaftspotential on EEG (myoclonus only). According to the presence of primary and secondary criteria, they defined diagnoses as clinically definite, clinically probable, and clinically possible. Primary criteria included factors suggesting a movement disorder inconsistent with organic disease (i.e., distractibility), excessive pain or fatigue, and previous exposure to neurologic disease (usually family history). Secondary criteria included multiple somatizations and obvious psychiatric disturbance. These criteria had a high sensitivity (83%) and specificity (100%) for the identification of "probable" FMD. Sensitivity of this scale was higher (97%) when considering "possible," with a specificity of 96% (Shill and Gerber, 2006).

However, this study had several limitations. One was the emphasis placed on the presence of psychologic factors which are not part of the FMD diagnosis and that others have argued should not influence the diagnosis (Espay et al., 2009). In this study these features enhanced the sensitivity and specificity of the criteria. There were also important methodologic concerns, such as the retrospective design, the lack of provided evidence that all FMD patients and controls were evaluated for all the features that were eventually used as diagnostic criteria (creating diagnostic suspicion bias), and finally, the fact that Shill and Gerber suggested that the diagnosis of FMD can be made without consideration of the neurologic symptoms, given the emphasis placed on the presence of psychologic factors. These concerns make the application of their criteria less useful (Voon et al., 2007).

A subsequent study attempted to assess diagnostic agreement in 14 clinicians who provided a dichotomous judgment (psychogenic or organic) following review of a video and standardized clinical information (Morgante et al., 2012). Both sets of clinical criteria (Fahn and Williams, 1988; Shill and Gerber, 2006) showed poor inter-rater agreement when considering the "possible"

Table 17.10

Levels of certainty for functional movement disorders

Fahn and Williams (1988) criteria	Proposed revision (Gupta and Lang, 2009)
1. Documented Remittance with suggestion, physiotherapy, psychotherapy, placebos, "while unobserved"	1. Documented (as in original)
2. Clinically established Inconsistent over time/incongruent with clinical condition + other manifestations: other 'false' signs, multiple somatizations, obvious psychiatric disturbance	2a. Clinically established plus other features (as in original) 2b. Clinically established minus other features: unequivocal features incompatible with organic disease with no features suggesting another underlying neurologic or psychiatric problem
3. Probable a. Inconsistent/incongruent with no other features b. Consistent/congruent + "false" neurological signs c. Consistent/congruent + multiple somatizations	1 + 2a + 2b = Clinically definite 3. Laboratory-supported definite Electrophysiologic evidence proving a psychogenic movement disorder (primarily in cases of tremor and myoclonus)
4. Possible Consistent/congruent + obvious emotional disturbance	

Data from Gupta and Lang (2009).

and "probable" judgment, but they yielded a substantial agreement when considering the "clinically definite" level, suggesting that only this level is useful for the diagnosis of FMD (Morgante et al., 2012).

In contrast, another recent study evaluating 29 videos of movement disorders on YouTube showed a high inter-rater agreement (inter-rater reliability coefficient = 0.89) as well as a high level of certainty (4.33 ± 0.60 = 86.6%) on the part of seven experts who independently reviewed them. However, there was no independent confirmation of the diagnosis in these cases (Stamelou et al., 2011).

The utility of laboratory testing in support of the clinical diagnosis (Morgante et al., 2012) has led to subsequent modifications adding the idea that the diagnosis of FMD can be laboratory-supported (adding a "laboratory-supported definite" category to the diagnostic criteria in a fashion similar to the field of multiple sclerosis) (Gupta and Lang, 2009). In particular, this category applies to electrophysiologic tests capable of supporting the diagnosis of functional/psychogenic tremor and functional/psychogenic myoclonus.

Gupta and Lang proposed a further revision of the Fahn and Williams' criteria. They noted the possibility of establishing a diagnosis of FMD with only the clinical findings ("clinically established minus other features"; i.e., "other false signs, multiple somatic symptoms, other psychiatric disturbances," required by Fahn and Williams' criteria, are not present) and proposed eliminating the "possible" category because it may represent an organic movement disorder with superimposed psychiatric symptoms (Table 17.10) (Schrag and Lang, 2005).

Some studies have focused on the diagnosis of specific FMDs. Van der Salm and colleagues (2013) designed a survey to assess selected functional hyperkinetic movement disorders (psychogenic jerks, myoclonus, or tics). When the diagnostic steps applied by experienced movement disorders physicians included a short video, medical history, neurologic exam, and neurophysiologic information, the agreement was moderate (κ value = 5.6 ± 0.1) and the diagnostic certainty was relatively high (3.5 ± 1.2) (where 1 = very uncertain and 5 = absolutely certain). Importantly, when psychiatric evaluation was added, it did not increase either the agreement or the certainty.

Diagnostic criteria focused on the different types of movement disorders

Functional tremor is the most frequent presentation of a FMD (in at least 50% of cases) (Factor et al., 1995; Cubo et al., 2005). The reliability of some measures for the diagnosis of functional tremor was investigated in order to distinguish it from essential tremor. The tapping task for distraction reached the highest sensitivity and specificity (both 73%), followed by distraction with serial 7 s, with a sensitivity of 58% and specificity of 84% (Kenney et al., 2007). Suggestibility with a tuning fork also seemed to be a good predictor for functional tremor; it showed a high specificity (88%) but a relatively low sensitivity (42%). On the other hand, entrainment seemed to be less predictive for the diagnosis of functional tremor (Kenney et al., 2007).

With respect to laboratory tests, one study found that the diagnosis of functional tremor required a combination of several tests to reach adequate sensitivity and specificity, since no single measure was sufficiently reliable to differentiate it from an organic tremor (Schwingenschuh et al., 2011). The following tests were included in the study: (1) incorrect tapping performance at 1 Hz, 3 Hz, and 5 Hz (1 point each); (2) entrainment, suppression, or pathologic frequency shift at 1 Hz, 3 Hz, and 5 Hz (1 point each); (3) pause or 50% reduction in amplitude of tremor with contralateral ballistic movements (1 point); (4) tonic coactivation before tremor onset (1 point); (5) coherence of bilateral tremors (1 point); and (6) increase of total power (as surrogate of tremor amplitude) with 500-g weight loading (1 point). Attributing a score to every laboratory measure, the authors devised a cut-off of 3 out of 10 points for a diagnosis of laboratory-supported functional tremor which had sensitivity and specificity of 100% in their sample of 13 patients with functional tremor and 25 patients with organic tremor. This tool was recently validated by the same group in a larger sample (38 patients with functional tremor and 73 with organic tremor), showing good inter-rater reliability, test–retest reliability, and very high sensitivity (89.5%) and specificity (95.9%) (Schwingenschuh et al., 2016).

More recently, van der Salm and colleagues (2014) found that 104 out of the 179 cases (58%) of propriospinal myoclonus in the literature were actually functional, concluding that an FMD is far more frequent than previously assumed. Based on their clinical experience and review of literature, they proposed specific diagnostic criteria for propriospinal myoclonus and suggested three categories: idiopathic, secondary, and functional. The proposed criteria for functional propriospinal were: (1) clinical clues (for instance, previous somatizations); (2) coexistence of facial movements or vocalizations (they don't concur with a spinal origin); (3) normal imaging of the spinal axis with no evidence of myelopathy; and (4) presence of Bereitschaftspotential or inconsistent electromyogram pattern. However, the latter can be absent or not recordable and caution is recommended (van der Salm et al., 2014).

Two recent studies proposed hints for the diagnosis of functional tics, a rarely reported phenotype (i.e., adult onset, inability to suppress the movements, lack of premonitory sensations). However, given the small sample size reported in both studies (9 patients in the first and 11 in the second), retrospective analysis, and no Bereitschaftspotential assessment to support a functional origin, these clues should be interpreted with caution and confirmed in larger studies (Baizabal-Carvallo and Jankovic, 2014; Demartini et al., 2015).

Likewise, a retrospective study explored the typical clinical characteristics of functional (psychogenic) paroxysmal movement disorders based on 26 cases. The authors found that, even though the phenotypic presentation can be highly diverse, 11 characteristics help in distinguishing this condition from the three classic forms of primary paroxysmal dyskinesias (paroxysmal kinesigenic dyskinesia, paroxysmal nonkinesigenic dyskinesia, and paroxysmal exercise-induced dyskinesia): (1) an adult age of onset; (2) the presence of paroxysmal tremor; (3) high within-subject phenomenologic variability; (4) marked increases in attack frequency and severity during examination; (5) highly variable attack duration; (6) numerous and unusual triggers; (7) alteration of responsiveness during attacks; (8) odd precipitating factors; (9) odd relieving maneuvers; (10) medically unexplained somatic symptoms; and (11) atypical response to medication. However, the reliability of these features has not been evaluated, since no control group with organic paroxysmal dyskinesias was included (Ganos et al., 2014).

Regarding functional chorea, there are not specific criteria, probably because of the very low frequency of this phenotype (Thomas and Jankovic, 2004).

Table 17.11

Rating scale for psychogenic movement disorders*

Part 1: Phenomena†	Part 2: Functions	Part 3: Total scores
Rest tremor	Gait	Total phenomenology score
Action tremor	Speech	Total function score
Dystonia		Total psychogenic movement disorder score (1+2)
Chorea		
Bradykinesia		
Myoclonus		
Cerebellar		
Ballism		
Athetosis		
Tics		
Severity	Duration	Incapacitation
0 = none	0 = none	0 = none
1 = minimal	1 = < 25% of the time	1 = minimal
2 = mild	2 = 25–50% of the time	2 = mild
3 = moderate	3 = 50–75% of the time	3 = moderate
4 = severe	4 = > 75% of the time	4 = severe

Modified from Hinson et al. (2005), with permission from John Wiley.

*Retaining the terminology of the original report.

†Body parts considered: upper face, lips/perioral, jaw, tongue, neck, head, left shoulder, right shoulder, left upper extremity, right upper extremity, left lower extremity, right lower extremity, trunk, other region

Rating scales for severity of functional movement disorders

To date, only one scale has been developed with the specific intention of rating the severity of FMD (Hinson et al., 2005). It includes 10 phenomena (rest tremor, action tremor, dystonia, chorea, bradykinesia, myoclonus, cerebellar incoordination, ballism, athetosis, and tics), anatomic distribution, severity, and duration, along with two functions (gait and speech), incapacitation due to the abnormal movement/function, and total severity score (Table 17.11).

Each phenomenon is scored as absent or present. When it is present, the severity of each phenomenon is scored from 0 (none) to 4 (severe), the duration factor is rated from 0 (none) to 4 (>75% of the time), and the incapacitation ranges from 0 (none) to 4 (severe).

This scale includes three scores: (1) the total phenomenology score: the sum of the severity, duration, and incapacitation rating of all phenomena in affected regions; (2) the total function score: the sum of the scores of duration and incapacitation rating for gait and/or speech; and (3) the total Psychogenic Movement Disorder score is obtained from the addition of 1 and 2.

This scale showed an excellent inter-rater reliability for the presence or absence of each phenomenon (κ range 0.63–0.86) and also showed a high rate of agreement when measuring total phenomenology (ICC = 0.87, KCC = 0.91), function (ICC = 0.89, KCC = 0.92) and total score (ICC = 0.88, KCC = 0.93). It also demonstrated the ability to capture changes due to a therapeutic intervention. Moreover, the mean total score showed a high correlation with the mean CGI (Pearson correlation = 0.79), supporting its validity as a measure of severity.

On the other hand, this scale is problematic as it combines all movement disorders rather than assessing isolated movement disorders. This results in long evaluation times and also the potential for overrating and underrating the severity of the disorder (e.g., a patient who has only tremors of moderate severity, present 75% of the time, with moderate incapacitation would score less than a patient with more than three different types of movement disorders but each with mild severity and a duration of less than 25% of the time and minimal incapacitation). Besides, there is no other gold standard to compare the scale to. Thus, simpler scales are warranted, permitting the evaluation of single movement disorder phenomena.

CONCLUDING REMARKS

In summary, functional neurologic disorders are common in clinical practice, and diagnosis should rely on the presence of positive signs. Clinical criteria have been proposed for PNES and FMD, whereas to date, no criteria exist for other neurologic presentations, namely weakness, sensory or gait disorders. On the other hand, there are a significant number of clinical signs that can be helpful in the diagnosis of these clinical presentations, but with some limitations that reduce their general validity.

In addition, although numerous signs have been validated for the diagnosis of PNES, the final diagnosis in generalized shaking events is provided by the gold-standard video-EEG monitoring during the episodes where the diagnosis relies on assessing positive signs captured during video as much as the negative EEG. In FMD, no gold standard exists; therefore, diagnosis relies on diagnostic criteria, which have been refined over time and which may be supplemented by laboratory findings in selected phenotypes. The phenomenology of FMD is broad; however, surprisingly, when each movement is studied in isolation (e.g., tremor, dystonia), clinical criteria have only been proposed for functional tremor, propriospinal myoclonus, tics, and paroxysmal dyskinesias. The Fahn and Williams' criteria were initially proposed for the diagnosis of functional/psychogenic dystonia but were subsequently applied to all FMDs.

The scales for PNES and FMD may be useful as severity measures, but still have some limitations. The recently proposed sensorimotor scale showed a high specificity for a score of only 4 out of 14 points, but was only tested in one study. Future studies designed to validate these scales in other cohorts with larger samples are needed. Furthermore, future studies should also assess which signs should be routinely evaluated as part of shorter, more concise, and easily applicable scales.

References

American Psychiatric Association (2000). Diagnostic and statistical manual of mental disorders (4th edn., text revision). American Psychiatric Association, Washington, DC.

American Psychiatric Association (2013). Diagnostic and statistical manual of mental disorders. 5th edn. American Psychiatric Association, Washington, DC.

Avbersek A, Sisodiya S (2010). Does the primary literature provide support for clinical signs used to distinguish psychogenic nonepileptic seizures from epileptic seizures? J Neurol Neurosurg Psychiatry 81 (7): 719–725.

Azar NJ, Tayah TF, Wang L et al. (2008). Postictal breathing pattern distinguishes epileptic from nonepileptic convulsive seizures. Epilepsia 49 (1): 132–137.

Babinski J (1900). Diagnostic différentiel de l'hémiplégie organique et de l'hémiplégie hystérique. Gazette des Hôpitaux de Paris 73: 533–537.

Babinski J (1907). De la pronation de la main dans l'hémiplégie organique. Rev Neurol (Paris) 15: 755.

Baik JS, Lang AE (2007). Gait abnormalities in psychogenic movement disorders. Mov Disord 22 (3): 395–399.

Baizabal-Carvallo JF, Jankovic J (2014). The clinical features of psychogenic movement disorders resembling tics. J Neurol Neurosurg Psychiatry 85 (5): 573–575.

Baker JH, Silver JR (1987). Hysterical paraplegia. J Neurol Neurosurg Psychiatry 50 (4): 375–382.

Barré J (1919). La manoeuvre de la jambe; Nouveau signe objectif des paralysies ou parésis dues aux perturbations du faisceau pyramidal. Presse Med 79: 793–795.

Bell WL, Park YD, Thompson EA et al. (1998). Ictal cognitive assessment of partial seizures and pseudoseizures. Arch Neurol 55 (11): 1456–1459.

Benbadis SR, Agrawal V, Tatum 4th WO (2001). How many patients with psychogenic nonepileptic seizures also have epilepsy? Neurology 57 (5): 915–917.

Benbadis SR, LaFrance Jr WC, Papandonatos GD et al. (2009). Interrater reliability of EEG-video monitoring. Neurology 73 (11): 843–846.

Blocq P (1888). Sur une affection caractérisée par de l'astasie et d'abasie, Vol. 43. Progrès Médical, Paris.

Bowlus WE, Currier RD (1963). A test for hysterical hemianalgesia. N Engl J Med 269: 1253–1254.

Brown MCL, Ramsay BE, Katz E et al. (1991). Characteristics of patients with nonepileptic seizures. J Epilepsy 4: 225–229.

Burneo JG, Martin R, Powell T et al. (2003). Teddy bears: an observational finding in patients with non-epileptic events. Neurology 61 (5): 714–715.

Chabrol H, Peresson G, Clanet M (1995). Lack of specificity of the traditional criteria for conversion disorders. Eur Psychiatry 10 (6): 317–319.

Chen DK, Graber KD, Anderson CT et al. (2008). Sensitivity and specificity of video alone versus electroencephalography alone for the diagnosis of partial seizures. Epilepsy Behav 13 (1): 115–118.

Chung SS, Gerber P, Kirlin KA (2006). Ictal eye closure is a reliable indicator for psychogenic nonepileptic seizures. Neurology 66 (11): 1730–1731.

Cianci V, Ferlazzo E, Condino F et al. (2011). Rating scale for psychogenic nonepileptic seizures: scale development and clinimetric testing. Epilepsy Behav 21 (2): 128–131.

Critchley M (1964). Psychiatric symptoms and parietal disease: differential diagnosis. Proc R Soc Med 57: 422–428.

Cubo E, Hinson VK, Goetz CG et al. (2005). Transcultural comparison of psychogenic movement disorders. Mov Disord 20 (10): 1343–1345.

Daum C, Aybek S (2013). Validity of the "Drift without pronation" sign in conversion disorder. BMC Neurol 13: 31.

Daum C, Hubschmid M, Aybek S (2014). The value of 'positive' clinical signs for weakness, sensory and gait disorders in conversion disorder: a systematic and narrative review. J Neurol Neurosurg Psychiatry 85 (2): 180–190.

Daum C, Gheorghita F, Spatola M et al. (2015). Interobserver agreement and validity of bedside 'positive signs' for functional weakness, sensory and gait disorders in conversion disorder: a pilot study. J Neurol Neurosurg Psychiatry 86: 425–430.

Demartini B, Ricciardi L, Pareés I et al. (2015). A positive diagnosis of functional (psychogenic) tics. Eur J Neurol 22527–e36.

DeToledo JC, Ramsay RE (1996). Patterns of involvement of facial muscles during epileptic and nonepileptic events: review of 654 events. Neurology 47 (3): 621–625.

Devinsky O, Sanchez-Villasenor F, Vazquez B et al. (1996). Clinical profile of patients with epileptic and nonepileptic seizures. Neurology 46 (6): 1530–1533.

Diukova G (2001). Sternocleidomastoid (SCM) muscle test in patients with hysterical and organic paresis. J Neurol Sci 187 (Suppl 1): S109. (PO312).

Diukova GM, Stoliarova AV (2001). Psychogenic disorders of stance and gait as seen in videotaping. Zh Nevrol Psikhiatr Im S S Korsakova 101 (12): 13–18.

Drazkowski JF, Chung SS (2010). Differential diagnosis of epilepsy. Continuum (Minneap Minn) 16 (3 Epilepsy): 36–56.

Ehrbar R, Waespe W (1992). Functional gait disorders. Schweiz Med Wochenschr 122 (22): 833–841.

Espay AJ, Goldenhar LM, Voon V et al. (2009). Opinions and clinical practices related to diagnosing and managing patients with psychogenic movement disorders: an international survey of movement disorder society members. Mov Disord 24 (9): 1366–1374.

Factor SA, Podskalny GD, Molho ES (1995). Psychogenic movement disorders: frequency, clinical profile, and characteristics. J Neurol Neurosurg Psychiatry 59 (4): 406–412.

Fahn S, Williams DT (1988). Psychogenic dystonia. Adv Neurol 50: 431–455.

Freud S (1895). Studies in hysteria. Hogarth Press, London.

Ganos C, Aguirregomozcorta M, Batla A et al. (2014). Psychogenic paroxysmal movement disorders – clinical features and diagnostic clues. Parkinsonism Relat Disord 20 (1): 41–46.

Gates JR, Ramani V, Whalen S et al. (1985). Ictal characteristics of pseudoseizures. Arch Neurol 42 (12): 1183–1187.

Geyer JD, Payne TA, Drury I (2000). The value of pelvic thrusting in the diagnosis of seizures and pseudoseizures. Neurology 54 (1): 227–229.

Goldstein LH, Mellers JD (2006). Ictal symptoms of anxiety, avoidance behaviour, and dissociation in patients with dissociative seizures. J Neurol Neurosurg Psychiatry 77 (5): 616–621.

Gould R, Miller BL, Goldberg MA et al. (1986). The validity of hysterical signs and symptoms. J Nerv Ment Dis 174 (10): 593–597.

Greer S, Chambliss L, Mackler L et al. (2005). Clinical inquiries. What physical exam techniques are useful to detect malingering? J Fam Pract 54 (8): 719–722.

Gupta A, Lang AE (2009). Psychogenic movement disorders. Curr Opin Neurol 22 (4): 430–436.

Hendrickson R, Popescu A, Dixit R et al. (2014). Panic attack symptoms differentiate patients with epilepsy from those with psychogenic nonepileptic spells (PNES). Epilepsy Behav 37: 210–214.

Henry TR, Drury I (1998). Ictal behaviors during nonepileptic seizures differ in patients with temporal lobe interictal epileptiform EEG activity and patients without interictal epileptiform EEG abnormalities. Epilepsia 39 (2): 175–182.

Hinson VK, Cubo E, Comella CL et al. (2005). Rating scale for psychogenic movement disorders: scale development and clinimetric testing. Mov Disord 20 (12): 1592–1597.

Jedrzejczak J, Owczarek K, Majkowski J (1999). Psychogenic pseudoepileptic seizures: clinical and electroencephalogram (EEG) video-tape recordings. Eur J Neurol 6 (4): 473–479.

Jordbru AA, Smedstad LM, Moen VP et al. (2012). Identifying patterns of psychogenic gait by video-recording. J Rehabil Med 44 (1): 31–35.

Keane JR (1986). Wrong-way deviation of the tongue with hysterical hemiparesis. Neurology 36 (10): 1406–1407.

Keane JR (1989). Hysterical gait disorders: 60 cases. Neurology 39 (4): 586–589.

Kenney C, Diamond A, Mejia N et al. (2007). Distinguishing psychogenic and essential tremor. J Neurol Sci 263 (1-2): 94–99.

King DW, Gallagher BB, Murvin AJ et al. (1982). Pseudoseizures: diagnostic evaluation. Neurology 32 (1): 18–23.

Knapp P (1891). Astasia-abasia. J Nerv and Ment Dis XVII 673–701.

Knutsson E, Martensson A (1985). Isokinetic measurements of muscle strength in hysterical paresis. Electroencephalogr Clin Neurophysiol 61 (5): 370–374.

Koehler PJ (2003). Freud's comparative study of hysterical and organic paralyses: how Charcot's assignment turned out. Arch Neurol 60 (11): 1646–1650.

LaFrance Jr WC, Baker GA, Duncan R et al. (2013). Minimum requirements for the diagnosis of psychogenic nonepileptic seizures: a staged approach: a report from the International League Against Epilepsy Nonepileptic Seizures Task Force. Epilepsia 54 (11): 2005–2018.

Lempert T, Brandt T, Dieterich M et al. (1991). How to identify psychogenic disorders of stance and gait. A video study in 37 patients. J Neurol 238 (3): 140–146.

Lombardi TL, Barton E, Wang J et al. (2014). The elbow flex-ex: a new sign to detect unilateral upper extremity non-organic paresis. J Neurol Neurosurg Psychiatry 85 (2): 165–167.

Magee KR (1962). Hysterical hemiplegia and hemianesthesia. Postgrad Med 31: 339–345.

Marcus H, Aldam P, Lennox G et al. (2010). Medically unexplained neurological symptoms. JRSM Short Rep 1 (3): 25.

McWhirter L, Stone J, Sandercock P et al. (2011). Hoover's sign for the diagnosis of functional weakness: a prospective unblinded cohort study in patients with suspected stroke. J Psychosom Res 71 (6): 384–386.

Morgante F, Edwards MJ, Espay AJ et al. (2012). Diagnostic agreement in patients with psychogenic movement disorders. Mov Disord 27 (4): 548–552.

Okun MS, Rodriguez RL, Foote KD et al. (2007). The "chair test" to aid in the diagnosis of psychogenic gait disorders. Neurologist 13 (2): 87–91.

Park JE, Maurer CW, Hallett M (2015). The "Whack-a-mole" sign in functional movement disorders. Mov Disord Clin Pract 2: 286–288.

Parra J, Iriarte J, Kanner AM (1999). Are we overusing the diagnosis of psychogenic non-epileptic events? Seizure 8 (4): 223–227.

Pierelli F, Chatrian GE, Erdly WW et al. (1989). Long-term EEG-video-audio monitoring: detection of partial epileptic seizures and psychogenic episodes by 24-hour EEG record review. Epilepsia 30 (5): 513–523.

Popkirov S, Grönheit W, Wellmer J (2015). A systematic review of suggestive seizure induction for the diagnosis of psychogenic nonepileptic seizures. Seizure 31: 124–132.

Ramani SV, Quesney LF, Olson D et al. (1980). Diagnosis of hysterical seizures in epileptic patients. Am J Psychiatry 137 (6): 705–709.

Reeves RR, Bullen JA (1994). Misuse of the face-hand test for psychogenic neurologic deficits. J Clin Psychiatry 55 (8): 363.

Rolak LA (1988). Psychogenic sensory loss. J Nerv Ment Dis 176 (11): 686–687.

Saygi S, Katz A, Marks DA et al. (1992). Frontal lobe partial seizures and psychogenic seizures: comparison of clinical and ictal characteristics. Neurology 42 (7): 1274–1277.

Schrag A, Lang AE (2005). Psychogenic movement disorders. Curr Opin Neurol 18 (4): 399–404.

Schwingenschuh P, Katschnig P, Seiler S et al. (2011). Moving toward "laboratory-supported" criteria for psychogenic tremor. Mov Disord 26 (14): 2509–2515.

Schwingenschuh P, Saifee TA, Katschnig-Winter P et al. (2016). Validation of "laboratory-supported" criteria for functional (psychogenic tremor). Mov Disord 31 (4): 555–562.

Sen A, Scott C, Sisodiya SM (2007). Stertorous breathing is a reliably identified sign that helps in the differentiation of epileptic from psychogenic non-epileptic convulsions: an audit. Epilepsy Res 77 (1): 62–64.

Sethi NK, Sethi PK, Torgovnick J (2010). Supine catch sign – a simple clinical test to differentiate between true and false (pseudo) radial nerve palsy. Clin Neurol Neurosurg 112 (5): 441–442.

Shill H, Gerber P (2006). Evaluation of clinical diagnostic criteria for psychogenic movement disorders. Mov Disord 21 (8): 1163–1168.

Slater JD, Brown MC, Jacobs W et al. (1995). Induction of pseudoseizures with intravenous saline placebo. Epilepsia 36 (6): 580–585.

Sonoo M (2004). Abductor sign: a reliable new sign to detect unilateral non-organic paresis of the lower limb. J Neurol Neurosurg Psychiatry 75 (1): 121–125.

Southard E (1919). Shell-shock and other neuropsychiatric problems. WM Leonard, Boston.

Stamelou M, Edwards MJ, Espay AJ et al. (2011). Movement disorders on YouTube – caveat spectator. N Engl J Med 365 (12): 1160–1161.

Stone J, Zeman A, Sharpe M (2002). Functional weakness and sensory disturbance. J Neurol Neurosurg Psychiatry 73 (3): 241–245.

Stone J, Warlow C, Sharpe M (2010). The symptom of functional weakness: a controlled study of 107 patients. Brain 133 (Pt 5): 1537–1551.

Stone J, LaFrance Jr WC, Brown R et al. (2011). Conversion disorder: current problems and potential solutions for DSM-5. J Psychosom Res 71 (6): 369–376.

Stone J, Carson A, Duncan R et al. (2012). Which neurological diseases are most likely to be associated with 'symptoms unexplained by organic disease'. J Neurol 259 (1): 33–38.

Stone J, Reuber M, Carson A (2013). Functional symptoms in neurology: mimics and chameleons. Pract Neurol 13 (2): 104–113.

Syed TU, Arozullah AM, Suciu GP et al. (2008). Do observer and self-reports of ictal eye closure predict psychogenic nonepileptic seizures? Epilepsia 49 (5): 898–904.

Syed TU, LaFrance Jr WC, Kahriman ES et al. (2011). Can semiology predict psychogenic nonepileptic seizures? A prospective study. Ann Neurol 69 (6): 997–1004.

Thomas M, Jankovic J (2004). Psychogenic movement disorders: diagnosis and management. CNS Drugs 18 (7): 437–452.

Tinazzi M, Simonetto S, Franco L et al. (2008). Abduction finger sign: a new sign to detect unilateral functional paralysis of the upper limb. Mov Disord 23 (16): 2415–2419.

Todd RB (1856). Clinical lectures on paralysis, certain diseases of the brain, and other affections of the nervous system. 2nd edn. Lecture 1, London. 20.

van der Salm SM, de Haan RJ, Cath DC et al. (2013). The eye of the beholder: inter-rater agreement among experts on psychogenic jerky movement disorders. J Neurol Neurosurg Psychiatry 84 (7): 742–747.

van der Salm SM, Erro R, Cordivan C et al. (2014). Propriospinal myoclonus: Clinical reappraisal and review of literature. Neurology 83 (20): 1862–1870.

Vinton A, Carino J, Vogrin S et al. (2004). "Convulsive" nonepileptic seizures have a characteristic pattern of rhythmic artifact distinguishing them from convulsive epileptic seizures. Epilepsia 45 (11): 1344–1350.

Voon V, Lang AE, Hallett M (2007). Diagnosing psychogenic movement disorders – which criteria should be used in clinical practice? Nat Clin Pract Neurol 3 (3): 134–135.

Vossler DG, Haltiner AM, Schepp SK et al. (2004). Ictal stuttering: a sign suggestive of psychogenic nonepileptic seizures. Neurology 63 (3): 516–519.

Walczak TS, Bogolioubov A (1996). Weeping during psychogenic nonepileptic seizures. Epilepsia 37 (2): 208–210.

Williams DT, Ford B, Fahn S (1994). Phenomenology and psychopathology related to psychogenic movement disorders. In: WJ Weiner, AE Lang (Eds.), Behavioural neurology in movement disorders. Raven Press, New York, pp. 231–257.

Yugue I, Shiba K, Ueta T et al. (2004). A new clinical evaluation for hysterical paralysis. (Phila Pa 1976) 29 (17): 1910–1913. discussion 1913.

Ziv I, Djaldetti R, Zoldan Y et al. (1998). Diagnosis of "non-organic" limb paresis by a novel objective motor assessment: the quantitative Hoover's test. J Neurol 245 (12): 797–802.

Handbook of Clinical Neurology, Vol. 139 (3rd series)
Functional Neurologic Disorders
M. Hallett, J. Stone, and A. Carson, Editors
http://dx.doi.org/10.1016/B978-0-12-801772-2.00018-7

Chapter 18

Functional limb weakness and paralysis

J. STONE[1]* AND S. AYBEK[2]

[1]*Department of Clinical Neurosciences, Centre for Clinical Brain Sciences, University of Edinburgh, Edinburgh, UK*

[2]*Neurology Service, Geneva University Hospitals and Laboratory for Behavioural Neurology and Imaging of Cognition, University of Geneva-Campus Biotech, Geneva, Switzerland*

Abstract

Functional (psychogenic) limb weakness describes genuinely experienced limb power or paralysis in the absence of neurologic disease. The hallmark of functional limb weakness is the presence of internal inconsistency revealing a pattern of symptoms governed by abnormally focused attention.

In this chapter we review the history and epidemiology of this clinical presentation as well as its subjective experience highlighting the detailed descriptions of authors at the end of the 19th and early 20th century. We discuss the relevance that physiological triggers such as injury and migraine and psychophysiological events such as panic and dissociation have to understanding of mechanism and treatment. We review many different positive diagnostic features, their basis in neurophysiological testing and present data on sensitivity and specificity. Diagnostic bedside tests with the most evidence are Hoover's sign, the hip abductor sign, drift without pronation, dragging gait, give way weakness and co-contraction.

INTRODUCTION

We begin with a review of the history of functional paralysis in terms of its conception and clinical description. This section is unusually long, but that is because the historic literature is arguably as relevant today as our current clinical studies. The wider context of thoughts on hysteria can be found elsewhere Chapters 1–4. We then summarize what is known about its epidemiology and the reliability of positive signs in this area (Daum et al., 2014a, b). Imaging, neurophysiology, other etiologic models, and treatment are covered in other chapters of this volume.

HISTORIC DESCRIPTIONS

Paralysis is perhaps the quintessential functional neurologic symptom, and one of the most dramatic and obvious examples of loss of function among all functional disorders.

Historic descriptions of functional paralysis are numerous. Arguably, one of the first is in Luke 5:18–25:

> *Some men came carrying a paralysed man on a mat and tried to take him into the house to lay him before Jesus. When they could not find a way to do this because of the crowd, they went up on the roof and lowered him on his mat through the tiles into the middle of the crowd, right in front of Jesus ... So he said to the paralysed man, "I tell you, get up, take your mat and go home." Immediately he stood up in front of them, took what he had been lying on and went home praising God.*

In medieval times, religious institutions across Europe collected examples of patients with paralysis who had been miraculously cured by shrines. Churches also provided rehabilitation for visiting pilgrims. At least some of the miracle cures could, however, have plausibly occurred because the original problem was functional paralysis. This one was said to have occurred in the 12th century in Reading, England.

> *Ysembla, a young girl, slept out in the open one summer and thereby disabled her body and lost*

*Correspondence to: Jon Stone, Department of Clinical Neurosciences, Centre for Clinical Brain Sciences, University of Edinburgh, Crew Rd, Edinburgh EH4 2 XU, UK. Tel: +44-131-537-1167, E-mail: jon.stone@ed.ac.uk

her agility. In fact, her left side from the sole of her foot to her shoulder had withered and lost all living movement. Her hand was shrunken and paralysed and hung motionless from her side close to her back. Her foot was bent round and, incapable of acting as a foot … In the church at Reading she threw herself on the pavement and, letting out the most piercing cries, screamed in all directions. She shook her head about, banged her head and dashed her body against the stone with so little consideration for herself that one might have thought that she wished to destroy herself … After three hours the cure started, her limbs coming back to life so that she moved from a sprawling to a proper posture … The girl then returned home completely cured (Kemp, 1970).

Hysteria was a common subject among 17th- and 18th-century medical writers such as Willis, Cheyne, and Whytt. Specific examples of paralysis are hard to find though before the 19th century.

Sir Benjamin Brodie (1783–1862) was surgeon to Queen Victoria and the first president of the General Medical Council. In 1837, he published his thoughts about "local hysterical affections." In describing hysterical paralysis, he made the following observation: "In hysterical paralysis, it is not that the muscles are incapable of obeying the act of volition, but that the function of volition is not exercised" (Brodie, 1837).

Like the other authors mentioned below, he had quite complex views about the causes of hysteria which encompassed moral, nutritional, social, and physiologic disturbance.

Robert Todd (1809–1860), a London physician, is famous for his description of hemiplegia after an epileptic fit ("Todd's paralysis"). In his 1854 book on paralysis, he also gives the first clear description of the monoplegic hysterical gait. "She drags the palsied limb after her, as if it were a piece of inanimate matter … the foot sweeps the ground as she walks" (Todd, 1854).

His view on the cause of "hysterical" paralysis, like others of the day, was multifactorial, incorporating moral aspects but also physiologic abnormalities in the nervous system. "I believe hysterical paralysis is caused by depraved nutrition of the nerves of the limb affected, or of some part of the centre of volition."

Paul Briquet (1796–1881) is credited with the first systematic study of hysteria in 1859 (Briquet, 1859). In his dissertation he reports that 120 of his 430 cases had paralysis and he also introduces the notion that this symptom is more common on the left (since in his sample the ratio was 7:2). Like Todd, Briquet adopted a multifactorial view about the causes of hysteria. He describes predisposing factors, including female sex, low intelligence, young age, and heredity. He thought personality (being impressionable, fearful, prone to intense feeling, affectionate) and childhood experience (too soft or too hard) were important predisposing factors. He lists 16 precipitating causes, mainly different types of life events (marital and family problems, bad news) but also illness (such as pneumonia) and overwork. He also mentions the importance of shock after witnessing unexpected events such as a death or a fire.

Despite this broad approach to hysteria he also thought a biologic mechanism may be important in hysterical paralysis, suggesting that this might correlate with "injection of capillary vessels in nerve centres in the brain."

Sir James Paget (1814–1899), of Paget's disease, wrote an influential article in the *Lancet* in 1873 entitled "Nervous mimicry," which he also called "neuromimesis" (Paget, 1873). He used this term to describe "unwilling imitation of organic disease … a serious affection, making life useless and unhappy and not shortening it." His pithy description of "neuromimetic paralysis," expanding on Brodie's, is increasingly quoted as an early piece of cognitive neuropsychology observation:

A girl who has will enough in other things to rule the house has yet not will enough in regard to her limbs to walk a step with them, though they are as muscular as ever in her life. She says, as all such patients do, "I cannot"; it looks like "I will not"; but it is "I cannot will" (Paget, 1873).

The contribution of Jean-Martin Charcot (1825–1893) to hysteria is explored in Chapter 2 of this volume. With respect to paralysis, his clinical observations, unlike some of those he made of hysterical seizures, hold up perfectly well. He gives us one of the earliest photographs of a patient with the functional "dragging" gait (Fig. 18.1), described earlier by Todd.

His view on the mechanism of functional paralysis, that there must be some kind of "dynamic or functional lesions" to account for the symptom of paralysis, has seen a renaissance in the era of functional brain imaging. Some authors have become confused over Charcot's views, not appreciating that he saw a physiologic mechanism as compatible with a psychologic etiology.

One of the most lasting contributions from this period can be found in the work of Pierre Janet (1859–1947), Charcot's assistant, who was later given his own psychologic laboratory at the Salpêtrière. Only two of his works are in English (Janet, 1901, 1907). They are evidence of extensive clinical experience combined with a meticulous approach to talking to patients.

Janet summarized his work in 1907 in the book *The Major Symptoms of Hysteria*. In it, he steers the middle ground between physiologic and psychologic explanations towards something approaching cognitive neuropsychology. Janet is interested more in mechanism than in general predisposition.

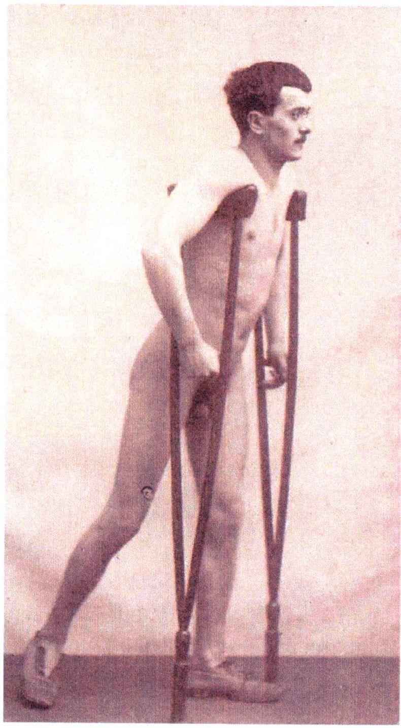
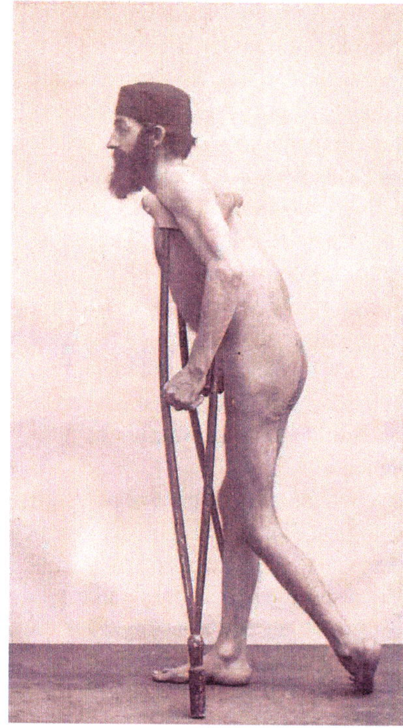

Fig. 18.1. Two patients from Charcot's *Nouvelle Iconographie de Salpêtrière* with "hysterical" hemiplegic gait (Charcot, 1888).

In the chapter on paralysis he places great weight on the frequency of "accidents" as precipitating factors: "they are always brought about by an accident which, while very slight in itself, is accompanied by a violent moral emotion and by disturbances of the imagination" (Janet, 1907).

It is worth recounting some of these "accidents," which include:

- minor injuries to the buttock or back, leading to lower-limb paralysis.
- fatigue of a limb from playing a musical instrument or painting a ceiling, leading gradually to paralysis.
- an "accident" which was not an actual accident at all, but one that was imagined to have happened, for example:

> *A man travelling by train had done an imprudent thing: while the train was running, he had got down on the step in order to pass from one door to the other, when he became aware that the train was about to enter a tunnel. It occurred to him that his left side, which projected, was going to be knocked slantwise and crushed against the arch of the tunnel. This thought caused him to swoon away but happily for him, he did not fall on the track, but was taken back inside the carriage, and his left side was not even grazed. In spite of this, he had a left hemiplegia (Janet, 1907).*

- a woman who developed hand paralysis at the moment of having to play the piano in public.
- a woman who dreamt at night that she was running away from a man, was exhausted and in her dream could not move. She then wakes up paralyzed.
- a woman who developed gradual-onset hemiplegia in her right side which she had been using to support her father who had just died
- after profound sleep.
- after a "convulsive fit."
- a nurse who thought she saw a ghost was frightened and felt her legs shake. Her legs then "gave way" and she became paraplegic.
- paraplegia after childbirth.

In describing the underlying psychology of hysterical paralysis and sensory loss, Janet is struck by the way that sensations and actions seem to be split off from patients' consciousness. He discusses examples of defects in mental imagery which he and others had observed:

> *Féré was one of the first who insisted on this point. "After having shut the patient's eyes," he says, "I ask her to try to represent to herself her left hand executing movements of extension and flexion. She is not able to do it. She can represent to herself her right hand making very complicated movements on the piano, but on her left, she has the sensation that her hand is lost in empty space. She cannot even represent to herself its form." I have verified this remark more than twenty times (Janet, 1907).*

Finally Janet discusses patients with selective paralysis. In astasia-abasia a patient has normal leg movements on the bed but is unable to walk. Patients who can run but can't walk, or move their lips but can't blow are also described. He uses these patients to show how certain systems of movements (what we would now call motor programs) can be selectively lost. Some of these patients may have had apraxia rather than hysteria. They still make the point that Janet was comfortable with the idea that a symptom could arise from a problem in a "system" that could not be accurately described as strictly psychologic or strictly anatomic. "The fact that a system is psychological should not cause us to conclude that it is not at the same time anatomical. On the contrary, the one involves the other" (Janet, 1907).

As supporters of psychoanalysis never tire of pointing out, Freud was a neurologist before he became a psychiatrist. One of his early papers was a description of the difference between organic and hysterical paralysis. It is hard to find anything in it which had not already been articulated elsewhere. Open any textbook of neurology around that time and there would usually be a hefty section on the diagnosis of hysteria. Even the celebrated notion that hysterical paralysis relates to the "idea of a limb" rather than anatomy had already been presaged by others, including Ross Reynolds (1869).

Gowers

Sir William Gowers' (1845–1915) magisterial chapter on hysteria in his single-volume textbook of neurology echoes others in this period who viewed the mechanism as a disturbance of the function of the nervous system which could affect men as well as women (Gowers, 1892).

> *The conditions of hemianaesthesia, paralysis and contracture must be regarded as the expression of a condition of restrained function (inhibition) or unrestrained activity, of certain cerebral centres, sensory and motor.*

The importance of normal physiology was stressed in terms of how symptoms might develop.

> *Paraplegia is excited by emotion with especial frequency. Even in health a sensation of weakness in the legs may be caused by sudden alarm, and this, in hysteria, may be followed by a progressive loss of power. It is common for the onset of persistent weakness to be preceded by occasional momentary "giving way of the legs," at once recovered from – a very characteristic feature.*

He also appreciated the importance of pain in precipitating paralysis: "Spinal pain is very common in these cases, and being increased by standing, may distinctly excite the paralysis."

Late 19th- and early 20th-century descriptions

Silas Weir Mitchell, the US neurologist, contributed a 132-page chapter on neurasthenia, hysteria, and traumatic neuroses to Dercum's *A Textbook on Nervous Diseases* in 1895 (Fig. 18.2). He made the following observation about hysterical paralysis:

> *It is especially likely to be caused or aggravated by a convulsion. Thus it may appear as a prodrome, and may persist after the fit for various periods. It may be caused by trauma – a not infrequent cause, and a most important one to be recognized ... Again hysterical paralysis may be caused by emotion, such as fright, anger, chagrin, or disappointed love (Dercum, 1895).*

Thomas Savill (1856–1910), a London physician, had rather biologic views about hysteria but also made a similar observation about the onset of patients with functional motor disorders, consistent with a view that some kind of nociceptive or altered experience ranging from mild dissociation to a dissociative nonepileptic attack could commonly trigger the symptoms:

> *If the patient is under careful observation at the time of onset, it will generally be found that cases of cerebral paresis, rigidity or tremor are actually initiated, about the time of onset, by a more or less transient hysterical cerebral attack...*
>
> *Affirmative evidence on this point is not always forthcoming unless the patient was at the time under observation, or is himself an intelligent observer. I found affirmative evidence of this point in 47/50 cases of hysterical motor disorder which I investigated particularly. Sometimes there was only a "swimming" in the head, or a slight syncopal or vertiginous attack, slight confusion of the mind, or transient loss of speech, but in quite a number there was generalised trepidation or convulsions (Savill, 1909).*

Paul Dubois, the Swiss neuropathologist, was a pioneer of cognitive therapy with his doctrine of "rational persuasion" and saw many patients with hysteria. He had this to say in 1909 about the role of emotional shock and the way in which physiologic states of paralysis might become persistent in a vulnerable individual. It elaborates a view on how psychologic factors can be grafted on to physiologic experiences:

> *There is generally no room for doubt when it is a question of hysterical paraplegia occurring suddenly under the influence of anger or spite...It is a result of a psychic shock, and is only an exaggeration of the feeling of motor helplessness*

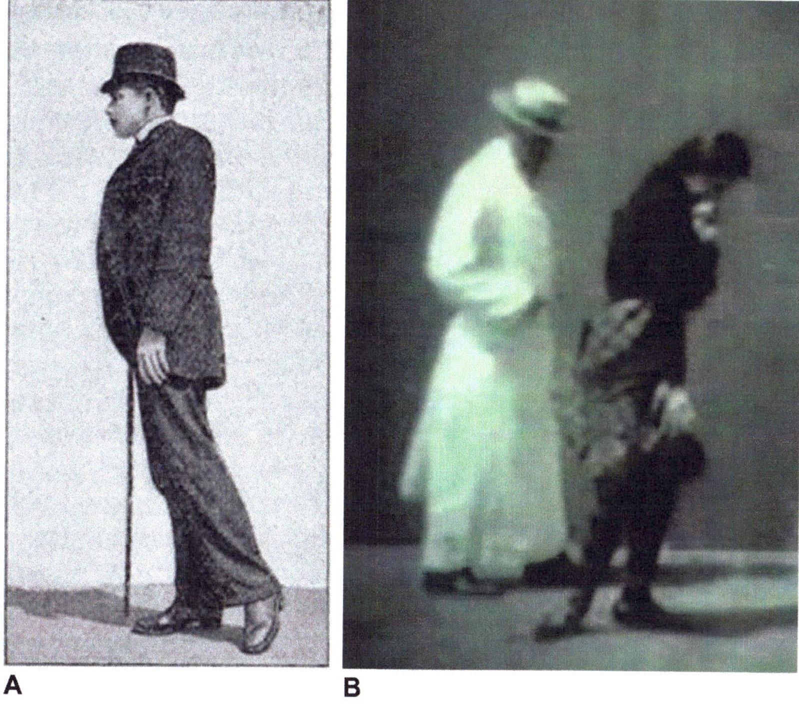

Fig. 18.2. (**A**) A case of traumatic hysterical paraplegia from Dercum's *A Textbook on Nervous Diseases by American Authors* (Dercum, 1895). (**B**) Hysterical hemiplegia (still) from a very early 1903 film by Romanian neurologist Marinescu (Barboi et al., 2004).

> *which takes possession of us under emotion and which we express by saying that "our legs give way under us!" Transient in the normal man the phenomenon becomes lasting in the hysterical patient who is always disposed to believe that the slightest functional disturbance is real (Dubois, 1909).*

The First World War and shellshock saw an increase in interest on hysteria and vigorous debate between those who believed in psychodynamic interpretations on one hand and those favoring a lack of moral fiber and cowardice on the other (discussed in Chapter 3 and by many authors, e.g., Wessely and Jones, 2005).

Ultimately the psychodynamic interpretations won out. For example, three books, *Functional Nerve Disease* (Miller, 1920), *The Pathology, Diagnosis and Treatment of Functional Nervous Diseases* (Bousfield, 1926) and *Functional Nervous Disorders* (Core, 1922), written during the 1920s, are heavily psychoanalytic despite their titles and their physician authors.

Explanations like this one were given regarding paralysis:

> *How can we regard a functional monoplegia as a primitive expression of thought? Gesture is primitive speech. A monoplegia is a gesture towards life, negative in character...It is not the arm as an anatomically or neurologically conceived structure that is involved, but it is the* thought *of the arm (Nicoll and Young, 1920).*

Mid to late 20th century

Once psychodynamic theories had taken hold there was remarkably little published research specifically on the clinical features and potential mechanism of functional paralysis over the latter half of the 20th century. Textbook descriptions became increasingly rare and less detailed (Stone et al., 2008). This began to change in the 1990s with the first functional imaging study of a "hysterical paralysis" (Marshall et al., 1997) along with better epidemiologic studies (Binzer et al., 1997; Crimlisk et al., 1998) (Fig. 18.3).

Early photographs often appeared unnecessarily sexualized, although most photographs of males and females at this time were taken nude.

EPIDEMIOLOGY

Prevalence and incidence

Population-based

Functional limb weakness usually requires diagnosis in secondary care by a neurologist. Population-based studies are therefore very difficult to perform and are likely to be strongly contaminated with other diagnoses. Older

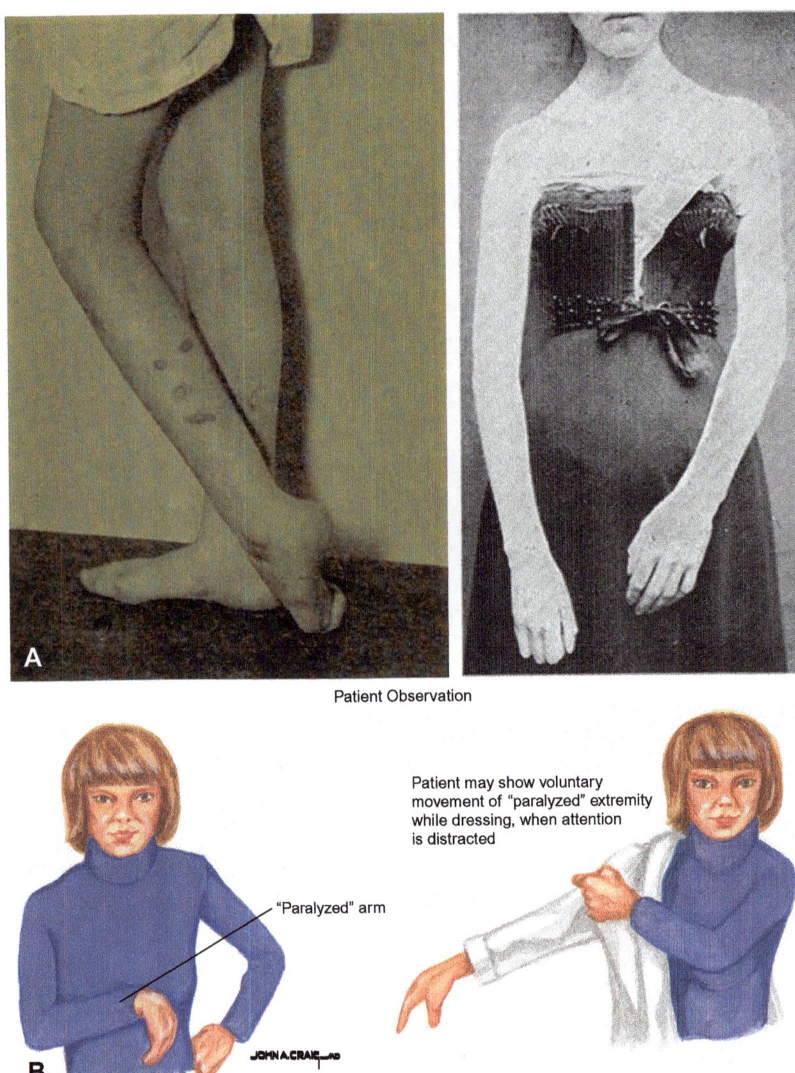

Fig. 18.3. (**A**) Depictions of functional weakness in a neurology textbook from the early 20th century. Right leg functional weakness with "self-inflicted burns" (left panel); Right functional arm weakness (right panel) (Purves-Stewart, 1911). (**B**) Illustration from 1970s text depicting inconsistency in arm movement (Weintraub, 1977).

studies from the St. Louis group who developed the concept of somatization disorder found a lifetime prevalence of an episode of unexplained paralysis in psychiatric patients, postpartum women, and medically ill patients to be high, at 7%, 9%, and 12% respectively (Farley et al., 1968; Woodruff, 1968; Woodruff et al., 1969). A study in Germany of 2050 people looked at a range of physical symptoms, asking patients to report symptoms for which there was no medical explanation (Rief et al., 2001). This reported a rate of 2% for "weakness," which was maintained in patients under the age of 45 (Rief, personal communication), although patients commonly use the term weakness to refer to generalized fatigue and limb heaviness as well as specific limb weakness.

Secondary care settings

In neurologic settings, Binzer et al.'s controlled study of 30 patients with recent-onset functional limb weakness in Sweden led to a minimum population incidence of 5/100 000 (Binzer et al., 1997). The study of one of the authors (JS) of 107 patients in Scotland with functional limb weakness equated to a minimum incidence of 3.7/100 000 (Stone et al., 2010b). Such numbers are similar to multiple sclerosis (3/100 000) and primary brain tumor (5/100 000).

Epidemiology within outpatient settings is discussed in more detail in Chapter 5. In our own study of 3781 neurology outpatients, approximately 15% had a functional or psychologic diagnosis and 5.5% had a primary diagnosis of a motor/sensory/seizure disorder. There were 45 patients with functional limb weakness (1.2%), and many more probably classified within a group labeled nonspecifically by neurologists as nonorganic ($n = 87$) (Stone et al., 2010a). Studies of neurology inpatients have suggested frequencies of functional paralysis between 1% and 18% (Schiffer, 1983; Marsden, 1986; Metcalfe et al., 1988; Ewald et al., 1994), and frequencies after back surgery of up to 3% (Janssen et al., 1995). These figures are likely to represent an underestimate given prevailing attitudes to the diagnosis of functional disorders over the time scales of these studies.

Age of onset and gender

Functional limb weakness has been reported in a wide range of ages, from children aged 5 up to the mid-70s. We have personally seen a case at the age of 83 with clearly positive clinical features. Looking at the main case series, the average age of onset is in the mid to late 30s (Ehrbar and Waespe, 1992; Binzer et al., 1997; Stone et al., 2010). This is in contrast to dissociative (nonepileptic) seizures, where age of onset averages mid-20s (Stone et al., 2004).

Analysis of gender across multiple studies shows heterogeneity. An analysis of seven studies comprising a total of 167 patients with functional limb weakness found an overall proportion of 48% female (Stone et al., 2004), but this was potentially biased because of studies from some military settings. In the studies where patients were clearly consecutive in secondary care there was a preponderance of females, although men are certainly not rare (%females: 80% ($n = 56$) (Stone et al., 2009b), 79% ($n = 107$) (Stone et al., 2010b), 64% ($n = 98$) (Gargalas et al., 2015), 62% ($n = 105$) (Nazir et al., 2005), and 60% ($n = 30$) (Binzer et al., 1997)).

CLINICAL FEATURES IN THE HISTORY

Subjective experience

Patients with functional limb weakness may present with nonspecific heaviness or weakness of a limb. Commonly, however, they have symptoms which are less common in other causes of limb weakness. They often describe symptoms of depersonalization for the affected limb, complaining that the limb feels as if it "isn't there" or "doesn't feel a part of me." They may complain that the limb is a "solid object" which feels as if it is "attached" or "stuck on" to them.

When the hand or arm is affected patient may often report frequently dropping things. Patients with neurologic disease may drop things too, but generally get a sense of how their limb will perform, whereas patients with functional limb weakness have quite variable weakness, so appear to drop things more often.

When there is functional leg weakness patients may report that they have to drag the leg and that it gives way at the knee. Such complaints lead some patients to orthopedic surgeons and investigations for knee instability.

Sensory symptoms, such as reduced sensation, are nearly universal in functional paralysis, perhaps reflecting the underlying mechanism of the symptom. Functional sensory symptoms are discussed in Chapter 24.

The neurologist Oliver Sacks described these symptoms in a book, *A Leg to Stand On* (1984), which recorded his experiences after experiencing a traumatic quadriceps rupture. One of the authors (JS) proposed that the book was a clear description of functional limb paralysis triggered by physical injury (Stone et al., 2012b):

> *I knew not my leg. It was utterly strange, not-mine, unfamiliar. I gazed upon it with absolute non-recognition ... The more I gazed at that cylinder of chalk, the more alien and incomprehensible it appeared to me. I could no longer feel it was "mine," as part of me. It seemed to bear no relation whatever to me. It was absolutely not-me and yet, impossibly, it was attached to me and even more impossibly, "continuous" with me (Sacks, 1984).*

Oliver Sacks, in an editorial reply (Sacks, 2012), did not agree that it was a functional disorder but did acknowledge that, "The sorts of complex perceptual and relational difficulties described in *A Leg to Stand On* are increasingly recognised as normal brain responses to peripheral injuries." In fact, his conception of the disorder, as a central effect of peripheral injury, maps on well to more modern biopsychosocial views of what functional paralysis is, and not well on to conceptions of hysteria as conceived in the 1970s when the injury occurred.

Distribution and laterality

Patterns of limb weakness can occur in any pattern, including triparesis. Unilateral symptoms, either hemiparesis or monoparesis, appear to be the commonest. Monoparesis was perhaps unusually overrepresented in some series (30%, $n = 30$) (Binzer et al., 1997); (37%, $n = 81$) (Lempert et al., 1990), although was not more common than controls with weakness due to neurologic disease in another study (16% vs. 24%) (Stone et al., 2010b). Clinically many patients who complain mostly of weakness in the arm or leg have mild weakness in the same limb. Lateralized symptoms occur in most patients (e.g., 79% (Stone et al., 2010b), 83% (Gargalas et al., 2015)). Patients with paraplegia or tetraplegia often have back pain and anecdotally more commonly have complete paralysis.

A systematic review of the laterality of functional limb weakness in 2002 involving 584 patients and 82 studies found that weakness was more common on the left (58%) in all studies. However, there was a suggestion of recruitment bias, because studies that set out to examine this question found a high frequency on the left (69%), whereas those that didn't found no difference (50%). Subsequent studies have tended to confirm that if there is a bias to left-sided symptoms it is small: 54% ($n = 107$) (Stone et al., 2010b); 59% ($n = 94$) (Gargalas et al., 2015); and 52% ($n = 105$) (Nazir et al., 2005).

Onset

Around half of patients with functional limb weakness present with sudden, stroke-like symptoms (Stone et al., 2012a). The rest present with more gradual-onset symptoms, making clinicians think more about multiple sclerosis or spinal lesions. The historic introduction to this chapter highlighted how commonly authors such as Pierre Janet commented on relevant physiologic, psychophysiologic, or pathologic triggers to functional paralysis, including injury, neurologic disease, panic attacks, dissociation, and dissociative (nonepileptic) seizures.

One of the authors of this chapter (JS) studied the mechanisms of onset among 107 patients with functional limb weakness, of whom 49 reported a sudden onset (Stone et al., 2012a). These historically reported triggers were found in modern-day patients and often overlapped with each other (Fig. 18.4). In addition, there were other

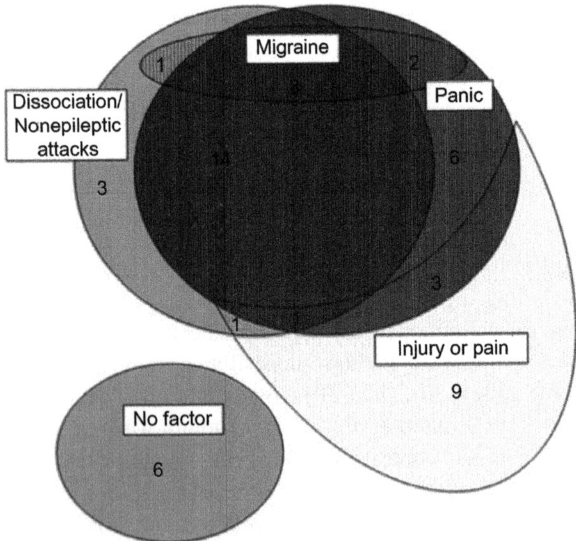

Fig. 18.4. Overlap of associated symptoms associated with onset of functional weakness in patients with sudden onset of symptoms ($n = 49$). (Reproduced from Stone et al., 2011, with permission.)

physiologic triggers such as sleep paralysis, prolonged bed rest, general anesthesia, and, in some cases, a health professional had noted the problem first.

Patients with functional paralysis can be reluctant to describe symptoms such as dissociation, which are hard to capture in words and may lead them to have concerns that they are "going mad." Conversely, if a clinician obtains information that during a panic attack or dissociative attack, the patient felt disembodied, it becomes relatively much easier to discuss how the paralysis has arisen as a residual effect of the episode. Hyperventilation during panic attack may also cause unilateral paresthesia (Blau et al., 1983), which, like migrainous paresthesia and heaviness, appears to form the stimulus for the development of functional limb weakness in some susceptible individuals.

Physical injury has a long history of association with functional neurologic disorders and is not uncommonly a trigger for functional limb weakness. A systematic review of 132 studies ($n = 869$ patients with functional motor or sensory symptoms) found 397 cases of functional limb weakness in which clinical features were described. A remarkable 41% of these cases had some kind of physical injury at onset (Stone et al., 2009a). Similarly high values were found for functional movement disorder (41%, $n = 397$) and even higher rates have been seen preceding functional/fixed dystonia (Schrag et al., 2004).

Complex regional pain syndrome (CRPS) is defined by a triggering physical injury. Weakness is one of the most common symptoms associated with the disorder (Veldman et al., 1993). When limb weakness, tremor, dystonia, or sensory disturbance has been subject to close scrutiny in CRPS, it is clear that it has the same qualities as functional limb weakness without pain (Birklein et al., 2000). New data on motor and sensory disturbances in CRPS are therefore likely to be relevant to patients with functional limb weakness also (Punt et al., 2013).

Such data need to be studied more carefully in neurologic disease, but the concept of a noxious stimulus triggering functional disorders is nonetheless one that can be useful when explaining and treating functional limb weakness (see Chapter 44).

Other functional disorders and symptoms

Like most functional neurologic symptoms, functional limb weakness rarely exists in isolation. In the case-control study of 107 patients with functional limb weakness vs. 46 controls with neurologic disease causing limb weakness, fatigue (82% vs. 65%), sleep disturbance (75% vs. 41%), pain (64% vs. 35%), memory symptoms (6% vs. 41%), gastrointestinal symptoms (49% vs. 20%), headache 40% vs. 9%, and back pain (36% vs. 17%) were all significantly more frequent in cases.

Dissociative nonepileptic attacks are reported in at least two series (14%) (Stone et al., 2010b); 23% (Crimlisk et al., 1998) at rates that are much higher than the general population, suggesting a shared etiology or mechanism.

Neurologic and other disease

Neurologic disease has long been known to be a powerful risk factor for functional disorders. In a study of 73 patients with mixed functional motor disorders (in which half were paralysis), 48% had a neurologic disease as well (Crimlisk et al., 1998). Half of these were peripheral neurologic disorders. Surgical comorbidity in the form of hysterectomy, appendicectomy, and cholecystectomy is common, often because of confounding with other functional disorders.

PHYSICAL SIGNS OF FUNCTIONAL LIMB WEAKNESS

The diagnosis of functional weakness should be made primarily on the basis of physical assessment. Below we list the many physical signs of functional weakness and in Table 18.1 provide data with respect to their sensitivity and specificity. The difficulty with nearly all of these studies is the lack of a gold standard for diagnosis. Thus it is likely that the test itself has often been used to make the diagnosis (diagnostic suspicion bias). The data should therefore be approached with caution, as indeed should be the case for any diagnostic sign in neurology. Preferably the diagnosis should be made using multiple positive features on assessment supported by a typical clinical picture.

General pitfalls of these tests are:

1. failure to consider that a patient who clearly has functional limb weakness may also have a comorbid neurologic disease.
2. failure to consider the influence of pain on the presentation. Pain also increases with abnormally focused attention and may result in a false-positive result.
3. patients with any condition may be keen to demonstrate that their problem is genuine by helping out the examiner.
4. cortical neglect and parietal lesions sometimes produce false positives.
5. mildly positive signs should be interpreted with caution.

General signs of functional limb weakness

Global pattern of weakness

One of the most striking features of functional limb weakness is the way in which all muscle groups are equally affected, unlike, for example, pyramidal, proximal, or distal patterns of weakness seen in neurologic disease processes.

Table 18.1

Sensitivity and specificity of functional sensory signs, using data from Daum et al. (2014a, b). Data should be interpreted with caution due to methodological issues described in text

Test	Sensitivity	Specificity	Positive predictive value	Number		Studies
				Case	Control	
Hoover's sign	63%	100%	99%	8	116	McWhirter et al. (2011)
	75%	100%	99%	16	17	Sonoo (2004)
	100%	100%	99%	8	11	Tinazzi et al. (2008)
	95%	86%	67%	63	7	Stone et al. (2010b)
	76%	100%	100%	17	18	Daum et al. (2014a)
Hip abductor sign	100%	100%	100%	16	17	Sonoo (2004)
Drift without pronation	93%	100%	93%	26	28	Daum and Aybek (2013)
	47%	100%	100%	19	20	Daum et al. (2014a)
Leg-dragging gait	11%	100%	100%	19	19	Daum et al. (2014a)
	8%	100%	100%	107	46	Stone et al. (2010b)
Give-way weakness	90%	100%	100%	20	20	Daum et al. (2014a)
	69%	98%	98%	107	46	Stone et al. (2010b)
	20%	95%	60%	15	40	Chabrol et al. (1995)
Co-contraction	40%	100%	100%	20	19	Daum et al. (2014a)
	20%	100%	100%	20	23	Baker and Silver (1987)

Give-way weakness

This is sudden loss of tone after an initial good/normal-strength response when a muscle is tested against resistance. To check that power is actually briefly normal, the instruction, "At the count of three, stop me from pushing: 3, 2, 1, push" may be helpful. Alternatively, apply very gentle pressure to the movement and gradually build up from imperceptible pressure to normal. Neurophysiologic studies of collapsing weakness have concluded that there is a relationship between muscle force and speed of movement: the slower the movement, the less force there is (Knutsson and Martensson, 1985). It is possible to dissect these differences neurophysiologically to form a clinical test, described below (van der Ploeg and Oosterhuis, 1991). The lack of development in this area may be due to the relative ease of making the diagnosis by a trained neurologist, although quantifiable diagnostic tests would be useful. This sign should be interpreted with caution when there is pain in the limb, especially in a joint. Myasthenia can sometimes appear to cause collapsing weakness.

Co-contraction

Co-contraction is important (and effortful) contraction of one muscle and its agonist resulting in almost no movement at the articulation. In a neurophysiologic study of 12 subjects with functional leg weakness, it was found that knee flexion was weaker than it would have been just with gravity (Knutsson and Martensson, 1985).

Motor inconsistency

Motor inconsistency is important difference of motor performance in different testing condition. For example:

- complete plegia of one limb when tested on the examination bed but strength maintained in that same leg when standing up and walking
- ability to use a hand to reach into a bag or tie shoelaces (Fig. 18.3)
- ability to stand on tiptoes or heels but very little ankle strength on the bed
- occasionally patients find that their weak limbs, when put into a certain position, will stay there – "pseudo waxy flexibility."

Inverse pyramidal weakness

In some patients a pattern of weakness occurs which is the opposite of pyramidal weakness, i.e., with weakness concentrated on the flexors in the arms and the extensors of the legs.

Signs of functional weakness in the face, neck, and arms

Functional facial spasm

This is discussed in detail in Chapter 31 and by Kaski et al. (2015). Functional facial spasm refers to contraction of orbicularis oculis on one side and/or hemiplatysmal contraction, leading to jaw deviation or a protruding lip. It can give the appearance of facial weakness, although it is actually a hyperkinetic movement disorder. This is a relatively common presentation and when it occurs is not only a clue to the nature of the facial symptoms (see Chapter 31), but also to the nature of the hemiparesis, which commonly presents ipsilateral to the facial symptoms.

Sternocleidomastoid test

In a stroke, sternocleidomastoid weakness is relatively unusual as the innervation is bilateral. However, if there is weakness then you would expect that to be of head turning to the contralateral side. In some patients with functional hemiparesis there is weakness of head turning to the ipsilateral side (Diukova et al., 2001).

Drift without pronation

The patient is asked to lift both arms in the air with forearms supinated and eyes closed to test for pronator drift. In functional arm weakness there may be downward drift but without pronation movement during the drift, as seen in patients with pyramidal lesions (Daum and Aybek, 2013) (Fig. 18.5).

The following tests have also been described but are generally of less utility.

Monrad–Krohn's cough test

This test evaluates the presence of involuntary contraction of the latissimus dorsi during cough but not during voluntary movement (the patient is asked to adduct the horizontally abducted extended arm against resistance).

Double crossed-arm pull test

In functional arm weakness there may be involuntary use of the weak arm when the examiner pulls the patient who is standing with crossed arms.

Finger abduction

This tests synkinetic (fifth-finger abduction) movement of the weak hand during abduction of the healthy fingers (contralateral hand) against resistance (Tinazzi et al., 2008). This may be useful in patients with complete paralysis of the hand.

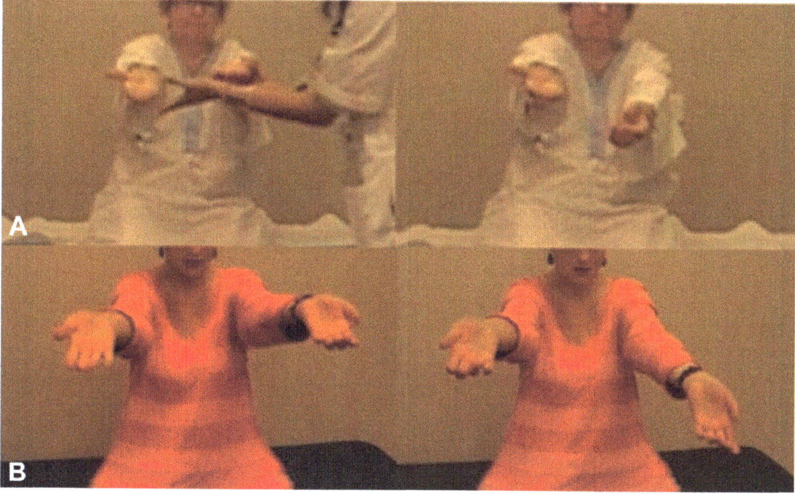

Fig. 18.5. Drift without pronation sign: (**A**) hand drift and pronation in organic pyramidal arm weakness; (**B**) hand drift without pronation in functional arm weakness.

The elbow flex-ex test

The elbow flex-ex test assesses involuntary elbow extension during contralateral flexion against resistance and/or involuntary elbow flexion during contralateral extension against resistance (Lombardi et al., 2014). Our experience with this test has been disappointing and we have not found it helpful.

"Make a fist" test

This test checks for discordance between voluntary hand extension, but intact involuntary dorsal extension when the patient makes a fist. Caution is necessary, as this inconsistency has been reported in upper motor neuron lesions.

Arm drop

This test is not advised but is often described. It is said that dropping the patient's own arm on to the patient's face will result, in functional weakness, in the arm avoiding the face, but in organic weakness in the arm dropping on the face. There are very few situations where this test is likely to add much. It involves inflicting a minor injury on patients with organic disease and in our previous experience may be positive in patients with functional limb weakness.

Bowlus maneuver

The Bowlus maneuver (see Chapter 24) may be used to test for altered sensation and movement. The patient is asked to cross the arms over at the wrist and intertwine the fingers. In some situations this may allow fingers to move better than they did normally and may be useful to show to the patient.

Signs of functional weakness in the trunk and legs

Hoover's sign

Hoover's sign is involuntary extension of the weak leg when the healthy contralateral leg is forced to flex against resistance (Fig. 18.6) (Hoover, 1908; Okun and Koehler, 2004). Other variants are also described: failure to flex the healthy hip when the patient is asked to extend the hip, and failure to see extension of the normal leg during hip flexion of the leg with functional weakness. Hoover's sign is often described with the patient supine but can be done just as effectively with the patient seated. Two quantitative studies have investigated this sign. The first used myometry to demonstrate the validity of the phenomenon (Ziv et al., 1998); the second used simple weighing scales (Diukova et al., 2013). The latter, which helpfully compared the sign in patients with neurologic leg weakness, patients with back pain, and healthy controls, suggested a cutoff ratio of 1.4:1 for involuntary to voluntary extension as strongly suggestive of functional leg weakness.

Hip abductor sign

This test reveals involuntary abduction of the weak leg during contralateral abduction against resistance (Fig. 18.7). This sign was first described by Raimiste (1912), but refined and tested by Sonoo (2004). It is less often positive than Hoover's sign but also provides

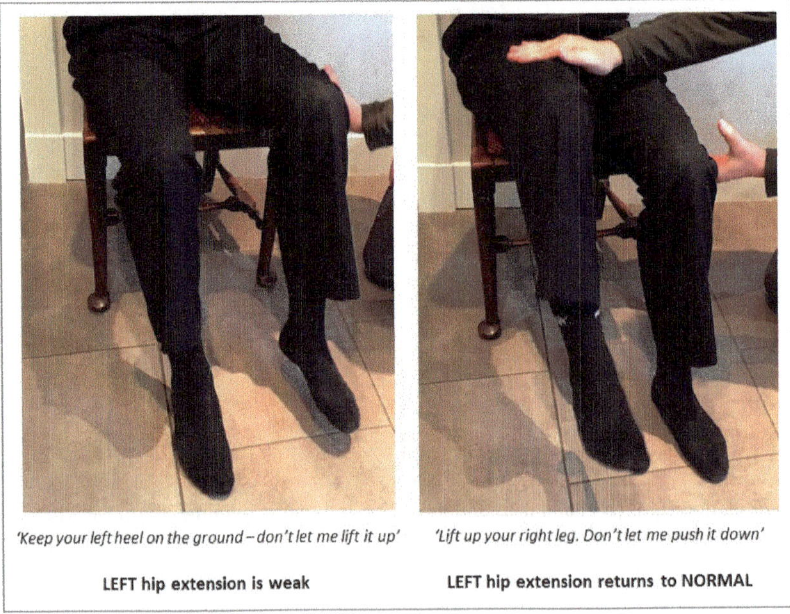

Fig. 18.6. Hoover's sign of functional leg weakness.

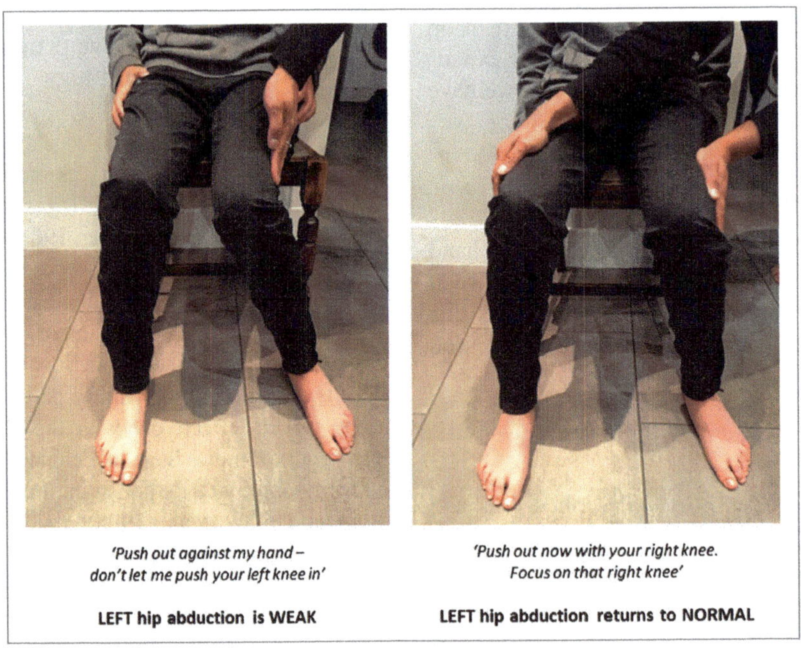

Fig. 18.7. Hip abductor sign.

a highly visible and understandable clinical sign which is often helpful in explanation and treatment.

Dragging monoplegic gait (Figs 18.1 and 18.2)

If functional leg weakness is marked, the patient will typically walk with a dragging gait in which the front part of the foot remains in contact with the floor through the step. The hip may be internally or externally rotated, although sometimes will remain in the normal position. Patients with this kind of gait may appear to hold the arm somewhat protected and flexed, even in the absence of pain, for reasons that they find hard to explain (Stone et al., 2010b).

The following tests have also been described but are generally of less utility.

Trunk–thigh test

In functional hemiparesis there may be no asymmetry observed in leg and shoulder movement when the patient sits from a lying position with arm crossed on chest. In organic hemiparesis the weak leg lifts up and the contralateral shoulder moves forwards (Babinski and Froment, 1918) (Fig. 18.8).

Spinal Injuries Center test

This can be useful in patients with paraplegia. With the patient supine the weak legs are passively put in a flexed position on the bed. In functional paraplegia they remain in that position instead of instantly falling to the side, as they usually do in organic paralysis (Yugue et al., 2004).

Barré sign (*manoeuvre de la jambe*)

The patient lies in a pronated position, legs flexed (knees touching the bed): the weak leg stays in position (instead of slowly falling, as in organic weakness) or instantly drops without any contraction of the hamstrings (Barré, 1937) (Fig. 18.9).

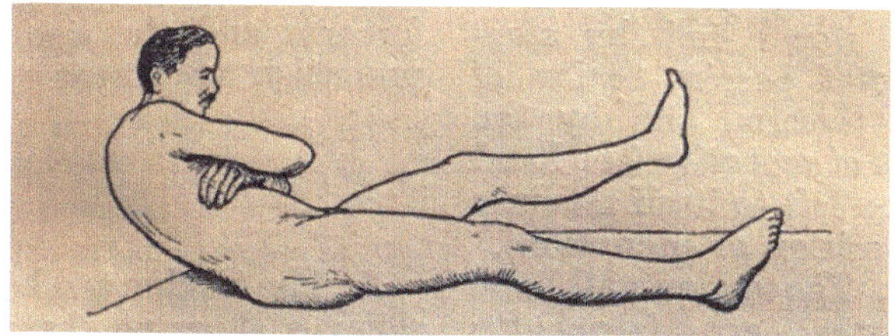

Fig. 18.8. Trunk–thigh test. In "organic" hemiplegia, as shown in the picture, the affected leg may be elevated as the patient attempts to sit up. In functional hemiplegia it is more likely to remain flat on the bed (Babinski and Froment, 1918).

Additional clinical findings in functional limb weakness

Many authors in the late 19th and early 20th century commented that reflex asymmetry was not that unusual in functional disorders. Co-contraction of muscles can attenuate deep tendon reflexes and lead to apparent asymmetry. Sometimes there is mild increase in tendon reflexes on the affected side, often in combination with heightened arousal or anxiety. Plantar responses may often be mute in patients with functional hemisensory loss and weakness.

A movement that at first sight appears to be clonus may actually be a form of pseudoclonus that again was well described in older literature (Fox, 1913). Clonus due to disease tends to get worse with maneuvers that direct attention elsewhere (e.g., the Jendrassik maneuver) whereas clonus in functional leg weakness resolves when the patient is asked to concentrate on copying externally cued rhythmic movement of the other foot.

Neurophysiologic tests of functional limb weakness

Neurophysiologic findings in functional disorders are discussed in detail in Chapter 6. Conventional neurophysiology in a patient with functional limb weakness should be normal, including central motor conduction time measured with transcranial magnetic stimulation (TMS) and peripheral nerve conduction studies. At least 11 studies of TMS have reported normal findings in patients with functional limb weakness (e.g., Meyer et al., 1992; Pillai et al., 1992; Janssen et al., 1995; Cantello et al., 2001; Stone and Sharpe, 2006), although one suggested some asymmetries at a group level in both patients with functional limb weakness (Liepert et al., 2009) and controls simulating weakness (Liepert et al., 2014). Electromyography may show a pattern of reduced recruitment equivalent to clinical "give-way" weakness.

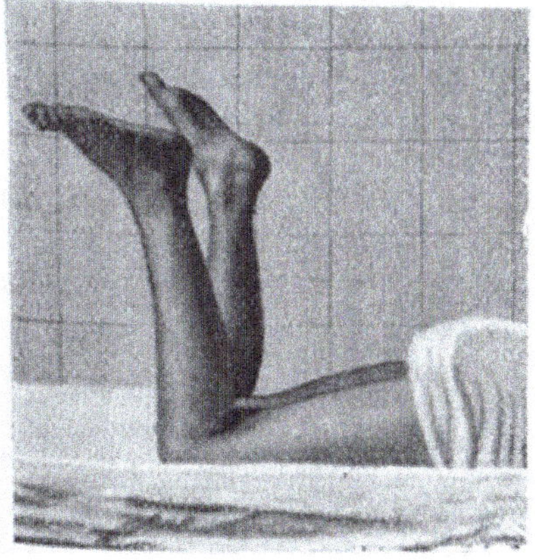

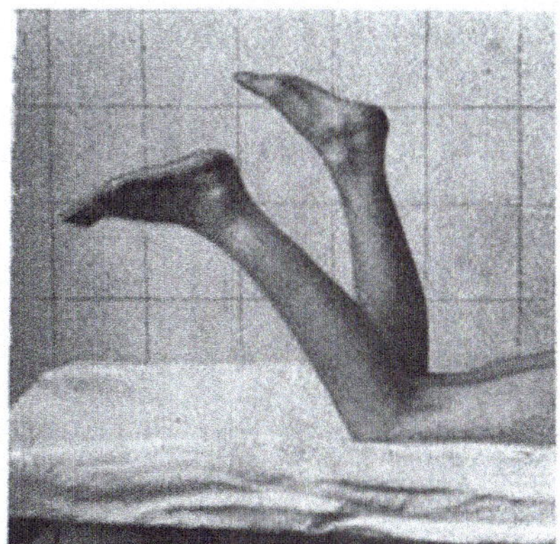

Fig. 18.9. *Manoeuvre de la jambe* (Barré, 1937). See text for details.

One additional study reported tests of a more positive nature to identify functional limb weakness. McComas et al. (1983) described using a single indirect stimulus of the tibial nerve superimposed on the patient's maximal voluntary contraction of ankle plantarflexion. In healthy subjects with submaximal contraction and patients with functional limb weakness an interpolated twitch was visible which disappeared in healthy controls during maximal contraction.

MECHANISM, ETIOLOGY, AND TREATMENT

Paralysis and limb weakness have been among the commonest symptoms to be studied using neurophysiologic and functional neuroimaging techniques. The data from these studies are discussed in Chapters 6 and 7. Treatment of functional neurologic disorders, including functional limb weakness, is discussed in detail in Chapters 44–51. The core elements of treatment are those of education, transparency (especially showing the patient the physical signs), physiotherapy specific for functional limb weakness, and psychotherapy where appropriate. Other treatments, including sedation, hypnosis, and TMS, may be appropriate in treatment-resistant patients who understand the diagnosis and are motivated to improve. What these additional treatments all have in common is the ability to show a patient that, whether chemically, hypnotically, or magnetically induced, a paralyzed limb can move.

CONCLUSION

Functional limb weakness is one of the commonest of the functional neurologic disorders. Relatively little attention has been paid to the clinical features, at least in the modern literature, although there are rich descriptions in older literature which are still valid.

There are characteristic features in the history and common comorbidities, but the diagnosis of functional limb weakness should be made primarily on the basis of the physical examination. A large number of maneuvers exist to aid the clinical diagnosis, which preferably should be shared with the patient as part of the physical and psychologic rehabilitation.

References

Babinski J, Froment J (1918). Hysteria or Pithiatism (trans. by JD Rolleston), University of London Press, London.

Baker JH, Silver JR (1987). Hysterical paraplegia. J Neurol Neurosurg Psychiatry 50: 375–382.

Barboi AC, Goetz CG, Musetoiu R (2004). The origins of scientific cinematography and early medical applications. Neurology 62: 2082–2086.

Barré JA (1937). Le syndrome pyramidal déficitaire. Rev Neurol (Paris) 67: 1–40.

Binzer M, Andersen PM, Kullgren G (1997). Clinical characteristics of patients with motor disability due to conversion disorder: a prospective control group study. J Neurol Neurosurg Psychiatry 63: 83–88.

Birklein F, Riedl B, Sieweke N et al. (2000). Neurological findings in complex regional pain syndromes – analysis of 145 cases. Acta Neurol Scand 101: 262–269.

Blau JN, Wiles CM, Solomon FS (1983). Unilateral somatic symptoms due to hyperventilation. BMJ 286: 1108.

Bousfield P (1926). The Pathology, Diagnosis and Treatment of Functional Nervous Diseases, Heinemann, London.

Briquet P (1859). Traité Clinique et thérapeutique de l'Hystérie. J.B. Ballière, Paris.

Brodie B (1837). Various forms of local hysterical affection. In: Lectures Illustrative of Certain Local Nervous Affections, Longmans, London.

Cantello R, Boccagni C, Comi C et al. (2001). Diagnosis of psychogenic paralysis: the role of motor evoked potentials. J Neurol 248: 889–897.

Chabrol H, Peresson G, Clanet M (1995). Lack of specificity of the traditional criteria of conversion disorders. Eur Psychiatry 10: 317–319.

Charcot J-M (1888). Nouvelle Iconographie de Salpêtrière. Clinique des Maladies du Système Nerveux, Lecrosnier et Babee, Paris.

Core D (1922). Functional Nervous Disorders: their Classification and Treatment, Wright, Bristol.

Crimlisk HL, Bhatia K, Cope H et al. (1998). Slater revisited: 6 year follow up study of patients with medically unexplained motor symptoms. BMJ (Clinical Research Ed.) 316: 582–586.

Daum C, Aybek S (2013). Validity of the "Drift without pronation" sign in conversion disorder. BMC Neurol 13: 31.

Daum C, Gheorghita F, Spatola M et al. (2014a). Interobserver agreement and validity of bedside "positive signs" for functional weakness, sensory and gait disorders in conversion disorder: a pilot study. J Neurol Neurosurg Psychiatry 86: 425–430.

Daum C, Hubschmid M, Aybek S (2014b). The value of "positive" clinical signs for weakness, sensory and gait disorders in conversion disorder: a systematic and narrative review. J Neurol Neurosurg Psychiatry 85: 180–190.

Dercum FX (1895). A Textbook on Nervous Disorders by American Authors, J. Pentland, Edinburgh.

Diukova GM, Stolajrova AV, Vein AM (2001). Sternocleidomastoid (SCM) muscle test in patients with hysterical and organic paresis. J Neurol Sci 187 (Suppl): S108.

Diukova GM, Ljachovetckaja NI, Begljarova MA et al. (2013). Simple quantitative analysis of Hoover's test in patients with psychogenic and organic limb pareses. J Psychosom Res 74 (4): 361–364.

Dubois P (1909). The psychic Treatment of Nervous Disorders, Funk & Wagnalls, New York.

Ehrbar R, Waespe W (1992). Funktionelle Gangstörungen. Schweiz Med Wochenschr 122: 833–841.

Ewald H, Rogne T, Ewald K et al. (1994). Somatization in patients newly admitted to a neurological department. Acta Psychiatr Scand 89: 174–179.

Farley J, Woodruff Jr RA, Guze SB (1968). The prevalence of hysteria and conversion symptoms. Br J Psychiatry 114: 1121–1125.

Fox CD (1913). The Psychopathology of Hysteria, Richard G. Badger, The Gorham Press, Boston.

Gargalas S, Weeks R, Khan-Bourne N et al. (2015). Incidence and outcome of functional stroke mimics admitted to a hyperacute stroke unit. J Neurol Neurosurg Psychiatry: 1–5.

Gowers WR (1892). Hysteria. In: A Manual of Diseases of the Nervous System, Churchill, London, pp. 903–960.

Hoover CF (1908). A new sign for the detection of malingering and functional paresis of the lower extremities. JAMA 51: 746–747.

Janet P (1901). The Mental State of Hystericals, Putnams, New York.

Janet P (1907). The Major Symptoms of Hysteria, Macmillan, London.

Janssen BA, Theiler R, Grob D et al. (1995). The role of motor evoked potentials in psychogenic paralysis. Spine 20: 608–611.

Kaski D, Bronstein Frcp AM, Edwards MJ et al. (2015). Cranial functional (psychogenic) movement disorders. Lancet Neurol 14: 1196–1205.

Kemp B (1970). The Miracles of the Hand of St James. Berkshire Archaeological Journal 65: 1–19.

Knutsson E, Martensson A (1985). Isokinetic measurements of muscle strength in hysterical paresis. Electroencephalogr Clin Neurophysiol 61: 370–374.

Lempert T, Dieterich M, Huppert D et al. (1990). Psychogenic disorders in neurology: frequency and clinical spectrum. Acta Neurol Scand 82: 335–340.

Liepert J, Hassa T, Tüscher O et al. (2009). Abnormal motor excitability in patients with psychogenic paresis. A TMS study. J Neurol 256: 121–126.

Liepert J, Shala J, Greiner J (2014). Electrophysiological correlates of disobedience and feigning-like behaviour in motor imagery. Clin Neurophysiol : Official Journal of the International Federation of Clinical Neurophysiology 125: 763–767.

Lombardi TL, Barton E, Wang J et al. (2014). The elbow flex-ex: a new sign to detect unilateral upper extremity non-organic paresis. J Neurol Neurosurg Psychiatry 85: 165–167.

Marsden CD (1986). Hysteria – a neurologist's view. Psychol Med 16: 277–288.

Marshall JC, Halligan PW, Fink GR et al. (1997). The functional anatomy of a hysterical paralysis. Cognition 64: B1–B8.

McComas AJ, Kereshi S, Quinlan J (1983). A method for detecting functional weakness. J Neurol Neurosurg Psychiatry 46: 280–282.

McWhirter L, Stone J, Sandercock P et al. (2011). Hoover's sign for the diagnosis of functional weakness: a prospective unblinded cohort study in patients with suspected stroke. J Psychosom Res 71: 384–386.

Metcalfe R, Firth D, Pollock S et al. (1988). Psychiatric morbidity and illness behaviour in female neurological in-patients. J Neurol Neurosurg Psychiatry 51: 1387–1390.

Meyer BU, Britton TC, Benecke R et al. (1992). Motor responses evoked by magnetic brain stimulation in psychogenic limb weakness: diagnostic value and limitations. J Neurol 239: 251–255.

Miller C (1920). Functional Nerve Disease: An Epitome of War Experience for the Practitioner, Frowde and Hodder & Stoughton, London.

Nazir F, Bone I, Lees KR (2005). Clinical predictors of medically unexplained stroke-like symptoms presenting to an acute stroke unit. Eur J Neurol 12: 81–85.

Nicoll M, Young J (1920). Psychoanalysis. In: C Miller (Ed.), Functional Nerve Disease, Frowde and Hodder & Stoughton, London, pp. 129–152.

Okun MS, Koehler PJ (2004). Babinski's clinical differentiation of organic paralysis from hysterical paralysis: effect on US neurology. Arch Neurol 61: 778–783.

Paget J (1873). Nervous mimicry. In: S Paget (Ed.), Selected Essays and Addresses by Sir James Paget, Longmans, Green, London.

Pillai JJ, Markind S, Streletz LJ et al. (1992). Motor evoked potentials in psychogenic paralysis. Neurology 42: 935–936.

Punt TD, Cooper L, Hey M et al. (2013). Neglect-like symptoms in complex regional pain syndrome: learned nonuse by another name? Pain 154: 200–203.

Purves-Stewart J (1911). The Diagnosis of Nervous Diseases. Arnold, London.

Raimiste J (1912). Deux signes d'hémiplegie organique du membre inférieur. Rev Neurol 125–129.

Reynolds JR (1869). Paralysis and other disorders of motion and sensation dependent on idea. BMJ i: 483–485.

Rief W, Hessel A, Braehler E (2001). Somatization symptoms and hypochondriacal features in the general population. Psychosom Med 63: 595–602.

Sacks OW (1984). A Leg to Stand On, Harper & Row, New York.

Sacks O (2012). The central effects of peripheral injury. J Neurol Neurosurg Psychiatry 83: 868.

Savill TD (1909). Lectures on Hysteria and Allied Vasomotor Conditions, Glaisher, London.

Schiffer RB (1983). Psychiatric aspects of clinical neurology. Am J Psychiatry 140: 205–207.

Schrag A, Trimble M, Quinn N et al. (2004). The syndrome of fixed dystonia: an evaluation of 103 patients. Brain : J Neurol 127: 2360–2372.

Sonoo M (2004). Abductor sign: a reliable new sign to detect unilateral non-organic paresis of the lower limb. J Neurol Neurosurg Psychiatry 73: 121–125.

Stone J, Sharpe M (2006). Functional paralysis and sensory disturbance. In: M Hallett, S Fahn, J Jankovic et al. (Eds.), Psychogenic Movement Disorders, Lippincott, Williams and Wilkins, Philadelphia, pp. 88–111.

Stone J, Sharpe M, Binzer M (2004). Motor conversion symptoms and pseudoseizures: a comparison of clinical characteristics. Psychosomatics 45: 492–499.

Stone J, Hewett R, Carson A et al. (2008). The "disappearance" of hysteria: historical mystery or illusion? J R Soc Med 101: 12–18.

Stone J, Carson A, Aditya H et al. (2009a). The role of physical injury in motor and sensory conversion symptoms: a systematic and narrative review. J Psychosom Res 66: 383–390.

Stone J, Carson A, Duncan R et al. (2009b). Symptoms "unexplained by organic disease" in 1144 new neurology out-patients: how often does the diagnosis change at follow-up? Brain : J Neurol 132: 2878–2888.

Stone J, Carson A, Duncan R et al. (2010a). Who is referred to neurology clinics? The diagnoses made in 3781 new patients. Clin Neurol Neurosurg 112: 747–751.

Stone J, Warlow C, Sharpe M (2010b). The symptom of functional weakness: a controlled study of 107 patients. Brain 133: 1537–1551.

Stone J, Warlow C, Sharpe M (2012a). Functional weakness: clues to mechanism from the nature of onset. J Neurol Neurosurg Psychiatry 83: 67–69.

Stone J, Perthen J, Carson AJ (2012b). "A Leg to Stand On" by Oliver Sacks: a unique autobiographical account of functional paralysis. J Neurol Neurosurg Psychiatry 83: 864–867.

Tinazzi M, Simonetto S, Franco L et al. (2008). Abduction finger sign: a new sign to detect unilateral functional paralysis of the upper limb. Mov Disord 23: 2415–2419.

Todd RB (1854). Clinical Lectures on Paralyses. Diseases of the Brain, and Other Affections of the Nervous System, J. Churchill, London.

van der Ploeg RJ, Oosterhuis HJ (1991). The "make/break test" as a diagnostic tool in functional weakness. J Neurol Neurosurg Psychiatry 54: 248–251.

Veldman PH, Reynen HM, Arntz IE et al. (1993). Signs and symptoms of reflex sympathetic dystrophy: prospective study of 829 patients. Lancet 342: 1012–1016.

Weintraub MI (1977). Hysteria. A clinical guide to diagnosis. Clin Symp 29: 1–31.

Wessely S, Jones E (2005). Shell Shock to PTSD: Military Psychiatry from 1900 to the Gulf War. Psychology Press, London.

Woodruff Jr RA (1968). Hysteria: an evaluation of objective diagnostic criteria by the study of women with chronic medical illnesses. Br J Psychiatry 114: 1115–1119.

Woodruff Jr RA, Clayton PJ, Guze SB (1969). Hysteria: an evaluation of specific diagnostic criteria by the study of randomly selected psychiatric clinic patients. Br J Psychiatry 115: 1243–1248.

Yugue I, Shiba K, Ueta T et al. (2004). A new clinical evaluation for hysterical paralysis. 29: 1910–1913.

Ziv I, Djaldetti R, Zoldan Y et al. (1998). Diagnosis of "non-organic" limb paresis by a novel objective motor assessment: the quantitative Hoover's test. J Neurol 245 (12): 797–802.

Handbook of Clinical Neurology, Vol. 139 (3rd series)
Functional Neurologic Disorders
M. Hallett, J. Stone, and A. Carson, Editors
http://dx.doi.org/10.1016/B978-0-12-801772-2.00019-9

Chapter 19

Functional tremor

P. SCHWINGENSCHUH[1] AND G. DEUSCHL[2]*
[1]*Department of Neurology, Medical University of Graz, Graz, Austria*
[2]*Department of Neurology, University Hospital Schleswig-Holstein, Campus Kiel, Kiel, Germany*

Abstract

Functional tremor is the commonest reported functional movement disorder. A confident clinical diagnosis of functional tremor is often possible based on the following "positive" criteria: a sudden tremor onset, unusual disease course, often with fluctuations or remissions, distractibility of the tremor if attention is removed from the affected body part, tremor entrainment, tremor variability, and a coactivation sign. Many patients show excessive exhaustion during examination. Other somatizations may be revealed in the medical history and patients may show additional functional neurologic symptoms and signs. In cases where the clinical diagnosis remains challenging, providing a "laboratory-supported" level of certainty aids an early positive diagnosis. In rare cases, in which the distinction from Parkinson's disease is difficult, dopamine transporter single-photon emission computed tomography (DAT-SPECT) can be indicated.

INTRODUCTION

Functional tremor (synonym: psychogenic tremor) is the commonest reported functional movement disorder, accounting for more than 50% of patients in published cohorts (Bhatia and Schneider, 2007). There has been a large variability in reporting of the incidence of functional tremor, ranging from a rare disorder to 11% of all tremor referrals to a movement disorder clinic (Deuschl et al., 1998). It has been repeatedly described since the First World War, when thousands of veterans suffered from functional tremor and other functional movement disorders. Two mechanisms of how the motor system may produce functional tremor have been proposed. The first one is just a repetitive voluntary movement as if a normal subject is mimicking a tremor. The second possibility uses the clonus mechanism, which can produce tremors during co-contraction of the extremities (Raethjen et al., 2004).

So far, there are no gold standards for diagnosing functional tremor apart from clinical criteria (Deuschl et al., 1998; Shill and Gerber, 2006; Gupta and Lang, 2009) and patients still often undergo a large number of diagnostic and therapeutic procedures until the final diagnosis is established. The importance of a positive diagnosis rather than one of exclusion has been repeatedly emphasized (Deuschl et al., 1998; Gupta and Lang, 2009; Edwards and Bhatia, 2012).

SYMPTOMS AND SIGNS

Although no single clinical finding is pathognomonic for functional tremor, several features are quite helpful. When making a diagnosis of a functional tremor, the overall clinical picture, including history and examination, needs to be taken into consideration (Table 19.1). History taking frequently reveals an unusual temporal profile with sudden tremor onset (Koller et al., 1989), which may be associated with a stressful life event or a preceding physical event (e.g., physical trauma, surgery, infection, or other illness) (Pareés et al., 2014). Variability in tremor severity with or without spontaneous remissions or a static disease course is characteristic. Variability of the body parts being affected is commonly reported (Edwards and Bhatia, 2012). Rarely, functional tremor presents as a paroxysmal movement disorder (Ganos et al., 2014).

*Correspondence to: Prof. Dr. Günther Deuschl, Department of Neurology, Christian-Albrechts-University Kiel, Arnold-Heller Str. 3, D-24105 Kiel, Germany. Tel: +49-431-5978707, Fax: +49-431-5978502, E-mail: g.deuschl@neurologie.uni-kiel.de

Table 19.1

Characteristics of functional tremor

Characteristics of functional tremor
Sudden onset, remissions, variability of affected body part
Unusual clinical combinations of rest, postural and kinetic tremors
Increased attention toward the affected limb
Improvement/suppression of tremor during distraction
Tremor entrainment
Tremor variability
Coactivation sign
Excessive exhaustion during examination
Somatization in the past history
Appearance of additional and unrelated neurologic signs

Functional tremor often has a complex clinical presentation with combinations of rest, postural and kinetic tremors that are unusual for most organic tremors. Hands and arms (usually in the absence of a finger tremor) are most frequently affected. Also tremors of the head, legs, trunk, and even the palate may occur (Edwards and Bhatia, 2012). Some patients present with a stance tremor, demonstrating irregular up-and-down movements mostly at low frequencies, which are often obviously functional (Deuschl et al., 1998).

The clue to distinguish a functional tremor from an organic tremor lies in a careful clinical examination by a neurologist experienced in movement disorders. In contrast to organic tremors, functional tremor is associated with increased attentional focus toward the affected limb during examination (van Poppelen et al., 2011). The majority of clinical tests used to positively diagnose a patient with a functional tremor rely on demonstrating a change of the tremor with distraction of attention away from the affected body part (Edwards and Bhatia, 2012).

Typically, tremor dramatically improves, subsides, or changes frequency and amplitude during distraction tasks. In some patients distractibility of the tremor may already become obvious during simple distractions such as history taking, performing arithmetic, or examining another body part. In others particular examination maneuvers are required. In clinical practice, a frequently used distraction task for a presumed functional arm tremor is performance of sudden ballistic movements with one hand, which will trigger a pause of tremor in the other hand. Performance of complex sequential finger movements or a finger-tapping task at a given frequency with the contralateral hand may induce tremor suppression or may help to demonstrate entrainment (i.e., adaptation to the frequency of the contralateral movements), which represents another clinical hallmark of functional tremor.

One pitfall that needs to be kept in mind is that distraction can only be successful when the level of attention toward the tremulous limb is sufficiently reduced by the distraction task. The "difficulty level" required may vary from patient to patient. If the task is too simple, this may be misinterpreted as nondistractability. If the patient is asked to perform a rhythm different from the tremor rhythm with the unaffected hand, it is important to command this rhythm and to constantly change this command in order to keep the "difficulty level" high. Also, tremor in different body parts warrants different distractors. For a leg tremor, a tapping task with the contralateral leg and for a head tremor an eye or tongue movement task may be helpful.

In some patients with functional tremor, distractibility cannot be demonstrated at least on clinical grounds, even if an adequate examination maneuver is used. Thus, functional tremor should not be excluded when persistence of tremor is found during distraction (Deuschl et al., 1998). If, on the other hand, the tremor is distractible, this is a strong indicator of functional origin. Sharing this "positive" sign with patients is often a powerful way of persuading them of the diagnosis (Stone and Edwards, 2012).

Another important characteristic of functional tremor is variability. Variability can present as change in frequency, amplitude, direction (e.g., change from a pronation/supination to a wrist flexion/extension pattern), or as fluctuation of anatomic tremor distribution. Such tremor variability sometimes occurs spontaneously when the patient is observed for a longer time period. In others it may only become obvious with a change in the level of attention towards the tremor (also see above). Tremor may increase when the attention is drawn to the affected limb, or when the patient is asked about it (Bhatia and Schneider, 2007). However, organic tremors can also have a variable amplitude influenced by the level of anxiety/exhaustion/position or may appear irregular in rhythm and may change direction (e.g., in the case of a dystonic head tremor). Hence tremor variability does not necessarily indicate functional tremor (Thenganatt and Jankovic, 2014).

Functional tremor may also show a "coactivation sign," i.e., some underlying antagonistic muscle activation whenever the tremor is present. If the increased muscle activation disappears, the tremor disappears too. This can be demonstrated during slow arrhythmic, passive movements – as rigidity is commonly tested. In functional tremor fluctuations or disappearance of muscle resistance and tremor may be observed (Deuschl et al., 1998).

Functional tremor is sometimes suggestible, and can vary in response to certain stimuli. One way to test for suggestibility is to apply a vibrating tuning fork to the affected body part and suggest that the vibrating stimulus may reduce the symptoms. Another way is to suggest that application of pressure on a certain "trigger point" with the examiner's finger may alter the tremor (Gupta and Lang, 2009; Thenganatt and Jankovic, 2014). The authors do not routinely test for suggestibility in their patients with presumed functional tremor as they may feel tricked by the examiner. If tests for suggestibility are used, we suggest explaining the findings to the patient immediately afterwards in order to avoid deception in the doctor–patient relationship.

In patients with functional tremor, voluntary movements can appear to be slow throughout the performance of rapid repetitive and alternating movements, but without the fatiguing and decreasing amplitude or the typical arrests that are seen in Parkinson's disease (Lang et al., 1995). In one study, patients with functional movement disorders (7 out of 13 patients had a tremor) performed an objective finger-tapping task significantly slower than patients with Parkinson's disease or other organic movement disorders (Criswell et al., 2010). Some patients with functional tremor seem to struggle and put more effort than needed into performing the tasks. During examination they may demonstrate exhaustion and excessive fatigue and may use their whole body in order to do a minor movement (Bhatia and Schneider, 2007; Thenganatt and Jankovic, 2014). Other patients with functional tremor apparently disregard their symptoms, despite showing a severe tremor on examination ("*la belle indifférence*"). However, the available evidence suggests that "*la belle indifférence*" does not discriminate between conversion symptoms/hysteria and symptoms of organic disease (Stone et al., 2006). Furthermore, patients with functional tremor have been shown to overestimate the percentage of waking hours they actually suffer from tremor, thus they fail to accurately perceive that they do not have tremor most of the day (Pareés et al., 2012).

In addition to findings typical of functional tremor, mentioned above, patients may have coexisting functional neurologic symptoms and signs that support the diagnosis of a functional tremor, such as positive features of functional weakness (e.g., Hoover's sign or give-away weakness), nonanatomic sensory loss, or convergence spasm and other dysconjugate oculomotor abnormalities (Gupta and Lang, 2009; Thenganatt and Jankovic, 2014). Some patients with functional tremor also have a functional gait disorder and sometimes respond in a theatrical way on postural stability testing and tandem walking. Careful history often reveals multiple other somatic symptoms, such as generalized fatigue, nonspecific pains, memory disturbance, and impaired vision (Bhatia and Schneider, 2007).

Clues from therapeutic responses suggesting a functional tremor include unresponsiveness to appropriate medications, response to placebos, and remission with psychotherapy.

Given the common co-occurrence of other functional disorders with organic diseases, e.g., epilepsy and nonepileptic seizures, co-occurrence of functional tremor and organic tremor should be considered. This phenomenon, also called functional overlay, has not been systematically investigated in tremor disorders so far (Edwards and Bhatia, 2012). However, one group proposed a particular susceptibility to develop functional symptoms in patients with Parkinson's disease (29/412 patients: 7%). Functional motor symptoms such as gait disorders or weakness were common, whereas functional tremor was not described (Onofrj et al., 2010). More recently, 11 patients with Parkinson's disease who developed a functional tremor ($n=7$), gait disorder ($n=3$), or fixed dystonia ($n=1$) were reported. The authors highlighted the importance of considering functional symptoms as a presenting feature as well as a cause of unexpected deterioration or treatment-refractory symptoms in Parkinson's disease (Pareés et al., 2013).

The positive clinical criteria mentioned above are based on a small number of prospective (Deuschl et al., 1998: $n=25$; McKeon et al., 2009: $n=33$) and retrospective (Koller et al., 1989: $n=24$; Kim et al., 1999: $n=25$; Jankovic et al., 2006: $n=127$) studies focusing on patients with functional tremor. One clinical study has systematically compared the effects of various provocative tests on patients with essential tremor and functional tremor using a standardized protocol (Kenney et al., 2007). Functional tremor was differentiated by negative family history, sudden onset, spontaneous remission, shorter duration of tremor, suggestibility, and distractibility. Interestingly, entrainment was not seen often in either tremor type. However, the method of evaluating entrainment (10 seconds of wrist extension and flexion in the unaffected arm) is probably not an adequate assessment of this feature (Gupta and Lang, 2009).

SUPPORTIVE ANCILLARY EXAMINATIONS

While functional tremor may be easily diagnosed in some cases, others remain challenging and diagnosis and appropriate treatment may therefore be delayed; this is thought to be a modifying factor regarding long-term outcome in these patients. In order to support an early and comfortable positive diagnosis of functional tremor, the development of laboratory-supported criteria has been suggested (Gupta and Lang, 2009).

A variety of electrophysiologic tests have been proposed to be useful in distinguishing patients with functional tremor from organic tremors (Brown and Thompson, 2001; Hallett, 2010). These include coactivation of antagonist muscles at the onset of tremor characterized by antagonist muscles tonically discharging approximately 300 ms before the onset of tremor bursts (Deuschl et al., 1998). In contrast to essential tremor and Parkinson's disease, there was an increase of tremor amplitudes in response to weighting the limb in a proportion of functional patients (Deuschl et al., 1998; Zeuner et al., 2003). Entrainment or an increase in variability and change of tremor frequency while tapping with the contralateral hand was described (O'Suilleabhain and Matsumoto, 1998). With the exception of orthostatic tremor, most patients with bilateral organic tremor have independent tremor rhythms in different extremities, while approximately half of the patients with functional tremor showed significant coherency between the two hands (Raethjen et al., 2004).

Furthermore, it has been shown that, in contrast to dystonic tremor patients with functional tremor, either show coherent oscillations in different limbs or the tremor can be entrained by contralateral rhythmic voluntary movements at a different frequency (McAuley et al., 1998; McAuley and Rothwell, 2004). In contrast to essential tremor and Parkinson's disease, tremor transiently stopped during a quick movement of the other hand (ballistic movement test) in functional tremor (Kumru et al., 2004).

A head-to-head comparison of the above-mentioned tests was performed in 13 patients with functional tremor and 25 patients with various organic tremors (Schwingenschuh et al., 2011). Test sensitivity and specificity of all separate tests varied between 33–77% and 84–100%, respectively. In order to strengthen the discriminative value of the electrophysiologic tests, a sum score for all performed tests (maximum 10 points) was calculated (Table 19.2). A combination of these electrophysiologic tests with a cutoff score of 3/10 points was able to distinguish functional and organic tremor with excellent sensitivity and specificity. Recently, this test battery was validated in a prospective study including 38 new patients with functional tremor and 72 new patients with organic tremors, yielding a test sensitivity of 89.5% and a specificity of 95.9%. The test battery can therefore be used to establish a "laboratory-supported" level of certainty in patients in whom uncertainty remains after clinical investigation. In patients in whom the clinical diagnosis of a functional tremor is more obvious, the test battery can still provide objective evidence and help convey the diagnosis to a patient (Schwingenschuh et al., 2016).

If the distinction between functional tremor (or functional parkinsonism) and Parkinson's disease causes difficulties, dopamine transporter single-photon emission computed tomography (DAT-SPECT) can be useful. Although data are limited, normal DAT-SPECT in functional tremor (or functional parkinsonism) is the rule, and a decreased striatal tracer uptake strongly suggests degenerative parkinsonism. However, a normal DAT-SPECT does not distinguish functional tremor (or functional parkinsonism) from benign tremor disorders such as essential or dystonic tremor or from nondegenerative parkinsonian disorders such as drug-induced or vascular parkinsonism (Kagi et al., 2010).

Table 19.2

Test battery* (Schwingenschuh et al., 2011, 2016)

Test battery	Sum score (maximum 10 points)
Incorrect tapping performance† (1, 3, 5 Hz)	Maximum 3 points
Entrainment, suppression, or pathologic frequency shift during tapping (1, 3, 5 Hz)	Maximum 3 points
Pause or significant amplitude/period decrement during ballistic movements (in at least 7/10 trials)	1 point
Tonic coactivation	1 point
Significant coherence in bilateral tremors	1 point
Increase of amplitude with loading	1 point

*The test battery (maximum sum score 10 points) was designed to distinguish patients with functional tremor from organic tremors. A sum score of $\geq$3 points indicates functional tremor.

†Incorrect tapping performance: patients were instructed to tap in time with a metronome at rates of 1, 3, and 5 Hz. Tapping performances beyond predefined ranges of 0.5–1.5 Hz, 2.5–3.5 Hz, and 4.5–5.5 Hz, respectively, were considered as incorrect.

References

Bhatia KP, Schneider SA (2007). Psychogenic tremor and related disorders. J Neurol 254: 569–574.

Brown P, Thompson PD (2001). Electrophysiological aids to the diagnosis of psychogenic jerks, spasms, and tremor. Mov Disord 16: 595–599.

Criswell S, Sterling C, Swisher L et al. (2010). Sensitivity and specificity of the finger tapping task for the detection of psychogenic movement disorders. Parkinsonism Relat Disord 16: 197–201.

Deuschl G, Koster B, Lucking CH et al. (1998). Diagnostic and pathophysiological aspects of psychogenic tremors. Mov Disord 13: 294–302.

Edwards MJ, Bhatia KP (2012). Functional (psychogenic) movement disorders: merging mind and brain. Lancet Neurol 11: 250–260.

Ganos C, Aguirregomozcorta M, Batla A et al. (2014). Psychogenic paroxysmal movement disorders – clinical features and diagnostic clues. Parkinsonism Relat Disord 20: 41–46.

Gupta A, Lang AE (2009). Psychogenic movement disorders. Curr Opin Neurol 22: 430–436.

Hallett M (2010). Physiology of psychogenic movement disorders. J Clin Neurosci 17: 959–965.

Jankovic J, Vuong KD, Thomas M (2006). Psychogenic tremor: long-term outcome. CNS Spectr 11: 501–508.

Kagi G, Bhatia KP, Tolosa E (2010). The role of DAT-SPECT in movement disorders. J Neurol Neurosurg Psychiatry 81: 5–12.

Kenney C, Diamond A, Mejia N et al. (2007). Distinguishing psychogenic and essential tremor. J Neurol Sci 263: 94–99.

Kim YJ, Pakiam AS, Lang AE (1999). Historical and clinical features of psychogenic tremor: a review of 70 cases. Can J Neurol Sci 26: 190–195.

Koller W, Lang A, Vetere-Overfield B et al. (1989). Psychogenic tremors. Neurology 39: 1094–1099.

Kumru H, Valls-Sole J, Valldeoriola F et al. (2004). Transient arrest of psychogenic tremor induced by contralateral ballistic movements. Neurosci Lett 370: 135–139.

Lang AE, Koller WC, Fahn S (1995). Psychogenic parkinsonism. Arch Neurol 52: 802–810.

McAuley J, Rothwell J (2004). Identification of psychogenic, dystonic, and other organic tremors by a coherence entrainment test. Mov Disord 19: 253–267.

McAuley JH, Rothwell JC, Marsden CD et al. (1998). Electrophysiological aids in distinguishing organic from psychogenic tremor. Neurology 50: 1882–1884.

McKeon A, Ahlskog JE, Bower JH et al. (2009). Psychogenic tremor: long-term prognosis in patients with electrophysiologically confirmed disease. Mov Disord 24: 72–76.

Onofrj M, Bonanni L, Manzoli L et al. (2010). Cohort study on somatoform disorders in Parkinson disease and dementia with Lewy bodies. Neurology 74: 1598–1606.

O'Suilleabhain PE, Matsumoto PE (1998). Time-frequency analysis of tremors. Brain 121: 2127–2134.

Pareés I, Saifee TA, Kassavetis P et al. (2012). Believing is perceiving: mismatch between self-report and actigraphy in psychogenic tremor. Brain 135: 117–123.

Pareés I, Saifee TA, Kojovic M et al. (2013). Functional (psychogenic) symptoms in Parkinson's disease. Mov Disord 28: 1622–1627.

Pareés I, Kojovic M, Pires C et al. (2014). Physical precipitating factors in functional movement disorders. J Neurol Sci 338: 174–177.

Raethjen J, Kopper F, Govindan RB et al. (2004). Two different pathogenetic mechanisms in psychogenic tremor. Neurology 63: 812–815.

Schwingenschuh P, Katschnig P, Seiler P et al. (2011). Moving toward "laboratory-supported" criteria for psychogenic tremor. Mov Disord 26: 2509–2515.

Schwingenschuh P, Saifee TA, Katschnig-Winter P et al. (2016). Validation of "laboratory-supported" criteria for functional (psychogenic) tremor. Mov Disord 31 (4): 555–562.

Shill H, Gerber P (2006). Evaluation of clinical diagnostic criteria for psychogenic movement disorders. Mov Disord 21: 1163–1168.

Stone J, Edwards M (2012). Trick or treat? Showing patients with functional (psychogenic) motor symptoms their physical signs. Neurology 79: 282–284.

Stone J, Smyth R, Carson A et al. (2006). La belle indifférence in conversion symptoms and hysteria: systematic review. Br J Psychiatry 188: 204–209.

Thenganatt MA, Jankovic J (2014). Psychogenic tremor: a video guide to its distinguishing features. Tremor Other Hyperkinet Mov (N Y) 4: 253.

Van Poppelen D, Saifee TA, Schwingenschuh P et al. (2011). Attention to self in psychogenic tremor. Mov Disord 26: 2575–2576.

Zeuner KE, Shoge RO, Goldstein SR et al. (2003). Accelerometry to distinguish psychogenic from essential or parkinsonian tremor. Neurology 61: 548–550.

Handbook of Clinical Neurology, Vol. 139 (3rd series)
Functional Neurologic Disorders
M. Hallett, J. Stone, and A. Carson, Editors
http://dx.doi.org/10.1016/B978-0-12-801772-2.00020-5

Chapter 20

Functional dystonia

D.A. SCHMERLER AND A.J. ESPAY*

Gardner Family Center for Parkinson's Disease and Movement Disorders, Department of Neurology, University of Cincinnati, Cincinnati, OH, USA

Abstract

Although currently lacking a sensitive and specific electrophysiologic battery test, functional (psychogenic) dystonia can sometimes be diagnosed with clinically definite certainty using available criteria. Certain regional phenotypes have been recognized as distinctive, such as unilateral lip and jaw deviation, laterocollis with ipsilateral shoulder elevation and contralateral shoulder depression, fixed wrist and finger flexion with relative sparing of the thumb and index fingers, and fixed foot plantar flexion and inversion. The pathophysiologic abnormalities in functional dystonia overlap substantially with those of organic dystonia, with similar impairments in cortical and spinal inhibition and somatosensory processing, but with emerging data suggesting abnormalities in regional blood flow and activation patterns on positron emission tomography and functional magnetic resonance imaging, respectively. Management of functional dystonia begins with compassionate and assertive debriefing of the diagnosis to ensure full acceptance by the patient, a critical step in enhancing the likelihood of success with physical rehabilitation, and psychodynamic or cognitive therapy. Physical therapy, with or without cognitive behavioral therapy, appears to be of benefit but has not yet been examined in a controlled fashion. While the prognosis remains grim for a substantial majority of patients, partly stemming from restricted mobility, delayed diagnosis, and inappropriate pharmacotherapy, early recognition and initiation of therapy stand to minimize iatrogenic harm and unnecessary laboratory investigations, and potentially reduce the long-term neurologic disability.

INTRODUCTION

Within the realm of functional (psychogenic) movement disorders (FMD), which may globally encompass 5–20% of patients in a movement disorder clinic, functional (psychogenic) dystonia (FD) is one of the commonest (Miyasaki et al., 2003). Making up nearly a third of all functional phenotypes, FD represents a uniquely challenging diagnosis, with regional expression involving virtually any body part (Lang and Voon, 2011). Because organic dystonia can exhibit bizarre features, the diagnosis of FD should only be made by an expert in movement disorders, capable of distinguishing the peculiarities of one disorder from those of the other. While fluctuations in severity and variation in tone with passive manipulation might suggest a functional etiology, these features might be variably present in organic dystonias and, thus, are not as helpful in ascertaining FD as they are for other functional phenotypes (Schrag and Lang, 2005). On the other hand, the measured use of suggestibility can serve as critical in inducing diagnostic incongruent phenomenologic changes. These are particularly valuable when magnification or abatement of the dystonic posture is brought on by the application of such nonphysiologic techniques as the placement of a vibrating tuning fork over the skull, the palpation of trigger points, or during or immediately after electric stimulation at just above the sensory threshold.

Because these and other examination techniques are not a standard part of the armamentarium of general neurologists, the diagnosis of FMD in general, and of FD in particular, is often delayed. Thus, these patients often come misdiagnosed to the attention of a specialized

*Correspondence to: Dr. Alberto J. Espay, University of Cincinnati Academic Health Center, 260 Stetson St., Suite 2300, Cincinnati OH 45267-0525, USA. Tel: +1-513-558-4035, Fax: +1-513-558-7015, E-mail: alberto.espay@uc.edu

movement disorders center, encumbered with iatrogenic complications, and accruing nearly twice the healthcare utilization rate and annual costs of medical care compared to their organic counterparts (Crimlisk et al., 2000; Ibrahim et al., 2009).

HISTORIC BACKGROUND

Dystonia was originally described as a functional disturbance of the brain without obvious pathology, as "*Krampfform mit hysterischen Symptomen*" or "form of spasm with hysterical symptoms" (Schwalbe, 1908; Munts and Koehler, 2010). Indeed, while early descriptions of dystonia assumed all cases to be "hysteric," at least some of the Jewish families from Eastern Europe described by Oppenheim, credited with coining the term dystonia, may have included members with familial DYT1 dystonia (Klein and Fahn, 2013). Nevertheless, the early descriptions of dystonia consistently highlighted its functional features until David Marsden's clinical evaluations suggested otherwise (Marsden, 1976). While Marsden correctly attributed many features hitherto believed hysteric as neurologic, he may have swung the pendulum too far to the organic end: he was highly reluctant to diagnose FD (Marsden, 1986).

Despite advances in neurophysiology and neuroimaging, the lack of diagnostic biomarkers for organic and functional disorders since the seminal descriptions has fueled a modern sort of backlash against FD in some corners (Schwartzman and Kerrigan, 1990). For instance, van Hilten and colleagues built an organic framework for posttraumatic pain and dysautonomia evolving into fixed dystonia, the most common FD phenotype, under the spectrum of complex regional pain syndrome type I (CRPS-I), previously known as reflex sympathetic dystrophy (van Rooijen et al., 2013a, b). One carefully reviewed series has shown that most of these CRPS-I patients exhibited features consistent with clinically definite FD (Verdugo and Ochoa, 2000). As will be reviewed later, however, the separation between organic dystonia and FD from an electrophysiologic perspective may not be as distinct as one would have assumed as late as the early 2000s, with many shared abnormalities identified between these disorders.

The development of diagnostic criteria for FD in 1988 (Fahn and Williams, 1988) became the first and most important frame of reference for clinical and research endeavors, and paved the way for moving away from a "diagnosis by exclusion" approach to one where a "documented" or "established" degree of certainty could be reached through the ascertainment of a combination of historic and examination findings, without need for further laboratory assessments. More recently, these criteria have been the subject of refinement efforts, most prominently with proposals for more (Shill and Gerber, 2006) or less (Gupta and Lang, 2009) reliance on psychogenic causation, and the inclusion of a laboratory-supported diagnostic category (Gupta and Lang, 2009).

Patient and physician disagreements on the very nomenclature of FMD may contribute to incomplete acceptance of the diagnosis and reduced likelihood of satisfactory outcomes (Edwards et al., 2014). In fact, there remains wide variability on how neurologists debrief patients about their FMD diagnosis (Espay et al., 2009). Most terms are nonspecific, may carry negative connotations, or presume underlying psychopathology (Stone et al., 2005). These and other factors, such as limited access to movement disorders expertise, have prompted a large proportion of patients with syndromic diagnoses (e.g., dystonia not otherwise specified) to post online videos portraying themselves as representing organic disorders (Stamelou et al., 2011).

DIAGNOSIS OF FUNCTIONAL DYSTONIA

While FD currently lacks a widely available laboratory signature, its diagnosis can sometimes be attained with clinically definite diagnostic certainty after careful neurologic examination (Peckham and Hallett, 2009; Espay and Lang, 2015). As with other FMDs, evidence must be mounted toward demonstrating internal inconsistency and disease incongruity. Laboratory tests need not be normal in order to confirm this diagnosis. The most common features of FD are its sudden onset and a fixed posture at rest, which offers marked resistance to passive manipulation. We have recently argued in favor of de-emphasizing the importance of psychiatric and historic features in the diagnosis of FMD, but the history of an abrupt appearance can be an exception given its importance in distinguishing it from the fixed dystonia of corticobasal syndrome (Espay and Lang, 2015). Additional clinical features may include little to no exacerbation with action, infrequent or absent response to sensory tricks, pain in the affected body parts, prompt resolution immediately after botulinum toxin injections or other nonphysiologic responses, and variable generalization to the rest of the body with intermittent episodes of exacerbation and/or appearance of associated FMD (Lang, 1995).

Fahn and Williams (1988) introduced four categories of diagnostic certainty: documented, clinically established, probable, and possible. However, the categories of possible and probable FD are less helpful in the clinic setting, as they still warrant excluding other diseases, and do not permit the favored inclusionary approach to the diagnosis. Also, because "obvious emotional disturbance" suffices for the diagnosis of possible FD, it renders this category of doubtful validity since

Table 20.1

Major distinctions between previously proposed categories of diagnostic certainty in the diagnosis of functional movement disorders

Criteria	Clinically definite*	Clinically probable†	Clinically possible‡
Fahn and Williams (Fahn and Williams, 1988; Williams et al., 1994)	Documented or Clinically established: Incongruent or inconsistent plus ≥1 of: 1. Other false signs 2. Multiple somatizations 3. Obvious psychiatric disturbance 4. Distractibility 5. Deliberate slowness	1. Distractibility 2. Other false signs 3. Multiple somatizations	Obvious emotional disturbance
Shill and Gerber (2006)	Proven or Primary criteria: 1. Excessive pain or fatigue 2. Previous exposure to a disease model 3. Potential for secondary gain Secondary criteria: 1. Multiple somatizations (other than pain and fatigue) 2. Obvious psychiatric disturbance	Example of probable (all four): 1. Excessive pain or fatigue 2. Previous exposure to a disease model 3. Multiple somatizations 4. Obvious psychiatric disturbance	Example of possible (all three): 1. Excessive pain or fatigue 2. Multiple somatizations 3. Obvious psychiatric disturbance
Gupta and Lang (2009)	Documented (as per Fahn and Williams) or Clinically established plus other features (as per Fahn and Williams) or Clinically established minus other features (i.e., unequivocal clinical features of functional movement disorder, incompatible with organic disease, without the other features required by the Fahn and Williams criteria)	Not endorsed	Not endorsed

Fahn and Williams:
*Inconsistent or incongruent movements plus any of the five listed here.
†Inconsistent or incongruent movements or one of the three listed here.
‡No requirement for movements to be inconsistent or incongruent in the presence of obvious emotional disturbance. The category of documented functional movement disorder is applied in cases of persistent relief by psychotherapy, suggestion, or placebo, or when movements disappear when unobserved.
Shill and Gerber:
*Movements that are inconsistent or three other primary criteria plus one secondary.
†Inconsistent movements or two other primary criteria plus two secondary.
‡Only one primary criterion and two secondary or two primary and one secondary (in none of these criteria is an inconsistent/incongruent movement mandatory).
Gupta and Lang:
*Inconsistent or incongruent movements plus Fahn and Williams' criteria for clinically documented or established with other features. Clinically established without other features indicates the presence of unequivocal clinical features of functional movement disorder incompatible with organic disease without the other features required by the Fahn and Williams' criteria. A laboratory-supported definite category is also suggested for tremor and myoclonus phenotypes. These criteria do not endorse "probable" and "possible" categories.
Modified from Espay and Lang (2015), with permission from Springer Science and Business Media.

this can be a feature of many organic disorders. Gupta and Lang (2009) suggested revisions to the diagnostic criteria, in part to account for this and other shortcomings, establish a clinically definite category from the combination of documented and clinically established, and recognized the aid of electrophysiology in ascertaining a laboratory-supported definite diagnosis of FD (Table 20.1).

Inconsistency (clinical features vary in severity or topographic distribution over time) and incongruence (signs are contrary to the pathophysiology or neuroanatomy of organic disorders) are the two most important elements forming the clinical diagnosis of all FMDs (Lang and Voon, 2011). Applicable to FD, incongruent features include fixed postures at onset, pain in affected body parts (beyond the cervical region), resistance to passive movements, false weakness, and nonanatomic sensory deficits; inconsistent features include a tendency to vary in distribution and severity spontaneously or with nonphysiologic interventions, and multiple somatizations that change over time (Fahn and Williams, 1988) (Table 20.2).

A laboratory-supported diagnosis of FD may be possible in cases of functional blepharospasm and some instances of fixed foot dystonia. The blink reflex, when assessed with paired supraorbital nerve stimuli, exhibits a normal recovery cycle (R2) in functional blepharospasm (Janssen et al., 2014), unlike its organic counterpart, where an abnormal R2 can be documented (Berardelli et al., 1985). An abnormal pattern of co-contraction of antagonist muscles in patients with fixed foot dystonia in the "pre-trial" for the "rest," "posture," and "move" conditions (a 30-second period between the verbal instruction of the forthcoming condition and the go signal for that condition) stands in contrast with the absence of such pre-trial co-contraction in both DYT1 dystonia patients and healthy controls (Mehta et al., 2013).

REGIONAL FUNCTIONAL DYSTONIA PHENOTYPES

Beyond general features helpful in distinguishing FD from organic dystonia (Table 20.3), a variety of highly specific phenotypes have been recognized in patients with focal phenotypes of FD (Fig. 20.1).

Table 20.2

Proposed diagnostic criteria for functional dystonia

Clinically definite functional dystonia if all are present	Supportive but neither necessary nor sufficient	Laboratory-confirmed
1. Rapid onset* 2. Fixed dystonia at rest 3. Variable resistance to manipulation and/or distractibility or absence when unobserved	1. Associated pain (except in cervical region) 2. Associated complex regional pain syndrome	1. Normal recovery of the blink reflex (functional blepharospasm) 2. Coactivation sign on surface electromyogram (fixed foot dystonia)

Modified from Espay and Lang (2015), with permission from Springer Science and Business Media.

*Sudden onset is the only historic feature considered "core" in fixed dystonia at rest, because fixed dystonia at rest can occur gradually in some organic disorders.

Table 20.3

Comparisons between organic dystonia and functional dystonia

	Organic dystonia	Functional dystonia
Onset	Insidious and evolving over months to years; posturing is action-induced at the outset	Sudden or evolving within a few days, posturing at rest from the outset
Precipitant	Not identifiable; traumatic history is rare and, when present, latency from injury to onset is longer	Minor trauma, work-related injury; very short latency to symptom onset
Course	Slow progression; paroxysms and remissions are rare; segmental extension is uncommon and leg involvement is virtually never present in adult-onset cases	Rapid progression to maximum severity, common paroxysms and remissions; segmental extension with leg involvement
Disability	Disability may occur after many years and individual coping strategies lessen its impact	Disproportionate to the extent of dystonia; litigation or compensation seeking is common
Passive manipulation	Little or no active resistance to passive movement	Often fixed, active resistance to passive movements of affected body parts; manipulation may trigger or exacerbate pain
Sensory tricks (*geste antagoniste*)*	Common	Absent or "paradoxic" (worsening upon touch)
Associated features	None or dystonic tremor	Functional limb weakness, functional hypoesthesia, other functional movement disorders
Response to therapy	Excellent response to botulinum neurotoxin	Usually poor; immediate placebo response with botulinum neurotoxin chemodenervation

*Sensory trick or *geste antagoniste* refers to the improvement in dystonic postures with the application of closed-loop sensory feedback.

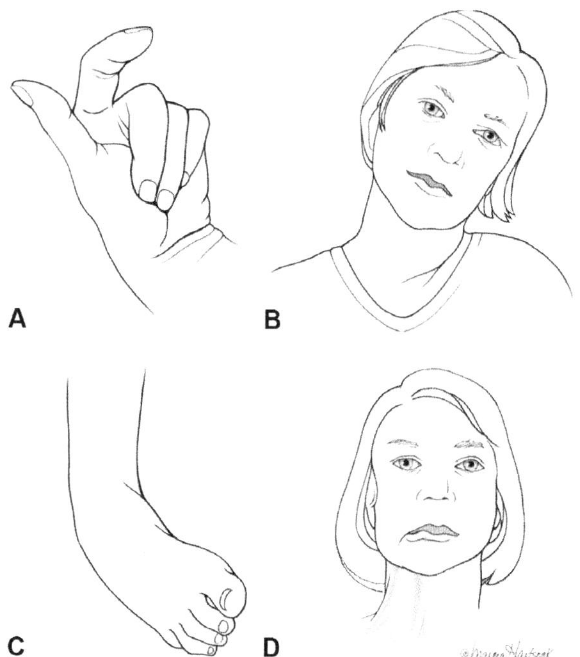

Fig. 20.1. Classic functional dystonia phenotypes. (**A**) Functional hand dystonia with preserved pincer function. (**B**) "Postraumatic painful torticollis," with fixed laterocollis, ipsilateral shoulder elevation, and contralateral shoulder depression. (**C**) Foot dystonia with fixed foot plantar flexion and inversion. (**D**) Functional facial dystonia with unilateral tonic jaw and lip deviation, often with ipsilateral platysma involvement.

Craniofacial region

Functional facial movement disorders exhibit tonic muscular spasms resembling dystonia and involving the lip, often pulling to one side (60.7%), eyelids (50.8%), perinasal region (16.4%), and forehead (9.8%) (Fasano et al., 2012). Tonic jaw deviation, with ipsilateral downward and lateral jaw pulling, is the most common phenotype, appreciated in 84.3% of 61 patients with FMD involving the craniofacial region (Fasano et al., 2012). Associated uni- or bilateral orbicularis oculi and platysma contraction are common associated features.

Cervical region

The most characteristic phenotype is the posttraumatic painful torticollis, of sudden appearance after (often trivial) trauma (Sa et al., 2003). It is characterized by predominant laterocollis, ipsilateral shoulder elevation, and contralateral shoulder depression. As organic cervical dystonia is never associated with contralateral shoulder depression, this phenomenologic feature of FD can serve (in addition to the fixed posturing) as a distinguishing clinical clue from its organic counterpart. The cervical posture is fixed from the outset and resistant to passive manipulation. Pain is a common associated feature, though it alone does not serve to distinguish from cervical dystonia (Schrag et al., 2004b). Spread of dystonia and accrual of additional functional disorders are common.

Foot

Fixed foot plantar flexion and inversion are the most common expressions of this adult-onset form of FD. Foot dystonia at rest (i.e., nonparoxysmal or exercise-induced) in adults is most often functional (Schrag et al., 2004a). An unusual variant in young adults is the functional "striatal toe" expressed as fixed first-toe extension and second- to fifth-toe flexion, whereby the first toe is resistant to forced flexion but undergoes spontaneous flexion when the examiner extends the second to fifth toes (Espay and Lang, 2011). Fixed foot dystonia may arguably be among the most malignant and refractory of functional phenotypes, with early and virtually permanent loss of ambulation. This may in part be due to the perception by patients of their foot posturing as straight (Stone et al., 2012). Residual ambulation tends to be associated with excessive effort (the "huffing and puffing" sign), disproportionate to the magnitude of objective disability (Laub et al., 2015). A sizable proportion of these patients may also develop secondary orthopedic abnormalities and dysautonomic features from disuse and immobility of the affected limb, although perhaps the reverse pattern may be more common: pain, CRPS diagnosis, then FD. A diagnosis of CRPS-I often distracts attention from the functional nature of the dystonia and arguably impedes initiation of appropriate treatment strategies.

Hand

Unlike idiopathic or poststroke brachial dystonia, FD affecting the hand leads to wrist and finger flexion of the second to fifth fingers with relative or complete sparing of the thumb and, in some instances, the index finger, thus preserving the important pincer function. In this variant of FD, digits four and five of the hand tend to be more affected than digits two and three, and the thumb least affected or not affected (Schrag et al., 2004a). This selective sparing of the thumb in the setting of rapid hand posturing is virtually pathognomonic of FD, though it can be involved in some patients. Again, here, the abruptness of the hand posturing is a necessary clinical clue that helps distinguish it from that evolving over months or years in dementia disorders, particularly those associated with the corticobasal syndrome (Godeiro-Junior et al., 2008), and severe autism (Turner et al., 2002).

PSYCHOPATHOLOGY

The question as to why anyone might develop FD, or any other FMD for that matter, is of fundamental importance. We understand conceptually that FMDs develop from a mismatch between patients' core beliefs and expectations and their environment and sensory data. This mismatch concept was first discussed by Janet in the late 1800s (Janet, 1889), and expanded upon by Freud, who felt that a psychologic dissociation was a defense mechanism, which provided an advantage or "secondary gain" (Freud et al., 1953). The mismatch, magnified by physical or emotional triggers, has been proposed to lead to the misattribution or misinterpretation of symptoms by the patient (Morgante et al., 2013). The largest series of FD demonstrated higher rates of dissociative (42%) and affective disorders (85%) (Schrag et al., 2004b). Other psychoemotional features identified in FD include childhood trauma, specifically greater emotional abuse and physical neglect, greater fear associated with traumatic events, and a greater number of traumatic episodes as compared with healthy volunteers and patients with focal hand dystonia, and controlling for depressive symptoms and sex (Kranick et al., 2011). Of importance, this series found no differences in the frequency of sexual abuse, physical abuse, and emotional neglect, parental bonding, self-reported personality traits, including neuroticism, and a measure of tendency to dissociation. In another series of 41 FD patients followed for a mean of 8 years, anxiety was documented in 41% and depression in 18% of this cohort; 18% scored within the range of dissociative/somatoform disorders (Ibrahim et al., 2009).

PATHOPHYSIOLOGY

Several studies have shown that some electrophysiologic features first identified in organic dystonia overlap with those of FD (Table 20.4). In general, three main pathophysiologic abnormalities have been identified in organic dystonia in the sensorimotor system: reduced excitability of cortical and spinal inhibitory circuits, impaired somatosensory processing and integration, and maladaptive plasticity in the sensorimotor cortex. Normal blink reflex in the first category and, tentatively, normal cortical plasticity in the last may serve to distinguish FD from organic dystonia.

Table 20.4

Tentative electrophysiologic abnormalities in organic and functional dystonias

	Organic dystonia	Functional dystonia
Blink reflex	Abnormal recovery cycle of the blink reflex (disinhibition of R2)	Normal recovery cycle of the blink reflex*
Cortical inhibitory circuits	Impaired intracortical inhibition (reduced resting short- and long-interval intracortical inhibition and cortical silent period)	
Spinal inhibitory circuits	Impaired intraspinal inhibition (increased cutaneous silent period)	
Somatosensory processing	Increased spatial and temporal discrimination thresholds	
Cortical plasticity	High cortical plasticity	Normal cortical plasticity*

*The blink reflex involves an early response (R1), ipsilateral to the stimulated supraorbital nerve, and a late bilateral response (R2). Normal recovery in the blink reflex and normal cortical plasticity (documented by paired associative stimulation) are the only two findings that may distinguish functional dystonia from organic dystonia patients.

This distinction remains tentative, as substantial overlap has been reported between these dystonia.

Cortical and spinal excitability

Cortical inhibition, as measured by resting short- and long-interval intracortical inhibition and cortical silent period, is reduced in patients with FD to an extent similar to patients with organic dystonia, both in the affected (Espay et al., 2006) as well as the unaffected limb (Avanzino et al., 2008). Spinal inhibition is similarly reduced in both FD and organic dystonia, as documented by an increased cutaneous silent period (Espay et al., 2006). Since the impairment of cortical and spinal inhibitory interneuronal systems is similar across functional and organic dystonia, it has been proposed that abnormal cortical excitability might represent an underlying trait predisposing to dystonia as a phenotype in general.

Somatosensory processing

Impairment in somatosensory processing identified by increased spatial and temporal discrimination thresholds in both affected and unaffected body parts in organic dystonia (Aglioti et al., 2003; Molloy et al., 2003) has also been documented in patients with FD (Morgante et al., 2011). Thus, as with the interpretation of the cortical and spinal inhibitory measures, abnormal somatosensory processing might represent a neurophysiologic trait predisposing to developing or maintaining a dystonic posture, with other, as yet unclear, variables turning the phenotype into FD or organic dystonia but not distinguishing between them.

Cortical plasticity

Cortical plasticity in sensorimotor circuits, tested with an electrophysiologic paradigm involving paired associative stimulation, was found to be abnormally high in organic dystonia (Quartarone et al., 2008) but normal in patients with FD (Quartarone et al., 2009). The lack of maladaptive plasticity in FD needs to be replicated by other groups before it can be of use in clinical and research settings.

Functional neuroimaging

One positron emission tomography study on 6 patients with right-foot FD showed abnormally increased blood flow in the cerebellum and basal ganglia, and a decrease in the primary motor cortex, compared to patients with organic dystonia exhibiting similar topographic involvement, who showed instead an increase in blood flow in the primary motor cortex, thalamus, and caudate nucleus (Schrag et al., 2013). These data suggested a cortical-subcortical differentiation between organic dystonia and FD in terms of regional blood flow. In a recently completed functional magnetic resonance imaging study using motor, basic emotion recognition, and intense-emotion stimuli tasks, there was hypoactivation in the posterior putamen bilaterally with simple motor and emotional stimuli and mixed hypo- and hyperactivation in key basal ganglia and cortical regions in response to intense emotional stimuli in FD patients compared with organic dystonia and healthy controls (Espay et al., preliminary data). These data suggest that specific impairments in stimulus-dependent emotion processing may underlie the generation and/or maintenance of FD or the psychologic comorbidities associated with FD. Additional studies will be needed to ascertain the extent to which these functional changes can be modified by available psycho- and physiotherapeutic modalities. Moreover, it is important to note that, while these imaging studies may show interesting group differences, they are not likely to be useful for diagnosis in the individual patient.

PROGNOSIS

The prognosis of patients with FD remains poor. Improvement is documented in fewer than 25% of patients, major remission in only 6%, and continued worsening in a third, with even new neuropsychiatric features emerging in some (Ibrahim et al., 2009). The co-diagnosis of CRPS at baseline was found to be an independent predictor of a worse outcome (Ibrahim et al., 2009). Other challenges that interfere with the management and recovery of these patients include ongoing litigation and incomplete acceptance of the diagnosis by the patient (Espay et al., 2009). The prognosis may be further compounded by long-term sedentarism and orthopedic complications. In the most severe cases, FD patients have sought amputation of the affected limb, suggesting a particularly malignant form of the disease associated with body integrity identity disorder (Edwards et al., 2011).

Given the poor response to available therapies, early and proper delivery of diagnosis remains critical for a positive outcome. Indeed, short duration of symptoms and high satisfaction with care have been shown to predict a positive outcome (Gelauff et al., 2014).

MANAGEMENT

Treatment of FD begins at the time of diagnostic debriefing, which ensures acceptance of the diagnosis. Exculpating the patient when delivering the diagnosis is the first therapeutic step, since it enhances the yield of therapy and improves prognosis (Salmon et al., 1999). Unfortunately, current treatments for FD are based on single case reports or small cohort studies. Therefore, we will summarize general therapeutic principles applicable to all FMD and only list promising reports specific to the management of FD.

General therapeutic principles

A multidisciplinary team approach has been advocated, with neurologists, psychiatrists, and physiotherapists. However, the neurologist is the only one with the appropriate training to diagnose FMD with clinically definite certainty and steer the therapy decisively away from additional laboratory investigations or pharmacotherapeutic trials. Dallocchio and colleagues (2010) suggested the acronym THERAPIST, modified here, as a reminder for the important elements in the management sequence for FMD, and, by extension, FD:

Terminology.
Hear out the patient.
Explain the diagnosis.
Reassure.
Address issues.
Prognosis.
Individualize.
Self-help.
Treat concurrent illnesses, if any.

The treating neurologist must clearly indicate the diagnosis and correct patient misconceptions, with the goal of helping patients accept the diagnosis and facilitating their embracing subsequent therapeutic efforts. The nomenclature to use during the diagnostic debriefing remains controversial, but a desire to reduce dualistic thinking and minimize potentially demeaning or pejorative language has led to the proposal of using the term functional (Edwards et al., 2014). It is important to emphasize that patients are not "crazy," are not "making up" their symptoms and deficits (i.e., they are "real"), and that their disability is as severe as that of neurodegenerative disorders (Anderson et al., 2007). Prior to introducing the treatment options, it is important to discuss any patient-related potential conflict of interest, which may prevent the success of therapy, such as disability proceedings, ongoing or anticipated litigation, and co-dependent relationship with spouse or caregiver.

Cognitive behavioral therapy

Cognitive behavioral therapy (CBT) had accrued substantial evidence in depression and anxiety before its recent translation for patients with FMD (Kroenke, 2007; LaFrance and Friedman, 2009). During CBT sessions, patients are guided toward the identification of their dysfunctional core beliefs (cognitive distortions) in order to disrupt the associated cognitive, emotional, and behavioral responses to past and ongoing stressors (Morgante et al., 2013). Pharmacologic treatment of comorbid depression and anxiety, if present, may enhance the odds of success (Feinstein et al., 2001; Lang and Voon, 2011). A consulting psychiatrist can help initiate a course of treatment for any relevant psychopathology with the support of the treating movement disorder specialist (Williams et al., 2005). Studies in psychogenic nonepileptic seizures have shown that selective serotonin reuptake inhibitors can induce nearly 50% reduction in event occurrence (LaFrance et al., 2010), a success rate that could plausibly be extrapolated to FD and other FMD. CBT remains to be formally examined for the treatment of FD.

Psychodynamic psychotherapy

Psychodynamic psychotherapy is another treatment modality potentially effective for FD. It may also be combined with antidepressant and/or anxiolytic treatment and is aimed at evaluating historical life experiences, especially in early life, and personality traits, and compares these to current life experiences and problematic emotions (Hinson et al., 2006).

Physical therapy

Physical therapy has been evaluated as a mechanism to treat functional gait disorders, including the ones associated with FD. In one study, patients with functional gait participated in a 3-week inpatient rehabilitation program with improvement upon completion and at 1 year following the study (Jordbru et al., 2014). While a physical therapy program has not been formally assessed in FD, Dallocchio and colleagues (2010) evaluated an exercise program in 5 FD patients (from a cohort of 16 total FMD patients), documenting substantial improvements in disability ratings in 3 of them, and one-third of the global cohort.

Motor reprogramming physiotherapy

A 1-week motor reprogramming physiotherapy program in 60 patients was developed at the Mayo Clinic for patients with a variety of FMDs, achieving nearly 60% improvement or remission (Czarnecki et al., 2012). Motor reprogramming "breaks down aberrant movements and postures into individual motor components and gradually reconstructs more normal motor patterns," reinforcing these patterns and ignoring inappropriate ones, thus forcing them into extinction (Czarnecki et al., 2012). While this therapeutic option appears promising, it is unclear whether its application to FD can be expected to be as successful (the authors did not specify how many patients had FD in their report). A controlled clinical trial examining this physiotherapy approach is needed.

FD-specific anecdotal experience

Van Nuenen et al. (2007) discussed the benefits of acupuncture applied to a single case with long-standing and refractory mixed FMD, which included FD. Hypnosis was reported to reduce symptoms in nearly two-thirds of FMD patients (though probably none with FD), with benefits persisting after 6 months (Moene et al., 2003). Therapeutic sedation with propofol was reported as useful in selected patients with severe FD, presumably prior to development of contractures (Stone et al., 2014). Motor cortex stimulation was also reported to rapidly improve a patient with fixed dystonia, previously treated with pallidal stimulation (Romito et al., 2007), although the possibility of a placebo response was not accounted for and this patient was not diagnosed as having FD prior to such intervention (Espay et al., 2007). Recently, repetitive transcranial magnetic stimulation was shown to reduce disability in patients with FMD, although this effort included no patients with FD (Pollak et al., 2014). Finally, low-dose naltrexone (Chopra and Cooper, 2013) and spinal cord stimulation with intrathecal baclofen therapy (Goto et al., 2013) have been reported to be of help in 2 and 4 FD-CRPS patients, respectively, but randomized controlled trials are unlikely to be designed for these therapies.

CONCLUSIONS AND FUTURE STEPS

FD is a major and often neglected source of disability among neurologic disorders. It can sometimes be diagnosed with clinically definite certainty using clinical examination findings alone, but is often very difficult. Ongoing and future research endeavors will focus on increasing the neurobiologic understanding of FD, further refining the pathophysiologic basis that distinguishes it from organic dystonia, and enhancing the yield of available treatment options in isolation or, most likely, in combination. Moving from "psychogenic" to "functional" dystonia (Edwards et al., 2014) is part of the basic building blocks of a long road ahead in improving the diagnosis and management of these patients.

References

Aglioti SM, Fiorio M, Forster B et al. (2003). Temporal discrimination of cross-modal and unimodal stimuli in generalized dystonia. Neurology 60: 782–785.

Anderson KE, Gruber-Baldini AL, Vaughan CG et al. (2007). Impact of psychogenic movement disorders versus Parkinson's on disability, quality of life, and psychopathology. Mov Disord 22: 2204–2209.

Avanzino L, Martino D, van de Warrenburg BPC et al. (2008). Cortical excitability is abnormal in patients with the "fixed dystonia" syndrome. Mov Disord 23: 646–652.

Berardelli A, Rothwell JC, Day BL et al. (1985). Pathophysiology of blepharospasm and oromandibular dystonia. Brain 108 (Pt 3): 593–608.

Chopra P, Cooper MS (2013). Treatment of complex regional pain syndrome (CRPS) using low dose naltrexone (LDN). J Neuroimmune Pharmacol 8: 470–476.

Crimlisk HL, Bhatia KP, Cope H et al. (2000). Patterns of referral in patients with medically unexplained motor symptoms. J Psychosom Res 49: 217–219.

Czarnecki K, Thompson JM, Seime R et al. (2012). Functional movement disorders: successful treatment with a physical therapy rehabilitation protocol. Parkinsonism Relat Disord 18: 247–251.

Dallocchio C, Arbasino C, Klersy C et al. (2010). The effects of physical activity on psychogenic movement disorders. Mov Disord 25: 421–425.

Edwards MJ, Alonso-Canovas A, Schrag A et al. (2011). Limb amputations in fixed dystonia: a form of body integrity identity disorder? Mov Disord 26: 1410–1414.

Edwards MJ, Stone J, Lang AE (2014). From psychogenic movement disorder to functional movement disorder: it's time to change the name. Mov Disord 29: 849–852.

Espay AJ, Lang AE (2011). The psychogenic toe signs. Neurology 77: 508–509.

Espay AJ, Lang AE (2015). Phenotype-specific diagnosis of functional (psychogenic) movement disorders. Curr Neurol Neurosci Rep 15: 556.

Espay AJ, Morgante F, Purzner J et al. (2006). Cortical and spinal abnormalities in psychogenic dystonia. Ann Neurol 59: 825–834.

Espay AJ, Chen R, Moro E et al. (2007). Fixed dystonia unresponsive to pallidal stimulation improved by motor cortex stimulation. Neurology 69: 1062–1063. author reply 1063.

Espay AJ, Goldenhar LM, Voon V et al. (2009). Opinions and clinical practices related to diagnosing and managing patients with psychogenic movement disorders: an international survey of movement disorder society members. Mov Disord 24: 1366–1374.

Fahn S, Williams DT (1988). Psychogenic dystonia. Adv Neurol 50: 431–455.

Fasano A, Valadas A, Bhatia KP et al. (2012). Psychogenic facial movement disorders: clinical features and associated conditions. Mov Disord 27: 1544–1551.

Feinstein A, Stergiopoulos V, Fine J et al. (2001). Psychiatric outcome in patients with a psychogenic movement disorder: a prospective study. Neuropsychiatry Neuropsychol Behav Neurol 14: 169–176.

Freud S, Strachey J, Freud A et al. (1953). The standard edition of the complete psychological works of Sigmund Freud, Hogarth Press, London.

Gelauff J, Stone J, Edwards M et al. (2014). The prognosis of functional (psychogenic) motor symptoms: a systematic review. J Neurol Neurosurg Psychiatry 85: 220–226.

Godeiro-Junior C, Felicio AC, Barsottini OG et al. (2008). Clinical features of dystonia in atypical parkinsonism. Arq Neuropsiquiatr 66: 800–804.

Goto S, Taira T, Horisawa S et al. (2013). Spinal cord stimulation and intrathecal baclofen therapy: combined neuromodulation for treatment of advanced complex regional pain syndrome. Stereotact Funct Neurosurg 91: 386–391.

Gupta A, Lang AE (2009). Psychogenic movement disorders. Curr Opin Neurol 22: 430–436.

Hinson VK, Weinstein S, Bernard B et al. (2006). Single-blind clinical trial of psychotherapy for treatment of psychogenic movement disorders. Parkinsonism Relat Disord 12: 177–180.

Ibrahim NM, Martino D, van de Warrenburg BP et al. (2009). The prognosis of fixed dystonia: a follow-up study. Parkinsonism Relat Disord 15: 592–597.

Janet P (1889). L'automatisme psychologique, Felix Alcan, Paris.

Janssen S, Veugen LC, Hoffland BS et al. (2014). Normal eyeblink classical conditioning in patients with fixed dystonia. Exp Brain Res 232: 1805–1809.

Jordbru AA, Smedstad LM, Klungsoyr O et al. (2014). Psychogenic gait disorder: a randomized controlled trial of physical rehabilitation with one-year follow-up. J Rehabil Med 46: 181–187.

Klein C, Fahn S (2013). Translation of Oppenheim's 1911 paper on dystonia. Mov Disord 28: 851–862.

Kranick S, Ekanayake V, Martinez V et al. (2011). Psychopathology and psychogenic movement disorders. Mov Disord 26: 1844–1850.

Kroenke K (2007). Efficacy of treatment for somatoform disorders: a review of randomized controlled trials. Psychosom Med 69: 881–888.

LaFrance Jr WC, Friedman JH (2009). Cognitive behavioral therapy for psychogenic movement disorder. Mov Disord 24: 1856–1857.

LaFrance WC, Keitner GI, Papandonatos GD et al. (2010). Pilot pharmacologic randomized controlled trial for psychogenic nonepileptic seizures. Neurology 75: 1166–1173.

Lang AE (1995). Psychogenic dystonia: a review of 18 cases. Can J Neurol Sci 22: 136–143.

Lang AE, Voon V (2011). Psychogenic movement disorders: past developments, current status, and future directions. Mov Disord 26: 1175–1186.

Laub HN, Dwivedi AK, Revilla FJ et al. (2015). Diagnostic performance of the "huffing and puffing" sign in functional (psychogenic) movement disorders. Mov Disord Clin Pract 2: 29–32.

Marsden CD (1976). Dystonia: the spectrum of the disease. Res Publ Assoc Res Nerv Ment Dis 55: 351–367.

Marsden CD (1986). Hysteria – a neurologist's view. Psychol Med 16: 277–288.

Mehta AR, Rowe JB, Trimble MR et al. (2013). Coactivation sign in fixed dystonia. Parkinsonism Relat Disord 19: 474–476.

Miyasaki JM, Sa DS, Galvez-Jimenez N et al. (2003). Psychogenic movement disorders. Can J Neurol Sci 30 (Suppl 1): S94–S100.

Moene FC, Spinhoven P, Hoogduin KA et al. (2003). A randomized controlled clinical trial of a hypnosis-based treatment for patients with conversion disorder, motor type. Int J Clin Exp Hypn 51: 29–50.

Molloy FM, Carr TD, Zeuner KE et al. (2003). Abnormalities of spatial discrimination in focal and generalized dystonia. Brain 126: 2175–2182.

Morgante F, Tinazzi M, Squintani G et al. (2011). Abnormal tactile temporal discrimination in psychogenic dystonia. Neurology 77: 1191–1197.

Morgante F, Edwards MJ, Espay AJ (2013). Psychogenic movement disorders. Continuum (Minneap Minn) 19: 1383–1396.

Munts AG, Koehler PJ (2010). How psychogenic is dystonia? Views from past to present. Brain 133: 1552–1564.

Peckham EL, Hallett M (2009). Psychogenic movement disorders. Neurol Clin 27: 801–819.

Pollak TA, Nicholson TR, Edwards MJ et al. (2014). A systematic review of transcranial magnetic stimulation in the treatment of functional (conversion) neurological symptoms. J Neurol Neurosurg Psychiatry 85: 191–197.

Quartarone A, Rizzo V, Morgante F (2008). Clinical features of dystonia: a pathophysiological revisitation. Curr Opin Neurol 21: 484–490.

Quartarone A, Rizzo V, Terranova C et al. (2009). Abnormal sensorimotor plasticity in organic but not in psychogenic dystonia. Brain 132: 2871–2877.

Romito LM, Franzini A, Perani D et al. (2007). Fixed dystonia unresponsive to pallidal stimulation improved by motor cortex stimulation. Neurology 68: 875–876.

Sa DS, Mailis-Gagnon A, Nicholson K et al. (2003). Posttraumatic painful torticollis. Mov Disord 18: 1482–1491.

Salmon P, Peters S, Stanley I (1999). Patients' perceptions of medical explanations for somatisation disorders: qualitative analysis. BMJ 318: 372–376.

Schrag A, Lang AE (2005). Psychogenic movement disorders. Curr Opin Neurol 18: 399–404.

Schrag A, Trimble M, Quinn N et al. (2004a). The syndrome of fixed dystonia: an evaluation of 103 patients. Brain 127: 2360–2372.

Schrag A, Trimble M, Quinn N et al. (2004b). The syndrome of fixed dystonia: an evaluation of 103 patients. Brain 127: 2360–2372.

Schrag AE, Mehta AR, Bhatia KP et al. (2013). The functional neuroimaging correlates of psychogenic versus organic dystonia. Brain 136: 770–781.

Schwalbe W (1908). Eine eigentumliche tonische Krampfform mit hysterischen, G Schade, Berlin.

Schwartzman RJ, Kerrigan J (1990). The movement disorder of reflex sympathetic dystrophy. Neurology 40: 57–61.

Shill H, Gerber P (2006). Evaluation of clinical diagnostic criteria for psychogenic movement disorders. Mov Disord 21: 1163–1168.

Stamelou M, Edwards MJ, Espay AJ et al. (2011). Movement disorders on YouTube – caveat spectator. N Engl J Med 365: 1160–1161.

Stone J, Smyth R, Carson A et al. (2005). Systematic review of misdiagnosis of conversion symptoms and "hysteria". BMJ 331: 989.

Stone J, Gelauff J, Carson A (2012). A "twist in the tale": altered perception of ankle position in psychogenic dystonia. Mov Disord 27: 585–586.

Stone J, Hoeritzauer I, Brown K et al. (2014). Therapeutic sedation for functional (psychogenic) neurological symptoms. J Psychosom Res 76: 165–168.

Turner G, Partington M, Kerr B et al. (2002). Variable expression of mental retardation, autism, seizures, and dystonic hand movements in two families with an identical ARX gene mutation. Am J Med Genet 112: 405–411.

Van Nuenen BF, Wohlgemuth M, Wong Chung RE et al. (2007). Acupuncture for psychogenic movement disorders: treatment or diagnostic tool? Mov Disord 22: 1353–1355.

van Rooijen DE, Marinus J, Schouten AC et al. (2013a). Muscle hyperalgesia correlates with motor function in complex regional pain syndrome type 1. J Pain 14: 446–454.

van Rooijen DE, Marinus J, van Hilten JJ (2013b). Muscle hyperalgesia is widespread in patients with complex regional pain syndrome. Pain 154: 2745–2749.

Verdugo RJ, Ochoa JL (2000). Abnormal movements in complex regional pain syndrome: assessment of their nature. Muscle Nerve 23: 198–205.

Williams DT, Ford B, Fahn S (1994). Phenomenology and psychopathology related to psychogenic movement disorders. In: WJ Weiner, AE Lang (Eds.), Behavioral neurology in movement disorders, Raven Press, New York.

Williams DT, Ford B, Fahn S (2005). Treatment issues in psychogenic-neuropsychiatric movement disorders. Adv Neurol 96: 350–363.

Handbook of Clinical Neurology, Vol. 139 (3rd series)
Functional Neurologic Disorders
M. Hallett, J. Stone, and A. Carson, Editors
http://dx.doi.org/10.1016/B978-0-12-801772-2.00021-7

Chapter 21

Functional jerks, tics, and paroxysmal movement disorders

Y.E.M. DREISSEN[1], D.C. CATH[2], AND M.A.J. TIJSSEN[1]*
[1]*Department of Neurology, University Medical Centre Groningen, Groningen, The Netherlands*
[2]*Department of Clinical and Health Psychology, Utrecht University/Altrecht, Utrecht, The Netherlands*

Abstract

Functional jerks are among the most common functional movement disorders. The diagnosis of functional jerks is mainly based on neurologic examination revealing specific positive clinical signs. Differentiation from other jerky movements, such as tics, organic myoclonus, and primary paroxysmal dyskinesias, can be difficult. In support of a functional jerk are: acute onset in adulthood, precipitation by a physical event, variable, complex, and inconsistent phenomenology, suggestibility, distractibility, entrainment and a Bereitschaftspotential preceding the movement. Although functional jerks and tics share many similarities, characteristics differentiating tics from functional jerks are: urge preceding the tic, childhood onset, rostrocaudal development of the symptoms, a positive family history of tics, attention-deficit hyperactivity disorder or obsessive-compulsive symptoms, and response to dopamine antagonist medication. To differentiate functional jerks from organic myoclonus, localization of the movements can give direction. Further features in support of organic myoclonus include: insidious onset, simple and consistent phenomenology, and response to benzodiazepines or antiepileptic medication. Primary paroxysmal dyskinesias and functional jerks share a paroxysmal nature. Leading in the differentiation between the two are: a positive family history, in combination with video recordings revealing a consistent symptom pattern in primary paroxysmal dyskinesias.

In this chapter functional jerks and their differential diagnoses will be discussed in terms of epidemiology, symptom characteristics, disease course, psychopathology, and supportive neurophysiologic tests.

INTRODUCTION

Jerky movements, including functional jerks, tics, and paroxysmal movement disorders, refer to a heterogeneous category of hyperkinetic movement disorders. The diagnosis of these jerky movements forms a true challenge for the clinician at the borderland between neurology and psychiatry (van der Salm et al., 2013). Over the last decade a paradigm shift has occurred towards a positive diagnosis of functional neurologic disorders instead of diagnosing by default after exclusion of all other possible diagnoses. More consensus seems to have been reached between psychiatrists and neurologists. First, the editors of the newest (fifth) edition of the *Diagnostic and Statistical Manual of Mental Disorders* (DSM-5, the standard psychiatric classification system) has incorporated "functional neurological symptom disorders" as a subcategory in the category of "conversion disorders," in line with the neurologic terminology (American Psychiatric Association, 2013). Second, the well-known diagnostic criteria of functional movement disorders (FMDs) by Fahn and Williams have been modified, leaving out psychologic disturbance, psychogenic signs, or multiple somatizations as a requirement for high diagnostic certainty (Fahn and Williams, 1988; Shill and Gerber, 2006; Gupta and Lang, 2009). Still, there is no pathognomonic sign or test, and diagnostic agreement between

*Correspondence to: Marina A.J. Tijssen, Department of Neurology AB 51, University Medical Centre Groningen (UMCG), Hanzeplein 1, PO Box 30.001, 9700 RB Groningen, The Netherlands. Tel: +31-50-3612400, E-mail: M.A.J.de.Koning-Tijssen@umcg.nl

clinicians in cases with lower diagnostic certainty (probable or possible) is poor to moderate (Morgante et al., 2012).

In a recent study the clinical decisions and accuracy of clinicians to establish the diagnosis of a jerky movement were tested (van der Salm et al., 2013). Interrater agreement on diagnoses of jerky movements was moderate (kappa $= 0.56 \pm 0.1$) between international movement disorder specialists. Remarkably, it appeared that best consensus was reached on the diagnosis of tics, and least consensus on the diagnosis of organic myoclonus, with FMDs scoring in between.

When can a jerky movement be considered as "functional"? How can FMD be discerned from tics on the one hand, and from myoclonic jerks on the other? In this chapter the differential diagnosis between functional jerks, myoclonus, tics, and primary paroxysmal dyskinesias (PxDs) is discussed, based on epidemiology, symptom characteristics, disease course, psychopathology, and neurophysiologic tests. We will start our chapter by defining functional jerks, myoclonus, and tics. In addition, functional paroxysmal movement disorders and their organic counterpart will be addressed.

EPIDEMIOLOGY AND CLINICAL PICTURE

Functional jerks

Epidemiology

Prevalence and incidence rates of functional jerks are largely unknown, due to diversity in the use of diagnostic criteria. Prevalence rates of FMD range between 0.24% and 3%, depending on whether they have been assessed in clinical or population-based samples (Factor et al., 1995; Stone et al., 2010). The higher prevalence rates at the upper end of this estimation are derived from specialized movement disorder clinics and are therefore an overestimation of the population prevalence. After functional tremor and dystonia, functional myoclonus or jerks represent the third most common diagnosis, comprising about 15% of all patients with FMDs (Factor et al., 1995; Hinson et al., 2005; Lang, 2006; Shill and Gerber, 2006). FMD (including functional jerks) can manifest at all ages, but mostly in adulthood, with mean age of onset ranging between 37 and 50 years (Factor et al., 1995; Williams et al., 1995). Women are more often affected than men, with female-to-male ratios ranging from 57% to 90% for females, although the male-to-female ratio seems to differ in specific subcategories of functional neurologic symptoms (Stone et al., 2010). For instance, functional jerks affecting the trunk (axial jerks) seem to affect men more often than women (van der Salm et al., 2014). Finally, little is known about clinical course. There is a clinical notion that the course is unfavorable (Gelauff et al., 2014), but this might be due to ascertainment bias, since all nonremitting cases are referred to specialized movement disorder clinics and the majority of spontaneously remitting cases are not seen.

Clinical picture

Consistent clinical features have been identified with respect to disease history and physical examination in functional jerks (Table 21.1) (Monday and Jankovic, 1993; Williams et al., 1995). Illness history often reveals an abrupt onset of symptoms, frequently preceded by a (minor) physical event (e.g., injury) or psychologic stressor, and subsequent rapid deterioration to maximal symptom severity (Monday and Jankovic, 1993; Factor et al., 1995; Williams et al., 1995; Pareés et al., 2014). The disease course is variable, with some patients experiencing a static course while others reveal fluctuations with complete remissions and sudden relapses. Often patients tend to overestimate the severity of their symptoms (Pareés et al., 2012). Previous episodes of somatization might be mentioned when interviewing on disease history and are of additional support in the diagnosis, but do not have high specificity, since functional and organic movement disorders seem to occur more often simultaneously than expected by chance (Ranawaya et al., 1990; Onofrj et al., 2010; Pareés et al., 2013a).

Clinically, functional jerks come in all shapes and sizes and can manifest everywhere in the body with focal, multifocal, segmental, axial, and generalized presentations (Monday and Jankovic, 1993; van der Salm et al., 2014). The localization of the jerks is an important factor in the differential diagnosis with tics and myoclonus. As a general rule of thumb, we find that axial jerks are likely to represent functional jerks, facial and neck jerks point more often towards tics, while limb and generalized jerks are more likely to reflect myoclonus (see below). Jerks might be present continuously or episodically (Monday and Jankovic, 1993; Ganos et al., 2014; van der Salm et al., 2014).

Functional jerks can increase with attention and decrease or disappear with (mental or motor) distraction or when patients are unobserved (Gupta and Lang, 2009); this feature is not specific for functional jerks though, and can occur in other movement disorders as well. The examiner, when asking the patient to perform a specific rhythmic task, might induce adaptation of the patient's jerks to the imposed frequency, a phenomenon called entrainment.

Abnormal stimulus sensitivity can be observed in FMDs, e.g., exaggerated tendon reflexes or excessive startle reactions. Other clinical signs frequently co-occur with FMD, including unexplained loss of muscle strength, sensory loss that is unexplained by any

Table 21.1

Clues in illness history, clinical examination, and additional features of functional jerks, tics, myoclonus, and primary paroxysmal dyskinesias

	Functional jerk	Tic	Myoclonus	Paroxysmal Dyskinesias
Clues in history				
Childhood onset	–	+	+/–	+
Positive family history	–	+	+/–	+
Acute onset	+	–	–	–
Precipitating physical event	+	–/+	–	–
Waxing and waning	+/–	+	–	–
Course characteristics	Static	↓ Adolescence	Static	↓ Adulthood
Premonitory urge	+/–	+	–	+/–
Persistence during sleep	–	+	+/–	–
Clinical examination				
Inconsistent	+	+/–	–	–
Rhythmic	+/–	–	+/–	–
Typical localization	Axial	Head/neck	Focal/segmental/axial/ generalized	Unilaterally
Entrainment	+	–	–	–
Temporal suppression	+/–	+	–	–
Suggestibility	+	+	–	–
Stimulus–sensitivity	+	–	+	+/–
Additional features				
Comorbid functional symptoms	+	–	–	+
Response medication	–	Antipsychotics	Benzodiazepines	Carbamazepine
Drastic response placebo	+	–	–	–
Psychopathology	+	+	+/–	–
Bereitschaftspotential	+	+/–	–	–

somatotopic organization, and pain (Monday and Jankovic, 1993; Gupta and Lang, 2009). Further supportive clues include marked response to placebo or suggestion, although, again, this is also observed in other movement disorders (Monday and Jankovic, 1993; Williams et al., 1995).

Since the frequency of functional jerks might vary and the nature of symptoms could be paroxysmal, it can be difficult to collect clues supportive of functional jerks during neurologic examination alone. Additional neurophysiologic testing, including a polymyographic electromyogram (EMG) and (if possible) electroencephalogram (EEG)-EMG with jerk-locked backaveraging in order to demonstrate a Bereitschaftspotential (BP) preceding the jerks, might be of particular use (Shibasaki and Hallett, 2006; van der Salm et al., 2012). This will be elaborated below.

Tics in the scope of Tourette's disorder

Epidemiology

The epidemiology of tics, i.e., movements seen in Tourette's syndrome and related disorders (denoted hereafter as "tics"), is well known: tics originate in most cases in childhood, with a mean age of onset of 5 years and male preponderance (male-to-female ratio 3:1) (Cath et al., 2011). This is in contrast with functional jerks, which usually start in adulthood (Monday and Jankovic, 1993; van der Salm et al., 2014). Tics are common in children, with prevalence estimates between 6% and 12%, but there is a sharp decline during adolescence in intensity and frequency of tics associated with maturation of the frontal lobes in adolescence (Singer, 2011). In sum, the prevalence (lifetime) of full-blown Tourette's syndrome ranges between 0.3% and 1%, depending on age of the study sample and rigor of sampling method used (Robertson et al., 2009). In contrast, functional jerks have unknown prevalence rates but are considered to be less common, and rare in children (Ferrara and Jankovic, 2008; Canavese et al., 2012). Most tics in adults do not cause much disability or the need to visit a physician. In contrast, functional jerks tend to increase in frequency in adults, causing distress and disability. Of note, tics in combination with functional tic-like jerks co-occur more often than expected by chance, and form a considerable diagnostic challenge for the treating physician (Barry et al., 2011). Patients with both functional jerks and tics are likely to be seen at movement disorder clinics.

Clinical picture

Tics are defined as sudden, rapid, repetitive, nonrhythmic, inapposite, irresistible muscle movements (motor tics) or vocalizations (vocal tics), which can be classified as simple or complex (Cath et al., 2011; Singer, 2011). Diagnosis of a tic disorder is solely made based on clinical examination, and with the aid of the Diagnostic Confidence Index (Robertson et al., 1999) or Yale Global Tic severity scale (Leckman et al., 1989). The fourth and fifth DSM (DSM-IV and DSM-5: American Psychiatric Association, 2000, 2013) and the 10th International Classification of Disease (ICD-10: World Health Organization, 2010) formulated diagnostic criteria for tic disorders, with Tourette's disorder (requiring at least two motor and one vocal tic) at the most severe end of the spectrum. The specific differentiation of a functional jerk from a tic can be challenging because of their overlapping clinical features (van der Salm et al., 2012, 2014); however, we will discuss clues supporting one or the other diagnosis below (Table 21.1).

The disease course in both tics and functional jerks is generally waxing and waning (Monday and Jankovic, 1993; Cath et al., 2011). Functional jerks often have abrupt onset and are precipitated by a physical event; this is not typical for tics (Tijssen et al., 1999; Cath et al., 2011).

Phenomenologically, motor tics are either simple – eye blinking, grimacing, nose/mouth twitches, and neck/shoulder jerks – or complex, portraying a sequence of movements, difficult to discern from more goal-directed compulsive movements (Fibbe et al., 2011). In general, motor tics are more stereotyped and less variable compared to functional jerks. Further, patients with tics sometimes tend to camouflage the movement by assimilating it into a purposeful movement, whereas patients with functional jerks are not inclined or able to hide their movements (Anderson et al., 2007; Cath et al., 2011; Pareés et al., 2013b).

Another important clinical feature of tics entails their localization: tics tend to develop following a rostrocaudal spread, usually starting in the face, with the face, neck, and shoulder region being mostly affected, as opposed to functional jerks that, except for axial jerks, lack a preferential localization (Monday and Jankovic, 1993; Cath et al., 2011; van der Salm et al., 2012, 2014).

Most patients with functional jerks are unable to voluntarily suppress symptoms, whereas patients with tics can usually suppress their tics for short periods of time. In adults, tics are usually experienced as intentional, self-directed movements performed in order to relieve inner tension, whereas functional jerks are characterized by their involuntary nature and lack of agency (Voon et al., 2010; Cath et al., 2011). As with functional jerks, tics might worsen due to emotional stress or fatigue but also with relaxation or excitement (e.g., while watching television). Decrease in intensity of functional jerks during a distracting arithmetic task supports the diagnosis. However, this can be seen in tic disorders as well (Cath et al., 2011).

Many adult patients (over 90%) experience a premonitory urge preceding the tic, which is often relieved by carrying out the tic (Cath et al., 2011). Although these premonitory urges have also been described in functional jerks (van der Salm et al., 2010, 2014), they are believed to be much less common. Moreover, tics are in up to 20% of cases accompanied by echophenomena such as echolalia and echopraxia (repetition of sounds or actions), and coprolalia (involuntary swearing). Echophenomena are usually not seen in functional jerks (Ganos et al., 2014).

To make things more complicated, "functional tics" have been described in a small group of patients (Baizabal-Carvallo and Jankovic, 2014; Demartini et al., 2015). Estimated to account for 2% of FMDs, functional tics are among the rarest phenomenologic expressions of FMD (Lang, 2006). The exact definition of a functional tic and its clinical differentiation from a functional jerk is not well established, and the diagnosis is solely based on illness history and assessment by movement disorder specialists. Typical tic features, such as premonitory sensations preceding the tic, childhood onset, rostrocaudal distribution, suppressibility, and positive family history, are lacking in functional tics. Moreover, there may be features in concordance with a functional origin, such as the inability to suppress the tic, striking disruption of normal movement – a.k.a. "blocking tics" – and the presence of other comorbid FMDs (Baizabel-Carvallo and Jankovic, 2014; Demartini et al., 2015). Finally, as described here above, the combination of tics and (tic-like) FMD seems to co-occur more often than expected when these disorders would be unrelated (Barry et al., 2011). To summarize, considering the scarceness of the occurrence of "pure" functional tics, this option is that this functional tic subtype is not considered as an independent phenotype but as an alternative expression of functional jerks, or as a phenomenon co-occurring with actual tics.

In terms of treatment and prognosis, tics and functional jerks differ. Outcome with respect to physical and psychologic disability is on average poorer in FMD (Gelauff et al., 2014) than in tics, since in the latter group a substantial proportion of patients (those with predominantly simple tics that have decreased in intensity during adolescence) has actually an excellent long-term prognosis (Cath and Ludolph, 2012). Prognosis of treatment in tics is favorable, both for behavior therapy (either habit reversal or exposure to premonitory urges with response prevention) (van de Griendt et al., 2013), with medium to large effect sizes (McGuire et al., 2013), as well as medication (dopamine D2-receptor antagonists), with small to medium effect sizes (Weisman et al., 2013). In our experience functional jerks usually do not react as well to behavior therapy, although evidence to support this statement is lacking.

Myoclonus

Epidemiology

Due to the very heterogeneous etiology of myoclonus, epidemiologic data are scarce. Myoclonus has a lifetime prevalence of 8.6 cases per 100 000 persons (Caviness et al., 1999). However, transient forms of myoclonus (e.g., drug-induced) are not included in these numbers (Yoon et al., 2008). In general, causes of myoclonus include physiologic, posthypoxic, toxic-metabolic, drug-induced, epileptic, neurodegenerative, and hereditary forms (for extensive overview, see Fahn, 2002; Dijk and Tijssen, 2010).

Clinical picture

Organic myoclonus (denoted hereafter as myoclonus) has to be considered in the differential diagnosis of functional jerks. The definition of a myoclonus is a brief, sudden, shock-like involuntary movement as the result of a muscle contraction (positive myoclonus) or the short interruption of tonic muscle activity (negative myoclonus) (Fahn et al., 1986).

To differentiate myoclonus from functional jerks, symptom onset provides a clue; myoclonus has an insidious symptom onset, whereas functional jerks often commence abruptly, possibly precipitated by a physical event (Table 21.1) (Factor et al., 1995; Williams et al., 1995; Dijk and Tijssen, 2010; Pareés et al., 2014). The disease course of myoclonus depends on its etiology. Generally, disease course is progressive (Dijk and Tijssen, 2010). This is in contrast with the course in functional jerks, where spontaneous remissions and abrupt re-emergence of symptoms are not uncommon (Monday and Jankovic, 1993). An exception with respect to progressiveness of disease course in myoclonus is formed by the metabolic and toxically induced forms of myoclonus. A positive family history in the hereditary forms of myoclonus (e.g., myoclonus-dystonia or hyperekplexia) is a strong positive clue.

At neurologic examination, myoclonus is usually a simple movement with a fixed pattern, lacking signs of distractibility or suggestibility (Dijk and Tijssen, 2010). This is in contrast with functional jerks, where complex movements, pattern variability, suggestibility, and alteration or decrease of symptoms with distraction are key features (Monday and Jankovic, 1993). In tics, distractibility and suppressibility play a substantial role, in contrast to myoclonus. Further, myoclonus does not show entrainment (adaptation of jerks to imposed rhythm), whereas entrainment (if present) is a very strong, almost pathognomonic feature of functional jerks. Both syndromes often reveal arrhythmic jerks, although there are some rare forms of myoclonus, e.g., segmental myoclonus (see below), revealing rhythmicity (Esposito et al., 2009).

Stimulus sensitivity, as well as triggering of symptoms by startling stimuli (visual, tactile, auditory), is seen in myoclonus and functional jerks. In myoclonus stimulus sensitivity is usually located in the limbs, whilst in functional jerks tactile stimulation of the trunk or testing of the tendon reflexes elicits the movements (Thompson et al., 1992; Williams et al., 1995; van der Salm et al., 2014). Further, premonitory urges form a clue: in functional jerks, sensations prior to the movement might be felt, whereas in myoclonus, premonitory urge is not a feature (van der Salm et al., 2010).

Functional jerks can manifest at different localizations and this strongly influences the approach and differential diagnosis of the jerks. The localization of the myoclonus – focal, segmental, axial, or generalized – strongly depends on the anatomic origin of the myoclonus and therefore, we will discuss the different forms of myoclonus shortly below with their differentiation from functional jerk.

Cortical myoclonus

When jerks manifest differentially in the limbs and in the face, especially if present simultaneously in hand and face, myoclonus of cortical origin should be considered. Causes of cortical myoclonus include posthypoxic, epileptic, and neurodegenerative diseases (Dijk and Tijssen, 2010). The jerks in cortical myoclonus are very brief and can be focal, multifocal, or generalized (Lozsadi, 2012). This is in contrast with functional jerks, which lack typical localization and have a longer burst duration (Brown and Thompson, 2001). Jerks in cortical myoclonus are stimulus-sensitive, e.g., myoclonus can often be triggered by movement, such as tapping the fingers (Dijk and Tijssen, 2010). Whereas functional jerks can be elicited by similar stimuli in some cases, they lack a typical stimulus-sensitive localization and show inconsistent patterns of movement.

With respect to treatment response, cortical myoclonus often responds well to levetiracetam or piracetam, although this is mainly based on expert opinion and small observational studies (class IV evidence) (Dijk and Tijssen, 2010).

Subcortical myoclonus

One of the most important forms of subcortical myoclonus is myoclonus-dystonia (DYT11), characterized by jerks of the proximal or distal upper limbs and trunk accompanied by mild dystonia (Foncke et al., 2006). This syndrome is caused by a SGCE gene mutation in 50% of cases (Peall et al., 2014). The onset of symptoms in childhood, alcohol-responsiveness, and often positive family history seen in myoclonus-dystonia can help distinguish it from functional jerks, but is similar to onset of tics. The high rate of comorbid psychiatric disorders in patients with myoclonus-dystonia, including anxiety, depression, and obsessive-compulsive disorder (OCD), might wrongly be considered as suggestive of a functional origin, although this pattern of psychiatric comorbidity would be in line with tic and not FMDs (van Tricht et al., 2012). The abundance of psychiatric comorbidity in myoclonus-dystonia might put the clinician on the wrong track of an FMD (Peall et al., 2015).

Brainstem myoclonus could be considered when generalized, synchronous, axially located myoclonus is seen (Dreissen and Tijssen, 2012). This form of myoclonus can be acquired, usually due to a cerebral hypoxic event, and is characterized by stimulus sensitivity over the limbs and elicitation by startling stimuli (Hallett, 2000; Beudel et al., 2014). A specific form of myoclonus originating in the caudal brainstem is hyperekplexia. This syndrome is caused by different gene mutations (e.g., GLRA1, Glyt2) engaged in the glycine neurotransmission pathway (Bakker et al., 2006; Davies et al., 2010; Dreissen et al., 2012).

Differentiation of hyperekplexia from functional startle-induced jerks can be helped by illness history evaluation: generalized (transient) stiffness at birth, and exaggerated nonhabituating startle reflexes followed by short-lasting generalized stiffness elicited by unexpected stimuli – both cardinal features in hyperekplexia. Further distinction between hyperekplexia and FMD can be made from neurophysiologic examination. As opposed to a physiologic startle response, seen in hyperekplexia, which is generated in the caudal brainstem and has a distinct recruitment pattern with short onset latencies (<100 ms), onset latencies of functional startle are generally > 100 ms, compatible with voluntary mimicking of a startle reaction (Thompson et al., 1992). Although there is little formal evidence, hyperekplexia is thought to respond well to clonazepam (Tijssen et al., 1997b; Bakker et al., 2009a).

Spinal myoclonus

Spinal myoclonus can be divided into spinal segmental myoclonus and propriospinal myoclonus. Jerks of one limb can be regarded as a manifestation of (segmental) spinal myoclonus. Herein muscles innervated by one or two contiguous spinal segments are affected, often as a consequence of a spinal lesion. As opposed to functional jerks, spinal segmental myoclonus is continuous, often rhythmic, and persists during sleep.

Propriospinal myoclonus is of particular interest, since an important paradigm shift has recently taken place in the diagnosis of this disorder. The majority of cases of idiopathic propriospinal myoclonus have recently been determined to be of functional origin, either because a BP (see below) was found preceding the jerks or the clinical course was strongly suggestive of a functional origin (van der Salm et al., 2010; Erro et al., 2013). Further, it was shown that the typical recruitment pattern as seen in propriospinal myoclonus could be mimicked voluntarily (Kang and Sohn, 2006). Moreover, the pathophysiology of symptomatic propriospinal myoclonus is poorly understood and heavily debated, since the correspondence between imaging and the neurophysiologic findings was not clear in most cases (Esposito et al., 2014). Yet the label propriospinal myoclonus, suggesting an organic origin in the propriospinal pathways of the spinal cord, is still widely used; therefore the descriptive term (functional) axial jerks might be better suited.

Axial functional jerks often start abruptly during middle age, with men being slightly more often affected than women (van der Salm et al., 2014). Phenomenology includes nonrhythmic flexion jerks of the trunk, hips, and knees, mostly present when supine. In a substantial proportion of patients, jerks are multifocal, with involvement of the face and/or neck, lacking the classic propriospinal stereotyped pattern (Erro et al., 2014b; van der Salm et al., 2014).

Disease course is variable, including spontaneous remissions, relapses, and complete resolution of symptoms in a substantial part (22%) of patients (van der Salm et al., 2014). Moreover, jerks show a high degree of inconsistency and variability over time and might show distractibility. Tactile stimulation of the abdomen can elicit jerks and patients are able to voluntarily suppress jerks in some cases (van der Salm et al., 2014). Premonitory urge is reported by some patients, together with vocalizations, resembling tics. However, they differ in disease history, including age at onset (middle age), lack of family history, and waxing and waning disease course, which is typical for a tic origin.

Red flags to suspect a very rare diagnosis of (secondary) propriospinal myoclonus due to a structural lesion of the spinal cord are clinical signs indicating a myelopathy such as urinary urgency, gait problems, abnormal reflexes, and sensory changes of the thorax wall. If a functional disorder is not considered based on clinical signs combined with neurophysiologic tests (see below) and a myelopathy is excluded, the diagnosis of idiopathic propriospinal myoclonus (or rather, axial jerks) remains. This term should be reserved for patients without a BP or any other signs of a functional cause (Shibasaki and Hallett, 2006; van der Salm et al., 2012).

Paroxysmal movement disorders

Epidemiology

Paroxysmal attacks of jerks sometimes elicited by triggers (e.g., loud noise) have been described as a specific entity together with other phenomenologies as functional paroxysmal movement disorders (FPMD) (Bressman et al., 1988; Fahn and Williams, 1988; Williams et al., 1995; Baik et al., 2009; Ganos et al., 2014). This distinction, however, might be arbitrary, since a paroxysmal nature and stimulus sensitivity in itself are typical characteristics of FMD.

Epidemiologic data on FPMD are scarce. In the largest case series, FPMD accounted for 10% of all patients referred with FMDs at a specialized movement disorder clinic (Ganos et al., 2014). The mean age at onset was 38.6 years, with a female predominance. FPMDs have also been reported in children (Bressman et al., 1988; Ferrara and Jankovic, 2008; Canavese et al., 2012), although caution is required, as potential non-FMDs may not have fully developed and one should be aware that organic movement disorders such as PxDs have sometimes been misdiagnosed as functional because of their bizarre and paroxysmal nature.

Differential diagnosis should include PxD, a rare, clinically heterogeneous group characterized by episodically occurring involuntary movements of brief duration (Bhatia, 2011; Erro et al., 2014a). They have been reported to account for 0.76% of all movement disorders and can either be inherited (largest group) or acquired (Blakeley and Jankovic, 2002). In this chapter we will only focus on inherited forms of PxDs, including paroxysmal kinesigenic dyskinesia, paroxysmal nonkinesigenic dyskinesia, and paroxysmal exercise-induced dyskinesia (Bhatia, 2001; Erro et al., 2014a). The primary PxDs all have their onset in the first or second decade of life and are caused by different gene mutations (PRRT-2 gene, MR-1 gene, GLUT-1 gene) (Erro et al., 2014a). PxDs can be differentiated from FPMDs based on a few features, which will be discussed below (Table 21.1).

Clinical picture

At clinical examination phenomenology can help distinguish between FPMD and PxD; attacks in FPMD include a broad range of involuntary movements, including dystonia, tremor, jerks, and complex movement disorders. FMPD symptoms often show great variability in symptom characteristics and attack duration, both between and within subjects (Ganos et al., 2014), in contrast to the PxD presentation with a consistent pattern of short-lasting attacks of dystonia, chorea, or ballism, or a mixture of these. For instance, tremor has never been described in primary PxD.

Usually FPMDs are not familial, in contrast to PxD. Coexistence, however, with organic movement disorders is described in a substantial proportion of patients (Ranawaya et al., 1990; Ganos et al., 2014).

Other features suggestive of a functional disorder are seen in FPMD as well, such as distractibility, entrainment, and aggravation during examination (Ganos et al., 2014). When symptoms manifest after age 20, this nearly always indicates a functional cause, since all forms of primary PxD manifest in the first two decades of life (Bhatia, 2011; Erro et al., 2014a). FPMDs, however, do occur in children, so age at onset is not always discriminating.

Precipitating physical or emotional events triggering symptoms have been reported in FPMD, including stress, but also loud noises, walking, and "feeling frightened" have been reported (Baik et al., 2009; Ganos et al., 2014). Not a trigger as such, but premonitory sensations or auras are reported in the majority of PxD patients and have been described as "butterflies in the stomach," "electricity in the head," or numbness or a tingling sensation in the limbs (fingers) (Bruno et al., 2004). Additionally, patients with FPMD might present with odd relieving maneuvers, such as focusing on the affected limb or exerting pressure on it. It is, however, not uncommon that functional and organic paroxysmal movement disorder co-occur, especially in the same or adjacent body part (Ranawaya et al., 1990; Ganos et al., 2014).

Further, the prognosis in FPMD is suggested to be favorable, in comparison with other FMDs, with strong responses not just to placebo and hypnotherapy but also physiotherapy and cognitive behavioral therapy. However, this is based on small sample sizes and low levels of evidence (Bressman et al., 1988; Baik et al., 2009; Ganos et al., 2014). The prognosis of PxD is static, disease is managed by avoiding triggers and treatment with anticonvulsive medication or ketogenic diet, and attacks tend to diminish with age.

If, despite clinical clues, there is still well-founded doubt, it can be helpful to perform video recordings to review the phenomenology and consistency of the attacks. Additionally, laboratory investigation, including genetic testing, can be performed (for further details, see Erro et al., 2014a).

Psychiatric comorbidity and psychopathology

Functional jerks

Psychiatric disturbances, traumatic life events, and their pathophysiologic meaning in FMD, and more specifically in functional jerks, have not been thoroughly investigated. This topic will be covered in a separate chapter and, therefore, we will focus on the differences in psychiatric disturbances between functional jerks, tics, and myoclonus.

Differential diagnosis with tics and myoclonus based on psychiatric comorbidity

When trying to distinguish a functional jerk from a tic or organic myoclonus, assessment of comorbid psychiatric disorders could be of help. In tic disorders, the two most prevalent psychiatric comorbidities, OCD and attention-deficit hyperactivity disorder (ADHD) occur most frequently (Cath et al., 2011), apart from impulsive disorder, sleep problems, and anxiety and depression (Freeman et al., 2000). OCD or obsessive-compulsive behavior is reported in 20–89% of tic disorder cases (Singer, 2011), and ADHD in up to 60% of patients (Stewart et al., 2006). These high rates of ADHD and OCD are not seen in functional jerks and the presence of these disorders actually makes it more likely that the movement disorder is organic. Other psychiatric disorders in tic disorder are less distinctive and encompass, amongst others, anxiety, depression, and sleep disorder (Robertson, 2000; Freeman, 2007), of which specifically depressive disorders might well be the consequence of suffering from a debilitating health condition.

In organic myoclonus, one distinct form of hereditary myoclonus, myoclonus-dystonia (DYT 11) is specifically associated with psychiatric comorbidity, such as OCD, anxiety disorders, and alcohol dependence (Foncke et al., 2009; van Tricht et al., 2012; Peall et al., 2013, 2015). Depression is also more prevalent, but appears to be secondary rather than primary in patients with myoclonus-dystonia (van Tricht et al., 2012; Peall et al., 2014).

Thus, although there is some overlap in comorbidity patterns between tics and myoclonus-dystonia, the psychiatric profile of patients with functional jerks is quite different from both tics and myoclonus and might be of additional value in the diagnosis.

PATHOPHYSIOLOGY OF FUNCTIONAL JERKS

The fascinating and yet incomprehensible feature of FMD and of functional jerks in particular is the discrepancy between several features (entrainment, distractibility, suppressibility, suggestibility, presence of a BP) of the movements, suggesting at least some intentional control on the one hand, and the uncontrollable and involuntary perception by patients on the other hand. Unraveling this mystery would be the key to understanding the pathophysiology of this disorder. It has been hypothesized that a discrepancy between predicted and actual information processed by the brain plays a key role in this matter (Edwards et al., 2012). Some functional imaging studies concerning functional tremor have been performed in which the temporoparietal junction, an area associated with the comparison of actual information and what is internally expected, is suggested to play a key role (this topic is covered in further details in Chapters 7 and 11) (Voon et al., 2010). However, no imaging studies have been performed so far in functional jerks, and therefore future studies need to elucidate whether similar mechanisms play a role in the neurobiology of functional jerks.

THE NEUROPHYSIOLOGIC EXAMINATION

Additional electrophysiologic investigation can be of particular help in the diagnosis of functional jerky movements (for an overview, see Table 21.2).

Since it is easily performed and can be distinctive in the differential diagnosis between functional jerks, tics, and myoclonus, recording the jerks with surface EMG is advised as a first step in order to establish the burst duration of the jerk. Contractions of less than 75 ms are generally considered unlikely to be of functional origin (Thompson et al., 1992; Edwards and Bhatia, 2012). The jerks in cortical myoclonus are very brief (<50 ms) (Lozsadi, 2012). All other forms of jerks, including subcortical myoclonus, tics, and functional jerks, reveal a longer burst duration, therefore it is of less distinctive value in the differential diagnosis.

A more extensive EMG registration, polymyographic EMG, enables evaluation of the pattern of muscle activation during a movement. It may aid in mapping the different characteristics in support of a functional jerk, such as an inconsistent recruitment pattern, entrainment, distractibility and stimulus sensitivity (Apartis, 2014). It can be especially helpful in the diagnosis of axial jerks. Typical electrophysiologic characteristics of axial jerks of propriospinal origin include a fixed pattern of synchronous muscle activation starting at the spinal generator (without involvement of the face), spreading up and down the spinal cord with slow conduction velocity (5–15 m/s) and burst duration of < 1000 ms (Chokroverty et al., 1992). The sensitivity and specificity of these findings are unknown. One should keep in mind that this pattern can even be mimicked by healthy volunteers (Kang and Sohn, 2006; van der Salm et al., 2014). However, most patients with functional axial jerks do not show this pattern.

Polymyography can also be used to study the stimulus-sensitive startle reflex. In order to differentiate between different startle disorders, measuring the whole-body auditory startle reflex is of value (Bakker et al.,

Table 21.2

Clinical neurophysiologic test characteristics in support of different jerky movement disorders

Neurophysiologic test	Characteristics	In support of
Surface EMG	Burst duration < 75 ms	Cortical myoclonus
	Burst duration > 75 ms	Tic, subcortical myoclonus, functional jerk
Polymyography	Inconsistent recruitment pattern, entrainment, distractibility	Functional jerk
Startle reflex	Inconsistent recruitment pattern, long-onset latencies (>100 ms)	Functional jerk
C-reflex	Long-loop reflex with latency of 40–45 ms	Cortical or subcortical reflex myoclonus
EEG-EMG with backaveraging	Cortical spike (latency 10–40 ms)	Cortical myoclonus
	Bereitschaftspotential (latency 1000–2000 ms)	Functional jerk*
EEG-EMG coherence analysis	Significant coherence between EEG and EMG	Cortical myoclonus
SSEP	Giant SSEP	Cortical myoclonus

*Can also occur in a minority of tic cases with shorter onset latencies (500–1000 ms) (van der Salm et al., 2012).
EMG, electromyogram; EEG, electroencephalogram; SSEP, somatosensory evoked potential.

2009b). Here, a fixed rostrocaudal recruitment pattern with short onset latencies (<100 ms) and habituating responses with repeated stimuli can be measured. Functional startle jerks are assumed to be characterized by extended onset latencies (>100 ms) and a variable recruitment pattern. However, except for one older study by Thompson et al. (1992), the auditory startle response has not been assessed in a systematic fashion in functional jerks so far. In hereditary hyperekplexia the startle reflex shows enlarged startle responses with normal onset latencies (Tijssen et al., 1997a). Reticular (brainstem) myoclonus shows a somewhat similar pattern as the startle reflex except for shorter latencies in the deep hand muscles (Brown et al., 1991; Beudel et al., 2014).

To classify reflex myoclonus of cortical or subcortical origin one could also study the so-called long-loop reflexes or C-reflex. The C-reflex is a discharge of the EMG 40–45 ms after stimulation of the median nerve in the same limb. Its presence is associated with hyperexcitability of the sensorimotor cortex and is often seen in cortical reflex myoclonus (Brown and Thompson, 2001; Cassim and Houdayer, 2006). However, enhanced long-loop reflexes can also be found in reticular reflex myoclonus. Further onset latencies show great intraindividual variability. Here again, distinction from stimulus-induced functional jerks can be made based on longer onset latencies (>100 ms).

EEG-EMG co-registration with backaveraging of the EEGs time-locked to the onset of the jerk might reveal a BP, or pre-movement potential (Shibasaki and Hallett, 2006). The BP is a slow negative cortical potential, with maximal amplitude over the central areas (Cz) starting about 2000–1000 ms prior to the jerk (Fig. 21.1). It is associated with self-initiated movement (Shibasaki and Hallett, 2006; van der Salm et al., 2012). A BP is not found in subcortical myoclonus (van der Salm et al., 2012), and therefore EEG-EMG registration with jerk-locked backaveraging is a good option to differentiate between myoclonus and functional jerks. A drawback of this procedure is that it is a time-consuming and technically difficult procedure, requiring at least 40 jerks for a good-quality recording. Although clinicians hardly ever use the BP to differentiate between the various movement disorders, and BP is not a diagnostic test as such, it is a strong positive clue in support of a functional jerk. In a small study assessing the presence of a BP preceding

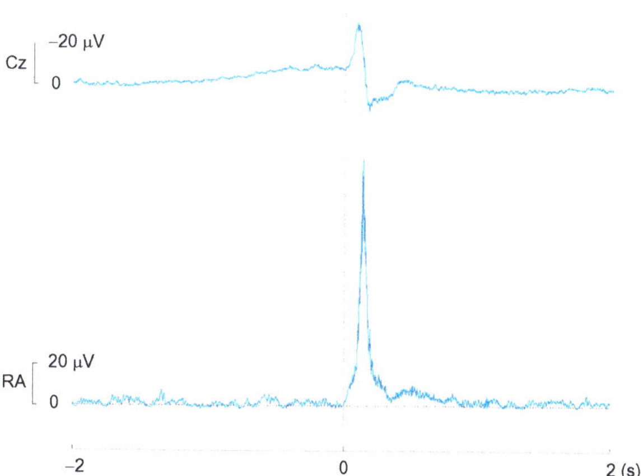

Fig. 21.1. Example of Bereitschaftspotential (BP) recording of a patient with axial jerks. The electromyogram was triggered at the onset of the rectus abdominis (RA) muscle. A premovement potential (BP) is seen starting about 1500 ms prior to the jerk, with maximal amplitude at the central cortical areas (Cz).

jerky movements, a BP was found in 25 of 29 patients with functional jerks, with a sensitivity and specificity of 0.86 (van der Salm et al., 2012). A BP was also found in a small proportion of patients with tics (6 of 14 patients), although it had a much shorter onset latency (500–1000 ms). These findings should be interpreted with caution, since a golden standard of functional jerks is lacking and clearcut criteria of a BP are absent.

In patients with cortical myoclonus, EEG-EMG back-averaging can also show a cortical correlate: a so-called cortical spike preceding myoclonus – with much shorter time delay (10–40 ms) than a BP (BP delay 1500–2000 ms) (Shibasaki and Hallett, 2005). Additional supportive electrophysiologic tests for cortical myoclonus include a giant somatosensory evoked potential, and with high frequent myoclonus, significant coherence between EEG-EMG can be found (Shibasaki and Hallett, 2005).

SUMMARY AND CONCLUSION

In this chapter we aimed to clarify different clinical jerky functional syndromes. Functional jerks show distinct positive clinical phenomena that we tried to highlight. Knowledge of the clinical and electrophysiologic characteristics of functional jerks, tics, myoclonus, and PxD helps to differentiate between the different types of jerks. In our opinion, FMDs and tic disorders represent movement disorders on the line between voluntary and involuntary movement. The exact etiologic relationship in this borderland between neurology and psychiatry needs to be further elucidated, i.e., does this comorbidity reflect one disorder being the consequence of the other, or shared multifactorial causes? Clinical neurophysiologic studies can be helpful in discriminating the different kind of jerks, although the sensitivity and specificity of these tests are largely lacking.

References

American Psychiatric Association (2000). Diagnostic and statistical manual of mental disorders (4th ed., text rev.), American Psychiatric Association, Washington, DC.

American Psychiatric Association (2013). Diagnostic and statistical manual of mental disorders (5th ed.), American Psychiatric Publishing, Arlington, VA.

Anderson KE, Gruber-Baldini AL, Vaughan CG et al. (2007). Impact of psychogenic movement disorders versus Parkinson's on disability, quality of life, and psychopathology. Mov Disord 22: 2204–2209.

Apartis E (2014). Clinical neurophysiology of psychogenic movement disorders: how to diagnose psychogenic tremor and myoclonus. Neurophysiol Clin 44: 417–424.

Baik JS, Han SW, Park JH et al. (2009). Psychogenic paroxysmal dyskinesia: the role of placebo in the diagnosis and management. Mov Disord 24: 1244–1245.

Baizabal-Carvallo JF, Jankovic J (2014). The clinical features of psychogenic movement disorders resembling tics. J Neurol Neurosurg Psychiatry 85: 573–575.

Bakker MJ, van Dijk JG, van den Maagdenberg AM et al. (2006). Startle syndromes. Lancet Neurol 5: 513–524.

Bakker MJ, Peeters EA, Tijssen MA (2009a). Clonazepam is an effective treatment for hyperekplexia due to a SLC6A5 (GlyT2) mutation. Mov Disord 24: 1852–1854.

Bakker MJ, Boer F, van der Meer JN et al. (2009b). Quantification of the auditory startle reflex in children. Clin Neurophysiol 120: 424–430.

Barry S, Baird G, Lascelles K et al. (2011). Neurodevelopmental movement disorders – an update on childhood motor stereotypies. Dev Med Child Neurol 53: 979–985.

Beudel M, Elting JWJ, Uyttenboogaart M et al. (2014). Reticular myoclonus: it really comes from the brainstem! Mov Disord Clin Pract 1: 258–260.

Bhatia KP (2001). Familial (idiopathic) paroxysmal dyskinesias: an update. Semin Neurol 21: 69–74.

Bhatia KP (2011). Paroxysmal dyskinesias. Mov Disord 26: 1157–1165.

Blakeley J, Jankovic J (2002). Secondary paroxysmal dyskinesias. Mov Disord 17: 726–734.

Bressman SB, Fahn S, Burke RE (1988). Paroxysmal non-kinesigenic dystonia. Adv Neurol 50: 403–413.

Brown P, Thompson PD (2001). Electrophysiological aids to the diagnosis of psychogenic jerks, spasms, and tremor. Mov Disord 16: 595–599.

Brown P, Thompson PD, Rothwell JC et al. (1991). A case of postanoxic encephalopathy with cortical action and brainstem reticular reflex myoclonus. Mov Disord 6: 139–144.

Bruno MK, Hallett M, Gwinn-Hardy K et al. (2004). Clinical evaluation of idiopathic paroxysmal kinesigenic dyskinesia: new diagnostic criteria. Neurology 63: 2280–2287.

Canavese C, Ciano C, Zibordi F et al. (2012). Phenomenology of psychogenic movement disorders in children. Mov Disord 27: 1153–1157.

Cassim F, Houdayer E (2006). Neurophysiology of myoclonus. Neurophysiol Clin 36: 281–291.

Cath DC, Ludolph AG (2012). Other psychiatric co-morbidities in Tourette syndrome. In: D Martino, JF Leckman (Eds.), Tourette Syndrome. Oxford University Press, New York.

Cath DC, Hedderly T, Ludolph AG et al. (2011). European clinical guidelines for Tourette syndrome and other tic disorders. Part I: assessment. Eur Child Adolesc Psychiatry 20: 155–171.

Caviness JN, Alving LI, Maraganore DM et al. (1999). The incidence and prevalence of myoclonus in Olmsted County, Minnesota. Mayo Clin Proc 74: 565–569.

Chokroverty S, Walters A, Zimmerman T et al. (1992). Propriospinal myoclonus: a neurophysiologic analysis. Neurology 42: 1591–1595.

Davies JS, Chung SK, Thomas RH et al. (2010). The glycinergic system in human startle disease: a genetic screening approach. Front Mol Neurosci 3: 8.

Demartini B, Ricciardi L, Parees I et al. (2015). A positive diagnosis of functional (psychogenic) tics. Eur J Neurol 22: e527–e536.

Dijk JM, Tijssen MA (2010). Management of patients with myoclonus: available therapies and the need for an evidence-based approach. Lancet Neurol 9: 1028–1036.

Dreissen YE, Tijssen MA (2012). The startle syndromes: physiology and treatment. Epilepsia 53 (Suppl 7): 3–11.

Dreissen YE, Bakker MJ, Koelman JH et al. (2012). Exaggerated startle reactions. Clin Neurophysiol 123: 34–44.

Edwards MJ, Bhatia KP (2012). Functional (psychogenic) movement disorders: merging mind and brain. Lancet Neurol 11: 250–260.

Edwards MJ, Adams RA, Brown H et al. (2012). A Bayesian account of 'hysteria'. Brain 135: 3495–3512.

Erro R, Bhatia KP, Edwards MJ et al. (2013). Clinical diagnosis of propriospinal myoclonus is unreliable: an electrophysiologic study. Mov Disord 28: 1868–1873.

Erro R, Sheerin UM, Bhatia KP (2014a). Paroxysmal dyskinesias revisited: a review of 500 genetically proven cases and a new classification. Mov Disord 29: 1108–1116.

Erro R, Edwards MJ, Bhatia KP et al. (2014b). Psychogenic axial myoclonus: clinical features and long-term outcome. Parkinsonism Relat Disord 20: 596–599.

Esposito M, Edwards MJ, Bhatia KP et al. (2009). Idiopathic spinal myoclonus: a clinical and neurophysiological assessment of a movement disorder of uncertain origin. Mov Disord 24: 2344–2349.

Esposito M, Erro R, Edwards MJ et al. (2014). The pathophysiology of symptomatic propriospinal myoclonus. Mov Disord 29: 1097–1099.

Factor SA, Podskalny GD, Molho ES (1995). Psychogenic movement disorders: frequency, clinical profile, and characteristics. J Neurol Neurosurg Psychiatry 59: 406–412.

Fahn S (2002). Overview, history, and classification of myoclonus. Adv Neurol 89: 13–17.

Fahn S, Williams DT (1988). Psychogenic dystonia. Adv Neurol 50: 431–455.

Fahn S, Marsden CD, Van Woert MH (1986). Definition and classification of myoclonus. Adv Neurol 43: 1–5.

Ferrara J, Jankovic J (2008). Psychogenic movement disorders in children. Mov Disord 23: 1875–1881.

Fibbe LA, Cath DC, van Balkom AJ (2011). Obsessive compulsive disorder with tics: a new subtype? Tijdschr Psychiatr 53: 275–285.

Foncke EM, Gerrits MC, van RF et al. (2006). Distal myoclonus and late onset in a large Dutch family with myoclonus-dystonia. Neurology 67: 1677–1680.

Foncke EM, Cath D, Zwinderman K et al. (2009). Is psychopathology part of the phenotypic spectrum of myoclonus-dystonia? A study of a large Dutch M-D family. Cogn Behav Neurol 22: 127–133.

Freeman RD (2007). Tic disorders and ADHD: answers from a world-wide clinical dataset on Tourette syndrome. Eur Child Adolesc Psychiatry 16 (Suppl 1): 15–23.

Freeman RD, Fast DK, Burd L et al. (2000). An international perspective on Tourette syndrome: selected findings from 3,500 individuals in 22 countries. Dev Med Child Neurol 42: 436–447.

Ganos C, Aguirregomozcorta M, Batla A et al. (2014). Psychogenic paroxysmal movement disorders – clinical features and diagnostic clues. Parkinsonism Relat Disord 20: 41–46.

Gelauff J, Stone J, Edwards M et al. (2014). The prognosis of functional (psychogenic) motor symptoms: a systematic review. J Neurol Neurosurg Psychiatry 85: 220–226.

Gupta A, Lang AE (2009). Psychogenic movement disorders. Curr Opin Neurol 22: 430–436.

Hallett M (2000). Physiology of human posthypoxic myoclonus. Mov Disord 15 (Suppl 1): 8–13.

Hinson VK, Cubo E, Comella CL et al. (2005). Rating scale for psychogenic movement disorders: scale development and clinimetric testing. Mov Disord 20: 1592–1597.

Kang SY, Sohn YH (2006). Electromyography patterns of propriospinal myoclonus can be mimicked voluntarily. Mov Disord 21: 1241–1244.

Lang A (2006). General overview of psychogenic movement disorders: epidemiology, diagnosis and prognosis. In: Psychogenic movement disorders – neurology and neuropsychiatry, Lippincott Williams & Wilkins, Philadelphia.

Leckman JF, Riddle MA, Hardin MT et al. (1989). The Yale Global Tic Severity Scale: initial testing of a clinician-rated scale of tic severity. J Am Acad Child Adolesc Psychiatry 28: 566–573.

Lozsadi D (2012). Myoclonus: a pragmatic approach. Pract Neurol 12: 215–224.

McGuire JF, Nyirabahizi E, Kircanski K et al. (2013). A cluster analysis of tic symptoms in children and adults with Tourette syndrome: clinical correlates and treatment outcome. Psychiatry Res 210: 1198–1204.

Monday K, Jankovic J (1993). Psychogenic myoclonus. Neurology 43: 349–352.

Morgante F, Edwards MJ, Espay AJ et al. (2012). Diagnostic agreement in patients with psychogenic movement disorders. Mov Disord 27: 548–552.

Onofrj M, Bonanni L, Manzoli L et al. (2010). Cohort study on somatoform disorders in Parkinson disease and dementia with Lewy bodies. Neurology 74: 1598–1606.

Pareés I, Saifee TA, Kassavetis P et al. (2012). Believing is perceiving: mismatch between self-report and actigraphy in psychogenic tremor. Brain 135: 117–123.

Pareés I, Saifee TA, Kojovic M et al. (2013a). Functional (psychogenic) symptoms in Parkinson's disease. Mov Disord 28: 1622–1627.

Pareés I, Kassavetis P, Saifee TA et al. (2013b). Failure of explicit movement control in patients with functional motor symptoms. Mov Disord 28: 517–523.

Pareés I, Kojovic M, Pires C et al. (2014). Physical precipitating factors in functional movement disorders. J Neurol Sci 338: 174–177.

Peall KJ, Smith DJ, Kurian MA et al. (2013). SGCE mutations cause psychiatric disorders: clinical and genetic characterization. Brain 136: 294–303.

Peall KJ, Kurian MA, Wardle M et al. (2014). SGCE and myoclonus dystonia: motor characteristics, diagnostic criteria and clinical predictors of genotype. J Neurol 261: 2296–2304.

Peall KJ, Kuiper A, de Koning TJ et al. (2015). Non-motor symptoms in genetically defined dystonia: homogenous groups require systematic assessment. Parkinsonism Relat Disord 21: 1031–1040.

Ranawaya R, Riley D, Lang A (1990). Psychogenic dyskinesias in patients with organic movement disorders. Mov Disord 5: 127–133.

Robertson MM (2000). Tourette syndrome, associated conditions and the complexities of treatment. Brain 123 (Pt 3): 425–462.

Robertson MM, Banerjee S, Kurlan R et al. (1999). The Tourette syndrome diagnostic confidence index: development and clinical associations. Neurology 53: 2108–2112.

Robertson MM, Eapen V, Cavanna AE (2009). The international prevalence, epidemiology, and clinical phenomenology of Tourette syndrome: a cross-cultural perspective. J Psychosom Res 67: 475–483.

Shibasaki H, Hallett M (2005). Electrophysiological studies of myoclonus. Muscle Nerve 31: 157–174.

Shibasaki H, Hallett M (2006). What is the Bereitschaftspotential? Clin Neurophysiol 117: 2341–2356.

Shill H, Gerber P (2006). Evaluation of clinical diagnostic criteria for psychogenic movement disorders. Mov Disord 21: 1163–1168.

Singer HS (2011). Tourette syndrome and other tic disorders. Handb Clin Neurol 100: 641–657.

Stewart SE, Illmann C, Geller DA et al. (2006). A controlled family study of attention-deficit/hyperactivity disorder and Tourette's disorder. J Am Acad Child Adolesc Psychiatry 45: 1354–1362.

Stone J, Carson A, Duncan R et al. (2010). Who is referred to neurology clinics? The diagnoses made in 3781 new patients. Clin Neurol Neurosurg 112: 747–751.

Thompson PD, Colebatch JG, Brown P et al. (1992). Voluntary stimulus-sensitive jerks and jumps mimicking myoclonus or pathological startle syndromes. Mov Disord 7: 257–262.

Tijssen MA, Voorkamp LM, Padberg GW et al. (1997a). Startle responses in hereditary hyperekplexia. Arch Neurol 54: 388–393.

Tijssen MA, Schoemaker HC, Edelbroek PJ et al. (1997b). The effects of clonazepam and vigabatrin in hyperekplexia. J Neurol Sci 149: 63–67.

Tijssen MA, Brown P, Morris HR et al. (1999). Late onset startle induced tics. J Neurol Neurosurg Psychiatry 67: 782–784.

van de Griendt JM, Verdellen CW, van Dijk MK et al. (2013). Behavioural treatment of tics: habit reversal and exposure with response prevention. Neurosci Biobehav Rev 37: 1172–1177.

van der Salm SM, Koelman JH, Henneke S et al. (2010). Axial jerks: a clinical spectrum ranging from propriospinal to psychogenic myoclonus. J Neurol 257: 1349–1355.

van der Salm SM, Tijssen MA, Koelman JH et al. (2012). The bereitschaftspotential in jerky movement disorders. J Neurol Neurosurg Psychiatry 83: 1162–1167.

van der Salm SM, de Haan RJ, Cath DC et al. (2013). The eye of the beholder: inter-rater agreement among experts on psychogenic jerky movement disorders. J Neurol Neurosurg Psychiatry 84: 742–747.

van der Salm SM, Erro R, Cordivari C et al. (2014). Propriospinal myoclonus: clinical reappraisal and review of literature. Neurology 83: 1862–1870.

van Tricht MJ, Dreissen YE, Cath D et al. (2012). Cognition and psychopathology in myoclonus-dystonia. J Neurol Neurosurg Psychiatry 83: 814–820.

Voon V, Gallea C, Hattori N et al. (2010). The involuntary nature of conversion disorder. Neurology 74: 223–228.

Weisman H, Qureshi IA, Leckman JF et al. (2013). Systematic review: pharmacological treatment of tic disorders – efficacy of antipsychotic and alpha-2 adrenergic agonist agents. Neurosci Biobehav Rev 37: 1162–1171.

Williams DT, Ford B, Fahn S (1995). Phenomenology and psychopathology related to psychogenic movement disorders. Adv Neurol 65: 231–257.

World Health Organization (2010). The ICD-10 classification of mental and behavioural disorders: clinical descriptions and diagnostic guidelines. World Health Organization, Geneva.

Yoon JH, Lee PH, Yong SW et al. (2008). Movement disorders at a university hospital emergency room. An analysis of clinical pattern and etiology. J Neurol 255: 745–749.

Handbook of Clinical Neurology, Vol. 139 (3rd series)
Functional Neurologic Disorders
M. Hallett, J. Stone, and A. Carson, Editors
http://dx.doi.org/10.1016/B978-0-12-801772-2.00022-9

Chapter 22

Psychogenic (functional) parkinsonism

M.A. THENGANATT AND J. JANKOVIC*

Parkinson's Disease Center and Movement Disorders Clinic, Department of Neurology, Baylor College of Medicine, Houston, TX, USA

Abstract

Psychogenic parkinsonism (PP), although often quite disabling, is one of the least commonly reported subtypes of psychogenic movement disorders. There are certain features that help distinguish PP from idiopathic Parkinson's disease, such as abrupt onset, early disability, bilateral shaking and slowness, nondecremental slowness when performing repetitive movements, voluntary resistance against passive movement without cogwheel rigidity, distractibility, "give-way" weakness, stuttering speech, bizarre gait, and a variety of behavioral symptoms. While the diagnosis of PP is clinical, functional imaging evaluating the integrity of nigrostriatal pathways can help distinguish PP from other types of parkinsonism. PP can coexist in patients with organic parkinsonism, adding to the challenge of making a diagnosis of PP. Being cognizant of the clinical signs of psychogenic movement disorders, including PP, will lead to earlier diagnosis and hopefully improved outcomes.

INTRODUCTION

Although often disabling, psychogenic parkinsonism (PP) is one of the least frequently reported psychogenic movement disorders (PMDs) (Jankovic and Hunter, 2011). PP presents as a constellation of symptoms, including rest tremor, slowness, and abnormal gait, and may be wrongly diagnosed as idiopathic Parkinson's disease (PD). Some patients have coexisting PD and PP, and distinguishing the two can be challenging. Features of the presenting history and physical examination should alert the examiner to the possible diagnosis of PP. In addition to the general features of PMDs (distractibility, variability, and suggestibility) (Thenganatt and Jankovic, 2014), the tremor, slowness, stiffness, and gait changes in PP have characteristic features that distinguish this diagnosis from PD (Jankovic, 2011; Jankovic and Hunter, 2011). Furthermore, other nonorganic signs seen in PMDs, such as give-away weakness, nonanatomic sensory loss, and convergence spasm, may be identified to support the diagnosis (Thenganatt and Jankovic, 2015). The aim of this chapter is to review the clinical characteristics of PP and highlight some of the phenomenologic features and ancillary testing that may be helpful in confirming the diagnosis.

EPIDEMIOLOGY

The overall prevalence of PP is not known, but in tertiary movement disorders clinics it has been reported to account for 1.5–7% of all PMDs (Factor et al., 1995; Thomas et al., 2006; Sage and Mark, 2015). A retrospective case series of PP at three movement disorders centers described 14 patients (7 men and 7 women) (Lang et al., 1995). The mean age at diagnosis was 48 years and the mean duration of symptoms prior to diagnosis was 5.3 years. All patients had marked impairment in functioning, and most were unable to return to work. A review of 9 PP cases (6 male, 3 female) found an age at onset of 50 years and a variable duration of symptoms (several months to 28 years) (Morgan et al.,

*Correspondence to: Joseph Jankovic, MD, Professor of Neurology, Distinguished Chair in Movement Disorders, Director of Parkinson's Disease Center, and Movement Disorders Clinic, Department of Neurology, Baylor College of Medicine, 7200 Cambridge, Suite 9A, MS: BCM 609, Houston TX 77030-4202, USA. Tel: +1-713-798-5998, Fax: +1-713-798-6808, E-mail: josephj@bcm.edu

2004). Four patients had a history of psychiatric disorder, including depression, bipolar and posttraumatic stress disorder, and 2 patients had a family history of PD. In a series of 32 patients diagnosed with PP at Baylor College of Medicine (Jankovic, 2011), 53% were female, in contrast to the well-recognized male predominance in PD. The mean duration of symptoms at diagnosis was 5.2 ± 1.2 years and the mean age at diagnosis was 48 ± 8.6 years. The mean education level of subjects was 14 ± 2.5 years and 13% were employed in the healthcare field.

PMDs, including PP, can have a marked impact on daily functioning, leading to considerable disability, comparable to that reported in neurodegenerative diseases. A study comparing 66 PMD patients with 704 PD patients demonstrated similar levels of reported disability between the two groups (Anderson et al., 2007). Mental health quality of life was reportedly worse in PMD patients, with higher levels of anxiety, depression, and somatization.

Somatoform disorders have been found to be higher in patients with PD and dementia with Lewy bodies compared with other neurodegenerative disorders, such as Alzheimer's disease, multiple system atrophy, progressive supranuclear palsy, and frontotemporal dementia (Onofrj et al., 2010). The symptoms included hypochondriasis motor or sensory conversion symptoms. These symptoms preceded the onset of PD and commonly recurred in follow-up.

CLINICAL HISTORY

The history of the initial presentation of symptoms and progression of disease, as well as other historic pieces of information, often support the diagnosis of PP. Patients with PP typically have an abrupt onset of symptoms, with maximum disease severity at onset (Lang et al., 1995). This can lead to severe disability, affecting employment and basic activities of daily living. A precipitating stressor, either physical or psychologic, may be identified. Often patients may not acknowledge or disclose a precipitant, but the absence of identifiable stress factors should not exclude the diagnosis of PP. Patients may have multiple somatic complaints, including pain, visual disturbance, and memory loss. They may also have depression, which they often deny (even in the presence of overt signs, including crying). There is often anxiety and irritability. Some may have a family history of tremor or PD. Among the patients reviewed at Baylor College of Medicine with PP, 28% had a family history of tremor or parkinsonism, 56% had a psychiatric disorder (most commonly depression), and 63% were on disability (Jankovic, 2011).

CLINICAL SIGNS

The clinical signs of PP have been described in small case series of patients, including varying numbers of patients (9–32) (Lang et al., 1995; Morgan et al., 2004; Benaderette et al., 2006; Jankovic, 2011) (Table 22.1). The tremor that occurs in PP often affects the dominant hand. It is often equally present in all states – rest, posture, and action – as opposed to the rest tremor in PD, which classically decreases with action. There is no brief pause in tremor when assuming an outstretched posture of the hands that is classically seen in the re-emergent tremor of PD (Jankovic et al., 1999). The tremor in PP often increases in intensity when asked about or when it is the focus of examination. The tremor is distractible, diminishing when performing movements with the opposite limb, doing mental calculations or while walking, especially when focusing on tandem gait. This is in contrast to the rest tremor in PD, which classically enhances when walking. The tremor in PP is often variable in frequency and direction, changing from pronation/supination to flexion/extension. When restricting a tremulous limb, the tremor may suddenly spread to another limb. In psychogenic tremor, the absence of finger tremor is a distinguishing feature from organic tremor (Deuschl et al., 1998; Thenganatt and Jankovic, 2014). The tremor in PP is similar to that seen in isolated psychogenic tremor.

Table 22.1

Clinical signs of psychogenic parkinsonism

Maximal symptom severity at onset with marked disability
Abrupt onset of tremor, often in dominant hand
Tremor present in all states – rest, posture, and kinetic
Lack of a re-emergent tremor
Tremor decreases in amplitude with distraction, including walking
Absence of finger tremor
Variability of tremor amplitude and frequency
Absence of cogwheel rigidity with active resistance
Increased resistance decreases with distracting maneuvers
Slowness without decrement or arrests in rapid successive movements
Excessive effort with sighing and grimacing with simple movements
Slow handwriting without micrographia
Abnormal speech with whispering, stuttering, gibberish, or "baby talk"
Markedly slow gait without freezing of gait
Signs of other psychogenic gait disorders, including astasia-abasia, buckling at the knees, and a "bouncy gait"
Excessive response to mild pull backwards with arms flailing, reeling back without falling

The slowness of movement in PP is often labored, with patients sighing, grimacing, and looking exhausted after the simplest of movements. While rapid successive movements may be slow, true bradykinesia with decrement in amplitude or arrests in movements is not seen (Morgan et al., 2004). Observing the patient throughout the encounter may demonstrate normal speed of movement with other activities. Writing may be of normal speed and does not have the classic micrographia seen in PD, including not having the decrement in size as the writing continues. When assessing tone, there is active resistance without cogwheeling (Lang et al., 1995). The resistance decreases with distraction maneuvers, the opposite of what occurs in PD. Speech abnormalities in PP include stuttering, whispering, gibberish, "baby talk," and foreign accents.

While the gait in PP may be slow and stiff with decreased arm swing, there is often no freezing of gait. The decreased arm swing does not improve with running, as can be seen in PD. Other features of a psychogenic gait may be present, such as astasia-abasia, buckling at the knees, and a bouncy gait. When testing for postural instability there is often an exaggerated response to the mildest pull, with arms flailing and reeling back without actually falling.

ANCILLARY TESTING

While the diagnosis of PP is largely clinical, ancillary testing, including nuclear imaging and neurophysiologic testing, can provide supporting information.

Dopamine transporter single-photon emission computed tomography (DaT-SPECT) involves a ligand that binds to the presynaptic dopamine transporter in the brain and can be used to evaluate dopamine deficiency seen in PD and atypical parkinsonism (multiple system atrophy, progressive supranuclear palsy, corticobasal degeneration), but not in PP (Gaig et al., 2006; Felicio et al., 2010; Ba and Martin, 2015; Rodriguez-Porcel et al., 2016). The commercially available DaT-SPECT in the USA should be performed at an experienced center, as the assessment of the scan is qualitative, not quantitative, and subject to interpretation. Thus, interpretation by clinicians without experience with DaT-SPECT scans can result in false-positive or false-negative results. While DaT-SPECT imaging is normal in PP and can help distinguish this disorder from PD, one must be aware of other parkinsonian and tremor disorders that can have normal scans, including vascular parkinsonism, drug-induced parkinsonism, dopa-responsive-dystonia, dystonic tremor, essential tremor, and fragile-X tremor ataxia syndrome (Menendez-Gonzalez et al., 2014). Furthermore, an abnormal DaT-SPECT does not rule out PP, as there are patients who may have a combination of PP and PD and thus an abnormal scan (Umeh et al., 2013). DaT-SPECT, along with neurophysiologic testing, can be especially useful when trying to distinguish patients with pure PP from those with a combination of PP and PD (Benaderette et al., 2006). While neurophysiologic testing can identify features of psychogenic tremor, it can also identify features of parkinsonian tremor that may not be appreciated by clinical examination (Thenganatt and Jankovic, 2014).

Neurophysiologic testing, using quantitative accelerometry and surface electromyography, is primarily available on a research basis but can provide information distinguishing PP from PD and other tremor disorders. Analysis of tremor amplitude has shown that loading the limb with increasing weight tends to increase tremor amplitude in psychogenic tremor, whereas in PD and other organic tremor, the amplitude decreases or remains the same (Deuschl et al., 1998). An analysis of tremor frequency demonstrated that the tremor in psychogenic patients had similar frequency in all affected limbs, while PD and essential tremor patients were more likely to have a frequency variation of greater than 0.1 Hz between limbs (O'Suilleabhain and Matsumoto, 1998). Furthermore, when performing voluntary movements with the contralateral limb, patients with psychogenic tremor were unable to maintain the tremor frequency; the tremor either entrained to the frequency of the voluntary movements or disappeared.

Another study evaluated the effect of finger tapping with the opposite limb on tremor and found greater variability in tremor frequency in psychogenic tremor patients compared to essential tremor and PD patients (Zeuner et al., 2003). In neuropsychiatric testing, finger tapping has been shown to be slower and more variable in malingering or psychogenic patients. Finger-tapping tests have been evaluated in patients with PMDs compared to organic movement disorders, including PD (Criswell et al., 2010). When asked to tap for 30-second trials, the psychogenic tremor patients had significantly lower finger-tapping scores (lower number of taps) when compared with essential tremor, dystonia, and PD patients.

While the administration of placebo to support a diagnosis of a PMD is controversial, it can provide helpful information that can help lead to an accurate diagnosis. Response to carbidopa 25 mg alone can be used as placebo, as it does not cross the blood–brain barrier. A dramatic improvement in symptoms after carbidopa would support a diagnosis of PP (Jankovic, 2011). However, response to placebo must be interpreted with caution, because even patients with organic disease such as PD can demonstrate placebo response (Lidstone et al., 2010).

The response to PD medications in PP can also provide useful information. Generally, PP patients do not demonstrate levodopa-induced dyskinesias as seen in PD patients. Furthermore, when medications such as dopamine agonists are withdrawn, they do not experience the dopamine withdrawal syndrome that can be seen in PD patients.

FUTURE DIRECTIONS

Currently, the diagnosis of PP is best made by movement disorder neurologists who are experts in PD and PMDs. As more neurologists become aware of the red flags that suggest PP, an earlier diagnosis of PP may be made without unnecessary investigations and treatment. The diagnosis of PP is especially important to recognize before more invasive therapies are implemented, such as deep-brain stimulation. Increasing recognition of the impact that PMDs, including PP, can have on quality of life, will hopefully lead to greater interest in the study and management of these patients by various healthcare providers, including neurologists, psychiatrists, and physiatrists.

References

Anderson KE, Gruber-Baldini A, Vaughan CG et al. (2007). Impact of psychogenic movement disorders versus Parkinson's on disability, quality of life, and psychopathology. Mov Disord 22: 2204–2209.

Ba F, Martin WR (2015). Dopamine transporter imaging as a diagnostic tool for parkinsonism and related disorders in clinical practice. Parkinsonism Relat Disord 21 (2): 87–94.

Benaderette S, Zanotti Fregonara P, Apartis E et al. (2006). Psychogenic parkinsonism: a combination of clinical, electrophysiological, and [(123)I]-FP-CIT SPECT scan explorations improves diagnostic accuracy. Mov Disord 21: 310–317.

Criswell S, Sterling C, Swisher L et al. (2010). Sensitivity and specificity of the finger tapping task for the detection of psychogenic movement disorders. Parkinsonism Relat Disord 16: 197–201.

Deuschl G, Koster B, Lucking CH et al. (1998). Diagnostic and pathophysiological aspects of psychogenic tremors. Mov Disord 13: 294–302.

Factor SA, Podskalny GD, Molho ES (1995). Psychogenic movement disorders: frequency, clinical profile, and characteristics. J Neurol Neurosurg Psychiatry 59: 406–412.

Felicio AC, Godeiro-Junior C, Moriyama TS et al. (2010). Degenerative parkinsonism in patients with psychogenic parkinsonism: a dopamine transporter imaging study. Clin Neurol Neurosurg 112: 282–285.

Gaig C, Marti MJ, Tolosa E et al. (2006). 123I-Ioflupane SPECT in the diagnosis of suspected psychogenic Parkinsonism. Mov Disord 21: 1994–1998.

Jankovic J (2011). Diagnosis and treatment of psychogenic parkinsonism. J Neurol Neurosurg Psychiatry 82 (12): 1300–1303.

Jankovic J, Hunter C (2011). Psychogenic parkinsonism. In: M Hallett, AE Lang, J Jankovic et al. (Eds.), Psychogenic Movement Disorders and Other Conversion Disorders. Cambridge University Press, Cambridge, pp. 14–19.

Jankovic J, Schwartz KS, Ondo W (1999). Re-emergent tremor of Parkinson's disease. J Neurol Neurosurg Psychiatry 67: 646–650.

Lang AE, Koller WC, Fahn S (1995). Psychogenic parkinsonism. Arch Neurol 52: 802–810.

Lidstone SC, Schulzer M, Dinelle K et al. (2010). Effects of expectation on placebo-induced dopamine release in Parkinson disease. Arch Gen Psychiatry 67: 857–865.

Menendez-Gonzalez M, Tavares F, Zeidan N et al. (2014). Diagnoses behind patients with hard-to-classify tremor and normal DaT-SPECT: a clinical follow up study. Front Aging Neurosci 6: 56.

Morgan JC, Mir P, Mahapatra RK et al. (2004). Psychogenic parkinsonism: clinical features of a large case series. Mov Disord 19: S345–S346.

Onofrj M, Bonanni L, Manzoli L et al. (2010). Cohort study on somatoform disorders in Parkinson disease and dementia with Lewy bodies. Neurology 74 (20): 1598–1606.

O'Suilleabhain PE, Matsumoto JY (1998). Time-frequency analysis of tremors. Brain 121 (Pt 11): 2127–2134.

Rodriguez-Porcel F, Jamali S, Duker AP et al. (2016). Dopamine transporter scanning in the evaluation of patients with suspected Parkinsonism: a case-based user's guide. Expert Rev Neurother 16 (1): 23–29.

Sage JI, Mark MH (2015). Psychogenic parkinsonism: clinical spectrum and diagnosis. Ann Clin Psychiatry 27 (1): 33–37.

Thenganatt MA, Jankovic J (2014). Psychogenic tremor: a video guide to its distinguishing features. Tremor Other Hyperkinet Mov (N Y) 4: 253.

Thenganatt MA, Jankovic J (2015). Psychogenic movement disorders. Neurol Clin 33: 205–224.

Thomas M, Vuong KD, Jankovic J (2006). Long-term prognosis of patients with psychogenic movement disorders. Parkinsonism Relat Disord 12: 382–387.

Umeh CC, Szabo Z, Pontone GM et al. (2013). Dopamine transporter imaging in psychogenic parkinsonism and neurodegenerative parkinsonism with psychogenic overlay: a report of three cases. Tremor Other Hyperkinet Mov (N Y) 3.

Zeuner KE, Shoge RO, Goldstein SR et al. (2003). Accelerometry to distinguish psychogenic from essential or parkinsonian tremor. Neurology 61: 548–550.

Handbook of Clinical Neurology, Vol. 139 (3rd series)
Functional Neurologic Disorders
M. Hallett, J. Stone, and A. Carson, Editors
http://dx.doi.org/10.1016/B978-0-12-801772-2.00023-0

Chapter 23

Functional gait disorder

V.S.C. FUNG*

Movement Disorders Unit, Department of Neurology, Westmead Hospital and Sydney Medical School, University of Sydney, Sydney, Australia

Abstract

Gait disorder is a common accompaniment of functional neurologic disorders. The diagnosis of a functional or psychogenic gait is complex. It requires a sound knowledge of the range of phenomenology observed in organic movement disorders, the ability to evaluate and diagnose nonmovement disorder neurologic symptoms and signs, but additionally knowledge of potential musculoskeletal causes of gait disturbance. A stepwise approach to the analysis of the phenomenology and separation into four (sometimes overlapping) psychogenic gait syndromes is suggested to aid diagnosis: (1) movement disorder mimics; (2) neurologic (nonmovement disorder) mimics; (3) musculoskeletal or biomechanical mimics; and (4) isolated disequilibrium or balance disorders. Accurate diagnosis can lead to effective therapy.

INTRODUCTION

Abnormal gait is a common feature in patients with psychogenic movement disorders, being the isolated syndrome in 5.7% and part of a mixed movement disorder in 36.6% of a series of 279 patients diagnosed at a movement disorder center (Baik and Lang, 2007). The diagnosis of a "psychogenic gait" should be based on the presence of positive clinical features, rather than a negative diagnosis that relies solely on vague concepts such as a "bizarre" or "unusual" gait which does not fit an organic gait recognized by the clinician. The ability to diagnose a psychogenic gait will be facilitated by a systematic approach to the clinical analysis of gait and balance.

NORMAL GAIT

Normal gait can be separated into two independent but interrelated components: equilibrium, which is the ability to assume and maintain an upright posture of the head and trunk, and locomotion, which is the ability to make steps in order to propel the body (Nutt et al., 1993).

In normal subjects during comfortable walking, the head and trunk are held erect. There is stability of the head and pelvis maximal in the vertical and anteroposterior planes, with greater instability in the mediolateral plane (Latt et al., 2008). Stability in the mediolateral plane increases if subjects walk more slowly or with a reduced cadence (steps/minute) compared with their comfortable speed.

Locomotion is achieved by alternate stepping movements of the legs. The motion of each leg can be divided into the stance and swing phases, which follow on from each other. Stance phase denotes the period when the foot is in contact with the ground, beginning with heel strike, moving to sole support, and ending with push-off with the toes. The swing phase begins with push-off, at which point the hip, knee, and ankle are flexed, the leg swings through with the toes clearing the ground, following which there is extension of the knee leading to heel strike and the beginning of the next stance phase. The left and right legs move out of phase with each other, with a brief time during which both feet contact the ground, referred to as the double-limb support phase. The arms swing freely by the sides in the direction of the opposite leg as an associated movement. The gait cycle is defined as the period of time between any two identical events (in the one leg) during walking (Murray et al., 1964; Whittle, 1996).

*Correspondence to: Victor Fung, MBBS, PhD, FRACP, Department of Neurology, Westmead Hospital, Westmead, NSW 2145, Australia. Tel: +61-298456793, Fax: +61-296356684, E-mail: vscfung@ozemail.com.au

The observation of the posture and plane of motion of the legs, arms, and trunk should be supplemented by observation of some additional movement parameters. Stride length is the distance from initial heel strike to the next heel strike of the same foot. Step length is the distance between the feet as one is in push-off and the other in heel strike. Stride width (or base) is the transverse distance between the center of the long axes of the feet during ground contact, and in normal subjects is narrow, with a mean value of approximately 8.0 cm. During normal aging, gait velocity reduces due to stride length reduction with maintained cadence, resulting in an increased stance phase and double-limb support time. However, stride width remains remarkably constant. Toe clearance during swing phase also does not significantly change with aging, with an average toe clearance of about 1 cm (Murray et al., 1964; Winter, 1983; Winter et al., 1990).

CHARACTERISTICS OF SOME CLASSIC ORGANIC GAITS

It is useful to analyze some features of classic organic gait disorders before analyzing the characteristics of some more complex gaits, both psychogenic and organic. The characteristics of some simple organic gait disorders are show in Table 23.1. Reading across the table provides a method of systematic clinical gait analysis. With the exception of cerebellar ataxic gait, a key feature of these gaits is consistency – in an individual patient, the trunk and legs, even if moving asymmetrically, have a stereotyped pattern of posture and movement during the stance and swing phases.

CHARACTERISTICS OF SOME COMPLEX ORGANIC GAITS

These gait disorders can be difficult to characterize and can be mistaken for psychogenic, because the clinical features of the gait in an individual can be variable rather than stereotyped, or can seem inconsistent or incongruent.

Isolated dystonic gait

Dystonia is defined as a movement disorder characterized by sustained or intermittent muscle contractions causing abnormal, often repetitive, movements, postures, or both (Albanese et al., 2013). In isolated dystonic gait, the abnormal posture may affect the legs, trunk, or both (as well as other body parts if the dystonia is multifocal or generalized). Dystonia is typically patterned (stereotyped), so that in the affected individual the abnormal posturing will consistently occur in the leg or trunk in the same phase of the gait cycle, although it can be different in different phases. For example, the ankle might invert and plantar flex at the beginning and middle of the swing phase, but evert or dorsiflex at the end of the swing phase just prior to heel strike. However, this will be the pattern each time that person walks. The abnormality in posture of the legs or trunk in a dystonic gait can be extreme and appear bizarre, leading to the erroneous conclusion of a psychogenic origin, but its stereotyped nature assists in differentiation between the two.

There are two aspects of a dystonic gait that can give the impression of inconsistency and lead to misdiagnosis of a psychogenic etiology. First, dystonic gait can be task-specific, so that abnormal posturing can vary or even be absent depending on whether the patient is walking forwards, backwards, running, or may even only be present when walking up or down stairs (Albanese, 2003). Second, dystonic gait can also be influenced by the patient adopting compensatory postures or maneuvers, for example, crawling instead of walking to avoid destabilizing truncal extension during walking (Trinh et al., 2014), or sensory or motor tricks (*gestes antagonistes*) (Ramos et al., 2014), for example, placing the palm of the hand on the anterior thigh while walking to reduce truncal flexion.

In patients with dystonia, despite the abnormal posturing, underlying balance and locomotive function during walking are usually well preserved. Therefore falls are rare unless the abnormal truncal or leg posturing is sufficient to push the patient's center of mass beyond the limits of stability. Frequent falling in the absence of a significant threat to the center of mass should raise suspicion that the dystonia is combined with additional motor pathology such as impaired postural reflexes from parkinsonism, cerebellar ataxia, or impaired ability to effect postural corrections from spasticity.

Gait in combined dystonia

It has been emphasized that a characteristic feature of an isolated dystonic gait is the stereotyped pattern of abnormal posturing during the gait cycle, even if the abnormal posturing or gait at first glance seems bizarre. However, if a dystonic gait is combined with another movement disorder (Albanese et al., 2013; Fung et al., 2013) that is unpredictable or random, then the gait can look both bizarre and inconsistent (Kim and Fung, 2011). Examples include a dystonic gait with superimposed chorea, tics, or stereotypies which can occur especially in the setting of Huntington disease or chorea-acanthocytosis, or if a dystonic gait is combined with cerebellar ataxia, which leads to random loss of balance with attempted corrections. The clue to the diagnosis of a combined dystonic gait is that an underlying stereotyped pattern of abnormal posturing can be observed, on which are

Characteristics of classic gait syndromes

Disorder	Standing balance	Truncal posture	Truncal sway	Leg posture	Stride length	Step height	Gait base	Symmetry	Cadence	Additional features
Parkinson's disease	Normal early, unstable late, with tendency to fall backwards	Flexed (stooped)	Normal	Flexed	Reduced	Reduced	Normal	Symmetric or mildly asymmetric. Can be very asymmetric if leg dystonia present during walking. Consistent pattern	Normal	May have freezing of gait (e.g., start hesitation, on turns, in doorways)
Cerebellar	Unstable with increased truncal sway or tremor	Normal	Increased	Normal	Variable	Variable, often reduced	Wide	Often asymmetric, variable	Reduced	Patients maintain widened base and often have increased double-limb support time during stance phase to increase stability in lateral plane. Base does not narrow and legs do not cross unless after stumble, e.g., during turning
Spastic paraparesis	Usually normal unless associated with significant pyramidal weakness	Normal	Normal	Extended at hips, knees, ankles often plantar flexed and inverted without change during gait phases	Reduced, with circumduction (abduction of the hip in an arc) of the leg during swing phase	Reduced, often with toe dragging	Normal or reduced with legs crossing ("scissoring")	Symmetric or mildly asymmetric. Consistent pattern	Reduced	Gait similar forwards or backwards
Antalgic	Normal	Normal or may be tilted to offload weight from antalgic leg	Increased to one side to offload weight from antalgic leg	Normal or asymmetric depending on whether mobility of painful leg is affected	Asymmetric, reduced in normal leg to reduce stance phase of antalgic leg, may be increased or decreased in antalgic leg depending on cause of pain	Reduced in normal leg to shorten swing phase, may be increased or decreased in antalgic leg depending on cause of pain	Normal or widened depending on cause of pain	Asymmetric due to reduced stance phase in antalgic leg. Consistent pattern	Normal or reduced	Testing weight bearing on one leg at a time (with support if necessary), and during passive movement of the hip, knee, and ankle when supine, can be helpful in confirming diagnosis
Trendelenburg	Normal when standing on both legs. Unstable when standing on affected leg due to weakness/instability of hip abduction, leading to dropping of contralateral pelvic rim and compensatory lateral tilt of body to ipsilateral side (Trendelenburg sign)	Abnormal during stance phase on affected leg due to weakness/ instability of hip abduction, leading to dropping of contralateral pelvic rim and compensatory lateral tilt of body to ipsilateral side	Increased during stance phase on affected leg due to weakness/ instability of hip abduction, leading to dropping of contralateral pelvic rim and compensatory lateral tilt of body to ipsilateral side	Adduction of affected hip during stance phase (due to pelvis/trunk tilting contralaterally)	Asymmetric, reduced in normal leg to reduce stance phase of unstable leg	Asymmetric, reduced in normal leg to reduce stance phase of unstable leg	Normal	Asymmetric due to reduced stance phase in unstable leg. Consistent pattern	Reduced	Look for Trendelenburg sign when standing on affected leg

superimposed the random movements that occur from the additional movement disorders.

Frontal ataxia

Pathology of the frontal lobes can impair stance, equilibrium, and locomotion in different ways, leading to gait abnormalities that range from appearing primarily parkinsonian with prominent reduced stride length and freezing of gait, to primarily ataxic with disequilibrium, widened gait base, and increased truncal sway (Thompson, 2012). The disequilibrium and increased truncal sway can be profound, leading to a highly variable gait pattern which can be confused with a psychogenic gait if other frontal signs are not prominent. The pattern of gait may also change with disease progression, adding further to apparent inconsistency and confusion with a psychogenic origin. The diagnosis relies on the presence of either other clinical or functional imaging evidence of frontal-lobe dysfunction, or evidence of structural pathology on neuroimaging.

PSYCHOGENIC GAIT

The preceding sections provide tools with which the clinician can now analyze gait and recognize some common and uncommon organic gaits. There have been a number of clinical features of psychogenic gait suggested by different authors (Table 23.2) (Keane, 1989; Lempert et al., 1991; Hayes et al., 1999; Baik and Lang, 2007). Many of the descriptors, however, overlap with terms used to describe organic phenomenology, and it is not always clear what aspects of the gait or other neurologic findings were used in making the diagnosis of psychogenicity. The sensitivity and specificity of specific symptoms and signs are, with few exceptions, unknown. None have perfect positive predictive value or specificity, so the diagnosis should never be made on a single feature. However, a helpful principle in the diagnosis of psychogenic illness is that, even if a single symptom or sign is inconclusive or nonspecific, the combined features of a patient's clinical syndrome (e.g., multiple medically unexplained symptoms (Hayes et al., 1999) or inconsistencies (Baik and Lang, 2007)) often make an underlying organic diagnosis implausible. For example, organic paroxysmal movement disorders can occur, but if a history of paroxysmal ataxic gait is combined with whole-body tremor as the dominant phenomenology, and there is a temporal course of daily attacks lasting hours for months at a time, interspersed with spontaneous remission for months, the syndrome becomes increasingly incongruent with any known organic paroxysmal movement disorder.

As with other psychogenic movement disorders, the diagnosis rests predominantly on the presence of inconsistency and/or incongruency in the symptoms (history) and signs (phenomenology).

Table 23.2

Characteristics of psychogenic gait

Phenomenology
Hemiparetic, paraparetic, ataxic, trembling, dystonic, truncal myoclonus, stiff-legged (robot), slapping (tabetic), camptocormia, fluctuation of impairment, excessive slowness of movements, hesitation, "psychogenic Romberg" test, "walking on ice" gait pattern, uneconomic postures with waste of energy, sudden buckling (with or without falls), astasia, vertical shaking tremor, pseudotaxia of the legs or the trunk, sudden sidesteps, flailing of the arms, dragging of the leg, continuous flexion of the toes, continuous extension of the toes, bizarre tremors, expressive behavior (grasping the leg, mannered posture of hands, suffering or strained facial expression, moaning, hyperventilation), exaggerated effort or fatigue, slowness, fluctuations, convulsive shaking, bizarre gait, exaggerated response to pull test or Romberg's test, improvement with distraction or worsening with suggestion, incongruent response to novel gait tasks, e.g., exaggerated slowness or effort during tandem gait or walking backwards, "tightrope" walking with exaggerated truncal sway while maintaining a narrow base, truncal instability with good targeting of nearby walls or furniture
Syndromic description
Hemiparetic, paraparetic, ataxic, trembling, dystonic, truncal myoclonus, stiff-legged (robot), slapping (tabetic), camptocormia, slow gait, astasia, buckling, pseudomyoclonus, rhythmic side-to-side rocking, fixed flexion of hips and knees, generalized tremor, walking on ice, tripping propulsion with falls, hesitation, monoparesis with dragging of the leg, unilateral limp, bilateral equinovarus posture of the feet, waddling in a squatting position, dragging along (like an exhausted wanderer in the desert), effortful, creeping, tightrope walking, hobbling, jigging hemiparetic, pseudoparkinsonian, scissoring

Adapted from Keane (1989), Lempert et al. (1991), Hayes et al. (1999), and Baik and Lang (2007).

History

Many of the red flags for psychogenic movement disorders in general also apply to psychogenic gait. An abrupt onset in the absence of any trauma or structural lesion is unusual for most organic movement disorders, especially if combined with a rapid escalation to severe impairment or disability, and was reported in 87.3% of patients with psychogenic gait in the series by Baik and Lang (2007). There may be a mismatch between impairment and disability, which can be in either direction (i.e., severe impairment yet little reported disability, or vice versa) (Hayes et al., 1999). Organic gait disorders are usually persistent rather than variable. Therefore a history of marked variability, whether short-term (e.g., able to walk from the car to the clinic but not from the waiting room into the consulting room) or long-term (sustained spontaneous remissions and exacerbations lasting days, weeks, or months) should suggest a psychogenic origin. Interestingly, a history of phenytoin intoxication was found to be a feature in one case series (Keane, 1989).

There are of course exceptions. Organic paroxysmal movement disorders can appear and disappear over minutes to hours, and it is necessary to be familiar with the clinical spectrum of the paroxysmal dyskinesias, ataxias, and paralyses. The majority of patients with these predominantly genetic disorders approximate one of the classic phenotypes, and marked differences between a patient's clinical presentation and these phenotypes should suggest the possibility of a psychogenic illness. Acquired organic movement disorders can also fluctuate spontaneously, with notable examples being inflammatory central (e.g., demyelination, stiff-man syndrome) or peripheral (e.g., myasthenia gravis, autoimmune neuromyotonia) nervous system disease, metabolic disease (e.g., hypoglycemia, including glucose transporter deficiency, or dopa-responsive dystonia) or drug-induced movement disorders (e.g., drug-induced asterixis causing a knee-buckling gait – although the loss of tone in asterixis is intermittent, brief, and shock-like, arising from loss of muscle tone from negative myoclonus, rather than variable in duration, sustained, or tremulous in psychogenic knee buckling).

Examination of gait (phenomenology)

As Table 23.2 indicates, the range of abnormalities observed in psychogenic gait is extremely wide. The approach to distinguishing organic from psychogenic gait disorders differs in some aspects from that used to diagnose other psychogenic movement disorders as gait is a complex motor and cognitive function which also commonly is impaired by nonneurologic (e.g., musculoskeletal or biomechanical) as well as neurologic dysfunction. Therefore a psychogenic gait may or may not be dominated by an actual psychogenic hyperkinetic or hypokinetic movement disorder. Where there is an obvious movement disorder such as tremor or dystonia (i.e., prominent abnormal posturing), the usual criteria used to distinguish organic from psychogenic origins of that phenomenology can be applied. Where the abnormal gait is dominated by other neurologic (e.g., weakness) or nonneurologic (e.g., antalgia) features, inconsistency of those features and/or incongruence with those other non-movement disorder gait disorders are still the keys to recognition of a psychogenic etiology.

The following stepwise approach can be useful in analyzing a gait disorder and deciding whether it is psychogenic:

1. During which part(s) of the gait cycle is the abnormality of movement occurring?
2. What is the nature of the abnormal movement? Is it abnormal posture, a superimposed involuntary movement, exaggeration or reduction in amplitude of a normal movement, or a combination of the above? Is it predominantly a manifestation of another impairment such as weakness, mechanical instability, or pain?
3. If abnormal posturing is present, does it occur consistently during each gait cycle? If it is inconsistent, can this be explained by superimposition of a random involuntary movement on to a consistent underlying abnormality in posture?
4. If the abnormal movements or postures are inconsistent and variable, can they be explained by a movement disorder that is random, such as choreoballism or ataxia?
5. If the abnormality of movement is inconsistent and incongruent with an unpredictable or random involuntary movement disorder, is it consistent or congruent with a different neurologic, musculoskeletal, or biomechanical impairment? If not, then a psychogenic cause should be considered.

The usefulness of analyzing gait by assessing specific components of the gait cycle is supported by a study of 19 normal and 66 organic gait disorder patients, in which a neural network using instrumental, four-dimensional measures of gait could be trained to identify normal, ataxic, spastic paraparetic, and parkinsonian gait patterns (Merello et al., 2012). The patients were successfully reclassified by the neural network into the same gait patterns when re-evaluated 3 months later. In contrast, 5 psychogenic patients showed a change in their quantitative gait parameters over 3 months, leading to classification by the neural network into different gait patterns at their initial and follow-up assessments, despite the clinical impression of their gaits being of no or slight change between visits. This study helps confirm the utility of inconsistency as a diagnostic tool. In an objective study of truncal sway, 12 patients with psychogenic gait and balance disturbance were shown to have increased overall sway parameters compared with 12 multiple sclerosis and 12 normal controls, as well as paradoxic reduction in sway with a distracting maneuver of recognizing a number being traced on their back by the examiner's finger (Wolfsegger et al., 2013). Mental distraction was also shown to paradoxically reduce sway in a study of patients with psychogenic lower-body sensorimotor disturbance or gait disorder compared with normal controls (Stins et al., 2015).

There are a couple of signs that have been studied for their diagnostic utility in psychogenic gait. "Huffing and puffing" signs (presence of huffing, grunting, grimacing, and breath holding while walking) were present in 44% of a cohort of 131 patients with clinically definite psychogenic gait (selected because of absence of pain in symptomatology) but minimal or absent in 37 organic gait disorder control patients, yielding 89–100% specificity (Laub et al., 2015). The presence of "huffing and puffing" signs increases the odds of a gait disorder being psychogenic by 13 times. In a preliminary report of the "chair test," 8/9 psychogenic gait patients were able to use their legs to propel themselves when seated on an office chair on wheels better than when walking, which was not observed in 9 patients with parkinsonian gait disorder (Okun et al., 2007). The authors caution that the utility of this sign needs to be confirmed with a larger study using objective measures. It is likely that patients with organic gait disorders affecting predominantly equilibrium rather than locomotion such as truncal ataxia, or with task specificity such as gait dystonia or freezing of gait, will also perform better mobilizing on a chair compared with walking.

Other less well-validated and somewhat subjective signs, which, although strictly speaking not movement disorder phenomenology, can be observed in psychogenic gait and rarely in organic gait disorders, are exaggerated slowness, repeated lurching towards the examiner, walls, or furniture but not towards open space, and repeated falling on to the knees.

Associated neurologic signs

Psychogenic gait may occur as the only impairment or disability, or in association with other movement disorders or nonmovement disorder neurologic symptoms and signs (Table 23.2) which also need to be evaluated according to their own merit (Stone and Carson, 2015).

Syndromes

Many of the syndromic descriptions which have been used to describe different psychogenic gaits are listed in Table 23.2. Jordbru et al. (2012) used videotape analysis of 30 consecutive patients with psychogenic gait and found that the clinical features proposed by Lempert et al. could be reduced to one of three patterns: limping of one leg, limping of two legs, and truncal imbalance, with high interrater reliability amongst the five raters who took part in the study. Table 23.3 lists some syndromic descriptions that can be applied to psychogenic gaits, most of which have organic counterparts. The different syndromic descriptions can be classified into one of four (albeit overlapping) categories. Categorizing the suspected psychogenic gait into one or more of these different categories can further assist in deciding what clinical tests or investigations are required to look for positive evidence of psychogenicity and to exclude potential underlying organic pathology: (1) movement disorder mimics; (2) neurologic (nonmovement disorder) mimics; (3) musculoskeletal or biomechanical mimics; and (4) isolated disequilibrium or balance disorders.

Table 23.3

Psychogenic gait syndromes

Psychogenic gait syndromes
Movement disorder mimics
Tremulous
Dystonic
Parkinsonian
Propulsive
Camptocormic
Choreoballistic
Ataxic
Spastic
Myoclonic
Collapsing (lower-limb asterixis)
Stiff-man syndrome/robotic
Neurologic (nonmovement disorder) mimics
Hemiparetic
Paraparetic
Sensory ataxic
Myopathic/waddling
Myopathic/cautious or parkinsonian
Myopathic/collapsing
Neuropathic (footdrop)
Musculoskeletal or biomechanical mimics
Antalgic (back pain)
Antalgic (sacroiliac/pelvis/hip pain)
Antalgic (knee or leg pain)
Trendelenburg (hip instability)
Hobbling
Isolated disequilibrium or balance disorders
Tightrope walking
Cautious/walking on ice/creeping

Movement disorder mimics

These psychogenic gaits are dominated by movement disorder phenomenology, such as tremor, myoclonus, or abnormal postures mimicking dystonia. The diagnosis relies on using the same criteria to distinguish psychogenic from organic phenomenology in nongait-related settings.

Neurologic (nonmovement disorder) mimics

Patients with psychogenic gait may have symptoms or impairment without an associated movement disorder, such as weakness that resembles central (e.g., hemiplegic, paraplegic) or peripheral (flaccid) nervous system disease, with or without hypertonia. Alternatively, patients may have nonmovement disorder neurologic symptoms or signs (e.g., sensory loss, speech disturbance) combined with movement disorder phenomenology.

Musculoskeletal or biomechanical mimics

Patients with psychogenic gait may report pain or limitation of movement localized to musculoskeletal structures, with or without neurologic symptoms or signs. It may be necessary to exclude musculoskeletal pathology through either cross-disciplinary consultation or imaging.

Isolated disequilibrium or balance disorders

Impaired equilibrium or balance is a common feature of both organic and psychogenic gait disorders. However, occasionally patients will have as their only symptom or impairment the inability to maintain a stable upright posture, which might occur only during standing (Baik and Lee, 2012), walking, or both. If occurring in isolation, without other neurologic features, the phenomenology observed during a psychogenic gait might consist only of what is judged subjectively as an exaggeration of normal compensatory maneuvers such as putting the arms out ("tightrope walking"), or marked reduction in the step height and stride length ("walking on ice"). In order to avoid reliance purely on the subjective assessment of whether the compensatory maneuvers are appropriate, observation of inconsistency or superadded positive features such as "huffing and puffing" is a major diagnostic clue. For example, as discussed above, sway may improve rather than worsen with mental distraction (Wolfsegger et al., 2013; Stins et al., 2015). Another form of inconsistency is when patients complain of poor balance or falls, yet display evidence of preserved or even skillful balance control by being able to maintain uneconomic postures (Lempert et al., 1991; Hayes et al., 1999) or continuous exaggerated truncal sway (astasia abasia) during stance or walking without actually falling.

Management

Treatment of psychogenic illness is reviewed comprehensively elsewhere in this volume and will not be reviewed in detail here. However, a recent randomized control trial of inpatient rehabilitation in 60 patients with psychogenic gait of less than 5 years' duration showed significant improvements in the Functional Independence Measure and Functional Mobility Scale, with good carry-over effects, being sustained at both 1 month and 1 year (Jordbru et al., 2014). Treatment was three-pronged, combining symptom explanation, positive reinforcement of normal function, and not positively reinforcing dysfunction, both during and between therapy sessions.

CONCLUSIONS

Gait disorder is a common accompaniment of functional illness, especially psychogenic movement disorders. The diagnosis of psychogenic gait is complex. It requires a sound knowledge of the range of phenomenology observed in organic movement disorders, the ability to evaluate and diagnose nonmovement disorder neurologic symptoms and signs, but additionally knowledge of potential musculoskeletal causes of gait disturbance. A stepwise approach to the analysis of the phenomenology and separation into four (sometimes overlapping) psychogenic gait syndromes is suggested to aid diagnosis: (1) movement disorder mimics; (2) neurologic (nonmovement disorder) mimics; (3) musculoskeletal or biomechanical mimics; and (4) isolated disequilibrium or balance disorders. Accurate diagnosis can lead to effective therapy.

References

Albanese A (2003). The clinical expression of primary dystonia. J Neurol 250: 1145–1151.

Albanese A, Bhatia K, Bressman SB et al. (2013). Phenomenology and classification of dystonia: a consensus update. Mov Disord 28: 863–873.

Baik JS, Lang AE (2007). Gait abnormalities in psychogenic movement disorders. Mov Disord 22: 395–399.

Baik JS, Lee MS (2012). Psychogenic balance disorders: is it a new entity of psychogenic movement disorders? J Mov Disord 5: 24–27.

Fung VS, Jinnah HA, Bhatia K et al. (2013). Assessment of patients with isolated or combined dystonia: an update on dystonia syndromes. Mov Disord 28: 889–898.

Hayes MW, Graham S, Heldorf P et al. (1999). A video review of the diagnosis of psychogenic gait: appendix and commentary. Mov Disord 14: 914–921.

Jordbru AA, Smedstad LM, Moen VP et al. (2012). Identifying patterns of psychogenic gait by video-recording. J Rehabil Med 44: 31–35.

Jordbru AA, Smedstad LM, Klungsoyr O et al. (2014). Psychogenic gait disorder: a randomized controlled trial of physical rehabilitation with one-year follow-up. J Rehabil Med 46: 181–187.

Keane JR (1989). Hysterical gait disorders: 60 cases. Neurology 39: 586–589.

Kim SD, Fung VS (2011). Unusual gait disorders. In: N Galvez-Jimenez, P Tuite, K Bhatia (Eds.), Uncommon Causes of Movement Disorders. Cambridge University Press, Cambridge.

Latt MD, Menz HB, Fung VS et al. (2008). Walking speed, cadence and step length are selected to optimize the stability of head and pelvis accelerations. Exp Brain Res 184: 201–209.

Laub HN, Dwivedi AK, Revilla FJ et al. (2015). Diagnostic performance of the "Huffing and Puffing" sign in psychogenic (functional) movement disorders. Mov Disord Clin Pract (Hoboken) 2: 29–32.

Lempert T, Brandt T, Dieterich M et al. (1991). How to identify psychogenic disorders of stance and gait. A video study in 37 patients. J Neurol 238: 140–146.

Merello M, Ballesteros D, Rossi M et al. (2012). Lack of maintenance of gait pattern as measured by instrumental methods suggests psychogenic gait. Funct Neurol 27: 217–224.

Murray MP, Drought AB, Kory RC (1964). Walking patterns of normal men. J Bone Joint Surg Am 46: 335–360.

Nutt JG, Marsden CD, Thompson PD (1993). Human walking and higher-level gait disorders, particularly in the elderly. Neurology 43: 268–279.

Okun MS, Rodriguez RL, Foote KD et al. (2007). The "chair test" to aid in the diagnosis of psychogenic gait disorders. Neurologist 13: 87–91.

Ramos VF, Karp BI, Hallett M (2014). Tricks in dystonia: ordering the complexity. J Neurol Neurosurg Psychiatry 85: 987–993.

Stins JF, Kempe CL, Hagenaars MA et al. (2015). Attention and postural control in patients with conversion paresis. J Psychosom Res 78: 249–254.

Stone J, Carson A (2015). Functional neurologic disorders. Continuum (Minneap Minn) 21: 818–837.

Thompson PD (2012). Frontal lobe ataxia. Handb Clin Neurol 103: 619–622.

Trinh B, Ha AD, Mahant N et al. (2014). Dramatic improvement of truncal tardive dystonia following globus pallidus pars interna deep brain stimulation. J Clin Neurosci 21: 515–517.

Whittle MW (1996). Clinical gait analysis: a review. Hum Mov Sci 15: 369–387.

Winter DA (1983). Biomechanical motor patterns in normal walking. J Mot Behav 15: 302–330.

Winter DA, Patla AE, Frank JS et al. (1990). Biomechanical walking pattern changes in the fit and healthy elderly. Phys Ther 70: 340–347.

Wolfsegger T, Pischinger B, Topakian R (2013). Objectification of psychogenic postural instability by trunk sway analysis. J Neurol Sci 334: 14–17.

Handbook of Clinical Neurology, Vol. 139 (3rd series)
Functional Neurologic Disorders
M. Hallett, J. Stone, and A. Carson, Editors
http://dx.doi.org/10.1016/B978-0-12-801772-2.00024-2

Chapter 24

Functional sensory symptoms

J. STONE[1]* AND M. VERMEULEN[2]

[1]*Department of Clinical Neurosciences, Centre for Clinical Brain Sciences, University of Edinburgh, Edinburgh, UK*

[2]*Department of Neurology, Academic Medical Center, Amsterdam, The Netherlands*

Abstract

Functional (psychogenic) sensory symptoms are those in which the patient genuinely experiences alteration or absence of normal sensation in the absence of neurologic disease. The hallmark of functional sensory symptoms is the presence of internal inconsistency revealing a pattern of symptoms governed by abnormally focused attention.

In this chapter we review the history of this area, different clinical presentations, diagnosis (including sensitivity of diagnostic tests), treatment, experimental studies, and prognosis.

Altered sensation has been a feature of "hysteria" since descriptions of witchcraft in the middle ages. In the 19th century hysteric sensory stigmata were considered a hallmark of the condition. Despite this long history, relatively little attention has been paid to the topic of functional sensory disturbance, compared to functional limb weakness or functional movement disorders, with which it commonly coexists.

There are recognizable clinical patterns, such as hemisensory disturbance and sensory disturbance finishing at the groin or shoulder, but in keeping with the literature on reliability of sensory signs in neurology in general, the evidence suggests that physical signs designed to make a positive diagnosis of functional sensory disorder may not be that reliable.

There are sensory symptoms which are unusual but not functional (such as synesthesia and allochiria) but also functional sensory symptoms (such as complete loss of all pain) which are most unusual and probably worthy of independent study.

INTRODUCTION

We begin with a review of the history of this area, moving on to a description of different types of sensory disturbance. We then summarize what is known about the reliability of sensory signs in this area, drawing heavily on the studies of Selma Aybek and colleagues (Daum et al., 2014a, b). Finally we discuss what is known about the pathophysiology of sensory symptoms and their treatment.

HISTORIC BACKGROUND

Freud stated in 1888 that, "In the middle ages, the discovery of anaesthetic and non-bleeding areas (stigmata diaboli) was regarded as evidence of witchcraft" (Freud, 1966). Although this is generally accepted, our search for primary material relevant to this was not fruitful. The "witches mark" was certainly often looked for; this was usually an accessory nipple or some skin lesion such as a wart or corn, which would have been more anasthetic and less likely to bleed. There were various trials by ordeal, such as picking a stone from boiling water to see if the wounds healed well (innocent) or festered (guilty). In England and Scotland, "common prickers" gave testimony on those suspected of witchcraft,

> *caused John Kincaid of Tranent [near Edinburgh], the common pricker, to exercise his craft upon her. He found two marks of the devil's making; for she could not feel the pin when it was put into either of the said marks, nor did the marks bleed when*

*Correspondence to: Jon Stone, Department of Clinical Neurosciences, Western General Hospital, Crew Rd, Edinburgh EH4 2 XU, UK. Tel: +44-131-537-1167, E-mail: jon.stone@ed.ac.uk

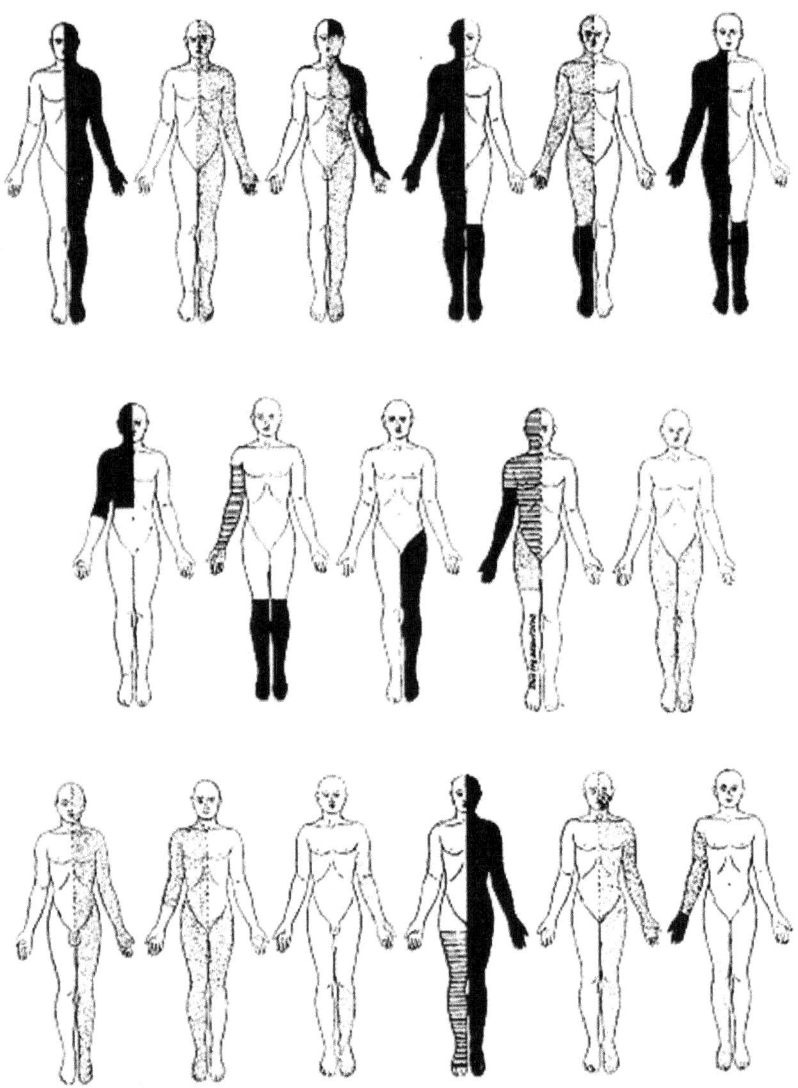

Fig. 24.1. Various types of "hysterical anesthesia." Total loss of sensation (black); shaded (more severe impairment); dotted areas (slight sensory loss). (Reproduced from Purves-Stewart, 1913.)

> *the pin was taken out again. When she was asked where she thought the pins were put in her, she pointed to a part of her body distant to the real place. They were pins of three inches in length (Pitcairn, quoted in Summers, 1926).*

From the 18th century onwards, descriptions of altered sensation in hysteria appear quite regularly in texts on the topic. Whytt, for example, writing about hysteria in 1767, wrote chapters on "an uncommon sense of cold or heat in different parts of the body, sometimes suddenly succeeding each other" and "pains in different parts of the body, suddenly moving from one place to another."

By the late 19th century there was quite intense interest in the various types of sensory disturbances seen in hysteria, and many textbooks of the time carry charts demonstrating patterns including hemisensory disturbance. Figure 24.1, from an early-20th-century textbook of neurology, indicates various patterns thought to be "hysterical" (Purves-Stewart, 1913).

The observation was made that such sensory disturbance could arise from the patients' own ideas (autosuggestion) or through suggestion by the physician, either informally or through hypnosis (heterosuggestion). There was a temporary vogue for using metals to cure hemisensory disturbance (metallotherapy) until it was discovered that wood and amyl nitrite did the same (Gowers, 1892). Often, it was observed that altered sensation arose accidentally through the way a physician spoke to the patient during the examination – "And do you feel numb here?" Generally speaking, the longer a patient is examined, the more abnormal areas would be found. Babinski was so impressed by this phenomenon that he asserted that all cases of hemisensory disturbance were a result of suggestion by physicians. He even wanted to change the name of hysteria to pithiatism (from the Greek "persuasion" and "curable") (Babinski and Froment, 1918). Others agreed, including Janet, although later he changed his mind on the basis of finding extensive anesthesia in patients apparently unaware of extensive sensory loss found on examination. He noted how it sometimes returned during chloroform anesthesia, when the patient was drunk, after a nonepileptic attack, or during sleep:

> *We have to take the patients by surprise at night, using all sorts of precautions not to wake them. We pinch them on the anaesthetic side. They groan, turn over, complain in their dream, or wake suddenly, exactly as a normal person would (Janet, 1907).*

Similar evidence that functional motor disorders improve during sleep has been published (Lauerma, 1993; Worley, 2002).

It was also realized that there was a close connection between sensory disturbance and weakness. Fox, for example, writing in 1913, commented that, "In the mind of the laity, paralysis must be accompanied necessarily by numbness; paralysis implying that the affected member must be numb and dead" (Fox, 1913). Hurst in 1920 asked medical students to simulate paralysis and found that many of them had areas of altered sensation that they had not been instructed to have and which conformed to patterns of altered and reduced sensation seen in hysteria. He proposed several situations in which hysteric anesthesia could occur, including: (1) suggestion by a physician; (2) anesthesia following an episode of stupor during which there is "profound inattention"; and (3) anesthesia beginning with a disease of the nervous system such as ulnar nerve irritation, but amplified by a functional disorder.

It was noted by several authors that cutaneous reflexes appeared to be altered in patients with hysteric sensory disturbance and this in turn suggested that there must be some form of psychophysiologic disturbance at work. For example, plantar responses have been found to be diminished in patients with hysteria by Allen (1935), and this is our experience also.

Dense anesthesia, including insensibility to pain, as occurs in some patients with functional sensory disturbance, is particularly thought provoking with respect to the physiology of the symptom. Some patients are able to experience a loss of sensation which goes beyond that which most people can imagine being able to sustain through effort or pretense. We have been impressed, for example, with the ability of some of our patients to tolerate very-high-amplitude peripheral nerve stimulation on the affected side. Nineteenth-century illustrations of patients with safety pins or long sharp objects through areas of anesthesia are in keeping with this clinical phenomenon, although claims that the patient didn't bleed or would be truly as cheerful, as depicted in Figure 24.2, are less plausible and speak more to theatric objectification of patients with hysteria at that time.

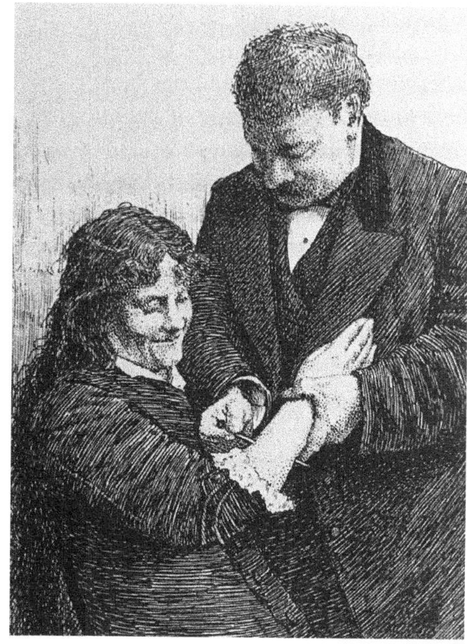

Fig. 24.2. Nineteenth-century illustration of "hysterical" anesthesia used to demonstrate complete absence of sensation (Regnard, 1887). The implausibility both of the lack of bleeding and the smiling nature of the subject in this drawing represent a theatric and objectified view of "hysteria," common at the time.

Conversely, pain is a frequently occurring symptom in patients with functional symptoms. Sollier (1897) produced a cartography of the main pain points on the body of women with functional symptoms. The zones were located above, on, and under the breast, between the ribs or just under the lower ribs, at the iliac crest, and at the site of the ovaries. According to Charcot, the ovaries were an important cause of pain and were often enlarged in patients with functional symptoms (Goetz, 1999). Jelgersma could not confirm this enlargement of the ovaries, which he explained by his difficulties with palpation in women with much pain of the ovaries. The observation of enlarged ovaries led to ovariectomy as a treatment for women with functional symptoms, but Charcot disapproved of this treatment (Goetz, 1999). In addition to the zones described by Sollier, Jelgersma (1926) mentioned the nasal cavity and the tympanic cavity.

Much of our knowledge of functional neurologic symptoms and their assessment emerged in the late 19th and early 20th century and has been passed on at the bedside to later generations of neurologists, which was for many of us the only way in which we were taught about this area. Textbooks of neurology had declining amounts of information on "hysteria" over the 20th century, with chapters on functional neurologic symptoms becoming increasingly rare and textbooks of psychiatry emphasizing (incorrectly) diagnosis by exclusion and psychologic mechanisms, not symptoms (Stone et al., 2008). In the absence of any recent systematic studies for this review, we have used British, French, German, and Dutch sources (Jelgersma, 1926) and combined this with our own experience in order to describe the phenomenology.

EPIDEMIOLOGY

"Sensory symptoms" appear as a category in many older studies of "hysteria" or "conversion symptoms," but usually with little other characterization. Typically, around one-third of patients are recorded as having these, usually in combination with other symptoms. The St. Louis group, in their original description of somatization disorder in 500 patients, recorded them in 25% (Guze et al., 1971). Other larger studies have recorded them in 43% ($n=43$) (Kapfhammer et al., 1992) and as low as 8% ($n=79$) (Wilson-Barnett and Trimble, 1985).

There are few published studies focusing on functional sensory symptoms. Toth (2003) described a case series of 34 patients with hemisensory syndrome: 74% were women, with a mean age of 35. Even this apparent series of sensory disturbance is a little deceptive. Twenty-five percent of the patients had unilateral heaviness of the limb as well as sensory disturbance. One-third had a sudden onset. In two-thirds it was gradual. Ipsilateral blurring of vision (asthenopia) was present in 28% and ipsilateral hearing loss in 16%. Toth reported persisting symptoms in only 20% of the 30 patients he followed up at 16 months. In a follow-up study of 60 patients with functional motor and sensory symptoms seen 12 years earlier, there was evidence of crossover between symptoms of weakness and numbness. Fifty-eight percent of those initially just complaining of altered sensation complained of weakness at follow-up (Stone et al., 2003).

A number of studies suggested that functional hemisensory symptoms were particularly likely to occur on the left. This fitted with various superficially attractive hypotheses drawing parallels with anosagnosia or *la belle indifférence*. A systematic review of laterality of functional motor and sensory symptoms in 121 studies with 1139 participants found that differences were only seen in studies ($n=395$) where laterality was an explicit aim of the study (66% on the left). In other studies ($n=553$) there was no difference with only 53% on the left (Stone et al., 2002) (Fig. 24.3). In fact, *la belle indifférence* itself is a sign without clear diagnostic value and in our experience often indicates a distressed patient "putting on a brave face" (Stone et al., 2006).

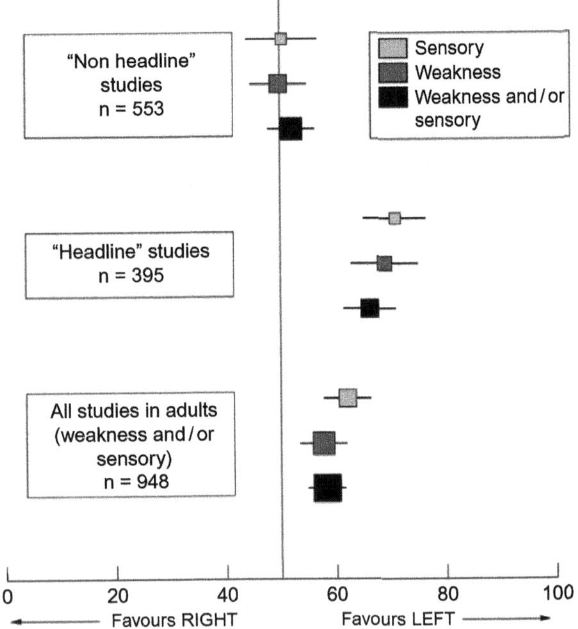

Fig. 24.3. Functional sensory symptoms appear to be more common on the left, but this seems to be a result of publication bias. There is no difference in studies where this was not the explicit aim of the study. n = numbers of patients; 121 studies in total. (Reproduced from Stone et al., 2002, with permission from BMJ Publishing Group.)

Studies in complex regional pain syndrome (CRPS) populations have demonstrated that a hemisensory syndrome or "whole-limb" sensory disturbance is quite common when looked for (Rommel et al., 1999). Sometimes the literature refers to them as "nondermatomal sensory abnormalities" (Mailis-Gagnon and Nicholson, 2010). In recent publications this type of sensory problem has been termed "neglect-like" (Lewis et al., 2007; Bultitude and Rafal, 2010), although others have pointed out that the symptom is different to neglect in that the patient pays attention to the affected limb and is hyperaware of the problem rather than unaware (Punt et al., 2013). In one study of 145 CRPS patients, sensory disturbance occurred in 88% of patients, with 36% reporting a glove-and-stocking distribution, hypoesthesia in 53%, and hyperesthesia in 17% (Birklein et al., 2000). Veldman et al. (1993) found hyperesthesia in 76% of 829 CRPS patients, as well as reduced proprioception and sometimes anesthesia dolorosa (pain in areas of numbness). Other studies of sensory disturbance in CRPS have shown significant response to placebo

(Verdugo and Ochoa, 1998). In their study Verdugo and Ochoa found that all 27 patients with CRPS with no nerve lesion had placebo responsiveness of their sensory disturbance. Tensions in this area have not been helped by equating functional disorders with malingering, which has led to entrenched positions. Arguably the field of functional sensory disorders has much to learn from the work already done on CRPS, and vice versa.

HYPOESTHESIA/SENSORY LOSS

Nature of symptoms

Patients are often not aware of their hypoesthesia. It is not unusual for them to notice this sensory impairment for the first time during the neurologic examination. However, some patients with hypoesthesia definitely do notice the symptom before presenting to medical services and come to clinic complaining that they have burnt themselves or that their limb "doesn't feel right."

The quality of the sensory impairment is variable. Most common is disturbance of pain sensation and in decreasing frequency it is the sensation of touch and temperature which is impaired. The intensity of the symptoms is also variable. There may be only a slight difference in touch or pinprick sensation between the left and the right side, but complete insensitivity to pain has also been observed. Patients may even lose the sensation of having an arm or leg, at which point the problem appears more like a loss of the "idea" of a limb rather than a cutaneous sensory problem. Lasègue (1864) described a situation when patients with functional sensory loss can only move an arm or leg when they look at it. They may find it difficult to say what the position of their arm is with eyes closed. Patients with fixed ankle dystonia have been observed to have similar difficulties knowing, with their eyes closed, whether their ankles were twisted or straight, typically either feeling that the foot "isn't there" or is in a normal straight position even when it patently isn't (Stone et al., 2012a). As with hypoesthesia, sometimes this observation is apparently new when we detect it and may be the result of suggestion, but other patients have told us that they had noticed it themselves but were reluctant to discuss it.

Distribution of symptoms

In some cases patients complain of generalized sensory loss over the whole body. This type of widespread sensory impairment is usually of short duration, but may recur during stressful events. Probably the most common sensory disturbance is hemisensory in nature. This may vary from a small area, often the face, to one side of the whole body. Patients commonly complain of feeling "cut in half" or "split down the middle." This is often more pronounced on the front of the trunk than the back. As found by Toth and described frequently in older texts (e.g., Gowers, 1892), there may be reduced vision (asthenopia) and, less commonly, reduced hearing on the same side. Numbness has a tendency to affect the arm and leg before the trunk. Sometimes sensory disturbance may mysteriously "flip" from one side to the other. A sensory level on the trunk should be a red flag for spinal demyelination or another type of spinal lesion.

Circumferential sensory deficit which ends at the top of the leg, with numbness extending down from the crease of the groin and posteriorly from the crease below the buttock, was described by Janet and Freud. Similar patterns may be seen in the arm, with sensory loss ending abruptly at the shoulder. Such distributions are often said to be "nonanatomic," although they are in keeping with the "idea of a limb." More limited forms of unilateral sock or glove circumferential sensory loss are also well described (Magee, 1962). In our personal experience, unless the patient spends a lot of time sitting on a hard bicycle seat (which can cause perineal nerve compression), has prostate pathology or, rarely, multiple sclerosis, complaints of a numb penis are usually functional.

Another distribution of sensory symptoms is irregular areas. Sensory impairment may be restricted to joints, for instance, shoulders or hips, or there is impairment of the whole foot or hand. In patients with irregular areas of sensory impairment, the boundaries between normal and abnormal are often difficult to establish. In these patients, the sensory disturbances have a distribution comparable with neither that in patients with peripheral neuropathies nor with that in patients with radicular segmental sensory loss. If there is a truncal deficit it may have only an anterior but not a posterior level. The sensory loss may extend over the boundaries between skin and mucosa, for instance, the conjunctiva, vagina, lips, and even the whole oral cavity.

Physical signs of functional sensory loss

In general terms, none of the signs described to diagnose functional sensory disturbance are that reliable, and have performed less well in controlled studies than signs for functional limb weakness or functional movement disorder. This is not surprising, since sensory signs generally have poor reliability and validity in the neurologic examination (Lindley et al., 1993). They rely on an interaction between doctor and patient and reporting of subjective phenomena. They are therefore prone to many forms of bias in their assessment, including problems with suggestion highlighted earlier. In addition, when sensory signs have been reported in previous studies there are several methodologic problems: (1) the diagnosis may have been made partly using the sign being reported, thus overinflating its utility (diagnostic suspicion bias); (2)

nearly all studies of these signs are unblinded (except for one study of interrater reliability (Daum et al., 2014a); (3) there are few studies, mostly with small numbers; and (4) sensory signs are especially liable to verbal misunderstanding. For example, in Janet's "say 'yes' when you feel it and 'no' when you don't" test, patients may think "no" means "feel it less." We describe the signs below and present data on sensitivity and specificity in Table 24.1, but these should be interpreted with great caution for these methodologic reasons.

1. Midline splitting of sensory deficit is suggestive of functional sensory symptoms. Midline splitting is defined by sensory loss with a clear edge on the midline. This midline splitting is considered typical for functional symptoms since in anatomic central lesions the trunk is either spared or sensory loss occurs a couple of centimeters from the midline because of crossover of cutaneous sensory nerves. The sensitivity of midline splitting appeared to be low, but this sign appears specific, particularly if thalamic lesions have been excluded (Rolak, 1988; Chabrol et al., 1995; Stone et al., 2010; Daum et al., 2014a).
2. Splitting of vibration sense has for a long time been a sign of functional sensory loss, since a tuning fork on the left or right side of the sternum or on the forehead is expected to be similar because of the bone conduction. However, although this sign is highly sensitive in patients with functional symptoms, the specificity is surprisingly too low (Rolak, 1988).
3. Nonanatomic sensory loss. Nonanatomic sensory loss has been described as a moderately sensitive and highly specific sign for functional sensory loss, although the quality of the study this is based on is particularly poor (Baker and Silver, 1987).
4. Inconsistency and nonreproducibility of sensory signs in repeated testing have been proposed as important characteristics of functional sensory symptoms (Baker and Silver, 1987; Chabrol et al., 1995), but these signs are difficult to define and therefore the diagnostic value is hard to evaluate. Some specific variants of this testing include:
   (a) Inconsistency between joint position sense and other signs may be informative. If the Romberg test and tandem walk are perfectly carried out in the absence of joint position sense, this supports the diagnosis of a functional disorder (Hayes et al., 1999).
   (b) An absent upper-limb position sense but normal finger-to-nose test with eyes closed is consistent with this diagnosis (Magee, 1962).

   Caution is especially warranted in the interpretation of inconsistencies of a subjectively reported phenomenon. Inconsistencies in sensory testing, for instance, may also be seen in patients with parietal lesions (Critchley, 1964) and complete instability to stand and walk without abnormalities of the legs in bed has also been seen in patients with thalamic lesions (Baik and Lang, 2007).
5. Below-chance performance. Sensory testing can be performed in such a way that the patient ought to score at least 50% by chance, for example by asking the patient to say whether the toe is going up or down during proprioception. Scores of 70% or 80% incorrect raise the suspicion of a functional

Table 24.1

Sensitivity and specificity of functional sensory signs. Data should be interpreted with caution due to methodologic issues, described in text

				Number		
Test	Sensitivity	Specificity	Positive predictive value	Case	Control	Studies
Midline splitting	20%	93%	40%	20	80	Rolak (1988)
	19%	98%	95%	107	46	Stone et al. (2010)
	26%	86%	40%	15	42	Chabrol et al. (1995)
	53%	100%	100%	17	14	Daum et al. (2014a)
Splitting of vibration	95%	14%	22%	20	80	Rolak (1988)
	38%	89%	89%	107	46	Stone et al. (2010)
	50%	88%	82%	18	16	Daum et al. (2014a)
Nonanatomic distribution	85%	95%	94%	20	20	Daum et al. (2014a)
	85%	100%	100%	20	23	Baker and Silver (1987)
Below-chance performance	15%	100%	100%	20	20	Daum et al. (2014a)
	10%	100%	100%	20	23	Baker and Silver (1987)

Adapted from Daum et al. (2014b), with permission from BMJ Publishing Group, adding data from Daum et al. (2014a).

sensory deficit and possibly even malingering but cannot confirm it. This is sometimes called "systematic failure" (Daum et al., 2014a). The principle of systematic failure has also been explored in a neurophysiologic setting using tactile threshold (Tegner, 1988) and a psychologic technique (Miller, 1986).

6. "Say 'yes' when you feel it and 'no' when you don't." Pierre Janet first described this sign (Janet, 1907). It is prone to error when the patient interprets "no" as "feeling it less." Patients may also figure out that the question is a trick and this could reduce trust between doctor and patient.
7. The Bowlus–Currier test. The patient is asked to place the palms of the hands together, thumbs down and wrists crossed. The fingers are interlocked and the patient is asked to rotate the hands and to bring them in front of the chest. Sensory testing starts with the fifth finger and goes on up to the thumb, the only uncrossed finger. The test is positive if the thumb of the normal side is reported to be hypoesthetic (Fig. 24.4) (Bowlus and Currier, 1963). This has been described as a test for malingering, although it is really no more so than any of the other tests described. Since functional disorders are dependent on idea, it would not be that surprising if the patient had the "idea" that a different part of the hand was numb during this test.
8. Sensory deficit sensitive to suggestion. The difficulty here is that symptoms in neurologic disease are also prone to suggestion. Chabrol et al. (1995), for example, found that 60% of patients with neurologic disease had this (vs. 60% of patients with functional disorders).

These studies highlight that, although these tests for functional sensory disturbance may have a reasonably sound basis, in practice there are many vagaries of sensory testing which tend to make them less valuable.

An examination of interrater reliability of these signs was carried out by Corinna Daum, Selma Aybek, and colleagues (Daum et al., 2014a). The study used videos of examination of 20 patients with functional disorders and 20 patients with organic disease in which a series of "functional" signs were performed and the viewers of the video were blinded to the diagnosis. In this study midline splitting and splitting of vibration sense both performed well with a good kappa and high specificity (greater than 90%) and reasonable sensitivity (40–50%), suggesting they can be used to support a diagnosis of functional disorders.

HYPERESTHESIA/PARESTHESIA AND PAIN

Patients with hyperesthesia and paresthesia typically complain about these symptoms more than those with hypoesthesia. Hyperesthesia is a common phenomenon in patients with functional neurologic symptoms. Hyperesthesia may be generalized and may occur as hemihyperesthesia. Literature on hyperventilation shows that hemisensory tingling can be induced experimentally in some people during hyperventilation (Brodtkorb et al., 1990; O'Sullivan et al., 1992). This is clinically relevant when considering physiologic triggers for hemisensory syndrome and functional limb weakness, which may

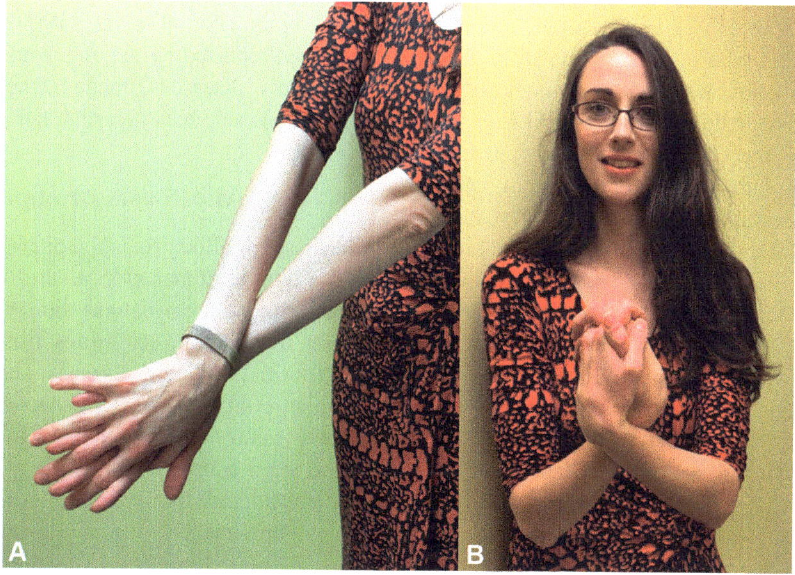

Fig. 24.4. Bowlus–Currier test for functional sensory loss in the hand.

include panic attacks, migraine, and dissociation (Stone et al., 2012b).

In the past, much attention has been given to hyperesthesia in the form of geometric segments or irregular areas. The geometric segments are often located around joints and are accompanied by contractures of muscles around the joint, whereas hypoesthesia comes with paresis of these muscles. These hyperesthesias around joints were often seen after physical trauma. In patients with functional symptoms the area of hyperesthesia is like a hood over the knee, hip, elbow, or shoulder. Slight touch of the skin is experienced as extremely painful (allodynia). This functional hyperesthesia has the tendency to expand and there are parallels again here with CRPS.

In the past problems with the knee after small traumas seem to have presented with high frequency to neurologists, especially in continental Europe, although now this is rarely the case (MV, personal observation). It was impossible to stretch the knee and movements of the knee were hardly possible. Pain was present from one finger under to one finger above the knee joint. Coxalgia or hip pain was another symptom to which much attention was given. These patients had a short period of limping, after which they became bedridden. The prognosis of the arthralgias was variable. According to Charcot, hyperesthesia was the last symptom that disappeared when more symptoms were present and if all symptoms had resolved the chance of recurrence was low. A case like this is presented in his lectures (Charcot, 1889).

If painful hyperesthesia is the only symptom, the diagnosis of small-fiber neuropathy should be considered (Themistocleous et al., 2014). In this type of neuropathy the sensory, often painful, symptoms begin in the feet and progress proximally, eventually involving the hands. Less typical onset of symptoms has been described in patients with demonstrated gain-of-function mutations of the genes *SCN 9A* or *SCN 10A*, mutations found in some patients with this type of neuropathy. Difficulties may arise when small-fiber neuropathy is diagnosed on the basis of skin biopsy. In this situation it can be unclear whether loss of nerve fibers occurs as a primary phenomenon or secondary to limb disuse in chronic pain. Paresthesia appears very commonly with many types of chronic pain syndrome, including those where there is a clear organic cause such as herpes zoster, but also those where there is no clear pathology, such as fibromyalgia. Hyperesthesia may be mixed with hyperalgesia and allodynia.

Sensory disturbance in CRPS has already been discussed. It now forms one of the accepted symptoms, and signs in the Budapest criteria (Harden et al., 2009). This means that a clinical diagnosis of CRPS can now be made on the basis of three symptoms and two signs. Two of these symptoms and two of the signs may be motor and sensory – both of which have been demonstrated repeatedly to share the same qualities as functional motor and sensory symptoms and signs (Verdugo and Ochoa, 1998, 2000; Birklein et al., 2000; Schrag et al., 2004).

UNUSUAL (BUT NONFUNCTIONAL) SENSORY SYMPTOMS

Some clinicians are tempted to make a diagnosis of functional disorder just because symptoms are weird or unusual. A good rule of thumb is that the more odd the symptoms are, the less likely they are to be functional.

Synesthesia

Synesthesia is when the experience of one sensory modality causes also an experience of another. For example, viewing letters or numbers causes the experience of colors (grapheme–color synesthesia) or listening to music causes the experience of seeing colors (Baron-Cohen et al., 1996; Blakemore et al., 2005). Synesthesia is relatively rare, but grapheme–color synesthesia occurs in 0.5–1% of the population (Ramachandran and Hubbard, 2001; Mulvenna et al., 2004) and is not a feature of a functional disorder.

Cenesthesias

Cenesthesias are abnormal bodily sensations which are perceived as totally different from sensations previously experienced and are therefore difficult for patients to communicate. This easily leads to the wrong conclusion that the symptoms are vague and therefore functional. Cenesthetic sensations may consist of very circumscript pain and of sensations of pulling, pressure, or movements in the brain (Podoll et al., 1999). These symptoms have been reported by patients with migraine, epilepsy, Parkinson's disease (Jimenez-Jimenez et al., 1997), and multiple sclerosis (Wurthmann et al., 1990).

Allesthesia or allochiria

Allesthesia or allochiria is the phenomenon that a touch on the contralesional side of the body is reported as occurring on the ipsilateral side (Obersteiner, 1881). Similar transferable sensations from left (affected) to right (normal) have been seen in audition and olfaction (Halligan et al., 1992). If allesthesia is present, a right parietal lesion should be looked for. We have already mentioned a couple of times that parietal lesions have to be considered, but a parietal lesion does not exclude the development of functional sensory symptoms superimposed on the lesion (Ramasubbu, 2002).

PATHOPHYSIOLOGY

Discussion of studies exploring the pathophysiology in functional sensory disorders using neurophysiology (Chapter 6) and functional imaging (Chapter 7) can be found elsewhere in this volume (Levy and Behrman, 1970; Moldofsky and England, 1975; Lorenz et al., 1998; Vuilleumier et al., 2001; Hoechstetter et al., 2002; Ghaffar et al., 2006; Egloff et al., 2009).

Evidence is converging towards a model in which symptoms arise from a physiologic or psychologic trigger (for example, hyperventilation, migraine, transient nerve compression) and are then perpetuated by abnormally focused attention in which a "top-down" expectation of the symptom overrides and modifies "bottom-up" sensory input (Edwards et al., 2012). Such ideas have a lot in common with those put forward by Janet, Charcot, and others at the end of the 19th and the beginning of the 20th century.

TREATMENT SPECIFIC FOR SENSORY SYMPTOMS

Treatment is discussed in detail elsewhere in this volume. Our personal experience is that reduced sensation often does not need specific treatment and it commonly co-occurs with weakness. Older textbooks frequently refer to successful treatment with faradization. In the modern era we have found a transcutaneous electric nerve stimulation machine, often turned up high, or in some cases peripheral nerve stimulation has provided a form of biofeedback, not only to see muscle contraction but also to experience new sensation in an anesthetic limb.

ACKNOWLEDGMENT

Thanks to Dr. Ingrid Hoeritzauer for demonstrating the Bowlus–Currier test in Figure 24.4.

References

Allen IM (1935). Observations on the motor phenomena of hysteria. J Neurol Psychopathol 16: 1–25.

Babinski J, Froment J (1918). Hysteria or Pithiatism, (trans. by JD Rolleston). University of London Press, London.

Baik JS, Lang AE (2007). Gait abnormalities in psychogenic movement disorders. Mov Disord 22: 395–399.

Baker JH, Silver JR (1987). Hysterical paraplegia. J Neurol Neurosurg Psychiatry 50: 375–382.

Baron-Cohen S, Burt L, Smith-Laittan F et al. (1996). Synaesthesia: prevalence and familiality. Perception 25: 1073–1079.

Birklein F, Riedl B, Sieweke N et al. (2000). Neurological findings in complex regional pain syndromes – analysis of 145 cases. Acta Neurol Scand 101: 262–269.

Blakemore SJ, Bristow D, Bird G et al. (2005). Somatosensory activations during the observation of touch and a case of vision-touch synaesthesia. Brain 128: 1571–1583.

Bowlus WE, Currier RD (1963). A test for hysterical hemianalgesia. New Engl J Med 269: 1253–1254.

Brodtkorb E, Gimse R, Antonaci F et al. (1990). Hyperventilation syndrome: clinical, ventilatory, and personality characteristics as observed in neurological practice. Acta Neurol Scand 81: 307–313.

Bultitude JH, Rafal RD (2010). Derangement of body representation in complex regional pain syndrome: report of a case treated with mirror and prisms. Exp Brain Res 204: 409–418.

Chabrol H, Peresson G, Clanet M (1995). Lack of specificity of the traditional criteria of conversion disorders. Eur Psychiatry 10: 317–319.

Charcot JM (1889). Clinical lectures on diseases of the nervous system (Volume 3), New Sydenham Society, London.

Critchley M (1964). Psychiatric symptoms and parietal disease: differential diagnosis. Proc R Soc Med 57: 422–428.

Daum C, Gheorghita F, Spatola M et al. (2014a). Interobserver agreement and validity of bedside "positive signs" for functional weakness, sensory and gait disorders in conversion disorder: a pilot study. J Neurol Neurosurg Psychiatry 86: 425–430.

Daum C, Hubschmid M, Aybek S (2014b). The value of "positive" clinical signs for weakness, sensory and gait disorders in conversion disorder: a systematic and narrative review. J Neurol Neurosurg Psychiatry 85: 180–190.

Edwards MJ, Adams RA, Brown H et al. (2012). A Bayesian account of "hysteria". Brain 135: 3495–3512.

Egloff N, Sabbioni MEE, Salathé C et al. (2009). Nondermatomal somatosensory deficits in patients with chronic pain disorder: clinical findings and hypometabolic pattern in FDG-PET. Pain 145: 252–258.

Fox CD (1913). The psychopathology of hysteria, Richard G. Badger, The Gorham Press, Boston.

Freud S (1966). Hysteria (published first in 1888). In: J Strachey, A Freud, A Strachey et al. (Eds.), The Standard Edition of the Complete Psychological Works of Sigmund Freud. Vol 1. Hogarth, London, pp. 37–59.

Ghaffar O, Staines WR, Feinstein A (2006). Unexplained neurologic symptoms: an fMRI study of sensory conversion disorder. Neurology 67: 2036–2038.

Goetz C (1999). Charcot and the myth of misogyny, Neurology 52: 1678–1686.

Gowers WR (1892). Hysteria. In: A Manual of diseases of the Nervous System, Churchill, London, pp. 903–960.

Guze SB, Woodrugg RA, Clayton PJ (1971). A study of conversion symptoms in psychiatric outpatients. Am J Psychiatry 128: 643–646.

Halligan PW, Marshall JC, Wade DT (1992). Left on the right: allochiria in a case of left visuo-spatial neglect. J Neurol Neurosurg Psychiatry 55: 717–719.

Harden RN, Bruehl S, Stanton-Hicks M et al. (2009). Proposed new diagnostic criteria for complex regional pain syndrome. Pain Med 10: 600.

Hayes MW, Graham S, Heldorf P et al. (1999). A video review of the diagnosis of psychogenic gait: appendix and commentary. Mov Disord 14: 914–921.

Hoechstetter K, Meinck H, Henningsen P et al. (2002). Psychogenic sensory loss: magnetic source imaging reveals normal tactile evoked activity of the human primary and secondary somatosensory cortex. Neurosci Lett 323: 137–140.

Hurst A (1920). The psychology of the special senses and their functional disorders, Henry Frowde, Hodder & Stoughton, Oxford University Press, London.

Janet P (1907). The major symptoms of hysteria, Macmillan, London.

Jelgersma J (1926). Leerboek der psychiatrie II, Scheltema & Holkema, Amsterdam.

Jimenez-Jimenez FJ, Orti-Pareja M, Gasalla T et al. (1997). Cenesthetic hallucinations in a patient with Parkinson's disease. J Neurol Neurosurg Psychiatry 63: 120.

Kapfhammer HP, Buchheim P, Bove D et al. (1992). Konverssionssymptome bei Patienten im psychiatrischen Konsiliardienst. Nervenarzt 63: 527–538.

Lauerma H (1993). Nocturnal limb movements in conversion paralysis. J Nerv Ment Dis 181: 707–708.

Lasègue C (1864). De l'anésthesie et de l'ataxie hystériques. Arch Gen Med 1: 385–402.

Levy R, Behrman J (1970). Cortical evoked responses in hysterical hemianaesthesia. Electroencephalogr Clin Neurophysiol 29: 400–402.

Lewis JS, Kersten P, McCabe CS et al. (2007). Body perception disturbance: a contribution to pain in complex regional pain syndrome (CRPS). Pain 133: 111–119.

Lindley RI, Warlow CP, Wardlaw JM et al. (1993). Interobserver reliability of a clinical classification of acute cerebral infarction. Stroke 24: 1801–1804.

Lorenz J, Kunze K, Bromm B (1998). Differentiation of conversive sensory loss and malingering by P300 in a modified oddball task. Neuroreport 9: 187–191.

Magee KR (1962). Hysterical hemiplegia and hemianaesthesia. Postgrad Med 31: 339–345.

Mailis-Gagnon A, Nicholson K (2010). Nondermatomal somatosensory deficits: overview of unexplainable negative sensory phenomena in chronic pain patients. Curr Opin Anaesthesiol 23: 593–597.

Miller E (1986). Detecting hysterical sensory symptoms: an elaboration of the forced choice technique. Br J Clin Psychol 25 (Pt 3): 231–232.

Moldofsky H, England RS (1975). Facilitation of somatosensory average-evoked potentials in hysterical anesthesia and pain. Arch Gen Psychiatry 32: 193–197.

Mulvenna C, Hubbard EM, Ramachandran VS et al. (2004). The relation between synaesthesia and creativity. J Cogn Neurosci (Suppl.16): 188.

Obersteiner H (1881). On allochiria: a peculiar sensory disorder. Brain 4: 153–163.

O'Sullivan G, Harvey I, Bass C et al. (1992). Psychophysiological investigations of patients with unilateral symptoms in the hyperventilation syndrome. Br J Psychiatry 160: 664–667.

Podoll K, Bollig G, Vogtmann T et al. (1999). Cenesthetic pain sensations illustrated by an artist suffering from migraine with typical aura. Cephalalgia 19: 598–601.

Punt TD, Cooper L, Hey M et al. (2013). Neglect-like symptoms in complex regional pain syndrome: Learned nonuse by another name? Pain 154: 200–203.

Purves-Stewart J (1913). Diagnosis of nervous diseases. Edward Arnold, London.

Ramachandran S, Hubbard EM (2001). Synaesthesia – a window into perception, thought and language. J Consciousness Stud: 3–34.

Ramasubbu R (2002). Conversion sensory symptoms associated with parietal lobe infarct: case report, diagnostic issues and brain mechanisms. J Psychiatry Neurosci 27: 118–122.

Regnard P (1887). Les maladies épidémiques de l'esprit; sorcellerie, magnétisme, morphinisme, délire des grandeurs, Plon-Nourrit, Paris.

Rolak LA (1988). Psychogenic sensory loss. J Nerv Ment Dis 176: 686–687.

Rommel O, Gehling M, Dertwinkel R et al. (1999). Hemisensory impairment in patients with complex regional pain syndrome. Pain 80: 95–101.

Schrag A, Trimble M, Quinn N et al. (2004). The syndrome of fixed dystonia: an evaluation of 103 patients. Brain 127: 2360–2372.

Sollier P (1897). Genèse et nature de l'hysterie. Recherche clinique et experimentales de psychophysiologie. Alcan, Paris.

Stone J, Sharpe M, Carson A et al. (2002). Are functional motor and sensory symptoms really more frequent on the left? A systematic review. J Neurol Neurosurg Psychiatry 73: 578–581.

Stone J, Sharpe M, Rothwell PM et al. (2003). The 12 year prognosis of unilateral functional weakness and sensory disturbance. J Neurol Neurosurg Psychiatry 74: 591–596.

Stone J, Smyth R, Carson A (2006). La belle indifférence in conversion symptoms and hysteria: systematic review. Br J Psychiatry 188: 204–209.

Stone J, Hewett R, Carson A et al. (2008). The "disappearance" of hysteria: historical mystery or illusion? J R Soc Med 101: 12–18.

Stone J, Warlow C, Sharpe M (2010). The symptom of functional weakness: a controlled study of 107 patients. Brain 133: 1537–1551.

Stone J, Gelauff J, Carson A (2012a). A "twist in the tale": altered perception of ankle position in psychogenic dystonia. Mov Disord 27: 585–586.

Stone J, Warlow C, Sharpe M (2012b). Functional weakness: clues to mechanism from the nature of onset. J Neurol Neurosurg Psychiatry 83 (1): 67–69.

Summers M (1926). The History of Witchcraft and Demonology. Routledge, Oxford.

Tegner R (1988). A technique to detect psychogenic sensory loss. J Neurol Neurosurg Psychiatry 51: 1455–1456.

Themistocleous AC, Ramirez JD, Serra J et al. (2014). The clinical approach to small fibre neuropathy and painful channelopathy. Pract Neurol 14: 368–379.

Toth C (2003). Hemisensory syndrome is associated with a low diagnostic yield and a nearly uniform benign prognosis. J Neurol Neurosurg Psychiatry 74: 1113–1116.

Veldman PH, Reynen HM, Arntz IE et al. (1993). Signs and symptoms of reflex sympathetic dystrophy: prospective study of 829 patients. Lancet 342: 1012–1016.

Verdugo RJ, Ochoa JL (1998). Reversal of hypoaesthesia by nerve block, or placebo: a psychologically mediated sign in chronic pseudoneuropathic pain patients. J Neurol Neurosurg Psychiatry 65: 196–203.

Verdugo RJ, Ochoa JL (2000). Abnormal movements in complex regional pain syndrome: assessment of their nature. Muscle Nerve 23: 198–205.

Vuilleumier P, Chicherio C, Assal F et al. (2001). Functional neuroanatomical correlates of hysterical sensorimotor loss. Brain 124: 1077–1090.

Whytt R (1767). Observations on the Nature, Causes, and Cure of those Disorders which have been commonly called Nervous, Hypochondriac, or Hysteric: to which are prefixed some Remarks on the Sympathy of Nerves, J. Balfour, Edinburgh.

Wilson-Barnett J, Trimble MR (1985). An investigation of hysteria using the Illness Behaviour Questionnaire. Br J Psychiatry 146: 601–608.

Worley G (2002). Diagnosis of psychogenic paralysis by observation of patient movement in sleep [comment]. J Neurol 249: 1322.

Wurthmann C, Daffertshofer M, Hennerici M (1990). Qualitativ abnorme Leibgefühle bei multipler Sklerose. Nervenarzt 61: 361–363.

Handbook of Clinical Neurology, Vol. 139 (3rd series)
Functional Neurologic Disorders
M. Hallett, J. Stone, and A. Carson, Editors
http://dx.doi.org/10.1016/B978-0-12-801772-2.00025-4

Chapter 25

Nonepileptic seizures – subjective phenomena

M. REUBER* AND G.H. RAWLINGS
Academic Neurology Unit, University of Sheffield, Sheffield, UK

Abstract

Psychogenic nonepileptic seizures (PNES) superficially resemble epileptic seizures or syncope and most patients with PNES are initially misdiagnosed as having one of the latter two types of transient loss of consciousness. However, evidence suggests that the subjective seizure experience of PNES and its main differential diagnoses are as different as the causes of these three disorders. In spite of this, and regardless of the fact that PNES are considered a mental disorder in the current nosologies, research has only given limited attention to the subjective symptomatology of PNES. Instead, most phenomenologic research has focused on the visible manifestations of PNES and on physiologic parameters, neglecting patients' symptoms and experiences.

This chapter gives an overview of qualitative and quantitative studies providing insights into subjective symptoms associated with PNES, drawing on a wide range of methodologies (questionnaires, self-reports, physiologic measures, linguistic analyses, and neuropsychologic experiments). After discussing the scope and limitations of these approaches in the context of this dissociative phenomenon, we discuss ictal, peri-ictal and interictal symptoms described by patients with PNES. We particularly focus on impairment of consciousness. PNES emerges as a clinically heterogeneous condition. We conclude with a discussion of the clinical significance of particular subjective symptoms for the engagement of patients in treatment, the formulation of treatment, and prognosis.

INTRODUCTION

Psychogenic nonepileptic seizures (PNES) superficially resemble epileptic seizures or syncope but are not associated with ictal electroencephalographic (EEG) discharges. They are episodes of impaired self-control associated with a range of motor, sensory, and mental manifestations. Studies using a wide range of different methodologies indicate that PNES are an experiential and behavioral response to internal or external stimuli (Reuber, 2009; Roberts and Reuber, 2014). The key symptoms of PNES, such as alterations in consciousness and the partial or complete loss of normal integration between memory, awareness of identity, and control of bodily movements, have increasingly been conceptualized as paroxysmal dissociative responses (Bowman, 2006).

Although different labels (including major hysteria and hysteroepilepsy) have been used to describe it, the clinical entity of what is today categorized as PNES has been recognized for a long time. However, especially since the introduction of synchronous video-EEG monitoring into routine care in the 1970s and 1980s, phenomenologic research about PNES has focused almost entirely on demonstrating the absence of the physiologic changes associated with epileptic seizures and on externally observable differences between PNES and epilepsy (Reuber, 2008). In contrast, the subjective symptomatology of PNES has largely been neglected, despite the current medical nosologies (*International Classification of Diseases*, 10th edition: ICD-10; *Diagnostic and Statistical Manual of Mental Disorders*, 5th edition: DSM-5) categorizing PNES as a mental disorder (World Health Organization, 1992; American Psychiatric Association, 2013). Given that PNES may be a dissociative phenomenon, the reasons for this neglect may not be limited to

*Correspondence to: Markus Reuber, MD, PhD, FRCP, Department of Neurology, Royal Hallamshire Hospital, Glossop Road, Sheffield, South Yorkshire S10 2JF, UK. Tel: +44-114-226-8763, E-mail: m.reuber@sheffield.ac.uk

the fact that visible PNES manifestations are easier to capture, objectify, analyze, and report than subjective experiences; they may also include that PNES usually involve subjective states or experiences that are particularly difficult for patients to share.

Nevertheless, research on the subjective experience of PNES is of great practical importance. Firstly, subjective symptoms may help with the differentiation of PNES and other paroxysmal disorders, especially epilepsy and syncope. Subjective PNES symptoms may also have implications for treatment. For example, the recognition of emotional triggers for PNES may help with patient engagement and an insight into the patient's subjective PNES experience is key to psychotherapeutic treatment, for instance, interventions which aim to enhance patients' tolerance of distress (LaFrance et al., 2013). Lastly, although this remains an area of ongoing study, patients' experiences of ictal and interictal states may co-determine their prognosis.

This chapter will review studies that have shed light on the subjective symptomatology of PNES using a range of different quantitative and qualitative approaches. The first section will focus on the methodologies that have been used to investigate subjective symptoms of PNES and outline their scope and limitations. The second section will address the temporal characteristics of subjective symptoms associated with PNES, i.e., differences between the ictal and the interictal state, including transition periods, warnings, triggers, and postictal symptoms. The third section will focus on alteration of consciousness, which is the key feature distinguishing PNES from other mental health problems more generally or other somatic symptom disorders more specifically. The fourth section will look at the clinical significance of subjective experiences, including diagnostic, therapeutic, and prognostic implications. The chapter will conclude with a discussion drawing on all previous sections and exploring what our current understanding of the subjective phenomenology of PNES tells us about the nature of this disorder.

METHODOLOGIC CONSIDERATIONS

In this section we discuss the methods used to study subjective PNES experiences, describing their merits and limitations. These are preliminary observations intended to provide readers with the ability better to judge the findings themselves, which will be discussed below.

Most studies examining PNES symptoms have used self-report questionnaires comparing the mean responses of different groups of participants, mainly patients with PNES and epilepsy, less commonly, healthy controls or other patient groups. This methodology has provided useful insights into the disorder and has been especially valuable in aiding the differentiation of PNES and epilepsy (and, to a much lesser extent, syncope). However, the narrow focus of this approach is prone to oversimplifying the complexity and heterogeneity of PNES disorders. Questionnaires only deliver the respondents' replies to their understanding of the exact questions asked; they give respondents little opportunity to qualify their responses or to communicate the finer subtleties of their experience.

The relative lack of studies involving other patient control groups than people with epilepsy also means that we know very little about differences in the subjective phenomenology of PNES and syncope or other mental disorders mainly characterized (at least in part) by subjective paroxysmal symptoms, such as panic disorder or posttraumatic stress disorder. Apart from the more general self-report limitation of social desirability biases (van de Mortel, 2008), there are also more specific problems with relying on the self-report of symptoms of a dissociative state. The neurobiologic mechanisms underpinning PNES may well interfere with patients' awareness of ictal symptom experiences, the storage and consolidation of ictal symptoms, memories, and postictal symptom recall (Bakvis et al., 2010; Roberts and Reuber, 2014). Last, but not least, patients may (at least prior to psychologic treatment) also be unwilling or emotionally unable to report unpleasant or unacceptable memories of PNES experiences, which must have been encoded successfully in long-term memory, and there is some evidence in support of this assertion, because patients are able to report them as psychologic treatment progresses (von Fabeck, 2010).

One well-established approach to getting around emotional blocks to the recall of unpleasant experiences has involved the use of hypnosis (Kihlstrom, 1985). Hypnosis was first used in somatoform disorders based on early theories suggesting that highly hypnotizable individuals are particularly prone to displaying "hysterical" symptoms (Schachter, 2011). Hypnosis has since been used in patients with PNES to aid the diagnostic differentiation from epilepsy and to contribute to treatment (Kuyk et al., 1999; Barry and Reuber, 2010). For instance, the phenomenon that patients who have had a PNES have a clearer recollection of ictal events under hypnosis than without hypnosis (and more complete recall than patients with epilepsy) has been used as a differential diagnostic method since World War I (Brown et al., 1999). Whilst this observation demonstrates that there is likely to be a significant difference between patients' actual PNES experience and their recall (or report) of ictal experiences, to date, hypnotic recall of subjective PNES symptoms has not been studied systematically. This means that we are currently unable to glean as much information about patients' PNES experiences from studies using hypnosis as this method might yield.

Insights about subjective PNES symptoms are also available from a number of studies that have employed conversation analysis and other qualitative linguistic methods to address clinical questions about the disorder. The fact that patients used their own words to describe their experiences in these studies makes the findings harder to categorize, but means that, at least potentially, these studies can provide a more highly differentiated understanding of patients' individual subjective seizure manifestations compared to questionnaires. Most of these studies aimed to identify aspects of patients' interactional behavior in clinical encounters with neurologists, which might help with the differential diagnosis of epilepsy and PNES. However, these studies, in which researchers focused specifically on how patients described their problems to the doctor, have also yielded interesting insights into the etiology and experience of PNES (Reuber et al., 2014). Especially the analysis of patients' use of metaphors and diagnostic labels has enhanced our understanding of the subjective seizure experiences of PNES and how these differ from those of patients with epilepsy (Plug et al., 2009, 2010, 2011). Metaphors hold particular importance in phenomenology research: Lakoff (1993) argues that metaphors hold particular importance in phenomenology research as they are surface representations of mental domains that allow us to understand abstract unstructured matter in a more concrete manner by applying older, preexisting concepts to new experiences. What is more, the examination of metaphors for seizure experiences used by patients in interactions with doctors are one example of how objective observations (such as interactional behavior or word choices) can provide clues about patients' subjective experience.

Clues about subjective PNES experiences can also be gathered from neuropsychologic experiments. Whilst there are obvious practical limitations to experimentation in the ictal state itself (which mean that no such studies have been undertaken to date), several studies have revealed important differences between patients with PNES or epilepsy in the interictal state, as well as between those with PNES, healthy controls, or volunteers with posttraumatic stress symptoms. On a group level, PNES patients have differed from these controls in terms of stimulus perception as well as cognitive, autonomic, and emotional stimulus processing. The differences that distinguish patients with PNES in the interictal state from the other groups listed may be less obvious or disabling than those that would be expected in the ictal state; however, their nature provides a plausible indication of the (much greater) differences, which might be observed in PNES patients during the ictal state. For instance, such studies found evidence for increased vigilance towards social stressors (Bakvis et al., 2009), an increased tendency to use avoidant responses to stressful stimuli (Bakvis et al., 2011), and a combination of an increased sensitivity to certain emotions with a reduced expressive response to the perceived emotion (Roberts et al., 2012). The findings from this type of research have been particularly enlightening when physiologic arousal levels were manipulated. However, given that none of these studies have captured PNES *per se,* the relationship between interictal findings and PNES remains inferential.

There is another important limitation of all studies investigating the subjective symptomatology of PNES. Temporal differences in terms of subjective symptoms are not limited to contrasts between ictal and interictal states but extend to differences of subjective PNES experiences between the earliest phases of the development of a PNES disorder and later stages, when PNES have become established and the seizure disorder has become more chronic. Unfortunately, very few studies have investigated or accounted for this factor, although there is a strong suspicion that the experience of PNES is dynamic and subject to change over the trajectory of the disorder's timeline. For instance, patients with PNES may originally experience typical panic attacks, but over time, symptoms of anxiety may diminish and manifestations of dissociation increase (Goldstein and Mellers, 2006). A study based on conversation analysis of a series of interviews with 4 patients with PNES undergoing inpatient or outpatient psychotherapy demonstrated that, as patients progressed through therapy, they used less projection, and fewer theoretic terms and preformed expressions such as "I feel really ill" to describe their PNES experiences. Instead, in their descriptions of PNES, they made increasing use of episodic reconstruction and more references to environmental stimuli or PNES-related subjective symptoms (von Fabeck, 2010).

These changes in patients' access to their PNES experiences mean that it would be best to describe subjective symptoms at different stages of the disorder rather than collating all patients together in one group. The fact that there is currently not enough evidence to pursue a more differentiated view does not mean that such an approach would not be more appropriate.

TEMPORAL CHARACTERISTICS OF SUBJECTIVE SYMPTOMS ASSOCIATED WITH PNES

Even in epilepsy, when seizure states are defined by ictal EEG changes that markedly differ from "background" EEG activity, there is debate about the exact timing of seizure onset and offset. Although patients with PNES tend to speak of their disorder as characterized by "seizures" (i.e., paroxysmal experiences) (Plug et al., 2009), the moment of transition from the interictal to the ictal state is often harder to define and associated with less dramatic physiologic arousal than the transition into an epileptic seizure (Ponnusamy et al., 2012). Nevertheless, we will use a temporal framework in this section, addressing subjective symptoms associated with PNES to discuss triggers, warnings, the ictal phase itself, post-ictal and interictal PNES manifestations.

PNES triggers

No research has specifically focused on subjective experiences of seizure triggers in patients with PNES. A study in which 100 patients with PNES (diagnosed by video-EEG) self-reported their experience of PNES manifestations demonstrated considerable heterogeneity of experiences of seizure triggers (measured by using a questionnaire listing 86 possible symptoms, including several questions relating to triggers or warnings). Only a small minority of patients (10%) stated that they were "always" aware of triggers, 57% were aware of triggers for some but not all of their PNES, and 31% claimed never to be aware of triggers. In the same study, 43% of patients stated that their PNES "always" "come on out of the blue without warning," 51% responded that at least some of their PNES came on in this way and 6% said this never happened. Whilst this study therefore suggested that PNES triggers may (at least at times) be experienced by just over one-half of patients, PNES witnesses questioned in the same study reported being aware of seizure triggers more often than patients themselves (Reuber et al., 2011) (this finding resonates with an observation made in a study in which the Illness Perception Scale-revisited was administered to patients with PNES and their caregivers and which demonstrated that caregivers of patients were more likely to perceive an association between psychologic factors (in particular, stress) and PNES than patients themselves) (Whitehead et al., 2015).

In an unpublished study in which a psychotherapist working in the Department of Neurology at the Royal Hallamshire Hospital, Sheffield, UK, prospectively questioned 58 consecutive patients with PNES attending a first appointment for psychotherapy about their symptoms (74% female, 19% reporting more than one type of PNES), 79% reported experiencing at least occasional PNES triggers. Recognized triggers included internal or external factors. The most commonly perceived triggers were emotional states (50%: feeling stressed, upset, anxious, aroused, neglected, nonspecific unwell). Bodily states (21%: illness, loss of sleep, feeling hot or cold, tiredness, pain, feeling dehydrated or exhausted after something energetic) and external stimuli (9%: crowded places, flashing lights, black and white patterns, blue light, flashing lights, smoke/flames/dogs/household objects acting as traumatic reminders, sun on surface, neon lights) were less commonly described potential triggers (S. Howlett, personal communication).

The facts that triggers cannot be recalled by all patients after all PNES and that about one-half of patients with PNES report having seizures from sleep do not mean that PNES are not always triggered by a particular internal or external stimulus (Duncan et al., 2004). Closer study of nocturnal PNES demonstrates that PNES happen when patients have actually been awake, and it is quite feasible that a completely "successful" dissociative response to an aversive trigger protects patients against the realization that they have difficulties with tolerating certain stimuli. In fact, one study demonstrated that, unlike in patients with epilepsy or healthy controls, patients with PNES showed discrepancies between a high number of explicitly self-reported anxiety symptom and normal implicit anxiety scores (measured by an Implicit Relational Assessment Procedure). This study suggests that, despite experiencing relatively high levels of anxiety symptoms, patients with PNES do not consider themselves as anxious individuals (Dimaro et al., 2014).

It is well recognized that PNES can be triggered during brief outpatient video-EEG recordings in a diagnostic setting with a number of provocation techniques, typically used in conjunction with verbal suggestion. Provocation with saline patches, vibration, and hypnosis has been described, but the most commonly used technique involves the suggestive intravenous injection of normal saline solution (Cohen and Suter, 1982). This procedure will provoke typical PNES in about three-quarters of patients (Reuber and Elger, 2003). However, over the last decade there have been increasing ethical concerns about the deceptive use of placebo to diagnose PNES (Bernat, 2010), and therefore, the combination of hyperventilation and photic stimulation with verbal suggestion has been proposed as a PNES provocation method instead. With this alternative method PNES can be triggered in about two-thirds of patients during a brief outpatient video-EEG recording (McGonigal et al., 2002).

Considering that a wide range of different stimuli seems to trigger PNES in the majority of patients, it is unlikely that the triggers used in these provocation procedures operate in a similar way to the highly specific stimuli that may trigger epileptic seizures (for instance, in musicogenic or photosensitive epilepsy). Instead, it is more likely that the provocation procedures for PNES cause physical or cognitive symptoms (for instance, physiologic arousal or anxiety) or anticipatory anxiety about a possible seizure, and that it is this state, combined with excessive distress avoidance tendencies, which triggers PNES in this setting.

Evidence for increased avoidance tendencies in patients with PNES comes from self-report and experimental studies. For instance, a study using the Multiple Experiential Avoidance Questionnaire demonstrated increased levels of avoidance compared to healthy controls and patients with epilepsy in terms of behavioral avoidance, distress aversion, procrastination, distraction, and repression (Dimaro et al., 2014). An experimental study by Bakvis et al. (2011) used an affect evaluation task to assess avoidance. In their study, patients had to respond to happy or angry faces by making arm movements in response to the facial expression which were either consistent or inconsistent with usually preferred motor responses (extending the arm in response to a negative stimulus like an angry face, flexing the arm in response to a positive stimulus like a happy face). The findings in a group of 12 patients with PNES and 20 healthy controls signaled an instinctive avoidant action tendency towards social threatening cues (slower flexion/"approach" movements to angry faces).

PNES warnings

Research on prodromal or warning symptoms of PNES is also very limited. The frequency with which prodromal or warning symptoms of PNES have been self-reported in patient cohorts varies widely, between 24% and 92% (Cohen and Suter, 1982; Gulick et al., 1982; Luther et al., 1982; Lancman et al., 1993; Vein et al., 1994; Goldstein et al., 2006). This wide range is likely to reflect differences in methodology and patient selection. Also, authors (and study participants) may not have separated clearly between "warning" and "ictal" symptoms. In the unpublished psychotherapy patient cohort mentioned above, 69% of patients reported symptoms that they (and the therapist) considered as seizure warnings (patients were able to report several warning symptoms, so the percentages add up to more than 100%). "Panic" (52% of patients) and "non-bodily panic" symptoms (38%) were reported most commonly, followed by "sensory non-panic" (24%) and "dissociative" symptoms (16%). The symptoms interpreted as indicating "panic" included dizziness, feeling hot, sweaty, shaky, panicky, light-headed, numb, tingly, cold, sick, nauseated, warm, clammy, as if going to pass out, short of breath, or frightened. The symptoms categorized as "bodily non-panic" included: muscle tightening or spasms, heavy-headedness, "thick" or "groggy" head, headache, head pain, feeling drained, weird, awkward, tired, lethargic, unable to stand up, as if falling asleep, drowsy, really ill, or as if energy was draining away. This category also included warnings such as limb weakness, beginning to stutter, developing slurred speech, or feeling the floor coming up. "Sensory non-panic" symptoms included white spots in peripheral vision, fuzzy eyesight, visual images moving sideways, spots and floaters, metallic or strange taste, taste of blood, horrible, strange, or burning smell or a high-pitched whine in ears. "Dissociative" symptoms included *déjà vu*, everything feeling distant, feeling as if stepping back, rushing past, as if things were slowing down, things going dark, and as if things were going distant (S. Howlett, personal communication).

The presence of particular subjective warning symptoms may depend on the subtype of PNES. A study based on a cluster analysis of patient-reported symptoms and seizure manifestations visible on video which had been rated by two independent experts suggested that PNES warnings were reported more often before "hyperkinetic prolonged attacks" (in 66.7% of cases) than in association with any of the other four semiologic subtypes ("dystonic attacks," "pauci-kinetic attacks," "pseudosyncope," and "axial dystonic prolonged attacks"). Sensory symptoms (34.5%) were only observed in "pauci-kinetic attacks" (Hubsch et al., 2011).

Clinical experience suggests that warning symptoms can last from seconds to many hours. Whilst most of these warning symptoms are unpleasant, patients may be more aware of the physical symptoms themselves than the fact that these symptoms are associated with emotional distress (or, indeed, that they may be symptoms of distress). In a study comparing ictal anxiety symptoms in patients with PNES and patients with epilepsy, both groups reported identical levels of cognitive or mental symptoms of anxiety; however, patients with PNES reported a significantly higher number of somatic anxiety symptoms (Goldstein and Mellers, 2006).

The fact that PNES warning states are subjectively distressing, even when patients may be unable to recognize or recall this fact, is supported by the observation that some patients admit to making a conscious effort in at least some of their PNES to black out and escape the sensation (Stone and Carson, 2013). This phenomenon of "willful submission" is perhaps not that surprising if PNES are a defense mechanism providing relief from a distressing emotional experience (the trigger), but also the aversive experience of anticipating the attack itself (and the fact that dissociation may be achieved in a way which appears subjectively "willful" to patients with PNES does, of course, not mean that the dissociation really was achieved by willed action or that the same dissociative mechanisms cannot also operate "automatically," i.e., without patients willing themselves to black out).

An effort not to contemplate the aversive experiences associated with PNES may also explain the observation made in sociolinguistic studies comparing diagnostic discussions between doctors and patients about epilepsy or PNES. Whereas patients with epilepsy tend to be very happy to give detailed first-person accounts of their seizure experiences, those with PNES have a tendency to avoid discussing their symptoms, and to show conversational phenomena termed "detailing blocking" and "focusing resistance" as manifestations of avoidance instead (Schwabe et al., 2007, 2008; Reuber et al., 2009).

Ictal symptoms

Behavioral manifestations tend to develop more gradually in PNES than in epileptic seizures (Meierkord et al., 1991; Syed et al., 2011). Whilst the speed of development of subjective symptoms in PNES has not been specifically examined, electrocardiographic studies also suggest that autonomic changes in epileptic seizures are typically more sudden than those seen in PNES (Opherk and Hirsch, 2002). Thus, it may be reasonable to assume that subjective symptoms also develop more slowly in PNES. Nevertheless, once the ictal PNES state has developed, it is associated with a significantly higher level of autonomic arousal than the resting state (even though arousal is less marked than that seen with epileptic seizures) (Ponnusamy et al., 2012).

The ictal state tends to last longer in PNES than in epilepsy (Luther et al., 1982; Ettinger et al., 1999b; Selwa et al., 2000). For example, one study based on the analysis of patients with epilepsy ($n=25$) and patients with PNES ($n=25$, actual number of recorded seizures was not disclosed) in a video-EEG unit showed that generalized tonic-clonic seizures lasted 50–92 seconds, whereas PNES lasted 20–805 seconds. Many PNES went on for more than 2 minutes (Gates et al., 1985). PNES continuing for over 30 minutes (also called pseudostatus or PNES status) occur in about one-third of patients, and more than one-quarter of patients diagnosed with PNES at epilepsy centers have received intensive care treatment for presumed status epilepticus at least once (Reuber et al., 2003c).

Evidence suggests that the ictal symptomatology of PNES is as heterogeneous as the preictal symptoms. Unfortunately, most studies do not separate clearly between preictal and ictal symptoms, so it is difficult to say how commonly patients are able to report subjective ictal symptoms. Only 19% of the 58 psychotherapy patients mentioned above could report any subjective ictal (as opposed to PNES warning) symptoms. Those who could report symptoms most commonly reported symptoms indicative of anxiety. Flashbacks, hallucinations, and dissociative symptoms were reported less frequently (S. Howlett, personal communication). In other studies, symptoms of anxiety were also most prominent: in the group of 100 patients with PNES studied by Reuber et al. (2011), patients most commonly reported disorientation (86%), fear (80%), and a feeling of disconnection (being conscious during the attack but unable to react to things: 77%) in at least some of their attacks. The next most common symptoms occurring in at least some attacks were rising bodily sensations (62%), nausea (59%), and a bad taste in the mouth (46%). Cognitive phenomena such as flashbacks (33%) and *déjà vu* (27%) were reported by fewer patients.

The questionnaire about ictal symptoms used in this study also included eight questions based on the Dissociative Experience Scale (DES) Taxon thought to reflect "pathological dissociation" experiences (Bernstein and Putnam, 1986; Waller et al., 1996). These eight symptoms were rarely endorsed: the proportion of people who reported that they were "always" or "frequently" present in their PNES ranged from 1% ("After an attack, I find things among my belongings which I don't remember buying") to 26% ("During an attack, I do not recognise my friends or family"), with the mean item response being 11%. In contrast, the number of people who reported that these symptoms were "never" or "rarely" present ranged from 43% ("During an attack, I do not recognise my friends or family") to 77% ("During an attack, I feel as if other people, objects, and the world are not real"), with the mean item response being 66.6%. This does not mean that the dissociative interpretation of PNES is incorrect. However, it shows that (for the majority of patients) the recalled ictal experience of PNES is materially different from the forms of dissociation captured by the DES Taxon.

Whilst this study showed that ictal PNES symptoms are very heterogeneous, it also demonstrated that symptom combinations are not randomly distributed. Reuber et al. (2011) used a correlation matrix to explore possible relationships between the DES Taxon, symptoms of anxiety, and other PNES symptoms. Significant positive correlations were seen between duration of seizures and seizures from reported sleep ($r=0.28$, $p=0.006$), seizure-related motor activity and seizures from reported sleep ($r=0.48$, $p<0.001$), flashbacks and anxiety ($r=0.44$, $p<0.001$), or dissociation ($r=0.66$, $p<0.001$), and between ictal symptoms of anxiety and dissociation ($r=0.53$, $p<0.001$).

A number of other studies have reported high levels of ictal anxiety symptoms in PNES as well: Vein et al. (1994) found that more than 90% of 15 patients with PNES reported experiencing dyspnea, palpitations, and dizziness during their attacks. Several other panic symptoms were reported by more than 70% of their patients. Another study (which did not distinguish between immediately pre-ictal, ictal, or immediately postictal symptoms) in which the authors compared the prevalence of 13 DSM-IV-TR (American Psychiatric Association, 2000) symptoms of panic disorder in 224 patients with PNES and 130 with epilepsy, showed that patients with PNES described more panic symptoms than those with epilepsy, allowing the authors to classify up to 80% of patients with PNES correctly on the basis of these symptoms alone. In this study symptoms possibly related to hyperventilation were much more common in patients with PNES and separated particularly clearly between the two patient groups (shortness of breath: 55.8% in PNES vs. 13.8% in epilepsy; paresthesia: 58.0% in PNES vs. 23.1% in epilepsy) (Hendrickson et al., 2014).

Galimberti et al. (2003) found evidence of ictal autonomic arousal in more than half of their patients with PNES (although far fewer reported ictal fear or other affective symptoms) and ictal anxiety symptoms may be even more frequent (100%) in adolescents with PNES (Witgert et al., 2005).

Information about the ictal PNES experience can also be taken from linguistic findings. A study using metaphor analysis showed that patients with PNES were more likely to conceptualize their seizures as a "state/place" that they "enter" or "cannot come out of" and where the attack is a "passive location" or "state." Patients with epilepsy, on the other hand, depicted the seizure as an external "active/force" or "event/situation" and an independently acting entity that acts on their body (Plug et al., 2009). This is in keeping with a study by Watson et al. (2002), who asked patients with PNES and patients with epilepsy, who had experienced an earthquake in Seattle (6.8 on Richter scale), how this related to their seizure experiences. Only patients with epilepsy thought that there were similarities between their experience of the earthquake (i.e., an external independent entity impacting on them) and their seizures.

Another linguistic study looked at the labels (i.e., nouns) patients chose to use for their paroxysmal events. This study also yielded results supporting the analysis of metaphoric conceptualizations. In a diagnostic conversation with a neurologist, unlike those with epilepsy, patients with PNES showed interactional resistance to the use of the term "seizure," although this was still the label they most commonly used (Plug et al., 2009). Resistance could, for instance, manifest as a patient choosing a different term than "seizure" in their answer when the doctor had used "seizure" in the question, as hesitation before the use of the word "seizure," or through the addition of statements like "or whatever you want to call them." Whilst not apparent from this study, the fact that the word "seizure" conveys the impression of a person being seized by an independently acting force may have been one explanation for this observation.

Postictal symptoms

Patients with PNES typically find it much easier to report postictal than ictal symptoms. In the study conducted by Reuber et al. (2011), involving 100 patients with PNES, 93% of patients said their muscles ached after the attack, 38% of patients said that they may wake from their attacks with a cut tongue, and 20% reported that they may have burned themselves after seizures. Similarly, in the series of psychotherapy patients reported above ($n=58$), 74% said that they had at least one postictal symptom (fatigue 45%, memory problems 22%, emotional symptoms 22%, headache/pain 18%, altered sensation 17%, confusion 9%, altered speech 3%). It may be that the preferential recall of postictal symptoms is a manifestation of the tendency of patients with PNES to highlight the consequences of their seizures rather than the seizure experiences themselves (Schwabe et al., 2007, 2008).

However, not all studies have found symptoms in the postictal phase after PNES to be reported as frequently: Ettinger et al. (1999b) looked at spontaneous responses to the question "What symptoms do you have after a seizure?" This question was intentionally left vague to avoid endorsing specific symptoms. All patients with epilepsy ($n=16$) reported having at least one postictal symptom, whereas 52% of 23 patients with PNES approached in this study had none ($p=0.001$). Patients with PNES also reported a significantly lower prevalence of headaches ($p=0.008$) and fatigue symptoms ($p=0.004$). Although there were no differences between the groups in terms of any other symptoms or confusion, the authors of this study came to the conclusion that the aftermath of epileptic seizures tends to be more disabling or distressing than that of PNES.

In keeping with this finding, most studies investigating autonomic functioning in the postictal state suggest that disturbances are more marked in patients with epilepsy than those with PNES. Azar et al. (2008), for instance, compared postictal respiration after epileptic seizures and PNES and reported that deep, loud breathing, including snoring lasting approximately 5 minutes after the seizure, is common in epilepsy, whereas, quiet, shallow, and short irregular breathing patterns lasting 1 minute postseizure were associated with PNES. These findings were replicated by another study showing that patients with PNES have higher median respiratory rates postictally compared to patients with epilepsy ($p=0.047$) and that abnormal respiration resolves more quickly after PNES than epileptic seizures (3.28 minutes compared to 6.34 minutes, $p<0.0001$) (Rosemergy et al., 2013).

Interictal symptoms

Many studies have explored symptoms in patients with PNES in the interictal state, although it is unlikely that the self-report methodology employed in most of these studies distinguished safely between symptoms, which are actually directly PNES-related, and symptoms not directly related to seizures. Another difficulty that arises with the interpretation of interictal symptoms in patients with PNES is the high level of symptoms usually attributed to other mental health disorders. Patients most commonly fulfill the diagnostic criteria for other somatic symptom (22–84%), other dissociative (22–91%), posttraumatic stress (35–49%), depressive (57–85%), or anxiety disorders (11–50%) (Reuber, 2008). The likely presence of comorbid disorders (or the manifestation of PNES as features of other mental health disorders) makes it difficult to separate between symptoms attributable to the interictal state of PNES and more or less coincidental symptoms of other conditions.

Having said that, many studies have demonstrated significant elevations of interictal anxiety symptoms in patients with PNES compared to population norms. In addition, the prevalence of clinical anxiety disorders in patients with PNES is about twice as high as in the general population (Galimberti et al., 2003; Tellez-Zenteno et al., 2007). However, neither clinical diagnoses of anxiety disorders nor self-reported interictal anxiety symptom have been found to be persistently higher in patients with PNES than in those with epilepsy (Tojek et al., 2000; Owczarek, 2003; Bewley et al., 2005; Hixson et al., 2006; Dimaro et al., 2014).

Findings have been similar for symptoms of dissociation. Patients with PNES report more symptoms than the general population or healthy controls but symptoms of dissociation have not been found consistently more frequently than in patients with epilepsy (Goldstein et al., 2000; Prueter et al., 2002; Reuber et al., 2003a; Lawton et al., 2008; Ito et al., 2009). However, one study demonstrated that significantly fewer symptoms of dissociation were reported by seizure-free PNES patients compared to those with continuing seizures ($p < 0.05$) (Kuyk et al., 2008). Another study showed that self-reported dissociative symptoms are a significant predictor of health-related quality of life (HRQoL) in patients with PNES. Mitchell et al. (2012) found a strong negative correlation of symptoms to HRQoL and dissociative symptoms ($r = -0.64$, $p < 0.05$). After taking account of depressive symptoms (58.1%), Mitchell et al. found that dissociative symptoms explained an additional 14.4% of the variance in HRQoL ($p < 0.001$).

Somatization (i.e., a higher number of somatic symptoms other than seizures) may be slightly more specific for PNES than symptoms of anxiety or dissociation, in the sense that it differentiates not only between patients with PNES and healthy controls, but also between patient groups with PNES or epilepsy (Owczarek, 2003; Reuber et al., 2003a). High numbers of other somatic symptoms have been found to characterize patients with PNES regardless of whether they belonged to one cluster characterized by high levels of psychopathology, alexithymia, and emotional regulation problems (identifying, accepting, and describing feelings, accessing adaptive regulatory strategies, performing goal-directed behaviors, and controlling feelings/actions) or another cluster with elevated depression scores but comparatively normal levels of alexithymia and emotion regulation (Uliaszek et al., 2012; Brown et al., 2013). What is more, Reuber et al. (2003a) found that high somatization scores were correlated with a PNES severity score once dissociation and psychopathology had been controlled for. A high number of somatic symptoms also predicted poor prognosis in a naturalistic long-term outcome study (Reuber et al., 2003b).

Last but not least, LaFrance and Syc (2009) observed a significant association between the increased reporting of physical symptoms and lower HRQoL ($r = -0.73$, $p < 0.001$). Commonly reported somatic symptoms included headaches, insomnia, and memory difficulties. In another study, a higher number of somatic symptoms correlated negatively with the physical health component summary of the Short Form 36 (a measure of HRQoL), but not with the mental health component ($r = -0.45$, $p < 0.001$) (Lawton et al., 2009). In this study, the "bodily pain" subscale was rated particularly highly by patients with PNES, prompting the discussion about whether pain is a symptom, a trigger, or part of a comorbid pain condition (e.g., fibromyalgia) in patients with PNES (Benbadis, 2005).

IMPAIRMENT OF CONSCIOUSNESS

In the context of seizure disorders, impairment of consciousness has been defined operationally as involving deficits in awareness and self-control or responsiveness (Lux et al., 2002). Although clinicians have applied the diagnosis of PNES when patients do not exhibit impairment of consciousness, awareness, self-control, or responsiveness, the apparent temporary reduction of the patient's level of consciousness is a key clinical feature of most PNES (Eddy and Cavanna, 2014). Much more than patients with epilepsy, those with PNES have been noted to highlight the complete and absolute nature of their impairment of consciousness when they talk about their seizures to a doctor. For instance, in linguistic studies patients with PNES showed a tendency to describe the gaps in their memory using uncontextualized negations, e.g., "I can't remember anything," or "I can't see, I can't hear, I can't move" (Schwabe et al., 2008; Plug and Reuber, 2009; Reuber et al., 2009). Caregivers may highlight patients' loss of awareness even more than patients themselves. In the self-report questionnaire study mentioned above, the 100 responses from patients with PNES were compared to responses from 86 caregivers. The caregivers' reports demonstrated that they considered patients' loss of awareness as more profound than the individuals experiencing PNES themselves (Reuber et al., 2011).

Having said this, there are several indicators suggesting that loss of awareness in PNES is rarely (if ever) complete. During their PNES, patients often display purposeful movements, for instance reaching out for objects or people around them, or moving items out of the way. Patients whose eyes are usually closed in PNES often show resistance to eye opening and may move their eyes away from an examination torch (Reuber and Kurthen, 2011). One study demonstrated that, during their seizures, 48% of patients with PNES but only 18% of patients with epilepsy were able to follow simple commands, such as "shake my hand" (Bell et al., 1998). Similarly, in another study, verbal or motor responses to a nurse or doctor who approached patients during video-EEG examinations were observed in 58% of patients with PNES (Hubsch et al., 2011).

The 58 consecutive patients mentioned previously, who were interviewed about their PNES symptoms in their first appointment with a psychotherapist, were asked specifically about awareness and responsiveness during their seizures. Of these patients, only 46% stated that they were neither aware nor responsive in their seizures, 38% said they were aware during their seizures, although they were unresponsive, 19% said they were unaware, but responsive, and 2% said they were aware and responsive (19% had more than one seizure type and 5% had seizures fitting more than one of these categories) (S. Howlett, personal communication).

Whether or not patients report impairment of consciousness or loss of awareness in their PNES may be associated with certain visible PNES manifestations. In the semiology cluster analysis mentioned previously, "pauci-kinetic" attacks were particularly likely to be associated with maintained responsiveness (96.6% of cases), whereas "pseudosyncope" typically involved unresponsiveness (85.7%) (Hubsch et al., 2011).

Content and level of ictal impairment of consciousness have been explored using self-report questionnaires. Ali et al. (2010) conducted a quantitative evaluation of subjective experiences of ictal consciousness in patients with epilepsy ($n = 66$) and patients with PNES ($n = 29$). Using a bi-dimensional model plotting general level of awareness versus specific contents of consciousness, patients with PNES exhibited less impaired conscious profiles demonstrating greater levels of responsiveness, contents, and quality of consciousness than those with a range of different epileptic seizure types.

Others have demonstrated that patients with PNES are more likely to be able to recall ictal experiences than those with epilepsy. For example, Devinsky et al. (1996) demonstrated that, when 16 patients with both epilepsy and PNES were asked to remember a word or phrase during seizures, 15 patients were unable to recall the item after an epileptic seizure, whereas 14 patients were able to recall it after a PNES. Another study compared recall before and after hypnotic induction, finding that 17 of 20 (85%) patients with PNES but no patients with epilepsy recovered accurate seizure memories. Similarly, patients' reports of ictal memories were noted to become more detailed during the course of psychotherapy (von Fabeck, 2010). Taken together, this evidence suggests the initial amnesia resulting from PNES is, at least in part, the result of a postictal retrieval deficit rather than a learning impairment during the seizures themselves (Kuyk et al., 1999). Having said that, an interictal study has demonstrated working-memory impairments in patients with PNES, which were further exaggerated by stress (Bakvis et al., 2010). This suggests that postictal memory gaps may result from a combination of different factors.

CLINICAL SIGNIFICANCE OF SUBJECTIVE PNES EXPERIENCE

Diagnostic implications

In PNES, like many other disorders, the differential diagnosis is crucial because the most effective treatments of PNES and the paroxysmal disorders that PNES could be mistaken for (mainly epilepsy and syncope) is very different. This is particularly true for the distinction of PNES, epilepsy, and syncope. Delayed or incorrect diagnoses are likely to lead to patients being subjected to inappropriate, ineffective, and potentially iatrogenic treatments. Despite impressive developments in brain imaging and improved access to video-EEG, the act of taking and interpreting patients' narrative of their subjective experience is, arguably, still the most important diagnostic tool in patients who have lost consciousness (Plug and Reuber, 2009; Malmgren et al., 2012).

A better understanding of the typical interictal, ictal, and peri-ictal symptom profiles of patients with PNES should improve the diagnostic process. Batteries of self-report questionnaires which included questions about interictal somatic and mental health symptoms have already been shown to distinguish accurately between PNES and epilepsy with a sensitivity and specificity of 85% (Syed et al., 2009). One study used the Paroxysmal Event Profile mentioned above to examine whether subjective experience profiles could be used to differentiate between the three commonest causes of transient loss of consciousness (TLOC). One hundred patients with definite epilepsy, 100 with proven PNES, and 100 with physiologically documented recurrent syncope completed the questionnaire, eliciting responses to 86 symptom prompts. Respondents rated symptoms on a five-point Likert scale (always to never). An initial exploratory factor analysis identified a five-factor structure based on 74/86 questionnaire items with loadings ≥ 0.4. In a confirmatory factor analysis goodness-of-fit statistics, including chi-square, root mean square error approximation, comparative fit index and Tucker Lewis index, were used to test the proposed model. The five resulting latent factors were named as "feeling overpowered," "sensory experience," "mind/body/world disconnection," "catastrophic experience," and "amnesia." Pairwise regression analysis based on these factors correctly classified 91% of patients with epilepsy versus those with syncope, 94% of those with PNES versus those with syncope, and 77% of those with epilepsy versus those with PNES. Thus, diagnostic distinction on the basis of symptoms was better between syncope and the other two common causes of recurrent TLOC than between epilepsy and PNES. These findings suggest that clusters of TLOC-associated symptoms can be used to direct patients to appropriate investigation and treatment pathways for syncope on the one hand, and seizures on the other, although additional information is required for definitive diagnoses, especially for the distinction between epilepsy and PNES (Reuber et al., in press).

In another analysis, the same dataset was used to explore whether the seven TLOC-associated panic symptoms included in the Paroxysmal Event Profile could differentiate between the PNES, syncope, and epilepsy groups ("During my attacks I feel very frightened"; "During my attacks I feel that something terrible might happen"; "During my attacks I am frightened that I am going to die"; "During my attacks I am frightened that I will lose control"; "During my attacks I am frightened that I will go crazy"; "During my attacks my heart pounds and I feel shaky and sweaty"; and "During my attacks I feel that I have to get out of the situation"). Patients with PNES reported more panic symptoms (median = 15.5) than those with epilepsy (median = 10, $p < 0.001$) and syncope (median = 9, $p < 0.001$). Panic symptoms were reported with similar frequency in the epilepsy and syncope groups ($p = 0.057$). Logistic regression demonstrated that differences in the subjective experience of panic could distinguish PNES from epilepsy and syncope (sensitivity 71.4%, specificity 65.6%), but not epilepsy from syncope (Rawlings et al., manuscript in preparation).

Links with etiology

Specific symptoms may also provide clues about etiologic factors. For example, Selkirk et al. (2008) demonstrated that patients with PNES who have a history of antecedent sexual abuse ($n = 64$) were more likely than those without this history ($n = 112$) to report emotional triggers (relative risk (RR), 1.46), attack prodromes (RR 1.33), urinary incontinence (RR 1.82), self-injuries (RR 1.81), nocturnal attacks (RR 1.42), internal experiences (RR 1.97), flashbacks (RR 3.9), and convulsions (RR 1.21) during their PNES. A logistic regression model based on these features correctly predicted whether sexual abuse had been reported in 77.5% of cases. The features accounted for 46.4% of the variance (R. Duncan, personal communication).

Treatment implications

A better understanding of subjective experiences is also likely to have implications for engagement and adherence to interventions. The engagement of patients with PNES in the treatment of choice, psychotherapy (LaFrance et al., 2013), is often difficult because patients perceive their disorder to be a "physical" rather than a "psychologic" problem (Whitehead et al., 2013).

For instance, several studies have demonstrated that patients who accept the diagnosis of PNES are more likely to have better treatment outcomes (Ettinger et al., 1999a; Duncan et al., 2014). It may well be easier for clinicians to convince patients (and caregivers) that they have PNES if the patient is aware of unpleasant warning symptoms, or at least of interictal mental health problems, and can accept that the seizures could be manifestations of arousal or distress (Thompson et al., 2009; Monzoni et al., 2011a, b). Indeed, there is one study which analyzed predictors of PNES cessation in 260 patients after the initial explanation of the diagnosis. This research demonstrated that those with evidence of anxiety and depression were 2.34 times more likely to become spell-free than those without symptoms of these disorders (McKenzie et al., 2010).

The identification of seizure triggers may also allow psychotherapists or other clinicians to assist patients in building up their tolerance of these stimuli. The presence of seizure warning symptoms and the retention of a degree of self-control during the PNES state may enable patients to learn seizure suppression or control techniques, such as distraction or sensory grounding approaches (Howlett and Reuber, 2009). The fact that HRQoL in patients with PNES is co-determined by other somatic and dissociative symptoms (as well as symptoms of depression) suggests that intervention aiming to reduce symptoms (or increase tolerance of these symptoms) rather than PNES themselves may improve patients' level of functioning (Birbeck and Vickrey, 2003; Szaflarski et al., 2003).

Prognostic implications

A naturalistic study of outcome in PNES (a mean of 4.1 years after diagnosis and 11.9 years after PNES manifestation) suggested that better prognosis was predicted by a number of factors characterized by subjective symptoms, including fewer additional somatoform complaints, lower numbers of other dissociative symptoms, and lower scores of the higher-order personality dimensions ("inhibitedness," "emotional dysregulation," and "compulsivity"), as measured by the Dimensional Assessment of Personality Pathology Brief Questionnaire. Outcome was also poorer in those patients whose seizures involved "loss" of consciousness (Reuber et al., 2003b). Similarly, another study found that outcome after 6 months was worse if patients had symptoms of major depression, dissociative and personality disorders, or new somatic symptoms after disclosure of diagnosis (Kanner et al., 1999). Whilst no study has been undertaken to provide a comprehensive assessment of the value of ictal, peri-ictal, or interictal symptoms associated with PNES for the prediction of outcome (and whilst much more differentiated approaches of capturing symptoms and using them to characterize particular types of PNES would be desirable), somewhat less robust observations show that at least some subjective symptoms experienced by patients with PNES are relevant to how likely they are to become free of their seizures in the longer term.

CONCLUSION

Despite the fact that PNES are considered a manifestation of mental disorder, the subjective symptoms associated with this disorder have received much less attention from researchers than visible or physiologic features. Whilst this chapter demonstrates the challenges involved in studying the symptoms of a dissociative phenomenon, it also shows that they should not be ignored or devalued. Most of the studies which form the basis of this discussion only explore subjective symptoms in passing whilst focusing on another facet of PNES. However, this chapter shows how aspects of the subjective phenomenology of PNES can improve the diagnostic process, provide insights into the etiology of PNES in individual patients, help to shape treatment formulations, and allow for a better prognostication of likely treatment outcomes. This suggests that further research focusing more specifically on subjective PNES symptoms and their clinical relevance would be entirely justified and may allow us to understand and treat this complex disorder more successfully in the future. Having said that, even the limited knowledge base about subjective symptoms in PNES available thus far allows us to draw some conclusions.

The current psychiatric nosologies separate dissociative seizures or conversion seizures as a specific somatic symptom disorder from other manifestations of psychopathology and medical disorders (World Health Organization, 1992; American Psychiatric Association, 2013). However, a closer examination of the symptoms that patients experience (including those which they may not be able to recall during a first interaction with a clinician) demonstrates how indistinct the boundaries between PNES, other dissociative symptoms, somatic symptoms, and anxiety disorders are. We are not arguing that the categoric classifications need to be abandoned. However, it would be a serious misunderstanding of the current categoric classification systems for clinicians or researchers to use particular diagnostic categories as rigid pointers to particular interventions. Treatment formulations are likely to work best if they take account of the full range of a patient's personal PNES symptomatology and experience.

Another borderline of PNES, which emerges as rather indistinct, is that between the ictal and the interictal state. The differences between seizures and the interictal state are considerably less distinct in PNES than in epileptic seizure disorders. The onset and offset of PNES are often difficult to determine and there is considerable overlap between interictal, peri-ictal, and (when they can be reported) ictal symptoms. This observation suggests that PNES themselves are only the tip of an iceberg of a more pervasive disorder of perception and emotion processing.

Previous studies have demonstrated that the etiology and visible phenomenology of PNES are heterogeneous (Reuber, 2009; Hubsch et al., 2011). This overview shows that the subjective PNES experience is also rather varied. There are marked differences, not only between different patients but also between one patient's experiences of different seizures. Nevertheless, it is possible to describe some subtypes of PNES disorders, probabilistically characterized by combinations of etiologic factors and clinical features. To date, at least two such subtypes have been suggested: (1) patients with symptoms of marked emotional dysregulation, high levels of psychopathology, distress, and dissociation as well as high levels of alexithymia; and (2) patients with increased depressive and somatic symptoms but no increased number of symptoms of emotional or mental health problems (Uliaszek et al., 2012; Brown et al., 2013). Future research may well distinguish between more subtypes requiring different therapeutic strategies and associated with different outcomes. For instance, research into the warnings of PNES has, so far, only looked at anxiety and physiologic arousal. However, clinical experience suggests that patients may also dissociate in response to feelings of guilt, shame, anger, and other aversive emotions or states or experiences (Griffith et al., 1998; Reuber et al., 2007, 2014).

We hope that the approach we have pursued in this chapter, integrating patients' subjective seizure experience with visible motor and measurable autonomic PNES manifestations but also with experimental insights into preconscious cognitive processing in the brain and relevant interictal findings, has not only demonstrated the scope of future PNES symptom research but also inspired readers to pay more attention to the subjective phenomenology of PNES in the meantime.

References

Ali F, Rickards H, Bagary M et al. (2010). Ictal consciousness in epilepsy and nonepileptic attack disorder. Epilepsy Behav 19: 522–525.

American Psychiatric Association (2000). Diagnostic and statistical manual of mental disorders (4th ed., text revision). American Psychiatric Association, Washington, DC.

American Psychiatric Association (2013). Diagnostic and statistical manual of mental disorders, American Psychiatric Association, Arlington, VA.

Azar NJ, Tayah TF, Abou-Khalil BW et al. (2008). Postictal breathing pattern distinguishes epileptic from nonepileptic convulsive seizures. Epilepsia 49: 132–137.

Bakvis P, Roelofs K, Kuyk J et al. (2009). Trauma, stress, and preconscious threat processing in patients with psychogenic nonepileptic seizures. Epilepsia 50: 1001–1011.

Bakvis P, Spinhoven P, Putman P et al. (2010). The effect of stress induction on working memory in patients with psychogenic nonepileptic seizures. Epilepsy Behav 19: 448–454.

Bakvis P, Spinhoven P, Roelofs K et al. (2011). Automatic avoidance tendencies in patients with psychogenic non epileptic seizures. Seizure 20: 628–634.

Barry J, Reuber M (2010). The use of hypnosis and linguistic analysis to discriminate between patients with psychogenic non-epileptic seizures and patients with epilepsy. In: S Schachter, C LaFrance (Eds.), Gates and Rowan's non-epileptic seizures. Cambridge University Press, Cambridge, pp. 82–90.

Bell WL, Park YD, Thompson EA et al. (1998). Ictal cognitive assessment of partial seizures and pseudoseizures. Arch Neurol 55: 1456–1459.

Benbadis Sr (2005). A spell in the epilepsy clinic and a history of "chronic pain" or "fibromyalgia" independently predict a diagnosis of psychogenic seizures. Epilepsy Behav 6: 264–265.

Bernat JL (2010). The ethics of diagnosing nonepileptic seizures with placebo infusion. Virtual Mentor 12: 854.

Bernstein EM, Putnam FW (1986). Development, reliability and validity of a dissociation scale. J Nerv Ment Dis 174: 727–735.

Bewley J, Murphy P, Mallows J et al. (2005). Does alexithymia differentiate between patients with nonepileptic seizures, patients with epilepsy, and nonpatient controls? Epilepsy Behav 7: 430–437.

Birbeck GL, Vickrey BG (2003). Determinants of health-related quality of life in adults with psychogenic nonepileptic seizures: are there implications for clinical practice? Epilepsia 44: 141.

Bowman ES (2006). Why conversion seizures should be classified as a dissociative disorder. Psychiatr Clin North Am 29: 185–211.

Brown P, van Der Hart O, Graafland M (1999). Trauma-induced dissociative amnesia in World War I combat soldiers. II. Treatment dimensions. Aust N Z J Psychiatry 33: 392–398.

Brown R, Bouska J, Frow A et al. (2013). Emotional dysregulation, alexithymia, and attachment in psychogenic nonepileptic seizures. Epilepsy Behav 29: 178–183.

Cohen RJ, Suter C (1982). Hysterical seizures – suggestion as a provocative EEG test. Ann Neurol 11: 391–395.

Devinsky O, Sanchezvillasenor F, Vazquez B et al. (1996). Clinical profile of patients with epileptic and nonepileptic seizures. Neurology 46: 1530–1533.

Dimaro LV, Dawson DL, Moghaddam NG et al. (2014). Anxiety and avoidance in psychogenic nonepileptic seizures: the role of implicit and explicit anxiety. Epilepsy Behav 33: 77–86.

Duncan R, Duncan M, Oto AJC et al. (2004). Pseudosleep events in patients with psychogenic non-epileptic seizures: prevalence and associations. J Neurol Neurosurg Psychiatry 75: 1009–1012.

Duncan R, Grahamb CD, Oto M (2014). Neurologist assessment of reactions to the diagnosis of psychogenic nonepileptic seizures: relationship to short- and long-term outcomes. Epilepsy Behav 41: 79–82.

Eddy CM, Cavanna AE (2014). Video- electroencephalography investigation of ictal alterations of consciousness in epilepsy and nonepileptic attack disorder: practical considerations. Epilepsy Behav 30: 24–27.

Ettinger AB, Devinsky O, Weisbrot DM et al. (1999a). A comprehensive profile of clinical, psychiatric, and psychosocial characteristics of patients with psychogenic nonepileptic seizures. Epilepsia 40: 1292–1298.

Ettinger AB, Weisbrot DM, Nolan E et al. (1999b). Postictal symptoms help distinguish patients with epileptic seizures from those with non-epileptic seizures. Seizure 8: 149–151.

Galimberti CA, Ratti MT, Murelli R et al. (2003). Patients with psychogenic nonepileptic seizures, alone or epilepsy-associated, share a psychological profile distinct from that of epilepsy patients. J Neurol 250: 338–346.

Gates JR, Ramani V, Whalen S et al. (1985). Ictal characteristics of pseudoseizures. Arch Neurol 42: 1183–1187.

Goldstein LH, Mellers J (2006). Ictal symptoms of anxiety, avoidance behaviour, and dissociation in patients with dissociative seizures. J Neurol Neurosurg Psychiatry 77: 616–621.

Goldstein LH, Drew C, Mellers J et al. (2000). Dissociation, hypnotizability, coping styles and health locus of control: characteristics of pseudoseizure patients. Seizure 9: 314–322.

Goldstein LH, Goldstein JDC, Mellers JDC (2006). Ictal symptoms of anxiety, avoidance behaviour, and dissociation in patients with dissociative seizures. J Neurol Neurosurg Psychiatry 77: 616–621.

Griffith J, Polles A, Griffith ME (1998). Pseudoseizures, families, and unspeakable dilemmas. Psychosomatics 39: 144–153.

Gulick TA, Spinks IP, King DW (1982). Pesudoseizures – ictal phenomena. Neurology 32: 24–30.

Hendrickson R, Popescu A, Dixit R et al. (2014). Panic attack symptoms differentiate patients with epilepsy from those with psychogenic nonepileptic spells (PNES). Epilepsy Behav 37: 210–214.

Hixson JD, Balcer LJ, Glosser G et al. (2006). Fear sensitivity and the psychological profile of patients with psychogenic nonepileptic seizures. Epilepsy Behav 9: 587–592.

Howlett S, Reuber M (2009). An augmented model of brief psychodynamic interpersonal therapy for patients with nonepileptic seizures. Psychotherapy 46: 125–138.

Hubsch C, Baumann C, Hingray C et al. (2011). Clinical classification of psychogenic non- epileptic seizures based on video- EEG analysis and automatic clustering. J Neurol Neurosurg Psychiatry 82: 955–960.

Ito M, Adachi N, Okazaki M et al. (2009). Evaluation of dissociative experiences and the clinical utility of the Dissociative Experience Scale in patients with coexisting epilepsy and psychogenic nonepileptic seizures. Epilepsy Behav 16: 491–494.

Kanner A, Parra J, Frey M et al. (1999). Psychiatric and neurologic predictors of psychogenic pseudoseizure outcome. Neurology 53: 933–938.

Kihlstrom JF (1985). Hypnosis. Annu Rev Psychol 36: 385.

Kuyk J, Spinhoven P, van Dyck R (1999). Hypnotic recall: a positive criterion in the differential diagnosis between epileptic and pseudoepileptic seizures. Epilepsia 40: 485–491.

Kuyk J, Siffels MC, Bakvis P et al. (2008). Psychological treatment of patients with psychogenic non-epileptic seizures: an outcome study. Seizure 17: 595–603.

LaFrance W, Syc S (2009). Depression and symptoms affect quality of life in psychogenic nonepileptic seizures. Neurology 73: 366–371.

LaFrance WC, Reuber M, Goldstein LH (2013). Management of psychogenic nonepileptic seizures. Epilepsia 54: 53–67.

Lakoff G (1993). The contemporary theory of metaphor. In: A Ortony (Ed.), Metaphor and Thought, 2nd edition. Cambridge University Press, Cambridge, pp. 202–251.

Lancman ME, Brotherton TA, Asconapé JJ et al. (1993). Psychogenic seizures in adults: a longitudinal analysis. Seizure 2: 281–286.

Lawton G, Baker G, Brown R (2008). Comparison of two types of dissociation in epileptic and nonepileptic seizures. Epilepsy Behav 13: 333–336.

Lawton G, Mayor R, Howlett S et al. (2009). Psychogenic nonepileptic seizures and health-related quality of life: the relationship with psychological distress and other physical symptoms. Epilepsy Behav 14: 167–171.

Luther JS, McNamara JO, Carwile S et al. (1982). Pseudoepileptic seizures – methods and video analysis to aid diagnosis. Ann Neurol 12: 458–462.

Lux S, Kurthen M, Helmstaedter C et al. (2002). The localizing value of ictal consciousness and its constituent functions – A video-EEG study in patients with focal epilepsy. Brain 125: 2691–2698.

Malmgren K, Reuber M, Appleton R (2012). Differential diagnosis of epilepsy. In: S Shorvon, M Cook, R Guerrini et al. (Eds.), Oxford Textbook of epilepsy and epileptic seizures. Oxford University Press, Oxford, pp. 81–94.

McGonigal A, Oto M, Russell AJC et al. (2002). Outpatient video EEG recording in the diagnosis of non-epileptic seizures: a randomised controlled trial of simple suggestion techniques. J Neurol Neurosurg Psychiatry 72: 549–551.

McKenzie P, Oto M, Russell A et al. (2010). Early outcomes and predictors in 260 patients with psychogenic nonepileptic attacks. Neurology 74: 64–69.

Meierkord H, Will B, Fish D et al. (1991). The clinical feature and prognosis of pseudo seizures diagnosed using video-ERG telemetry. Neurology 41: 1643–1646.

Mitchell JW, Ali F, Cavanna AE (2012). Dissociative experiences and quality of life in patients with non-epileptic attack disorder. Epilepsy Behav 25: 307–312.

Monzoni CM, Duncan R, Grünewald R et al. (2011a). How do neurologists discuss functional symptoms with their patients: a conversation analytic study. J Psychosom Res 71: 377–383.

Monzoni CM, Grünewald R, Reuber M et al. (2011b). Are there interactional reasons why doctors may find it hard to tell patients that their physical symptoms may have emotional causes? A conversation analytic study in neurology outpatients. Patient Educ Couns 85: e189–e200.

Opherk C, Hirsch LJ (2002). Ictal heart rate differentiates epileptic from non-epileptic seizures. Neurology 58: 636–638.

Owczarek K (2003). Somatisation indexes as differential factors in psychogenic pseudoepileptic and epileptic seizures. Seizure 12: 178–181.

Plug L, Reuber M (2009). Making the diagnosis in patients with blackouts: it's all in the history. Pract Neurol 9: 4–15.

Plug L, Sharrack B, Reuber M (2009). Seizure metaphors differ in patients' accounts of epileptic and psychogenic nonepileptic seizures. Epilepsia 50: 994–1000.

Plug L, Sharrack B, Reuber M (2010). The use of diagnostic labels by patients with epileptic or non- epileptic seizures. Appl Linguist 31: 94–114.

Plug L, Sharrack B, Reuber M (2011). Metaphors in the description of seizure experiences: common expressions and differential diagnosis. Lang Cogn 3: 209–233.

Ponnusamy A, Marques J, Reuber M (2012). Comparison of heart rate variability parameters during complex partial seizures and psychogenic nonepileptic seizures. Epilepsia 53: 1314–1321.

Prueter C, Schultz-Venrath U, Rimpau W (2002). Dissociative and associated psychopathological symptoms in patients with epilepsy, pseudoseizures, and both seizure forms. Epilepsia 43: 188–192.

Rawlings G, Jamnadas-Khoda J, Broadhurst M, et al. (manuscript submitted). Panic symptoms in transient loss of consciousness: frequency and diagnostic value in the differentiation of psychogenic nonepileptic seizures, epilepsy and syncope. Manuscript in preparation.

Reuber M (2008). Psychogenic nonepileptic seizures: answers and questions. Epilepsy Behav 12: 622–635.

Reuber M (2009). The etiology of psychogenic non-epileptic seizures: toward a biopsychosocial model. Neurol Clin 27: 909–924.

Reuber M, Elger CE (2003). Psychogenic nonepileptic seizures: review and update. Epilepsy Behav 4: 205–216.

Reuber M, Kurthen M (2011). Consciousness in non-epileptic attack disorder. Behav Neurol 24: 95–106.

Reuber M, House A, Pukrop R et al. (2003a). Somatization, dissociation and general psychopathology in patients with psychogenic non-epileptic seizures. Epilepsy Res 57: 159–167.

Reuber M, Pukrop R, Bauer J et al. (2003b). Outcome in psychogenic nonepileptic seizures: 1 to 10- year follow- up in 164 patients. Ann Neurol 53: 305–311.

Reuber M, Pukrop R, Mitchell AJ et al. (2003c). Clinical significance of recurrent psychogenic nonepileptic seizure status. J Neurol 250: 1355–1362.

Reuber M, Howlett S, Khan A et al. (2007). Non-epileptic seizures and other functional neurological symptoms: predisposing, precipitating, and perpetuating factors. Psychosomatics 48: 230–238.

Reuber M, Monzoni C, Sharrack B et al. (2009). Using interactional and linguistic analysis to distinguish between epileptic and psychogenic nonepileptic seizures: a prospective, blinded multirater study. Epilepsy Behav 16: 139–144.

Reuber M, Jamnadas-Khoda J, Broadhurst M et al. (2011). Psychogenic nonepileptic seizure manifestations reported by patients and witnesses. Epilepsia 52: 2028–2035.

Reuber M, Micoulaud-Franchi JA, Micoulaud-Franchi E et al. (2014). Comment ce que disent les patients peut nous renseigner sur leurs crises non épileptiques psychogènes. Neurophysiol Clin 44: 375–388.

Reuber M, Chen M, Jamnadas-Khoda J, et al. (2016). Value of patient-reported symptoms in the differential diagnosis of transient loss of consciousness. Neurology (in press).

Roberts NA, Reuber M (2014). Alterations of consciousness in psychogenic nonepileptic seizures: emotion, emotion regulation and dissociation. Epilepsy Behav 30: 43–49.

Roberts NA, Burleson MH, Weber DJ et al. (2012). Emotion in psychogenic nonepileptic seizures: responses to affective pictures. Epilepsy Behav 24: 107–115.

Rosemergy I, Frith R, Herath S et al. (2013). Use of postictal respiratory pattern to discriminate between convulsive psychogenic nonepileptic seizures and generalized tonic-clonic seizures. Epilepsy Behav 27: 81–84.

Schachter SC (2011). Evidence-based Management of Epilepsy. TFM Publishing, Shrewsbury, UK.

Schwabe M, Howell SJ, Reuber M (2007). Differential diagnosis of seizure disorders: a conversation analytic approach. Soc Sci Med 65: 712–724.

Schwabe M, Reuber M, Schondienst M et al. (2008). Listening to people with seizures: how can linguistic analysis help in the differential diagnosis of seizure disorders? Commun Med 5: 59–72.

Selkirk M, Duncan R, Oto M et al. (2008). Clinical differences between patients with nonepileptic seizures who report antecedent sexual abuse and those who do not. Epilepsia 49: 1446–1450.

Selwa L, Geyer J, Nikakhtar N et al. (2000). Nonepileptic seizure outcome varies by type of spell and duration of illness. Epilepsia 41: 1330–1334.

Stone J, Carson AJ (2013). The unbearable lightheadedness of seizing: wilful submission to dissociative (non-epileptic) seizures. J Neurol Neurosurg Psychiatry 84: 822–824.

Syed T, Arozullah A, Loparo K et al. (2009). A self-administered screening instrument for psychogenic nonepileptic seizures. Neurology 72: 1646–1652.

Syed T, Lafrance W, Kahriman E et al. (2011). Can semiology predict psychogenic nonepileptic seizures? A prospective study. Ann Neurol 69: 997–1004.

Szaflarski JP, Hughes C, Szaflarski M et al. (2003). Quality of Life in Psychogenic Nonepileptic Seizures, MA, USA, Boston.

Tellez-Zenteno JF, Patten SB, Williams J et al. (2007). Psychiatric comorbidity in epilepsy: a population-based analysis. Epilepsia 48: 2336–2344.

Thompson R, Isaac C, Rowse G et al. (2009). What is it like to receive a diagnosis of nonepileptic seizures? Epilepsy Behav 14: 508–515.

Tojek TM, Lumley M, Barkley G et al. (2000). Stress and other psychosocial characteristics of patients with psychogenic nonepileptic seizures. Psychosomatics 41: 221–226.

Uliaszek AA, Prensky E, Baslet G (2012). Emotion regulation profiles in psychogenic non-epileptic seizures. Epilepsy Behav 23: 364–369.

van de Mortel T (2008). Faking it: social desirability response bias in self- report research. Aust J Adv Nurs 25: 40–48.

Vein AM, Djukova GM, Vorobieva OV (1994). Is panic attack a mask of psychogenic seizures? A comparative analysis of phenomenology of psychogenic seizures and panic attacks. Funct Neurol 9: 153–159.

von Fabeck F (2010). Zur Dynamik narrativer (Re-) Konstruktionen im Behandlungsverlauf dissoziativer Patienten, Bielefeld Doctoral Thesis, Kurzvorstellung Elisabeth Gütlich, Germany.

Waller NG, Putnam FW, Carlson EB (1996). Types of dissociation and dissociative types: a taxometric analysis of dissociative experiences. Psychol Methods 1: 300–321.

Watson N, Doherty M, Dodrill C et al. (2002). The experience of earthquakes by patients with epileptic and psychogenic nonepileptic seizures. Epilepsia 43: 317–320.

Whitehead K, Kandler R, Reuber M (2013). Patients' and neurologists' perception of epilepsy and psychogenic nonepileptic seizures. Epilepsia 54: 708–717.

Whitehead K, Stone J, Norman P et al. (2015). Differences in relatives' and patients' illness perceptions in functional neurological symptom disorders compared with neurological diseases. Epilepsy Behav 42: 159–164.

Witgert ME, Wheless JW, Breier JI (2005). Frequency of panic symptoms in psychogenic nonepileptic seizures. Epilepsy Behav 6: 174–178.

World Health Organization (1992). The ICD-10 classification of mental and behavioural disorders: clinical descriptions and diagnostic guidelines. World Health Organization, Geneva.

Handbook of Clinical Neurology, Vol. 139 (3rd series)
Functional Neurologic Disorders
M. Hallett, J. Stone, and A. Carson, Editors
http://dx.doi.org/10.1016/B978-0-12-801772-2.00026-6

Chapter 26

Nonepileptic seizures – objective phenomena

W. CURT LAFRANCE JR.[1]*, R. RANIERI[2], AND A.S. BLUM[3]
[1]*Division of Neuropsychiatry and Behavioral Neurology, Rhode Island Hospital, Providence, RI, USA*
[2]*Department of Psychiatry, Università degli Studi di Milano, Ospedale San Paolo, Milan, Italy*
[3]*Department of Neurology, Rhode Island Hospital, Brown University, Providence, RI, USA*

Abstract

This chapter describes the evaluation process for the diagnosis of psychogenic nonepileptic seizures (PNES), which is determined based on concordance of the composite evidence available, including historic and physical exam findings, seizure semiology, and ictal/interictal electroencephalogram (EEG). No single clinical feature is pathognomonic of PNES. The diagnosis of PNES can be at times challenging, such as when seizure documentation on video-EEG cannot be readily achieved. A multicomponent approach to the diagnosis of PNES, with use of all available evidence, may facilitate diagnosis and then care of patients with PNES. Emerging evidence supports the use of symptom identification by the patient as part of the treatment of these patients. With advances in diagnostic methods and criteria, the diagnosis of PNES can be made reliably.

INTRODUCTION

Seizures can be divided into three major categories: epileptic seizures (ES) caused by abnormal (epileptiform) neuronal firing, physiologic nonepileptic events caused by a coincident medical process leading to a seizure, or psychogenic nonepileptic seizures (PNES), a conversion (or functional) disorder. PNES are a common somatoform disorder, presenting like ES or sometimes like syncope, with paroxysmal, time-limited alterations in motor, sensory, autonomic, and/or cognitive signs and symptoms, while lacking video-electroencephalogram (vEEG) epileptiform activity (Gates, 2000). PNES occur across cultures and continents and the semiologies are described similarly across ethnicities and cultures (LaFrance et al., 2013). The majority of patients with PNES have been exposed to a traumatic situation or conflict, or overwhelming emotion in the recent or remote past (Bowman and Markand, 1996). How mental processes lead to the physical presentation of seizures remains unknown; however, as a conversion disorder diagnosis, PNES are an involuntary somatic expression of that stressor or distress, with or without the awareness of "being stressed," associated with predisposing, precipitating, and perpetuating factors (LaFrance and Devinsky, 2002). PNES may significantly affect an individual's quality of life (LaFrance and Syc, 2009), impact psychosocial functioning, and are associated with significant costs to the healthcare system (Martin et al., 1998).

DIAGNOSIS

A staged approach to PNES diagnosis addresses these issues. Levels of diagnostic certainty were developed, including possible, probable, clinically established, and documented diagnosis, based on the availability of history, witnessed event, and investigations, including vEEG (LaFrance et al., 2013). vEEG recording of the event is the gold standard in investigating the diagnosis of PNES, and establishing PNES vs. ES or syncope (Syed et al., 2011). The challenge of differentiating between scalp-negative ictal EEGs with frontal-lobe ES and PNES can be aided by semiologic differences between the two (LaFrance and Benbadis, 2011), by their

*Correspondence to: W. Curt LaFrance Jr., MD, MPH, Rhode Island Hospital, Brown University, 593 Eddy Street, Providence RI 02903, USA. Tel: +1-401-444-3534, Fax: +1-401-444-3298, E-mail: william_lafrance_jr@brown.edu

onset in wake only versus sleep ± wake onsets, by the degree of stereotypy of the semiologies encountered in any individual patient and complemented by the interictal EEG tracing.

The diagnosis of PNES is confirmed by recording events typical of PNES with simultaneous video and EEG, finding an absence of ictal EEG changes (and the presence of normal awake EEG rhythms) before, during, and after the event. Levels of diagnostic certainty are based on history, semiology, and studies consistent with PNES and are ranked as documented, clinically established, probable, and possible (LaFrance et al., 2013). Validation of the recorded event by an eyewitness as being typical of those occurring in daily life provides assurance of ictal capture. Individuals can have more than one type of seizure. If clinical descriptions suggest more than one event pattern variety, then capturing each distinct semiologic event type must, if possible, be recorded, in order to see if a patient has more than one PNES semiology, or if the patient has both epilepsy and PNES. Because vEEG is not available worldwide, or for every patient, a description of a directly witnessed seizure or one recorded with home video and provided to the evaluator is also valuable.

SEMIOLOGY

A plethora of semiologic signs has been suggested to distinguish PNES from ES, and tables listing semiologic elements and comparing their frequency in ES versus PNES have been published (Avbersek and Sisodiya, 2010; Mostacci et al., 2011; Syed et al., 2011; Dhiman et al., 2013). The semiologic subdivisions of seizures in PNES may be less important for outcomes. Caregiver reports and event semiologies are frequently not comparable (Syed et al., 2011), so it is important to distinguish if what was recorded matches eyewitness reports. Many patients with mixed PNES/ES and their caregivers have difficulty differentiating between their PNES and ES (Gordon et al., 2014).

No single feature is pathognomonic for PNES (Goldstein and Mellers, 2012). An estimated 10–30% of patients with PNES have coexisting ES (Benbadis et al., 2001). PNES are one of the most common disorders diagnosed in epilepsy monitoring unit (Benbadis et al., 2004; Salinsky et al., 2011). The majority of patients with recurrent seizures are initially presumed to have epilepsy and are commonly treated with antiepileptic drugs (Reuber et al., 2002), which do not benefit PNES and may exacerbate them (Niedermeyer et al., 1970).

CLASSIFICATION

Several classifications of nonepileptic seizures pattern have been published based on ictal semiology (Meierkord et al., 1991; Gröppel et al., 2000; Seneviratne et al., 2010; Hubsch et al., 2011; Szabo et al., 2012; Dhiman et al., 2013). Seizures may affect one or more of the domains of alertness, sensorial, autonomic, or motor. Similar to epilepsy, many patients with PNES also have auras, a subjective warning symptom they may experience before having a seizure. Auras typically consist of sensory symptoms and are brief and consistent over time in the same patient. Just as in epilepsy, there are different types of auras for PNES. Examples include visual auras, which consist of a visual hallucination or illusion, gustatory auras, auditory auras, or pain. Patients may describe experiencing sensorial symptoms, not only as an aura, but also during the seizure or just during the ictus itself (see Chapter 25).

ES also may be classified based upon ictal semiology.

Four major categories of ES have been described by Lüders et al. (1998): autonomic, dialeptic, motor, and other (special).

1. An autonomic seizure is defined as an episodic alteration of an autonomic function documented by appropriate monitoring.
2. A dialeptic (from the Greek, *dialeipein*, to interrupt) seizure's main manifestation is an alteration of consciousness without motor accompaniment. In this category are coma-like states ("catatonic"), falls/drops, or lack of response to external stimuli.
3. A motor seizure can be simple, in which the movements are basic (whole-body rigidity or flaccidity; flexion/extension or low-amplitude and high-speed side-to-side movements of the head/neck/limbs); or can be complex, in which the movements have more complex characteristics. They could resemble natural body movements but are inappropriate for the situation. Examples include limb movements, violent thrashing, grabbing, or kicking movements.
4. Special seizures are those that cannot be classified in the categories above. Most are inhibitory or negative motor seizures.

The patient may experience affective or emotional behavioral phenomena (including grimacing, weeping, grunting, moaning, and screaming) not only before the seizure but also, or even only, during the event. Mixed patterns are common and represent a combination of two or more subtypes within a single patient.

One group proposed new categories for PNES classification (Dhiman et al., 2013), improving upon the previous classification mentioned above and modeled on the reported epilepsy classification. The definition and description of the proposed categories of PNES are summarized in Table 26.1.

The most widespread clinical patterns of PNES observed include "convulsive" or "thrashing," wherein

Table 26.1

A proposal for categories for the new classification of psychogenic epileptic seizures

Type	Definition	Semiologic characteristics
I. Abnormal motor response A. Hypermotor	Episode characterized by movement of the whole body (head, neck, limbs, and trunk); pelvic thrusting Trunk: opisthotonic posturing Synchronous/asynchronous Rhythmic/arrhythmic With or without response to external stimuli	1. Out-of-phase limb movements 2. Violent thrashing/grabbing/ kicking/punching movements 3. Whole-body rigidity 4. Whole-body jerky movements
B. Partial motor	Episode characterized by the involvement of a part of the body (either head and neck or limbs (upper or lower limbs, unilateral/bilateral), trunk) Combination of the above but not all together Synchronous/asynchronous Rhythmic/arrhythmic With or without response to external stimuli	1. Head and neck: side-to-side, flexion/extension movements 2. Limbs: flexion/extension abduction/adduction movements, jerking 3. Facio-pharyngeo-respiratory: coughing, gagging, hyperventilation
II. Affective/ emotional behavior phenomena	Psychic manifestations	Weeping, grimacing, screaming, moaning, grunting
III. Dialeptic type	"Coma-like state," no response to external stimuli	Coma-like state, fall, flaccidity
IV. Nonepileptic aura	Subjective feeling during the attack without any external manifestations	Dizziness, pressing "alarm button" himself/herself
V. Mixed pattern	A. Hypermotor + affective/emotional behavior phenomena B. Hypermotor + dialeptic type C. Hypermotor + nonepileptic aura D. Partial motor + affective/emotional behavior phenomena E. Partial motor + dialeptic type F. Partial motor + nonepileptic aura G. Affective/emotional behavior phenomena + dialeptic type H. Affective/emotional behavior phenomena + nonepileptic aura I. Dialeptic type + nonepileptic aura	See above

Reproduced from Dhiman et al. (2013), with permission from the publisher.

the subject becomes unresponsive with variable movements of limbs, head, and trunk (usually tremors); and "swoon/catatonic/syncope-like," wherein patients fall down and lie still, with eyes closed and unresponsive. A significant minority of patients have "dialeptic" or "absence"-like events, with the predominant symptomatology consisting of an alteration in consciousness. Another type of semiology, the "swoon" type of PNES, is more often confused with vasovagal or cardiac syncope, and tilt table testing and/or prolonged heart rhythm recordings can help identify these paroxysmal cardiovascular physiologic nonepileptic mimics of ES (Benbadis and Chichkova, 2006).

A study comparing vEEG-based diagnosis with individual semiologic signs reported by seizure witnesses identified video-documented semiologic signs that are clinically and statistically significant for distinguishing PNES and ES. The majority of signs associated with PNES and ES signs were not sensitive or specific and were not significantly associated with seizure type (Syed et al., 2011). Six signs, however, best differentiated the two seizure types during vEEG: for epilepsy: abrupt-onset, postictal confusion/sleep, eye opening or widening at onset, and for PNES: eye flutter, preserved awareness, and others can intensify or alleviate (highlighted in boxes in Figures 26.1 (for PNES) and 26.2 (for ES)).

OTHER CHARACTERISTICS TO HELP CLINICIANS DIFFERENTIATE PNES FROM ES

Other clinical factors have been considered to distinguish PNES from ES. Duration of PNES is longer than ES on

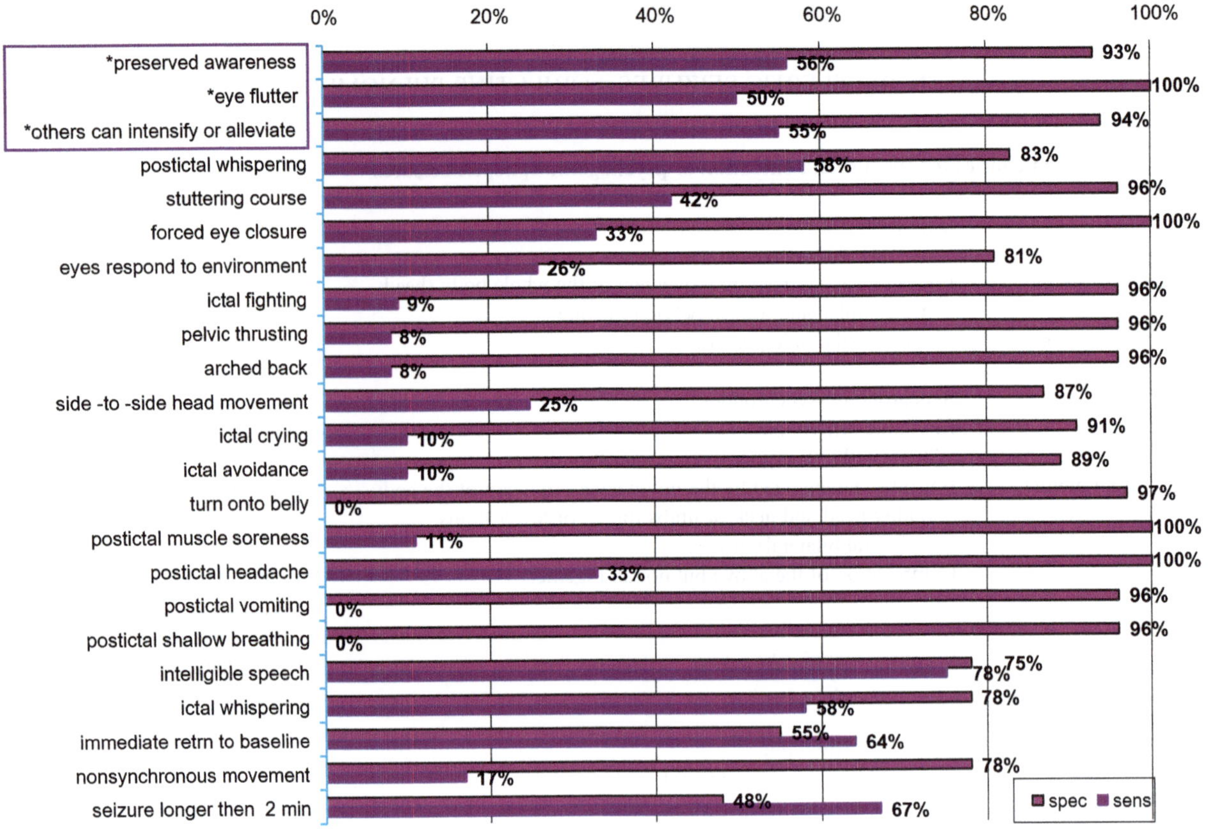

0%
20%
40%
60%
80%
100%
*preserved awareness 93% 56%
*eye flutter 100% 50%
*others can intensify or alleviate 94% 55%
postictal whispering 83% 58%
stuttering course 96% 42%
forced eye closure 100% 33%
eyes respond to environment 81% 26%
ictal fighting 96% 9%
pelvic thrusting 96% 8%
arched back 96% 8%
side -to -side head movement 87% 25%
ictal crying 91% 10%
ictal avoidance 89% 10%
turn onto belly 97% 0%
postictal muscle soreness 100% 11%
postictal headache 100% 33%
postictal vomiting 96% 0%
postictal shallow breathing 96% 0%
intelligible speech 78% 75%
ictal whispering 78% 58%
immediate retrn to baseline 55% 64%
nonsynchronous movement 78% 17%
seizure longer then 2 min 48% 67%
spec sens

Fig. 26.1. Subject-level sensitivity and specificity of video-documented signs for identification of psychogenic epileptic seizures (PNES) (based on 36 PNES from 12 subjects). Values are derived from original cohort, except for the four PNES signs that were tested in the validation cohort. $*p<0.05$, according to seizure-level analysis (generalized estimating equations) in original and validation cohorts. sens, sensitivity; spec, specificity. (Reproduced from Syed et al., 2011, with permission.)

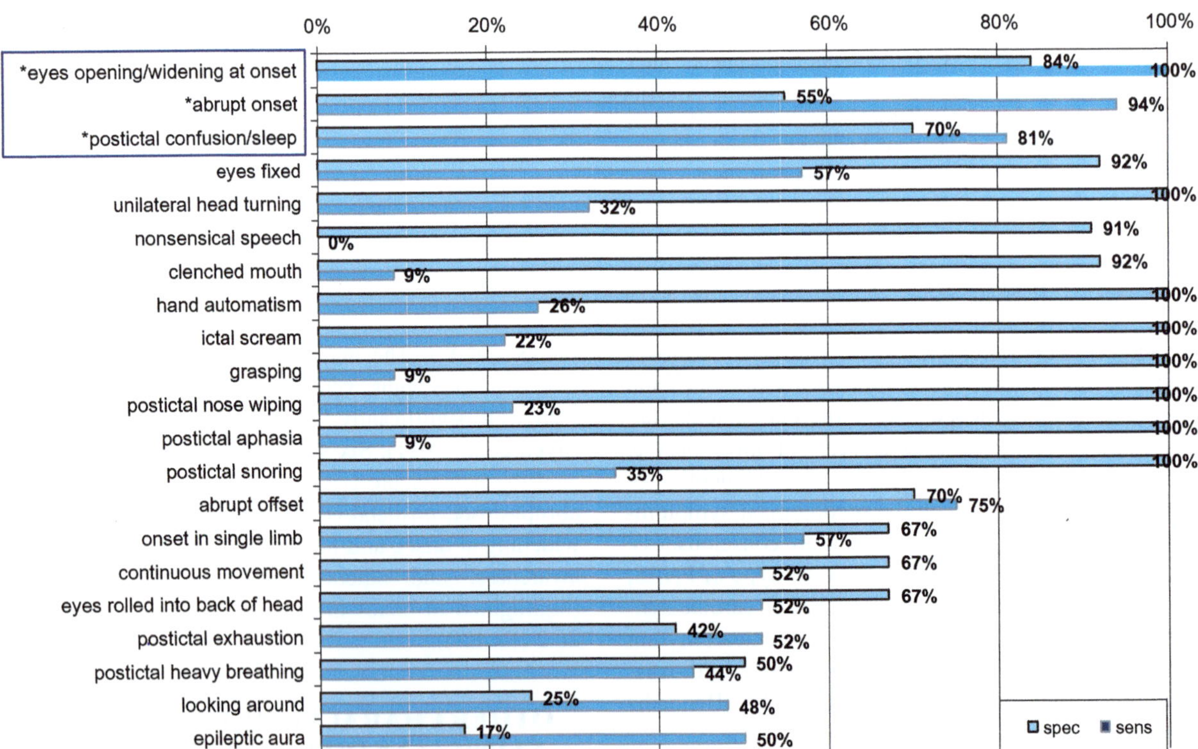

Fig. 26.2. Subject-level sensitivity and specificity of video-documented signs for identification of epileptic seizures (ES) (based on 84 ES from 23 subjects). Values are derived from original cohort, except for the four ES signs that were tested in the validation cohort. $*p<0.05$ according to seizure-level analysis (generalized estimating equations) in original and validation cohorts. sens, sensitivity; spec, specificity. (Reproduced from Syed et al., 2011, with permission.)

average, and seizures lasting longer than 2 minutes with semiology consistent with PNES should be examined for the possibility of PNES. A sudden motionless unresponsive episode with eyes closed lasting 2 minutes or more is pathognomonic of PNES, as well. Seizures with a duration of >10 minutes that are not consistent with status epilepticus semiology more strongly suggest PNES. Out-of-phase limb movements and side-to-side head movements, especially with coordinated alternating agonist and antagonist activity, are also highly suggestive of PNES. Vocalization in PNES occurs during or after seizures, and may be complex, with affective content. In contrast, vocalization in ES usually occurs at seizure onset, and is primitive (e.g., grunting) (Devinsky et al., 2011; Dhiman et al., 2013).

Semiology can help reduce diagnostic delay of PNES if eyewitnesses can recall and report whether or not seizure-specific signs have actually occurred in patients' seizures. Unfortunately, seizure witnesses provide unreliable accounts of seizure semiology (Syed et al., 2011). Practitioners can educate family members to carefully observe seizure onset, including patients' eyes, and to assess their level of awareness. For example, by observing patient responses to verbal commands during seizures, they may increase report accuracy. It is also relevant for family to assess their interaction with patients during subsequent seizures to see if, in fact, seizures consistently intensify or subside in response to others' prompts. Acquisition of home video recordings of seizures is of value and may lessen the need to rely on eyewitness reports and should be encouraged.

Other clinical features may also raise the suspicion of PNES. Three-fourths of patients with PNES are women in civilian studies. Up to 50% of patients report a precipitating event for their seizures. Many patients with PNES have other psychogenic neurologic disorders. Up to 70% of patients report antecedent trauma, which is of a sexual nature in up to 40% (Bowman and Markand, 1996). Current or previous mental health and psychosocial problems such as posttraumatic stress disorder, other anxiety disorders, dissociative disorders, depression, personality disorders, and pain symptoms are frequently encountered in patients with PNES (Kanner et al., 2012). Medical comorbidities (Dixit et al., 2013), chronic pain (Gazzola et al., 2012), and somatic complaints (Testa et al., 2011) are also common in PNES.

Another difference between patients with PNES and ES is the age of onset of the seizures, with older mean age of onset in the PNES group (onset in 20s in PNES and teens in ES) (Ettinger et al., 1999; Hoepner et al., 2014). Event frequency is higher in patients with PNES than those with epilepsy (Jedrzejczak et al., 1999). Recurrent hospital admissions with apparent status, daily convulsive events, or the predisposition to have seizures in medical settings, such as in scanners and during consultations, suggest PNES (McGonigal et al., 2002). Lengthy periods of apparent remission from seizures followed by relapse and resumption of frequent events may be more consistent with PNES. None of these are pathognomonic of PNES, as ES can present similarly. As noted above, the combination of history, semiology, and EEG/vEEG establishes the PNES diagnosis.

A variety of physical triggers can be associated with ES or syncope; however, some, such as change in lighting conditions and visual activities that are not usually associated with ES or syncope, may be reported by patients with PNES (LaFrance et al., 2013). Conventional activation procedures, including photic stimulation and hyperventilation, can provoke PNES during EEG recording (Leis et al., 1992), along with provoking seizures in specific forms of epilepsy.

There are few data about the different characteristics of the ictal events in patients who have both ES and nonepileptic seizures, compared with those who have only a single type of seizure. Table 26.2 enumerates symptoms occurring in patients with ES, PNES, or both.

Some studies have tried to associate personality types with semiologic subtypes of PNES. Psychologic tests can help to identify and characterize psychopathology in patients with PNES and sometimes are administered during vEEG monitoring. Neuropsychologic batteries and personality measures, however, do not distinguish patients with PNES from those with epilepsy (Harden et al., 2009; Tremont et al., 2012).

There are a few published studies based upon analysis of the Personality Assessment Inventory (PAI), a self-report personality survey assessing dimensions of adult psychopathology. PAI profiles of groups with PNES or with epilepsy were clinically elevated on somatic complaints, anxiety, depression, schizophrenia, and borderline personality features. Patients with PNES were characterized by higher levels of alexithymia (Myers et al., 2013) and scored higher than those with ES on somatic complaints and stress on the Somatic Complaints subscales of Conversion (SOM-C) and Somatization (SOM-S) and in the Physiological Anxiety subscale. The Health Concerns scale did not differ between PNES and ES, but both groups had higher levels of concern about their well-being compared to the healthy population.

Other centers have used the Minnesota Multiphasic Personality Inventory-2 (MMPI-2) to examine a relationship between semiology and psychologic profiles and are mostly negative. These studies are small in size (catatonic: $n=4$, minor motor: $n=6$, major motor: $n=21$) and have not yet been validated (Griffith et al., 2007). Also of note is that the MMPI-2 differences are not able to distinguish between individuals with ES and those with PNES.

Table 26.2

Semiologic and exam features that can help distinguish psychogenic nonepileptic seizures from epileptic seizures

Distinguishing semiologic or exam features	Psychogenic nonepileptic seizures	Epileptic seizures
Emergence out of EEG-confirmed sleep	Rare	Common
Concurrent tongue biting (severe, side of tongue) and urinary incontinence	Rare	Common after GTC
Ictal dystonic posture with contralateral automatisms	Not present	Occurs in mesial TLE
Ictal figure-of-four sign	Not present	Occurs in TLE
Ictal fencing posture	Not present	Occurs in mesial FLE
Ictal grasping (gripping of an object with one hand or both hands)	Rare	Occurs in FLE and TLE
Postictal stertorous breathing	Not present	Common after GTC
Postictal nose rubbing	Not present	Occurs in TLE
Impaired corneal reflex	Not present	Common after GTC
Extensor plantar response	Not present	Common after GTC
Closed eyelid during peak of ictus	Very common	Rare
Gradual onset and prolonged duration	Common	Rare
Undulating motor activity	Common	Very rare
Asynchronous limb movements	Common	Rare
Side-to-side head shaking	Common	Rare
Ictal or postictal whispering/stuttering	Common	Rare
Ictal signs of emotional distress (e.g., grimacing, weeping)	Common	Rare
Pelvic thrusting	Sometimes	Rare
Memory recall for period of unresponsiveness	Sometimes	Rare
Resisted eyelid opening	Common	Very rare
Guarding of hand dropping over face	Common	Rare

Modified from Benbadis and LaFrance (2010).
EEG, electroencephalogram; GTC, generalized tonic-clonic seizures; TLE, temporal-lobe epilepsy; FLE, frontal-lobe epilepsy.

CONCLUSIONS

In summary, the differential diagnosis of PNES can be quite challenging; however, eyewitness history, reviewing the event through home video, and vEEG monitoring yield a higher level of confidence in establishing the diagnosis. Recognizing more subtle presentations of ES from PNES, especially ES associated with frontal-lobe epilepsy, can be problematic. Such frontal-lobe ES usually consists of short-duration events with stereotyped tonic posturing and with the ictus arising out of electrographic sleep and may be easily misdiagnosed as PNES (LaFrance and Benbadis, 2011).

Specific PNES seizure semiology may be less helpful to understanding its proximate causes or to informing its treatment, but semiology is especially relevant to distinguishing ES from nonepileptic seizures. Another significant aspect of semiology relates to aura identification, which can be potentially quite valuable for treatment of PNES. Recovery is possible when patients take control of their seizures by learning how to cope with their personal trauma or emotion and addressing fear and anxiety (LaFrance and Wincze, 2015). To achieve that goal and to reduce seizure frequency, the patient can learn to identify and recognize prodromal symptoms, auras, and major life stressors. At the onset of the seizure, the patient can implement the tools learned in therapy to hopefully stop the seizure from progressing, or to prevent seizures altogether (Reiter et al., 2015). The treatment of PNES is covered in more depth in Chapter 27.

REFERENCES

Avbersek A, Sisodiya S (2010). Does the primary literature provide support for clinical signs used to distinguish psychogenic nonepileptic seizures from epileptic seizures? J Neurol Neurosurg Psychiatry 81 (7): 719–725.

Benbadis SR, Chichkova R (2006). Psychogenic pseudosyncope: an underestimated and provable diagnosis. Epilepsy Behav 9 (1): 106–110.

Benbadis SR, LaFrance Jr WC (2010). Chapter 4. Clinical features and the role of video-EEG monitoring. In: SC Schachter, WC LaFrance Jr (Eds.), Gates and Rowan's Nonepileptic Seizures, Cambridge University Press, Cambridge, pp. 38–50.

Benbadis SR, Agrawal V, Tatum 4th WO (2001). How many patients with psychogenic nonepileptic seizures also have epilepsy? Neurology 57 (5): 915–917.

Benbadis SR, O'Neill E, Tatum WO et al. (2004). Outcome of prolonged video-EEG monitoring at a typical referral epilepsy center. Epilepsia 45 (9): 1150–1153.

Bowman ES, Markand ON (1996). Psychodynamics and psychiatric diagnoses of pseudoseizure subjects. Am J Psychiatry 153 (1): 57–63.

Devinsky O, Gazzola D, LaFrance Jr WC (2011). Differentiating between nonepileptic and epileptic seizures. Nat Rev Neurol 7 (4): 210–220.

Dhiman V, Sinha S, Rawat VS et al. (2013). Semiological characteristics of adults with psychogenic nonepileptic seizures (PNESs): an attempt towards a new classification. Epilepsy Behav 27 (3): 427–432.

Dixit R, Popescu A, Bagic A et al. (2013). Medical comorbidities in patients with psychogenic nonepileptic spells (PNES) referred for video-EEG monitoring. Epilepsy Behav 28 (2): 137–140.

Ettinger AB, Devinsky O, Weisbrot DM et al. (1999). A comprehensive profile of clinical, psychiatric, and psychosocial characteristics of patients with psychogenic nonepileptic seizures. Epilepsia 40 (9): 1292–1298.

Gates JR (2000). Epidemiology and classification of non-epileptic events. In: JR Gates, AJ Rowan (Eds.), Non-Epileptic Seizures, Butterworth-Heinemann, Boston, pp. 3–14.

Gazzola DM, Carlson C, Rugina A et al. (2012). Psychogenic nonepileptic seizures and chronic pain: a retrospective case-controlled study. Epilepsy Behav 25 (4): 662–665.

Goldstein LH, Mellers JD (2012). Recent developments in our understanding of the semiology and treatment of psychogenic nonepileptic seizures. Curr Neurol Neurosci Rep 12 (4): 436–444.

Gordon PC, Valiengo Lda C, Proenca IC et al. (2014). Comorbid epilepsy and psychogenic non-epileptic seizures: how well do patients and caregivers distinguish between the two? Seizure 23 (7): 537–541.

Griffith NM, Szaflarski JP, Schefft BK et al. (2007). Relationship between semiology of psychogenic nonepileptic seizures and Minnesota Multiphasic Personality Inventory profile. Epilepsy Behav 11 (1): 105–111.

Gröppel G, Kapitany T, Baumgartner C (2000). Cluster analysis of clinical seizure semiology of psychogenic nonepileptic seizures. Epilepsia 41 (5): 610–614.

Harden CL, Jovine L, Burgut FT et al. (2009). A comparison of personality disorder characteristics of patients with nonepileptic psychogenic pseudoseizures with those of patients with epilepsy. Epilepsy Behav 14 (3): 481–483.

Hoepner R, Labudda K, May TW et al. (2014). Distinguishing between patients with pure psychogenic nonepileptic seizures and those with comorbid epilepsy by means of clinical data. Epilepsy Behav 35: 54–58.

Hubsch C, Baumann C, Hingray C et al. (2011). Clinical classification of psychogenic non-epileptic seizures based on video-EEG analysis and automatic clustering. J Neurol Neurosurg Psychiatry 82 (9): 955–960.

Jedrzejczak J, Owczarek K (1999). Majkowski J Psychogenic pseudoepileptic seizures: clinical and electroencephalogram (EEG) video-tape recordings. Eur J Neurol 6 (4): 473–479.

Kanner AM, Schachter SC, Barry JJ et al. (2012). Depression and epilepsy, pain and psychogenic non-epileptic seizures: clinical and therapeutic perspectives. Epilepsy Behav 24 (2): 169–181.

LaFrance Jr WC, Benbadis SR (2011). Differentiating frontal lobe epilepsy from psychogenic nonepileptic seizures. Neurol Clin 29 (1): 149–162. ix.

LaFrance Jr WC, Devinsky O (2002). Treatment of nonepileptic seizures. Epilepsy Behav 3 (5 Supplement 1): S19–S23.

LaFrance Jr WC, Syc S (2009). Depression and symptoms affect quality of life in psychogenic nonepileptic seizures. Neurology 73 (5): 366–371.

LaFrance Jr WC, Wincze J (2015). Treating Nonepieptic Seizures: Therapist Guide, Oxford University Press, New York.

LaFrance Jr WC, Baker GA, Duncan R et al. (2013). Minimum requirements for the diagnosis of psychogenic nonepileptic seizures: a staged approach: a report from the International League Against Epilepsy Nonepileptic Seizures Task Force. Epilepsia 54 (11): 2005–2018.

Leis AA, Ross MA, Summers AK (1992). Psychogenic seizures: ictal characteristics and diagnostic pitfalls. Neurology 42 (1): 95–99.

Lüders H, Acharya J, Baumgartner C et al. (1998). Semiological seizure classification. Epilepsia 39 (9): 1006–1013.

Martin RC, Gilliam FG, Kilgore M et al. (1998). Improved health care resource utilization following video-EEG-confirmed diagnosis of nonepileptic psychogenic seizures. Seizure 7 (5): 385–390.

McGonigal A, Oto M, Russell AJ et al. (2002). Outpatient video EEG recording in the diagnosis of non-epileptic seizures: a randomised controlled trial of simple suggestion techniques. J Neurol Neurosurg Psychiatry 72 (4): 549–551.

Meierkord H, Will B, Fish D et al. (1991). The clinical features and prognosis of pseudoseizures diagnosed using video-EEG telemetry. Neurology 41 (10): 1643–1646.

Mostacci B, Bisulli F, Alvisi L et al. (2011). Ictal characteristics of psychogenic nonepileptic seizures: what we have learned from video/EEG recordings – a literature review. Epilepsy Behav 22 (2): 144–153.

Myers L, Matzner B, Lancman M et al. (2013). Prevalence of alexithymia in patients with psychogenic non-epileptic seizures and epileptic seizures and predictors in psychogenic non-epileptic seizures. Epilepsy Behav 26 (2): 153–157.

Niedermeyer E, Blumer D, Holscher E et al. (1970). Classical hysterical seizures facilitated by anticonvulsant toxicity. Psychiatr Clin (Basel) 3 (2): 71–84.

Reiter J, Andrews D, Reiter C et al. (2015). Taking Control of Your Seizures: Workbook, Oxford University Press, New York.

Reuber M, Fernandez G, Bauer J et al. (2002). Diagnostic delay in psychogenic nonepileptic seizures. Neurology 58 (3): 493–495.

Salinsky M, Spencer D, Boudreau E et al. (2011). Psychogenic nonepileptic seizures in US veterans. Neurology 77 (10): 945–950.

Seneviratne U, Reutens D, D'Souza W (2010). Stereotypy of psychogenic nonepileptic seizures: insights from video-EEG monitoring. Epilepsia 51 (7): 1159–1168.

Syed TU, LaFrance Jr WC, Kahriman ES et al. (2011). Can semiology predict psychogenic nonepileptic seizures? A prospective study. Ann Neurol 69 (6): 997–1004.

Szabo L, Siegler Z, Zubek L et al. (2012). A detailed semiologic analysis of childhood psychogenic nonepileptic seizures. Epilepsia 53 (3): 565–570.

Testa SM, Lesser RP, Krauss GL et al. (2011). Personality Assessment Inventory among patients with psychogenic seizures and those with epilepsy. Epilepsia 52 (8): e84–e88.

Tremont G, Smith MM, Bauer L et al. (2012). Comparison of personality characteristics on the Bear-Fedio Inventory between patients with epilepsy and non-epileptic seizures. J Neuropsych Clin Neurosc 24 (1): 47–52.

Handbook of Clinical Neurology, Vol. 139 (3rd series)
Functional Neurologic Disorders
M. Hallett, J. Stone, and A. Carson, Editors
http://dx.doi.org/10.1016/B978-0-12-801772-2.00027-8

Chapter 27

Psychogenic nonepileptic seizures: EEG and investigation

R. DUNCAN*
Department of Neurology, University of Otago and Department of Neurology, Christchurch Hospital, Christchurch, New Zealand

Abstract

In the investigation of psychogenic nonepileptic seizures (PNES), the main differential diagnoses are between convulsive PNES and tonic-clonic seizures, between swoon PNES and syncope, and between pseudoabsence PNES and absence seizures. For the best diagnostic certainty, events must be captured, ideally using video-electroencephalogram (EEG), including an electrocardiographic channel. The "video" part of video-EEG allows EEG changes (or lack of them) to be interpreted in the appropriate clinical context. When the diagnosis is based on less good data (e.g., video alone or EEG alone), then the limitations and constraints of the tests should borne in mind, and a lesser degree of certainty must be accepted. Tests such as serum prolactin (PRL) level and postictal EEG should be regarded as adjunctive rather than definitive. Excluding additional epilepsy with a good probability is not possible using investigations alone. In particular, one standard interictal EEG recording is of little value in excluding additional epilepsy, though multiple or prolonged recordings may offer additional sensitivity.

INTRODUCTION

Commonly used operational definitions of psychogenic nonepileptic seizures (PNES) stipulate that they resemble or may be mistaken for epileptic seizures (Lesser, 1996), the implication being the differential diagnosis is with epileptic seizures. This is partly true, but a more precise statement of the differential diagnosis would be:

1. The main differential diagnosis of convulsive-type PNES is a tonic-clonic seizure.
2. The main differential diagnosis of swoon-type (fall down, lie still, eyes closed, unresponsive) PNES is probably not any type of epileptic seizure, but syncope, either vasovagal or cardiac.
3. The main differential diagnosis of "pseudoabsence"-type PNES is an absence or complex partial seizure.

This chapter is written with these differential diagnoses in mind.

Confirming the diagnosis of paroxysmal disorders can be challenging, as tests that are carried out between events or attacks are generally of limited use. Those tests that are most sensitive and specific require that the event in question be recorded on video, electroencephalogram (EEG), electrocardiogram (ECG), or some combination of those. As we will see below, it is essential to understand that the results of such tests must be interpreted in the clinical context, particularly in the light of the clinical semiology of the recorded event. In many patients with PNES, it is surprisingly easy to record events. However, some patients have events less frequently, or tend not to have them in observed or monitored settings. In that case, the diagnosis may have to rest on some less-than-ideal combination of test data and clinical data.

In principle, nonetheless, investigational strategy should start from the point of attempting to obtain the best data: video-EEG-ECG recordings of as many events as possible. When this is difficult to achieve and compromise is being considered, it is useful to remember that it is not just the doctor who has to be convinced. Patients with PNES and their relatives are not always receptive to the diagnosis, so test data that are less than ideal may be enough for the doctor but may fail to convince patients

*Correspondence to: Roderick Duncan, MD, PhD, FRCP, University of Otago, Christchurch, New Zealand, Department of Neurology, Christchurch Hospital, Private Bag 4710, Christchurch 8001, New Zealand. Tel: +64-33-640-940, E-mail: Roderick.Duncan@cdhb.health.nz

or relatives, potentially making management difficult. In this regard, video-EEG data (which, for the rest of this chapter, will be assumed to include an ECG channel) is unequivocally best. It can be straightforwardly and honestly presented to patients and relatives as gold standard and, if a few known situations are excluded, watertight.

INPATIENT VIDEO-EEG MONITORING

The diagnosis of PNES is best confirmed by recording events simultaneously on video and EEG/ECG, finding an absence of ictal EEG changes (and, importantly, the presence of normal awake EEG rhythms) before, during, and after the event. With the exception of sinus tachycardia (which is often seen in association with convulsive PNES), the same applies to ECG rhythm.

If these conditions are met, a positive diagnosis of the recorded event can be made in the great majority of cases. To state the obvious, in order to identify EEG rhythms during an event, the EEG must be visible through movement artefact. This is not always so in convulsive PNES, nor in epileptic seizures. Nonetheless, gaps in movement artefact usually allow identification of EEG rhythms during at least part of a convulsive event, and the immediate emergence of normal rhythms (or not) when movements cease is often sufficient to confirm the diagnosis. It is probably worth stating that this applies equally to "pseudoabsence"-type PNES, seen in a minority of patients (Duncan and Oto, 2008). Any epileptic seizure resulting in the semiologic picture of "motionless unresponsive stare" would straightforwardly be expected to show clear EEG change. Therefore, a normal awake EEG during such an event excludes epileptic seizure.

There are a few uncommon, but well-known, clinical situations where the absence of EEG change during an event does not necessarily indicate PNES, or where video-EEG data should be interpreted with particular care:

Simple partial seizures

Simple partial seizures, consisting of jerking movements restricted to a small part of the musculature, or consisting of a subjective experience only, are not usually accompanied by detectable surface EEG change (Kanner et al., 1990). The diagnostic problem is, however, much simplified by the fact that these are not clinical forms usually taken by PNES. In some patients, especially those with a learning difficulty, simple partial seizures that manifest as ictal experiences (such as abdominal auras, auditory experiences, or fear) may cause distress and provoke behaviors that may be mistaken for PNES (Devinsky and Gordon, 1998). If that is suspected, investigational strategy would then be to record multiple examples of the events in question. Such simple partial seizures often vary in the extent of their propagation, and eventually one may be recorded that is sufficiently severe to show some surface EEG change (in which event the video will often show a more clinically obvious seizure).

Hypermotor frontal-lobe seizures

Hypermotor frontal-lobe seizures (HFLS) are often not associated with detectable EEG change at the surface, either because change is not present or because the EEG is obscured by movement artefact. However, when video data are available, the difficulty is much less: as with simple partial seizures, the clinical semiology of HFLS is quite different from that of PNES (Kanner et al., 1990; Saygi et al., 1992). They often arise exclusively from sleep, and they are much shorter than PNES (tens of seconds, rather than minutes or tens of minutes): one study found that the ranges of duration of PNES and HFLS not only differed but did not overlap. The movements in HFLS are semi-coordinated, with high-amplitude movements of proximal musculature (producing wild, flailing, or kicking movements): tremors (the main movement associated with convulsive PNES) are usually absent. Thus, while the EEG may not immediately identify these events as seizures, the video usually does.

"Swoon"-type events

It is less common to record "swoon"-type events in the video-EEG unit, whether they are due to PNES, vasovagal syncope, or cardiac syncope (most will be due to PNES). Epileptic seizure is not usually in the differential diagnosis for clinical reasons (see Introduction, above), and cardiac syncope can be easily excluded by the ECG. However, the distinction between PNES and vasovagal syncope may occasionally be difficult. The EEG flattens or slows during many (Amirati et al., 1998), but not all, syncopal events, and the changes may be subtle. The ECG will usually show a period of sinus bradycardia, but again the change may not be clearcut. In that event, the diagnosis will rest on clinical features obtained from the history and from the video recording. The clinical duration of the recorded event is often helpful. In vasovagal syncope, once the patient is horizontal, rapid recovery is the rule, within seconds or tens of seconds. Swoon-type PNES usually last a number of minutes, sometimes tens of minutes (Gates et al., 1991; Jedrzejczak et al., 1999).

Tilt table testing

Some patients with a swoon presentation may undergo (or have undergone) tilt table testing, with the aim of confirming or refuting a diagnosis of vasovagal syncope. It is wise to evaluate the results of this carefully in the context of suspected PNES. The prevalence of syncope in the general population is high, much higher than PNES. It is therefore not uncommon to provoke vasovagal syncope in a patient with swoon-type PNES: if care is not taken to ensure that the symptomatology (especially prodromal symptoms and duration of loss of consciousness) of the provoked event matches that of the events occurring in everyday life (see below), then swoon-type PNES can be misdiagnosed as vasovagal syncope.

The need to capture habitual events

Crucially, the investigating doctor must always remember that video-EEG data relate directly only to the event that has been recorded. A positive identification of an event can be extrapolated to events occurring in daily life by showing the video recording to an eyewitness, by comparing video recordings to eyewitness accounts, and by ensuring that the subjective manifestations of the event are recognized by the patient as what always occurs. In the literature, the phrase "habitual event" is often used. In reality, "only event" might be a better term. You should seek to establish that the recorded event is the one that the patient *always* has. A report even of one event among many that does not correspond to the recorded event raises the possibility of a dual diagnosis. A second event type, even if single or rare, should be evaluated carefully and recorded if possible (see below).

In summary, the video part of video-EEG must not be forgotten. Recordings should be evaluated in the context of the clinical form taken by the events. Care must be taken in the video-EEG evaluation of any event that does not correspond with common PNES semiology, or that is not associated with amnesia reported by the patient, nor with observed unresponsiveness (i.e., when simple partial seizure might be clinically credible). Events that appear strange and bizarre are in fact quite likely to be epileptic (usually, but not always, HFLS), even if not accompanied by visible EEG change.

THE USE OF VIDEO-EEG IN PRACTICE

Video-EEG recording is usually carried out in the setting of an epilepsy monitoring unit. When considering the duration of monitoring, some factors should be taken into consideration. The majority of patients with PNES will produce an event within the first few hours of video-EEG recording (Ettinger et al., 1999), and monitoring beyond 2 days probably stands a rather low chance of capturing PNES, if that is the main diagnostic suspicion. If there is a clinical indication of additional epileptic seizures, or if antiepileptic drugs (AEDs) have to be withdrawn, then a longer monitoring period will be required. To maximize yield, ordinary provocation techniques can be used: photic stimulation and hyperventilation are useful for provoking both epileptic seizures and PNES (McGonigal et al., 2002). The use of other induction techniques, ranging from simple verbal suggestion to injection of saline, may improve the rate of capture of PNES (McGonigal et al., 2002, 2004; Benbadis et al., 2004; Varela et al., 2007). Ethical concerns have been raised with saline injections and placebo wipes (Stagno and Smith, 1997), but the routine activation procedures (Benbadis et al., 2000) are uncontroversial. The same applies to simple verbal suggestion techniques if the patient is clearly informed of what is being done and why (this does not seem to prevent patients from having events during recording: McGonigal et al., 2002). Preliminary data evaluating video-EEG monitoring at home suggest that this might be useful in some patients (Brunnhuber et al., 2014), though as yet experience is limited.

Short-duration outpatient video-EEG monitoring

Before arranging to admit the patient to hospital, two alternative ways of obtaining "ideal" data should be considered, depending on the clinical indication and on what is available.

First, it is often useful to carry out a routine outpatient EEG recording, preferably with a video monitor (increasingly, this is standard in EEG systems). Up to 30% of patients suspected of having PNES will have a diagnostic event during a standard EEG recording, especially if the standard activating procedures are used (McGonigal et al., 2002). The data are easiest to interpret if an eyewitness to the patient's events is present, and efforts should be made to ensure this is the case, so that even if video is not available, then the clinical identity of the event and its compatibility with previous events can be established. Of course, a routine EEG may also helpfully provide interictal evidence of epilepsy (see below).

Second, if appropriate skills are available, it may be worth carrying out a standard outpatient EEG recording with the addition of some simple verbal suggestion to increase the probability of recording a PNES (McGonigal et al., 2002, 2004; Benbadis et al., 2004; Varela et al., 2007). A randomized controlled trial of such simple techniques added to standard EEG with hyperventilation and photic stimulation suggested that they added approximately 30% to diagnostic yield and can avoid hospital admission in up to half of patients (McGonigal et al., 2004). The technique used in that study consisted of some simple reinforcement at the point of referral for the test (i.e., the referring doctor emphasized the probability that the patient would have an event at the time of the test – since shown to be effective in increasing yield: Hoepner et al., 2013), the technician going through the subjective semiology of the events with the patient at the time of the test, and giving simple encouragement to focus on symptoms during the recording, in particular during hyperventilation. Even when a full event is not captured, in many patients the initial symptoms of the events can be convincingly reproduced by hyperventilation, sometimes allowing a diagnosis to be made if other data are sufficiently supportive.

If no event is recorded using short outpatient video-EEG with suggestion, should you then go on to longer-term video-EEG? Clinical experience suggests that there is a low probability of capturing an event in that circumstance, but longer-term recording may nonetheless be indicated if a diagnosis of epilepsy remains in play. An epileptic seizure may be captured, and the multiple circadian interictal EEG recordings offered by a period of video-EEG probably have the best chance of detecting interictal evidence of epilepsy (see below).

Home video monitoring

If video-EEG is not available or fails to capture an event, then the next best option is to attempt to capture events on video or on EEG alone. Video recording is of course widely available to patients and their relatives, and it has become common in clinical practice for patients to attend the first consultation already supplied with a smartphone containing a video recording of the event, especially if events are frequent. This can allow a positive identification of the events in many cases, especially when events include motor activity (King et al., 1982; Chen et al., 2008). One important limitation of home video recordings is that they seldom capture the whole of the event, and almost never capture the beginning of them, for obvious practical reasons. It is important to bear in mind, in this context, that the postictal phase of epileptic seizures can involve some rather PNES-like behaviors. The obvious example of this is that patients may lie still and unresponsive for some time after an epileptic seizure, especially, but not exclusively, a major one. Thus, a video may seem to have captured a swoon-type PNES, but has missed the preceding epileptic seizure. In the worst case, the eyewitness may not actually have seen the beginning of the attack, so any indication of a preceding seizure is lacking. Therefore, the video recording may show the patient lying still, unresponsive (i.e., semiology compatible with PNES), but you do not know whether that "behavior" is all the event consists of, or whether it has been preceded by semiology compatible with an epileptic seizure.

Ambulatory EEG monitoring

Ambulatory EEG recording is not very widely used in the differential diagnosis of epileptic seizures and PNES. This is mainly because of the lack of clinical correlation for the EEG. This can be overcome to a degree if the patient has relatives who are capable of keeping a good event diary, and have given detailed event descriptions. If some home video footage of events is also available, then that can provide a reasonably secure diagnosis in many cases. Ambulatory EEG is particularly useful in patients who have attacks in certain situations only. The most common of such situations is in teenagers who may have attacks only at school. The other situation in which ambulatory EEG may be useful is in the relative minority of patients with PNES who appear to behave as if they are avoiding a diagnosis, with frequent (e.g., daily or more) events outside hospital but none when monitored in hospital. Some such patients do not have events on ambulatory monitoring, even when the reported event frequency is many per day. If this happens repeatedly, the doctor may have to infer the diagnosis from the absence of a credible medical reason for such an event pattern.

Serum prolactin estimation

Elevated serum PRL can provide useful adjunctive evidence in distinguishing convulsive PNES from tonic-clonic seizures. The absence of postictal PRL rise predicts PNES with a mean sensitivity to PNES of 89% across the studies (Cragar et al., 2002) and serum PRL levels are elevated in 88% of cases of generalized tonic-clonic seizures. False-positive PRL tests may occur in patients on dopamine antagonists, tricyclic antidepressants, breast stimulation, and syncope. False negatives can occur in patients on dopamine agonists, with status epilepticus (PRL rise may not persist with repeated or continuous seizures: Bauer, 1996), with frontal-lobe and some complex partial seizures. Equivocal rises in prolactin level are common, so the test should be based on a minimum twofold rise 10–20 minutes after the event, compared with several hours later (or beforehand, if possible).

The error rate in this test is such that it should probably be thought of as a "suspicion-raising" test, or an adjunctive test that can be used when better data are not available. It would be difficult, for example, to convincingly communicate the diagnosis of PNES to a skeptical patient or relative on the basis of clinical opinion and a test with an error rate of 11% or 12%.

Postictal EEG recording

Postictal EEG recording should also be thought of as an adjunctive or suspicion-raising test. There are no good data on its sensitivity or specificity as a test to distinguish PNES from epileptic seizures. Usually, however, tonic-clonic and complex partial seizures are followed by a period of slowing of EEG rhythms, relative to the interictal record. Slowing of EEG rhythms is more likely to be seen if the recording is very soon (minutes) after the seizure, if the seizure has been prolonged, or if there have been multiple seizures. Therefore the suspicion of PNES is stronger when the EEG is normal in those circumstances. For obvious reasons, this test is more useful and reliable when positive than when negative.

Additional epilepsy: using EEG as a screening test

With earlier recognition of PNES, many patients now present before being started on AEDs. Few such patients turn out to have additional epilepsy (Duncan et al., 2011), and unless there is clinical reason to suspect it (e.g., from attack descriptions), then screening for additional epilepsy using interictal EEG is probably unwise: the positive predictive value of EEG is low in this type of population, so screening in the absence of clinical indication will yield few positives (in this context, "positive" tests being restricted to those showing epileptiform abnormalities), and a relatively high proportion of those positives will be false positives.

In the more general population of patients with longstanding PNES, approximately 10–15% turn out to have additional epilepsy (Benbadis et al., 2001), rising to approximately 30% if the patient has a learning disability (Duncan and Oto, 2008). This PNES population, therefore, has a higher prevalence of epilepsy than the normal population, so a positive EEG is more likely to occur, and is more likely to be a true positive. Many such patients have already had one or more interictal EEG recordings by the time a diagnosis of PNES is considered but, if not, it is a reasonable initial test for additional epilepsy, remembering that a negative result is uninformative (see below).

Additional epilepsy – using EEG to exclude it

To what degree can normal interictal EEG exclude epilepsy? This probably depends on the duration of the recording: long or repeated interictal EEG recordings and the inclusion of sleep periods all increase the sensitivity of EEG in the diagnosis of epilepsy (Faulkner et al., 2012), and will likely increase its negative predictive value. Four or 5 days of video-EEG gives a large sample of interictal EEG, as well as a number of prolonged sleep recordings. While this gives the best available investigational evidence of the absence of epilepsy, the exact negative predictive value of the absence of epileptiform activity during a 5-day (or shorter) video-EEG monitoring period is unknown, and it needs to be borne in mind that approximately 8% of patients with epilepsy are thought never to have interictal discharges (Goodin and Aminof, 1984). Importantly, some drugs may suppress interictal epileptiform discharges, particularly in primary generalized epilepsies. This includes sodium valproate and levetiracetam, barbiturates, and benzodiazepines (Pedley et al., 2003; Van Cott and Brenner, 2003). The last two are associated with specific withdrawal problems, including a risk of withdrawal epileptic seizures. It may be necessary to monitor EEG during and after withdrawal, particularly if a primary generalized epilepsy is a possibility. Examples of EEG in a patient with both PNES and epilepsy are shown in Figure 27.1.

Overinterpretation of nonepileptiform interictal EEG abnormalities

The above figures for specificity and sensitivity of EEG are based on the finding of epileptiform abnormalities. False-positive errors increase with overinterpretation of nonspecific abnormalities, a well-known problem and one of the most common reasons for diagnostic error in patients thought to have refractory epilepsy (Smith et al., 1992; Benbadis and Tatum, 2003; Benbadis, 2007). Straightforwardly nonspecific EEG abnormalities should be ignored in the present context.

THE VALUE OF MEDIUM-TERM RESIDENTIAL MONITORING

In some countries there exist medium-term assessment centers that allow extended EEG monitoring and observation, with withdrawal of AEDs where appropriate. These facilities are of most value where shorter-term video-EEG monitoring and other measures have failed to produce a diagnosis, when AEDs have to be withdrawn in patients in whom the risk of additional epilepsy is difficult to define, or where behavioral problems make diagnosis difficult (Duncan and Oto, 2010). Particularly useful in this context are monitoring systems that use ambulatory EEG sets in conjunction with synchronized closed-circuit television recording throughout the center. This allows extended monitoring periods, during which the patient can move freely in all areas under video surveillance.

CONCLUSIONS

A range of tests can be used to support or confirm the diagnosis of PNES, but the results of those tests must be interpreted in their clinical context. The ideal test is video-EEG, though the choice of test is often modified by practical circumstance, and the investigating doctor needs to have a flexible approach. While EEG can help in diagnosing additional epilepsy, exclusion of additional epilepsy is not possible on investigational grounds alone.

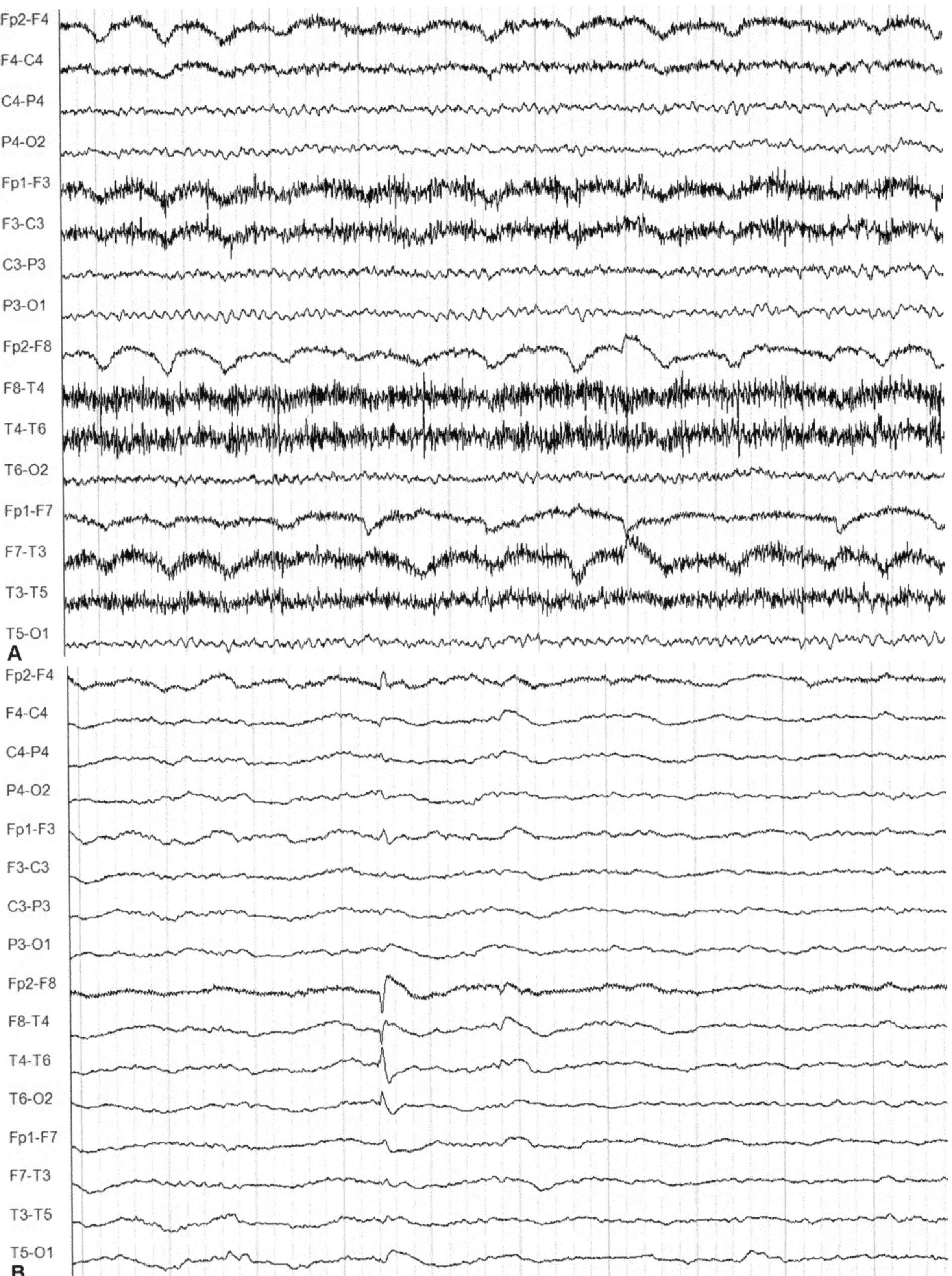

Fig. 27.1. (**A**) Sample of electroencephalogram (EEG) several minutes into a prolonged convulsive psychogenic non-epileptic attacks. Major divisions are 1 second. Note muscle artefact with rhythmic displacement of baseline due to patient movement, particularly in channels Fp2-F4, Fp1-F3, F3-C3, F8-T4, T4-T6, F7-T3, and T3-T5. Alpha rhythm (indicating wakefulness) can nonetheless be seen intermittently in the posterior channels, particularly C4-P4, P4-O2 and P3-O1 and T5-O1. The captured event was identified as her usual clinical type. (**B**) Sample of EEG during sleep in the same patient, showing a clear spike discharge over the right hemisphere, centering on the frontotemporal leads, phase reversing between F8-T4 and T4-T6. Major divisions are 1 second. Patient history had suggested the possibility of a second event type that had not occurred recently, with a description more suggestive of complex partial seizure.

REFERENCES

Amirati F, Colivicci F, Di Battista G et al. (1998). Electroencephalographic correlates of vasovagal syncope induced by head up tilt testing. Stroke 29: 2347–2351.

Bauer J (1996). Epilepsy and prolactin in adults: a clinical review. Epilepsy Res 24: 1–7.

Benbadis SR (2007). Errors in EEGs and the misdiagnosis of epilepsy: importance, causes, consequences, and proposed remedies. Epilepsy Behav 11: 257–262.

Benbadis SR, Tatum WO (2003). Overintepretation of EEGs and misdiagnosis of epilepsy. J Clin Neurophysiol 20: 42–44.

Benbadis SR, Johnson K, Anthony K et al. (2000). Induction of psychogenic nonepileptic seizures without placebo. Neurology 55: 1904–1905.

Benbadis SR, Agrawal V, Tatum WO (2001). How many patients with psychogenic nonepileptic seizures also have epilepsy? Neurology 57: 915–917.

Benbadis SR, Siegrist K, Tatum WO et al. (2004). Short term outpatient EEG video with induction in the diagnosis of psychogenic seizures. Neurology 63: 1728–1730.

Brunnhuber F, Amin D, Nguyen Y et al. (2014). Development, evaluation and implementation of video-EEG telemetry at home. Seizure 23: 338–343.

Chen DK, Graber KD, Anderson CT et al. (2008). Sensitivity and specificity of video alone versus electroencephalography alone for the diagnosis of partial seizures. Epilepsy Behav 13: 115–118.

Cragar DE, Berry DT, Fakhoury TA et al. (2002). A review of diagnostic techniques in the differential diagnosis of epileptic and nonepileptic seizures. Neuropsychol Rev 12: 31–64.

Devinsky O, Gordon E (1998). Epileptic seizures progressing into nonepileptic conversion seizures. Neurology 51: 1293–1296.

Duncan R, Oto M (2008). Psychogenic non-epileptic seizures in patients with learning disability: comparison with patients with no learning disability. Epilepsy Behav 112: 183–186.

Duncan R, Oto M (2010). Managing psychogenic nonepileptic seizures in patients with epilepsy. In: S Schachter, LaFrance (Eds.), Rowan & Gates Nonepileptic Seizures, Cambridge University Press, Cambridge, pp. 247–252.

Duncan R, Razvi S, Mulhearn S (2011). Newly presenting psychogenic nonepileptic attacks: incidence, population characteristics and early outcome from a prospective audit of a First Seizure Clinic. Epilepsy Behav 20: 308–311.

Ettinger AB, Devinsky O, Weisbrot DM et al. (1999). Headaches and other pain symptoms among patients with psychogenic non-epileptic seizures. Seizure 8: 424–426.

Faulkner HJ, Arima H, Mohamed A (2012). Latency to first interictal discharge in patients with outpatient ambulatory EEG. Clin Neurophysiol 123: 1732–1735.

Gates JR, Luciano D, Devinsky O (1991). The classification and treatment of nonepileptic events. In: O Devinsky, WH Theodore (Eds.), Epilepsy and behavior, Wiley-Liss, New York, pp. 251–263.

Goodin DS, Aminoff MJ (1984). Does the interictal EEG have a role in the diagnosis of epilepsy? The Lancet 323: 837–839.

Hoepner R, Labudda K, Schoendienst M et al. (2013). Informing patients about the impact of provocation methods increases the rate of psychogenic nonepileptic seizures during EEG recording. Epilepsy Behav 28: 457–459.

Jedrzejczak J, Owczarek K, Majkowski J (1999). Psychogenic pseudoepileptic seizures: clinical and electroencephalogram (EEG) video-tape recordings. Eur J Neurol 6: 473–479.

Kanner AM, Morris HH, Luders H et al. (1990). Supplementary motor seizures mimicking pseudoseizures: some clinical differences. Neurology 40: 1404–1407.

King DW, Gallagher BG, Murvin AJ et al. (1982). Pseudoseizures: diagnostic evaluation. Neurology 32: 18–23.

Lesser RP (1996). Psychogenic seizures. Neurology 46: 1499–1507.

McGonigal A, Oto M, Russell AJ et al. (2002). Outpatient video EEG recording in the diagnosis of non-epileptic seizures: a randomised controlled trial of simple suggestion techniques. J Neurol Neurosurg Psychiatr 72: 549–551.

McGonigal A, Russell AJ, Mallik AK et al. (2004). Use of short term video EEG in the diagnosis of attack disorders. J Neurol Neurosurg Psychiat 75: 771–772.

Pedley TA, Mendiratta A, Walkczak TS (2003). Seizures and epilepsy. In: JS Ebersole, TA Pedley (Eds.), Current practice of clinical electroencephalography, 3rd edn. Williams & Wilkins, Philadelphia, PA, pp. 510–512.

Saygi S, Katz A, Marks DA et al. (1992). Frontal lobe partial seizures and psychogenic seizures: a comparison of clinical and ictal characteristics. Neurology 42: 1274–1277.

Smith D, Defalla BA, Chadwick DW (1992). The misdiagnosis of epilepsy and the management of refractory epilepsy in a specialist clinic. Q J Med 92: 15–23.

Stagno SJ, Smith ML (1997). The use of placebo in diagnosing psychogenic seizures: who is being deceived? Semin Neurol 17: 213–218.

Van Cott AC, Brenner RP (2003). Drug effects and toxic encephalopathies. In: JS Ebersole, TA Pedley (Eds.), Current practice of clinical electroencephalography, 3rd edn. Lippincott Williams & Wilkins, Philadelphia, PA, pp. 464–467.

Varela HL, Taylor DS, Benbadis SR (2007). Short-term outpatient EEGvideo monitoring with induction in a Veterans Administration population. J Clin Neurophysiol 24: 390–391.

Handbook of Clinical Neurology, Vol. 139 (3rd series)
Functional Neurologic Disorders
M. Hallett, J. Stone, and A. Carson, Editors
http://dx.doi.org/10.1016/B978-0-12-801772-2.00028-X

Chapter 28

Functional coma

L. LUDWIG[1], L. McWHIRTER[2], S. WILLIAMS[2], C. DERRY[2], AND J. STONE[3]*

[1]*Departments of Clinical Neurosciences and of Rehabilitation Medicine, NHS Lothian and Centre for Clinical Brain Sciences, University of Edinburgh, Edinburgh, UK*

[2]*Department of Clinical Neurosciences, Western General Hospital, Edinburgh, UK*

[3]*Department of Clinical Neurosciences, Centre for Clinical Brain Sciences, University of Edinburgh, Edinburgh, UK*

Abstract

Functional coma – here defined as a prolonged motionless dissociative attack with absent or reduced response to external stimuli – is a relatively rare presentation.

In this chapter we examine a wide range of terms used to describe states of unresponsiveness in which psychologic factors are relevant to etiology, such as depressive stupor, catatonia, nonepileptic "pseudostatus," and factitious disorders, and discuss the place of functional or psychogenic coma among these.

Historically, diagnosis of functional coma has sometimes been reached after prolonged investigation and exclusion of other diagnoses. However, as is the case with other functional disorders, diagnosis should preferably be made on the basis of positive findings that provide evidence of inconsistency between an apparent comatose state and normal waking nervous system functioning. In our review of physical signs, we find some evidence for the presence of firm resistance to eye opening as reasonably sensitive and specific for functional coma, as well as the eye gaze sign, in which patients tend to look to the ground when turned on to one side. Noxious stimuli such as Harvey's sign (application of high-frequency vibrating tuning fork to the nasal mucosa) can also be helpful, although patients with this disorder are often remarkably unresponsive to usually painful stimuli, particularly as more commonly applied using sternal or nail bed pressure. The use of repeated painful stimuli is therefore not recommended. We also discuss the role of general anesthesia and other physiologic triggers to functional coma.

INTRODUCTION

The silent and unresponsive patient, by definition unable to tell us what has happened or is happening, triggers alarm and anxiety in health professionals. Exclusion of key organic causes such as overdose, intoxication, metabolic disturbance, or seizure is understandably the priority in the first instance. However, failure to consider and test for functional coma at an early stage may lead to ongoing investigation and intervention beyond the point of helpfulness, even leading to harm, from repeated painful stimuli to invasive ventilation.

This chapter aims to review the literature on functional coma, discusses terminology in overlapping conditions, and evaluates helpful physical signs. A full discussion of the differential diagnosis of coma in general can be found elsewhere, but some conditions that may cause particular confusion with functional coma are discussed.

TERMINOLOGY, ASSESSMENT, AND DIFFERENTIAL DIAGNOSIS

> *Consciousness is the state of awareness of the self and the environment and coma is its opposite (Plum and Posner, 1972).*

Coma can be defined by both lack of awareness and lack of response to external stimulation. However, as awareness is subjective, and difficult to measure even in

*Correspondence to: Dr. Jon Stone, Department of Clinical Neurosciences, Western General Hospital, Edinburgh EH4 2XU, UK. Tel: +44-131-537-1167, E-mail: Jon.Stone@ed.ac.uk

organic coma, apparent unconsciousness (usually motionless, with eyes closed) and unresponsiveness to external stimulation are more clinically useful defining features. The widely used Glasgow Coma Scale uses eye opening, motor and vocal response as proxy measures of vigilance and responsiveness (Teasdale and Jennett, 1974).

Stupor, along with terms like obtundation, is variously defined as "a state of baseline unresponsiveness which requires vigorous stimuli to achieve arousal from coma" (Berger, 2016) or a state between coma and alertness. It is hard to find a generally agreed definition of what stupor is, so ideally should perhaps be avoided, but it nonetheless remains a useful term for the kinds of states described in this article.

Assessment of any patient in a state of coma, or unarousable unresponsiveness, involves taking a history and performing a general and focused neurologic examination. While the patient in a comatose state will be unable to provide a history, obtaining a description of the onset of coma and preceding events from witnesses, and when possible speaking to friends and family regarding the patient's past medical, psychiatric, and drug history is essential. Review of medical notes often provides vital additional information. Finally, targeted investigations may be helpful both in terms of excluding important treatable causes of coma, and in making a positive diagnosis.

A full general medical examination can provide critical diagnostic clues to the cause of coma, such as the presence of fever, hypertension, meningism, or bruising, and other signs of physical injury. It may also provide other potentially relevant information from a relative, such as evidence of intravenous drug use or deliberate self-harm.

A careful neurologic examination is vital, and often yields valuable diagnostic information, which may enable a positive diagnosis of a range of causes of coma, including functional coma. Key features of the neurologic examination include: eye movements (including an assessment of the oculovestibular reflex); pupillary reflexes; motor responses to a range of stimuli, including voice and pain (looking for evidence of hemiparesis, decorticate or decerebrate posturing); and limb reflexes, including plantar responses. A range of maneuvers described specifically for the testing of functional coma are discussed in detail later in this review.

Finally, targeted investigations are often, though not invariably, required. The most widely used investigations include: blood tests, for evidence of metabolic disturbance or the presence of drugs or toxins; brain imaging, for structural brain lesions; lumbar puncture, primarily for evidence of infection; and electroencephalogram (EEG), for evidence of abnormal cerebral function, including seizures or status epilepticus.

Coma has many potential causes, and a full review of these is beyond the scope of this chapter. In general terms, however, these can generally be grouped under the following headings: (1) structural brain lesions; (2) acute metabolic-endocrine derangement; (3) diffuse neuronal dysfunction; and (4) psychogenic unresponsiveness (Wijdicks, 2010). Structural brain lesions will often, though by no means invariably, be associated with localizing neurologic signs, such as pupillary and eye movement abnormalities, and abnormalities of motor function such as hemiparesis or reflex asymmetry. Diffuse neuronal dysfunction is often associated with "hard" abnormalities on neurologic examination, including decerebrate or decorticate posturing in response to pain. Metabolic and drug-related causes of coma can often be rapidly identified by a full history and the use of targeted blood tests. The examination findings are typically symmetric and nonfocal. In contrast, in patients with unresponsiveness of functional origin, there will be no "hard" neurologic localizing signs, and initial investigations will be normal or noncontributory. However, the absence of diagnostic findings on examination and investigation does not, in and of itself, confirm the diagnosis of a functional cause. It is important that positive features of functional coma are sought, and these are considered in detail later in this chapter. Targeted investigations may also be necessary to exclude other causes; although in some patients a confident diagnosis of functional coma can be made with few, if any, investigations, these are essential when diagnostic uncertainty exists.

Most common medical causes of coma should be identifiable with careful examination and appropriate standard investigations, and should not be confused with functional coma. However, some conditions warrant specific consideration in the differential diagnosis of functional stupor and coma, as they may not be associated with clear localizing neurologic signs and initial investigations may be normal. Brainstem lesions can cause the syndromes of locked-in syndrome and akinetic mutism, which are an important consideration; sometimes the neurologic signs can be subtle in these conditions, and plain computed tomography (CT) scanning may not detect early brainstem vascular changes. Careful clinical evaluation is vital, particularly in the identification of subtle cranial nerve abnormalities and limb signs, and specific imaging (such as CT angiography or magnetic resonance imaging (MRI)) may be necessary if this is suspected. Drug misuse may cause apparent coma of unknown cause without localizing neurologic signs and with normal basic investigations, and should be considered and tested for early. Rarer conditions, such as Klein–Levin syndrome, autoimmune encephalitis, and hemiplegic migraine may present with coexistent psychiatric or unexplained physical symptoms and normal baseline investigations. Functional coma should not be considered simply a diagnosis of exclusion, but a positive diagnosis, with recognizable clinical features. However, the inconsistent terminology used in the literature about psychogenic unresponsiveness can lead to confusion. In some places different presentations are described using similar terms, whereas in other places similar presentations are described using different terminology. Particular confusion arises in the use of the term psychogenic, commonly applied both to conditions arising as a result of mental illness (such as depressive stupor) and to quite distinct states of sudden motionless unresponsiveness seen in patients with functional coma. For the purposes of this chapter we group the main causes of psychogenic unresponsiveness as follows:

1. functional coma
2. functional stupor
3. nonepileptic pseudostatus epilepticus (i.e., a prolonged nonepileptic seizure)

(items 1–3: also called psychogenic, conversion, or hysterical)

4. stupor in catatonia, depression, or mania
5. factitious/malingered unresponsiveness/coma.

FUNCTIONAL STUPOR AND COMA (INCLUDING NONEPILEPTIC PSEUDOSTATUS)

CASE 28.1. A 39-year-old woman presented with recurrent severe migraine, anxiety, and social withdrawal. She developed a severe migraine with increasing drowsiness. Her family reported that she appeared more and more "spaced out" before apparently going to sleep. The family found that they could not wake her and called an ambulance. On assessment she had normal physiologic and biochemical parameters; her eyes were closed but resisting eye opening; there was no response to painful stimuli such as nail bed or sternal pressure. MRI, EEG, lumbar puncture, and extensive testing for metabolic and autoimmune disorders were negative. Within 5 days she improved. Over the next few years she had several similar episodes. Between episodes she complained of fatigue, migraine, and anxiety but never had any psychotic symptoms.

To our knowledge the term functional stupor has not often been used in the literature so far; a corresponding condition has historically been called hysterical stupor. Dissociative stupor also appears in the 10th edition of the *International Classification of Diseases* (ICD-10: World Health Organization, 1992) as a name for the same phenomenon.

We consider functional stupor and coma to lie on a continuum of degrees of unresponsiveness. Functional stupor is a disorder of action and response rather than vigilance and wakefulness, and eyes may be open; at the other extreme of this continuum in functional coma there is total unresponsiveness, usually but not always with the eyes closed. The essence of functional stupor or coma is as follows:

1. a time-limited state that resembles stupor or coma with impaired responsiveness to external stimuli, such as pain lasting longer than 30 minutes
2. unequivocal evidence that brain function is analogous to a waking state during this state, but usually accompanied by subsequent amnesia of events by the subject
3. experienced by the patient as a genuine and involuntary problem
4. not explained better by a comorbid psychiatric disorder such as catatonia, depression, or mania.

Within this category we would also include the patient said to have nonepileptic ("pseudo") status. This condition manifests itself as a dissociative/psychogenic nonepileptic seizure lasting 30 minutes or longer, or as several repetitive or continuous nonepileptic seizures without recovery in between (Dworetzky et al., 2015), normally characterized by limb/body shaking, commonly with closed eyes, but at times still responsive to noxious stimuli (Reuber et al., 2000b). Here, a clinical concern of status epilepticus with impaired consciousness can lead to patients receiving treatment in intensive care unnecessarily, with associated risk of iatrogenic harm from procedures, drug exposure, and hospital-acquired infection (Reuber et al., 2003; Dworetzky et al., 2015). Up to 30% of patients with dissociative/psychogenic nonepileptic seizures actually have episodes of motionless unresponsiveness which resemble syncope more than seizures (Meierkord et al., 1991; Wadwekar et al., 2014). Therefore a prolonged version of this type of event will naturally resemble coma rather than status epilepticus (although nonconvulsive status epilepticus may also present like this).

We therefore suggest that functional coma can helpfully be considered alongside prolonged dissociative nonepileptic seizures (nonepileptic status) and be defined as a prolonged motionless dissociative attack with reduced or absent response to external stimuli.

A final type of disorder that may overlap with functional coma is a condition that has variously been described as pervasive refusal syndrome, pervasive autonomic withdrawal syndrome, and resignation syndrome. This rare, but life-threatening, disorder is primarily seen in children, is more common in girls than in boys, and has been described in refugee populations in Sweden (Sallin et al., 2016). The condition is characterized by progressive social withdrawal, school refusal, food refusal, and weight loss, and partial or complete refusal in two or more of the following domains: mobilization, speech, and attention to personal care; typically the patient regresses back through stages of development in a reverse chronologic fashion. No underlying organic or psychiatric condition accounts for the severity of the symptoms (Thompson and Nunn, 1997). The condition has been considered as a manifestation of depression, a form of learned helplessness, a response to trauma, or a conversion disorder. More recently, in the absence of clear evidence of voluntary "refusal" in most patients, Nunn et al. (2014) have reconceptualized the condition as one of overactivation of both the sympathetic and parasympathetic nervous system: pervasive autonomic withdrawal syndrome. However, although patients might present with mutism, most are still responsive and able to engage to an extent sufficient to distinguish from functional coma, only rarely progressing to states of almost complete unresponsiveness.

The term stupor refers to a clinical presentation that is the result of psychiatric illness, such as catatonia (often in the context of schizophrenia), severe depression, or rarely, mania. In functional stupor as a milder presentation of functional coma there will be no such underlying severe psychiatric illness, but the patient presents to medical services with a relatively sudden and unexplained unresponsive state. Below we attempt to standardize what is meant by these definitions and to discuss clinical case examples.

STUPOR IN PSYCHIATRIC DISORDERS, SUCH AS DEPRESSION, MANIA, AND CATATONIA

CASE 28.2. DEPRESSIVE STUPOR

A 76-year-old man presented to hospital with impaired responsiveness and confusion. His eyes were open but he only spoke a few words. He was a retired and highly respected hospital consultant and his illness had led to many visits from senior colleagues suggesting rare and unusual neurologic causes for his illness. Investigations were normal for age. It was noted, however, that his affect was flat and a history was obtained of previous major depressive illness occurring at the time of retirement. His family agreed that he had been progressively more depressed prior to the onset of the illness. He received a course of six electroconvulsive therapy (ECT) treatments, following which he made a substantial recovery back to independent living and indeed working at a high level.

Stupor arising due to primary psychiatric illness is an important differential, a state of mutism and akinesis despite usually apparent wakefulness and vigilance. When stupor occurs in severe depression, there is usually a clear background of recent depressive symptoms: feelings of emptiness, anhedonia, and psychomotor retardation, with or without low mood. The following features may help in distinguishing depressive from functional stupor: (1) in depressive stupor the eyes still may variously respond to surrounding events; (2) the onset of depressive stupor is usually rather slow (e.g., Johnson (1984) reported on cases with depressive stupor whose mutism and akinesia developed over 2 weeks or even within 3 months); (3) the stuporous state may develop out of psychomotor retardation, often with a degree of diurnal variation, being worse in the morning; and (4) patients' altered state of consciousness may change due to specific treatment of the underlying psychiatric illness. In depressive stupor, for example, there is often a good response to ECT, with antidepressant medication also helpful (Johnson, 1984). Crawford (1972), however, pointed out that, even if psychiatric illness is present, organic disease could be the actual cause of the stupor.

CASE 28.3. CATATONIA

A 45-year-old man with an established diagnosis of schizophrenia, on depot antipsychotic medication, became more socially withdrawn than usual after an increase in dose triggered by worsening of auditory hallucinations. He was admitted to an acute psychiatric ward, where he could frequently be observed standing in uncomfortable-looking positions for long periods of time. His facial appearance was staring and expressionless, and he responded, between episodes of motionlessness, with brief muddled phrases or words. On examination, resting tone was increased in all four limbs, without cogwheeling, and his arms would remain in the positions the examiner had placed them in for several minutes. Regular diazepam was commenced, with some gradual improvement over 2 weeks, and ultimately a change in antipsychotic medication brought recovery to baseline.

A further type of psychiatric stupor is seen in the context of catatonia. Catatonia is a common syndrome, depending on how it is defined, and has been found in about 10% of acutely ill psychiatric inpatients (Taylor and Fink, 2003). The definition and classification of catatonia, however, have varied, with arguably overinclusive diagnostic criteria, leading to doubts about their specificity. For example, one study suggested that 73% of acutely ill medical and psychiatric patients met *Diagnostic and Statistical Manual of Mental Disorders*, fifth edition (DSM-5: American Psychiatric Association, 2013) criteria for catatonia (Wilson et al., 2015). In addition, it is possible that many historic diagnoses of catatonia of psychiatric origin were in fact cases of autoimmune encephalitis, catatonia being a recognized feature of, for example, *N*-methyl-D-aspartate receptor antibody encephalitis (Barry et al., 2011).

The key feature of catatonia is muscle rigidity that is abolished by voluntary movement, and this often occurs alongside associated disorders of motor initiation and control, such as waxy flexibility and adoption of abnormal postures. Other potential symptoms include mutism, staring, agitation, Gegenhalten, stereotypy, mannerisms, grimacing, echolalia, echopraxia, and agitation. Catatonia is most common in patients with schizophrenia and severe depression, but can also occur in mania, autism, and in some organic conditions. A high percentage of patients are said to have a temporary response to benzodiazepines – in contrast to functional coma, which, in our experience, tends to get worse with benzodiazepine administration, perhaps because it accentuates dissociation. Some of these features clearly overlap with those of delirium. Catatonia may present with or without stupor but not without motor features. Catatonic syndromes can also occur due to organic causes (Hurwitz, 2011). Terms such as comatoid catatonia (Bender and Feutrill, 2000) and catatonic coma (Freudenreich et al., 2007) have been used to describe patients presenting with clinical features of functional coma while lacking any actual catatonic symptoms, and this leads to further confusion in a field with already uncertain boundaries.

Other conditions arising as complications of psychotropic drug administration and causing reduced consciousness may be included in the initial differential when patients with severe mental illness present in this state. Neuroleptic malignant syndrome is a rare and serious medical complication of treatment with antipsychotic medication, with muscle rigidity, impaired cognition or consciousness, hyperthermia, and autonomic instability. Plasma creatinine kinase and white cells are elevated, aiding differentiation of the condition from catatonia. Another distinct condition, the serotonin syndrome, can arise after overdose of serotonergic medications such as antidepressants. Although the serotonin syndrome can lead to coma, additional clinical signs, including tremor, myoclonus, diaphoresis, hyperreflexia, hypertension, hyperthermia, and seizures, together with history of serotonergic medication excess, should aid differentiation from primary psychiatric or functional causes.

FACTITIOUS UNRESPONSIVENESS

CASE 28.4. FACTITIOUS DISORDER

A 53-year-old man on trial for historic charges of child sexual abuse collapsed in court and was admitted to the neurology ward in an apparently comatose state. There was clear evidence of a "functional coma," with normal response to stimulation of the nasal mucosa with a tuning fork (Harvey's sign, discussed below) and eyes closed with resistance to eye opening. The comatose state lasted 12 hours, following which he rapidly recovered and returned to prison. On recovery he had Ganser-type answers – that is, answering "approximate" answers to very simple questions to which nearly everyone should know the answer, such as "What is two plus two?" "Five" Later he admitted to a prison psychiatrist that he had deliberately faked the episode as he was finding the experience in court intolerable.

The possibility of intentional feigning of unconsciousness should also be considered among the differentials in cases of unexplained unconsciousness and unresponsiveness, although clear evidence of feigning can be difficult or impossible to obtain and positive signs of functional coma do not exclude feigned symptoms. Factitious disorder is differentiated from malingering, in that, where malingering of symptoms is for clear purposes of personal gain, there are no such external rewards in factitious disorder. Our own personal experience across a range of functional disorders is that extreme presentations, such as complete paralysis or coma, whilst often genuine, are a "red flag" for the possibility of factitious symptoms and so *a priori* we might expect a higher incidence of willful exaggeration in this patient group. On the other hand more extreme symptoms can also be a red flag for more severe comorbidity, especially personality disorder and previous abuse. We have met patients with functional coma who appeared to have an entirely genuine and distressing experience with no obvious potential for material gain. It seems reasonable to assume there may be a spectrum of willful exaggeration that patients may move across over time, even during a single episode. However, it is not reasonable to assume that all patients in a functional coma are willfully exaggerating.

In seven out of 25 reviewed cases there was evidence of willful exaggeration (Hopkins, 1973; Henry and Woodruff, 1978; Albrecht et al., 1995). However, two of these articles were published with titles including terms such as pretending and factitious, suggesting bias within the selection and interpretation of the presented cases. In these cases evidence for conscious simulation was either derived from the observation that patients were looking around when felt unwatched or on the basis of the patients' comments after regaining consciousness. One patient even admitted that she produced the fits of unconsciousness when faced with stress (Henry and Woodruff, 1978).

FUNCTIONAL COMA: CLINICAL FEATURES AND REVIEW OF PUBLISHED CASES

For the rest of this chapter we concentrate on the phenomenon of functional coma as defined above, reviewing reported cases for clinical features, prevalence, and treatment. Twenty-five cases were derived from 12 reviewed case reports (presenting more than one case at times: Table 28.1). These case reports were sometimes explicitly published in order to promote a certain positive sign (such as the eye gaze test) or aimed to present cases pretending coma. The indication of a proportion (e.g., 10/25 cases) should be therefore understood as a reflection of a tendency presented in the scarce literature – prone to bias of selection and interpretation.

Diagnostic classification

In DSM-5, functional coma best falls under 300.11 "Conversion Disorder/Functional Neurological Symptom Disorder with attacks or seizures." In ICD-10 we would suggest that functional coma aligns best to a diagnosis of dissociative convulsions (F44.5) or dissociative stupor (F44.2).

Etiology

Since most case reports of this presentation use the term psychogenic coma, it is not surprising that they have emphasized psychologic triggers. Downs et al. (2008) define psychogenic coma as "a manifestation of a psychiatric illness which presents as a state of unresponsiveness without organic cause." Plum and Posner (1972) described the process of diagnosing psychogenic coma in two steps. Firstly, they state that neurologic signs have to be inconsistent with expected anatomic or physiologic patterns; secondly, the emotional background and current psychologic problems must provide sufficient evidence for the diagnosis. Hurwitz (2011) emphasizes that a psychogenic etiology does not imply that unresponsiveness is under willed control. However, psychologic etiology, specifically a response to a psychologic stressor or life event, is assumed in much of the reviewed literature.

More recently, etiologic models and DSM-5 (Stone et al., 2011) have moved away from a view that psychologic stressors or life events are always relevant in functional neurologic disorders. In functional coma and unresponsiveness, medical procedures and the experience of anesthesia may also be important in determining the nature of symptoms. So, for example, it may be that an individual who is generally susceptible to functional or dissociative symptoms finds himself or herself in a dissociative state triggered by the experience of a particular physiologic stimulus, such as dissociative symptoms induced by anesthesia, or feelings of profound lethargy accompanying migraine. These triggers may in some patients be sufficient to induce symptoms, especially if those symptoms are habitual in the absence of any other recent stressful event (Stone et al., 2012; Pareés et al., 2014). Downs et al. (2008) present a case of postanesthesia psychogenic coma with a review of literature. Reuber et al. (2000a) similarly report on 5 cases of postoperative nonepileptic status.

Prevalence

Plum and Posner (1972) presented data on 500 patients initially diagnosed with "coma of unknown etiology" – only 8 of these patients were finally diagnosed with "psychiatric coma," 4 (0.8%) of whom had a "conversion reaction" and with 2 cases each (0.4%) of depression and catatonic stupor. In a more recent study, Weiss et al. (2012) presented data on the causes of coma in 2189 patients treated over 8 years at an intensive care unit. Only 0.3% were diagnosed with psychogenic coma, although this was a proportion of all coma and not just coma of initially unknown origin. Beside these studies, the recent literature consists mainly of case reports, suggesting that the occurrence of functional coma is rare.

In 1907 Janet described hysteric states of unresponsiveness, "fits of sleep" or a "hysteric patient in lethargy," occurring as frequently as "hysterical convulsions." Changing terminology makes comparative analysis of historic data difficult, but it is also unclear whether the frequency of functional coma has decreased over the last 100 years or whether cases are just less likely to be recognized or reported.

The ambiguous use of multiple terms for states of nonorganic unconsciousness may also have led to a historic and current underestimation of the occurrence of all such cases, including of functional coma. We speculate that a clear definition of functional coma, that of a prolonged motionless, unresponsive, dissociative attack with positive diagnostic features, could lead to increased recognition and better management.

Diagnosis

(Positive) clinical signs

A prompt diagnosis based on positive clinical signs may require some clinical experience but is essential to prevent unnecessary ongoing investigation and interventions with associated risks of iatrogenic harm, costs, and distress. A summary of physical signs reported to be useful in the diagnosis of functional coma is shown in Table 28.2. What the positive signs of functional coma have in common is that they indicate (briefly) a normal voluntary nervous system that is inconsistent with the comatose presentation of the patient.

Some authors have observed that, in patients with functional unresponsiveness, the eyes deviate towards the ground, and when the patient is rolled to the opposite side the eyes deviate again to the ground on that side. Other case reports have supported the use of this "eye gaze sign" (Henry and Woodruff, 1978; Dhadphale,

Table 28.1

Summary of published case reports

Author	Gender	Age (years)	Relevant psychiatric/ medical history	Assumed trigger	Clinical features	Duration	Positive signs	Reversed	Stated final diagnosis and additional comments
Albrecht et al. (1995)	F	36	Prolonged post-op paresis after GA 7 years previously, conversion disorder, histrionic personality traits	GA	Unresponsive to sternal rub	>90 minutes		Cold calorics (nystagmus, nausea, "What did you have to do that for?")	Factitious disorder
	F	32	No psychiatric history	GA	No memory of syncope-like episode			Placebo (injection of 1 ml Ringer's solution.)	Factitious disorder
Baxter and White (2003)	M	20	Substance abuse	PS	Intermittent periods of consciousness	3 days	Eyes closed, resisted eye opening, fluttering eyelids, Bell's phenomenon, positive hand drop test, normal cold caloric response	Spontaneous	Coma due to dissociative disorder not otherwise specified/ psychogenic coma
Bender and Feutrill (2000)	M	24	Episode of paranoid ideas 3 years earlier	PS	Muscle tone flaccid			Electroconvulsive therapy	Catatonic coma
Dhadphale (1980)	M	16	Seizure after a fall 6 years ago, "bizarre behavior" over 3 days	PS	Stuporose	4 days	Positive eye gaze test	Abreaction with diazepam	Hysterical stupor due to emotional stress. Followed up with supportive psychotherapy. Recurrence after eight months resolved with same treatment.
	M	35	"Religious guilt"			48 hours	Positive eye gaze test	Intravenous thiopentone	Author recommends the eye gaze test

Continued

Table 28.1

Continued

Author	Gender	Age (years)	Relevant psychiatric/ medical history	Assumed trigger	Clinical features	Duration	Positive signs	Reversed	Stated final diagnosis and additional comments
Downs et al. (2008)	F	28	Progressive dysphagia, hypothyroidism, PTSD, personality disorder	GA	Avoidance of light, no spontaneous movements, unresponsive to pain	16 hours	Positive hand drop test. Positive oculocephalic reflexes	Spontaneously	Psychogenic coma following upper endoscopy
Freudenreich et al. (2007)	M	27	Paranoid schizophrenia, minor head trauma, polysubstance abuse	Psychiatric illness	Eyes closed, no spontaneous movements, unresponsive to pain		Bell's phenomenon when eyelids were opened against minimal resistance, positive hand drop test	Intravenous benzodiazepines	Catatonic coma
Haller et al. (2003)	F	31	No psychiatric history reported	GA	Unresponsive to pain	~3 hours	Resisted eye opening	Lorazepam	Dissociative stupor
Henry and Woodruff (1978)	M(3), F(3)	14–45	Psychosocial problems in 2 of 6 cases	Not stated	Nonepileptic attacks rather than coma, described in 2 cases. Unresponsive to pain in 1 case	1–40 hours	Eye gaze sign in all cases	Intravenous saline solution in one case. Remark within earshot that the "fit would be expected to wear off" in one case, spontaneous resolution or ongoing attacks in other cases	'No organic basis', no diagnosis, 'no organic basis', no diagnosis, 'she told how she produced the attacks when confronted by stressful situations', 'attention seeking behaviour'. The authors recommend the eye gaze test

Hopkins (1973)	M (3), F (3)	18–60	Sexual abuse in family (1), self-harm (1), financial difficulties and paranoid delusions (schizophrenia or anxiety state considered) (1), depression and atrophy of the left hemisphere (1). Multiple other functional symptoms (1)	PS (3), psychiatric illness (2), unclear (2)	Unresponsive to painful stimuli (6)		Eyelids closed (5) but seen to flutter (1), resistance to eye opening (1), Bell's phenomenon (1), "shining a light in his eyes caused him to curl up vigorously" (1)	Spontaneously (3), followed by tears (1), when burr holes were made without anaesthetic on one occasion and after IV phenobarbitone and methylamphetamine on two further occasions (1), after suggestion ('he was told it was time to wake up, and he did so') (1)	Title of paper 'Pretending to be unconscious' reflects emphasis, with the author finding 'conscious simulation' in one case and 'method of escaping from an intolerable situation' in the others
Maddock et al. (1999)	M	36	Depression and self-harm	GA	Unresponsive to painful stimuli	~4 hours	Flickering of closed eyelids, eye gaze sign	Occluding the patient's airway	Postoperative coma due to hysterical conversion
Orr and Glassman (1985)	F	17	Depression	GA	Unresponsive to light pain		Eyes closed, eye gaze sign	Ammonia capsule was broken and placed beneath the nose and the patient opened her eyes and began to cry	Hysterical conversion following general anaesthesia
	F	23	Previous alcohol misuse	GA			Eyes closed, eye gaze sign	Spontaneous	Hysterical conversion following general anaesthesia.
Stone and Sharpe (2006)	F	27	Extensive psychiatric history, self-harm, depression, probable personality disorder, sexual abuse, termination of pregnancy	GA				Sedation with propofol	Functional coma following general anaesthesia

M, male; F, female; GA, general anesthesia; PS, psychosocial stress; PTSD, posttraumatic stress disorder.

Table 28.2

Clinical signs in functional coma

	Physical sign	Description	Differential: Functional	Differential: Organic	Notes
	Positive signs inconsistent with organic coma				
1	Eye gaze test	Patient's gaze is observed while turning the patient on to one side of his or her body and then to the other side	Eyes deviate tonically toward the floor. When turned over to the other side eyes again deviate downwards to the floor	No spontaneous eye movements, roving eye movements, or fixed gaze	Suggested by some authors (Henry and Woodruff, 1978; Dhadphale, 1980), but not confirmed by others (Plum and Posner, 1972). In one case gaze deviated persistently upward (Maddock et al., 1999)
2	Tightly shut eyelids	Examiner attempts to open the closed eyelids	Eyelids resist actively and usually close rapidly when they are released (Plum and Posner, 1972)	Slow, steady closure of passively opened eyelids (cannot be mimicked voluntarily.) (Plum and Posner, 1972)	Plum and Posner, 1972; Stone and Sharpe, 2006 Only helpful where the eyes are shut; this may not always be the case
3	Bell's phenomenon when opening eyelids	Examiner attempts to open the closed eyelids	Eyes roll up on attempted eye opening	Should not occur	Hopkins, 1973; Baxter and White, 2003
4	Harvey's sign	High-frequency tuning fork (440–1024 Hz) is applied to the mucosa overlying the nasal septum (Larner, 2010)	Reaction to surprisingly painful (but harmless) stimulus	No reaction	Maddock et al., 1999; Harvey, 2004; Stone and Sharpe, 2006
5a	Hand drop test towards the face	Protective reflexes; one arm is raised, held in front of the face and is dropped towards the face	Patient avoids self-injury: hand falls to the side of rather than on to the patient's face	No protective reflex: hand falls to face	Popular (Baxter and White, 2003; Freudenreich et al., 2007; Downs et al., 2008), but not reliable, since patients may withstand painful stimuli, including from their own hand. (Stone and Sharpe, 2006; Wijdicks, 2010) Rate of descent (below) may be more specific
5b	Hand drop test – rate of descent	Hand is lifted by examiner and dropped from height but not towards face. Examiner observes the rate of descent of the hand	Transient retention of tone	Hand falls rapidly like a "dead weight"	May be a more useful sign than whether it drops on the patient's face (Stone and Sharpe, 2006)
6	Noxious stimuli	Painful stimuli applied to sternum, nail bed, or using tetanic stimulation of ulnar nerve	Patient withdraws from stimuli	Only limb withdrawal at best (often with reflex motor movements) (Wijdicks, 2010)	Again, this may not be a particularly specific test for functional coma: "these patients tolerate extraordinary degrees of pain" (Maddock et al., 1999), especially to nail bed or sternum pressure

Table 28.2

Continued

	Physical sign	Description	Differential: Functional	Differential: Organic	Notes
	Signs used to demonstrate normal brain function in coma				
7	Oculocephalic reflex (doll's eyes maneuver)	The patient's eyes are held open and the head is quickly turned from side to side and held briefly still at the end of each turn. If the brainstem is intact, the eyes rotate to the opposite side to the direction of head rotation before returning gradually to midposition. A similar pattern is seen with the head for vertical eye movements when the head is flexed and extended	May or may not be present (Plum and Posner, 1972)	Positive if brainstem is intact (although "on rare occasions the oculocephalic reflex may be intact even when oculovestibular reflexes are abolished," particularly in low lateral brainstem lesions (Plum and Posner, 1972)	Reported as positive in case of functional coma after endoscopy (Downs et al., 2008) A positive result (i.e., intact reflexes) is nonspecific, only indicating that the brainstem is intact
8	Cold caloric oculovestibular reflex	Examiner introduces iced water into the ear canal to stimulate the tympanic membrane	Nystagmus lasting 1–2 minutes with the quick component away from the irrigated ear (Downs et al., 2008). Nausea and vertigo	Brainstem lesion – no nystagmus. Organic coma with intact brainstem – tonic deviation towards the irrigated side (Campbell and DeJong, 2005)	Plum and Posner, 1972; Albrecht et al., 1995; Baxter and White, 2003; Downs et al., 2008 Distinguishes brainstem lesion from other neurological causes but does not distinguish functional from organic coma with intact brainstem

1980; Orr and Glassman, 1985; Maddock et al., 1999). Another case report, however, described upwards deviation of the gaze (Maddock et al., 1999).

Tightly shut eyes that resist attempts at eye opening are widely accepted as a positive sign of functional coma (4/25 cases: Hopkins, 1973; Baxter and White, 2003; Haller et al., 2003; Freudenreich et al., 2007). Once they have been opened, the eyelids usually close rapidly; steady and slow eye closure occurs in organic coma states and cannot be produced voluntarily. This is obviously not helpful in more unusual cases, particularly of functional stupor, where the eyes may be open (Hopkins, 1973; Hurwitz, 2011). Fluttering eyelids have been reported by some authors (Hopkins, 1973; Maddock et al., 1999; Baxter and White, 2003), as well as eyes rolling upwards when opened against resistance (Bell's phenomenon) (Hopkins, 1973; Baxter and White, 2003; Freudenreich et al., 2007), and, rarely, light sensitivity (Hopkins, 1973; Downs et al., 2008).

Peter Harvey, a London neurologist, described a sign that he considered helpful in the diagnosis of functional coma. He came across it accidentally one day when idling as a medical student. He discovered that the application of a tuning fork (440–1024 Hz) to the inside of the nostril causes a surprisingly adverse but harmless sensation (Harvey, 2004). Noxious stimuli in general (e.g., applied to sternum, nail bed, and ulnar nerves) have been used widely in order to diagnose and reverse the altered state of consciousness in a functional comatose patient. However, in many cases it has been reported that functional patients at times tolerate a surprisingly high degree of pain (Hopkins, 1973; Maddock et al., 1999) (in 12 out of 25 cases this was explicitly mentioned, whereas in only one case an unresponsiveness towards light pain was reported, suggesting that the patient withdrew from higher degrees of pain: Orr and Glassman, 1985). In addition, patients with dissociative (nonepileptic) seizures sometimes report being able to feel noxious stimuli but being unable to respond. Use of excessively painful stimuli (which can also cause bruising) should therefore be reconsidered. Aside from being ethically questionable, repeated application of painful stimuli without response is neither sensitive nor specific for diagnosis of functional coma. Absent response to pain should rather be noted alongside other features as a qualitative characteristic of the individual state of detachment.

The hand drop test, examining semireflex protective movements occurring when the patient's hand is lifted above and dropped towards the face, received a positive appraisal in three papers (Baxter and White, 2003; Freudenreich et al., 2007; Downs et al., 2008), but remained questioned in other. Jackson (2000) argued that, since patients with functional coma tolerate surprisingly painful stimuli, a negative hand drop sign (that is, where the hand is allowed to fall directly on to the face) represents tolerance of only minor discomfort and is unlikely to be helpful. In addition, our own experience is that the hand may fall to the side of the face in organic coma because of the mechanics of the arm, depending on how the test is done. However, observations of the speed of the hand's descent may be more helpful, with transient retention of tone slowing the drop and therefore suggesting a degree of physiologic wakefulness (Stone and Sharpe, 2006). Other signs that can be used to identify the absence of disease might support such positive findings, but are not sufficient in themselves. The doll's-eyes maneuver, testing the oculocephalic reflex, is discussed rather vaguely (Downs et al., 2008). In particular, it is worth noting that the oculocephalic reflexes can be preserved in the absence of oculovestibular reflexes in certain cases of organic coma (Plum and Posner, 1972).

The oculovestibular reflex, tested by ice-water calorics, has been considered useful by some authors (Plum and Posner, 1972; Albrecht et al., 1995; Baxter and White, 2003; Downs et al., 2008). In functional coma, a person is presumed to be physiologically awake (although the individual's subjective experience may be otherwise). In a person who is physiologically awake, ice water in one ear induces nystagmus, with the fast component in the opposite direction of the ear thus stimulated. In contrast, in coma due to organic damage, nystagmus may be absent or abnormal during ocular vestibular reflex testing (Plum and Posner, 1972), and a tonic deviation towards the irrigated side may be seen (Campbell and DeJong, 2005). While a "normal awake" response, with nystagmus, is expected and typically seen in functional coma, this finding may also occur in some organic forms of coma. In particular, nystagmus can be preserved in coma due to metabolic encephalopathy (Maccario et al., 1972). The reliability of this "normal awake" response in other forms of encephalopathy (such as in an autoimmune encephalitis) has not, to our knowledge, been studied, and so its overall value is uncertain. In our opinion, therefore, a "normal awake" caloric response is supportive of a functional cause for coma in the correct clinical context, but in isolation is not definitive.

EEG

The primary role of the EEG in coma is in excluding the possibility of nonconvulsive status, and it is also sometimes used for prognostication for organic forms of coma, with certain EEG patterns (such as burst suppression and isoelectric EEG) being associated with poor prognosis (Poothrikovil et al., 2015; Sivaraju et al., 2015).

EEG may also have a role in the positive diagnosis of functional coma. Patients with functional coma usually have a normal awake EEG pattern, containing responsive alpha rhythms and other features typical of waking state (Cartlidge, 2001), in contrast to most forms of coma. However, while a normal awake EEG is inconsistent with many forms of coma (such as that resulting from a structural cortical lesion, or due to a toxic or metabolic encephalopathy), it can be seen in certain situations. In particular, patients with brainstem lesions may be associated with little in the way of EEG abnormality, and in locked-in syndrome the EEG may be entirely normal.

To our knowledge there are no systematic studies of EEG in functional coma. While the EEG is typically reported as normal in functional conditions such as dissociative seizures (Gedzelman and LaRoche, 2014), the possibility that an intense dissociative state, as seen in functional coma, might cause some EEG changes cannot be entirely excluded. Moreover, EEG abnormalities are common in the general population. Nonspecific abnormalities occur in up to 10% of the general population; frankly epileptiform discharges are reported in 0.5% of normal healthy adults (Gregory et al., 1993), and up to 3% of psychiatric inpatients (Zivin and Marsan, 1968), and in a higher proportion of individuals with psychiatric disorders, probably related (at least in part) to medication (Amann et al., 2003). The presence of minor EEG abnormalities in a patient with unresponsiveness does not, therefore, necessarily exclude a diagnosis of functional coma, and EEG findings should always be interpreted with care.

In summary, therefore, while a normal awake EEG pattern in a patient in a comatose state is highly suggestive of functional coma, and a markedly abnormal EEG is highly suggestive of an "organic" etiology, exceptions can occur. While EEG can therefore be a very useful diagnostic test, the findings must be interpreted within the context of the overall clinical presentation.

Treatment and prognosis

Treatment begins with identification of the diagnosis. None of the signs described above are entirely sensitive or specific, and some have been dismissed as "tricks," with writers, including Jackson (2000), stating that patients' knowledge of the test leads to conscious modification of the response. For example, it is suggested that the hand drop test only works if the patient is unaware of the test. Baxter and White (2003) warn that physicians may find themselves in engaging in a battle to outwit the patient or to "catch the patient out."

However, Jackson's suggestion is not in accordance with clinical experiences elsewhere in the field of functional disorders. Hoover's sign of functional lower-limb weakness, for example, had been similarly viewed as a "trick," but can be usefully shared as a helpful demonstration to the patient of symptom reversibility during the consultation (Stone and Edwards, 2012). Although the challenges are different in an unresponsive patient, the reported benefits of supportive suggestion in reversing functional coma suggest to us that, in certain cases, demonstration of physiologic wakefulness alongside calm reassurance may be beneficial (Hopkins, 1973; Baxter and White, 2003). The clinician could, for example, talk to the patient as if he or she is awake while carrying out the procedures described above.

Recovery from functional coma is inevitable, although recurrence is not unusual. In 8 out of 25 reported cases, the comatose state had occurred repeatedly or more than once (Hopkins, 1973; Henry and Woodruff, 1978; Stone and Sharpe, 2006; Downs et al., 2008). This mirrors experience in patients with recurrent pseudostatus epilepticus (Reuber et al., 2003). Three out of 11 cases presented by Downs et al. (2008) regained consciousness spontaneously.

Literature on the treatment of functional coma is scarce. Patients may require nasogastric feeding, and intravenous fluids for several days in some cases. There are considerable iatrogenic risks to such a state, including venous thrombosis, hospital-acquired infection, and complications from intravenous and other lines. Cold caloric testing was reported to bring about reversal of the unconscious state in 1 patient when used as a diagnostic investigation (Albrecht et al., 1995). In another patient who tolerated extreme degrees of pain, occlusion of the patient's airway was described as a dramatic and successful but ethically questionable way to "wake" the patient from the state of coma (Maddock et al., 1999).

Sedation with propofol was successful in one reported case of functional coma. One explanation for this success would be that excessive executive inhibitory mechanisms, speculated as important in functional neurologic disorders, are disrupted by induction of anesthesia (Stone et al., 2014). Supportive suggestion, reported as helpful in a patient with nonepileptic status (Jagoda et al., 1995), may also be of benefit. Baxter and White (2003) recommended the provision of a gentle recovery in a supportive manner, since severe underlying psychologic distress must be assumed . Historically, barbiturates such as sodium amytal and, more recently, benzodiazepines have been used in a similar manner alongside suggestion, and with some success in the treatment of conversion disorders, including conditions with mutism and amnesia (Poole et al., 2010).

CONCLUSION

Functional coma can be defined as a prolonged, motionless, dissociative attack during which the patient is unresponsive and usually has the eyes closed. Overlapping diagnoses include nonepileptic status and functional (historically, hysteric) stupor. Additional psychiatric or motor features may point to a diagnosis of stupor in depression or mania, or of catatonia with stupor in schizophrenia, depression, or mania.

The diagnosis should be made on the basis of clinical history and positive clinical signs and not as a diagnosis of exclusion: although, clearly, there are numerous potentially serious causes that must be considered and investigated appropriately. Perhaps the greatest difficulty is in excluding feigning, either as malingering or in the context of factitious disorder.

We suggest that, as well as assessing the role of life events and psychosocial factors, attention should be paid towards recent medical or surgical interventions; in particular, the experience of general anesthesia may act as a "trigger" for functional coma and similar dissociative states such as nonepileptic status.

We consider that diagnostic importance should be given to those clinical signs that on the whole only occur in functional coma. Such positive signs include, according to the limited literature, tightly shut eyes that resist opening, a deviated eye gaze as described, Harvey's sign, and Bell's phenomenon. Of additional value are signs that indicate the absence of an organic cause, such as intact oculocephalic and oculovestibular reflexes, the presence of normal deep tendon reflexes, and a normal EEG. Prolonged and repeated painful stimuli should not be applied, since a high tolerance to pain has been reported in this group of conditions.

References

Albrecht RF, Wagner SRIV, Leicht CH et al. (1995). Factitious disorder as a cause of failure to awaken after general anesthesia. Anesthesiology 83 (1): 201–204.

Amann BL, Pogarell O, Mergl R et al. (2003). EEG abnormalities associated with antipsychotics: a comparison of quetiapine, olanzapine, haloperidol and healthy subjects. Hum Psychopharmacol 18 (8): 641–646.

American Psychiatric Association (2013). Diagnostic and statistical manual of mental disorders. 5th edn. American Psychiatric Association, Washington, DC.

Barry H, Hardiman O, Healy DG et al. (2011). Anti-NMDA receptor encephalitis: an important differential diagnosis in psychosis. Br J Psychiatr 199 (6): 508–509.

Baxter CL, White WD (2003). Psychogenic coma: case report. Int J Psychiatry Med 33 (3): 317–322.

Bender KG, Feutrill J (2000). Comatoid catatonia. Aust New Zeal J Psychiatr 34 (1): 169–170.

Berger JR (2016). Stupor and coma. In: RB Daroff, J Jankovic, JC Mazziotta et al. (Eds.), Neurology in Clinical Practice, 7th edn. Elsevier, London.

Campbell WW, DeJong RN (2005). DeJong's the Neurologic Examination, Lippincott, Williams and Wilkins, Philadelphia.

Cartlidge N (2001). States related to or confused with coma. J Neurol Neurosurg Psychiatry 71 (Suppl 1): i18–i19.

Crawford JP (1972). Organic or psychogenic stupor. Br J Psychiatr 120 (558): 592.

Dhadphale M (1980). Eye gaze diagnostic sign in hysterical stupor. Lancet 2 (8190): 374–375.

Downs JW, Young PE, Durning SJ (2008). Psychogenic coma following upper endoscopy: a case report and review of the literature. Mil Med 173 (5): 509–512.

Dworetzky BA, Weisholtz DS, Perez DL et al. (2015). A clinically oriented perspective on psychogenic nonepileptic seizure-related emergencies. Clin EEG Neurosci 46 (1): 26–33.

Freudenreich O, McEvoy JP, Goff DC et al. (2007). Catatonic coma with profound bradycardia. Psychosomatics 48 (1): 74–78.

Gedzelman ER, LaRoche SM (2014). Long-term video EEG monitoring for diagnosis of psychogenic nonepileptic seizures. Neuropsychiatr Dis Treat 10: 1979–1986.

Gregory RP, Oates T, Merry RT (1993). Electroencephalogram epileptiform abnormalities in candidates for aircrew training. Electroencephalogr Clin Neurophysiol 86 (1): 75–77.

Haller M, Kiefer K, Vogt H (2003). Dissoziativer Stupor als Ursache fur postoperative Bewusstlosigkeit. Anaesthesist 52 (11): 1031–1034.

Harvey P (2004). Harvey's 1 and 2. Pract Neurol 3 (4): 178–179.

Henry JA, Woodruff GH (1978). A diagnostic sign in states of apparent unconsciousness. Lancet 2 (8096): 920–921.

Hopkins A (1973). Pretending to be unconscious. Lancet 302 (7824): 312–314.

Hurwitz TA (2011). Psychogenic unresponsiveness. Neurol Clin 29 (4): 995–1006.

Jackson AO (2000). Faking unconsciousness. Anaesthesia 55 (4): 409.

Jagoda A, Richey-Klein V, Riggio S (1995). Psychogenic status epilepticus. J Emerg Med 13 (1): 31–35.

Janet P (1907). The major symptoms of hysteria, Macmillan, London.

Johnson J (1984). Stupor: a review of 25 cases. Acta Psychiatr Scand 70 (4): 370–377.

Larner AJ (2010). A Dictionary of Neurological Signs, Springer Science & Business Media, Berlin.

Maccario M, Backman JR, Korein J (1972). Paradoxical caloric response in altered states of consciousness. Clinical and EEG correlations in toxic metabolic encephalopathies. Neurology 22 (8): 781–788.

Maddock H, Carley S, McCluskey A (1999). An unusual case of hysterical postoperative coma. Anaesthesia 54 (7): 717–718.

Meierkord H, Will B, Fish D et al. (1991). The clinical features and prognosis of pseudoseizures diagnosed using video-EEG telemetry. Neurology 41 (0028-3878 SB - A SB - M): 1643–1646.

Nunn KP, Lask B, Owen I (2014). Pervasive refusal syndrome (PRS) 21 years on: a re-conceptualisation and a renaming. Eur Child Adolesc Psychiatr 23 (3): 163–172.

Orr DL, Glassman AS (1985). Conversion phenomenon following general anesthesia. J Oral Maxillofac Surg 43 (10): 817–819.

Pareés I, Kojovic M, Pires C et al. (2014). Physical precipitating factors in functional movement disorders. J Neurol Sci 338 (1–2): 174–177.

Plum F, Posner JB (1972). The diagnosis of stupor and coma. Contemp Neurol Ser 10: 1–286.

Poole NA, Wuerz A, Agrawal N (2010). Abreaction for conversion disorder: systematic review with meta-analysis. Br J Psychiatr 197 (2): 91–95.

Poothrikovil RP, Gujjar AR, Al-Asmi A et al. (2015). Predictive value of short-term EEG recording in critically ill adult patients. Neurodiagn J 55 (3): 157–168.

Reuber M, Enright SM, Goulding PJ (2000a). Postoperative pseudostatus: not everything that shakes is epilepsy. Anaesthesia 55: 74–78.

Reuber M, Enright SM, Goulding PJ (2000b). Postoperative pseudostatus: not everything that shakes is epilepsy. Anaesthesia 55 (0003-2409 SB - AIM SB - IM): 74–78.

Reuber M, Pukrop R, Mitchell AJ et al. (2003). Clinical significance of recurrent psychogenic nonepileptic seizure status. J Neurol 250 (0340-5354 (Print)): 1355–1362 (Print).

Sallin K, Lagercrantz H, Evers K et al. (2016). Resignation syndrome: catatonia? culture-bound? Front Behav Neurosci 10: 7.

Sivaraju A, Gilmore EJ, Wira CR et al. (2015). Prognostication of post-cardiac arrest coma: early clinical and electroencephalographic predictors of outcome. Intensive Care Med 41 (7): 1264–1272.

Stone J, Edwards M (2012). Trick or treat? Showing patients with functional (psychogenic) motor symptoms their physical signs. Neurology 79 (3): 282–284.

Stone J, Sharpe M (2006). Functional symptoms in neurology: case studies. Neurol Clin 24 (2): 385–403.

Stone J, LaFrance WC, Brown R et al. (2011). Conversion disorder: current problems and potential solutions for DSM-5. J Psychosom Res 71 (1879-1360 (Electronic)): 369–376. Electronic.

Stone J, Warlow C, Sharpe M (2012). Functional weakness: clues to mechanism from the nature of onset. J Neurol Neurosurg Psychiatry 83 (1): 67–69.

Stone J, Hoeritzauer I, Brown K et al. (2014). Therapeutic sedation for functional (psychogenic) neurological symptoms. J Psychosom Res 76 (2): 165–168.

Taylor MA, Fink M (2003). Catatonia in psychiatric classification: a home of its own. Am J Psychiatr 160: 1233–1241.

Teasdale G, Jennett B (1974). Assessment of coma and impaired consciousness. A practical scale. Lancet 2 (7872): 81–84.

Thompson SL, Nunn KP (1997). The pervasive refusal syndrome: the RAHC experience. Clin Child Psychol Psychiatry 2 (1): 145–165.

Wadwekar V, Nair PP, Murgai A et al. (2014). Semiologic classification of psychogenic non epileptic seizures (PNES) based on video EEG analysis: do we need new classification systems? Seizure 23 (3): 222–226.

Weiss N, Regard L, Vidal C et al. (2012). Causes of coma and their evolution in the medical intensive care unit. J Neurol 259 (7): 1474–1477.

Wijdicks EFM (2010). The bare essentials: coma. Pract Neurol 10 (1): 51–60.

Wilson JE, Niu K, Nicolson SE et al. (2015). The diagnostic criteria and structure of catatonia. Schizophr Res 164 (1-3): 256–262.

World Health Organization (1992). International Statistical Classification of Diseases and Related Health Problems, 10th Revision (ICD-10). WHO, Geneva.

Zivin L, Marsan CA (1968). Incidence and prognostic significance of "epileptiform" activity in the EEG of non-epileptic subjects. Brain 91 (4): 751–778.

Handbook of Clinical Neurology, Vol. 139 (3rd series)
Functional Neurologic Disorders
M. Hallett, J. Stone, and A. Carson, Editors
http://dx.doi.org/10.1016/B978-0-12-801772-2.00029-1

Chapter 29

Functional and simulated visual loss

M. DATTILO[1], V. BIOUSSE[2,3], B.B. BRUCE[2,3,4], AND N.J. NEWMAN[2,3,5]*

[1]*Department of Ophthalmology, SUNY Downstate Medical Center, Brooklyn, NY, USA*

[2]*Department of Ophthalmology, Emory University Hospital, Emory University School of Medicine, Atlanta, GA, USA*

[3]*Department of Neurology, Emory University Hospital, Emory University School of Medicine, Atlanta, GA, USA*

[4]*Department of Epidemiology, Rollins School of Public Health, Emory University, Atlanta, GA, USA*

[5]*Department of Neurological Surgery, Emory University Hospital, Emory University School of Medicine, Atlanta, GA, USA*

Abstract

Nonorganic visual loss (NOVL) is the cause of a large number of referrals to neurologists and ophthalmologists and is a frequent area of overlap between neurologists, ophthalmologists, and psychiatrists. NOVL is the presence of visual impairment without an organic cause for disease despite a thorough and comprehensive investigation. A diagnosis of NOVL requires both the absence of any findings on examination and proof of the integrity and functioning of the visual system. Although sometimes a challenging diagnosis to make, there are a number of techniques and maneuvers which can be utilized fairly easily, either at the bedside or in the clinic, to help determine if a patient has NOVL. In some instances specialized testing, such as formal visual field testing, optical coherence tomography, visual evoked responses, electroretinogram, and various imaging modalities (magnetic resonance imaging) are performed to help determine if the cause of visual loss is organic or nonorganic. Once a diagnosis of NOVL is made, treatment centers around reassurance of the patient, close follow-up, and, if necessary, referral to a psychiatrist, as these patients may have underlying psychiatric disorders and a preceding strong emotional event leading to the current symptoms, and may be more likely to develop depression and anxiety.

INTRODUCTION

Functional or nonorganic disease is a common source of referral to neuro-ophthalmologists (Henningsen et al., 2003; Reuber et al., 2005; Stone et al., 2005), and falls within the categories of "conversion disorder" and "factitious disorder" (American Psychiatric Association and American Psychiatric Association DSM-5 Task Force, 2013).

Patients diagnosed with visual loss related to conversion disorder or factitious disorder exhibit visual symptoms suggesting a medical condition. Although no medical or physical cause for their symptoms can be identified, their symptoms are associated with significant distress and dysfunction. All of these patients typically undergo an extensive and exhaustive workup, usually performed by a variety of specialists, to rule out organic diseases (Weller and Wiedemann, 1989; Felber et al., 1993; Villegas and Ilsen, 2007), which rarely produces a unifying physical diagnosis and leaves the patient and physician dissatisfied and frustrated (Kathol et al., 1983a, c; Keltner et al., 1985; Thompson, 1985). This situation is particularly difficult when patients with organic disease exaggerate their symptoms (so-called "functional overlay"), which is a very common problem in neuro-ophthalmology.

Differentiating between patients who are intentionally feigning disease to assume the sick role or for secondary gain versus those whose symptoms are not intentionally produced is difficult and remains in the realm of the psychiatrist (Bruce and Newman, 2010; Newman and Biousse, 2014). Since the focus of this chapter is on

*Correspondence to: N.J. Newman, Department of Ophthalmology, Emory University Hospital, Emory University School of Medicine, Atlanta GA 30322, USA. E-mail: OPHTNJN@emory.edu

visual loss without anatomic or organic cause, the term nonorganic visual loss (NOVL) will be used throughout this chapter to include all patients who present with visual loss without a definitive anatomic or organic cause irrespective of whether the symptoms described are intentionally produced or outside of the patient's conscious control.

As an aside, it is important to note that care must be taken with medical documentation as there are medicolegal consequences derived from the diagnoses and medical billing codes used in patients' charts. For example, certain diagnoses, such as malingering, will preclude patients from receiving compensation and certain services in some states in the USA (Lessell, 2011); additionally, driving often becomes illegal for patients with documented visual loss.

NONORGANIC VISUAL LOSS

One area where the fields of neurology, ophthalmology, and sometimes psychiatry overlap is the patient with visual disturbances or visual loss. Neurologists and ophthalmologists are frequently asked to evaluate patients with unexplained visual loss. A proportion of these patients will have NOVL (Schlaegel and Quilala, 1955; Kirk and Saunders, 1977; Berlin et al., 1983; Kathol et al., 1983a, c; Stone et al., 2005; Villegas and Ilsen, 2007; Incesu, 2013). Differentiating between organic visual loss and NOVL has important therapeutic, medical, and legal ramifications (Mavrakanas and Schutz, 2009; Lessell, 2011).

Simply stated, NOVL is visual impairment in the absence of any biologic or physical cause for the visual impairment. This implies a normal ophthalmologic examination, absence of abnormal laboratory values which can cause visual disturbances, and normal imaging of the orbit and brain. As with all nonorganic diseases, the diagnosis of NOVL requires the absence of findings on examination. However, this is not sufficient; the physician must prove the integrity and functioning of the visual system prior to diagnosing a patient with only NOVL (Bruce and Newman, 2010; Newman and Biousse, 2014).

Patients with NOVL frequently are referred to neurologists and neuro-ophthalmologists after detailed ophthalmologic examination fails to find a cause for the reported symptoms (Kathol et al., 1983b; Miller, 2011). Up to 12% of patients who present to an ophthalmologist with visual loss are diagnosed with NOVL and these cases can represent up to 5% of the referrals to neurologists (Schlaegel and Quilala, 1955; Kathol et al., 1983b, c; Villegas and Ilsen, 2007; American Psychiatric Association and American Psychiatric Association DSM-5 Task Force, 2013; Incesu, 2013). The scope of the problem is likely larger than is reported in the current literature, because of the frequent coexistence of organic visual loss and NOVL in the same patient. It has been reported that 16–53% of patients presenting with NOVL also have organic disease with abnormal findings on neuro-ophthalmologic examination (Bain et al., 2000; Scott and Egan, 2003; Ney et al., 2009; Incesu and Sobaci, 2011).

NOVL can occur at any age and in either gender. In general, there is a female predominance. Children more frequently present with bilateral symmetric visual loss, while adults present with monocular or binocular visual loss (Behrman and Levy, 1970; Kathol et al., 1983c; Weller and Wiedemann, 1989; Clarke et al., 1996; Griffiths and Eddyshaw, 2004; Lim et al., 2005; Toldo et al., 2010; Gupta et al., 2011; Munoz-Hernandez et al., 2012; Pula, 2012). Despite the strict definition of NOVL requiring the absence of any physical cause for vision loss, it is critical to realize that patients believed to have NOVL can have underlying visual pathology and patients with organic visual pathology can have concomitant NOVL. Therefore, a thorough investigation must be undertaken to rule out any and all causes of visual loss, lest we do our patients a disservice and possibly fail to diagnose a treatable condition.

Neurologists and neuro-ophthalmologists are in a unique position when it comes to evaluating a patient suspected of having NOVL because the visual system follows specific anatomic guidelines and principles which are typically not well known to the patient (Bruce and Newman, 2010; Newman and Biousse, 2014). For example, lesions in certain areas of the visual pathways produce characteristic visual field deficits which can be used to localize the lesion (Fig. 29.1). These patterns of visual field loss are not intuitively known to the patient and would be nearly impossible to reproduce without either extensive knowledge of the visual system or an organic cause for the visual field loss. Additionally, the visual system is unique in that most parameters of the visual system are either directly observable (e.g., pupils, eye movements) or are quantifiable (e.g., visual acuity, color vision) (Bruce and Newman, 2010; Newman and Biousse, 2014). Therefore, using objective tests, it is usually possible to identify nonorganic responses and prove, unequivocally, the integrity of the visual system.

EVALUATION

Any evaluation of a visual disturbance must begin with determining whether the disturbance is monocular or binocular. Monocular visual disturbances are localized to the parts of the visual system anterior to the optic chiasm (i.e., optic nerve, orbit, and globe). Binocular visual disturbances typically localize at the optic chiasm or

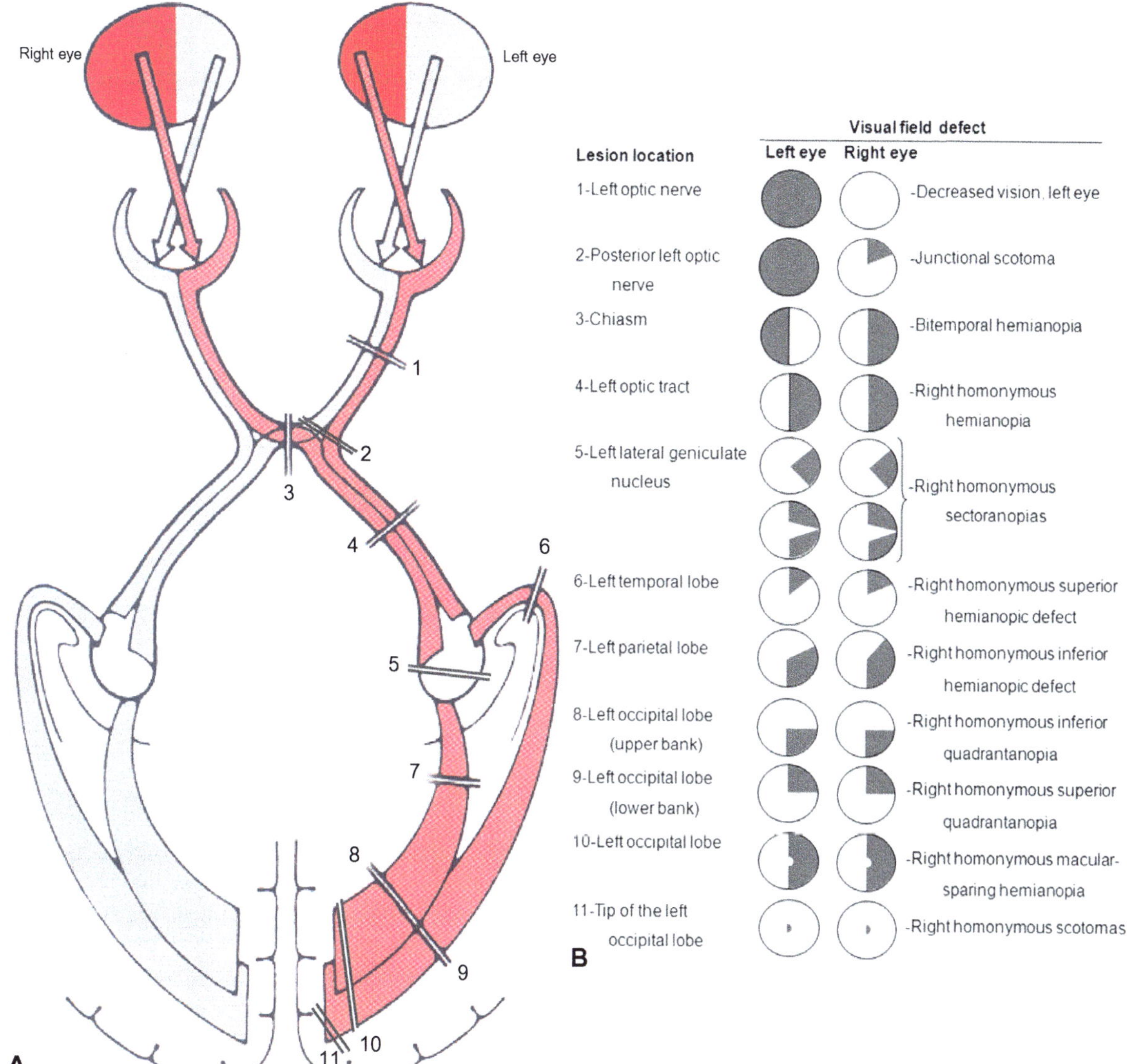

Fig. 29.1. Visual pathway anatomy and characteristic visual field defects. (**A**) Schematic depicting the anatomy of the intracranial visual pathways with lesions of the visual pathway noted at the numbered locations (1–11). The representation from each hemiretina (nasal and temporal) is depicted as well, with the temporal retina of the left eye and the nasal retina of the right eye projecting to the visual pathway of the left side of the brain, and vice versa. Also depicted is the decussation of nerve fibers from the optic nerve at the optic chiasm. (**B**) Schematic depicting the representative visual field defects arising from the corresponding lesions shown in (**A**). (Reproduced with permission from Biousse and Newman, 2009, pp. 42–43.)

posterior to the optic chiasm, although bilateral ocular or optic nerve lesions can also produce binocular visual loss.

As with any patient, the examination initially starts with observation of the patient in the waiting room, while in the examination room, and while navigating an unfamiliar environment (as the patient traverses the waiting room on the way to the examination room) (Villegas and Ilsen, 2007; Incesu, 2013; Rota et al., 2014). For example, the observation of a patient wearing sunglasses indoors, the "sunglasses sign," without an obvious ophthalmic reason for light sensitivity, is highly suggestive of NOVL. It has been reported that the sensitivity and specificity of the "sunglasses sign" for NOVL is 0.46 and 0.995, respectively. The use of sunglasses in the ophthalmologist's office increased the probability of NOVL from 0.043 to 0.079 (Bengtzen et al., 2008). In addition, in a patient describing profound bilateral visual loss, observation of the patient in a novel environment is useful, since the ability to track objects and navigate new environments should be severely impaired. Patients with NOVL may avoid walking into objects or maneuver a new environment with ease, whereas this would be impossible for a person with truly profound vision loss in both eyes. Patients with NOVL describing "blindness" or profound visual impairment in both eyes may also be observed to track objects while sitting in the waiting room or the physician in the examination room (Incesu, 2013).

MONOCULAR VISION LOSS

Monocular vision loss represents the ideal testing situation, since it is difficult for the patient to separate out what each eye sees individually (Bruce and Newman, 2010; Newman and Biousse, 2014). Truly monocular patients can still navigate a new environment with ease as long as there is useful vision in the unaffected eye. However, observation does have a role in the NOVL patient who complains of monocular vision loss. For example, these patients may attempt to close one eye during examination to simulate their complaint of monocular vision loss (Bruce and Newman, 2010; Newman and Biousse, 2014). Patching the good eye (with a taped patch) of a patient with presumed profound monocular visual loss and observing the patient's behavior during the interview can be helpful. The success of many of the tests that will be presented in the rest of this chapter depends, in part, on the ability of the examiner to use sleight of hand, appropriate banter, and misdirection, much in the same way an illusionist misdirects an audience with hand or body motions or distracts the audience with skillfully engaging banter (Bruce and Newman, 2010; Newman and Biousse, 2014).

Tests of stereopsis are a good way to prove useful binocular vision. Good stereopsis requires good vision in each eye individually and the ability to use the eyes in unison (fusion) (Levy and Glick, 1974; Bruce and Newman, 2010; Newman and Biousse, 2014). When performing stereopsis with a patient suspected of monocular NOVL, the examiner should describe the test in a way that is truthful but does not give away the examiner's true intent, such as saying, "This is a test of your ability to see in 3D." Table 29.1 shows the association between stereopsis and visual acuity in each eye for the degree of stereopsis recorded (Levy and Glick, 1974).

Similarly, using glasses with colored lenses (one green lens and one red lens) or glasses with lenses which are polarized in different directions can help unmask the NOVL patient. Using specially designed eye charts with alternating green and red letters, in the former case, or with polarized letters, in the latter case, can allow the examiner to test the vision in each eye separately without the patient's knowledge (Levy and Glick, 1974; Bruce and Newman, 2010; Newman and Biousse, 2014). In the case of using colored lenses, the patient will only be able to see red letters through the red lens and green letters through the green lens. Similarly, polarized lenses only allow light through them that is projected in the same axis as the lenses and no light will be seen if the axis of the light is 90° away from the axis of lens polarization.

Table 29.1

Relationship of Snellen visual acuity and stereopsis*

Stereopsis (arc seconds)	Visual acuity in each eye (Snellen)
40	20/20
43	20/25
52	20/30
61	20/40
89	20/50
94	20/70
124	20/100
160	20/200

Adapted from Biousse and Newman (2009), pp. 7 and 503.
*Stereopsis, measured in arc seconds from a standard Titmus test, is listed in the left-hand column. The corresponding minimum Snellen visual acuity necessary to obtain a given score on Titmus testing is listed in the right-hand column. A mismatch between visual acuity and stereopsis, i.e., worse visual acuity than would be suggested by the corresponding Titmus test score, is suggestive of nonorganic visual loss.

Testing stereopsis and/or using glasses with colored lenses or polarized lenses are excellent choices in the NOVL patient reporting decreased vision in only one eye, because they work on principles that are typically not known to our patients. They allow the patient to keep both eyes open yet actually test each eye individually without altering/manipulating the vision in the "better-seeing" eye, they are quantifiable, and they can be replicated accurately among examiners.

A newly designed pocket eye card, developed for use with patients suspected of NOVL, contains objects of progressively decreasing size, but the minimum visual acuity necessary to see the largest objects on the card is the same as the visual acuity needed to see the smallest objects. Patients with organic visual loss are able to identify all objects on the eye card, while patients with NOVL have a tendency to only identify the larger objects (Mojon and Flueckiger, 2002; Pula, 2012).

Another quantifiable test for determining vision in the reportedly worse eye is to fog (add a moderately high plus lens in front of) the "better-seeing" eye, effectively reducing the vision in that eye. The best vision obtained from the patient will then equal the vision from the non-fogged, "bad" eye (Miller, 1973; Kramer et al., 1979; Smith et al., 1983; Keltner et al., 1985; Thompson, 1985; Bienfang and Kurtz, 1998). Although fogging typically requires the use of a phoropter, a specialized piece of equipment used for refraction in ophthalmology practices, holding up a loose lens in front of the patient has the same effect. Alternatively, fogging glasses can be made from over-the-counter reading glasses, where one lens of a moderately high-power pair of reading glasses (e.g., +3.50 D) is removed and replaced with either a low-power plus lens (e.g., +0.25 D) or a lens without any refractive power (plano). These glasses can then be placed on to the patient to obtain a quantifiable measure of vision from the eye in question. These tests have the advantage of not only being able to disprove dysfunction of the involved eye, but to quantifiably demonstrate the degree of function in that eye, thereby allowing the examiner to diagnose NOVL.

Less quantitative maneuvers also exist, such as the prism test or binocular visual field test. In the prism test an object, such as a letter on the eye chart, is presented to the patient and each eye is sequentially occluded. The object chosen for the test should be the largest object that the patient reports being able to see with the "good" eye but unable to see with the "bad" eye. A prism (e.g., 4-D prism) is placed vertically over the "good" eye and the patient is asked if he or she sees two objects (Bienfang and Kurtz, 1998; Golnik et al., 2004; Chen et al., 2007; Bruce and Newman, 2010; Pula, 2012; Newman and Biousse, 2014). If the patient sees two objects, then the examiner has proven useful vision in the "bad" eye. A truly monocular patient would never be able to see two objects on a prism test.

A variation on this test involves occluding the "bad" eye and bisecting the visual axis of the "good" eye with a prism producing monocular diplopia in the "good" eye. The patient is then asked to open the "bad" eye and the prism is quickly shifted to completely cover the "good" eye (ideally, without the patient being aware that the prism has been moved). In patients with extremely poor vision in one eye, no diplopia will be present. However, a patient with NOVL will still claim to have diplopia (Incesu, 2013). This is a useful variation of the prism test but does involve some sleight of hand and may be uncovered by the astute patient with NOVL. Although these tests are useful skills to have, one premise is that the "bad" eye must have profoundly worse vision than the "good" eye. These tests are not useful for patients complaining of subtle vision loss in one eye.

In patients claiming vision worse than 20/400 in one eye, an optokinetic nystagmus (OKN) drum can be used to assess vision in the "bad" eye. Once the "good" eye is occluded, the OKN drum is rotated in front of the patient. The presence of the appropriate fast and slow phase of nystagmus in response to the OKN drum in the "bad" eye demonstrates a visual acuity of at least 20/200 (Weller and Wiedemann, 1989; Bienfang and Kurtz, 1998; Bruce and Newman, 2010; Newman and Biousse, 2014).

The binocular visual field test, another test best utilized with patients complaining of profound monocular vision loss, works by mapping the physiologic blind spot on formal visual field testing. With both eyes open the physiologic blind spot should not be apparent on the visual field display. However, if one eye has profound vision loss, then the blind spot will be present, even with both eyes open. The caveat is that mapping the blind spot even with one eye occluded requires the patient to have good fixation on the specified target throughout the test. If the patient is unable to fixate on the target then the blind spot will not be mapped even in a person with good visual acuity (Bruce and Newman, 2010; Newman and Biousse, 2014).

Testing pupillary responses is essential in patients with monocular visual loss. The lack of a relative afferent pupillary defect (RAPD or Marcus Gunn pupil) implies functioning of the visual system from the retina to the optic chiasm. Ocular diseases responsible for profound visual loss are obvious on examination. When the ocular examination is normal, profound monocular visual loss suggests an optic neuropathy and an RAPD should be obvious. Occult retinal disorders must not be missed in this situation. Posterior to the optic chiasm, up to the level of the lateral geniculate body, a lesion of the optic tract will produce a subtle contralateral RAPD (Bruce and Newman, 2010; Newman and Biousse, 2014).

The tests described in the following section on binocular visual loss can also be applied to patients with monocular visual loss; however, in patients with monocular visual loss, the "good" eye must be occluded in order to prove useful vision in the "bad" eye. Astute patients with NOVL may tailor their responses to the eye being tested. Careful misdirection and sleight of hand are sometimes necessary to get a reliable examination in these situations.

BINOCULAR VISION LOSS

Proving NOVL in patients with binocular visual loss can be more difficult than in patients with monocular visual loss (Bruce and Newman, 2010; Newman and Biousse, 2014). Several methods are helpful in assessing the patient with binocular vision loss. Some rely on the suggestibility of the patient or innate ocular and visual reflexes, while others rely on the physiology of the brain, not well known by most patients, to prove the existence of a functioning visual system.

One test with reportedly high sensitivity and specificity for NOVL is to record the patient's visual acuity at the full distance from the eye chart (20 feet) and at half the distance to the eye chart (10 feet). Frequently patients with NOVL will report the same visual acuity at both distances. The visual system is designed in such a way that the recorded vision at 10 feet should be twice as good as it is at 20 feet. For example, a normal patient with a Snellen

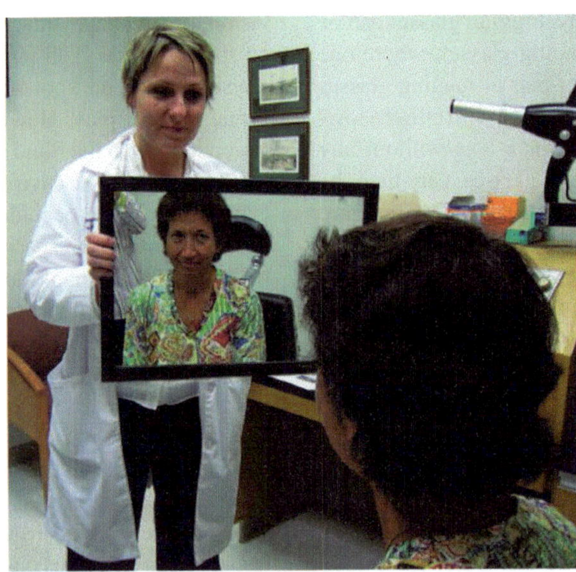

Fig. 29.2. The mirror test. A large mirror is held in front of the patient and the patient is instructed to look straight ahead into the mirror. The mirror is slowly rotated in front of the patient and the patient's eye movements are observed. Patients with markedly decreased vision will not follow their own image in the mirror. However, patients with nonorganic visual loss will follow their own image in the mirror. This test can be performed with both eyes open if the patient claims severe bilateral visual loss or, with each eye patched, to determine the response to the motion of the mirror in each eye separately. (Reproduced with permission from Biousse and Newman, 2009, p. 505.)

eye chart visual acuity of 20/200 at 20 feet should read the 20/100 line at 10 feet; however, NOVL patients will typically read to the same visual acuity line at 20 and 10 feet (Zinkernagel and Mojon, 2009; Bruce and Newman, 2010; Newman and Biousse, 2014).

Another test, which relies on the ability to engage the patient and the patient's suggestibility, is to have the patient begin reading the eye chart at the lowest possible acuity line (20/10). The examiner must give the patient a great deal of time on each line and must also provide constant encouragement and prodding, with statements like, "You should be able to read this line. I'm going to make the letters larger for you so they will be easier for you to read. Give me your best guess for all of the letters on the line." Not infrequently, people with NOVL will be able to accurately read the 20/20 to 20/30 line on the eye chart (Bruce and Newman, 2010; Pula, 2012; Newman and Biousse, 2014). However this test is not useful in the patient who is obviously intentionally feigning vision loss.

Less quantifiable tests also exist which can be used to at least prove the presence of vision in a patient reporting profound visual loss (i.e., counting fingers vision to no light perception vision). As mentioned above in the section on monocular vision loss, an OKN drum can also be used in a patient claiming profound visual loss in both eyes. One eye should be occluded and the OKN drum presented to the nonoccluded eye. The test should then be repeated in the other eye. If each eye shows the appropriate fast and slow phase of nystagmus, then vision $\geq$20/200 has been established (Weller and Wiedemann, 1989; Bienfang and Kurtz, 1998; Bruce and Newman, 2010; Newman and Biousse, 2014).

Additionally, the mirror test can be performed. In this test a large mirror is held in front of the patient and slowly rotated back and forth in the vertical axis in front of the patient (Fig. 29.2). It is very difficult for a seeing patient to avoid following his/her image in the mirror (Kramer et al., 1979; Smith et al., 1983; Bruce and Newman, 2010; Miller, 2011; Newman and Biousse, 2014). Also, patients can be asked to look at their own hand or to touch their two extended index fingers together (Fig. 29.3) or to touch the tip of their own extended finger to their nose (finger-to-nose test) (Weller and Wiedemann, 1989; Villegas and Ilsen, 2007; Bruce and Newman, 2010; Newman and Biousse, 2014). Truly blind patients will be able to perform these tasks with ease, as they rely on proprioception and not on visual acuity or the presence of vision. Since these tests appear to require a functioning visual system, the patient with NOVL likely will perform poorly on these tests. These patients may be noted to stare in obscure directions when asked to look at their own hand, intentionally avoiding where they are holding their hand. Similarly, they likely will not be able to touch the tips of their index fingers together or to touch their nose with their index finger.

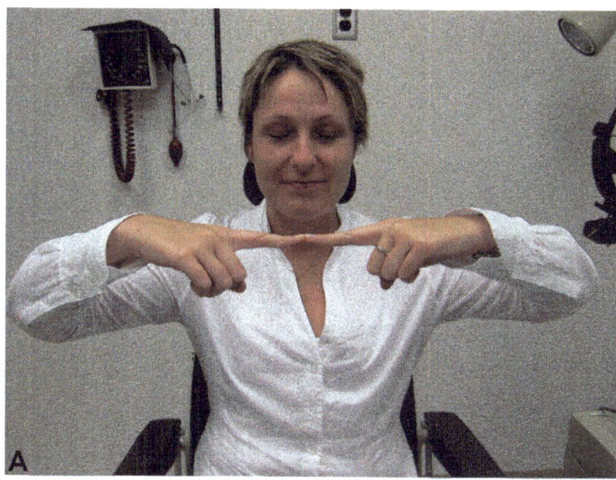

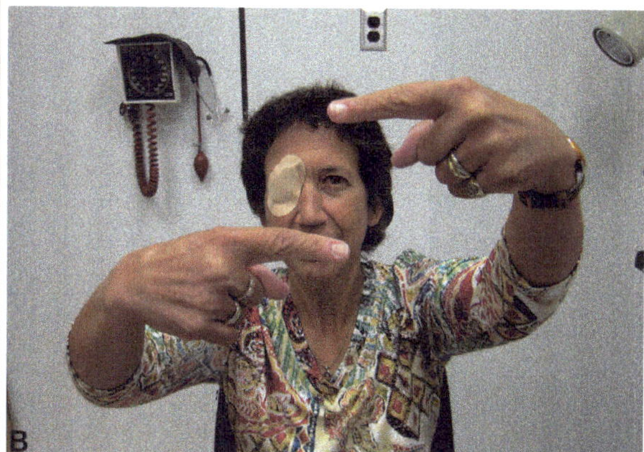

Fig. 29.3. Finger-to-finger test. The patient is asked to extend the arms and then extend the index finger of each hand. With the good eye patched, or both eyes open if claiming severe bilateral visual loss, the patient is asked to bring the tips of the index fingers together. Though this test seems to rely on the presence of a functioning visual system, the test actually relies on proprioception and not visual acuity. As in (**A**), truly blind patients or normal individuals with both eyes closed can easily bring the tips of their index fingers together. However, patients with nonorganic visual loss will oftentimes struggle to bring the tips of their fingers together or be completely unable to perform the task (**B**). (Reproduced with permission from Biousse and Newman, 2009, p. 504.)

VISUAL FIELD LOSS

In addition to vision loss, NOVL can take the form of visual field changes. The most common visual field change seen in patients with NOVL is a constricted visual field (tunnel vision) (Linhart, 1956; Keane, 1979, 1998). Although the visual field may appear to be severely constricted, these patients may be observed to navigate novel environments (i.e., the waiting room or examination room) without difficulty. On visual field testing (confrontation, tangent screen (Fig. 29.4), Goldmann), patients with NOVL often do not show an appropriate increase in the size of the visual field with increasing distance from the target objects (Kramer et al., 1979; Keltner et al., 1985; Thompson et al., 1996; Pineles and Volpe, 2004; Villegas and Ilsen, 2007; Bruce and Newman, 2010; Hsu et al., 2010; Miller, 2011; Incesu, 2013; Newman and Biousse, 2014). Normal physiology of the visual system is such that, as the distance to an area or point of reference is doubled, your field of vision also doubles. Additionally, Goldmann perimetry may show overlap of isopters (which does not occur physiologically), indicating that smaller, dimmer objects are seen further in the periphery than are larger, brighter objects (Linhart, 1956).

Patients with NOVL may also plot out a continuous spiral pattern or other nonphysiologic patterns, such as a star pattern or, in rare instances, shapes of animals, on kinetic visual field testing (Linhart, 1956; Keane, 1979, 1998; Keltner et al., 1985; Thompson, 1985; Weller and Wiedemann, 1989; Barris et al., 1992; Graf, 1999; Bain et al., 2000; Pineles and Volpe, 2004; Villegas and Ilsen, 2007; Bruce and Newman, 2010; Hsu et al., 2010; Miller, 2011; Incesu, 2013; Newman and Biousse, 2014) (Fig. 29.5).

In addition to the above-mentioned patterns, other visual field patterns can be seen in patients with NOVL, though they are much less common (Smith and Baker, 1987; Thompson et al., 1996; Keane, 1998). Monocular temporal hemianopias, if believed to be nonorganic in origin, can be evaluated by performing a binocular visual field. In patients with NOVL, the hemianopia may persist even when testing the patient while both eyes are open (Keane, 1979, 1982; Martin, 1998; Yoneda et al., 2013). In a patient with organic disease causing a monocular temporal hemianopia, when the visual field is repeated with both eyes open, the good eye will compensate, at least partially, if not completely, for the decreased visual field in the bad eye, resulting in a fuller field with binocular testing as compared to monocular testing (Miller, 2011; Incesu, 2013). Similar is the patient claiming profound vision loss in one eye with good vision in the other eye. Someone with organic disease will show recovery of all or part of the monocular visual field defect when tested with both eyes open, while the patient with NOVL may show a nonphysiologic constriction of the visual field or preservation of visual field loss on the side of the "bad" eye, even with binocular visual field testing (Fig. 29.6). This test requires the patient to be cooperative and concentrate on the specified fixation target.

An alternative to testing the visual field with each eye separately and then with both eyes open is to test each

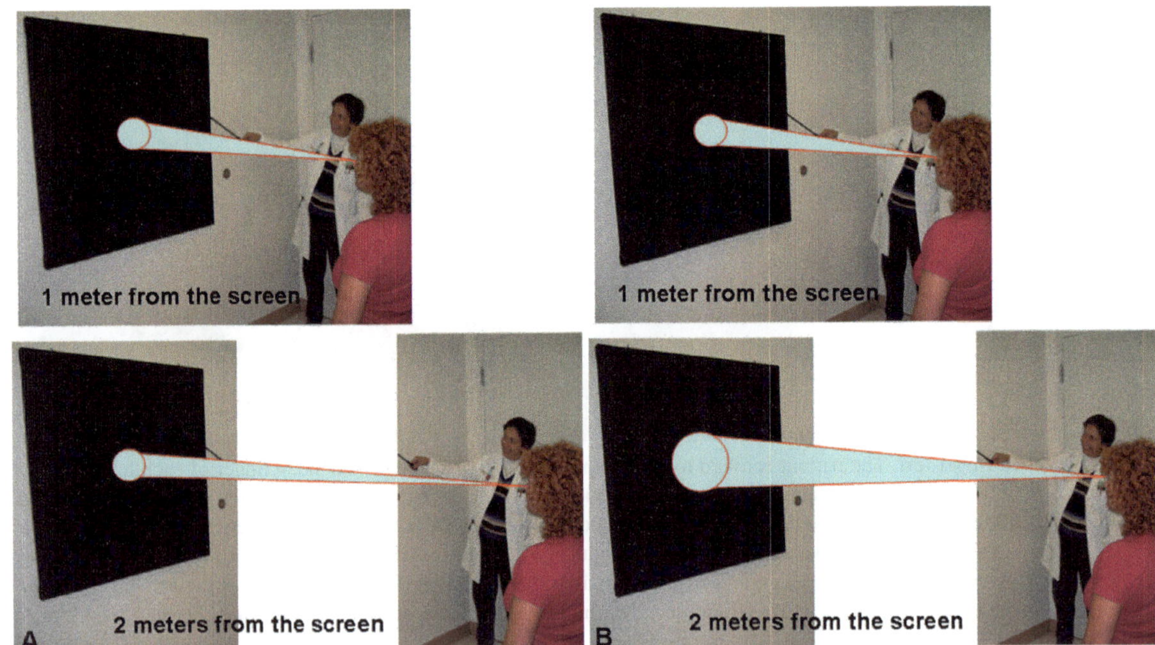

Fig. 29.4. Nonphysiologic visual field constriction on tangent screen. The patient's visual field is initially tested at the standard testing distance (i.e., 1 meter on tangent screen testing (**A**) or in a standard visual field machine (not shown)). A large proportion of patients with nonorganic visual loss (NOVL) will show a constricted visual field (**A**). The test is then repeated at double the distance (i.e., 2 meters on tangent screen testing (**B**) or with reverse telescopic lenses in a standard visual field machine (not shown)). The physiology of the visual system is such that doubling the distance to a target in a visual field test will double the size of the visual field. However, in patients with NOVL, doubling the distance to the target will not produce the appropriate increase in size of the visual field (**B**). (Reproduced with permission from Biousse and Newman, 2009, p. 507.)

eye separately while the patient has both eyes open. This technique was described by Martin (1998): two fixation targets were placed on the automated static perimeter and a piece of cardboard was placed in between the patient's eyes, effectively separating the visual fields of each eye, and allowing the visual field of each eye to be tested independently while the patient has both eyes open (Martin, 1998). The patient is initially told that only the good eye is being tested and the visual fields for both eyes are plotted. The test is then repeated and the patient is told that only the bad eye is being tested. Patients with NOVL consistently perform worse in both visual fields when they believe that the bad eye is being tested (large intertest difference in visual field thresholds but minimal intereye threshold difference). Conversely, patients with organic monocular visual field tests perform similarly (similar threshold values) whether they are told that the "good" or "bad" eye is being tested. Patients with an organic cause for their visual field loss have a large intereye threshold difference but minimal intertest difference. Normal individuals have low intertest and low intereye differences. Although this test requires special equipment, it has the advantage of proving a normal visual field in the reportedly "bad" eye, thereby proving NOVL.

Another characteristic sign of NOVL is pattern reversal on subsequent manual kinetic visual field testing. In this test the subject has the visual field test performed first on the right eye and then on the left eye in standard fashion. As an example, we will assume that the right eye showed a spiral pattern on Goldmann visual field testing suggestive of NOVL, and a normal or nonspiral pattern in the left eye. On a subsequent visit, the same type of visual field test should be repeated, with the only difference being that the left eye is tested first. Reversal of the visual field pattern, i.e., spiral pattern seen in the left eye and nonspiral pattern in the right eye, is a classic sign of NOVL, since this would never occur physiologically and no organic disease process is known to cause visual field patterns to transfer between eyes (Incesu, 2013).

Additionally, manual kinetic perimetry allows the investigator to move the location of the fixation target. If the fixation target is moved, then the location of visual field defects should move a corresponding distance and in the same direction as the new fixation target. NOVL patients may map out the visual field deficit in the exact same location as the initial test (Lim et al., 2005; Incesu, 2013).

Another method of assessing visual field loss in a patient suspected of NOVL is to have the patient quickly

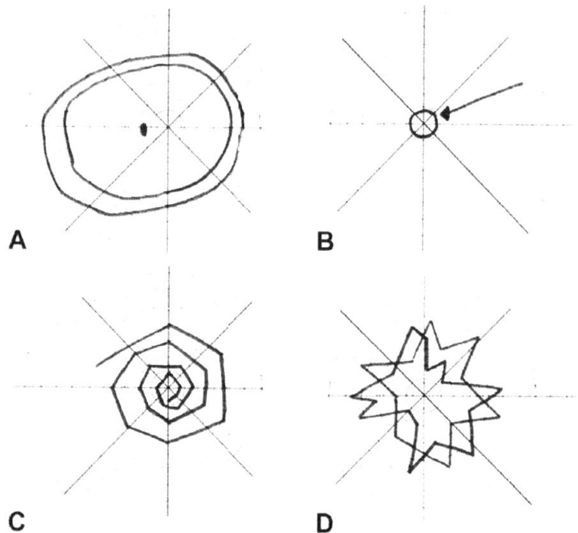

Fig. 29.5. Representative Goldmann visual fields depicting a normal visual field (**A**) and examples of visual fields seen in nonorganic visual loss (NOVL) (**B–D**). (**A**) Representative visual field from a normal patient. Note the progressively larger visual field seen with larger, brighter stimuli. (**B**) Representative visual field showing nonphysiologic constriction of visual field seen in NOVL. In contrast to the normal patient, there is no increase in the size of the visual field with increasing size and/or intensity of the visual stimulus. (**C**) Representative visual field from a patient with NOVL demonstrating a spiral pattern. (**D**) Representative visual field from a patient with NOVL demonstrating a star-shaped pattern. In this visual field note the overlapping or crossing of isopters on the Goldmann visual field, indicative of a nonphysiologic visual field.

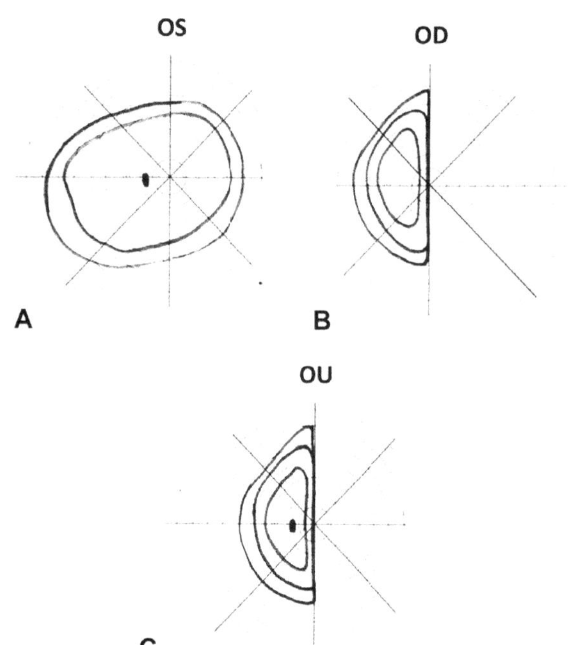

Fig. 29.6. Representative Goldmann visual field from a patient claiming a monocular visual field deficit. (**A**) Representative visual field from the patient's left eye (OS) showing a normal visual field. (**B**) Representative visual field of the right eye (OD) demonstrating a temporal visual field deficit. (**C**) Visual field performed with both eyes open, showing preservation of the temporal visual field deficit, as seen in (**B**). In a patient with true organic pathology producing the visual field deficit shown in (**B**), performing the visual field with both eyes open would compensate, at least in part, if not completely, for the visual field deficit in the right eye and produce a more normal visual field. Patients with nonorganic visual loss can show nonphysiologic preservation of monocular visual field deficits on binocular visual field testing.

look from a finger on one of the examiner's hand to a finger on the examiner's other hand. Initially the two fingers are held close together, in the patient's reported visual field. The fingers are slowly separated as the patient is asked to continue looking quickly from one finger to the other finger. A patient with NOVL will be able to perform this task with one saccade required to fixate on each finger, even when the fingers are slowly moved out of the reported visual field. In contrast, a patient with organic visual field loss will require more than one saccade, possibly two, three, or more saccades, to be able to quickly fixate on the finger that has been moved outside of the patient's visual field (Zinkernagel et al., 2009; Bruce and Newman, 2010; Incesu, 2013; Newman and Biousse, 2014).

Although static automated perimetry might be problematic in determining if a patient has NOVL due to inconsistent patient responses and the learning curve required to produce reliable, repeatable tests, in some cases they may be useful in the diagnosis of NOVL (Macleod et al., 1994; Frisen, 2014). However the methods used to analyze the fields are different from the standard method used to analyze visual fields. One characteristic that suggests NOVL on automated static perimetry is a change in the pattern of the visual field loss between examinations, e.g., tunnel vision on the initial exam in the right eye, which changes to a hemianopia on repeat testing at a future date. The presence of "threshold spikes," isolated areas within an area of visual field loss that show better-than-average threshold levels, in random locations within a visual field defect, is indicative of nonorganic visual field loss (Frisen, 2014). These spikes may be seen at the border zones of visual field deficits in patients with organic visual field loss but they have not been reported to occur within the central area of the visual field loss with organic pathology. These "threshold spikes" are not detectable in the gray-scale perimetric maps, but are detectable in the numeric maps for the total and pattern deviation. These spikes lend themselves to numeric quantification and cutoff values for determining if a spike is present can be objectively defined (e.g., deviation > 3 dB above neighboring depressed levels) (Frisen, 2014).

Certain visual field patterns are highly suggestive of organic disease, such as central scotomas, bitemporal hemianopias, and arcuate defects (Scott and Egan, 2003; Incesu, 2013; Frisen, 2014). Most patients are not well-enough versed in the visual system and its physiology to be able to spontaneously produce these types of visual field patterns, which typically require a detailed workup as to the cause of the visual field loss (Ghate et al., 2014). However, it recently has been shown that healthy, visual field-naïve patients can reliably simulate neurologic visual field defects after having been shown pictures of the visual field defect to simulate (Ghate et al., 2014). Hemianopias and quadrantanopias were more easily and more reliably produced and reproduced than enlarged blind spots, cecocentral scotomas, or paracentral scotomas (Thompson et al., 1996; Ghate et al., 2014). Since it has been shown that visual field defects suggestive of organic pathology (e.g., central scotomas, cecocentral scotomas) can be simulated reliably by people without true organic disease, information garnered form visual fields needs to be viewed in the entire clinical context and not in isolation. The appropriate workup needs to be performed based on the individual's complaints and entire clinical presentation, with visual fields being only a piece of the entire puzzle.

In conclusion, even if patients are not complaining of visual field loss, testing visual fields in patients believed to have NOVL is still a useful endeavor because most patients with NOVL will have visual field patterns that can provide further evidence supporting a diagnosis of NOVL.

IMAGING AND ANCILLARY TESTING

Although a thorough clinical examination with the appropriate techniques as outlined above will usually be sufficient to prove normal functioning of the visual system and the presence of NOVL, there are some cases where other testing modalities will need to be employed in order to definitively prove normal anatomy and functioning of the visual system and diagnose a patient with NOVL. These ancillary tests (e.g., magnetic resonance imaging (MRI), optical coherence tomography, visual evoked potentials (VEPs), electroretinograms (ERGs)) are excellent for determining if an organic pathology exists from the retina to the visual cortex. The one caveat is that these tests require, to some degree, the active participation and cooperation of the patient (Weinstein et al., 1991; Bobak et al., 1993; Bienfang and Kurtz, 1998; Saitoh et al., 2001). For example, VEP measures the brain activity in the visual cortex in response to visual stimuli that appear and disappear or that reverse. The stimuli can either be simple patterns, such as a checkerboard pattern, or more complex images, such as the image of a face or complex scene (Kramer et al., 1979; Weinstein et al., 1991; Bobak et al., 1993). A normal VEP test with normal and symmetric latency and amplitude of responses in a patient reporting severe monocular visual loss is inconsistent with an organic cause of visual loss (Kramer et al., 1979; Nakamura et al., 2001).

Similarly, multifocal VEP can also be used to objectively assess visual fields. In a patient reporting constriction of visual fields, and even demonstrating constricted visual fields on perimetric testing, a normal multifocal VEP essentially proves a full visual field and diagnoses NOVL in these patients (Petersen and Airas, 1985; Hood et al., 2003; Raghunandan and Buckingham, 2008; Bhatt, 2013; Incesu, 2013; Yoneda et al., 2013). Because voluntary changes or obliteration of the evoked responses is not only possible but not uncommon, and may even be undetected by trained observers, an abnormal test is not helpful in deciphering which patients have true organic disease versus those patients with NOVL (Bobak et al., 1993; Saitoh et al., 2001).

Similarly, with pattern and multifocal ERGs, tests of the electric response of the retina to a flash or pattern of light (Weinstein et al., 1991), a normal symmetric test makes severe organic dysfunction of the retina unlikely, while an abnormal test is not beneficial in making the determination between organic and nonorganic disease (Kramer et al., 1979; Weinstein et al., 1991). Certain ancillary tests evaluate only certain aspects of the visual system; the flash ERG, for example, evaluates the function of cells in the outer retinal layers (e.g., photoreceptor cells, ganglion cells), while the pattern ERG detects abnormalities in the inner retina, such as the ganglion cell layer and the optic nerve (Weinstein et al., 1991). Although an abnormal test indicates organic dysfunction in the part of the visual system being tested, it does not rule out dysfunction in other areas of the visual system (such as the optic nerve, optic tracts, or brain proper in the case of the flash ERG).

Neuroimaging may also be employed to assess the anatomic integrity of certain parts of the visual system, such as looking for brain lesions which may account for vision or visual field complaints. These studies may help rule out infarction or mass lesions which may be responsible for the reported symptoms. Although no functional imaging modality can be used to diagnose, or potentially even add evidence towards a diagnosis of NOVL, a common pattern on functional MRI and positron emission tomography scanning has been reported in a few cases to show decreased activity in certain parts of the visual cortex while showing increased activity in other brain locations (Werring et al., 2004; Harris, 2005; Stone et al., 2005; Becker et al., 2013).

However, as with the ancillary studies listed above, negative studies do not establish a diagnosis of NOVL and not all positive studies indicate a diagnosis of NOVL. It is necessary to correlate the findings of a positive study with the reported symptoms, since, as technology advances and imaging studies obtain higher resolution, the likelihood of asymptomatic "incidentalomas" also increases. Remember, NOVL is never a diagnosis of exclusion; it is of utmost importance to prove the presence and normal functioning of an intact visual system.

MANAGEMENT

Management of patients with NOVL is difficult and can be frustrating for both the physician and the patient. It is not uncommon for patients to be misdiagnosed and subject to repeat examinations (Henningsen et al., 2003; Reuber et al., 2005; Rosendal et al., 2005). If NOVL is proven, the patient should be informed that no pathologic cause for the symptoms was found. Occasionally, detailing the conditions which have been ruled out may be helpful to the patient (Barris et al., 1992; Reuber et al., 2005; Stone et al., 2005). Care should be taken to avoid portraying to patients that their symptoms are not "real" or that they are lying; this is especially true with the malingering patient, who may become confrontational. As a general rule, it is important to reassure the patient, and emphasize the potential for recovery (Kathol et al., 1983a, c; Smith et al., 1983; Thompson, 1985; Barris et al., 1992; Bain et al., 2000; Lim et al., 2005; Stone et al., 2005). Not uncommonly, it is discovered that a strong emotional event preceded the onset of the visual disturbances. Although psychiatric consultation is often helpful, this option may be difficult to introduce at the time of initial evaluation in the eye clinic or the neurology office. Spontaneous improvement is common and a psychiatric evaluation may not always be necessary, as literature suggests that a large proportion of patients with NOVL do not have an underlying psychiatric disorder (Kathol et al., 1983a, b, c). However, the physician does need to be aware of certain "red flags" which should prompt consultation with a psychiatrist, such as a history of psychiatric disorder, history of psychologic trauma, evidence of sexual or physical abuse, or lack of resolution of symptoms over time (Porteous and Clarke, 2009).

In addition, patients with self-reported visual loss or visual dysfunction are two to four times more likely to become depressed compared with people with normal visual function (Morse, 2013), likely due to a loss of independence and the inability to independently perform routine tasks of daily living with progressively worsening vision, whether organic in nature or perceived (Chou, 2008; Mojon-Azzi et al., 2008; Rees et al., 2010; Kempen et al., 2012; Morse, 2013; Zhang et al., 2013). There is a direct relationship between the severity of visual dysfunction and the severity and prevalence of depression; as patients report more and worse visual dysfunction, the severity and prevalence of depression in this group rise (Zhang et al., 2013). Since there is a frequent association between NOVL and psychiatric disorders such as depression and anxiety, high suspicion for these conditions should be maintained and the appropriate referrals made (Sharpe, 2002; Henningsen et al., 2003; Reuber et al., 2005; Stone et al., 2005).

CONCLUSIONS

Neurologists and ophthalmologists frequently interact with patients with suspected NOVL. As detailed above, based on the patient's complaints, certain easily performed bedside or office examination techniques coupled with certain ancillary tests can be used to prove normal functioning of the visual system. However, in every case of visual loss, referral should be made to an ophthalmologist or neuro-ophthalmologist to exclude occult organic ophthalmologic causes for the patient's symptoms. Referral to a psychiatrist may also be warranted to assess for underlying psychosocial pathology causing or caused by the reported visual dysfunction. Working together, the neurologist and ophthalmologist should be well equipped to either uncover an organic cause for the patient's symptoms or prove functioning of the visual system beyond that reported by the patient. In the end it is our job to do no harm to our patients and to approach each patient with an open mind as we look for organic, treatable causes for our patient's symptoms and, if no organic cause is found, to assess for and treat the potential underlying mental or psychosocial causes.

DISCLOSURES

This manuscript was supported in part by an unrestricted departmental grant (Department of Ophthalmology) from Research to Prevent Blindness, New York, NY, and by the National Institutes of Health/National Eye Institute (NIH/NEI) core grant P30-EY006360 (Department of Ophthalmology).

B.B. Bruce received research support from the NIH/NEI grant K23-EY019341.

N.J. Newman received the Research to Prevent Blindness Lew R. Wasserman Merit Award.

References

American Psychiatric Association and American Psychiatric Association Dsm-5 Task Force (2013). Diagnostic and statistical manual of mental disorders: DSM-5. American Psychiatric Association, Washington, D.C.

Bain KE, Beatty S, Lloyd C (2000). Non-organic visual loss in children. Eye (Lond) 14 (Pt 5): 770–772.

Barris MC, Kaufman DI, Barberio D (1992). Visual impairment in hysteria. Doc Ophthalmol 82: 369–382.

Becker B, Scheele D, MOESSNER R et al. (2013). Deciphering the neural signature of conversion blindness. Am J Psychiatry 170: 121–122.

Behrman J, Levy R (1970). Neurophysiological studies on patients with hysterical disturbances of vision. J Psychosom Res 14: 187–194.

Bengtzen R, Woodward M, Lynn MJ et al. (2008). The "sunglasses sign" predicts nonorganic visual loss in neuro-ophthalmologic practice. Neurology 70: 218–221.

Berlin RM, Ronthal M, Bixler EO et al. (1983). Psychiatric symptomatology in an outpatient neurology clinic. J Clin Psychiatry 44: 204–206.

Bhatt D (2013). Electrophysiology for ophthalmologist (A practical approach). J Clin Ophthalmol Res 1: 45–54.

Bienfang DC, Kurtz D (1998). Management of functional vision loss. J Am Optom Assoc 69: 12–21.

Biousse V, Newman NJ (2009). Neuro-Ophthalmology Illustrated, Thieme, New York, NY.

Bobak P, Khanna P, Goodwin J et al. (1993). Pattern visual evoked potentials in cases of ambiguous acuity loss. Doc Ophthalmol 85: 185–192.

Bruce BB, Newman NJ (2010). Functional visual loss. Neurol Clin 28: 789–802.

Chen CS, Lee AW, Karagiannis A et al. (2007). Practical clinical approaches to functional visual loss. J Clin Neurosci 14: 1–7.

Chou KL (2008). Combined effect of vision and hearing impairment on depression in older adults: evidence from the English Longitudinal Study of Ageing. J Affect Disord 106: 191–196.

Clarke WN, Noel LP, Bariciak M (1996). Functional visual loss in children: a common problem with an easy solution. Can J Ophthalmol 31: 311–313.

Felber SR, Ettl AR, Birbamer GG et al. (1993). MR imaging and proton spectroscopy of the brain in posttraumatic cortical blindness. J Magn Reson Imaging 3: 921–924.

Frisen L (2014). Identification of functional visual field loss by automated static perimetry. Acta Ophthalmol 92: 805–809.

Ghate D, Bodnarchuk B, Sanders S et al. (2014). The ability of healthy volunteers to simulate a neurologic field defect on automated perimetry. Ophthalmology 121: 759–762.

Golnik KC, Lee AG, Eggenberger ER (2004). The monocular vertical prism dissociation test. Am J Ophthalmol 137: 135–137.

Graf MH (1999). Information from false statements concerning visual acuity and visual field in cases of psychogenic visual impairment. Graefes Arch Clin Exp Ophthalmol 237: 16–20.

Griffiths PG, Eddyshaw D (2004). Medically unexplained visual loss in adult patients. Eye (Lond) 18: 917–922.

Gupta V, Singh A, Upadhyay S et al. (2011). Clinical profile of somatoform disorders in children. Indian J Pediatr 78: 283–286.

Harris JC (2005). A Clinical Lesson at the Salpêtrière. Arch Gen Psychiatry 62: 470–472.

Henningsen P, Zimmermann T, Sattel H (2003). Medically unexplained physical symptoms, anxiety, and depression: a meta-analytic review. Psychosom Med 65: 528–533.

Hood DC, Odel JG, Winn BJ (2003). The multifocal visual evoked potential. J Neuroophthalmol 23: 279–289.

Hsu JL, Haley CM, Foroozan R (2010). Target visual field: a technique to rapidly demonstrate nonorganic visual field constriction. Arch Ophthalmol 128: 1220–1222.

Incesu AI (2013). Tests for malingering in ophthalmology. Int J Ophthalmol 6: 708–717.

Incesu AI, Sobaci G (2011). Malingering or simulation in ophthalmology-visual acuity. Int J Ophthalmol 4: 558–566.

Kathol RG, Cox TA, Corbett JJ et al. (1983a). Functional visual loss. Follow-up of 42 cases. Arch Ophthalmol 101: 729–735.

Kathol RG, Cox TA, Corbett JJ et al. (1983b). Functional visual loss: I. A true psychiatric disorder? Psychol Med 13: 307–314.

Kathol RG, Cox TA, Corbett JJ et al. (1983c). Functional visual loss: II. Psychiatric aspects in 42 patients followed for 4 years. Psychol Med 13: 315–324.

Keane JR (1979). Hysterical hemianopia. The 'missing half' field defect. Arch Ophthalmol 97: 865–866.

Keane JR (1982). Neuro-ophthalmic signs and symptoms of hysteria. Neurology 32: 757–762.

Keane JR (1998). Patterns of hysterical hemianopia. Neurology 51: 1230–1231.

Keltner JL, May WN, Johnson CA et al. (1985). The California syndrome. Functional visual complaints with potential economic impact. Ophthalmology 92: 427–435.

Kempen GI, Ballemans J, Ranchor AV et al. (2012). The impact of low vision on activities of daily living, symptoms of depression, feelings of anxiety and social support in community-living older adults seeking vision rehabilitation services. Qual Life Res 21: 1405–1411.

Kirk C, Saunders M (1977). Primary psychiatric illness in a neurological out-patient department in North East England. An assessment of symptomatology. Acta Psychiatr Scand 56: 294–302.

Kramer KK, La Piana FG, Appleton B (1979). Ocular malingering and hysteria: diagnosis and management. Surv Ophthalmol 24: 89–96.

Lessell S (2011). Nonorganic visual loss: what's in a name? Am J Ophthalmol 151: 569–571.

Levy NS, Glick EB (1974). Stereoscopic perception and Snellen visual acuity. Am J Ophthalmol 78: 722–724.

Lim SA, Siatkowski RM, Farris BK (2005). Functional visual loss in adults and children patient characteristics, management, and outcomes. Ophthalmology 112: 1821–1828.

Linhart WO (1956). Field findings in functional disease; report of 63 cases. Am J Ophthalmol 42: 75–84.

Macleod JDA, Manners RM, Heaven CJ et al. (1994). Visual field defects: how easily can they be fabricated using the automated perimeter? Neuro-Ophthalmology 14: 185–188.

Martin TJ (1998). Threshold perimetry of each eye with both eyes open in patients with monocular functional (nonorganic) and organic vision loss. Am J Ophthalmol 125: 857–864.

Mavrakanas NA, Schutz JS (2009). Feigned visual loss misdiagnosed as occult traumatic optic neuropathy: diagnostic guidelines and medical-legal issues. Surv Ophthalmol 54: 412–416.

Miller BW (1973). A review of practical tests for ocular malingering and hysteria. Surv Ophthalmol 17: 241–246.

Miller NR (2011). Functional neuro-ophthalmology. Handb Clin Neurol 102: 493–513.

Mojon DS, Flueckiger P (2002). A new optotype chart for detection of nonorganic visual loss. Ophthalmology 109: 810–815.

Mojon-Azzi SM, Sousa-Poza A, Mojon DS (2008). Impact of low vision on well-being in 10 European countries. Ophthalmologica 222: 205–212.

Morse AR (2013). Vision function, functional vision, and depression. JAMA Ophthalmol 131: 667–668.

Munoz-Hernandez AM, Santos-Bueso E, Saenz-Frances F et al. (2012). Nonorganic visual loss and associated psychopathology in children. Eur J Ophthalmol 22: 269–273.

Nakamura A, Akio T, Matsuda E et al. (2001). Pattern visual evoked potentials in malingering. J Neuroophthalmol 21: 42–45.

Newman N, Biousse VR (2014). Diagnostic approach to vision loss. Continuum (Minneap Minn) 20: 785–815.

Ney JJ, Volpe NJ, Liu GT et al. (2009). Functional visual loss in idiopathic intracranial hypertension. Ophthalmology 116 (1808–1813): e1.

Petersen J, Airas K (1985). Testing of concentric visual field constriction by means of scotopic visually evoked potentials. Graefes Arch Clin Exp Ophthalmol 223: 66–68.

Pineles SL, Volpe NJ (2004). Computerized kinetic perimetry detects tubular visual fields in patients with functional visual loss. Am J Ophthalmol 137: 933–935.

Porteous AM, Clarke MP (2009). Medically unexplained visual symptoms in children and adolescents: an indicator of abuse or adversity? Eye (Lond) 23: 1866–1867.

Pula J (2012). Functional vision loss. Curr Opin Ophthalmol 23: 460–465.

Raghunandan A, Buckingham RS (2008). The utility of clinical electrophysiology in a case of nonorganic vision loss. Optometry 79: 436–443.

Rees G, Tee HW, Marella M et al. (2010). Vision-specific distress and depressive symptoms in people with vision impairment. Invest Ophthalmol Vis Sci 51: 2891–2896.

Reuber M, Mitchell AJ, Howlett SJ et al. (2005). Functional symptoms in neurology: questions and answers. J Neurol Neurosurg Psychiatry 76: 307–314.

Rosendal M, Olesen F, Fink P (2005). Management of medically unexplained symptoms. BMJ 330: 4–5.

Rota E, Gallo A, Papaleo A et al. (2014). Functional neuroimaging correlates of medically unexplained vision loss. Psychosomatics 55: 200–204.

Saitoh E, Adachi-Usami E, Mizota A et al. (2001). Comparison of visual evoked potentials in patients with psychogenic visual disturbance and malingering. J Pediatr Ophthalmol Strabismus 38: 21–26.

Schlaegel Jr TF, Quilala FV (1955). Hysterical amblyopia; statistical analysis of forty-two cases found in a survey of eight hundred unselected eye patients at a state medical center. AMA Arch Ophthalmol 54: 875–884.

Scott JA, Egan RA (2003). Prevalence of organic neuro-ophthalmologic disease in patients with functional visual loss. Am J Ophthalmol 135: 670–675.

Sharpe M (2002). Medically unexplained symptoms and syndromes. Clin Med 2: 501–504.

Smith TJ, Baker RS (1987). Perimetric findings in functional disorders using automated techniques. Ophthalmology 94: 1562–1566.

Smith CH, Beck RW, Mills RP (1983). Functional disease in neuro-ophthalmology. Neurol Clin 1: 955–971.

Stone J, Carson A, Sharpe M (2005). Functional symptoms in neurology: management. J Neurol Neurosurg Psychiatry 76 (Suppl 1): i13–i21.

Thompson HS (1985). Functional visual loss. Am J Ophthalmol 100: 209–213.

Thompson JC, Kosmorsky GS, Ellis BD (1996). Field of dreamers and dreamed-up fields: functional and fake perimetry. Ophthalmology 103: 117–125.

Toldo I, Pinello L, Suppiej A et al. (2010). Nonorganic (psychogenic) visual loss in children: a retrospective series. J Neuroophthalmol 30: 26–30.

Villegas RB, Ilsen PF (2007). Functional vision loss: a diagnosis of exclusion. Optometry 78: 523–533.

Weinstein GW, Odom JV, Cavender S (1991). Visually evoked potentials and electroretinography in neurologic evaluation. Neurol Clin 9: 225–242.

Weller M, Wiedemann P (1989). Hysterical symptoms in ophthalmology. Doc Ophthalmol 73: 1–33.

Werring DJ, Weston L, Bullmore ET et al. (2004). Functional magnetic resonance imaging of the cerebral response to visual stimulation in medically unexplained visual loss. Psychol Med 34: 583–589.

Yoneda T, Fukuda K, Nishimura M et al. (2013). A case of functional (psychogenic) monocular hemianopia analyzed by measurement of hemifield visual evoked potentials. Case Rep Ophthalmol 4: 283–286.

Zhang X, Bullard KM, Cotch MF et al. (2013). Association between depression and functional vision loss in persons 20 years of age or older in the United States, NHANES 2005-2008. JAMA Ophthalmol 131: 573–581.

Zinkernagel SM, Mojon DS (2009). Distance doubling visual acuity test: a reliable test for nonorganic visual loss. Graefes Arch Clin Exp Ophthalmol 247: 855–858.

Zinkernagel MS, Pellanda N, Kunz A et al. (2009). Saccade testing to distinguish between non-organic and organic visual-field restriction. Br J Ophthalmol 93: 1247–1250.

Handbook of Clinical Neurology, Vol. 139 (3rd series)
Functional Neurologic Disorders
M. Hallett, J. Stone, and A. Carson, Editors
http://dx.doi.org/10.1016/B978-0-12-801772-2.00030-8

Chapter 30

Functional eye movement disorders

D. KASKI[1,2] AND A.M. BRONSTEIN[1,2]*

[1]*Division of Brain Sciences, Department of Neuro-otology, Imperial College London, London, UK*

[2]*Department of Neuro-otology, The National Hospital for Neurology and Neurosurgery, London, UK*

Abstract

Functional (psychogenic) eye movement disorders are perhaps less established in the medical literature than other types of functional movement disorders. Patients may present with ocular symptoms (e.g., blurred vision or oscillopsia) or functional eye movements may be identified during the formal examination of the eyes in patients with other functional disorders. Convergence spasm is the most common functional eye movement disorder, but functional gaze limitation, functional eye oscillations (also termed "voluntary nystagmus"), and functional convergence paralysis may be underreported. This chapter reviews the different types of functional eye movement abnormalities and provides a practical framework for their diagnosis and management.

INTRODUCTION

An assessment of eye movements constitutes an important part of the neurologic examination in patients with movement disorders as it can help identify cortical, subcortical, and sometimes low-order oculomotor abnormalities that may assist the distinction between the various parkinsonian, cerebellar, or cognitive syndromes. Abnormal eye movements, however, are perhaps an underrecognized feature of patients with functional (psychogenic) neurologic symptoms (Fasano et al., 2012; Fekete et al., 2012). As a consequence of this, the prevalence of functional eye movement disorders is largely unknown. Such patients may present overtly with a complaint suggestive of an eye movement disorder (e.g., double vision) or, most commonly, a patient with other functional neurologic symptoms (e.g., functional gait disorder) may be found to have functional eye movement abnormalities only on formal examination. As with other motor disturbances such as weakness or tremor, they are particularly amenable to objective clinical assessment (in contrast to a subjective report of sensory symptoms).

Whereas it is usually very difficult to trigger organic paroxysmal eye movement disorders in the clinic, many positive signs of a functional eye movement disorder will be present during the consultation (discussed below) (Kaski et al., 2015). When such positive signs are present, one can make a more confident diagnosis. Therefore, if the eye movement abnormality is not immediately apparent when examining a patient with a suspected functional eye movement disorder, it can sometimes be induced by sustained contraction of ocular muscles (e.g., longer than 10 seconds), as in patients with convergence spasm (see below) (Fasano et al., 2012).

Functional eye movement disorders typically have an abrupt onset, there is a fluctuation or disappearance of symptoms and signs with distraction, symptoms worsen in situations of physical stress or emotional anxiety, and symptomatic improvement can be seen with suggestion or placebo (Factor et al., 1995; Rommelfanger, 2013).

In this chapter we review the common symptoms and clinical signs of functional eye movement disorders to provide a practical diagnostic and management framework.

*Correspondence to: Adolfo M. Bronstein, MD, PhD, FRCP, Neuro-otology Unit, Charing Cross Hospital, London W6 8RF, UK. Tel: +44-20-3311-7523, E-mail: a.bronstein@imperial.ac.uk

THE EYE MOVEMENT EXAMINATION

A full eye movement examination should include an assessment of voluntary and reflexive eye movements, including vergence (the simultaneous movement of both eyes to maintain or obtain a single image on the fovea), saccades, pursuit, the vestibulo-ocular reflex, and optokinetic nystagmus. The examination of the eyes, however, should begin from the moment the patient sits down in front of you in the consultation room. This is the "informal" or "casual" examination, and is a key aspect of the eye movement examination, particularly in patients with a suspected functional eye movement symptom where there may be a discrepancy between the casual and formal examinations. Table 30.1 summarizes the different type of eye movements and how these can be assessed clinically at the bedside (Kaski et al., 2015).

EPIDEMIOLOGY

There are no studies that have systematically evaluated the prevalence of functional eye movement disorders. Convergence spasm is the most commonly reported functional eye movement disorder, occurring in as many as 69% of functional movement disorder cases in one study of 13 patients (Fekete et al., 2012). This study also suggested that as many as 4 of 11 healthy controls had convergence spasm during formal oculomotor assessment (Fekete et al., 2012), but this is at odds with our own clinical experience (Kaski et al., in press). We find that functional eye movement disorders are rare in the general population; for example, none of 47 medical students who underwent formal eye movement examination as part of control data for an ongoing study had evidence of convergence spasm (or other functional eye movement problems).

FUNCTIONAL EYE MOVEMENT SYNDROMES

Table 30.2 lists the common functional eye movement disorders that we have encountered in general neurology and specialist neuro-otology clinics.

Functional convergence spasm

Convergence is required to shift gaze from a distant target to a near one. Convergence spasm refers to the abnormal persistence of this movement when the patient is no longer fixating on a near target. Patients with convergence spasm may complain of blurred vision when looking in the distance following near fixation. Patients may also report intermittent blurred vision that temporarily corrects by "crinkling" the eyelids, and intermittent diplopia. Symptoms usually last seconds but patients may describe them as continuous, as one episode may follow another.

Convergence spasm is elicited by instructing the patient to look at a near object (e.g., 10 cm) that is then moved to the extremes of lateral gaze. Abduction would normally overcome the convergence response, but in convergence spasm one or both eyes remain adducted with strong medial rectus contraction (Fig. 30.1 and Video 30.1). Consequently, patients with convergence spasm are often erroneously thought to have unilateral or bilateral abducens nerve palsies (Cogan and Freese, 1955; Keane, 1982; Faucher and De Guise, 2004). Convergence spasm can be differentiated from an abducens nerve palsy (Leigh and Zee, 2006) by the presence of miosis developing at the same time as the convergence in convergence spasm (Fig. 30.1), and normal abduction of the affected eye during rapid, small-amplitude passive head turns (head impulse test), optokinetic stimuli, or doll's-eye manoeuvre (Kaski et al., in press). Examining the eyes in low-lighting conditions (or with the use of oculography) may help visualize pupillary responses.

Convergence spasm, also termed spasm of the near reflex, has been described in organic pathology (Rutstein and Galkin, 1984), although this is rare. Reported organic causes include lesions of the diencephalic–mesencephalic junction (thalamic esotropia) (Gomez et al., 1988), Wernicke–Korsakoff syndrome (Herman, 1977), posterior fossa lesions (Dagi et al., 1987; Mossman et al., 1990), epilepsy (Shahar and Andraus, 2002), and phenytoin toxicity (Guiloff et al., 1980).

The clinician should place the finding of convergence spasm in the wider clinical context and should be cautious not to overinterpret convergence spasm in otherwise healthy subjects (Fekete et al., 2012), given that convergence is under both reflex and voluntary oculomotor control, and is thus the only dysconjugate ocular movement that can be initiated voluntarily (Duke-Elder and MacFaul, 1974).

Functional convergence paralysis

Convergence paralysis or insufficiency describes a complete or partial failure, respectively, of convergence. Here, diplopia occurs only at near fixation, adduction is normal, and the patient is unable to converge when a visual target is presented at close range. Patients will often report difficulty reading with blurring of vision.

Differentiating organic from a functional convergence paralysis represents a greater clinical challenge than diagnosing convergence spasm because there is an absence of movement rather than the generation of a complex oculomotor action. There may, however, be some clues. Thus, convergence will always be absent in organic convergence paralysis (as may also occur in normal aging). In functional convergence paralysis, convergence movements may be observed during the

Table 30.1

Voluntary and reflexive eye movements

Type of eye movement	Bedside assessment	Role of eye movement	Features	Relevance to functional eye movement disorders
Voluntary eye movements				
Fixation	Ask patient to look straight at a target (finger, or tip of a pen) held directly in front of and at approx. 40 cm from the patient's nose	To visualize a static object of interest	Assess for nystagmus or opsoclonus. If nystagmus is present, note the type of oscillation (fast and slow phases, jerk nystagmus), the plane of the oscillation, and the direction of the fast phase. Assess blink rate and eyelid abnormalities	Functional eye oscillations ("voluntary nystagmus"); "chaotic" saccades (functional opsoclonus); convergence spasm
Range of eye movements	Take the fixation target to the extremes of view: right, left, up, and down	Turn eyes to objects outside central fixation	Look to see whether each eye moves fully in all directions, and ask about diplopia	Functional gaze limitation, with effortful expressions, increased blink rate, and pain on eye movements
Smooth pursuit	Hold a target 40 cm away from the patient's nose and move it slowly in horizontal, and then vertical planes	Allows clear vision of small, slow-moving objects	Smooth tracking eye movements may appear "broken" in patients with cerebellar disease. Pursuit is deemed abnormal, qualitatively, when too many catch-up saccades are present	There may be a normal horizontal and vertical range of movements despite an apparent inability to move the eyes during saccades or when testing range of movements
Saccades	Provide the patient with two fixation targets spaced $\pm 30°$ right–left, or up–down, and instruct the patient to look from one to another	Shift gaze from one target to another	Assess the latency (how quickly movements are initiated), velocity (how fast the movement is), and metrics (under- or overshooting the target)	This may reveal a functional limitation that can be overcome with reflexive eye movements. Saccades may be normal during the casual examination
Convergence	Bring an accommodative target (e.g., pen, finger) slowly along the sagittal plane towards the bridge of the patient's nose	Fixate near targets (e.g., reading)	Smooth movement of the eyes with simultaneous pupillary constriction	May trigger convergence spasm, during which pupillary constriction will be present
Doll's-head eyes	Instruct the patient to keep gaze on your nose whilst gently rotating the head horizontally, then vertically	Gently places the eyeball in extreme positions within the orbit, without shifting gaze (it is VOR mediated, see below)	Smooth movement of the eyes in the opposite direction to the head movement	Used to overcome a functional limitation of gaze
Reflexive eye movements				
Vestibulo-ocular reflex (VOR)	Instruct the patient to fixate on your nose, and then rotate the patient's head very rapidly to one side with a small-amplitude movement (= head-impulse tests)	Stabilizes the eyes during fast head movements	A head turn to the patient's right tests the right horizontal VOR. The normal response consists of a compensatory eye movement to the left, which occurs without delay (<16 ms)	Used to overcome a functional limitation of gaze

Continued

Table 30.1

Continued

Type of eye movement	Bedside assessment	Role of eye movement	Features	Relevance to functional eye movement disorders
Optokinetic nystagmus	Tested using a small drum upon which are placed vertically oriented alternating black and white stripes. Rotate drum in front of the patient in either the horizontal or vertical plane, and observe the eyes	Allows the eye to follow continuous motion when the head is stationary	Alternating slow-phase eye movements (pursuit system) towards the direction of visual motion, with fast phases (saccades) to recenter gaze	Used to overcome a functional limitation of gaze
Ocular counteroll	The head is tilted laterally towards one shoulder; the patient is asked to keep his/her eyes on your nose	This maneuver generates a compensatory vestibular nystagmus to preserve vision during the head movement (termed ocular counter-roll)	The fast phases of the nystagmus beat in the direction of the head movement and are generated by the same saccadic mechanisms that produce vertical saccades	To assess the integrity of saccadic pathways in patients with a suspected functional limitation of upward gaze

Table 30.2

Functional eye movement disorders

Condition	Presenting symptoms	Examination findings	Distinguishing features from organic disease
Functional eye oscillations ("voluntary nystagmus")	Episodes of oscillopsia lasting 3–20 seconds	Binocular conjugate high-frequency oscillations without a slow phase	Often triggered by examination; convergence at onset of nystagmus; brief episodes though can be recurrent
Functional convergence paralysis	Inability to fixate near objects; difficulty reading; blurred vision	Adduction is normal, but the patient is unable to converge when a visual target is presented at close range	Convergence movements may be observed during the casual examination when the patient is performing other near tasks such as looking at wristwatch or phone
Functional gaze limitation	Inability to move the eyes in a given (or multiple) directions; diplopia; headache	Variability in the degree of ocular movements, particularly with distraction; normal saccades during casual examination	Effortful facial expression; eyelid fluttering; variable limitation of gaze; absent frontalis corrugation on attempted upgaze
Convergence spasm	"Eye spasm"; oscillopsia; diplopia; difficulty concentrating	One or both eyes remain adducted with strong medial rectus contraction, when a near-fixation target is moved further away	Miosis during convergent effort. Brief episodes triggered by clinical examination
Functional tonic gaze deviation	Sustained (usually upward) gaze, with blurred vision, intermittent diplopia, or functional blindness	Recurrent tonic conjugate gaze deviation, that may be brief (seconds to minutes) or persistent	Distractible; inability to suppress movements volitionally (usually possible in organic oculogyric crisis)
Functional opsoclonus	Abnormal eye movements (usually noticed by others first)	Excessive saccades in multiple directions and planes	Intermittent bursts of saccades; distractible; not present during sleep

"casual examination" when the patient is performing other near tasks such as reading. A more formal method of detecting a functional abnormality is to test fusional convergence using prisms, and this can be done by experienced optometrists and ophthalmologists. This tests the patient's ability to "control" a latent or intermittent ocular misalignment, and may induce convergence in such patients. Note that convergence may be absent in the older healthy population.

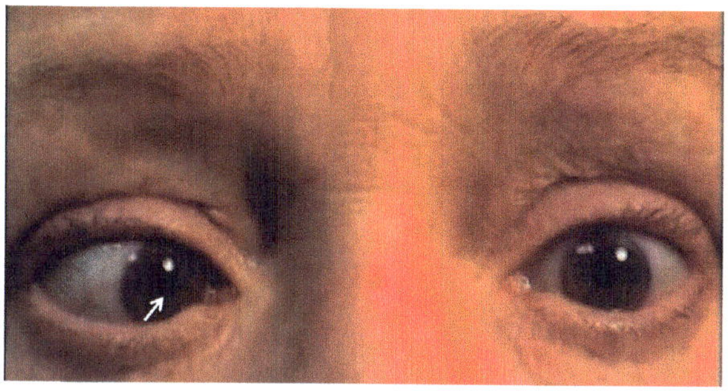

Fig. 30.1. Convergence spasm following accommodative effort in the right eye in a male patient, showing associated pupillary constriction in the right eye (white arrow), ruling out an abducens nerve palsy.

Functional limitation of gaze

Functional gaze limitation rarely presents as a primary complaint but rather manifests on formal testing of eye movements in patients with other functional movement symptoms. Patients may have eyelid fluttering on attempted eye movements, and commonly have effortful facial expressions exclusively during the examination (Video 30.2). Many patients will also report pain on eye movements, with a tendency to avoid moving the eyes on the formal examination (Video 30.2), but no apparent discomfort during casually observed saccades. There may be inability to move the eyes in a single direction (and, more often, all directions), sometimes with diplopia despite conjugate eye movements.

Gaze limitation is a feature of organic supranuclear gaze palsies. Functional gaze limitation can be distinguished from organic supranuclear palsies by the presence of normal saccades in the casual examination, and variability in the degree of ocular movements, particularly with distraction. Pursuit movements can be normal in organic supranuclear gaze palsies (e.g., progressive supranuclear palsy), particularly with large targets (Seemungal et al., 2003), but in a functional gaze limitation it may produce an optokinetic response as the patient's gaze is recentered when the eyes move with the visual scene. Patients with functional gaze limitation will often report an inability to perform smooth pursuit, although "breakthrough" smooth slow phases can often be detected. More importantly, most organic causes of supranuclear gaze palsy will be accompanied by slow saccades, which are not seen in functional symptoms. Furthermore, in organic supranuclear palsies there is frontalis overactivity, whereas in functional vertical gaze limitation the eyebrows typically do not elevate during attempted upward gaze, and there will be absence of frontalis corrugation (Bruno et al., 2013) (Video 30.3).

Functional eye oscillations

Approximately 8% of college students can produce voluntary nystagmus at will (Zahn, 1978), often done as a "party trick." Thus, the term "voluntary nystagmus" refers to a high-frequency (approximately 10 Hz), low-amplitude (approximately 4°) eye oscillation (Video 30.4) that can be voluntarily initiated and terminated (Fig. 30.2) (Friedman and Blodget, 1955; Wist and Collins, 1964; Blair et al., 1967), and is more common in children. There is usually a convergent effort at the onset of movement. Functional eye oscillations (also termed "functional nystagmus") refers to this same phenomenon when experienced as an involuntary symptom with oscillopsia (oscillation of the visual scene), blurred vision, and difficulty concentrating. Functional eye oscillations are usually confined to horizontal oscillations. The oscillations may be superimposed on smooth-pursuit movements, and may also be accompanied by a head tremor (Lee and Gresty, 1993) as well as eyelid flutter (Bassani, 2012).

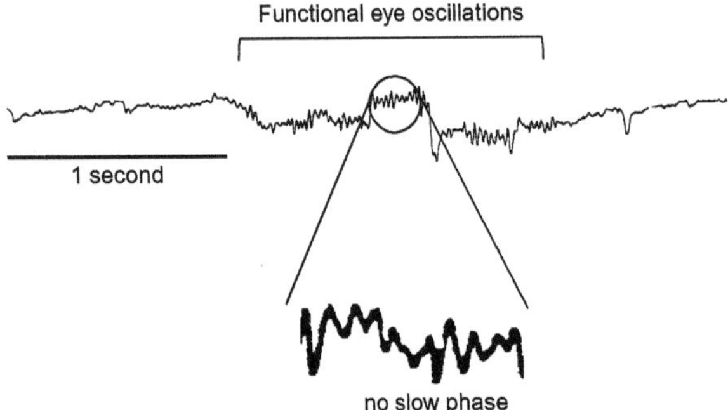

Fig. 30.2. Electro-oculographic trace in a patient with functional eye oscillations. Note that in this patient the ocular oscillations were brief, lasting approximately 1.5 seconds, without slow phases, and are therefore not strictly speaking nystagmic in nature.

Given the nature of the eye movements, patients with functional eye oscillations present with oscillopsia. The nystagmus may be easily triggered by the routine eye movement examination, typically on convergence, but may not be present during the casual examination. There is typically convergence at the onset of the oscillations (Video 30.4), as well as diminution in their intensity and frequency with repeated examination.

Whilst the appearance of functional eye oscillations is usually characteristic and a positive diagnosis can be made on clinical examination alone, the main differential diagnosis is organic ocular flutter (Blair et al., 1967). Ocular flutter is defined as intermittent bursts of rapid (10–15 Hz) conjugate, horizontal saccades without an intersaccadic interval. Typically, functional eye oscillations cannot be maintained for more than 25 seconds, often less (Zahn, 1978), whereas flutter is more persistent, present during the casual examination, and is usually accompanied by additional oculomotor signs of the cerebellar type, such as broken pursuit, downbeat nystagmus, or hypermetric saccades. Other differential diagnoses and their features are listed in Table 30.3.

Another differential diagnosis for intermittent oscillopsia is superior oblique myokymia (Hoyt and Keane, 1970). This consists of repetitive spasmodic contractions of the superior oblique muscle that affects one eye only. The episodes of oscillopsia and unsteadiness (secondary to the disorienting paroxysmal oscillopsia) occur multiple times in the day, often with no specific trigger. Given the paroxysmal nature, the ocular movements are usually difficult to observe in the clinic. In contrast, functional eye oscillations, which is the main differential diagnosis, is more readily triggered. Vestibular paroxysmia is a condition that is characterized by brief (milliseconds to seconds) attacks of vestibular symptoms involving vertigo, oscillopsia and imbalance, thought to arise from neurovascular cross-compression of the vestibular nerve and an offending vessel. This should also be considered in patients presenting with intermittent oscillopsia. The nystagmus (in any plane) is again very rarely observed clinically due to the brevity of the attacks.

Of note, it is not unusual to see patients with simultaneous convergence spasm and functional eye oscillations, likely related to an initial convergence effort required to elicit both these conditions. Despite the apparent sinusoidal appearance of the eye movement waveform when formally recorded, voluntary nystagmus (and functional eye oscillations) reflects the behavior of

Table 30.3

Organic eye movement disorders that may resemble functional nystagmus

Condition	Clinical features	Cause	Distinguishing features from functional eye oscillations
Superior oblique myokymia	Brief (seconds) uniocular episodes of oscillopsia, occurring multiple times per day. High-frequency spasmodic contractions of the superior oblique muscle (torsional [rotatory] ocular oscillation with intorsion)	Possible neurovascular compression of IVth nerve at root entry zone	Uniocular; difficult to elicit during a clinic consultation due to paroxysmal nature
Vestibular paroxysmia	Brief (milliseconds to seconds) attacks of vestibular deficits, including vertigo oscillopsia and imbalance. May see brief nystagmus, in any plane	Possible neurovascular compression of VIIIth nerve. Often idiopathic	Rare to see nystagmus due to brevity of attacks, and paroxysmal nature
Ocular flutter	Very frequent visual blurring or oscillopsia. Intermittent bursts of rapid (10–15 Hz) conjugate, horizontal saccades without an intersaccadic interval	Cerebellar or brainstem pathology	Persistent bursts of abnormal eye oscillation; associated pyramidal, brainstem or cerebellar signs; persists during eyelid closure
Opsoclonus	Continuous (or almost continuous) oscillopsia. Rapid, chaotic, conjugate saccadic movements of the eyes in horizontal, vertical, and torsional planes	Neuroblastoma or paraneoplastic syndromes	Persist during eyelid closure and sleep

the saccadic system with normal saccadic movements alternating in direction (Nagle et al., 1980). Oculographic recordings can therefore be of diagnostic use to distinguish functional eye oscillations from other organic eye movement abnormalities.

Functional opsoclonus

Opsoclonus is a saccadic oscillation without intersaccadic intervals, consisting of conjugate multidirectional saccades occurring in random directions with varying amplitudes (Leigh and Zee, 2006). Baizabal-Carvallo and Jankovic (2016) have described 5 patients with functional opsoclonus, and 2 of these patients also had brief oculogyric crisis or ocular flutter. We have observed functional opsoclonus in patients with functional head tremor, with nystagmus that has the oculographic characteristic of voluntary nystagmus (Lee and Gresty, 1993), and in association with functional limitation of gaze (Video 30.3). Organic opsoclonus has a large differential that includes paraneoplastic disorders, autoimmune, infectious, metabolic, and toxic disorders (Baizabal-Carvallo et al., 2013; Lemos and Eggenberger, 2013). However organic opsoclonus persists during eyelid closure and sleep, whereas this type of functional eye movement does not. In addition, functional opsoclonus is usually distractible, such that performing a secondary motor task will temporarily abolish the ocular movements.

Functional tonic eye deviation (oculogyric crisis)

Oculogyric crisis refers to spasms of extraocular muscles leading to tonic eye deviation (usually upward), with each spasm lasting from seconds to several hours; the entire episode may last up to several weeks or months (Poston and Frucht, 2008). Oculogyric crisis was originally described in patients with encephalitis lethargica, but these days are more commonly observed after exposure to a variety of medications (e.g., antiemetics, antidepressants, and antipsychotics) that cause acute dystonic reactions or tardive phenomena (Thenganatt and Jankovic, 2015). The temporal association of oculogyric crisis with other functional movement disorders is a strong clue to its underlying etiology (Kaski and Bronstein, 2016). Other features of functional tonic eye deviation are the inability to transiently overcome the crisis volitionally (patients with organic oculogyric crisis frequently can), and the abolition of the abnormal movements with distraction. Functional oculogyric crisis can be brief (a few seconds), or more persistent, in which case it is usually associated with photophobia and eyelid closure (sometimes resulting in functional blindness: Baizabal-Carvallo and Jankovic, 2016).

Functional diplopia

Diplopia may be a symptom of a functional eye movement disorder. For example, most patients with convergence spasm will report double vision. Organic diplopia is typically binocular (disappears when one eye is covered) and is the result of dysconjugate gaze. Thus, there will be a limitation of movement of one or more ocular muscles, which may be confirmed clinically, or using a Hess chart. Asking the patient to look in the direction of the suspected weak muscle will increase the diplopia (e.g., right lateral gaze for a right lateral rectus weakness) in organic disease. Monocular diplopia, in the appropriate clinical context, should raise the possibility of functional disease but it can also be due to ocular pathology, e.g., retinal disease, refractive errors, abnormalities of the cornea and lens, and, more rarely, of visual cortex lesions (Meadows, 1973). The presence of true monocular diplopia, where two separate and equal images of an object are seen with one eye only, almost always indicates a functional disorder (Newman, 1993).

Although the clinical examination usually suffices, where there remains diagnostic confusion, oculographic recordings showing brief high-frequency oscillations during convergence may help clarify the origin of the diplopia (e.g., functional eye oscillations; Fig. 30.2).

MANAGEMENT OPTIONS

Treatment options are based on case series, case reports, and expert opinion consensus, but general principles can be drawn from the treatment of other functional movement disorders, as there are no randomized controlled trials in functional eye movement disorders. Given that functional eye movement disorders may only become apparent on formal examination, they do not typically cause disability, and medications are therefore rarely necessary.

The management of patients with functional eye movement disorders begins with a positive clinical diagnosis and clear explanation of the nature of the problem to the patient (Peckham and Hallett, 2009). Motor signs can form an important part of the explanation of the diagnosis to the patient, such as using pictures or videos from eye movement recordings to explain how limitation of gaze during eye movement examination disappears when a patient is distracted (Stone and Edwards, 2012). It can be helpful to emphasize that, although the abnormal eye movements are experienced as involuntary, the eye muscles themselves are under voluntary control. Our own experience indicates that an explanation that the oculomotor pathways are intact, and that eye movements can be normalized through practice, usually results in symptomatic improvement. It is important to identify and address any environmental, psychologic, or physical triggers that may have precipitated or exacerbated the problem (Edwards et al., 2012). For example, we often encounter teenagers with brief paroxysmal oscillopsia (functional nystagmus) in the context of "tired eyes," lack of sleep, and anxiety when revising for university admission exams. Anxiety from parents and doctors alike, and unnecessary (normal) investigations tend to worsen the clinical situation. This specific scenario appears to have a good prognosis with a convincing explanation and may in some patients be the only treatment necessary.

Exercises from an optometrist may be helpful in some patients if they know that the purpose is to relax a movement pathway that has become overactive. Symptomatic benefit in convergence spasm has also been reported in small patient groups with cycloplegic agents (e.g., atropine drops) that cause temporary paralysis of the ciliary muscles in combination with reading glasses (Cogan and Freese, 1955), and miotic agents that are given as placebo (Moore and Stockbridge, 1973; Christoff and Christiansen, 2002), although the evidence for functional eye movement disorders is anecdotal.

Further research in this field will require epidemiological studies and better clinical phenotyping to help understand the scale of the problem, improve diagnostic accuracy, and perhaps make use of evolving technology to allow patients both to capture intermittent eye movement problems and as a form of biofeedback for monitoring treatment outcomes.

References

Baizabal-Carvallo JF, Jankovic J (2016 Jan 21). Psychogenic ophthalmologic movement disorders. J Neuropsychiatry Clin Neurosci. appineuropsych15050104 (epub ahead of print).

Baizabal-Carvallo JF, Stocco A, Muscal E et al. (2013). The spectrum of movement disorders in children with anti-NMDA receptor encephalitis. Mov Disord 28: 543–547.

Bassani R (2012). Images in clinical medicine. Voluntary nystagmus. New Engl J Med 367 (9): e13.

Blair CJ, Goldberg MF, Von Noorden GK (1967). Voluntary nystagmus. Electro-oculographic findings in four cases. Arch Ophthalmol 77 (3): 349–354.

Bruno E, Mostile G, Dibilio V et al. (2013). Clinical diagnostic tricks for detecting psychogenic gaze paralysis. Eur J Neurol 20 (8): e107–e108.

Christoff A, Christiansen SP (2002). Spasm of the near reflex: treatment with miotics revisited. Am Orthopt J 52: 110–113.

Cogan DG, Freese Jr CG (1955). Spasm of the near reflex. AMA Arch Ophthalmol 54 (5): 752–759.

Dagi LR, Chrousos GA, Cogan DC (1987). Spasm of the near reflex associated with organic disease. Am J Ophthalmol 103 (4): 582–585.

Duke-Elder S, MacFaul PA (1974). System of ophthalmology, Kimpton, London.

Edwards MJ, Adams RA, Brown H et al. (2012). A Bayesian account of 'hysteria'. Brain 135: 3495–3512.

Factor SA, Podskalny GD, Molho ES (1995). Psychogenic movement disorders: frequency, clinical profile, and characteristics. J Neurol Neurosurg Psychiatry 59 (4): 406–412.

Fasano A, Valadas A, Bhatia KP et al. (2012). Psychogenic facial movement disorders: clinical features and associated conditions. Mov Disord 27 (12): 1544–1551.

Faucher C, De Guise D (2004). Spasm of the near reflex triggered by disruption of normal binocular vision. Optom Vis Sci 81 (3): 178–181.

Fekete R, Baizabal-Carvallo JF, Ha AD et al. (2012). Convergence spasm in conversion disorders: prevalence in psychogenic and other movement disorders compared with controls. J Neurol Neurosurg Psychiatry 83 (2): 202–204.

Friedman MW, Blodget Jr RM (1955). Voluntary ocular fibrillation. Am J Ophthalmol 39 (1): 78–80.

Gomez CR, Gomez SM, Selhorst JB (1988). Acute thalamic esotropia. Neurology 38 (11): 1759–1762.

Guiloff RJ, Whiteley A, Kelly RE (1980). Organic convergence spasm. Acta Neurol Scand 61 (4): 252–259.

Herman P (1977). Convergence spasm. Mt Sinai J Med 44 (4): 501–509.

Hoyt WF, Keane JR (1970). Superior oblique myokymia. Report and discussion on five cases of benign intermittent uniocular microtremor. Arch Ophthalmol 84 (4): 461–467.

Kaski D, Bronstein AM, Edwards MJ et al. (2015). Cranial functional (psychogenic) movement disorders. Lancet Neurol 14 (12): 1196–1205.

Kaski D, Bronstein AM (2016). Functional (psychogenic) saccadic oscillations and oculogyric crises—authors' reply. Lancet Neurol 15 (8): 791–792.

Kaski D, Pradhan V, Bronstein AM (in press). The clinical features of functional (psychogenic) eye movement disorders. J Neurol Neurosurg Psychiatry.

Keane JR (1982). Neuro-ophthalmic signs and symptoms of hysteria. Neurology 32 (7): 757–762.

Lee J, Gresty M (1993). A case of "voluntary nystagmus" and head tremor. J Neurol Neurosurg Psychiatry 56 (12): 1321–1322.

Leigh RJ, Zee DS (2006). The neurology of eye movements. 3rd edn. Oxford University Press, New York.

Lemos J, Eggenberger E (2013). Saccadic intrusions: review and update. Curr Opin Neurol 26: 59–66. 15.

Meadows JC (1973). Observations on a case of monocular diplopia of cerebral origin. J Neurol Sci 18 (2): 249–253.

Moore S, Stockbridge L (1973). Another approach to the treatment of accommodative spasm. Am Orthopt J 23: 71–72.

Mossman SS, Bronstein AM, Gresty MA et al. (1990). Convergence nystagmus associated with Arnold-Chiari malformation. Arch Neurol 47 (3): 357–359.

Nagle M, Bridgeman B, Stark L (1980). Voluntary nystagmus, saccadic suppression, and stabilization of the visual world. Vision Res 20 (8): 717–721.

Newman NJ (1993). Neuro-ophthalmology and psychiatry. Gen Hosp Psychiatry 15 (2): 102–114.

Peckham EL, Hallett M (2009). Psychogenic movement disorders. Neurol Clin 27 (3): 801–819. vii.

Poston KL, Frucht SJ (2008). Movement disorder emergencies. J Neurol 255 (Suppl 4): 2–13.

Rommelfanger KS (2013). Opinion: a role for placebo therapy in psychogenic movement disorders. Nat Rev Neurol 9 (6): 351–356.

Rutstein RP, Galkin KA (1984). Convergence spasm – two case reports. J Am Optom Assoc 55 (7): 495–498.

Seemungal BM, Faldon M, Revesz T et al. (2003). Influence of target size on vertical gaze palsy in a pathologically proven case of progressive supranuclear palsy. Mov Disord 18 (7): 818–822.

Shahar E, Andraus J (2002). Near reflex accommodation spasm: unusual presentation of generalized photosensitive epilepsy. J Clin Neurosci 9 (5): 605–607.

Stone J, Edwards M (2012). Trick or treat? Showing patients with functional (psychogenic) motor symptoms their physical signs. Neurology 79 (3): 282–284.

Thenganatt MA, Jankovic J (2015). Psychogenic movement disorders. Neurol Clin 33: 205–224.

Wist ER, Collins WE (1964). Some characteristics of voluntary nystagmus. Arch Ophthalmol 72: 470–475.

Zahn JR (1978). Incidence and characteristics of voluntary nystagmus. J Neurol Neurosurg Psychiatry 41 (7): 617–623.

Handbook of Clinical Neurology, Vol. 139 (3rd series)
Functional Neurologic Disorders
M. Hallett, J. Stone, and A. Carson, Editors
http://dx.doi.org/10.1016/B978-0-12-801772-2.00031-X

Chapter 31

Functional facial and tongue movement disorders

A. FASANO[1,2]* AND M. TINAZZI[3]

[1]*Morton and Gloria Shulman Movement Disorders Clinic and the Edmond J. Safra Program in Parkinson's Disease, Toronto Western Hospital and Division of Neurology, University of Toronto, Toronto, Ontario, Canada*

[2]*Krembil Research Institute, Toronto, Ontario, Canada*

[3]*Department of Neurological and Movement Sciences, University of Verona, Italy*

Abstract

Functional movement disorders (FMDs) affecting the eyelids, tongue, and other facial muscles are often underrecognized because their phenomenology has not been fully characterized. Nevertheless, these disorders are more common than previously thought. In this chapter we will discuss the phenomenology as well as the clinical and instrumental diagnosis of facial FMDs. Facial FMDs should be considered when a patient exhibits any combination of the following features: (1) fixed unilateral facial contractions, especially with lower lip, with or without ipsilateral jaw involvement, of maximal severity at onset; (2) inconsistent features such as changes in side and pattern during or between examination; (3) associated somatoform or nonphysiologic sensory or motor findings; (4) reduction or abolition of facial spasm with distraction; (5) response to suggestion or psychotherapy; (6) rapid onset and/or spontaneous remissions; and (7) normal neurologic examination. Supportive features are young age, female gender, and associated medical conditions such as depression, headaches, facial pain, fibromyalgia, or irritable-bowel syndrome.

Finally, the differential diagnosis with the organic counterparts will be also addressed, particularly with respect to blepharospasm, oromandibular dystonia, and hemifacial spasm.

INTRODUCTION

Many systemic and neurologic conditions may involve the facial musculature and functional movement disorders (FMDs) are not an exception. While eye disorders have historically received more attention and are covered in Chapter 30, FMDs affecting the eyelids, tongue, and other facial muscles are often underrecognized. Nevertheless, facial involvement – occurring either alone or in combination with other FMDs – is more common than previously thought (Fasano et al., 2012).

Facial FMDs have been already described in the early literature of the 19th century. The first description was probably formulated by Charcot in 1887 as "unilateral hysterical facial spasm." One year later, Gowers (1888) described the "hysterical" tonic contracture of the facial muscles. These entities entered subsequent textbooks as "glosso-labial hemispasm" (Babinski, 1918) and their description was enriched by important features, such as the variable involvement of other facial muscles, such as eyelids or platysma. During the same years, the terms "hook-like appearance" (Babinski, 1918) or "hysterical spasm" (Hurst, 1920) were used to describe the tongue of patients with other FMDs.

After these early descriptions, facial FMDs were largely neglected for almost a century. Over the last two decades, the increased awareness of facial FMDs has contributed to a reappraisal of prior literature (Fasano et al., 2012). In fact, while organic dystonia has originally been mischaracterized as functional, the reverse situation has occurred in the recent past. For example, some atypical facial disorders have been anecdotally reported as representing rare phenotypes of focal dystonia (Tan and Jankovic, 2001; Kleopa

*Correspondence to: Alfonso Fasano, MD, Morton and Gloria Shulman Movement Disorders Clinic, Toronto Western Hospital, 399 Bathurst St, 7 Mc412, Toronto, ON, M5T 2S8, Canada. Tel: +1-416-603-5800 ext 5961, E-mail: alfonso.fasano@uhn.ca

and Kyriakides, 2004; Wohlgemuth et al., 2005; de Entrambasaguas et al., 2007). However, given the inconsistency, incongruence with known organic conditions, associated features, and response to treatment of these disorders, we have recently proposed that they may be better classified as FMDs (Fasano et al., 2012).

EPIDEMIOLOGY

Functional blepharospasm has been reported in 0.3% (Williams et al., 1995) to 7% (Factor et al., 1995) of all types of FMDs, in 20% of the total population of blepharospasm followed by a single center (Gazulla et al., 2015), and in 22% of a consecutive series of 50 patients in a botulinum neurotoxin clinic (Schwingenschuh et al., 2011).

Functional unilateral spasms of the eyelid were initially described as "psychogenic pseudoptosis" (Hop et al., 1997) and subsequently as "psychogenic" hemifacial spasm (HFS). HFS was initially described by Tan and Jankovic (2001) in 5 of 210 consecutive patients (2.4%) referred for the evaluation of HFS; a subsequent updated retrospective chart review performed in the same center found that 7.4% of all the cases referred for HFS had a functional etiology (Yaltho and Jankovic, 2011). A similar entity was later described by other authors (Tarsy et al., 2006; Stone and Carson, 2010).

More recently, we sought to examine a large series of FMD patients with involvement of the orofacial region followed up in seven tertiary movement disorder centers and found that facial FMDs represent 16.3% of all the FMD cases seen during the examined period (Fasano et al., 2012).

In conclusion, although no study has specifically addressed the epidemiology of facial FMDs, we can conclude that this condition is much more common than previously recognized.

CLINICAL FEATURES

Like many other FMDs, facial involvement is generally characterized by an episodic onset, highly variable course, inconsistency of presentation over time, higher prevalence in women and young-adult population, and association with other conditions (atypical facial pain, migraine) as well as other FMDs (speech problems or, more frequently, weakness or dystonia ipsilateral to the most affected hemiface) (Fasano et al., 2012; Morgante et al., 2013).

In the largest series of facial FMDs published so far, a total of 61 patients (92% females; mean age at onset of 37 ± 11.3 years and mean disease duration of 6.7 ± 6.9 years) were further characterized and a common clinical picture emerged, affecting predominantly young women (9:1 female-to-male ratio). In detail, phasic or tonic muscular spasms resembling dystonia were documented in all patients, most commonly involving the lips (60.7%), followed by eyelids (50.8%), perinasal region (16.4%), and forehead (9.8%) (Fig. 31.1). Symptom onset was abrupt in most cases (80.3%), with at least one precipitating psychologic stress or trauma identified in 57.4%. Therefore, the most common type of facial FMD is muscle overactivity. In this context, three basic patterns can be recognized: (1) bilateral contraction of orbicularis oculis (OOc) resembling blepharospasm or, less commonly, eyelid-opening apraxia; (2) unilateral contraction of OOc and/or orbicularis oris (OOr), resembling HFS; and (3) variable association of unilateral and bilateral signs also involving OOr and resembling oromandibular dystonia.

By contrast, functional weakness (or inability to move facial muscles) is extremely rare and is characterized by unilateral or bilateral palpebral ptosis, which is variable or improves in response to unusual stimuli, features already recognized more than a century ago (Preston, 1897; Hurst, 1920).

Bilateral involvement of orbicularis oculis

A series of 8 patients (5 women, mean age 42.5 years) with isolated functional blepharospasm has recently been published (Gazulla et al., 2015). Spontaneous remission took place in 4 cases, while the remaining patients experienced prolonged symptomatic relief from administration of placebo (saline injections). The authors also described a sign not seen in the organic counterpart of the condition: the contraction of corrugator and procerus muscles in the absence of spasm of the OOc (Gazulla et al., 2015) (Fig. 31.2A). The narrowing of eyelid fissure and frowning of the eyebrows during eyelid spasms is instead seen in organic blepharospasm and this is known as the "Charcot sign" (Fig. 31.2B).

Other clinical features described in functional blepharospasm are: (1) a sustained asymmetry (only described in the initial phases of organic blepharospasm); (2) changes in pattern and side of predominant eye closure; (3) the association with other ocular symptoms not seen in organic blepharospasm (sudden visual loss, oculogyria, or bilateral ocular convergence) (Fekete et al., 2012); and (4) sudden onset of spasms, whereas blepharospasm is usually preceded by increased blinking at rest (Bentivoglio et al., 2006). Although the improvement/resolution of symptoms during distracting maneuvers (e.g., while performing arithmetic calculations aloud) may help the diagnosis of FMD, such a feature should be cautiously interpreted in functional blepharospasm, because talking aloud usually decreases the severity/frequency of spasms in organic blepharospasm as well (Bentivoglio et al., 2006). Although of note, the presence of a *geste antagoniste* (or sensory trick) has been reported also in functional dystonias (Morgante et al., 2013).

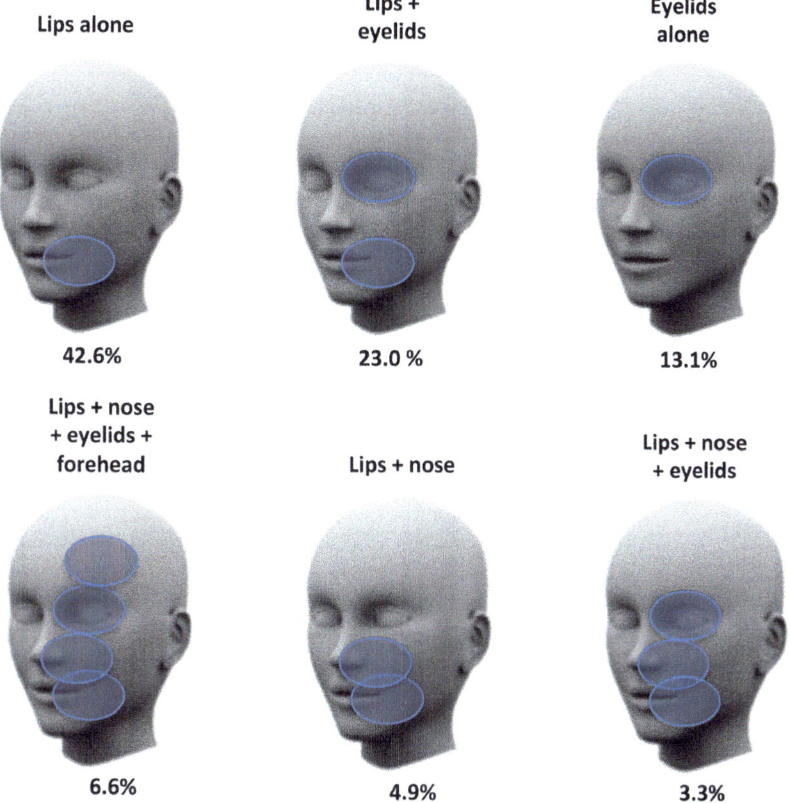

Fig. 31.1. The distribution of facial muscle involvement at the latest follow-up visit in the series by Fasano et al. (2012). Isolated lip involvement was the most frequent pattern (43%), followed by lips and eyelids (23%), and eyelids alone (13%). Platysma was involved in 61% of patients. Other, less common combinations were also present.

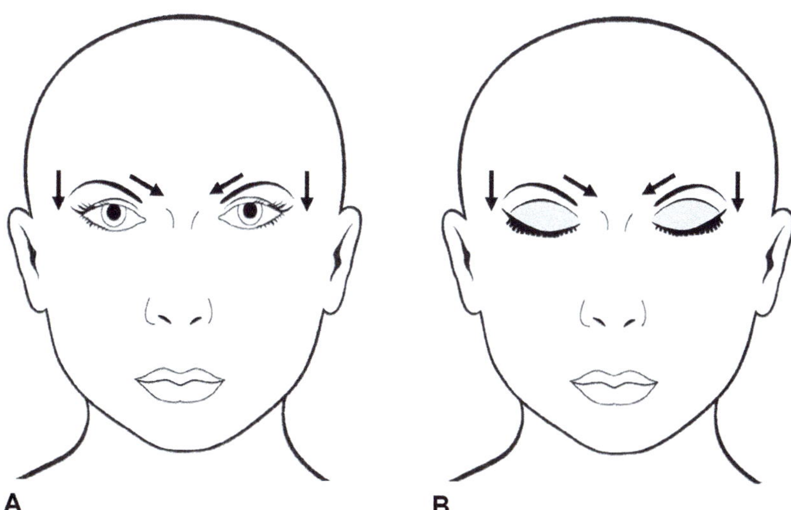

Fig. 31.2. The narrowing of eyelid fissure and frowning of the eyebrows due to the contraction of corrugator and procerus muscles in the absence of spasm of the orbicularis oculis is seen in functional patients (**A**), whereas patients with blepharospasm (**B**) also have eyelid spasms ("Charcot sign").

In our experience, 3 cases with functional blepharospasm reported a *geste antagoniste*, 1 at the second visit, after having received information on the phenomenon during the first visit (Fasano et al., 2012).

The differential diagnosis of bilateral involvement of OOc is wide (Table 31.1). Sometimes contraction of OOc is mistaken for ptosis, especially by nonneurologists, who may formulate a diagnosis of myasthenia gravis,

Table 31.1

Differential diagnosis of organic facial movement disorders

Face site	Diagnosis	Clinical features in comparison to facial FMDs
Bilateral and symmetric conditions		
Eyelids	Blepharospasm	Isolated dystonia, bilaterally affecting the eyelids and surrounding muscles; it may be slightly asymmetric (especially at onset) and is generally preceded by an increased blink rate
Peribuccal muscles	Parkinson's disease tremor	Jaw, lip, and tongue tremor (5 Hz) accompanied by the other signs of the disease
	"Rabbit syndrome"	High-frequency tremor of the lips and perioral muscles due to chronic neuroleptic treatment
Tongue	Essential tremor of the tongue	Tremor has the same frequency (4–8 Hz) of hand tremor (when present), with therapeutic benefit from ethanol or propranolol
	Isolated tremor of the tongue	It may present as an initial finding of essential tremor. Transient tongue tremor has been reported to occur as an isolated side-effect of neuroleptics, brain tumors, metabolic conditions (such as liver cirrhosis, Wilson's disease), infections (e.g., in neurosyphilis the so-called "trombone tongue") or head injury (e.g., the "galloping tongue," in which there is a peculiar episodic slow 3-Hz tremor beginning as posterior midline focal tongue contractions)
	Primary lingual dystonia	Represents an isolated task-induced dystonia induced by speaking and characterized by protrusion. It may be associated with the involvement of other body sites, such as larynx
	Lingual protrusion dystonia	Tongue protrusion sometimes associated with feeding dystonia is frequently seen in heredodegenerative diseases, including pantothenate kinase-associated neurodegeneration, Lesch–Nyhan syndrome, Wilson's disease and, especially, chorea-acanthocytosis, in which it represents a disease hallmark. It may be also seen in postanoxic and tardive dystonia
	Lingual myoclonus	It is a very rare entity that has been associated with an underlying abnormality, such as Arnold–Chiari malformation, craniovertebral junction abnormalities, brainstem ischemia, or systemic lupus erythematosus
Peribuccal muscles and jaw	Oromandibular dystonia	Usually bilateral and associated with masticatory and speech dystonia
	Oculomasticatory myorhythmia	A rare condition characterized by relatively fast and continuous slow-frequency muscle twitches associated with cerebral Whipple's disease
	Geniospasm	Isolated and benign contractions of mentalis muscle with an onset in childhood; it is usually hereditary
Asymmetric conditions		
Hemiface (upper and lower portion)	Idiopathic hemifacial spasm	Contractions are normally synchronous and shock-like (it is a peripheral myoclonus). They affect one hemiface, usually eyelid and surrounding muscles; the corner of the mouth and the forehead are commonly involved (see text for the "other Babinski sign")
	Facial nerve palsy with synkinetic aberrant reinnervation	Involuntary movements also triggered by voluntary movements involving movements adjacent to previously weak muscles
Hemiface (lower portion)	Hemimasticatory spasm	Involves muscles of mastication only. Only one side is affected
Variable distribution		
Facial tic		Brief movements associated with premonitory sensations, urge to move in a patterned response. Other tics are usually present
Facial myoclonus in focal seizures		Very fast muscular twitching, EEG evidence of cortical discharge
Facial myokymia		Occasional eye or face twitching is common in the general population and made worse with fatigue or caffeine. It may also occur in brainstem lesions (e.g., multiple sclerosis) and other neurologic diseases affecting the nerve excitability

Adapted from Yaltho and Jankovic (2011) and Silverdale et al. (2008), with permission from John Wiley.
FMDs, functional movement disorders; EEG, electroencephalogram.

also given the asymmetry and variability of presentation. Patients with paroxysmal facial FMDs resembling tics usually do not acknowledge voluntary control, urge, or relief of urge after the movements (Fasano et al., 2012). Moreover, these patients never feature fast movements, as seen in tics.

Although it represents a rarer phenotype, functional patients can also present the inability to open their eyes, thus resembling "eyelid-opening apraxia" (Kerty and Eidal, 2006). Usually, the strength of patients' eye closure varies depending on the force exerted against the eyelids by the examiner, which is a very useful diagnostic clue. This disorder has to be differentiated from catatonia because functional patients are otherwise responsive and actually complain about the symptom.

Unilateral involvement of orbicularis oculis and/or oris

Pseudoptosis was the term originally used to describe this condition (Hop et al., 1997), but it is no longer used, as a real ptosis is not accompanied by spasm around the eye (Stone, 2002). The few other cases of "pseudoptosis" reported share common features, such as acute onset, young age, common involvement of the left side, and response to placebo (Peer Mohamed and Patil, 2009; Matsumoto et al., 2012; Bagheri et al., 2015).

When spasms are tonic without any phasic component, the picture may resemble a "unilateral blepharospasm," which was already considered functional by definition in 1898 (Wood, 1898).

Sometimes unilateral OOc contraction is also present, thus resembling HFS. In a recent series of functional HFS (Yaltho and Jankovic, 2011), almost all patients were women (15 of 16); mean age at onset and disease duration of symptoms were 37.4 ± 19.5 and 1.7 ± 2.2 years, respectively. These patients presented findings incongruent with HFS or facial dystonia, such as acute onset of symptoms, nonprogressive course, fluctuations in symptom severity, spontaneous improvement, and other inconsistent signs.

Facial spasms are characterized by upward or lateral deviation of the corner of the mouth (Tan and Jankovic, 2001; Yaltho and Jankovic, 2011). Platysma is also commonly contracted and may contribute to the downward deviation of one corner of the mouth (Fig. 31.3A). The corner of the mouth may also be elevated compared to the other side, a condition previously termed "smirk" (Tarsy et al., 2006); in this situation the OOc is nearly always contracted as well (Fig. 31.3B).

The most common pattern of facial FMDs consists of tonic, sustained, lateral, and/or downward protrusion of one side of the lower lip with ipsilateral jaw deviation, as found in 84.3% of the largest series published so far (Fasano et al., 2012) (Fig. 31.3B). In this series, ipsi- or contralateral OOc spasms and excessive platysma contraction occurred in isolation or combined with fixed lip dystonia (60.7%). Paroxysmal (65%) or fixed (26%) eyelid involvement occurred mostly unilaterally with alternating sides (65%). The right side was affected twice as often as the left (Fasano et al., 2012).

The differential diagnosis of unilateral facial movement disorder (Yaltho and Jankovic, 2011) is also wide (Table 31.1). Most organic conditions involve brief myoclonic twitches in facial muscles rather than the sustained contractions seen in patients with functional disorders. The duration of spasm also helps the differential diagnosis between epileptic twitches and paroxysmal facial FMDs. On the other hand, longer episodes of paroxysmal facial FMDs may be confused with tics, especially given the observation that these patients may also have premonitory symptoms that are abolished by paroxysmal movements, a phenomenon that is also seen in patients with dissociative (nonepileptic) seizures (Stone and Carson, 2013).

In addition, the vast majority of patients with facial FMDs display a variable degree of face asymmetry, as some muscles pull sideways. However, the same clinical picture may be actually caused by weakness of contralateral hemiface, as pointed out by Babinski at the beginning of the 20th century (Babinski, 1918). For example, eyebrows can be pulled down during an overcontraction of OOc, but clinicians may also wonder if there is unilateral weakness of the frontalis muscle. Therefore, assessing the strength of facial muscles is the first step in the evaluation of these patients.

The unilateral involvement of facial muscles is common to facial FMDs and HFS. However, unlike the synchronous myoclonic jerks seen in HFS (Tan and Jankovic, 1999), most patients with facial FMDs show asynchronous, generally tonic, contractions. In addition, in HFS there may be elevation of frontalis on the same side as OOc involvement; this is called Babinski's "other" sign and has a specificity of 100% (Stamey and Jankovic, 2007; Devoize, 2011). This sign was not found in any of the functional patients with asymmetric spasm of OOc, who, rather, had the eyebrow rising contralateral to the closing eye (Fasano et al., 2012) (Fig. 31.4). Furthermore, these functional patients do not report facial spasms during sleep (Yaltho and Jankovic, 2011; Fasano et al., 2012), a condition present in up to 80% of HFS patients (Wang and Jankovic, 1998). Finally, most functional patients had lower-face involvement at onset, in contrast to the isolated lid involvement typically present at onset in HFS.

Functional facial movements can often be triggered by examination of eye movements or by asking the patients to sustain muscular contraction of the face.

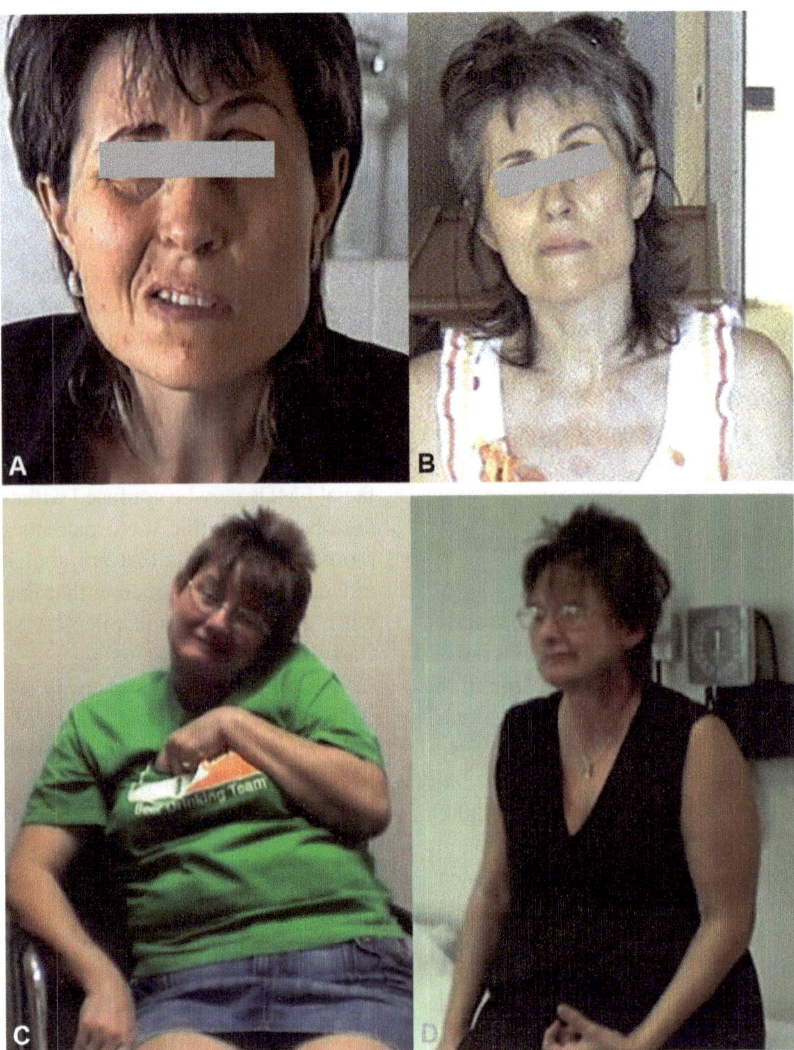

Fig. 31.3. (A) The involvement of the lower lip with downward deviation at the angle of the mouth is a very common pattern of facial functional movement disorders (FMDs); in this situation the orbicularis oculis is nearly always contracted as well. (B) Variability of clinical presentation in the same patient displayed in (A). (C) Patient with facial FMD and fixed dystonia of ipsilateral upper limb. (Courtesy of Dr. Alberto Espay, University of Cincinnati, USA.) (D) Variability of clinical presentation in the same patient displayed in (D).

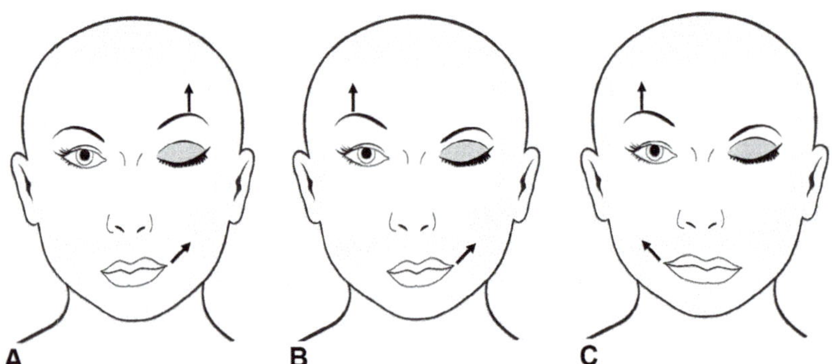

Fig. 31.4. The unilateral involvement of facial muscles is common to hemifacial spasm (HFS) (A) and facial functional movement disorders (B and C). However, in HFS there may be elevation of frontalis on the same side as orbicularis oculis (Babinski's "other" sign: A). This sign is not found in functional patients with asymmetric spasm of orbicularis oculis, who, rather, had the eyebrow rising contralateral to the closing eye (B and C).

On the other hand, clinicians should bear in mind that voluntary facial movement may also exacerbate HFS (documented in up to 39% of patients: Wang and Jankovic, 1998) or synkinetic movements seen after facial palsy (secondary HFS). For example, contraction of OOc in facial FMDs can sometimes be triggered or increased by asking the patient to elevate the eyebrows or look up, a phenomenon also seen in patients with HFS.

"Unilateral dystonia of the jaw" is uncommon and was first reported in 1986 by Thompson and colleagues in a small series. In retrospect, at least one of these patients was subsequently diagnosed as having a functional etiology (Fasano et al., 2012). Indeed, apart from masticatory spasm, whose clinical features are easily recognizable (e.g., the association with facial hemiatrophy: Esteban et al., 2002), few references to unilateral jaw spasms are to be found in the literature and several of these have clinical features that might support their reclassification as a facial FMD (Thompson et al., 1986; Jacome, 2001; Kleopa and Kyriakides, 2004; Wohlgemuth et al., 2005; de Entrambasaguas et al., 2007).

Finally, other entities not to overlook are nonneurologic conditions. Examples include local/mechanical disorders of the mandible or temporomandibular joint or ophthalmic conditions that can trigger the ipsilateral contraction of corrugator, procerus, and OOc muscle; the occurrence of local pain and functional impairment (e.g., difficulties with chewing) helps the differential diagnosis.

Bilateral involvement of orbicularis oris

In contrast to the more common involvement of upper facial muscles in organic cranial movement disorders, the involvement of the lower face appears to be characteristic of facial FMDs (Fabbrini et al., 2009).

Bilateral involvement of OOr is nevertheless rare, as it was documented in a minority (15.7%) of patients of a large series of facial FMDs; alternating sides was even rarer (3.3%) (Fasano et al., 2012). Bilateral involvement has been observed in 7 of 16 patients with a reported diagnosis of functional HFS (Yaltho and Jankovic, 2011). The phenomenology is in general the one of fixed dystonia, often associated with tongue involvement (see below).

Unlike organic oromandibular dystonia, most subjects had asymmetric facial involvement and absence of *gestes antagonistes*. The majority of these patients had no involvement of speech, which is commonly seen in oromandibular dystonia and has been reported in other series of FMDs (Hallett et al., 2012). Moreover, FMDs are usually present at rest, in contrast to task-specific dystonias affecting perioral muscles (e.g., embouchure dystonia) (Frucht et al., 2001).

Fixed dystonia of the oromandibular region has been reported to result from peripheral facial injury (Sankhla et al., 1998) and may develop within hours to months after dental procedures (Schrag et al., 1999). Such onset is in keeping with observations in patients with limb FMDs, in whom local traumas are often precipitating factors (Parcés et al., 2014). In addition, these atypical cranial dystonias exhibit persistent pain and dysesthesia, reminiscent of the limb complex regional pain syndrome, which is also suggestive of a functional etiology (Bhatia et al., 1993).

Tongue involvement

A variety of FMDs can involve the tongue, although these are rarer than other facial disorders and generally seen in the context of other body part involvement.

Little has been written on functional orolingual dystonia. Tongue deviation caused by a tonic contraction is the most common condition, almost always associated with other, generally ipsilateral, FMDs. The tongue may be involved by many organic disorders and particularly weakness; in this respect, "wrong-way" tongue deviation is helpful to diagnose functional tongue deviations (Keane, 1986). In fact, in organic weakness the tongue deviates on protrusion towards the affected side, the same side generally associated with facial weakness. By contrast, a tongue deviation towards the side of the facial pulling (i.e., contralateral to the facial weakness) has been originally described by Gowers as "wrong-way" tongue deviation (Gowers, 1888) (Fig. 31.5).

A recent work has evaluated the clinical features of tongue dyskinesias in patients with FMDs resembling tics (Baizabal-Carvallo and Jankovic, 2014): the coexistence of other functional conditions (e.g., pseudoseizures) and the lack of benefit from medical treatment (tetrabenazine and haloperidol) supported the diagnosis.

The spectrum of orolingual tremors has been reviewed by Silverdale and colleagues (2008), who also proposed a classification system helping the differential diagnosis (Table 31.1). Functional tongue tremor represents a rare variant, sometimes seen in the context of palatal tremor (see below). Speech can be variably affected by tongue disorders and in some cases "stuttering" speech has been described (Silverdale et al., 2008).

Palate involvement

Palate involvement is rarely seen in conjunction with other functional disorders but it can be selectively seen in the so-called "palatal tremor," particularly in its "essential" form. Essential palatal tremor occurs without any overt central nervous pathology and is characterized by rhythmic movements of the soft palate (tensor veli palatini), usually with an ear click that can be heard by the examiner. The tensor contraction is visible as a movement of the roof

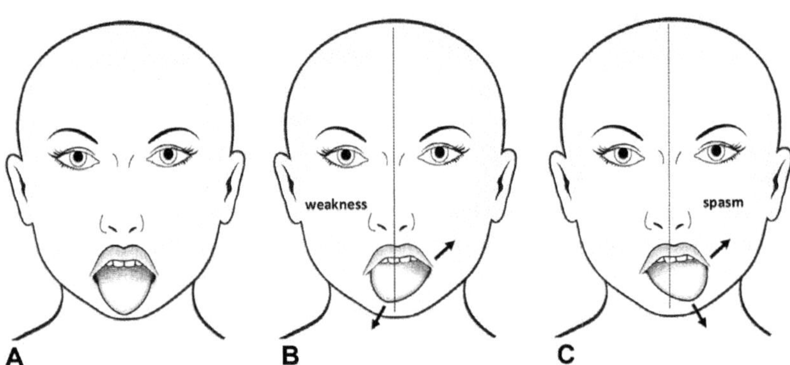

Fig. 31.5. (**A**) Normal symmetric face with protruded tongue. (**B**) In case of unilateral facial weakness (on the right side in this example), the contralateral side of the face is pulling due to the tonic contraction of the spared hemiface; in this context, patients may have ispilateral tongue weakness, meaning that the tongue deviates on the same side when protruded due to the active contraction of the spared hemitongue. (**C**) In case of unilateral facial functional spasm (on the left side in this example), patients may have the tongue deviated on the same side ("wrong-way" tongue).

of the palate (Deuschl et al., 1994b). The pathophysiology of essential palatal tremor has been unknown for many years (Deuschl et al., 1994b), but after the initial reports of functional patients (Williams, 2004; Pirio Richardson et al., 2006), recent case series found evidence that some cases might represent tics or a voluntary/special motor skill (Zadikoff et al., 2006), whereas the vast majority are functional (Stamelou et al., 2012). These patients occasionally demonstrate extrapalatal movement involving the jaw, tongue, and floor of the mouth (Zadikoff et al., 2006). In some cases, a good response to placebo has been reported (Baik et al., 2008).

Symptomatic palatal tremor represents the organic counterpart of essential palatal tremor. It is characterized by the rhythmic movements of the soft palate (levator veli palatini), clinically visible as a rhythmic movement of the edge of the palate (Deuschl et al., 1994a). Other brainstem-innervated or extremity muscles can be involved and are the source of disability (e.g., due to oscillopsia in case of extraocular muscle involvement) (Masucci et al., 1984). Symptomatic palatal tremor typically follows a brainstem/cerebellar lesion with a variable delay and is often associated with a cerebellar syndrome. Degenerative forms also exists, as in progressive ataxia with palatal tremor (Samuel et al., 2004), *GFAP* gene mutation (Alexander's disease), neuroferritinopathy or SCA20; a reversible form caused by celiac disease has been also described.

Associated conditions

In a series of 61 facial FMD patients, associated body regions involved included upper limbs (29.5%), neck (16.4%), lower limbs (16.4%), and trunk (4.9%) (Fasano et al., 2012). Dystonia was the most frequent phenotype of extrafacial sites (58%), followed by tremor (14%) and other jerks (10%). When present, limb involvement was ipsilateral to the facial involvement (Fig. 31.3C). Along with the motor symptoms, patients complained of a number of comorbidities (e.g., atypical pain or psychiatric conditions), further corroborating the functional etiology (Table 31.2). In this sample depression is the most common associated condition, with a much higher prevalence than observed in the same age group of women in the general population (38% vs. 4%: Olsen et al., 2004). By contrast, although very common, the prevalence of tension-type headache was not higher than reported in cohorts without FMDs but with similar age and gender distribution (Schwartz et al., 1998).

DIAGNOSIS

As for most FMDs, functional facial disorders have no definitive test or biomarker; however, rather than excluding similar organic conditions, the diagnosis can be reliably made applying "positive" diagnostic clinical criteria, (Hallett et al., 2012). In fact, a prompt diagnosis based on phenomenology will avoid the extensive diagnostic workup characteristic of a diagnosis-of-exclusion approach, prevent unnecessary costly investigations, and permit the institution of appropriate physical, psychologic, and medical therapy (Gupta and Lang, 2009).

In the series by Fasano et al. (2012), the vast majority of these cases received a "positive" diagnosis rather than a diagnosis based on the exclusion of organic diseases. Diagnosis of FMDs was made according to the criteria of Fahn and Williams (Williams et al., 1995) and Gupta and Lang (2009). Notably, not all patients could fulfill a psychiatric diagnostic entity as conversion disorder (*Diagnostic and Statistical Manual*, fourth edition (DSM-IV): American Psychiatric Association, 1994) was diagnosed in 40.7%, somatization disorder in 9.8%, and malingering in 4.9% (Fasano et al., 2012).

The diagnosis of FMD is based on the inconsistency and incongruity of the observed phenomenology. The

Table 31.2

Medical conditions associated and features supporting a functional etiology in the cohort of patients published by Fasano et al. (2012)

Medical condition associated with facial FMDs*	%
Depression	38.0
Tension headache	26.4
Migraine	25.9
Anxiety	18.0
Fatigue	17.6
Fibromyalgia	9.8
Hypertension	4.9
Temporomandibular joint dysfunction	3.9
Irritable-bowel syndrome	3.8
Hearing loss	3.7
Feature supporting a functional etiology	%
Historic information	
Employed in allied health professions	28.0
History of minor trauma	26.8
Exposure to a disease model	18.5
History of physical abuse	4.3
History of sexual abuse	2.1
Clinical course	
Rapid onset	96.7
Nonprogressive course	85.2
Remissions	21.3
Suggestibility	
Movements decrease with distraction	89.6
Placebo effect†	89.5
Movements increase with attention	86.0
Resolution when the patient feels unobserved	61.1
Ability to trigger or relieve the abnormal movements‡	36.4
Disability	
Functional disability out of proportion to exam findings	47.2
Selective disability§	28.1
Secondary gain¶	20.3
Accompanying features	
Other somatizations†	49.2
False sensory complaints**	34.4
Deliberate slowness of movements	27.9
False (give-away) weakness†	18.0
Delayed and excessive startle response to a stimulus	1.6
Self-inflicted injuries	0.0

*Other, less common (1 case each), conditions were: breast cancer, hypothyroidism, ovary dermoid cyst, otosclerosis, miscarriage, spina bifida occulta, thoracic outlet syndrome, cervical cancer treated with radiation, gastroesophageal reflux disease, osteoarthritis, morbid obesity, intestinal malabsorption.

†See text for details.

‡By using nonphysiologic interventions (e.g., trigger points on the body, tuning fork).

§Defined as disability limited only to specific activities of daily living.

¶Defined as ongoing or pending litigation, disability benefits, release from personal/legal/social/employment responsibilities, and/or increased personal attention.

**For example, blurred vision, pain, numbness or sense of swelling not following anatomy (whole or half body, ipsilateral hand and foot).

FMDs, functional movement disorders.

former refers to the variability over time, which can be spontaneous or triggered by suggestibility maneuvers (Fig. 31.3C and D and 31.6). These are not sensible but highly specific: a nonphysiologic or placebo maneuver (most often a vibrating tuning fork or a pen light) improved 16% and worsened 10% of 19 cases of facial FMDs to whom it was applied (Fasano et al., 2012).

Incongruity refers to a presentation not fulfilling any of the known medical conditions. For instance, in some instances the pattern of abnormal movement was very complex and did not fall into any of the better-defined movement disorders affecting the face. Examples included the unilateral isolated spasm of platysma (rarely seen and only in HFS and some tics), tongue deviation in absence of weakness, or an alternating involvement of hemifaces (although possible in the rare patients with bilateral HFS: Holds et al., 1990). Furthermore, the diagnosis is usually more secure when the patient has more than one functional symptom; a typical example is when the patient has motor symptoms in the upper and lower halves of the face as well as in the ipsilateral arm and/or leg. Several clinical signs can assist the physician in confirming the diagnosis on clinical grounds (see below).

A variety of other features may suggest a functional cause (Table 31.3) (Monday and Jankovic, 1993; Factor et al., 1995; Lang et al., 1995; Williams et al., 1995; Kim et al., 1999; Tan and Jankovic, 2001; Hinson and Haren, 2006; Shill and Gerber, 2006; Gupta and Lang, 2009; Stone and Carson, 2011). Comorbidities, and particularly psychiatric conditions, may also support a functional etiology, but their role is limited and sometimes confusing. In fact, around 30% of patients with FMD report no psychiatric disorder and, on the other hand, psychiatric disorders, particularly obsessive compulsive disorder, are common in diseases affecting the basal ganglia. Recognizing the difficulties inherent in deciding whether psychologic problems are causative, coincidental, or a reaction, the latest revision of the DSM regarded them as having low diagnostic reliability and so removed them from diagnostic criteria (American Psychiatric Association, 2013).

Electrophysiologic studies can also support the diagnosis (laboratory-supported diagnosis) (Gupta and Lang, 2009), although it should be acknowledged that these studies may also disclose abnormal findings in patients with FMDs (Thompson et al., 1986; Kang and Sohn, 2006).

A normal blink reflex study has been reported in 9 patients with "presumed psychogenic" blepharospasm, in contrast to patients with organic blepharospasm (Schwingenschuh et al., 2011). These findings have been confirmed in another series of 10 patients with facial FMDs (Fasano et al., 2012). In addition, sensorimotor plasticity has been found normal in functional

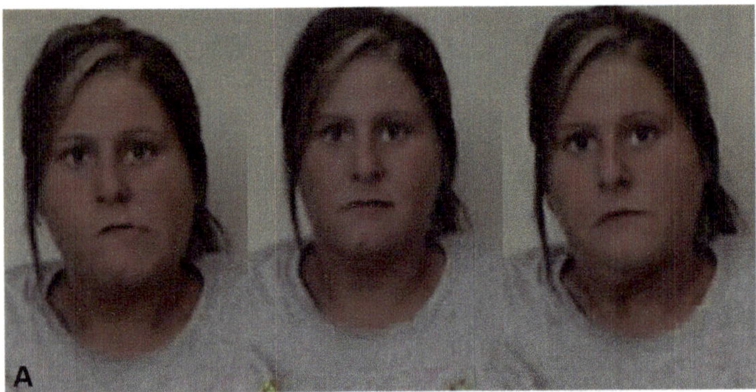

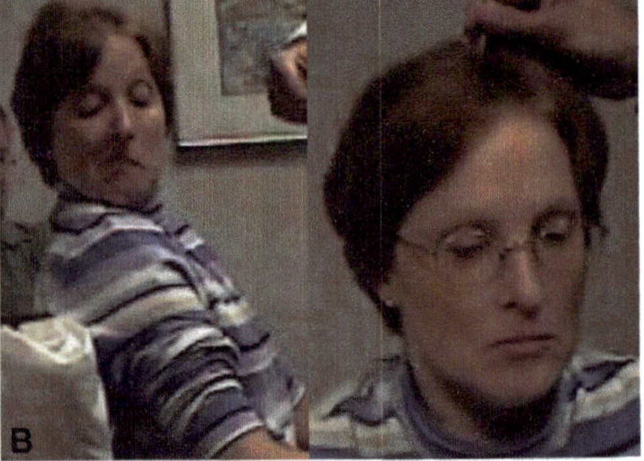

Fig. 31.6. The variability of presentation over time (**A**) or the effect of suggestibility maneuvers (**B**) in 2 patients with facial functional movement disorder. (Courtesy of Dr. Alberto Espay, University of Cincinnati, USA.)

Table 31.3

Features distinguishing organic vs. functional oromandibular and facial dystonia

	Organic	Functional
Onset and progression	Gradual, slow progression	Sudden onset, static course
Sensory tricks	May be present	Rarely present
Most common distribution	Lips	Jaw, eyelids
Most common sidedness	Bilateral	Unilateral
Platysma involvement	Very rare, bilateral	Common, ipsilateral
OOc and frontalis muscle involvement (if present)	OOc and frontalis, ipsilateral	OOc and frontalis, contralateral*
Dystonic pattern	Phasic	Tonic
Dystonic exacerbation	Action-induced	Paroxysmal, maximum at rest
Dystonic spread	Segmental to cervical region	Segmental or multifocal
Evolution	Slowly progressive, no spontaneous exacerbations or remissions	Fluctuations in severity, spontaneous exacerbation and remissions
Pain	Usually absent	Often present

Reproduced from Fasano et al. (2012).
*If orbicularis oculi (OOc) present in isolation, it most often occurred contralateral to the affected lip/jaw.

blepharospasm in contrast to the organic counterparts (Quartarone et al., 2009).

Electrophysiologic examination may also help in distinguishing HFS from other abnormal facial movements by demonstrating ephaptic impulse transmission between different facial nerve branches (Valls-Sole, 2002). Indeed, a neurophysiologic hallmark of HFS is the spread of the blink reflex responses elicited by supraorbital nerve stimulation to muscles other than the OOc.

In our hands, electromyogram or motion capture systems using facial markers are helpful in order to document the effects of distractibility maneuvers, placebo, or spontaneous inconsistency.

DIFFERENTIAL DIAGNOSIS

Many systemic and neurologic conditions may involve the facial musculature. Table 31.1 indicates the commonest causes and the clinical features that help distinguish them from functional disorders. From tetanus to blepharospasm, most are characterized by muscular spasms (Thompson et al., 1986). While some are easily recognizable, sometimes the differential diagnosis can be challenging. For example, diagnosing dystonia following minor peripheral injury remains a major source of controversy in this field given the functional features exhibited by these patients (Lang and Chen, 2010).

MANAGEMENT

Little is known about the course and treatment response of facial FMDs. In a series of facial FMDs, the course was variable in 47% of patients; spontaneous remissions were reported in 13 subjects (21%), with recurrence in 2 patients after 2 weeks and 10 years (Fasano et al., 2012).

The management of facial FMDs can be challenging and disappointing, especially when using pharmacologic approaches, as treatments usually used for the organic

Table 31.4

Treatments used in patients with facial functional movement disorders enrolled in the series by Fasano et al. (2012)

Nonpharmacologic	*n*	Pharmacologic	*n*
Psychotherapy	5	Antidepressant	15
Cognitive-behavioral therapy	2	Botulinum neurotoxin	14
Hypnosis	1	Benzodiazepines	9
Acupuncture	1	Anticholinergic	2
Other*	6	Neuroleptics†	1
None	38	Other‡	20
		None	6

*Including physiotherapy, massage, chiropractic treatment.
†Prescribed after onset of functional movement disorder.
‡Including antiepileptics, baclofen, and morphine derivative.

counterparts are ineffective and only expose the patient to the risk of side-effects. In a series of 55 patients with facial FMDs, medical and/or nonpharmacologic treatments caused no improvement (56%) or even worsening (20%) (Table 31.4); only 20% of these patients improved after treatment (botulinum neurotoxin injection at therapeutic doses was effective in 5 cases, antidepressants in 3, antiepileptics in 2, and psychotherapy in 1) (Fasano et al., 2012). Low doses of botulinum neurotoxin can be also effective for the treatment of palatal tremor (Eryilmaz et al., 2015).

As for other functional disorders, the treatment of facial FMDs starts with a positive clinical diagnosis and explanation to the patient. Motor signs can form an important part of the explanation of the diagnosis to patients. This step alone can produce major therapeutic benefit, and may in some patients be the only treatment necessary (Morgante et al., 2013). For others, treatment has to be individualized within a rehabilitative approach consisting of education, physical therapy, and cognitive-behavioral therapy. In keeping with what has been observed in functional tremor affecting the limbs, entrainment test can be successfully used as a treatment for facial functional tremor, as in the case of palatal tremor (Kern and Lang, 2015).

References

American Psychiatric Association (1994). Diagnostic and statistical manual of mental disorders, 4th ed. American Psychiatric Association, Washington, DC.

American Psychiatric Association (2013). Diagnostic and Statistical Manual of Mental Disorders, Fifth Edition (DSM-5), American Psychiatric Association, Arlington, VA, USA.

Babinski JJFF (1918). Hysteria or Pithiatism, University of London Press, London.

Bagheri A, Abbasnia E, Pakravan M et al. (2015). Psychogenic unilateral pseudoptosis. Ophthal Plast Reconstr Surg 31: e55–e57.

Baik JS, Lyoo CH, Lee JH et al. (2008). Drug-induced and psychogenic resting suprahyoid neck and tongue tremors. Mov Disord 23: 746–748.

Baizabal-Carvallo JF, Jankovic J (2014). The clinical features of psychogenic movement disorders resembling tics. J Neurol Neurosurg Psychiatry 85: 573–575.

Bentivoglio AR, Daniele A, Albanese A et al. (2006). Analysis of blink rate in patients with blepharospasm. Mov Disord 21: 1225–1229.

Bhatia KP, Bhatt MH, Marsden CD (1993). The causalgia-dystonia syndrome. Brain 116 (Pt 4): 843–851.

Charcot JM (1887). Leçons sur les Maladies du Système Nerveux faites à la Salpêtrière, A. Delahaye, Paris.

de Entrambasaguas M, Plaza-Costa A, Casal J et al. (2007). Labial dystonia after facial and trigeminal neuropathy controlled with a maxillary splint. Mov Disord 22: 1355–1358.

Deuschl G, Toro C, Hallett M (1994a). Symptomatic and essential palatal tremor. 2. Differences of palatal movements. Mov Disord 9: 676–678.

Deuschl G, Toro C, Valls-Sole J et al. (1994b). Symptomatic and essential palatal tremor. 1. Clinical, physiological and MRI analysis. Brain 117: 775–788.

Devoize JL (2011). Neurological picture. Hemifacial spasm in antique sculpture: interest in the 'other Babinski sign'. J Neurol Neurosurg Psychiatry 82: 26.

Eryilmaz A, Basal Y, Gunel C et al. (2015). Successful treatment of essential palatal tremor lasting over a long term with a rare application of botulinum toxin in a child. Iran J Child Neurol 9: 75–77.

Esteban A, Traba A, Prieto J et al. (2002). Long term follow up of a hemimasticatory spasm. Acta Neurol Scand 105: 67–72.

Fabbrini G, Defazio G, Colosimo C et al. (2009). Cranial movement disorders: clinical features, pathophysiology, differential diagnosis and treatment. Nat Clin Pract Neurol 5: 93–105.

Factor SA, Podskalny GD, Molho ES (1995). Psychogenic movement disorders: frequency, clinical profile, and characteristics. J Neurol Neurosurg Psychiatry 59: 406–412.

Fasano A, Valadas A, Bhatia KP et al. (2012). Psychogenic facial movement disorders: clinical features and associated conditions. Mov Disord 27: 1544–1551.

Fekete R, Baizabal-Carvallo JF, Ha AD et al. (2012). Convergence spasm in conversion disorders: prevalence in psychogenic and other movement disorders compared with controls. J Neurol Neurosurg Psychiatry 83: 202–204.

Frucht SJ, Fahn S, Greene PE et al. (2001). The natural history of embouchure dystonia. Mov Disord 16: 899–906.

Gazulla J, Garcia-Rubio S, Ruiz-Gazulla C et al. (2015). Clinical categorization of psychogenic blepharospasm. Parkinsonism Relat Disord 21: 325–326.

Gowers WR (1888). A manual of diseases of the Nervous System, J & A Churchill, London.

Gupta A, Lang AE (2009). Psychogenic movement disorders. Curr Opin Neurol 22: 430–436.

Hallett M, Lang AE, Jankovic J et al. (2012). Psychogenic Movement Disorders and Other Conversion Disorders, Cambridge University Press, Cambridge, UK.

Hinson VK, Haren WB (2006). Psychogenic movement disorders. Lancet Neurol 5: 695–700.

Holds JB, Anderson RL, Jordan DR et al. (1990). Bilateral hemifacial spasm. J Clin Neuroophthalmol 10: 153–154.

Hop JW, Frijns CJ, van Gijn J (1997). Psychogenic pseudoptosis. J Neurol 244: 623–624.

Hurst A (1920). The psychology of the special senses and their functional disorders, Oxford University Press, London.

Jacome DE (2001). Dracula's teeth syndrome. Headache 41: 892–894.

Kang SY, Sohn YH (2006). Electromyography patterns of propriospinal myoclonus can be mimicked voluntarily. Mov Disord 21: 1241–1244.

Keane JR (1986). Wrong-way deviation of the tongue with hysterical hemiparesis. Neurology 36: 1406–1407.

Kern DS, Lang AE (2015). Successful treatment of functional palatal tremor: insights into pathogenesis and management. Mov Disord 30: 875–876.

Kerty E, Eidal K (2006). Apraxia of eyelid opening: clinical features and therapy. Eur J Ophthalmol 16: 204–208.

Kim YJ, Pakiam AS, Lang AE (1999). Historical and clinical features of psychogenic tremor: a review of 70 cases. Can J Neurol Sci 26: 190–195.

Kleopa KA, Kyriakides T (2004). A novel movement disorder of the lower lip. Mov Disord 19: 663–666.

Lang AE, Chen R (2010). Dystonia in complex regional pain syndrome type I. Ann Neurol 67: 412–414.

Lang AE, Koller WC, Fahn S (1995). Psychogenic parkinsonism. Arch Neurol 52: 802–810.

Masucci EF, Kurtzke JF, Saini N (1984). Myorhythmia: a widespread movement disorder. Clinicopathological correlations. Brain 107 (Pt 1): 53–79.

Matsumoto H, Shimizu T, Igeta Y et al. (2012). Psychogenic unilateral ptosis with ipsilateral muscle spasm of orbicular oculi. Acta Med Indones 44: 243–245.

Monday K, Jankovic J (1993). Psychogenic myoclonus. Neurology 43: 349–352.

Morgante F, Edwards MJ, Espay AJ (2013). Psychogenic movement disorders. Continuum (Minneap Minn) 19: 1383–1396.

Olsen LR, Mortensen EL, Bech P (2004). Prevalence of major depression and stress indicators in the Danish general population. Acta Psychiatr Scand 109: 96–103.

Pareés I, Kojovic M, Pires C et al. (2014). Physical precipitating factors in functional movement disorders. J Neurol Sci 338: 174–177.

Peer Mohamed BA, Patil SG (2009). Psychogenic unilateral pseudoptosis. Pediatr Neurol 41: 364–366.

Pirio Richardson S, Mari Z, Matsuhashi M et al. (2006). Psychogenic palatal tremor. Mov Disord 21: 274–276.

Preston G (1897). Hysteria and certain allied conditions, P. Blakiston, Philadelphia.

Quartarone A, Rizzo V, Terranova C et al. (2009). Abnormal sensorimotor plasticity in organic but not in psychogenic dystonia. Brain 132: 2871–2877.

Samuel M, Torun N, Tuite PJ et al. (2004). Progressive ataxia and palatal tremor (PAPT): clinical and MRI assessment with review of palatal tremors. Brain 127: 1252–1268.

Sankhla C, Lai EC, Jankovic J (1998). Peripherally induced oromandibular dystonia. J Neurol Neurosurg Psychiatry 65: 722–728.

Schrag A, Bhatia KP, Quinn NP et al. (1999). Atypical and typical cranial dystonia following dental procedures. Mov Disord 14: 492–496.

Schwartz BS, Stewart WF, Simon D et al. (1998). Epidemiology of tension-type headache. JAMA 279: 381–383.

Schwingenschuh P, Katschnig P, Edwards MJ et al. (2011). The blink reflex recovery cycle differs between essential and presumed psychogenic blepharospasm. Neurology 76: 610–614.

Shill H, Gerber P (2006). Evaluation of clinical diagnostic criteria for psychogenic movement disorders. Mov Disord 21: 1163–1168.

Silverdale MA, Schneider SA, Bhatia KP et al. (2008). The spectrum of orolingual tremor – a proposed classification system. Mov Disord 23: 159–167.

Stamelou M, Saifee TA, Edwards MJ et al. (2012). Psychogenic palatal tremor may be underrecognized: reappraisal of a large series of cases. Mov Disord 27: 1164–1168.

Stamey W, Jankovic J (2007). The other Babinski sign in hemifacial spasm. Neurology 69: 402–404.

Stone J (2002). Pseudo-ptosis. Pract Neurol 2: 364–365.

Stone J, Carson A (2010). Psychogenic/dissociative/functional facial symptoms – a case report. J Neurol Neurosurg Psychiatry 81: e8–e9.

Stone J, Carson A (2011). Functional neurologic symptoms: assessment and management. Neurol Clin 29 (1–18): vii.

Stone J, Carson AJ (2013). The unbearable lightheadedness of seizing: wilful submission to dissociative (non-epileptic) seizures. J Neurol Neurosurg Psychiatry 84: 822–824.

Tan EK, Jankovic J (1999). Bilateral hemifacial spasm: a report of five cases and a literature review. Mov Disord 14: 345–349.

Tan EK, Jankovic J (2001). Psychogenic hemifacial spasm. J Neuropsychiatry Clin Neurosci 13: 380–384.

Tarsy D, Dengenhardt A, Zadikoff C (2006). Psychogenic facial spasm (the smirk) presenting as hemifacial spasm. In: M Hallett, S Fahn, J Jankovic et al. (Eds.), Psychogenic Movement Disorders, Lippincott Williams & Williams, Philadelphia.

Thompson PD, Obeso JA, Delgado G et al. (1986). Focal dystonia of the jaw and the differential diagnosis of unilateral jaw and masticatory spasm. J Neurol Neurosurg Psychiatry 49: 651–656.

Valls-Sole J (2002). Facial palsy, postparalytic facial syndrome, and hemifacial spasm. Mov Disord 17 (Suppl 2): S49–S52.

Wang A, Jankovic J (1998). Hemifacial spasm: clinical findings and treatment. Muscle Nerve 21: 1740–1747.

Williams DR (2004). Psychogenic palatal tremor. Mov Disord 19: 333–335.

Williams DT, Ford B, Fahn S (1995). Phenomenology and psychopathology related to psychogenic movement disorders. Adv Neurol 65: 231–257.

Wohlgemuth M, Pasman JW, de Swart BJ et al. (2005). Movement disorder of the lower lip. Mov Disord 20: 1085–1086.

Wood C (1898). The methods employed in examining the eyes for the detection of hysteria. JAMA 31: 1136–1138.

Yaltho TC, Jankovic J (2011). The many faces of hemifacial spasm: differential diagnosis of unilateral facial spasms. Mov Disord 26: 1582–1592.

Zadikoff C, Lang AE, Klein C (2006). The 'essentials' of essential palatal tremor: a reappraisal of the nosology. Brain 129: 832–840.

Handbook of Clinical Neurology, Vol. 139 (3rd series)
Functional Neurologic Disorders
M. Hallett, J. Stone, and A. Carson, Editors
http://dx.doi.org/10.1016/B978-0-12-801772-2.00032-1

Chapter 32

Functional auditory disorders

D.M. BAGULEY[1]*, T.E. COPE[2], AND D.J. McFERRAN[3]

[1]*Department of Audiology, Cambridge University Hospitals, Cambridge, UK*

[2]*Department of Neurology, Cambridge University Hospitals, Cambridge, UK*

[3]*Department of Otolaryngology, Colchester Hospital University, Colchester, UK*

Abstract

There are a number of auditory symptom syndromes that can develop without an organic basis. Some of these, such as nonorganic hearing loss, affect populations similar to those presenting with functional somatosensory and motor symptoms, while others, such as musical hallucination, affect populations with a significantly different demographic and require different treatment strategies. Many of these conditions owe their origin to measurably abnormal peripheral sensory pathology or brain network activity, but their pathological impact is often due, at least in part, to overamplification of the salience of these phenomena. For each syndrome, this chapter briefly outlines a definition, demographics, investigations, putative mechanisms, and treatment strategies. Consideration is given to what extent they can be considered to have a functional basis. Treatments are in many cases pragmatic and rudimentary, needing more work to be done in integrating insights from behavioral and cognitive psychology to auditory neuroscience. The audiology literature has historically equated the term functional with malingering, although this perception is, thankfully, slowly changing. These disorders transcend the disciplines of audiology, otorhinolaryngology, neurology and psychiatry, and a multidisciplinary approach is often rewarding.

INTRODUCTION

This chapter outlines the disparate collection of auditory symptoms that can be considered to have a functional basis, at least in some cases. They transcend the disciplines of audiology, otorhinolaryngology, neurology, and psychiatry. Many of these conditions owe their origin to measurably abnormal peripheral sensory pathology or brain network activity, but their pathological impact is often due, at least in part, to overamplification of the salience of these phenomena.

Some of the conditions we describe, such as nonorganic hearing loss (NOHL), appear to affect a similar demographic and are amenable to similar psychological interventions to those functional disorders affecting motor or somatosensory systems that are commonly encountered in neurology clinics. Others, such as musical hallucination (MH), affect strikingly different population groups. As in those functional disorders affecting motor and sensory symptoms, it has only been in relatively recent years that we have come to recognize these conditions as truly disabling.

NONORGANIC HEARING LOSS

Definition

The situation in which patients may behave as if they have a significant hearing loss, both in general communication and on pure-tone audiometry, that is not borne out by specialized or objective testing, has a varied terminology. The descriptors malingering and feigning have been used clinically, possibly deriving from early reports of such behavior in wartime (Peck, 2012), and assume intentionality. The term psychogenic hearing loss makes an assumption that this is an exclusively

*Correspondence to: David M. Baguley, Audiology (94), Cambridge University Hospitals, Hills Road, Cambridge CB2 0QQ, UK. Tel: +44-1223-217594, E-mail: dmb29@cam.ac.uk

psychological disorder. Functional hearing loss and NOHL are less loaded, and thus are preferable.

Demographics

Information regarding the epidemiology of NOHL is extremely sparse. There have been estimates that up to 30% of individuals claiming compensation for noise-induced hearing loss have some nonorganic component to their complaint (Peck, 2012). The presentation is familiar to all audiologists and otolaryngologists, but no systematic study of prevalence and incidence has been undertaken.

The patient population with NOHL is varied, but there are some classic presentations. Teenagers, said to be more often girls than boys (Peck, 2012), may claim poor hearing but demonstrate inconsistent extent of hearing loss. Individuals claiming compensation for industrial or accidentally caused hearing loss may wish the extent of the loss to appear greater than it is. Some adults may receive secondary gain from being thought to have a hearing loss, whether in terms of support from family/friends, from the state, or greater respect and identity; recognition of this gain might not be conscious.

Investigations

Pure-tone audiometry is required in any consideration of hearing loss but it should be remembered that the audiogram is a threshold test of signal detection and does not adequately represent real-world hearing abilities. In NOHL an audiologist can use specific techniques to obtain audiometric thresholds: these may include presenting the stimuli at random, nonpredictable intensities, or only presenting at low intensities.

Specialized behavioral tests exist, the most common example being the Stenger test, which exploits the principle that if stimuli are presented simultaneously to each ear, only the louder will be perceived. A tone is presented at 10 dB above audiometric threshold to one ear, and 20 dB below the admitted threshold in the other, this latter tone then being raised in steps until the patient ceases responding, that point approximating the threshold in that ear.

Objective (physiological) hearing testing, in the form of auditory evoked potentials and otoacoustic emission testing, has largely replaced the behavioral testing approaches. It does require patient compliance for extended test periods, but can glean ear- and frequency-specific physiological thresholds. Cortical auditory evoked potentials require the patient to be alert, and are attenuated with general anesthesia (Simpson et al., 2002). Auditory brainstem responses (ABRs) persist under general anesthesia and natural sleep, and frequency-specific test protocols are now in use, rather than the traditional wide frequency band click stimuli.

Is it functional?

Austen and Lynch (2004) proposed a model that considered the following factors: motivating factors that may be observed, the type of gain (including financial or role), the degree of intention, and the consistency of response to testing.

They hypothesized that three categories of disorder occur: malingering, factitious, and conversion. It was considered that individuals might move between these categories, and that management strategies would be different for each. This model has been influential and widely adopted, despite retaining pejorative vocabulary, but no further systematic research has been undertaken.

It is almost tautologic but nonetheless important to indicate that NOHL is functional in some cases, though in others there may be intentional aspects to the behaviors.

Treatment strategies

There are indications that NOHL may be a marker for psychological problems (Austen and Lynch, 2004), so the approach to treatment has to include vigilance to such issues, but to avoid overreaction. The present consensus is to avoid confrontation, and to create an expectation of recovery. Where there is secondary gain, psychology support to meet those needs in other forms may be of use, and where conversion disorder is evident, psychiatric support should be sought.

DISORDERS OF AUDITORY PROCESSING

Definition

Auditory processing disorder (APD) encompasses a range of developmental and acquired disorders that affect auditory analysis and cannot be directly explained by structural pathology in the brain or cochlea or generalized cognitive deficit. Patients typically have normal auditory threshold sensitivity but have difficulty identifying speech (Keith, 2000) and/or nonspeech sounds (Rosen, 2005; Moore, 2006). The usual presenting complaint is an impaired ability to hear speech in background noise in comparison to their peers. APD may coexist with peripheral hearing loss, complicating diagnosis (Moore et al., 2013). The auditory discrimination difficulties are especially marked in challenging listening environments, when target sounds are brief, masked, or degraded (ASHA, 1996; Jerger and Musiek, 2000). The diagnosis encompasses a number of overlapping clinical syndromes (Jerger and Musiek, 2000; Hind, 2006), and its underlying pathological basis is poorly understood. Of those children complaining of symptoms consistent with APD, only around 5% have an underlying structural or other obvious neurological cause (Chermak and Musiek, 1997).

Demographics

There remains debate about whether the diagnosis of APD should be confined to that small group of children who have difficulties restricted to the processing of complex sounds, or whether it can be invoked for individuals with multimodal perceptual processing difficulties (Cacace and McFarland, 2005). When defined broadly, APDs are a common group of conditions, affecting up to 7% of children (Bamiou et al., 2001), but only a small proportion of this group will seek a medical opinion.

Investigations

In APD pure-tone audiometry is often, but not always, normal. ABRs can be helpful in disambiguating APD from its key differential diagnosis, auditory neuropathy / dyssynchrony, in which the presenting symptom may also be problems with complex sound processing. In APD one would expect ABRs to mirror pure-tone audiometry and outer hair cell function (i.e., to be normal if peripheral function is normal), while in auditory neuropathy ABRs are significantly disrupted (Starr et al., 1996; Berlin et al., 2003).

Middle latency responses and cortical responses to unexpected stimuli (mismatch negativity: Garrido et al., 2009) are rarely measured in clinical practice (Emanuel et al., 2011). While some authorities have proposed that these responses, which are generated higher in the auditory pathway, might provide objective evidence of a processing abnormality (Sharma et al., 2006), their sensitivity and specificity are not well established.

Auditory psychophysical tests form the cornerstone of assessment for APD, but no gold-standard test battery has been established (Moore et al., 2013). The most commonly applied battery of tests is called SCAN (Bensimon et al., 2009), and versions exist for children under 12 (SCAN-C: Keith, 2000), as well as adolescents and adults (SCAN-A: Keith, 1995). It comprises four subtests assessing the perception of: (1) words presented monaurally in background noise; (2) acoustically degraded single words; (3) dichotic single words; and (4) sentences.

It is heavily linguistically based, and population norms vary significantly between countries and ethnic background (Dawes and Bishop, 2007). Because of this, many centers supplement SCAN with nonlinguistic tests of auditory processing, commonly assessing performance in temporal and pitch processing, as well as sequence analysis and binaural integration. It is also important to assess global cognitive function with a battery of standard neuropsychological tests.

Is it functional?

A particular diagnostic challenge is the disambiguation of APD from more general deficits of attentional processes such as attention deficit hyperactivity disorder and, indeed, these conditions frequently coexist (Riccio et al., 1994). The interplay of attention and auditory processing is complex and variable. Performance on objective tests of auditory processing is strongly affected by inattention, especially in young children (Moore et al., 2008). Some have argued that this process underlies the majority of deficits in APD, while others point to cases where auditory processing is impaired despite intense concentration by the listener. As such, a functional component is present in many cases of APD.

Treatment strategies

Intervention in APD focuses on auditory training in combination with compensatory environmental and behavioral modification. There is no universally agreed strategy for auditory training, and both computer-based and face-to-face strategies are employed, but it is generally more effective if it involves audiovisual integration of meaningful sound stimuli (Loo et al., 2010). There is preliminary evidence that these methods modestly improve both behavioral performance and neural encoding of auditory information (Russo et al., 2005), especially if the deficit affects only one ear (Moncrieff and Wertz, 2008). For school- and university-age patients, educational support, sound reinforcement, and personal FM systems (frequency-modulated radio devices that allow teachers to communicate directly with pupils) can be of benefit. In general, APD improves with age, but it can persist into adulthood or develop *de novo* in elderly individuals (Cooper and Gates, 1991).

TINNITUS

Definition

Tinnitus is a common symptom that is surprisingly difficult to define unambiguously. One regularly used definition is that tinnitus is the conscious perception of an auditory sensation in the absence of a corresponding external stimulus. This definition could include the auditory hallucinations of psychotic illness but in practice these are excluded. Other symptoms that comply with this definition and are sometimes seen as subtypes of tinnitus include musical hallucination (see below) and pulsatile tinnitus. The latter is a rhythmic percept and, if synchronous with the heart beat, a vascular origin is likely; if asynchronous, myoclonus of the middle-ear muscles or palatal muscles is likely. The sound of pulsatile tinnitus can occasionally be perceived by external measuring equipment, in which case it is designated as objective. Most tinnitus, however, can only be heard by the sufferer and is classified as subjective. Commonly perceived sounds include buzzing, ringing, whistling or humming, and the sensation may be localized in one or both ears, or inside the head. A small number of people perceive tinnitus as an external sound.

Demographics

Epidemiological studies have estimated the prevalence of tinnitus in Europe, Asia, Africa, and North America, mostly producing rates between 10 and 15% of the adult population (Baguley et al., 2013). The largest study so far was undertaken in the UK as part of the National Study of Hearing in England (Davis and El Rafaie, 2000). With a study population of 48 313, this gave a tinnitus prevalence of 10.1%, with 2.8% describing the tinnitus as at least moderately annoying and 0.5% reporting that it had a severe effect on their ability to lead a normal life.

Prevalence in men and women is broadly similar. Tinnitus prevalence increases with age up to the seventh decade of life, with some studies showing the prevalence continuing to rise beyond that point, whereas others demonstrate a plateau or even a decline (see Baguley et al., 2013 for review). It is unusual for children to spontaneously complain about tinnitus but, when appropriate questions are asked, the prevalence of tinnitus experience in childhood seems similar to that in adulthood. Tinnitus is more common in people who have had significant noise exposure, and more common in those with hearing loss. However, the relationship between hearing loss and tinnitus is controversial: it is possible to have tinnitus with a normal audiogram and the degree of any hearing loss correlates poorly with tinnitus impact. There are few longitudinal incidence studies and it is difficult to draw conclusions, though one study demonstrated that tinnitus severity generally lessens rather than worsens with time (Nondahl et al., 2010). Tinnitus is seen as part of several otological diseases, including otosclerosis, Ménière's disease, and tumors of the cerebellopontine angle. Tinnitus has several comorbidities: the most common are disorders of loudness perception (discussed below) and other forms of impaired sound tolerance; anxiety, depression, and temporomandibular joint dysfunction are also seen in association.

Investigations

Audiometry is the main (and often the only) investigation required for tinnitus patients. A pure-tone audiogram aids otological diagnosis, determines those who need further investigations, and helps to direct subsequent management strategies. Measuring middle-ear function using tympanometry is often useful, as many patients with tinnitus complain of a feeling of aural fullness or blockage; normal tympanometry results exclude a diagnosis of eustachian tube dysfunction at the time of testing. Audiometric equipment can be used to try and match the pitch and loudness of tinnitus (Cope et al., 2011), but this is time consuming and does not usually help with treatment. Patients with unilateral or asymmetric tinnitus, an asymmetric audiogram, or associated unexplained neurological symptoms should undergo magnetic resonance imaging (MRI).

The most commonly found pathology in association with tinnitus is a vestibular schwannoma, which can be missed by computed tomography. For those with variants of tinnitus, particularly pulsatile tinnitus, more complex investigative algorithms are required. Tinnitus-specific questionnaires can help to assess the impact of tinnitus, the present instrument of choice being the Tinnitus Functional Index (Meikle et al., 2012).

There is an association between tinnitus and anxiety and depression, and in assessing a patient with tinnitus, some awareness of these symptoms and assessment of severity is indicated.

Is it functional?

There are subtypes of tinnitus, particularly pulsatile tinnitus, in which the symptom is associated with real noise of vascular or muscular origin. Such cases have hitherto generally not been regarded as functional. Recent observational studies, however, have suggested that at least some cases of both middle-ear myoclonus and palatal myoclonus may have a functional basis and hence any associated tinnitus could be regarded as functional (Stamelou et al., 2012; Ellenstein et al., 2013). For the majority of cases of tinnitus the percept is nonpulsatile and not associated with any internal sound source. Such tinnitus has paradoxes: tinnitus is possible with normal audiometry; most people with hearing loss do not have tinnitus; the extent of any hearing loss does not correlate well with tinnitus severity; tinnitus can occur even after the auditory nerve has been severed. But can tinnitus occur with a completely normal peripheral auditory system? Even those patients who have a normal pure-tone audiogram may have subtle cochlear deficits, and using tools such as extended-range audiometry, threshold-equalizing noise testing, or distortion product otoacoustic emission testing supports the view that the patients with tinnitus are more likely to have defects within the cochlea than audiometrically matched non-tinnitus controls (Weisz et al., 2006; Fabijańska et al., 2012).

There are, however, some tinnitus patients who appear to have tinnitus in the presence of normal cochlear function: a study that used extended-range audiometry to investigate 18 people who had tinnitus with a normal conventional audiogram found that 6 of the 18 subjects had high-frequency hearing as good as or better than the control group (Shim et al., 2009). Certainly, aural pathology on its own cannot fully explain symptom variability, giving rise to a theory that the pathophysiology of tinnitus is a two-stage process with an ignition occurring anywhere in the auditory system and then a process of promotion within the central auditory system (Baguley, 2006). Suggestions regarding the central mechanisms include the sequelae of deafferentation, namely increased spontaneous neural firing, cortical map reorganization, or increased neural synchrony. Overall, the evidence suggests an experience-dependent abnormal central analysis of peripheral information, remarkably concordant with evolving views of functional motor and somatosensory phenomena (Edwards et al., 2012).

Treatment strategies

In a small proportion of cases a specific treatment may be possible: examples include stapedectomy for people with tinnitus in association with otosclerosis, or embolization of an arteriovenous fistula that has caused pulsatile tinnitus. For the vast majority of cases of tinnitus there is no specific curative treatment, and management is largely supportive and empirical. Explanation, reassurance, and education may be all that is required. Correcting any associated hearing loss with hearing aids is anecdotally helpful, even if the hearing loss is mild and not causing significant communication problems (Sereda et al., 2015). Sound therapy is often utilized – either adding low-level sound to the patient's environment or giving the patient a wide-band, ear-level sound generator (masker) to wear. There are also combination devices that marry a sound generator to a hearing aid. Despite being widely used there is little scientific evidence to support sound therapy in tinnitus management (Hobson et al., 2012). Relaxation training may be offered, particularly to those who report that their tinnitus increases when stressed.

Psychological treatments have the best evidence base for effective tinnitus management, particularly cognitive-behavioral therapy (CBT) (Martinez-Devesa et al., 2010; Hesser et al., 2011), though recently mindfulness meditation (Philippot et al., 2012) and acceptance and commitment therapy (Westin et al., 2011) have also been positively assessed. Several protocols have been devised that use a range of the above modalities in combination in a structured framework. These include tinnitus retraining therapy (Jastreboff and Hazell, 1993), progressive audiologic tinnitus management (Myers et al., 2014), and tinnitus activities treatment (Tyler et al., 2007): there is limited evidence that this approach is helpful. Many drugs have been investigated, but none is currently recommended for the treatment of tinnitus. Similarly, although several other treatment modalities such as repetitive transcranial magnetic stimulation, transcranial direct current brain stimulation, and low-level laser therapy have been studied experimentally, none is in widespread clinical usage.

MUSICAL HALLUCINATION (MH)

Definition

Hallucination is the experience of a percept without a causal external stimulus. MH is therefore more than simply having a tune "stuck in your head" (an earworm), as it must have a compelling sense of reality. Indeed, patients commonly present to our services having first erroneously complained to police or local council services about their neighbors' antisocial music playing, and some still believe the source to be external when assessed in clinic. MH is typically experienced as short fragments of simple melodies – often from music heard regularly and familiar from youth, and especially from hymns and carols (Griffiths, 2000; Warner and Aziz, 2005). Lyrics may or may not be heard, but it is phenomenologically and demographically distinct from verbal hallucination (in which voices are heard) and has different neural correlates (Izumi et al., 2002).

Demographics

MH is much less common than tinnitus (described above). To date there have been no robust prevalence studies in large unselected populations. Amongst 3678 general psychiatric admissions, only 0.16% reported MHs (Fukunishi et al., 1998); this comprised 6 cases, of whom 5 were female, 3 were hearing-aid users, and 3 elderly. In the at-risk group of elderly individuals with hearing impairment, prevalence in small samples ranges from 0.8% (Cole et al., 2002) to 3.6% (Teunisse and Olde Rikkert, 2012). A salutary lesson on the subjectivity of survey questions comes from Goycoolea et al. (2007), who report "spontaneous musical sensations" in 39.4% of a group of 150 otolaryngologists and 97% of a group of 100 musicians.

There is a female preponderance of approximately 3:1, even accounting for the fact that women live to an older age and are more likely to live alone in old age (Cope and Baguley, 2009). Socially isolated individuals with hearing loss are more likely to be affected. MH is more common in those over 60, but there is no apparent increase in risk beyond this (Berrios, 1990); it is unclear to what extent age is an independent factor, and how much it is merely co-associated with hearing loss, vascular and neurological pathologies, social isolation, and pharmacological treatment.

Investigations

There is an association between MH and hearing loss, and initial investigation should always include measurement of audiometric thresholds. While organic brain pathology in a number of regions can give rise to MH, and some form of brain imaging should be performed to rule out a structural lesion, this is normally unrevealing. Paroxysmal MH as a primary manifestation of epilepsy is very rare (Couper, 1994), and electroencephalography should only be performed if there are other grounds for clinical suspicion. More intensive investigation for organic brain disease should be triggered by transient visual disturbances, disabling dizziness, severe headache, abnormal speech or neurological examination, or an audible carotid bruit.

A mental state examination should be performed, primarily assessing mood. Depression is common in MH, affecting around a third of elderly sufferers (Aizenberg et al., 1987). This should be probed for in the history, and treatment of depression can often improve MH. It is unclear whether this occurs simply through reducing social isolation or whether the interplay is more complex. MH is also common in patients with obsessive compulsive disorder (OCD): patients with OCD have an approximately 40% lifetime risk of experiencing MH, although most patients with MH do not have OCD. MH is, however, exceedingly rare in patients with schizophrenia and related psychoses (Hermesh et al., 2004).

Is it functional?

An attractive model for the pathogenesis of MH relies on the concept of peripheral and central "disinhibition" (Griffiths, 2000). Reduced auditory inputs (due to hearing loss and social isolation) combine with reduced inhibition from higher centers to increase the "gain" of association auditory cortex. This leads to an increasing tendency to interpret "system noise" as musical, and imagined musical imagery (earworms) as perceptually salient. Mechanistically, this can be understood within a "predictive coding" framework (Kumar et al., 2014a); as the sensory signal becomes degraded and prior expectations become more precise, perceptual inference is abnormally shifted. Although the underlying causes differ, as noted above, this mechanism bears a striking resemblance to the evolving understanding of functional somatosensory and motor phenomena (Edwards et al., 2012).

Treatment strategies

Although the framework for understanding MH is similar to that of functional sensory and motor phenomena, it has a number of underlying drivers that should be addressed before psychological therapies are considered. Specifically, hearing loss should be corrected and, if possible, social isolation and low mood addressed. It should be stressed that MH is not a sign of dementia or psychosis, as this is a common concern amongst patients, and a thorough explanation of symptoms should be provided. If an underlying cause is suspected, treatment of this can often resolve MH, but beyond this, there is little consensus regarding optimal therapy. While the literature most commonly reports pharmacological success with antipsychotics and anticholinesterases, before embarking on this course it should be borne in mind that MH is often not particularly distressing and, after reassurance that it does not signify more concerning pathology, patients are often happy to coexist with their musical experiences.

LOW-FREQUENCY NOISE COMPLAINT

Definition

A small number of individuals have a persistent complaint of low-frequency noise (LFN) in their environment (usually the home), causing them severe physical and emotional distress. In comparison with patients with tinnitus, those with LFN complaint are insistent that the source is external rather than internal. Complainants tend to describe humming or rumbling, often accompanied by a feeling of pressure on the ears or vibration in the body – a common descriptor would be that of a "distant engine." When acoustic measurements are undertaken, an LFN signal can be identified in only 30% of cases (and in such cases there is hope of a noise control solution), leaving uncertainty about the etiology of the LFN perception in the majority of cases (Moorhouse et al., 2005). The incidence of LFN in homes where there is no LFN complaint is unknown.

The distress of the LFN complainant can be severe and on occasion debilitating. Physical agitation can be marked, as can the emotional reaction, including fear and aversion to the home environment, and a component of hypervigilance to LFN can be observed. The LFN is perceived to be worse at night, and may lead to insomnia, and affected individuals may resort to sleeping in a car away from their property. One individual is usually affected in a household, but in some cases a partner or relative may develop some awareness of LFN at some later date. In rare circumstances many members of a community may complain of LFN (Pedersen et al., 2008). Complainants often have a definite belief about the source of the LFN, and this may include a component of the agent causing the LFN (e.g., a company or local council) being dismissive or antagonistic. Suggestions that there may be a tinnitus component to the percept may be met with dismay and disbelief. Reports of this phenomenon have been noted in the UK (Tempest, 1989), the Netherlands (Oud, 2012), Denmark (Møller and Lydolf, 2002), and Sweden (Persson and Rylander, 1988).

Demographics

Data on the epidemiology of LFN complaint are very sparse. Surveys of complainants have indicated that this phenomenon is more likely to be reported in middle age, with a mean age of 55 reported (Pedersen et al., 2008). Two-thirds of LFN complainants are female (Leventhall, 2003).

Investigations

There are two aspects to the investigation of LFN complaint: that of the individual, and of the environment. Regarding the individual, otoscopic and audiometric examination is required, as is a careful history for tinnitus, hyperacusis, and for anxiety and depression both prior to, and associated with, the LFN. An assessment should be made of the risk the individual represents to him- or herself (e.g., self-harm, or physical harm due to sleeping outside the home) and to any others that the patient believes are involved in generating the noise or disinclined to make it cease.

Testing low-frequency hearing thresholds (e.g., below 250 Hz) is not feasible in most clinical environments. When it has been performed in laboratory conditions, LFN complainants are found to have normal LF thresholds, but when asked to set acceptable levels, do so at a lower intensity than noncomplainers (Leventhall et al., 2008).

A structured protocol for the environmental investigation in an LFN complaint is available (Moorhouse et al., 2005), produced in the UK to support environmental health officers involved in such cases and ensure definitive investigation. Appropriate specialist recording equipment is needed, and should run through several nights. When no LFN source is identified, complainants often opine that the recording was done on an occasion when the LFN was unexpectedly absent.

Is it functional?

In a LFN complaint where no noise source is found, there are at least two possibilities:

1. that the individual has an LF tinnitus, and mistakenly attributes this to an external source
2. that the individual has become sensitized to environmental LF sound, and is experiencing some form of LF hyperacusis.

Understanding of the mechanisms by which the distress has arisen rests upon the more classic presentations of tinnitus and hyperacusis, specifically the links between the auditory brain and systems of learning, vigilance, and threat reaction.

An alternative model of heightened awareness of LFN was proposed by Salt and Hullar (2010), who contended that outer hair cells in the cochlea may be activated by low-frequency sound at subthreshold levels, and that in certain conditions an individual may become aware of that stimulus. Whilst this theory has not been substantiated with physiological evidence, the possibility that LFN complainants may be experiencing a psychophysical phenomenon rather than a heightened or over-vigilant response to environment sound should not be discounted.

Treatment strategies

Acoustic masking of LFN is not feasible as most masking devices have little output below 250 Hz. Informational masking (i.e., utilizing an alternative sound that has properties that capture the attention of the auditory brain) may have a role, specifically the use of rain/ocean-type environmental sounds at the bedside throughout the night. Hearing aids may fulfill this function during the day.

Three studies have investigated the benefits of CBT-like interventions. Leventhall et al. (2008) evaluated sessions in a small group ($n=9$) involving information, imaginal exposure exercises, and relaxation, delivered by an experienced psychotherapist, with moderate benefits. Similar material was used in book and online formats in a larger study ($n=27$ completers from a group of $n=46$ who agreed to participate), with similar results, though no intention-to-treat analysis was undertaken (Leventhall, 2009). Moorhouse et al. (2015) trialed a treatment protocol delivered by audiologists including information, attentional masking and relaxation – benefits were positive but modest. No data regarding long-term benefit are available. We are unaware of studies evaluating the efficacy of CBT in LFN complaint.

DISORDERS OF LOUDNESS PERCEPTION

Definition

Disorders of sound tolerance fall into two categories: dislike of sound above a certain intensity and dislike of particular sounds irrespective of their level. Terminology is confusing and still developing. Hyperacusis is a word used both as a blanket term to cover all types of impaired sound tolerance and to define a specific subtype. When used in the specific instance, hyperacusis refers to a dislike of all sounds above a certain level. Recruitment is a condition seen in association with significant sensorineural hearing loss in which rising sound intensity causes a greater than normal rise in perceived loudness.

Misophonia is a strong dislike of certain sounds, irrespective of their level, and is discussed separately. Phonophobia is a variant of misophonia in which the dominant emotion is fear. These definitions have recently been challenged and a new classification of loudness hyperacusis, annoyance hyperacusis, fear hyperacusis, and pain hyperacusis has been proposed (Tyler et al., 2014). Different types of impaired sound tolerance may coexist in the same patient.

Demographics

There are very few epidemiological studies regarding impaired loudness tolerance. Studies in Sweden (Andersson et al., 2002) and Poland (Fabijanska et al., 1999) showed a hyperacusis prevalence of 8.6% and 15.2% of their adult populations respectively. Neither of these studies attempted to assess the severity or impact of the symptom. A study in Brazil (Coelho et al., 2007) found a hyperacusis prevalence of 3.2% in the pediatric population. There is a strong comorbidity of hyperacusis and tinnitus: 40% of people with tinnitus as their main complaint report some degree of hyperacusis, whereas 86% of those who present with hyperacusis will also describe tinnitus.

Investigations

The investigation of patients with impaired sound tolerance is largely the same as for patients with tinnitus (see above), with a few additional caveats. Tympanometry, particularly when used to estimate stapedial reflex thresholds, involves significant sound levels and MRI scanning is notoriously noisy. Patients with impaired sound tolerance need careful counseling prior to such tests and if necessary the test should be deferred or a quieter alternative sought. Loudness tolerance can be estimated using standard audiologic equipment to measure the loudest sounds that the patient can tolerate at particular frequencies (loudness discomfort levels). Because of the sound levels involved, such tests run significant risk of distressing the patient and any clinical benefit is usually outweighed by the risk of losing the patient's trust.

Is it functional?

Hyperacusis is occasionally associated with facial nerve palsies which cause loss of the ear's protective stapedial reflex. In such cases, because the symptom is associated with a demonstrable lesion, it cannot be regarded as functional. The vast majority of cases of hyperacusis, however, are not associated with structural pathology. Although various pathophysiological mechanisms have been suggested, the cause remains unknown. Some theories are directed at the auditory periphery but many focus on the central auditory system, proposing similar mechanisms to those seen in tinnitus (see above). It therefore seems likely that impaired loudness tolerance has a functional basis in at least a proportion of cases.

Treatment strategies

Education and reassurance are important treatment components. In particular, many patients with significant hyperacusis protect themselves from sound by seeking quiet environments or by wearing sound-attenuating devices. Although this seems sensible, it is hypothesized to result in increased central auditory gain, which exacerbates the problem. Careful reintroduction of sound is one of the mainstays of hyperacusis treatment. Sound therapy can be used to improve sound tolerance using continuous low-level sound in a technique called recalibration or by slowly increasing sound in a technique called desensitization. As with tinnitus, protocols been developed that use several treatment modalities in a structured way. These include tinnitus retraining therapy (see section on tinnitus, above) and hyperacusis activities treatment (Tyler et al., 2009). Psychological treatments, particularly CBT, have been tried with some benefit (Jüris et al., 2014).

MISOPHONIA

Definition

Misophonia is a disorder of the emotional processing of specific sounds, and can be literally translated as "hatred of sound" (Jastreboff and Jastreboff, 2001). Background sounds that would be generally described as perhaps mildly irritating, such as eating, noisy breathing, and typing, produce a strong sense of anger, and either aggressive or aversive behavior in sufferers (Schroder et al., 2013). This effect is distinguished from hyperacusis in that it is restricted to particular sounds, individual to each sufferer, and does not relate to the spectral properties of the auditory stimulus that contribute to the general unpleasantness of sounds such as nails on a chalkboard (Kumar et al., 2012), although these conditions can coexist (Jastreboff and Jastreboff, 2015). It should be emphasized that the dominant emotion is almost always anger and therefore misophonia is not a true phobia, but many sufferers will adopt avoidance behaviors for situations where trigger sounds might occur.

Demographics

Age of onset is variable, but symptoms often emerge in childhood or adolescence and persist into adulthood (Kumar et al., 2014b), with an average latency before formal diagnosis of 25 years. This is likely to be an underestimate, as it only records that minority of sufferers seeking medical assessment. Males and females appear equally likely to be affected. Approximately 50% of sufferers have anankastic (obsessive compulsive) personality traits, but true OCD and other psychiatric comorbidities are rare (Schroder et al., 2013).

Investigations

There are no reports of misophonia arising as a result of organic brain pathology, so unless there are other grounds for clinical suspicion, routine brain imaging is not necessary. Mental state examination should be performed as the detection of psychiatric comorbidities or personality traits can be useful in tailoring the treatment approach.

Is it functional?

The exact mechanisms of misophonia are unclear, and are a topic of ongoing investigation (Kumar et al., 2014b). Trigger sounds are associated with abnormal autonomic effects that do not generalize to visual stimuli (such as a video of chewing gum) (Edelstein et al., 2013). Current conceptualizations rely on repetitive minor annoyances associated with sounds and culminating in pathological emotional valence (LeDoux, 2000), but evidence of this from the patient history is rarely present (Schroder et al., 2013).

Treatment strategies

There are no randomized controlled trials of treatment methods. Explanation and validation of the condition can be helpful. Pragmatic strategies such as using noise-canceling headphones at mealtimes can be employed. Beyond this, currently employed strategies involve habituation and retraining therapies similar to those used in tinnitus and hyperacusis (Jastreboff and Jastreboff, 2015), as well as CBT and other psychological interventions.

ACOUSTIC SHOCK

Definition

Acoustic shock (also known as acoustic shock syndrome or acoustic shock disorder) describes a group of symptoms seen in people who have been exposed to sudden unexpected sounds. Initially recognized in people working in call centers using headsets, the symptom cluster has also been seen following exposure to a variety of other sound sources, particularly when the causative sound is generated close to the ear. The commonest symptom reported is pain in or close to the ear, followed by tinnitus, hyperacusis, balance disturbance, hypervigilance, and sleep disturbance (Milhinch, 2002). The level of the causative sound seems relatively unimportant compared to its rise time: it seems to be the suddenness rather than the loudness that is the issue. Hearing loss occurs in fewer than 1 in 5 people with acoustic shock and when it does happen it does not necessarily have the characteristics of noise-induced hearing loss.

Demographics

There are no reliable epidemiological data regarding acoustic shock. Initial reports were from Australia, Denmark, and the UK, but anecdotally the symptom is recognized globally.

Investigations

The investigation of a patient with suspected acoustic shock is the same as for patients with tinnitus or disorders of loudness perception (see above).

Is it functional?

Suggestions for the pathophysiology of acoustic shock include cochlear damage, tonic contraction of the tensor tympani muscle (Westcott, 2006), or psychological mechanisms. In many cases there is no measurable deficit within the peripheral auditory system, suggesting that a functional origin is likely. There have, however, been suggestions that at least some cases are attributable to malingering (Hooper, 2014).

Treatment strategies

Treatment is largely the same as for disorders of loudness perception (see above). If the acoustic shock occurred in a call center environment, adjustments to the patient's job may be required. Electronic devices to try and suppress causative sounds and limit overall sound exposure while maintaining speech clarity have been developed for telecommunications equipment within call centers.

CONCLUSION

There are a number of auditory symptoms that appear to have a functional component, some of which affect similar populations to those with functional neurological symptoms, whilst others affect very specific populations (notably MH and misophonia). Understanding in this area is emergent, and treatments are in many cases pragmatic and rudimentary, needing more work to be done in integrating insights from behavioral and cognitive psychology to auditory neuroscience. The audiology literature has historically equated the term functional with malingering, and more work needs to be done in developing interest and expertise in these conditions.

References

Aizenberg D, Modai I, Roitman M et al. (1987). Musical hallucinations, depression and old-age. Psychopathology 20: 220–223.

Andersson G, Lindvall N, Hursti T et al. (2002). Hypersensitivity to sound (hyperacusis): a prevalence study conducted via the internet and post. Int J Audiol 41: 545–554.

ASHA (1996). Central auditory processing: current status of research and implications for clinical practice. Am J Audiol 5: 41–54.

Austen S, Lynch C (2004). Non-organic hearing loss redefined: understanding, categorizing and managing non-organic behaviour. Int J Audiol 43: 449–457.

Baguley DM (2006). What progress have we made with tinnitus? The Tonndorf lecture 2005. Acta Otolaryngol Suppl 556: 4–8.

Baguley DM, Andersson GA, McFerran D et al. (2013). Tinnitus: a multidisciplinary approach, 2nd edn. Wiley-Blackwell, Oxford.

Bamiou DE, Musiek FE, Luxon LM (2001). Aetiology and clinical presentations of auditory processing disorders – a review. Arch Dis Child 85: 361–365.

Bensimon G, Ludolph A, Agid Y et al. (2009). Riluzole treatment, survival and diagnostic criteria in Parkinson plus disorders: the NNIPPS study. Brain 132 (Pt 1): 156–171.

Berlin CI, Hood L, Morlet T et al. (2003). Auditory neuropathy/dys-synchrony: diagnosis and management. Ment Retard Dev Disabil Res Rev 9: 225–231.

Berrios GE (1990). Musical hallucinations – a historical and clinical study. Br J Psychiatry 156: 188–194.

Cacace AT, McFarland DJ (2005). The importance of modality specificity in diagnosing central auditory processing disorder. Am J Audiol 14: 112–123.

Chermak GD, Musiek FE (1997). Central auditory processing disorders. New perspectives, Singular, San Diego, CA.

Coelho CB, Sanchez TG, Tyler RS (2007). Hyperacusis, sound annoyance, and loudness hypersensitivity in children. Prog Brain Res 166: 169–178.

Cole MG, Dowson L, Dendukuri N et al. (2002). The prevalence and phenomenology of auditory hallucinations among elderly subjects attending an audiology clinic. Int J Geriatr Psychiatry 17: 444–452.

Cooper Jr JC, Gates GA (1991). Hearing in the elderly – the Framingham cohort, 1983–1985: Part II. Prevalence of central auditory processing disorders. Ear Hear 12: 304–311.

Cope TE, Baguley DM (2009). Is musical hallucination an otological phenomenon? A review of the literature. Clin Otolaryngol 34: 423–430.

Cope TE, Baguley DM, Moore BC (2011). Tinnitus loudness in quiet and noise after resection of vestibular schwannoma. Otol Neurotol 32: 488–496.

Couper J (1994). Unilateral musical hallucinations and all that jazz. Aust N Z J Psychiatry 28: 516–519.

Davis A, El Rafaie A (2000). Epidemiology of tinnitus. In: RS Tyler (Ed.), Tinnitus handbook, Singular, Thomson Learning, San Diego, CA, pp. 1–23.

Dawes P, Bishop DV (2007). The SCAN-C in testing for auditory processing disorder in a sample of British children. Int J Audiol 46: 780–786.

Edelstein M, Brang D, Rouw R et al. (2013). Misophonia: physiological investigations and case descriptions. Front Hum Neurosci 25: 7.

Edwards MJ, Adams RA, Brown H et al. (2012). A Bayesian account of 'hysteria'. Brain 135: 3495–3512.

Ellenstein A, Yusuf N, Hallett M (2013). Middle ear myoclonus: two informative cases and a systematic discussion of myogenic tinnitus. Tremor Other Hyperkinet Mov (N Y) 15: 3.

Emanuel DC, Ficca KN, Korczak P (2011). Survey of the diagnosis and management of auditory processing disorder. Am J Audiol 20: 48–60.

Fabijanska A, Rogowski M, Bartnik G et al. (1999). Epidemiology of tinnitus and hyperacusis in Poland. In: J Hazell (Ed.), Proceedings of the Sixth International Tinnitus Seminar. The Tinnitus and Hyperacusis Centre, Cambridge, UK, pp. 569–571.

Fabijańska A, Smurzyński J, Hatzopoulos S et al. (2012). The relationship between distortion product otoacoustic emissions and extended high-frequency audiometry in tinnitus patients. Part 1: normally hearing patients with unilateral tinnitus. Med Sci Monit 18: CR765–CR770.

Fukunishi I, Horikawa N, Onai H (1998). Prevalence rate of musical hallucinations in a general hospital setting. Psychosomatics 39: 175.

Garrido MI, Kilner JM, Stephan KE et al. (2009). The mismatch negativity: a review of underlying mechanisms. Clin Neurophysiol 120: 453–463.

Goycoolea MV, Mena I, Neubauer SG et al. (2007). Musical brains: a study of spontaneous and evoked musical sensations without external auditory stimuli. Acta Oto-Laryngol 127: 711–721.

Griffiths TD (2000). Musical hallucinosis in acquired deafness. Phenomenology and brain substrate. Brain 123: 2065–2076.

Hermesh H, Konas S, Shiloh R et al. (2004). Musical hallucinations: Prevalence in psychotic and nonpsychotic outpatients. J Clin Psychiatry 65: 191–197.

Hesser H, Weise C, Westin VZ et al. (2011). A systematic review and meta-analysis of randomized controlled trials of cognitive behaviour therapy for tinnitus distress. Clin Psychol Rev 31: 545–553.

Hind SE (2006). Survey of care pathway for auditory processing disorder. Audiol Med 7: 12–24.

Hobson J, Chisholm E, El Refaie A (2012). Sound therapy (masking) in the management of tinnitus in adults. Cochrane Database Syst Rev: CD006371.

Hooper RE (2014). Acoustic shock controversies. J Laryngol Otol 128 (Suppl 2): S2–S9.

Izumi Y, Terao T, Ishino Y et al. (2002). Differences in regional cerebral blood flow during musical and verbal hallucinations. Psychiatry Res 116: 119–123.

Jastreboff PJ, Hazell JWP (1993). A neurophysiological approach to tinnitus: clinical implications. Br J Audiol 27: 7–17.

Jastreboff MM, Jastreboff PJ (2001). Components of decreased sound tolerance: hyperacusis, misophonia, phonophobia. ITHS News Lett 2: 5–7.

Jastreboff PJ, Jastreboff MM (2015). Treatments for decreased sound tolerance (hyperacusis and misophonia). Semin Hear 35: 105–120.

Jerger J, Musiek F (2000). Report of the consensus conference on the diagnosis of auditory processing disorders in school-aged children. J Am Acad Audiol 11 (9): 467–474.

Jüris L, Andersson G, Larsen HC et al. (2014). Cognitive behaviour therapy for hyperacusis: a randomized controlled trial. Behav Res Ther 54: 30–37.

Keith RW (1995). Development and standardization of SCAN-A: test of auditory processing disorders in adolescents and adults. J Am Acad Audiol 6 (4): 286–292.

Keith RW (2000). Development and standardization of SCAN-C test for auditory processing disorders in children. J Am Acad Audiol 11: 438–445.

Kumar S, von Kriegstein K, Friston K et al. (2012). Features versus feelings: dissociable representations of the acoustic features and valence of aversive sounds. J Neurosci 32: 14184–14192.

Kumar S, Sedley W, Barnes GR et al. (2014a). A brain basis for musical hallucinations. Cortex 52: 86–97.

Kumar S, Hancock O, Cope T et al. (2014b). Misophonia: a disorder of emotion processing of sounds. J Neurol Neurosurg Psychiatry 85 (8): e3.

LeDoux JE (2000). Emotion circuits in the brain. Annu Rev Neurosci 23: 155–184.

Leventhall G (2003). A review of published research on low frequency noise and its effects, technical report. Defra, London.

Leventhall G (2009). Development of a course in computerised cognitive behavioural therapy aimed at relieving the problems of those suffering from noise exposure, in particular, exposure to low frequency noise (NANR 237). Interim Report, Defra, London.

Leventhall G, Benton S, Robertson D (2008). Coping strategies for low frequency noise. J Low Freq Noise Vibr Active Contr 27: 35–52.

Loo JH, Bamiou DE, Campbell N et al. (2010). Computer-based auditory training (CBAT): benefits for children with language- and reading-related learning difficulties. Dev Med Child Neurol 52: 708–717.

Martinez-Devesa P, Perera R, Theodoulou M et al. (2010). Cognitive behavioural therapy for tinnitus. Cochrane Database Syst Rev: CD005233. Issue.

Meikle MB, Henry JA, Griest SE et al. (2012). The tinnitus functional index: development of a new clinical measure for chronic, intrusive tinnitus. Ear Hear 33: 153–176.

Milhinch JC (2002). Acoustic shock injury: real or imaginary, AudiologyOnline, available at http://www.audiologyonline.com/articles/acoustic-shock-injury-real-or-1172 (accessed 28 November 2015).

Møller H, Lydolf M (2002). A questionnaire survey of complaints of infrasound and low frequency noise. J Low Freq Noise Vibr 21: 53–65.

Moncrieff DW, Wertz D (2008). Auditory rehabilitation for interaural asymmetry: preliminary evidence of improved dichotic listening performance following intensive training. Int J Audiol 47: 84–97.

Moore DR (2006). Auditory processing disorder (APD): definition, diagnosis, neural basis, and intervention. Audiol Med 4: 4–11.

Moore DR, Ferguson MA, Halliday LF et al. (2008). Frequency discrimination in children: perception, learning and attention. Hear Res 238: 147–154.

Moore DR, Rosen R, Bamiou DE et al. (2013). Evolving concepts of developmental auditory processing disorder (APD): A British Society of Audiology APD Special Interest Group 'white paper'. Int J Audiol 52: 3–13.

Moorhouse A, Waddington D, Adams M (2005). Field trials of proposed procedure for the assessment of low frequency noise complaints (NANR45), Defra, London.

Moorhouse A, Baguley D, Husband T (2015). UK-wide support infrastructure for low frequency noise sufferers ('LFN network'). Defra NANR271, London.

Myers PJ, Griest S, Kaelin C et al. (2014). Development of a progressive audiologic tinnitus management program for veterans with tinnitus. J Rehabil Res Dev 51: 609–622.

Nondahl DM, Cruickshanks KJ, Wiley TL et al. (2010). The ten-year incidence of tinnitus among older adults. Int J Audiol 49: 580–585.

Oud M (2012). Low-frequency noise: a biophysical phenomenon. In: Conf. proc. Noise, Vibrations, Air quality, and Field & Building, Nieuwegein, The Netherlands, Available at: http://home.kpn.nl/oud/publications/OudM_ProcGTLGG2012.pdf (accessed 28 November 2015).

Peck JE (2012). Pseudohypacusis: false and exaggerated hearing loss, Plural Publishing, San Diego.

Pedersen CS, Møller H, Waye KP (2008). A detailed study of low-frequency noise complaints. J Low Freq Noise Vibr Active Contr 27: 1–33.

Persson K, Rylander R (1988). Disturbance from low-frequency noise in the environment: a survey among the local environmental health authorities in Sweden. J Sound Vib 121: 339–345.

Philippot P, Nef F, Clauw L et al. (2012). A randomized controlled trial of mindfulness-based cognitive therapy for treating tinnitus. Clin Psychol Psychother 19: 411–419.

Riccio CA, Hynd GW, Cohen MJ et al. (1994). Comorbidity of central auditory processing disorder and attention-deficit hyperactivity disorder. J Am Acad Child Adolesc Psychiatry 33: 849–857.

Rosen S (2005). "A riddle wrapped in a mystery inside an enigma": defining central auditory processing disorder. Am J Audiol 14: 139–142.

Russo NM, Nicol TG, Zecker SG et al. (2005). Auditory training improves neural timing in the human brainstem. Behav Brain Res 156: 95–103.

Salt AN, Hullar TE (2010). Responses of the ear to low frequency sounds, infrasound and wind turbines. Hear Res 268: 12–21.

Schroder A, Vulink N, Denys D (2013). Misophonia: diagnostic criteria for a new psychiatric disorder. PLoS One 8 (1).

Sereda M, Hoare DJ, Nicholson R et al. (2015). Consensus on hearing aid candidature and fitting for mild hearing loss, with and without tinnitus: Delphi review. Ear Hear 36: 417–429.

Sharma M, Purdy SC, Newall P et al. (2006). Electrophysiological and behavioral evidence of auditory processing deficits in children with reading disorder. Clin Neurophysiol 117: 1130–1144.

Shim HJ, Kim SK, Park CH et al. (2009). Hearing abilities at ultra-high frequency in patients with tinnitus. Clin Exp Otorhinolaryngol 2: 169–174.

Simpson TP, Manara AR, Kane NM et al. (2002). Effect of propofol anaesthesia on the event-related potential mismatch negativity and the auditory-evoked potential N1. Br J Anaesth 89 (3): 382–388.

Stamelou M, Saifee TA, Edwards MJ et al. (2012). Psychogenic palatal tremor may be underrecognized: reappraisal of a large series of cases. Mov Disord 27: 1164–1168.

Starr A, Picton TW, Sininger Y et al. (1996). Auditory neuropathy. Brain 119 (Pt 3): 741–753.

Tempest W (1989). A survey of low frequency noise complaints received by local authorities in the United Kingdom. J Low Freq Noise Vibr 8: 45–49.

Teunisse RJ, Olde Rikkert MGM (2012). Prevalence of musical hallucinations in patients referred for audiometric testing. Am J Geriatr Psychiatry 20: 1075–1077.

Tyler RS, Gogel SA, Gehringer AK (2007). Tinnitus activities treatment. Prog Brain Res 166: 425–434.

Tyler RS, Noble W, Coelho C et al. (2009). Tinnitus and hyperacusis. In: J Katz, R Burkard, L Medwetsky et al. (Eds.), Handbook of Clinical Audiology, 6th edn. Lippincott Williams and Wilkins, Baltimore.

Tyler RS, Pienkowski M, Rojas Roncancio E et al. (2014). A review of hyperacusis and future directions: part i. definitions and manifestations. Am J Audiol 23: 402–419.

Warner N, Aziz V (2005). Hymns and arias: musical hallucinations in older people in Wales. Int J Geriatr Psychiatry 20: 658–660.

Weisz N, Hartmann T, Dohrmann K et al. (2006). High-frequency tinnitus without hearing loss does not mean absence of deafferentation. Hear Res 222 (1–2): 108–114.

Westcott M (2006). Acoustic shock injury (ASI). Acta Otolaryngol Suppl 556: 54–58.

Westin VZ, Schulin M, Hesser H et al. (2011). Acceptance and commitment therapy versus tinnitus retraining therapy in the treatment of tinnitus: a randomised controlled trial. Behav Res Ther 49: 737–747.

Handbook of Clinical Neurology, Vol. 139 (3rd series)
Functional Neurologic Disorders
M. Hallett, J. Stone, and A. Carson, Editors
http://dx.doi.org/10.1016/B978-0-12-801772-2.00033-3

Chapter 33

Functional speech disorders: clinical manifestations, diagnosis, and management

J.R. DUFFY*
Division of Speech Pathology, Mayo Medical School, Rochester, MN, USA

Abstract

Acquired psychogenic or functional speech disorders are a subtype of functional neurologic disorders. They can mimic organic speech disorders and, although any aspect of speech production can be affected, they manifest most often as dysphonia, stuttering, or prosodic abnormalities. This chapter reviews the prevalence of functional speech disorders, the spectrum of their primary clinical characteristics, and the clues that help distinguish them from organic neurologic diseases affecting the sensorimotor networks involved in speech production. Diagnosis of a speech disorder as functional can be supported by sometimes rapidly achieved positive outcomes of symptomatic speech therapy. The general principles of such therapy are reviewed.

INTRODUCTION

Changes in speech can be the first or only sign or symptom of neurologic disease, and it is well established that the identification of specific patterns of speech breakdown can contribute to lesion localization and a narrowing of diagnostic possibilities. Speech is also susceptible to a wide variety of psychologic, emotional, and maladaptive influences that can alter its character in a way that can raise concerns about organic or structural neurologic disease. Recognition of such speech disturbances as functional (or psychogenic) can contribute substantially to neurologic differential diagnosis. The often rapidly successful behavioral management of functional speech disorders (FSDs) can increase diagnostic confidence and contribute to the recovery and well-being of affected individuals.

FSDs are the focus of this chapter. Their symptoms and signs and the distinctions between them and the lesion-based neurologic speech deficits they may mimic will be emphasized, as will general principles of behavioral management. The broad psychologic and neurobiologic explanations for FSDs are similar to those associated with functional neurologic disorders in general. They are addressed elsewhere in this volume.

THE SPECTRUM OF FUNCTIONAL SPEECH DISORDERS

FSDs can be considered a symptom subcategory of functional movement disorders, but they by no means form a homogeneous set of characteristics. Although they are most frequently manifest as voice disorders (dysphonias) in general medical and ear, nose, and throat practices (functional dysphonias are addressed in Chapter 34), speech can go awry in many other ways.

Table 33.1 summarizes the distribution of different FSDs, excluding isolated functional dysphonias, based on approximately 10 years of data from the Mayo Clinic Speech Pathology practice. Stuttering-like dysfluencies were the most frequent single FSD, accounting for about one-third of cases; this is consistent with the relative predominance of acquired functional stuttering among reports of FSDs in the literature, and with the predominance of stuttering-like dysfluencies among FSDs in patients with functional movement disorders (Baizabel-Carvallo and Jankovic, 2015). Although not nearly as common as functional dysphonias, acquired functional stuttering is probably more frequently mistaken as a sign of neurologic disease than functional dysphonia.

*Correspondence to: Joseph R. Duffy, Ph.D., BC-ANCDS, Consultant Emeritus, Speech Pathology, Mayo Medical School, Rochester MN 55905, USA. Tel: +1-507-282-1093, E-mail: jduffy@mayo.edu

Table 33.1

Distribution of acquired functional speech disorders in Mayo Clinic Speech Pathology practice, excluding isolated functional voice disorders ($n = 240$)

Primary speech characteristics	Percentage of cases
Stuttering-like dysfluency	34
Articulation deficits	11
Prosodic abnormalities (including foreign accent)	10
Other (abnormal resonance, infantile speech, psychotic language)	11
Mixed (two or more of above categories)	34

Relatively isolated abnormalities of articulation (distortions, substitutions, additions, or omissions of speech sounds) accounted for 11% of cases. Ten percent of the cases had abnormalities of prosody (rhythm, stress, intonation), including prosodic variations perceived as a foreign accent (foreign-accent syndrome (FAS)). Eleven percent had a variety of infrequently occurring problems such as infantile speech, abnormal resonance, and psychotic language. Finally, about one-third of the cases had combined deficits (e.g., stuttering plus articulation and prosodic abnormalities). These data illustrate the heterogeneity of FSDs while highlighting the relative predominance of stuttering and prosodic disturbances. Functional stuttering and FAS can be particularly challenging diagnostically because, broadly defined, they can also be caused by structural brain injury. However, virtually any of the broad categories of FSDs can raise concerns about organic neurologic disease.

PREVALENCE

Although frequently ignored and often not emphasized, functional speech and cranial nerve deficits have been recognized for years as possible manifestations of functional movement disorders (e.g., Hinson and Haren, 2006; Keane, 2006). Thus, for example, in 1922 Henry Head observed that "disorders of speech were amongst the commonest hysterical affections due to the strain of war" (p. 827). Although their incidence and prevalence have not been established, in some studies about one-quarter to more than half of patients with functional movement disorders have had speech abnormalities among their symptoms (Hinson et al., 2005; Saifee et al., 2012; Baizabel-Caravallo and Jankovic, 2015). They certainly are not uncommon in speech pathology practices in tertiary care centers where speech pathologists work closely with neurologists. Excluding functional dysphonias, during a 3-year period in the Mayo Clinic Speech Pathology practice (a division in the Department of Neurology), 3% ($n = 128$) of patients with acquired communication disorders received a primary speech diagnosis of acquired psychogenic/nonorganic speech disorder; most of them were seen as part of an outpatient medical or neurology workup in which neurologic disease was a diagnostic consideration (Duffy, 2013).

EXAMINATION AND DIFFERENTIAL DIAGNOSIS

Neurologic motor speech disorders (MSDs) include the dysarthrias, of which there are several types, and apraxia of speech. By definition, MSDs reflect organic abnormalities in brain regions and networks involved in the planning, programming, control, or execution of speech. There is overlap among the speech features associated with the different types of MSDs but they are perceptually distinguishable to experienced clinicians because each type has a relatively distinct pattern of abnormalities. The distinctive patterns of MSDs establish the "rules of the game" for differential diagnosis and the boundaries beyond which FSDs lie. Just as the presentation of some functional movement disorders unambiguously violates the rules for organic neuromotor disturbances, while others straddle the boundaries of the distinction, so too can some FSDs unambiguously violate the rules for MSDs, while others generate clinical diagnostic uncertainty. The ability to make such distinctions relies heavily on clinical experience with a variety of both MSDs and FSDs.

The speech characteristics associated with MSDs and FSDs can be similar and they can co-occur. In some cases, a FSD represents a psychologic or maladaptive physical response to organic neurologic disease or one or more of its outward signs. For example, stuttering-like dysfluencies can emerge as a conscious or subconscious "biding time" strategy in aphasic patients who are trying to retrieve a word. In others, functional and organic neurologic speech disorders can coexist as relatively independent entities, or the FSD might be driven by frustrations or anxiety associated with an MSD (e.g., functional stuttering might occur in a person with spastic-ataxic dysarthria associated with traumatic brain injury).

Information gleaned from the history which is incongruent with that commonly associated with neurologic disease or that identifies psychiatric, psychologic, or psychosocial variables that may explain the symptoms is as relevant to the assessment of FSDs as they are to functional neurologic disorders in general. These broad general assessment and history-taking issues are addressed in Chapter 15 and will not be reviewed here in any detail.

Answers to the following questions that can be derived from speech examination are often important to the diagnosis of a FSD. Table 33.2 summarizes clinical observations that contribute to the identification of FSDs.

Can the abnormal speech pattern be classified neurologically?

As is true for functional neurologic disorders in general, when examination results are incongruent with expectations for neurogenic or other structural speech deficits, the possibility that the disorder is functional must be considered. FSDs rarely mimic apraxia of speech but they often raise questions about flaccid (lower motor neuron), spastic (upper motor neuron, usually bilateral), ataxic (cerebellar control circuit), or hypokinetic or hyperkinetic (usually basal ganglia control circuit) dysarthrias, or combinations of them. Discrepancies from the speech patterns associated with the dysarthrias may reflect a functional disturbance or a functional contribution to an organic MSD. In patients with known neurologic disease, or an established lesion locus, incongruity between the abnormal speech pattern and the disease or lesion locus, even if the abnormal speech pattern fits well with a particular dysarthria type, should raise the possibility of an FSD.

Are observations of the oral mechanism consistent with the speech and/or oral mechanism abnormalities typically associated with neurologic disease?

Unlike organic MSDs in which abnormal oral mechanism findings (e.g., facial asymmetry, lingual atrophy or fasciculations, drooling, involuntary movements, pathologic oral reflexes, nonverbal oral apraxia) are usually congruent with expectations about speech, FSDs often depart from them.

Is the speech deficit consistent?

With few exceptions, organic speech abnormalities, unlike FSDs, are consistent during examination. Examples of exceptions to this rule are flaccid dysarthria that emerges only after speech stress testing in myasthenia gravis; paroxysmal ataxic dysarthria associated with multiple sclerosis or channelopathies; and dysarthria brought on or exacerbated by rapid speech rate in action myoclonus. Some patients with FSDs demonstrate considerable inconsistency during examination or by their or others' report.

Is the speech deficit suggestible or subject to distractibility?

MSDs do not fluctuate significantly as a function of suggestion or distraction. In contrast, the speech of some individuals with FSDs will deteriorate or improve under such conditions.

Does speech fatigue in a lawful manner?

MSDs, with the exception of the flaccid dysarthria associated with myasthenia gravis, as noted above, do not fatigue dramatically during speech assessment, even when considerable speaking is required. In addition, the pattern of fatigue-related speech breakdown in myasthenia gravis is very consistent with increasing weakness (e.g., the emergence or worsening of breathiness, hypernasality, or imprecise lingual articulation). In contrast, the "fatigue" that emerges in some people with FSDs whose chief complaint is weakness or fatigue is often in the direction of increased muscle contraction (e.g., emergence of strained voice quality or exaggerated facial posturing during speech).

Is the speech deficit reversible?

Although MSDs can improve with speech therapy, the improvement is rarely rapidly dramatic. In contrast, a substantial percentage of individuals with FSDs associated with conversion disorder or effects of life stresses respond rapidly and dramatically to symptomatic treatment during the evaluation session or a subsequent therapy session provided by a speech-language pathologist who is experienced in working with FSDs (see section on management, below). This symptom reversibility rules out an MSD and confirms the diagnosis of an FSD.

BROAD CATEGORIES OF FUNCTIONAL SPEECH DISORDERS

Stuttering

Acquired stuttering can result from organic neurologic disease or from psychologic/functional influences (Lundgren et al., 2010; Duffy, 2013); malingered stuttering has also been reported (e.g., Seery, 2005).

Acquired neurologic stuttering secondary to central nervous system disease is most often called "neurogenic stuttering." It is typically characterized by repetition, silent blocking, or prolongation of sounds or syllables that interrupt the flow of speech. On the basis of speech characteristics alone, acquired neurogenic stuttering can be difficult to distinguish from developmental stuttering (Van Borsel and Tallieu, 2001). Stroke and traumatic brain injury are the most frequent presumed etiologies but it has been associated with numerous other causes, such as drug toxicity and neurodegenerative disease, as well as cases without identifiable lesions or a specific neurologic diagnosis (see reviews by Rosenbek, 1984; Helm-Estabrooks, 1993; or Duffy, 2013).

Although the literature suggests neurogenic stuttering can occur in the absence of other speech or language disturbances, it is much more often associated with aphasia,

Table 33.2

Clinical clues to the presence of a functional speech disorder (FSD)

Primary speech abnormality	Clinical findings
General (possible in any FSD)	Abnormal speech pattern is incompatible with common motor speech disorder types (various dysarthria types, apraxia of speech) Abnormal speech pattern is incongruous with known lesion locus or working neurologic diagnosis Nonspeech oral mechanism findings are incompatible with abnormal speech pattern or with organic neurologic disease. For example: • Give-way weakness of jaw or tongue • Wrong-way tongue deviation • Lower-face downward retraction simulating central facial droop/weakness (Fasano et al., 2012) • Dyskinetic jaw, face, or tongue movements evident on steady posture tasks but not evident during other tasks, including speech Inconsistencies during examination or within history, such as: • Irregular or slow speech alternating motion rates (e.g., rapid repetition of "puhpuhpuh") in the absence of irregularities or slowness on other speech tasks • Variable severity across examination activities (e.g., conversation, reading, repetition, emotionally laden topics) • Amplification of symptoms when patient is aware that examiner is attending closely to speech • Complaint or presence of symptom fluctuation as a function of setting, specific listeners, certain stimuli (e.g., noise, odors), or self-proclaimed "spells" without physiologic correlates Suggestibility – amplification of symptoms when examiner suggests a simple task may be challenging Distractibility – presence of normal speech, reduced speech symptom severity, or reduced accompanying abnormalities (e.g., facial retraction or grimacing) during casual conversation or small talk, or when the patient addresses a topic enthusiastically Paradoxic fatigability – when weakness is suspected, deterioration of speech that is not compatible with increasing weakness but rather reflects increased muscle activity (e.g., emergence of strained voice; amplification of abnormal oromotor movement during speech) Indifference to or denial of speech abnormality that is easily recognized by others Severe speech deficits relative to severity of neurologic injury (e.g., mild traumatic brain injury), or known locus of lesion (e.g., single, unilateral lacunar stroke) Speech abnormality is accompanied by "broken English" or telegraphic expressive language (e.g., "Me go store," "Can't speak, talking hard"), in absence of aphasia. Most often evident in functional stuttering and foreign accent, but can occur in other FSD types Modifiability – resolution or near-normalization of speech in one or two symptomatic therapy sessions
Stuttering	Excessive variability – long stretches of fluent speech interspersed with periods of significant stuttering (or vice versa) Excessive consistency – stuttering on every sound, syllable, or word Struggle behavior during dysfluent speech (e.g., facial grimacing, neck extension) Absence of aphasia, dysarthria, or apraxia of speech
Prosody	Modifiability – the ability to produce another accent with relative ease on request in cases of functional foreign accent Absence of history of or current aphasia, dysarthria, or apraxia of speech Infantile/childlike prosody, especially if accompanied by infantile affective facial expression and gestures
Articulation	Lingual, jaw, or face weakness on nonspeech tasks out of proportion to articulatory imprecision Wrong-way tongue deviation if hemiparesis present
Resonance	Inconsistency of hypernasality Consistent hypernasality or nasal emission on only one or a small number of consonant sounds

apraxia of speech, or dysarthria (usually hypokinetic dysarthria), and in fact may be a direct manifestation of those problems. Because of its frequent association with aphasia and apraxia of speech it frequently is tied to left-hemisphere lesions, but associations with right-hemisphere, posterior fossa, and subcortical lesions have been reported. It tends to be more persistent with bilateral or multifocal lesions. It is quite possible that some reported cases of neurogenic stuttering, particularly those without other speech or language disturbances or identifiable lesions, actually had a functional basis. It has been suggested, for example, that severe stuttering (or language difficulty) following mild traumatic brain injury is very unusual and should raise suspicions about functional or psychogenic etiology (Binder et al., 2012).

Acquired stuttering also has long been recognized as a possible manifestation of a conversion disorder (e.g., Head, 1922), but most of what is known about functional stuttering (often termed "psychogenic stuttering") is derived from single case studies or small cases series (e.g., Wallen, 1961; Deal, 1982; Attanasio, 1987; Deal and Doro, 1987; Brookshire, 1989; Duffy, 1989; Roth et al., 1989; Mahr and Leith, 1992; Binder et al., 2012). A useful summary of its demographic and clinical features can be derived from the largest study of acquired functional stuttering to date (Baumgartner and Duffy, 1997), which retrospectively summarized relevant clinical data for 49 people without evidence of neurologic disease and 20 people with evidence of neurologic disease who developed stuttering-like dysfluencies that were diagnosed as psychogenic. Men and women were equally represented in each of the two groups. Average age of onset was in the mid-40s but about 15% of cases in each group were over 60. The stuttering had been present for days to years in both groups (median of approximately 3 months). More than 80% of cases in each group had additional symptoms that raised the possibility of organic neurologic disease. Within the group with confirmed neurologic disease, traumatic brain injury, seizure disorder, and degenerative neurologic disease were the most common diagnoses (each of those diagnoses represented 25% of the group). A minority of the cases (30%) had prior or current evidence of aphasia, apraxia of speech, or dysarthria. Among the 25% of patients with neurologic disease and 41% of patients without neurologic disease who were seen for psychiatric evaluation, conversion reaction, anxiety or hysterical neurosis, and depression were the most frequent psychiatric diagnoses in both groups.

There were no obvious meaningful differences in the type of dysfluencies between the two groups. Sound and syllable repetitions were by far the most common dysfluency but a wide variety of additional dysfluencies were noted (e.g., hesitations or blocking, prolongations, whole-word repetitions). An important finding was the presence of effortful physical struggle (oral, limb, torso, head) during speech in a majority of cases, as well as a "broken English" pattern (e.g., "Me not talk right") that accompanied the dysfluencies in a minority of patients; the latter characteristics do not occur in neurogenic stuttering alone. Most relevant to the validity of the diagnosis of the stuttering as functional, about 70% of symptomatically treated patients in both groups improved rapidly and dramatically during one or two sessions of speech therapy.

FOREIGN-ACCENT SYNDROME AND OTHER PROSODIC DISTURBANCES

Neurologic disease can induce a rare and unusual speech pattern with articulatory and prosodic features that lead to a perception of an often not reliably identified regional or foreign accent. Known as FAS, or pseudoforeign accent or dialect, its perceptual characteristics are heterogeneous and not linked to any specific language. The perception of an accent reflects changes in vowel and consonant production, and alterations in stress, rhythm, and intonation, all features that contribute to the "true" accent associated with any language.

Although FAS was described over 100 years ago, uncertainty persists about whether it represents an unusual variant of apraxia of speech (a speech-planning or programming disturbance) or a distinct problem of linguistic prosody with a single underlying explanatory mechanism and neural substrate (Aronson, 1990; Coelho and Robb, 2001; Blumstein and Kurowski, 2006; Aronson and Bless, 2009). Among the scores of cases that have been reported, many have had right-sided weakness, and aphasia and/or apraxia of speech are frequently present. Stroke (predominantly left-hemisphere) is the presumed etiology in about 70% of cases, and traumatic brain injury in about 20% of cases, but FAS also has been associated with multiple sclerosis (Bakker et al., 2004; Chanson et al., 2009), left-hemisphere tumor (Abel et al., 2009; Tomasino et al., 2013), primary progressive aphasia (Luzzi et al., 2008) and, perhaps, other neurodegenerative conditions (Katz et al., 2012). (See Duffy, 2013, for a more detailed summary of etiologies and speech characteristics associated with neurogenic/organic FAS.)

Of importance in the context of this chapter are the facts that FAS can emerge in individuals without identified organic etiology and that it may be functional, including in some individuals with confirmed neurologic disease (Gurd et al., 2001). Perusal of cases reported as lesion-based FAS suggests that the problem might in fact have been functional, and a number of published cases of FAS show strong evidence that the accent was functional (e.g., conversion disorder, psychosis) (e.g., Van Borsel et al., 2005; Verhoven et al., 2005; Reeves et al., 2007; Haley et al., 2010).

On the basis of the accent alone, functional versus neurogenic FAS may not be reliably distinguished. The most important diagnostic clues probably lie in the company kept by the accent (history, symptoms, or signs) or in the variability of the accent during examination.

Evidence of or a history of aphasia, dysarthria, or apraxia of speech would be common in organic FAS and uncommon in functional FAS. Inconsistency in the accent would be more in keeping with functional FAS. A useful diagnostic task for any case of FAS is to ask patients to imitate an accent other than their presenting accent, preferably one they indicate they have been able to produce in the past. Patients with organic FAS cannot do this without great effort, if at all. Nor can many patients with functional FAS, but the ability to do this with relative ease should be taken as a strong sign of functional FAS because the volitional production of an accent requires considerable motor speech control. Finally, as is the case for any FSD, rapid resolution of the accent with symptomatic therapy would confirm a diagnosis of functional FAS.

Not all FSDs that affect prosody are perceived as a foreign accent. Some patients have a childlike or infantile speech pattern, or a pattern of prosodic variation that is simply perceived as unusual or bizarre, or at least unlike prosodic abnormalities associated with dysarthria or apraxia of speech, or the aprosodia (Ross, 1981) that may occur with right-hemisphere pathology.

OTHER MANIFESTATIONS OF FUNCTIONAL SPEECH DISORDERS

FSDs can affect speech in ways beyond fluency and accent. Why FSDs take different forms of expression is uncertain. Possible explanations include: somatic compliance, in which the functional symptom is directed by the locus of an organic problem (e.g., a traumatic neck injury leads to functional dysphonia versus oral surgery, which leads to lingual articulation problems or hypernasality) or, relatedly, hypervigilance, in which excessive attention to normal somatic stimuli, perhaps from an injured structure, interferes with normal functioning of that structure. In other cases, prior exposure to or beliefs about the effects of illness may help prime symptom locus (e.g., stroke or brain injury often causes speech problems).

Articulation abnormalities

When FSDs predominantly or exclusively affect articulation they are usually secondary to reduced jaw, face, or tongue movements in a manner suggestive of weakness, or they are secondary to abnormal, seemingly involuntary movements of those structures. In general, they need to be distinguished from effects of structural lesions, such as tumors or traumatic injuries (e.g., oral surgery, accidents), lower motor neuron weakness of cranial nerves V, VII, or XII, or hyperkinetic dysarthria secondary to dystonia, chorea, or tremor. When isolated, they may be associated with a history of physical trauma to speech structures (e.g., oral surgery, intubation). Pending litigation can complicate diagnosis because of possible secondary gain or malingering. Conversion or somatization disorders are probably more frequent causes of functional articulation disorders than are "simple" responses to life stresses (Duffy, 2013); abnormal articulation, characterized by pervasive glottal stop substitutions, has been reported in Munchausen syndrome (Kallen et al., 1986).

Articulatory distortions associated with dysarthria or apraxia of speech can range from subtle to severe, whereas functional articulation problems usually are not subtle. Error sounds, when the tongue is the main symptom locus, are often those associated with persistent developmental error sounds or those portrayed negatively in the media (i.e., /r/, /l/, and /s/). This is not necessarily helpful to differential diagnosis because those sounds are also among the most susceptible to genuine tongue weakness. However, distortion of only a single sound would be uncommon in any MSD. Lingual atrophy or fasciculations are often evident if the hypoglossal nerve is involved; obviously, those signs should not be present if the articulation problem is only functional. It would be unusual for significant articulatory distortions on multiple sounds, combined with poor performance on jaw, face, or lingual strength tasks suggestive of weakness, to be present without dysphagia or difficulties with chewing or saliva control. It can be very difficult to distinguish between functionally based bizarre posturing or movements of the jaw, face or tongue from focal speech-induced dystonia affecting those structures, although patients with genuine dystonia benefit from sensory tricks (e.g., a bite block, tongue blade, or piece of gum managed by the tongue during speech) more often than do those with functional movement disorders that affect articulation.

Resonance abnormalities

Although rare, an FSD can be manifest as relatively isolated hypernasality, which can be difficult to distinguish from that which can occur in flaccid dysarthria. However, hypernasality due to palatal weakness rarely occurs in isolation (i.e., without voice abnormalities or dysphagia) unless the cause is myasthenia gravis. Oral or sinus surgery, or uvulectomy for obstructive sleep apnea, may serve as a somatic compliance trigger or conversion disorder in some cases. Functional hyponasality (an abnormal lack of nasal resonance) is probably extremely rare and should be considered only after patulous eustachian tube (Aronson and Bless, 2009) and upper pharyngeal or nasal obstruction have been ruled out.

Mixed and related abnormalities

A substantial percentage of patients with FSDs have a combination of speech abnormalities (Table 33.1). It is not uncommon, for example, to encounter patients with various combinations of abnormal speech breathing patterns, dysphonia, abnormal prosodic variations (including foreign accent), stuttering-like dysfluencies, slow or rapid or variable speaking rate, and sound substitutions, additions, omissions, distortions, or, sometimes, excessively precise articulation.

Although they go beyond the scope of this chapter, functional neurologic disorders can also be manifest in language behavior that can resemble or raise suspicions about aphasia, alexia, or agraphia (Lecours and Vanier-Clément, 1976; DiSimoni et al., 1977; Marshall, 2004). It is not uncommon for patients with FSDs also to have language or cognitive complaints that affect communication. Such deficits would fall under the heading of functional disorders of cognition (see Chapter 35).

MANAGEMENT

Treatment of FSDs ideally is best deferred until the medical/neurologic workup has been completed and possible organic causes for the speech disturbance have been ruled out. Nonetheless, assuming patients are not firmly convinced their symptoms have an organic basis, it is not uncommon for speech therapy to be successful during the initial speech examination, before all other diagnostic tests have been completed. When the case, dramatic improvement of speech may make some medical tests unnecessary or may help focus the remaining workup more efficiently. It may also open the door to improvement of other functional motor symptoms.

Principles for symptomatic management of functional neurologic disorders are applicable to FSDs. They are addressed in the latter chapters in this book. In general, the histories surrounding the development of FSDs, their specific speech characteristics, and the heterogeneity of associated organic and psychologic variables across patients preclude a one-size-fits-all approach to therapy (Duffy, 2013).

Although speech therapy for FSDs is predominantly symptomatic, it seems crucial that symptomatic efforts be made in a context in which the clinician first conveys an appropriate degree of confidence that there are not likely any neurologic or other medical factors that preclude the possibility of a successful outcome of the patient's concerted efforts during therapy. Patients should be encouraged to feel confident that, with the clinician's assistance to improve their speech, good outcomes sometimes can be achieved relatively quickly.

There are a multitude of specific techniques for modifying speech. Detailing them is not important in this context (see Duffy, 2013, for a more detailed review). The "theme" and general sequence of techniques for FSDs often include the following:

1. Identify for patients their primary abnormal speech features (e.g., strained voice, sound repetitions, facial grimacing) and establish that they represent a barrier to speaking normally and need to be modified.
2. Have them imitate some very simple sounds or words that either approximate normal or at least are produced differently than the baseline behavior (e.g., slowly prolong instead of rapidly repeating a sound or word), with initial praise for anything that represents change.
3. Gradually have them self-correct errors without assistance, with praise for their initial recognition of an "error" and any attempt at self-correction, and express optimism that this is a crucial step to overall improvement.
4. When appropriate, use physical contact to provide feedback (e.g., touch the face to identify the locus of abnormality if it is moved abnormally during speech attempts.
5. Gradually shape their improved response efforts to longer utterances.
6. When speech begins to improve consistently, accelerate enthusiasm, withdraw touch, and ask them to self-correct consistently.
7. Gradually move to longer, more natural reading or conversational speech.
8. As improvement occurs, have them estimate the degree to which speech is advancing to 100% normal, and ask how they are feeling about their ability to control their speech and the effort required to do so.

When symptomatic therapy is successful, and especially when it is rapidly successful, it is very important to develop with patients an explanation they can provide to others about the nature of the problem they had and the reasons for the improvement. At least part of the latter explanation should include the belief that improvement has occurred because of motivated, concerted hard work on their part to achieve control over a problem that had not previously been under their control. These issues should be discussed again in the presence of significant others whenever possible.

This general process of symptomatic treatment and subsequent explanation for success sometimes can be accomplished in one or two sessions, although multiple sessions may be required in many cases. In our practice, if observable progress is not evident within two sessions, therapy is discontinued with an option to restart if changes in other aspects of management suggest improved readiness to benefit from therapy.

Although there are no controlled trials regarding behavioral management of FSDs, case studies and case series have documented that therapy can be effective for a substantial proportion of affected individuals, at least in the short term, sometimes rapidly and dramatically so, and at least to a degree that permits confidence that the speech disturbance is functional. In the previously discussed retrospective study of 49 patients with acquired functional stuttering in the absence of neurologic disease (Baumgartner and Duffy, 1997), among 21 patients (43%) who were treated symptomatically, 48% achieved normal speech during the diagnostic evaluation or one additional therapy session; an additional 29% of treated patients improved to nearly normal in one or two sessions. In addition, in a group of 20 patients with acquired functional stuttering who did have evidence of neurologic disease (30% of whom had evidence of aphasia, apraxia of speech, or dysarthria), among the 11 patients who were treated (55% of the group), 45% improved to normal in one or two sessions, and another 18% improved to near normal. The similar response to treatment between the groups with and without neurologic disease suggests that the presence of organic disease does not preclude successful speech therapy for acquired functional stuttering and that behavioral treatment for it can/should be undertaken in the diagnostic session (Sapir and Aronson, 1990). Note, however, that absence of a rapidly dramatic treatment effect does not, by itself, preclude longer-term therapy with a goal of resolving the FSD. There are reports of positive treatment outcomes for patients with a diagnosis of (probable) psychogenic stuttering who responded well to longer-term therapy (Brookshire, 1989; Mahr and Leith, 1992).

The success of speech therapy is likely not confined to functional stuttering. There are no data or face validity reasons to suggest that success should vary as a function of the specific abnormal speech characteristics (e.g., stuttering versus foreign accent). This receives some support from an unpublished review of 92 consecutive cases with a wide variety of FSDs (excluding isolated functional dysphonia) that were seen recently in the Division of Speech Pathology at Mayo Clinic. Therapy was undertaken during the diagnostic session and/or one subsequent therapy session for 54% of the patients. Speech returned to normal or was markedly improved in 50% of those patients. An additional 18% of treated patients returned to normal or were markedly improved in three to eight therapy sessions. These positive results (and those reported by Deal, 1982; Duffy, 1989; Roth et al., 1989; Tippett and Siebens, 1991) are similar to those reported for psychogenic voice disorders, including some cases with coexisting neurologic disease (e.g., Sapir and Aronson, 1985, 1987; Aronson, 1990; Stemple, 1993). This success rate is also comparable to that reported by Czarnecki et al. (2011) for 60 patients with chronic functional nonspeech movement disorders who participated in a 1-week intensive motor reprogramming rehabilitation program.

There are several variables that weigh against but do not necessarily preclude the success of symptomatic speech therapy. For example, when the FSD is unpredictably episodic or spell-like, the speech abnormalities may not be evident at the time of therapy, or may vary from normal to abnormal during treatment, leaving all parties uncertain about the effect of therapy. When severe pain, especially in the head, neck, or face, is part of the presentation, the pain may preclude focused effort by the patient and may reduce the degree to which therapeutic touch, gentle massage, or manipulation of speech structures can be successful. When the speech problem is not a high patient priority on a long list of somatic complaints or ongoing psychosocial stressors, or when serious psychopathology is present, speech therapy beyond attempts during the diagnostic session may be contraindicated or deferred. When the patient is unwavering in a belief that the FSD and any accompanying functional neurologic symptoms have an organic basis, speech therapy should be deferred until the patient is receptive to the possibility that behavioral therapy may be of benefit. And, as is occasionally the case, if a patient denies the presence of speech abnormality, speech therapy is unlikely to be beneficial (Czarnecki et al., 2011; Duffy, 2013).

CONCLUSION

Acquired FSDs can mimic organic disorders of speech and challenge differential diagnosis of neurologic disease. They are most often manifest as dysphonia, stuttering, or prosodic abnormalities, but any aspect of speech production can be affected. Numerous clinical clues can help distinguish them from manifestations of organic neurologic diseases and diagnosis of a FSD can be supported by the sometimes rapidly achieved positive outcome of symptomatic speech therapy. Although high-level evidence is limited, available data suggest that speech therapy can be effective in a significant percentage of cases. Future efforts in the area of FSDs should include refining criteria for their reliable diagnosis, identifying the active ingredients of effective treatments and best predictors of outcomes, and acquiring higher-quality evidence about which interventions are most effective in the short and long term.

References

Abel TJ, Hebb AO, Silbergeld DL (2009). Cortical stimulation mapping in a patient with foreign accent syndrome: case report. Clin Neurol Neurosurg 111: 97–101.

Aronson AE (1990). Clinical voice disorders, 3rd edn. Thieme, New York.

Aronson AE, Bless DM (2009). Clinical voice disorders, 4th edn. Thieme, New York.

Attanasio JS (1987). A case of late-onset or acquired stuttering in adult life. J Fluency Disord 12: 287–290.

Baizabal-Carvallo JF, Jankovic J (2015). Speech and voice disorders in patients with psychogenic movement disorders. J Neurol 262: 2420–2424.

Bakker JI, Apeldoorn S, Metz LM (2004). Foreign accent syndrome in a patient with multiple sclerosis. Can J Neurol Sci 31: 271–272.

Baumgartner J, Duffy JR (1997). Psychogenic stuttering in adults with and without neurologic disease. J Med Speech-Lang Pathol 5: 75–95.

Binder LM, Spector J, Youngjohn JR (2012). Psychogenic stuttering and other nonorganic speech and language abnormalities. Arch Clin Neuropsychol 27: 557–568.

Blumstein SE, Kurowski K (2006). The foreign accent syndrome: a perspective. J Neurolinguist 19: 346–355.

Brookshire RH (1989). A dramatic response to behavior modification by a patient with rapid onset of dysfluent speech. In: N Helm-Estabrooks, JL Aten (Eds.), Difficult diagnoses in communication disorders, College-Hill Press, Boston, pp. 3–12.

Chanson JB, Kremer S, Blanc F et al. (2009). Foreign accent syndrome as a first sign of multiple sclerosis. Multiple Scler 15: 1123–1125.

Coelho CA, Robb MP (2001). Acoustic analysis of foreign accent syndrome: an examination of three explanatory models. J Med Speech Lang Pathol 9: 227–242.

Czarnecki K, Thompson JM, Seime R et al. (2011). Functional movement disorders: successful treatment with a physical therapy rehabilitation protocol. Parkinsonism Relat Disord 18: 247–251.

Deal JL (1982). Sudden onset of stuttering: a case report. J Speech Hear Disord 47: 301–304.

Deal JL, Doro JM (1987). Episodic hysterical stuttering. J Speech Hear Disord 52: 299–300.

DiSimoni FG, Darley FL, Aronson AE (1977). Patterns of dysfunction in schizophrenic patients on an aphasia battery. J Speech Hear Disord 42: 498–513.

Duffy JR (1989). A puzzling case of adult onset stuttering. In: N Helm-Estabrooks, JL Aten (Eds.), Difficult diagnoses in communication disorders, College-Hill Press, Boston, pp. 13–22.

Duffy JR (2013). Motor speech disorders: substrates, differential diagnosis, and management, Elsevier, St. Louis.

Fasano A, Valadas A, Bhatia KP et al. (2012). Psychogenic facial movement disorders: clinical features and associated conditions. Mov Disord 27: 1544–1551.

Gurd JM, Coleman JS, Costello A et al. (2001). Organic or functional? A new case of foreign accent syndrome. Cortex 37: 715–718.

Haley KL, Roth HL, Helm-Estabrooks N et al. (2010). Foreign accent syndrome due to conversion disorder: Phonetic analyses and clinical course. J Neurolinguist 23: 1–16.

Head H (1922). An address on the diagnosis of hysteria. BMJ 1: 827–829.

Helm-Estabrooks N (1993). Stuttering associated with acquired neurological disorders. In: RF Curlee (Ed.), Stuttering and related disorders of fluency, Academic Press, St Louis, pp. 205–219.

Hinson VK, Haren WB (2006). Psychogenic movement disorders. Lancet Neurol 5: 695–700.

Hinson VK, Cubo E, Comella C et al. (2005). Rating scale for psychogenic movement disorders: scale development and clinimetric testing. Mov Disord 20: 1592–1597.

Kallen D, Marshall RC, Casey DE (1986). Atypical dysarthria in Munchausen syndrome. Br J Disord Commun 21: 377–380.

Katz WF, Garst DM, Briggs RW et al. (2012). Neural basis of the foreign accent syndrome: a functional magnetic resonance imaging case study. Neurocase 18: 199–211.

Keane JR (2006). Functional diseases affecting the cranial nerves. In: JH Noseworthy (Ed.), second edition. Neurological therapeutics: principles and practice, vol. 2. Informa Healthcare, Andover, UK, pp. 2197–2204.

Lecours AR, Vanier-Clément M (1976). Schizophasia and jargonaphasia: a comparative description with comments on Chaika's and Fromkin's respective looks at "schizophrenic" language. Brain Lang 3: 516–565.

Lundgren K, Helm-Estabrooks N, Klein R (2010). Stuttering following acquired brain damage: a review of the literature. J Neurolinguist 23: 447–454.

Luzzi S, Viticchi G, Piccirilli M et al. (2008). Foreign accent as the initial sign of primary progressive aphasia. J Neurol Neurosurg Psychiatry 79: 79–81.

Mahr G, Leith W (1992). Psychogenic stuttering of adult onset. J Speech Hear Res 35: 283–286.

Marshall RC (2004). Speech disorders in adults, psychogenic. In: RD Kent (Ed.), The MIT encyclopedia of communication disorders. MIT Press, Cambridge MA, pp. 186–189.

Reeves RR, Burke RS, Parker JD (2007). Characteristics of psychotic patients with foreign accent syndrome. J Neuropsychiatry Clin Neurosci 19: 70–76.

Rosenbek J (1984). Stuttering secondary to nervous system damage. In: RF Curlee, WH Perkins (Eds.), Nature and treatment of stuttering: new directions, College-Hill Press, San Diego, CA, pp. 31–48.

Ross ED (1981). The aprosodias: functional-anatomic organization of the affective components of language in the right hemisphere. Arch Neurol 38: 561–569.

Roth CR, Aronson AE, Davis LJ (1989). Clinical studies in psychogenic stuttering of adult onset. J Speech Hear Disord 54: 634–646.

Saifee TA, Kassavetis P, Parées I et al. (2012). Inpatient treatment of functional motor symptoms: a long-term follow-up study. J Neurol 259: 1958–1963.

Sapir S, Aronson AE (1985). Aphonia after closed head injury: aetiologic considerations. Br J Disord Commun 20: 289–296.

Sapir S, Aronson AE (1987). Coexisting psychogenic and neurogenic dysphonia: a source of diagnostic confusion. Br J Disord Commun 22: 73–80.

Sapir S, Aronson AE (1990). The relationship between psychopathology and speech and language disorders in neurologic patients. J Speech Hear Disord 55: 503–509.

Seery CH (2005). Differential diagnosis of stuttering for forensic purposes. Am J Speech Lang Pathol 14: 284–297.

Stemple JC (1993). Voice therapy: clinical studies, Mosby, St Louis.

Tippett DC, Siebens AA (1991). Distinguishing psychogenic from neurogenic dysfluency when neurologic and psychologic factors coexist. J Fluency Disord 16: 3–12.

Tomasino B, Marin D, Maieron M et al. (2013). Foreign accent syndrome: a multimodal mapping study. Cortex 49: 18–39.

Van Borsel J, Tallieu C (2001). Neurogenic stuttering versus developmental stuttering: an observer judgment study. J Commun Disord 34: 385–395.

Van Borsel J, Janssens L, Santens P (2005). Foreign accent syndrome: an organic disorder? J Commun Disord 38: 421–429.

Verhoven J, Mariën P, Engelborghs S et al. (2005). A foreign speech accent in a case of conversion disorder. Behav Neurol 16: 225–232.

Wallen V (1961). Primary stuttering in a 28-year-old adult. J Speech Hear Disord 26: 394–395.

Handbook of Clinical Neurology, Vol. 139 (3rd series)
Functional Neurologic Disorders
M. Hallett, J. Stone, and A. Carson, Editors
http://dx.doi.org/10.1016/B978-0-12-801772-2.00034-5

Chapter 34

Functional voice disorders: clinical presentations and differential diagnosis

J. BAKER*
Speech Pathology and Audiology, School of Health Sciences, Flinders University, Adelaide, Australia

Abstract

In this chapter, an overview of the heterogeneous group of functional voice disorders is given, including the psychogenic voice disorder (PVD) and hyperfunctional or muscle tension voice disorder (MTVD) subgroups. Reference is made to prevalence and demographic data, with empiric evidence for psychosocial factors commonly associated with the onset and maintenance of these disorders. Clinical features that distinguish between the different presentations of PVD and MTVD are described. While there are some shared characteristics, key differences between these two subgroups indicate that PVD more closely resembles the psychogenic movement disorders and a range of other functional neurologic disorders.

Assessment procedures and auditory-perceptual features of the voice that distinguish these disorders from the neurologically based voice disorders are discussed, with case examples highlighting ambiguous features that may influence differential diagnosis. The clinical profiles of PVD and MTVD affirm approaches to clinical management by speech-language pathologists that integrate symptomatic behavioral voice therapy with "top-down" models of counseling or psychotherapy. They also support the proposition that PVD may be construed as a subtype of functional neurologic disorders.

INTRODUCTION

In addition to our expressive and receptive language, voice and resonance, articulation, fluency, and prosodic features are the major elements of human speech production. When any one of these elements changes even moderately, our ability to communicate can be compromised. Impairments in these key domains of speech production may herald early signs of structural and organic changes to particular neurophysiologic systems in the body. This may affect a person's ability to participate in normal communication activities, with implications for overall physical and mental health.

However, alterations to aspects of voice and speech may also occur in the absence of structural organic or neurologic changes sufficient to account for these changes. They may appear under innocuous circumstances that seem to bear little or no relation to the nature or severity of the symptoms, they may reflect temporary psychobiologic responses to everyday occurrences, or may develop in association with both acute threat and more chronically stressful situations. Under any or all of these scenarios, these changes may precipitate objective signs and self-reported symptoms that indicate the development of a "nonorganic," "psychogenic," or "functional" disorder of speech or voice.

Where these signs and symptoms indicate the onset of a functional speech disorder they may manifest as psychogenic stuttering, as aberrant patterns of articulation displayed as individual features, or as unusual articulation in combination with abnormal prosody to produce childlike speech patterns in adults, or functional foreign-accent syndrome. These disorders are addressed in Chapter 33.

Alternatively, other signs and symptoms may manifest as a functional voice disorder (FVD). This is a large heterogeneous group of "nonorganic" voice disorders

*Correspondence to: Dr. Jan Baker, 22 Howard Terrace, Hazelwood Park, South Australia 5066, Australia. Tel: +1-61-8-8361-3141, E-mail: Janet.Baker@flinders.edu.au

where the dysphonia may present in the form of a muscle tension voice disorder (MTVD), often referred to as a hyperfunctional voice disorder. These disorders are associated with strained patterns of phonation characterized by "excessive laryngeal musculoskeletal activity, force, or tension" (Roy, 2008, p. 195), and generally develop in response to high vocal demands. This may present in the form of MTVD without pathology, or in the form of MTVD with minor pathology, such as vocal nodules or contact ulcers. Retaining these disorders within the MTVD subgroup is not to deny the organic nature of these small benign lesions, but reflects the fact that these tissue changes have arisen in response to hyperfunctional vocal behaviors, as defined above.

Other FVDs may present as a psychogenic voice disorder (PVD). This may occur in the form of a conversion reaction aphonia or dysphonia; as a puberphonia or mutational falsetto, as seen in adolescent and adult males; and, under rare circumstances, as a psychogenic adductor spasmodic dysphonia (ADSD). While there are some shared features between PVD and MTVD, the different clinical presentations within the PVD subgroup demonstrate more marked similarities to the psychogenic movement disorders and other functional neurologic disorders that are the focus of this handbook. For these reasons, a greater emphasis will be placed upon the PVD subgroup than MTVD.

Some of the voice disorders from the two subgroups mentioned above may appear to be similar to those arising from structural or neurologic disease and may even co-occur with a neurologic disorder. However, there are unique and distinctive features that clearly differentiate PVD and MTVD from one another and from their organic and neurogenic counterparts. Therefore, being able to identify, diagnose, and explain the essential nature of these functional communication disorders is fundamental to the clinical practice for speech-language pathologists and otolaryngologists. These processes determine approaches to intervention and provide a necessary platform for patients to gain a genuine understanding about their troubling condition. Significantly, too, these processes contribute directly to medical, neurologic, and psychiatric differential diagnoses (Duffy, 2013).

COMPLEXITIES OF LARYNGEAL FUNCTION

In setting out to describe and understand the possible mechanisms that may account for FVD and the processes involved in differential diagnosis, it is relevant to appreciate the structural positioning of the larynx in relation to other systems within the body and to recognize several vital functions of the laryngeal valve over and above those involved in the production of phonation (Aronson and Bless, 2009). Since the larynx is connected inferiorly to the respiratory system and superiorly to the supraglottic structures of the vocal tract and the oral cavity, differential diagnosis requires assessment of all these components (Stemple et al., 2014). This is not only relevant to our understanding of normal laryngeal function, but may shed further light on the possible symbolic meaning of "nonorganic" disordered function.

Other vital roles of the laryngeal valve

Other vital functions of the laryngeal valve entail preservation of the airway during respiration, protection of the airway from foreign substances during breathing or swallowing, and fixation of the thorax for effort closure during throat clearing, coughing, vomiting, or sneezing. The laryngeal sphincter is also closed firmly to stabilize the thorax during weight bearing, lifting, pushing, defecation, or parturition, and as a stress response in preparing the body for "fight or flight." These vital roles are achieved by interactions between opening and closing of the three anatomic levels of the laryngeal valve which comprise the aryepiglottic sphincter, the ventricular bands, and the true vocal folds.

While all of these are normal activities and functions, excessive constriction at any or all of these three levels of the laryngeal valve may indicate abnormal levels of intrinsic muscular tension. During laryngoscopic examination these involuntary postures are frequently described as excessive anterior/posterior constriction of the aryepiglottic folds, overinvolvement of the false vocal folds, and marked medial compression of the true vocal folds. They may occur during voluntary efforts to phonate, during both quiet speaking and singing activities and particularly with projection of the voice.

These laryngeal and supralaryngeal postures may be evident to some degree in patients with organic voice disorders (OVD) as well as FVD, and in this sense they are not necessarily diagnostic (Behrman et al., 2003; Sama et al., 2001). However, in the more severe presentations, such as a PVD following a traumatic event, or where a PVD in the form of a mutational falsetto has become habituated, this tight closure of the sphincter may completely obliterate the view of the true vocal folds, limiting phonation altogether (Baker et al., 2013).

Communicative role of the voice and as a reflection of personal identity

The other crucial function of the laryngeal valve is in producing voice for communication. At the more primitive levels the voice is engaged in making noises and expressing raw emotions such as groaning, crying, laughing, intimidating, and luring. For more sophisticated vocal activities requiring higher levels of cortical function, the voice is integral to speech, enabling the communication of intentions, thoughts, and feelings, and the more creative activities of singing and oratory.

The distinctive features of a person's voice as reflected in the auditory-perceptual patterns of pitch, quality, intensity, and intonation all serve to differentiate one person from another, reflecting age, gender, education and intelligence, aspects of personality, and sociocultural background. These unique characteristics also lie at the heart of one's personal identity, and strongly affirm each person's sense of self (Rosen and Sataloff, 1997; Aronson and Bless, 2009; Bickford et al., 2013). It is through the use of our voice that we portray our most basic emotions of anger, sadness, fear, and joy, and with further refinements, our voices can convey the more subtly nuanced emotions of shame, humiliation, derision, uneasiness, affection, and humor (Mathieson, 2001). Somewhat ironically, the voice above all other aspects of human verbal communication can signify the psychologic levels of meaning and what is truly meant, often belying the ostensible message conveyed through our carefully chosen words.

Voice as an indicator of physical and mental health

A further aspect to the communicative role of the voice is that even subtle alterations to the pitch, quality, or intonation may reflect a response to psychologic stress, or early signs of changes to a person's physical and mental health. These changes in the form of an aphonia or dysphonia may suggest: an organic illness such as upper respiratory tract infection; a mass lesion on the vocal folds; damage to the laryngeal cartilages; an imbalance in endocrine function; a disturbance to the innervation of the laryngeal muscles secondary to neurologic disease; or psychiatric mood disorder such as anxiety or depression. The sensitivity of the voice in responding to stress and emotional expression, and the links between various laryngeal control mechanisms and the limbic system renders the voice particularly vulnerable to the development of the different clinical manifestations of either PVD or MTVD.

TERMINOLOGIES AND DIAGNOSTIC CLASSIFICATION

Terminology and the diagnostic classification of voice disorders remain problematic, and there are many terminologies used in relation to the "nonorganic" or "functional" voice disorders. Some of these diagnostic terms have a strong behavioral emphasis, suggesting that dysfunctional vocal behaviors and laryngeal muscle tension patterns are causally related. The others terms clearly imply that disturbed psychologic processes are fundamental to etiology (Tables 34.1 and 34.2).

It could be argued that some of the "related disorders" in both Tables 34.1 and 34.2 might not necessarily sit comfortably in the FVD classification, because they may not be construed as disorders of the voice in the strict sense of the word. However, they are included here because they are often listed in well-established diagnostic classification systems within the "functional" or "psychogenic" categories; they can present in association with an aphonia or dysphonia; and serious psychologic issues are considered germane to their clinical presentation.

It can also be seen that some of these terms are no longer evident in the more recent literature, but many are still used, often indiscriminately or without clear definitions.

Table 34.1

Diagnostic terminologies with a behavioral emphasis

Functional voice and related disorders*
Behavioral emphasis
Muscle tension dysphonia
Muscle misuse voice disorder
Hyperfunctional dysphonia
Hypofunctional dysphonia
Phonasthenia/vocal fatigue
Ventricular phonation
Paradoxical vocal fold dysfunction
Globus pharyngis*
Chronic/habitual cough*
Hyperventilation syndrome*

*Disorders that might not be construed as disorders of the voice in the strict sense of the word.

Table 34.2

Diagnostic terminologies with a psychologic emphasis

Functional voice and related disorders*
Psychologic emphasis
Psychogenic voice disorder
Conversion reaction aphonia/dysphonia
Hysteric aphonia/dysphonia
Medically unexplained voice disorders
Mutational falsetto or puberphonia
Phononeurosis/war neurosis of the larynx
Iatrogenic
Globus hystericus*
Psychogenic cough*
Gender dysphoria/transsexualism*
Immature speech/childlike voice in adults*
Psychogenic and/or elective mutism*

*Disorders that might not be construed as disorders of the voice in the strict sense of the word.

These inconsistencies in nomenclature and conceptual frameworks have led to the development of several diagnostic classification systems aiming to redress these problems (Mathieson, 2001; Rammage et al., 2001; Verdolini et al., 2006; Baker et al., 2007; Butcher et al., 2007; Aronson and Bless, 2009). Each of these classification systems provides helpful clues to differential diagnosis between functional, organic, and neurologic voice disorders. In this chapter I will refer to the terminologies used in the Diagnostic Classification System for Voice Disorders, which has been shown to be reliable in distinguishing between FVD and OVD and between PVD and MTVD subtypes (Baker et al., 2007) (Table 34.3).

Table 34.3

Diagnostic terminologies and operational guidelines from the Diagnostic Classification System for Voice Disorders (Baker et al., 2007)

Organic voice disorder

Organic voice disorder (OVD) refers to an aphonia/dysphonia due to mass lesions, structural changes to the vocal folds or cartilaginous structures, or interruption to the neurologic innervations of the laryngeal mechanism. Psychosocial factors often arise in response to, or may aggravate, the situation

Functional voice disorder

Functional voice disorder (FVD) refers broadly to an aphonia/dysphonia where there is no organic pathology, or if there is, it is either insufficient to account for the nature and severity of the voice disorder, or is considered secondary to the functional problem. There are two main subdivisions within the FVD classification: muscle tension voice disorder and psychogenic voice disorder.

Muscle tension voice disorder

Muscle tension voice disorder (MTVD) refers to a dysphonia that develops gradually as a result of psychologic processes that lead to patterns of dysregulated vocal behaviors that over time may result in secondary organic changes such as vocal nodules, polyps, or contact ulcers, and which are generally amenable to resolution through behavioral change. Whilst psychosocial factors play a role in the onset or aggravation of the dysphonia, they may appear secondary to the vocal trauma produced by hyperfunctional vocal behavior patterns

Psychogenic voice disorder

Psychogenic voice disorder (PVD) refers to an aphonia/dysphonia that occurs as a result of disturbed psychologic processes where there is a sudden or intermittent loss of volitional control over the initiation and maintenance of phonation in the absence of structural or neurologic pathology sufficient to account for the dysphonia. Symptom incongruity and reversibility are demonstrated, and psychosocial factors are often linked to onset. While muscle tension patterns may be observed, these are secondary to the psychologic processes operating

CLINICAL VOICE EVALUATION AND DIFFERENTIAL DIAGNOSIS

The assessment of voice disorders is usually carried out by an otolaryngologist and speech-language pathologist and may be undertaken either individually or together in a voice analysis clinic. On the basis of the initial consultation additional referrals may be made to specialists from neurology, clinical psychology, psychiatry, endocrinology, respiratory medicine, oncology, and gastroenterology and, in some cases, to a specialist singing teacher with expertise in voice disorders associated with the performing voice.

The assessment process involves the following: indirect laryngoscopy and videostroboscopy; objective acoustic measures; standard oromotor speech examination; functional assessment of the voice and speech with attention to auditory-visual-kinesthetic-perceptual features of articulation, respiration, phonation voice, and resonance. It also includes the detailed case history and psychosocial interview with self-ratings by the patient in relation to the impact of the voice disorder on quality of life.

In the sections below, emphasis will be given to the laryngeal and functional assessment of the voice and those clinical features that differentiate between the MTVD and PVD subgroups. Brief reference is made to precipitating or predisposing psychosocial factors that support these different clinical profiles of MTVD and PVD. Clinical examples are then given in order to illustrate how these clinical profiles may contribute to the differential diagnosis between FVD and the neurologic voice disorders.

Laryngeal and functional assessment of the voice

The laryngoscopic examination and auditory-perceptual changes to the voice may indicate organic changes such as mass lesions on the vocal folds (e.g., intubation granuloma); alterations to the cartilaginous structures (e.g., subluxation of the arytenoid cartilage); or interruption to the neurologic innervation of the larynx (e.g., unilateral vocal fold palsy following damage to the recurrent laryngeal nerve). Any of these conditions may prevent efficient and symmetric adduction of the vocal folds and cause a dysphonia.

However, differential diagnosis is not just one of exclusion, and the process is more complex where neurologic voice disorders are involved. For example, seemingly similar changes to the voice quality may suggest either an FVD or an acquired or progressive neurologic disorder of the central nervous system leading to a dysarthria, a laryngeal dystonia, or an apraxia of phonation. Similarly, auditory-perceptual changes as manifested in a PVD can easily be confused with those associated with early signs of myasthenia gravis. Further, the various neurologic voice disorders will rarely be confined to the phonation alone. Rather, they will exhibit the particular features associated with the different types of neurologic motor speech disorders according to neurologic levels of involvement and will reflect perceptually distinct patterns of abnormalities to respiration, articulation, phonation, and resonance.

Aronson and Bless (2009) propose that these neurologic voice disorders may manifest as: flaccid, pseudobulbar, and hypokinetic dysphonias; ataxic, choreic, or dystonic dysphonias; organic essential tremor; paroxysmal bursts of voice, as shown in Tourette syndrome; or as disorders of higher cortical control over phonation such as akinetic mutism, foreign-accent syndrome, and frontal-lobe syndrome. Comprehensive and detailed descriptions of the specific voice and speech patterns associated with the different neurologic voice disorders are presented in a number of excellent texts (Mathieson, 2001; Aronson and Bless, 2009; Duffy, 2013; Stemple et al., 2014).

Differential diagnosis may be even more challenging where it is necessary to distinguish between neurologic voice disorders and those in the FVD subgroups of MTVD and PVD, or under circumstances where they may co-occur. These distinctions are not trivial and have important implications for intervention and therapeutic outcomes. A number of clinical features that differentiate between these groups are shown in Table 34.4.

Table 34.4

Clinical features of vocal symptoms and signs that differentiate between neurologic and functional voice disorders

Functional voice disorders (FVDs)		Organic voice disorders (OVDs)
Psychogenic voice disorders (PVDs)	Muscle tension voice disorders (MTVDs)	Neurologic voice disorders (NVDs)
Aphonia or dysphonia with loss of voluntary control over initiation and maintenance of phonation despite normal structure and potential for normal function	Dysphonia typically associated with hyperfunctional vocal patterns in efforts to meet high vocal demands of social and vocational activities	Mass lesions, structural changes to the vocal folds or cartilaginous structures, or interruption to the neurologic innervations of the laryngeal mechanism
Aphonia with normal or tight whisper Dysphonia that may be breathy, high-pitched falsetto, low-pitched and hoarse, diplophonia (two tones)	Altered pitch and quality in association with raised larynx, vocal fatigue, pain or discomfort, and sensitivity of the thyrohyoid laminae	Quality of voice depends on pathology
Symptoms are inconsistent and incongruent with normal structure and function Symptom variability and reversibility	Symptoms consistent with patterns of intrinsic laryngeal tension leading to hyper-/hypoadduction observed during laryngoscopy	Symptoms are consistent and congruent with the site of neurologic lesion and extent of the neurologic damage as observed during oromotor speech and voice examination and laryngoscopy
Onset is generally sudden	Onset is generally gradual (except after acute phonotrauma to vocal folds)	Onset may be sudden but generally gradual
Course of the dysphonia is variable with intermittent episodes of normal voice, aphonia/dysphonia depending on topic of conversation, social or emotional context	Course of the dysphonia is generally consistent More variability in vocal quality occurs where vocal demands increase and as vocal misuse patterns persist	Course of disorder consistent with pathology
Globus sensation is commonly reported	Globus sensation may be reported	Globus sensation is not generally reported
Exaggerated facial, lip, tongue, and respiratory movements may be used in efforts to achieve phonation. These "struggle behaviors" may resemble articulatory or phonatory apraxia	Speech is normal	Usually "embedded" as one symptom of a dysarthria, dystonia, apraxia of voice/speech or frontal-lobe mutism
MTP may be inferred or observed. A/P constriction of the aryepiglottic folds and FVF may obliterate sight of true folds	MTPs are evident and over time may cause secondary organic changes, e.g., edema, vocal nodules, polyps. A/P constriction of aryepiglottic folds and FVF are often present	MTP may be observed in efforts to compensate for neurologic symptoms of laryngeal muscle weakness or incoordination. FVF constriction may reflect efforts to compensate

Continued

Table 34.4

Continued

Functional voice disorders (FVDs)		Organic voice disorders (OVDs)
Psychogenic voice disorders (PVDs)	Muscle tension voice disorders (MTVDs)	Neurologic voice disorders (NVDs)
Normal or improved phonation cannot be voluntarily produced, but may be "leaked" unconsciously or during reflex activities such as laugh or cough; automatic nonpropositional utterances such as counting, days of the week or singing; when deliberately facilitated by distraction with vocal (but nonverbal) strategies	Improved phonation can be elicited by reflex activities such as yawn, laugh, or cough, and with voluntary attention to suggested strategies that promote deconstriction of the extrinsic and intrinsic laryngeal musculature	Normal or significantly improved phonation cannot generally be achieved with patient efforts or facilitating techniques

Modified and adapted from the operational guidelines in the Diagnostic Classification System of Voice Disorders (Baker et al., 2007).
MTPs, muscle tension patterns; A/P, anterior posterior; FVF, false vocal folds.

MUSCLE TENSION VOICE DISORDERS – CLINICAL FEATURES

Subtypes within the MTVD classification

- MTD type 1: with no secondary pathology
- MTD type 2a: with secondary pathology, e.g., vocal nodule
- MTD type 2b: with secondary pathology, e.g., diffuse erythema, chronic laryngitis
- MTD type 2c: with secondary pathology, e.g., Reinke's edema.

These subtypes are based upon those described by Morrison et al. (1986), reflecting increasing degrees of benign vocal pathology induced by hyperfunctional vocal patterns over time. The clinical features described below are applicable across all subtypes.

Clinical features of MTVD

The clinical features of MTVD are reflected in dysfunctional vocal behaviors such as excessive, atypical, or abnormal laryngeal movements that lead to hyperadduction or hypoadduction of the true vocal folds. These patterns of vocal misuse that characterize MTVD develop in association with strenuous speaking, projecting over distance or ambient noise, excessively loud or aggressive screaming, or singing with inappropriate vocal skill or technique. Onset is usually gradual, and the course of the dysphonia as reflected in vocal quality remains relatively consistent except under circumstances where vocal demands are more extreme.

Initial observation

Initial observation may reveal tension in the head and shoulders, with visible cording of the extrinsic laryngeal muscles and a raised position of the larynx. Palpation of the larynx will often reveal minimal thyrohyoid space, marked sensitivity of the thyrohyoid laminae on palpation, and rigidity of the larynx during efforts to gently move the larynx side to side. Respiratory patterns show a tendency to raised chest and clavicular breathing.

Laryngoscopic examination

Laryngoscopic examination of the structure and function of the vocal folds and supralaryngeal structures is carried out during quiet respiration, cough, voluntary production of sustained vowels, sung tones, and conversational speech. A diagnosis of MTVD requires the exclusion of organic or neurologic pathology sufficient to account for the nature and severity of the dysphonia. Even where hyperfunctional phonatory patterns have led to small changes to the vocal folds, such as redness, swelling, or benign lesions such as vocal nodules, the diagnosis of a functional MTVD will still hold.

The patterns of intrinsic laryngeal muscles commonly observed during laryngoscopic examination include medial compression of the true vocal folds, anterior–posterior constriction of the aryepiglottic sphincter, and involvement of the false vocal folds. In some extreme cases this overactivity of the false vocal folds may prevent visualization of the true vocal folds or become habituated and lead to ventricular dysphonia characterized by a low-pitched, rough, and effortful phonation.

Perception of MTVD

Perceptually MTVD presents as a dysphonia and may be breathy, hoarse, rough, strained, or harsh, with excessively high or low habitual pitch, and reduced vocal range and flexibility. Most often, the voice is somewhat driven and loud, but in other cases it may be strained and unusually quiet. It is significant to note that, while auditory-perceptual changes to the voice alert others to the presence and severity of an MTVD, patients often complain firstly about kinesthetic symptoms. These may include the effort of producing and sustaining phonation, a tightness at the level of the sternal notch, vocal fatigue, tickle in the throat, cough, pain, or a sensation of "lump in the throat" (Stemple et al., 2014).

Related signs

Related signs that often occur in association with MTVD are globus (Lee and Kim, 2012), chronic or habitual cough, and hyperventilation syndrome, all of which share a number of similarities with their organic counterparts (Mathers-Schmidt, 2001; Vertigan et al., 2007a, b). However, when arising directly in relation to the MTVD, these laryngeal and respiratory symptoms often abate with behavioral and psychologic interventions, confirming their "functional" etiology.

Co-occurrence of MTVD

Co-occurrence of MTVD with other organic, neurologic, or psychiatric conditions is commonly noted. Patients often report onset of MTVD shortly after an upper respiratory tract infection (that may or may not have been medically verified). It may also develop postoperatively, or as a form of compensation for structural or neurologic problems. For instance, ventricular dysphonia may occur as a "substitution valve" for phonation in association with a unilateral vocal fold paralysis.

Normal or improved phonation

Normal or improved phonation can be elicited by reflex activities such as yawn, laugh, or cough, along with many other behavioral strategies designed to promote less effortful voice production. This process may be achieved quite readily, but generally involves a number of sessions to help the person reduce constriction of extrinsic and intrinsic laryngeal musculature and to master more efficient coordination between respiration, phonation, and resonance.

Prognosis

Prognosis is generally very good for MTVD, with positive outcomes often achieved gradually over three to six sessions. In some cases, especially where deeply entrenched patterns of muscle tension persist, if complex issues related to worker's compensation are operating (such as with teachers), or where the necessary changes to lifestyle are difficult to achieve, generalization may take many months. For more complete resolution, and in order to avoid recurrence, appropriate levels of counseling by the speech-language pathologist will be integrated with the direct voice work. Here attention will be given to the patient's overall health, vocal demands, work environment, performance conditions, lifestyle, and other psychosocial issues that may be impinging.

PSYCHOGENIC VOICE DISORDERS – CLINICAL FEATURES

Subtypes within the PVD classification

- PVD type 1: aphonia (including mutism)
- PVD type 2: dysphonia
- PVD type 3: psychogenic ADSD
- PVD type 4: puberphonia or mutational falsetto (in adolescent or adult males).

The four main PVD groups are loosely based on those recommended by Aronson and Bless (2009), with some slight differences. For instance, voice disorders associated with transsexualism are not included, because in this author's opinion gender dysphoria is a psychiatric condition where any kind of voice problem may develop in response to an individual seeking to modify the voice in keeping with the person's altered gender status. Similarly, elective mutism as distinct from psychogenic mutism is not included here as this reflects a conscious decision not to speak, rather than a loss of volitional control over initiating voice in the context of speech.

Clinical features of PVD

The clinical features of PVD in general are demonstrated in a loss of voluntary control over the initiation and maintenance of normal phonation in the absence of structural or neurologic pathology to explain this problem. It may present as a total loss of voice in the form of an aphonia or as unusual manifestations of dysphonia that are inconsistent with the normal laryngoscopic findings. The aphonia or dysphonia may also be dispersed with intermittent normal phonation that inadvertently "leaks out" during vegetative behaviors, such as coughing, grunting, laughing, or crying. These sounds may not be recognized as normal voice by the patient. These disorders are thought to develop in response to unconscious psychologic processes leading to a difficulty with "willed movement," as described by Haggard (2008). This loss of voluntary control over the initiation of phonation and the production of unusual forms of dysphonia distinguishes PVD from the more behaviorally based MTVD and from the neurologic voice disorders.

Onset of PVD

Onset is generally sudden but it can also develop over several hours, where the patient reports a gradual deterioration of the voice, starting with a mild hoarseness and fading to a complete aphonia. The course of PVD can be highly variable and in one conversation many qualitative changes in the character of the dysphonia or severity of the symptoms can occur. While PVD sometimes resolves spontaneously, it more commonly remains for many days and weeks, sometimes for months, and in rare cases for years.

Symptom incongruity and reversibility

Symptom incongruity and reversibility are the main clinical features that distinguish PVD from MTVD, and from the organic or neurologic voice disorders. These clinical features are typically demonstrated in other functional neurologic disorders (Hallett et al., 2011; Stone et al., 2012). Basing the diagnosis on these positive features also allows for the diagnosis of psychogenic voice symptoms co-occurring with a neurologic voice disorder (Sapir and Aronson, 1985, 1987; Baker, 2016).

Life events and stress are common in PVD and important for formulation and treatment; however, their absence should not preclude a diagnosis of PVD. This is in keeping with the recently published *Diagnostic and Statistical Manual for Mental Disorders,* fifth edition (DSM-5: American Psychiatric Association, 2013), where it is no longer a requirement for clinicians to identify psychologic factors in association with conversion reaction symptoms.

Symptom incongruity

Symptom incongruity noted during laryngoscopic examination may reveal a severe dysphonia despite a healthy larynx and the potential for normal vocal fold adduction. Symptom incongruity often reflects somatic compliance in association with a pre-existing organic or neurogenic disorder. It may also be demonstrated where the pitch or quality of the voice is inappropriate in relation to a person's age, gender, physical structure, and general health, or it may be suspected when causal explanations have a poor fit with the case history. Several case examples that illustrate symptom incongruity might include:

1. a woman of 48 years old presenting with psychogenic aphonia 2 months after successful thyroplasty for medialization of a paralyzed vocal fold
2. a man of 64 years old, who is tall, heavily built, and renowned for his deep and resonant voice as a radio announcer presenting with sudden onset of a puberphonia characterized by "flutey" falsetto phonation a full octave above his normal range
3. a woman of 58 years presenting with a tightly strained and variable dysphonia that her general practitioner attributes to too much singing in her local choir. Case history reveals singing has never caused a voice problem before and that her dysphonia developed within 1 hour of her daughter ringing to let her know that she had been diagnosed with uterine cancer.

Symptom reversibility

Symptom reversibility is one of the most important clinical features of PVD. For instance, during laryngoscopic examination, an aphonia or severe dysphonia may be reflected in abnormal patterns of glottic closure (posterior chink, bowed, or elliptic), and overinvolvement of the false vocal folds as the patient makes an effort to initiate and sustain phonation. The potential for symptom reversibility can then be established when the patient is asked to clear the throat, or to cough, or if informal comments made by the specialists prompt the patient to laugh. These reflex activities can generally facilitate normal adduction of the vocal folds with brief moments of normal phonation and often with simultaneous retraction of the false vocal folds. Despite the fact that patients often revert to their aphonic or dysphonic voice immediately after the laryngoscopic examination, the spontaneous and inadvertent production of normal voice during these vegetative behaviors serves to eliminate frank organic or neurologic voice disorders and supports a likely diagnosis of PVD.

Symptom reversibility may also be demonstrated during the case history and psychosocial interview or during informal conversation, perhaps with another family member. The discerning listener will hear squeaks or glimpses of normal phonation that "leak out" on occasional syllables, words, or phrases, often in relation to more emotionally charged topics and according to the social and interpersonal context. If the patient cries or laughs, normal phonation will almost certainly be heard.

Symptom reversibility may also be elicited and distractibility noted during specific activities designed to trigger normal vocal fold movement and phonation, even if only involuntarily and fleetingly. Throughout these attempts to initiate normal phonation, exaggerated facial, lip, tongue, and respiratory movements may be used. These often manifest as struggle behaviors that are out of proportion to the actual physical effort required and may resemble similar struggle behaviors that are often seen in association with articulatory or phonatory apraxia of neurogenic origin. A selection of strategies often used by speech-language pathologists to facilitate normal

Table 34.5

Clinical strategies to demonstrate symptom reversibility and distractibility

Vegetative behaviors accompanied by sound
- Coughing and throat clearing
- Yawn followed by a sigh (as if with genuine relief)
- Short whimpering sounds (as if a small distressed animal such as a kitten)
- Grunting or groaning (as if in pain)
- Gargling with a firm sound (firstly with water, then simulated without water)

Playful prelinguistic vocal sounds that we might enjoy with a young infant
- Blowing raspberries, waggling the tongue while making happy sounds
- Gently patting the patient's back while s/he sighs out "ah" (as if with comfort)
- Patient patting his/her own chest firmly while sighing out (as if with relief)
- Sirening quietly down the scale using nasal sounds such as /m/ /n/ or /ng/
- Producing a low-pitched glottal fry at the very bottom of the vocal range
- Giggling or laughing (as if in absolute delight)

Automatic phrases and utterances with minimal communicative responsibility
- Counting and reciting the days of the week
- Singing "Happy birthday" or favorite song
- Respond with short "mm," "OK," "uh huh" (as in response to question)

phonation and to categorically affirm symptom reversibility is shown in Table 34.5.

The clinician needs to give respectful explanations to the patient about the reasons for suggesting the use of these young, playful, or unusual sounds and activities, and it is particularly relevant to invite the patient to imbue these sounds with emotions such as relief, humor, comfort, affection, or distress. Practitioners also need to be prepared to model these activities for the patient. It is frequently the case that if the clinician joins the patient, and makes the same sounds with a firm voice, this has the effect of masking the patient's attempts. This process serves to interrupt the person's auditory feedback loop that may make the individual overly sensitive and critical of his or her own attempts, and helps to decrease levels of anxiety. Some patients will be very relieved to hear evidence of their normal voice emerging, but others may immediately tighten and further inhibit their normal phonation. It is important to emphasize that these activities can be very helpful in demonstrating symptom reversibility and distractibility, even in facilitating the return of normal vocal function. However, this does not mean that the PVD has been resolved.

Perception of PVD

Perceptually PVD is characterized by the full range of aberrations in vocal quality, pitch, and loudness, as previously outlined in relation to MTVD. These abnormal perceptual features can vary significantly within one utterance or across the span of a conversation, with shifts between "falsetto," "ventricular," "strangled," or "diplophonic" (two tones at the same time) phonation. These extremes of variation are not consistent with abnormality of structure or neurologic disease.

PVD most frequently presents as an aphonia with either a normal or tight whisper, or as a dysphonia with segments of whispered or breathy voice alternating between high-pitched or low-pitched cracks in the voice, roughness, hoarseness, and strain. It may also present as a psychogenic mutism where the patient makes no attempt to use speech at all or mouths words silently. This is not to be confused with an elective mutism where the patient consciously chooses not to speak in some environments, but can readily speak in others (e.g., with a pet parrot or with a total stranger).

PVD may also manifest as a psychogenic ADSD characterized by markedly strained or strangled vocal quality, with phonation breaks and apparent "spasmodic arrests" seen in neurologically based ADSD. Some patients will demonstrate a tremulousness on sustained vowels, but this is an atypical approximation of what would be observed with the rhythmic and regular pulse of a neurologic tremor. (Clinical examples highlighting criteria for differential diagnosis in situations such as this are presented later in this chapter.)

In adolescent or mature males, PVD may present as a puberphonia or mutational falsetto. This disorder is characterized by high-pitched, breathy, falsetto voice with irregular pitch breaks. The falsetto phonation is weak, and it is difficult to project over noise or distance. Most significantly, it is usually produced a full octave above the normal pitch and modal voice appropriate to the person. In younger adolescent males, psychosexual conflicts during transition through pubertal changes may be significant (despite normal hormonal development). In others, previous success as a boy soprano, which often fosters a strong sense of identity and prestige, may lead the young person to subconsciously hold on to his prepubescent voice and resist the normal changes expected with maturity (Aronson, 1990; Baker, 2002a). PVD may also present in adult males who have previously had a perfectly normal voice with sudden onset of puberphonia. This can be very embarrassing and the presentation is similar to other conversion reaction voice disorders (Baker, 1998).

Signs and symptoms of PVD

Related signs and symptoms of PVD are similar to those found in relation to MTVD, as detailed above. The troubling symptom of globus pharyngis is reported most commonly, and in some cases, symptoms of chronic/habitual cough may meet the diagnostic criteria for a conversion reaction or psychogenic cough. This is relatively unusual, and the quality of the cough is different from a chronic cough related to upper respiratory hypersensitivity or disease. It may sound more like a "bark" that is produced by vibrations of the trachea below the level of the true vocal folds. Variability with this psychogenic cough will be evident in different emotional or interpersonal contexts.

Co-occurrence of PVD

Co-occurrence of PVD may be noted following upper respiratory tract infection, minor injury to the larynx, or postoperatively for a condition related to the head and neck but not in any way implicating the structure and function of the vocal folds. PVD may also develop in association with a pre-existing structural, psychiatric, or neurologic condition. In such cases the specific nature of the voice symptoms often indicates a degree of somatic compliance in association with these pre-existing conditions.

Normal or improved phonation

Normal or improved phonation is usually achieved with clinician-assisted strategies as suggested above, usually in the first session. This is integrated with counseling and further sessions to ensure generalization outside the clinical setting. In some cases this may take numerous sessions over weeks or months. If the patient is not able to achieve normal voice, second opinion, supervision, or referral for psychotherapy may be required.

Prognosis of PVD

Prognosis for PVD is generally good. This is especially so if referral for assessment and treatment is made shortly after onset of symptoms; if normal voice is readily restored; and if insights about the essential nature of the disorder are embraced. More effective resolution is achieved if issues related to stressful life situations have been resolved and more effective ways of coping have been integrated.

In rare cases that fulfill the diagnostic criteria for a "classic" conversion reaction voice disorder, prognosis is more uncertain and efforts may need to be sustained for many months (Baker, 2003; Butcher et al., 2007). Prognosis is often poor if diagnosis is delayed, if assessment procedures are overly confounded with unnecessary medical investigations that tend to affirm an organic etiology, or if therapy cannot be offered shortly after initial consultation by the therapist. Poor outcomes are also likely if treatment can only be offered very sporadically and if due attention is not given to the psychologic stresses underpinning the problem (Kollbrunner et al., 2010). Under these circumstances dysphonic symptoms are likely to become habituated and psychologic issues arising in response to the voice disorder may become firmly entrenched.

ETIOLOGY

Patterns of excessive extrinsic and intrinsic laryngeal muscle tension underpin the different presentations of FVD and heavy vocal demands across occupational, social, or performance settings are key issues for many, especially those with MTVD. In addition, recent upper respiratory tract infection and poor general health are often reported prior to onset of FVD (MacKenzie et al., 2001; O'Hara et al., 2011).

Etiologic studies in relation to FVD have focused upon a range of psychosocial factors such as stressful life events and difficulties preceding onset, and dispositional features such as personality traits, emotional expressiveness, and different ways of coping. It is recognized that psychosocial issues are not limited to individuals with FVD, but they are not related to the development of organic or neurologic voice disorders to the same extent. Rather, they may act as trigger events or develop in response to these conditions (Aronson and Bless, 2009). Findings throughout the literature for psychosocial factors in relation to FVD are similar to those associated with the functional neurologic disorders discussed elsewhere in this handbook, but those related to FVD frequently suggest issues pertaining to verbal communication.

For instance, in a recent case study (Baker et al., 2013), the Life Events and Difficulties Schedule (Brown and Harris, 1978) was used to investigate psychosocial factors that may differentiate between a group of women with FVD ($n=73$), a group with OVD ($n=55$), and a control group with normal voices ($n=66$). Analysis of the same variables was then carried out for the PVD ($n=37$) and MTVD ($n=36$) subgroups within the FVD cohort. The empirical data showed that significantly more women with FVD were likely to experience stressful life events and difficulties in the 12 months prior to onset than those in the other groups. No significant differences were noted between the PVD and MTVD subgroups. Amongst the events and

Table 34.6

Number of women who experienced at least one severe life event, major difficulty, COSO event or difficulty or COSO difficulty with PITS in research period

	FVD (n=73)		OVD (n=55)		Control (n=66)		
	n	%	*n*	%	*n*	%	*p*-value
Severe event	54	74.0	12	21.8	9	13.6	<0.001
Major difficulty	17	23.3	6	10.9	3	4.5	0.004
Severe COSO event	40	54.8	5	9.1	6	9.1	<0.001
COSO with PITS	26	35.6	2	3.6	4	6.1	<0.001

COSO, conflict over speaking out; PITS, powerless in the system; FVD, functional voice disorder; OVD, organic voice disorder (Baker et al., 2013).

difficulties reported, some situations were traumatic, involving violent sexual assault, serious illness, or death of close ties. Others were associated with disintegration of significant relationships and loss of social support. Importantly, many of these stressful incidents were characterized by conflict over speaking out and a sense of powerlessness or futility (Table 34.6).

These findings support previous studies revealing difficulties with the expression of negative emotion during interpersonal conflicts and the heavy burden of responsibility in the family or workplace (House and Andrews, 1988; Aronson, 1990; Andersson and Schalen, 1998; Butcher et al., 2007). They also echo early narrative accounts of conversion reaction aphonia experienced by soldiers during World War I, where the men often described overwhelming fatigue and a sense of futility in returning to the front with no hope of making any difference (Smurthwaite, 1919; Sokolowsky, 1944; Barker, 1991).

However, in some cases, as shown in Table 34.6, no such incidents were reported. These findings reflect clinical practice where, even if such incidents are suspected, it is not always possible to elicit evidence of psychologically stressful events. Furthermore, in some cases, after what appears to be successful resolution of the dysphonia, factors related to psychologic distress may not have been identified (Baker, 2003). These phenomena have also been recognized in relation to other functional neurologic disorders (Stone et al., 2011).

Dispositional features of patients with FVD have also been shown to contribute to the different clinical presentations of MTVD and PVD (Roy and Bless, 2000a, b; Dietrich and Verdolini Abbott, 2008, 2012; Baker and Lane, 2009; Dietrich et al., 2012). For example, patients with MTVD are more likely to be extraverted and driven to action and achievement, whereas those with PVD are prone to introversion and behavioral inhibition, with elevated health concerns in association with abnormal illness behaviors (van Mersbergen et al., 2008; Roy, 2011; Baker et al., 2014). Contrary to assumptions that individuals with psychogenic or conversion reaction disorders invariably manifest bland denial and *la belle indifférence*, most patients with PVD seen by speech-language pathologists do not fit this profile. They more frequently express very real concerns about their voice disorder and express marked relief when it has resolved. While very few patients with FVD are diagnosed with frank psychiatric disorders, many are vulnerable to elevated levels of anxiety and depression (House and Andrews, 1987; White et al., 1997; Baker, 1998; Millar et al., 1999; Roy and Bless, 2000a; Mirza et al., 2003; Seifert and Kollbrunner, 2005; Willinger et al., 2005; Dietrich et al., 2008). This personality profile is typical of patients presenting with somatoform and other medically unexplained conditions (Deary et al., 2007; Deary and Miller, 2011; O'Hara et al., 2011; Miller et al., 2014).

The major theoretic models that seek to explain the development of FVD emphasize how interactions between these psychosocial factors may lead to a range of behavioral, cognitive, affective, and neurophysiologic responses. Although the precise mechanisms underlying the different clinical presentations are not yet fully understood, recent studies have shown how specific psychobiologic markers of stress may be reflected in autonomic nervous system reactivity, and how this may impact upon vocal function (Demmink-Geertman and Dejonckere, 2002, 2008; Helou, 2014). Others, using a functional magnetic resonance imaging paradigm, have shown a relationship between trait stress reactivity and the possible role of the limbic system in the central neural control of vocalization (Dietrich et al., 2012). A comprehensive account of the different theoretic models for FVD and implications for clinical management is presented by Baker (2016).

PREVALENCE

Studies from several Western countries show that prevalence of voice problems ranges from 3% to 17% in the general population (Roy et al., 2004a; Russell et al., 2005; Aronson and Bless, 2009), with estimates of 3–4% in Australian society (Russell, 1999). Anecdotal estimates suggest a substantially higher prevalence of FVD in comparison to OVD across these general populations. People in occupations where the voice is the primary tool of trade are more prone to voice disorders, and teachers are three to five times more likely to have voice problems such as MTVD than the general population (Pemberton, 2010).

Prevalence in relation to gender and age

Women are twice as likely to seek help for voice problems than men (Roy et al., 2005b; Russell et al., 2005) and women comprise 76% of referrals to voice specialists (Morton and Watson, 1998). Across all FVD groups, women are more likely to present than men in ratios of at least 2:1 (Gerritsma, 1991; White et al., 1997). In the PVD subgroups that include conversion reaction aphonia/dysphonia, females present more often than males at a ratio of 8:1 (Wilson et al., 1995; Baker, 2002b, 2008; Aronson and Bless, 2009). Exceptions to this pattern are found where adolescent and adult males present with a mutational falsetto or puberphonia as a subtype of PVD.

Ages of women with FVD across the general population and occupational groups reveal a high prevalence peaking between 40 and 60 years of age (Russell et al., 1998; Roy et al., 2004a, b; Pemberton et al., 2009).

BIOGRAPHIC DETAILS FOR INDIVIDUALS WITH FUNCTIONAL VOICE DISORDERS

There is a surprising paucity of data about the individuals with FVD other than details related to age and gender (Baker, 2008). In the case-control study cited above (Baker et al., 2013), efforts were made to redress this problem by gathering more comprehensive biographic information about participants. These findings showed that women with FVD in comparison to those with OVD were more likely to be educated to higher levels, and to work full-time in teaching, and in jobs with managerial, professional, or supervisory responsibilities. There were no significant differences between the groups for marital status, family constellation, or family of origin. The majority of women were in some form of conjugal relationship with one to three children.

However, there was a difference between groups for any experience of sexual abuse, violence, or strangulation in their lifetime (FVD 36/73 = 49% vs. OVD 18/55 = 33%). Some of these experiences had occurred during their formative years, others during the 12 months prior to onset of their dysphonia. To the best of our knowledge, these are the first data related to sexual abuse and violence in a cohort of women with voice disorders. We also found statistically significant differences between the PVD ($n = 37$) and MTVD ($n = 36$) subgroups for age (51 vs. 43 years, $p = 0.004$), education (38% vs. 72% tertiary education, $p < 0.011$), and any experience of sexual abuse in their lifetime (43% vs. 19%, $p = 0.03$).

DIAGNOSTIC DILEMMAS BETWEEN FUNCTIONAL AND NEUROLOGIC VOICE DISORDERS

The clinical features outlined above provide broad clinical profiles that distinguish the FVD subgroups of MTVD and PVD from one another, and these may differentiate between the neurologic voice disorders. Many of the features described above are clearly inconsistent with an organic and neurologic etiology.

However, diagnostic dilemmas often arise where precipitating factors preceding onset defy usual patterns, where auditory-perceptual and kinesthetic symptoms are quite similar or ambiguous in their presentation and course, or where vocal symptoms persist despite therapeutic interventions that are generally successful in helping patients to resolve their voice disorder. Detailed clinical profiles and case studies with clues to differential diagnosis for a range of psychogenic and neurologic voice disorders are presented in several excellent publications (Mathieson, 2001; Verdolini et al., 2006; Aronson and Bless, 2009; Duffy, 2013). For the purposes of this chapter, I now highlight some of these ambiguous features that may be manifested in some of the MTVD or PVD subtypes that may also be seen in specific neurologic voice disorders.

FUNCTIONAL VOICE DISORDERS VERSUS NEUROLOGIC VOICE DISORDERS

Example 1

A diagnosis of MTVD may be given following apparently normal laryngoscopy examination and auditory perceptual assessment characterized by weak and breathy vocal quality, reduced vocal loudness, marked difficulty in raising the pitch, and sensory symptoms of vocal fatigue, tickle in the throat, with an increased tendency to cough and globus sensation.

These features resemble those associated with unilateral damage to the external branch of the superior laryngeal nerve leading to sensory loss in the laryngopharynx, accounting for the irritability in the throat, and motor impairment to the cricothyroid muscle that explains difficulties in raising the pitch of the voice. This condition is rare and, as there is no definitive laryngoscopic profile, it is a diagnosis that is often missed (Stemple et al., 2014). Recent studies suggest that epiglottic petiole deviation to the side of the cricothyroid muscle weakness during high-pitched voice production is an important diagnostic sign (Roy et al., 2009, 2011).

Example 2

An MTVD may present as a dysphonia characterized by strained and breathy vocal quality, reduced vocal loudness and pitch range, with associated vocal fatigue.

These features may also be present with unilateral recurrent laryngeal nerve paralysis causing weakness of the intrinsic laryngeal muscles leading to strained breathy voice, with reduced vocal tone, rate, and range of movement during both adduction and abduction. Other perceptual features that help to distinguish laryngeal nerve paralysis from MTVD are a weak or a strained diplophonic cough, difficulty in sustaining a vowel beyond several seconds, and a marked reduction in length of phrases or sentences with a need to take frequent breaths. Audible laryngeal stridor may be heard during effortful struggles to inhale, especially when the person is attempting to project over noise. Such features are not typical of an MTVD.

Example 3

MTVD or PVD may manifest as a severe hyperfunctional dysphonia with excessively strained and effortful phonation, a pattern of harsh glottal attack on initiating phonation, occasional phonation breaks, self-reported sensations of effort in producing the voice, and observable extrinsic and intrinsic laryngeal muscle tension.

Where vocal hyperfunction is so extreme, and where this contributes to an unusual "strangled" quality, a neurologic laryngeal dystonia or ADSD may be suspected. It is generally accepted that ADSD is a focal dystonia reflected in involuntary muscle spasms at the different levels of the laryngeal sphincter that may include the true and false vocal folds and the supraglottic structures. While these structures may appear to be normal at rest, the abnormal spasmodic movements are induced by efforts to initiate phonation during speech. The precise neurologic processes that lead to this disorder are yet to be determined (Ludlow, 2011); however, it is thought these involuntary laryngospasms may originate with a disruption within the extrapyramidal system, possibly as a result of abnormality in the neurotransmitters in the basal ganglia (Mathieson, 2001; Aronson and Bless, 2009).

Perceptually this neurologic voice disorder is characterized by strained, strangled, staccato, and effortful phonation during task-induced connected speech. The voice stoppages and momentary pitch changes occur primarily on voiced aspects of speech, such as vowels and voiced consonants. For instance, in a sentence like "Annie ate apricots every day," marked spasms take place on each of the open vowels, and on the voiced consonant in the word "day." Approximately one-third of individuals with spasmodic dysphonia also have voice tremor that makes the pitch and loudness of the voice oscillate at 5 Hz during vowels. This is particularly obvious in a sustained vowel such as /a/, as in the word "car."

Phonation during emotional expression, such as laughing, crying, singing, and even shouting, is not affected and brief periods of normal phonation in spontaneous speech may be heard. These irregularities might lead the clinician to suspect a PVD in the form of a psychogenic ADSD; however, in association with the other symptoms they are entirely consistent with a neurologic presentation. Use of the voice in conversational speech is extremely effortful and patients complain of fatigue and tightness in the neck, back, and shoulders, and report shortness of breath in association with efforts to phonate. The process of differential diagnosis between severe MTVD and ADSD can be very difficult; however, several auditory-perceptual features have been empirically verified as diagnostic markers that may operate to provoke greater severity of symptoms of ADSD and to distinguish reliably between ADSD and MTVD. For instance:

1. Task-specific use of connected speech versus prolonged vowels is more likely to provoke symptoms in ADSD than MTVD (Roy et al., 2005a).
2. Task-specific phonetic loading of assessment tasks with all voiced phonemes is more likely to increase severity of symptoms in ADSD, and is not likely to occur with MTVD (Roy et al., 2007).
3. The frequency and duration of phonatory breaks within a word are greater across both parameters for ADSD than for MTVD (Roy et al., 2008).

Several other factors may assist with differential diagnosis. For instance, symptoms related to ADSD have generally persisted for up to a year or more before diagnosis is made. Further, while ADSD may present as an isolated disorder restricted to the larynx, it is often seen in association with other neurologic conditions, such as essential tremor, or other dystonias, such as blepharospasm, torticollis, or Meige's syndrome. In addition, modification of vocal behaviors with attention to psychosocial factors facilitates successful resolution of many MTVDs, but numerous studies have shown these approaches are not effective with ADSD. As proposed by Duffy (2013, p. 339), "resolution of the dysphonia with symptomatic/behavioral therapy can rule out a neurologic SD."

Example 4

A diagnosis of PVD may be given following auditory-perceptual assessment revealing a breathy dysphonia with reduced loudness and complaints about vocal fatigue and general tiredness. Laryngoscopy may indicate that vocal fold movements appear to be normal during cough and brief automatic utterances, with mild bowing and hypoadduction during volitional speech tasks.

These features may also be present in the early stages of myasthenia gravis. Such symptoms may initially appear to be confined to the voice, affecting only phonation and resonance with a weak, breathy voice and hypernasal resonance. As the disease progresses, it leads to general body weakness and fatigue and may also be reflected in early signs of a flaccid dysarthria affecting articulation and resonance. One of the key auditory-perceptual markers for myasthenia gravis is the rapid deterioration in the voice with sustained voice use. Such changes are markedly evident when the patient is asked to count rapidly and vigorously from 1 to 100, but rapid fatigue may occur within the first 4–5 seconds of sustained phonation. Furthermore, temporary improvement in the voice is audible after brief voice rest or cessation of voice use, and is notably improved by intravenous Tensilon. These patterns are not typical of PVD.

A number of excellent case reports serve to illustrate the clinical profiles of patients who may present with symptoms resembling those associated with either PVD or myasthenia gravis. These studies highlight the complex interactions that take place between the equivocal physical and auditory-perceptual symptoms, concomitant psychosocial factors that may be operating under both conditions, and the processes involved in differential diagnosis (Aronson, 1971; Ball and Lloyd, 1971).

Example 5

A diagnosis of PVD in the form of a stress-related dysphonia characterized by weak and breathy voice may present in an elderly person following the death of a spouse. Laryngoscopic findings may show normal structure of the vocal folds with symmetric adductor and abductor movements, but incomplete closure of the vocal fold, accounting for the breathy quality. Low affect and monotonous intonation may suggest a profound grief reaction or depression as the basis for her PVD.

These features may also be early signs of Parkinson's disease, where further signs of hypokinetic dysarthria and hypokinesia are likely to develop as the disease progresses. Low affect, monotonous intonation, and emotional lability in association with depression are all features of this neurologic dysarthrophonia.

MANAGEMENT

It is not within the scope of this chapter to discuss treatment, but many of the principles of management for functional speech and other neurologic disorders are applicable (these are addressed in Chapter 33). This starts with the initial consultation that encompasses a detailed assessment, case history, psychosocial interview, and explanation of the diagnosis. While many are very puzzled about the fact that their dysphonia is not organically or neurologically based and may even challenge a psychogenic or functional diagnosis, provided the explanation is given with sensitivity and transparency, these patients often report feeling empowered by their new insights. This deeper understanding helps to obviate recurrence, and if it does happen, patients are less likely to be so anxious, knowing that they can do something about it. For these reasons, appropriate levels of "top-down" models of counseling by the speech-language pathologist are often combined with direct voice work.

At the most basic level, therapy involves attention to basic principles of vocal hygiene and direct therapeutic techniques to optimize vocal function by modifying aberrant vocal behaviors. However, at all levels of the therapeutic intervention, beginning with the diagnostic interview, clinicians join with their patients in addressing the psychosocial issues (Baker, 2008). It is now recognized that better outcomes are achieved when patients understand the possible associations between psychosocial and emotional factors, as these may have contributed to their voice disorder. It has also been shown that integrating counseling or psychotherapeutic models such as cognitive-behavior therapy or systems and family therapy with traditional approaches to treatment helps patients to deal more effectively with negative emotions in response to stressful situations or to learn new ways of coping (Butcher et al., 1987, 1993; Baker, 1998; Deary and Miller, 2011; Miller et al., 2014). Where psychologic issues are thought to be too complex or beyond the professional scope of clinicians, supervision or working in collaboration with mental health colleagues is recommended.

CONCLUSION

FVDs that include both MTVD and PVD subgroups affect individuals across all ages, and have profound effects on people's lives. Differential diagnosis is often challenging, especially where auditory-perceptual, kinesthetic, and visual symptoms may resemble those seen in organic neurologic voice disorders, and especially under those circumstances where functional and organic conditions may coexist. While there is now empiric evidence that shows how a number of psychosocial factors may contribute to the onset and different clinical presentations of MTVD and PVD, understanding the neuropsychologic processes that underpin the loss of voluntary control over the initiation of phonation, or the inhibition of normal phonation under conditions of psychologic distress, is still a challenge. Recent brain imaging studies in relation to other functional neurologic disorders may hold the key (Aybek et al., 2008, 2014; Cojan et al., 2009; van Beilen et al., 2010; Voon et al., 2010; Stone et al., 2011; Carson et al., 2012).

References

American Psychiatric Association (2013). Diagnostic and statistical manual of mental disorders DSM-5, American Psychiatric Association, Washington, DC.

Andersson K, Schalen L (1998). Etiology and treatment of psychogenic voice disorder: results of a follow-up study of thirty patients. J Voice 12: 96–106.

Aronson AE (1971). Early motor unit disease masquerading as psychogenic breathy dysphonia: a clinical case presentation. J Speech Hear Disord 36: 115–124.

Aronson AE (1990). Psychogenic voice disorders. Clinical voice disorders: An interdisciplinary approach, 3rd edn. Thieme, New York.

Aronson AE, Bless DM (2009). Clinical voice disorders. Thieme, New York.

Aybek S, Kanaan RA, David AS (2008). The neuropsychiatry of conversion disorder. Curr Opin Psychiatry 21: 275–280.

Aybek S, Nicholson TR, Zelaya F et al. (2014). Neural correlates of recall of life events in conversion disorder. JAMA Psychiatry 71: 52–60.

Baker J (1998). Psychogenic dysphonia: peeling back the layers. J Voice 12: 527–535.

Baker J (2002a). Persistent dysphonia in two performers affecting the singing and projected speaking voice: a report on a collaborative approach to management. Logoped Phoniatr Vocol 27: 179–187.

Baker J (2002b). Psychogenic voice disorders-heroes or hysterics? A brief overview with questions and discussion. Logoped Phoniatr Vocol 27: 84–91.

Baker J (2003). Psychogenic voice disorders and traumatic stress experience: a discussion paper with two case reports. J Voice 17: 308–318.

Baker J (2008). The role of psychogenic and psychosocial factors in the development of functional voice disorders. Int J Speech Lang Pathol 10: 210–230.

Baker J (2016). Psychosocial perspectives on the management of voice disorders, Compton Publishing, Devon, UK.

Baker J, Lane RD (2009). Emotion processing deficits in functional voice disorders. In: K Izdebski (Ed.), Emotions in the human voice. Plural Publishing, San Diego.

Baker J, Ben-Tovim DI, Butcher A et al. (2007). Development of a modified diagnostic classification system for voice disorders with inter-rater reliability study. Logoped Phoniatr Vocol 32: 99–112.

Baker J, Ben-Tovim DI, Butcher A et al. (2013). Psychosocial risk factors which may differentiate between women with functional voice disorder, organic voice disorder, and control group. Int J Speech Lang Pathol 15: 547–563.

Baker J, Oates J, Leeson E et al. (2014). Patterns of emotional expression and responses to health and illness in women with functional voice disorders (MTVD) and a comparison group. J Voice 28: 762–769.

Ball JRB, Lloyd JH (1971). Myasthenia gravis as hysteria. Med J Aust 4: 259–261.

Barker P (1991). Regeneration. Penguin, London.

Behrman A, Dahl LD, Abramson AL et al. (2003). Anterior-posterior and medial compression of the supraglottis: signs of nonorganic dysphonia or normal postures? J Voice 17: 403–410.

Bickford J, Coveney J, Baker J et al. (2013). Living with the altered self. Int J Speech Lang Pathol 15: 324–333.

Brown GW, Harris TO (1978). Social origins of depression, Tavistock Publications, London.

Butcher P, Elias A, Raven R et al. (1987). Psychogenic voice disorder unresponsive to speech therapy: psychological characteristics and cognitive-behaviour therapy. Br J Disord Commun 22: 81–92.

Butcher P, Elias A, Raven R (1993). Psychogenic voice disorders and cognitive behaviour therapy. Singular, San Diego, CA.

Butcher P, Elias A, Cavalli L (2007). Understanding and treating psychogenic voice disorder: a CBT framework, Wiley, Chichester.

Carson AJ, Brown R, David AS et al. (2012). Functional (conversion) neurological sysmptoms: research since the millennium. J Neurol Neursurg Psychiatry 83: 842–850.

Cojan Y, Waber L, Carruzzo A et al. (2009). Motor inhibition in hysterical conversion paralysis. Neuroimage 47: 1026–1037.

Deary V, Miller T (2011). Reconsidering the role of psychosocial factors in functional dysphonia. Curr Opin Otolaryngol Head Neck Surg 19: 150–154.

Deary V, Chalder T, Sharpe M (2007). The cognitive behavioural model of medically unexplained symptoms: a theoretical and empirical review. Clin Psychol Rev 27: 781–797.

Demmink-Geertman L, Dejonckere PH (2002). Non-habitual dysphonia and autonomic dysfunction. J Voice 4: 549–559.

Demmink-Geertman L, Dejonckere PH (2008). Neurovegetative symptoms and complaints before and after voice therapy for nonorganic habitual dysphonia. J Voice 22: 315–325.

Dietrich M, Verdolini Abbott K (2008). Psychobiological framework of stress and voice. In: K Izdebski (Ed.), Emotions in the Human Voice, Vol. 2. Plural Publishing, San Diego, CA.

Dietrich M, Verdolini Abbott K (2012). Vocal function in introverts and extraverts during a psychological stress reactivity protocol. J Speech-Lang Hear Res 55: 973–987.

Dietrich M, Verdolini Abbott K, Gartner-Schmidt J et al. (2008). The frequency of perceived stress, anxiety, and depression in patients with common pathologies affecting voice. J Voice 22: 472–487.

Dietrich M, Andreatta RD, Jiang Y et al. (2012). Preliminary findings on the relation between the personality trait of stress reaction and the central neural control of vocalization. IJSLP 14: 377–389.

Duffy JR (2013). Motor speech disorders: Substrates, differential diagnosis, and management. Elsevier, St. Louis.

Gerritsma EJ (1991). An investigation into some personality characteristics of patients with psychogenic aphonia and dysphonia. Folia Phoniatr 43: 13–20.

Haggard P (2008). Human Volition: towards a neuroscience of will. Nat Rev Neurosci 9: 934–946.

Hallett M, Lang A, Jankovic J et al. (Eds.), (2011). Psychogenic movement disorders and other conversion disorders. Cambridge University Press, Cambridge.

Helou LB (2014). Intrinsic laryngeal muscle response to a speech preparation stressor: Personality and autonomic predictors, PhD doctoral dissertation, University of Pittsburgh.

House A, Andrews HB (1987). The psychiatric and social characteristics of patients with functional dysphonia. J Psychosom Res 31: 483–490.

House A, Andrews HB (1988). Life events and difficulties preceding the onset of functional dysphonia. J Psychosom Res 32: 311–319.

Kollbrunner J, Menet A, Seifert E (2010). Psychogenic aphonia: no fixation even after a lengthy period of aphonia. Swiss Med Wkly 140: 12–17.

Lee BE, Kim GH (2012). Globus pharyngeus: a review of its etiology, diagnosis and treament. World J Gastroenterol 18: 2462–2471.

Ludlow CL (2011). Spasmodic dysphonia: a laryngeal control disorder specific to speech. J Neurosci 31: 793–797.

MacKenzie K, Millar A, Wilson JA et al. (2001). Is voice therapy an effective treatment for dysphonia? BMJ 2001: 658–661.

Mathers-Schmidt BA (2001). Paradoxical vocal fold motion: a tutorial on a complex disorder and the speech-language pathologist's role. Am J Speech Lang Pathol 10: 111–125.

Mathieson L (2001). Greene and Mathieson's: The voice and its disorders. Whurr Publishing, London.

Millar A, Deary IJ, Wilson JA et al. (1999). Is an organic/functional distinction psychologically meaningful in patients with dysphonia? J Psychosom Res 46: 497–505.

Miller T, Deary V, Patterson J (2014). Improving asscess to psychological therapies in voice disorders: a cognitive behavioural therapy model. Curr Opin Otolaryngol Head Neck Surg 22: 201–205.

Mirza N, Ruiz C, Baum ED et al. (2003). The prevalence of major psychiatric pathologies in patients with voice disorders. ENT J 82: 808–812.

Morrison MD, Nichol H, Rammage L (1986). Diagnostic criteria in functional dysphonia. Laryngoscope 94: 1–8.

Morton V, Watson DR (1998). The teaching voice: problems and perceptions. LPV 23: 133–139.

O'Hara J, Miller T, Carding P et al. (2011). Relationship between fatigue, perfectionism, and functional dysphonia. Otolaryngol Head Neck Surg 144: 921–926.

Pemberton C (2010). Voice injury in teachers: Voice care prevention programs to minimise occupational risk. Available online at http://www.parliament.vic.gov.au/images/stories/committees/etc/PL_Submissions/pemberton 201108.pdf (accessed September 2015).

Pemberton C, Oates J, Russell A (2009). Cost effective provision of vocal hygiene information: Preliminary evaluation of the Voice Care for Teachers Package as a prevention tool. In: Occupational Voice Symposium: Protecting your voice in the workplace. London.

Rammage L, Morrison M, Nichol H (2001). Management of the voice and its disorders, Singular Publishing, San Diego, CA.

Rosen DC, Sataloff RT (1997). Psychology of voice disorders. Singular Publishing, San Diego, CA.

Roy N (2008). Assessment and treatment of musculoskeletal tension in hyperfunctional voice disorders. IJSLP 10: 195–209.

Roy N (2011). Personality and voice disorders. In: TL Eadie (Ed.), Perspectives on Voice and Voice Disorders, ASHA, Rockville, ML.

Roy N, Bless DM (2000a). Toward a theory of the dispositional bases of functional dysphonia and vocal nodules: Exploring the role of personality and emotional adjustment. In: RD Kent, MJ Ball (Eds.), The handbook of voice quality measurement, Singular Publishing, San Diego, CA.

Roy N, Bless DM (2000b). Personality traits and psychological factors in voice pathology: a foundation for future research. J Speech Lang Hear Res 43: 737–748.

Roy N, Merrill R, Thibeault S et al. (2004a). Voice disorders in teachers and the general population: effects on work performance, attendance, and future career choices. J Speech Lang Hear Disord 47: 542–551.

Roy N, Merrill RM, Thibeault S et al. (2004b). Prevalence of voice disorders in teachers and the general population. J Speech Lang Hear Res 47: 281–293.

Roy N, Gouse M, Mauszycki SC et al. (2005a). Task specificity in adductor spasomodic dysphonia versus muscle tension dysphonia. Laryngoscope 115: 311–316.

Roy N, Merrill R, Gray SD et al. (2005b). Voice disorders in the general population: prevalence, risk factors, and occupational impact. Laryngoscope 115: 1988–1995.

Roy N, Mauszycki SC, Merrill RM et al. (2007). Toward improved differential diagnosis of adductor spasmodic dysphonia and muscle tension dysphonia. Folia Phoniatr Logop 59: 83–90.

Roy N, Whitchurch M, Merrill RM et al. (2008). Differential diagnosis of adductor spasmodic dysphonia and muscle tension dysphonia using phonatory break analysis. Laryngoscope 118: 2245–2253.

Roy N, Barton M, Smith ME et al. (2009). An in vivo model of acute ESLN paralysis: laryngoscopic findings. Laryngoscope 119: 1017–1032.

Roy N, Smith M, Houtz D (2011). Laryngoscopic features of external superior laryngeal nerve denervation: revisiting a century old controversy. Ann Otol Rhinol Laryngol 120: 1–8.

Russell A (1999). Voice problems in teachers: Prevalence and prediction, PhD, La Trobe University.

Russell A, Oates J, Greenwood KM (1998). Prevalence of voice problems in teachers. J Voice 4: 467–479.

Russell A, Oates J, Greenwood K (2005). Prevalence of self-reported voice problems in the general population in South Australia. Adv Speech Lang Pathol 7: 24–30.

Sama A, Carding PN, Price S et al. (2001). The clinical features of functional dysphonia. Laryngoscope 111: 458–463.

Sapir S, Aronson AE (1985). Aphonia after closed head injury. Br J Disord Commun 20: 289–296.

Sapir S, Aronson AE (1987). Coexisting psychogenic and neurogenic dysphonia: a source of diagnostic confusion. Br J Disord Commun 22: 73–80.

Seifert E, Kollbrunner J (2005). Stress and distress in non-organic voice disorders. Swiss Med Wkly 135: 387–397.

Smurthwaite H (1919). War neuroses of the larynx and speech mechanism. J Laryngol Otol 13–20.

Sokolowsky RR (1944). War aphonia. J Speech Disord 9: 193–208.

Stemple JC, Roy N, Klaben BK (2014). Clinical voice pathology, Plural Publishing, San Diego, CA.

Stone J, LaFrance WC, Brown R et al. (2011). Conversion Disorder: current problems and potential solutions for DSM-5. J Psychosom Res 71: 369–376.

Stone J, Warlow C, Sharpe M (2012). Functional weakness: clues to mechanism from the nature of onset. J Neurol Neurosurg Psychiatry 83: 67–69.

van Beilen M, Vogt BA, Leenders KL (2010). Increased activation in cingulate cortex in conversion disorder: What does it mean? J Neurol Sci 289: 155–158.

van Mersbergen M, Patrick C, Glaze L (2008). Functional dysphonia during mental imagery: testing the trait theory of voice disorders. J Speech Lang Hear Res 51: 1405–1423.

Verdolini K, Rosen CA, Branski RC (Eds.), (2006). Classification Manual for Voice Disorders – I. Laurence Erlbaum, New Jersey.

Vertigan AE, Theodoros DG, Gibson PG et al. (2007a). Voice and upper airway symptoms in people with chronic cough and paradoxical vocal fold movement. J Voice 21: 361–383.

Vertigan AE, Theodoros DG, Winkworth A (2007b). Perceptual voice characteristics in chronic cough and paradoxical vocal fold movement. Folia Phoniatr Logop 59: 256–267.

Voon V, Brezing C, Gallea C et al. (2010). Emotional stimuli and motor conversion disorder. Brain 133: 1526–1536.

White A, Deary IJ, Wilson JA (1997). Psychiatric disturbance and personality traits in dysphonic patients. Eur J Disord Commun 32: 307–314.

Willinger U, Volkl-Kernstock S, Aschauer HN (2005). Marked depression and anxiety in patients with functional dysphonia. Psychiatry Res 134: 85–91.

Wilson JA, Deary IJ, MacKenzie K (1995). Functional dysphonia. Not 'hysterical' but seen mainly in women. BMJ 311: 1039–1040.

Handbook of Clinical Neurology, Vol. 139 (3rd series)
Functional Neurologic Disorders
M. Hallett, J. Stone, and A. Carson, Editors
http://dx.doi.org/10.1016/B978-0-12-801772-2.00035-7

Chapter 35

Psychologic/functional forms of memory disorder

J. GRIEM[1]*, J. STONE[2], A. CARSON[3], AND M.D. KOPELMAN[1]

[1]*Institute of Psychiatry, Psychology and Neuroscience, King's College London, London, UK*

[2]*Department of Clinical Neurosciences, Centre for Clinical Brain Sciences, University of Edinburgh, Edinburgh, UK*

[3]*Departments of Clinical Neurosciences and of Rehabilitation Medicine, NHS Lothian and Centre for Clinical Brain Sciences, University of Edinburgh, Edinburgh, UK*

Abstract

In this chapter, we discuss the wide variety of patients who may attend a memory clinic or other health services presenting with memory symptoms but who do not have dementia. These diagnoses may include a wide range of neurologic and neuropsychiatric disorders; in this chapter we will focus on other causes of memory symptoms which may be labeled psychologic or functional, or be more obviously part of an established psychiatric disorder. We describe the differential categorization recently posited by Stone et al. (2015), and consider important aspects of assessment and management in these cases.

INTRODUCTION

Walking into a room only to forget why, or feeling frozen on the spot when you cannot remember your PIN code when it is your turn to pay are examples of everyday forgetfulness we have all experienced. These little memory slips do not usually indicate any form of memory problem, and in fact they are relatively normal. McCaffrey and colleagues (2006) emphasized that it is important to consider the base rate, or the average rate, of this everyday subjective forgetfulness in a given population, which might indicate how "normal" it is. For example, it was shown that the rate of forgetfulness increases with age in the healthy aging population, and may correlate as well with other factors such as depression and subjective health (Commissaris et al., 1998; Montejo et al., 2011). More importantly, the base rate might also be useful for clinicians in identifying when the rate of subjective forgetfulness becomes abnormal (McCaffrey et al., 2003).

Increasingly, individuals may be more aware of both their own subjective forgetfulness as well as general memory disorders like dementia, and may seek medical advice if worried. This may in part be due to rising media coverage focusing on the risks, causes, symptoms, and prognosis or outcome of dementia, which of course is helpful for those who actually have or develop dementia, but may be causing unnecessary anxiety in those who do not (Stone et al., 2015). The increasing media coverage reflects a current trend in memory research: much research and clinical work is focused on studying dementia, leading to advances in identifying and screening for dementia, and the associated benefit of recognizing it earlier (Stone et al., 2015). Services for dementia are often located in geriatric or psychogeriatric departments. The bulk of patients seen in these clinics are over 65 and roughly two-thirds are estimated to be diagnosed with some form of dementia (Lindesay et al., 2002; Banerjee et al., 2007). However the rates of dementia diagnosed in memory clinics that serve younger populations is considerably lower, with figures of around 30–40% from Liverpool and Sheffield in the UK (Stone et al., 2015).

So what about those individuals with subjective memory complaints who do not end up with a dementia diagnosis? Importantly, there are many cases who have neurologic or neuropsychiatric disorders (Kopelman and Crawford, 1996; Kopelman, 2002). Other patients have memory problems which cannot be explained by a progressive neurologic disease like dementia or other underlying neurologic pathologies like head injuries, and often do not involve other general cognitive

*Correspondence to: Ms Julia Griem, Academic Unit of Neuropsychiatry, 3rd Floor, South Wing, Block D, St Thomas's Hospital, Westminster Bridge Road, London SE1 7EH, UK. E-mail: julia.griem@kcl.ac.uk

problems (Kopelman and Crawford, 1996; Kopelman, 2002; Stone et al., 2015). Stone and colleagues (2015) suggested this is a separate group of individuals who have a large range of varying memory problems above the base rate, often not age-related, which impede everyday independent functioning. Such individuals are often referred to memory clinics from a variety of sources, but due to a lack of adequate diagnostic and therapeutic understanding and/or limited specialist availability, they may not receive the attention or management they need (Kopelman and Crawford, 1996; Hejl et al., 2002; Stone et al., 2015).

As is evident, both research and clinical work in this group of individuals is relatively limited. Nevertheless, recent attempts at studying and evaluating memory clinics and this group of individuals with nondementia memory complaints exist. This is both in terms of understanding their demographics and referral reasons (Kopelman and Crawford, 1996), and in terms of developing a more reliable system for identification, etiology, diagnosis, and treatment of their problems which can be used in services (Stone et al., 2015).

MEMORY CLINICS

Existing studies of memory clinics

Since the emergence of memory clinics in the 1980s, the number has substantially increased (Passmore and Craig, 2004). Lindesay and colleagues (2002) characterized services of 58 memory clinics across the UK and Ireland and found that clinics largely focus on specialist assessment, provision of information and advice, and initiating and monitoring treatment and management for memory problems. In recent years increasing efforts have been made in many countries to improve the availability of memory services, national health programs like the Memory Service National Accreditation Programme (MSNAP) have further increased the awareness and potentially the availability of memory services, and they generally aim to set standard guidelines clinics should follow in order not to miss patients who might develop dementia, and not to overlook patients who need other support (Doncaster et al., 2011). In an analysis of memory services in a local area of London, Banerjee and colleagues (2007) found that 33% of patients did not receive a clinical diagnosis. Further evaluation is needed to see whether the memory complaints of these individuals have underlying or associated causes which are poorly understood in the geriatric dementia-focused environment. There may be an overemphasis on dementia which limits knowledge, understanding, and available assessment and management of other forms of memory problems.

Many memory services, especially those located in geriatric/psychogeriatric environments, are structured for identifying and managing dementia. However, other memory services are located in general medical or neurologic outpatient clinics. Luce and colleagues (2001) compared an old-age psychiatry service with a general memory clinic and found that patients in general memory clinics were younger and manifested a wider range of complaints. Nevertheless, the main difference was in the age of dementia detection, rather than in the identification of other nondementia problems. More clinics are now targeting the under-65 age group (Luce et al., 2001; Doncaster et al., 2011). These clinics have been found to have fewer dementia diagnoses, with rates declining from 40% in 2006 to 24% in 2010 (Menon and Larner, 2010). Blackburn and colleagues (2013) found that the number of neurologic etiologies or diagnoses for memory problems in their clinic decreased from 65% to 45% between 2004 and 2012, and suggested that the number of psychiatric memory disorder diagnoses had increased.

Menon and Larner (2010) indicated that many individuals without dementia diagnoses are simply the "worried well" – those who, due to increased awareness of dementia and its devastating consequences, are overly careful and worried about their everyday memory problems. Other studies have also reported 30% of patients in a memory clinic as either "memory complainers (no diagnosis)" or "neurotic/mood disorder" (Stone et al., 2015). Although there is evidently a change in the approach to memory problems in the clinic, receiving a "memory complainer" diagnosis is not very helpful for a patient. It should be acknowledged that there is a danger in dismissing patients as the "worried well" and this carries a risk because important but subtle neurologic or neuropsychiatric causes may be missed. Further research into understanding, assessing, and managing memory problems unrelated to dementia is clearly required.

Patients in memory clinics – a range of different disorders

In a discussion on functional/psychologic memory symptoms from a neurology clinic perspective, Stone and colleagues (2015) devised a suggested differential diagnosis of symptoms which might be functional in nature. Beyond dissociative amnesia, psychologically based memory problems are relatively poorly recognized in diagnostic manuals like the *International Classification of Diseases* (ICD-10: World Health Organization, 2010), and the *Diagnostic and Statistical Manual of Mental Disorders,* 5th edition (DSM-5: American Psychiatric Association, 2013) (where it is not included within the definition of conversion disorder). Therefore, differentiating symptoms may guide assessment and appropriate management of psychogenic/functional symptoms to a better extent than previous evidence. Nevertheless, there is some overlap between the symptoms, such that the categories are not entirely mutually exclusive, but are likely to have dissociable causes, treatments, and outcomes.

Stone et al. (2015) have suggested a differential diagnosis for a subgroup of these nondementia memory complaints which includes patients with psychiatric memory symptoms. Psychologically based or functional memory symptoms are genuine and distressing complaints or signs of memory problems, which might mimic disease symptoms, but cannot be explained by an underlying neurologic etiology or disease. In some cases, they might be associated with psychologic factors like depression or anxiety (Kopelman and Crawford, 1996). Stone et al. (2015) suggested the term functional is used similarly as in other diagnoses like functional movement disorder (Reuber et al., 2007). They claimed this group of individuals is much neglected, and must be understood better in terms of their diagnosis, especially as some symptoms may be reversible if identified correctly (Hejl et al., 2002; Koepsell and Monsell, 2012). Stone et al. (2015) aimed to develop a suggested differential diagnosis of the memory symptoms in order to make suggestions for more positive diagnostic and treatment approaches. This might be helpful in guiding memory clinics on patients who do not have dementia. It should, however, be remembered that there are numerous other causes of memory loss that are neither dementia nor variants of functional disorders and those too must be considered.

NEUROLOGIC CAUSES OF MEMORY SYMPTOMS OTHER THAN DEMENTIA

In any discussion of memory disorders, it should be acknowledged that symptoms can arise from a wide variety of different neurologic or neuropsychiatric causes other than neurodegenerative dementias. There may be a past history of head injury, human immunodeficiency virus (HIV) infection, or deficiencies in vitamins B_1 and B_{12}, or thyroid function. The person may be drinking more than, or taking substances which, s/he does not readily admit to. There may be a sleep disorder. The client may be in the very earliest stages of a dementia, i.e., before the patient fulfills diagnostic criteria even for mild cognitive impairment. Particularly important issues to consider are as follows.

Diseases other than dementia causing memory disorders

In dementia-focused memory clinics, other neurologic disease etiologies may be overlooked more easily. Kopelman (2002) has distinguished between transient or discrete episodes of memory loss, as in the transient global amnesia syndrome, transient epileptic amnesia, or a confusional state, and more persistent memory disorders, which include the amnesic syndrome and milder forms of memory disorders (falling short of a diagnosis of amnesic syndrome) – for example, in multiple sclerosis, autoimmune encephalitis, paraneoplastic disorders, central nervous system infections, and metabolic disorders (including hypoxic brain damage). Additionally, other general medical disorders like obstructive sleep apnea can lead to memory problems, associated with concentration deficits.

Memory symptoms secondary to alcohol/ substance abuse or prescribed medication

There are many cases of memory problems secondary to alcohol misuse or dependence, resulting in memory and other cognitive problems, which do not strictly fulfill criteria for the alcoholic Korsakoff syndrome (Royal College of Psychiatrists, 2014). Other cases may arise from misuse of cannabis or other substances. Memory symptoms following prescribed medication, such as opiates for severe, sometimes chronic, pain as well as medications, including those for psychiatric disorders like depression, may also lead to memory problems.

Patients with psychiatric symptoms who actually go on to develop dementia

This category should be considered if a patient presents with memory problems but does not receive a dementia diagnosis. There is always a risk that a small proportion of individuals with apparently psychologic or "functional" symptoms with or without anxiety and depression may go on to develop a form of dementia or another neurologic disease. In these situations, the disorder is probably best considered a prodrome in the same way as an anxiety or depressive disorder can be the prodrome to a dementia syndrome. Such prodromes appear not to be limited to memory complaints and the authors have had a small number of patients with clear functional paresis who went on to develop frontotemporal dementia within 12 months; it may, of course, be coincidence, but viewed in retrospect it appears likely the symptom has been prodromal. This is best monitored by follow-up assessment of a patient, especially if memory problems persist throughout attempted management and treatment of a psychiatric diagnosis. Advances in neuroimaging and cerebrospinal fluid analysis might aid clinicians in distinguishing between individuals with apparently psychologic or functional symptoms and individuals with early, prodromal dementia, although ultimately the diagnosis of dementia is likely to remain a clinical decision.

PSYCHOLOGICAL/FUNCTIONAL CAUSES OF MEMORY SYMPTOMS

Memory symptoms as part of depression/ anxiety

As Commissaris et al. (1998) and Montejo et al. (2011) have identified, forgetfulness in individuals correlates with the presence of depression. Indeed, depression and anxiety are defined according to several symptoms, including fatigue, poor sleep, and poor concentration (Vaccarino et al., 2008). In healthy elderly individuals, the frequency of subjective memory complaints is associated with subsyndromal depression as well as anxiety (Balash et al., 2013). In fact, memory problems or poor memory and concentration are part of diagnostic criteria for major depression, as well as generalized anxiety disorder in the DSM. Fischer and colleagues (2008) compared depressed and nondepressed individuals without neurological diseases, substance abuse, or psychosis, and found that subjective memory complaints were significantly higher in the group diagnosed with major depression disorder.

Subjective memory problems associated with depression or anxiety may not become apparent from objective neuropsychologic testing (Fischer et al., 2008). Although this might result from poor sensitivity of the neuropsychologic tests, it may also suggest that individuals with depression or anxiety have an impaired expectation of their memory. Hence, they come to memory clinics with subjective memory complaints. Neuropsychologic testing should certainly not be the only approach in diagnosing memory complaints – a good history and mental-state evaluation are essential. Merema et al. (2013) suggested that both depression and memory complaints are linked by the presence of high neuroticism, suggesting that there might not be a direct causal relationship between depression/anxiety and memory complaints. On the other hand, memory symptoms are associated with, and may be a part of, an underlying depression or anxiety disorder. Additionally, increased awareness about or sensitivity towards memory problems (due to impaired memory expectation) may lead to subjective increase in depression or anxiety symptoms. If this is the case, then identification of this underlying problem is crucial in evaluating the nature and prognosis of the memory problem.

Patients with major depression tend to show overgeneralization in their memory (i.e., they cannot deal with specifics) and have difficulties with accessing positive memories (Nandrino et al., 2002). The mechanisms underpinning memory impairment in depression have not been fully elucidated. It is well recognized that depression is associated with reduced hippocampal volume (Videbech and Ravnkilde, 2004) and it is hard in principle to believe that this is not relevant. However, the significance of reduced hippocampal volume, and even whether it is a state or trait phenomenon, remains a subject of debate (Burt et al., 1995; MacQueen, 2009; MacQueen et al., 2003). Furthermore there is debate over whether subjective memory loss is truly a memory disorder or whether it relates more to attentional and, to a lesser extent, executive problems (Marazziti et al., 2010). However, more recent models are teasing apart some of these contradictions and appear promising – linking hippocampal pathology to glucocorticoid metabolism and to aspects of memory function (Nestler et al., 2002; Becker and Wojtowicz, 2007).

Aside from formal diagnoses of a depressive disorder, anxiety syndrome, or posttraumatic stress disorder, there may be transient life stresses – in marriage or relationships, at work, or in study – which do not fit a formal ICD-10 category, but which can be very important, and for which there is help readily available, if the stress is identified, in the form of counseling or cognitive-behavioral therapy.

"Normal" memory symptoms that become the focus of attention or anxiety

As indicated by studies of forgetfulness in the healthy population (Commissaris et al., 1998; Montejo et al., 2011; Balash et al., 2013), everyday forgetting is relatively common. Some individuals may be referred to memory clinics because of a strong focus or attention on these normal, everyday memory symptoms. Stone et al. (2015) suggested this may be due to one of three following reasons: (1) high subjective expectations for memory ability; (2) high subjective expectation of memory services, demanding management of normal memory complaints; or (3) referral by inexperienced or worried general practitioners. In any event, this group of individuals should not be neglected. Sometimes, simply reassuring people that their memory is "normal" is all that is needed, but more often this is not the case and clinicians need to remember that, whilst the memory may be normal, the degree of worry is not.

Health anxiety about dementia/memory

Health anxiety is the phenomenon by which individuals are overly sensitive, worried, or anxious about their own health, and may base their anxiety somewhat on assumptions about possible illnesses (Marcus et al., 2007). In some, any sign of a health problem (as small as a sneeze) might be taken very seriously, and may lead to a constant concern that the person is unwell or developing a serious disease. More commonly there is a background propensity to health anxiety that is particularly focused on a specific disorder. In severe cases, individuals like this were traditionally categorized as suffering from hypochondriasis or somatization disorder. Such focusing can usually be understood either temporally or diagnostically by exploration of a patient's illness experience and beliefs; i.e., there may be a long-term anxiety owing to a family history of dementia, or during a period of work-related stress, exposure to an newspaper article or a personal experience of dementia in a relative may completely alter how a "normal" memory failure is interpreted. We would predict the risk of this will increase with the heightened awareness and increased media attention on dementia in recent years. This is one potential explanation for the increased rates of "not dementia" diagnoses being reported from memory clinics. Thus, a person may appear at a memory clinic with increased health anxiety about developing dementia when simply showing normal rates of forgetfulness. This may also be partly due to a dysfunctional belief about dementia or memory (Marcus et al., 2007). Again, this diagnosis should not be neglected, as there are some successful therapeutic approaches described (Taylor and Asmundson, 2004). In Kopelman's terminology (Kopelman and Crawford, 1996), such patients are said to have "anxiety about memory" or "subjective memory complaints."

Memory symptoms as part of another functional disorder

Similar to the relatively high presence of depression in various psychiatric and medical disorders (Vaccarino et al., 2008), memory problems and subjective memory complaints are associated with various other disorders, such as fibromyalgia, chronic fatigue syndrome, irritable-bowel syndrome, and dissociative nonepileptic seizures. Concentration and sleep may also be impaired in these disorders, and increased subjective memory problems in this context have previously been described (Kopelman and Crawford, 1996; Grace et al., 1999). These disorders are believed to be mediated by a heightened, overly precise attentional focus on the affected body part (Edwards et al., 2012). If excess attention and processing power are being used in this way, then given the limited processing capacity of the brain, these systems cannot be doing their normal tasks, and the end result will be the perception of memory and concentration impairment. This finding is ubiquitous in functional motor symptoms to the extent that, if not present, one should at least question a functional etiology for the motor symptom.

Psychogenic memory disorder as an isolated symptom

Stone et al. (2015) reserved "isolated functional memory disorder" to describe patients who have greater everyday forgetfulness than normal which cannot be explained on the basis of comorbid anxiety or depressive symptoms, and impacts the individual's social and occupational functioning. Stone et al. (2015) argued that strong internal inconsistencies in memory reporting and day-to-day function and within neuropsychologic testing itself are core features of a functional memory disorder.

Kopelman (2002) has distinguished between what he calls global and situation-specific psychogenic amnesia. In global psychogenic amnesia, the person forgets all of his/her previous memories, and this is often accompanied by a loss of the sense of personal identity, as in a fugue state or so-called focal retrograde amnesia. In situation-specific psychogenic amnesia, there is simply a gap in the memory for a stressful event or incident, as in posttraumatic stress disorder, victims of crime (such as rape or child sexual abuse), and occasionally in offenders themselves.

In some cases, the history reveals a very time-specific retrograde (mostly autobiographic) amnesia preceding a particular time point or age, accompanied by intact anterograde memory (although in epilepsy cases, it is arguable that the deficit itself was in anterograde encoding, which then leaves an amnesic gap, reported as a retrograde gap historically). There may be a loss of personal identity, and the patients appear perplexed or even confused. Whilst neurologically caused amnesias characteristically show a temporal gradient by which older memories are recalled better than newer memories, psychogenic cases sometimes show a "reversed" temporal gradient. A fugue state consists of a sudden loss of all autobiographic memories, together with the sense of personal identity, often accompanied by a period of wandering, lasting a few hours or days (up to 4 weeks) (Schacter et al., 1982; Kopelman, 1987, 2002).

Kopelman (2002) created a model of psychogenic retrograde amnesia which incorporated the influence of precipitating stressors and current mood state (as well as the influence of any previous transient memory disorder) (Fig. 35.1). The maladaptive interplay of these factors was hypothesized to activate frontal inhibitory mechanisms, which prevent the retrieval of past autobiographic memories, and (if severe) personal semantic knowledge (identity) as well. This may result in the person appearing perplexed and lacking in affect, rather than depressed or aroused. Although s/he appears to be functioning normally in the environment, perhaps because of a relatively preserved medial temporal/diencephalic system, the latter cannot be functioning completely normally, because events which happened during the fugue are forgotten on recovery. There are functional imaging findings consistent with this model (Anderson et al., 2004; Kikuchi et al., 2009).

EXAGGERATION/MALINGERING OF MEMORY SYMPTOMS

Memory complaints may be exaggerated or malingered, sometimes (but not always) in the context of a legal

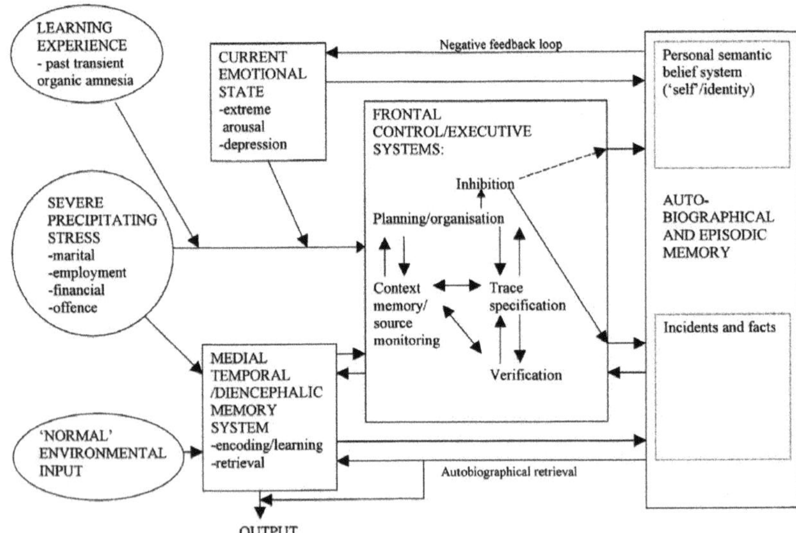

Fig. 35.1. The proposed model of retrograde (psychogenic) amnesia created by Kopelman (2002). It shows the interplay between psychologic and social factors, and frontal/executive inhibitory mechanisms, which prevent autobiographic memory retrieval and, in extreme cases, knowledge of personal identity. (Reproduced from Kopelman, 2002.)

claim. Malingering and factitious disorders are best identified by determining a marked discrepancy between what an individual says s/he can do (I can't read a newspaper) and what s/he is subsequently observed to do (seen reading a newspaper). Importantly, a discrepancy between the patient's subjectively reported difficulties (I can't remember anything, my memory is awful) and the subjectively reported function (I'm able to do my complex administrative job without any complaint) is not evidence of exaggeration. This is evidence that the patient has difficulty making an objective self-report. The same internal inconsistencies may be present on assessment.

Symptom validity/effort testing may be useful to assess the patient. These are tests in which even patients with moderate dementia or brain injury should perform reasonably well, and at least at chance level. Failure of effort testing is not always proof of conscious exaggeration. Some patients appear to "exaggerate to convince" health professionals there is a problem, consciously or otherwise. It is likely that exaggeration of genuine symptoms is far more prevalent than frank malingering. We also do not fully understand the preconscious component in the development of memory symptoms and it is unwise to impute a sinister motive in an area of such complexity. These issues are discussed in detail by Silver (2012).

APPROACHES TO ASSESSMENT

A good neuropsychiatric history and mental-state assessment are always required (Kopelman, 1994). The presence of other psychologically based disorders, especially functional neurologic disorders, should be a "red flag," but it is important to make a diagnosis on the basis of the memory symptoms themselves. Speaking to informants and follow-up are often crucial for accurate diagnosis. Neuropsychologic testing is also very important. A range of neuropsychologic memory tests has been validated in different contexts, and can usually indicate the nature of memory problems in a more quantitative way than can be described subjectively by an individual. An increasing range of symptom validity tests is now available (Merten and Merckelbach, 2013).

Table 35.1 summarizes some factors which may indicate memory problems particularly of a psychologic/functional rather than neurologic origin. However, these factors are not in themselves conclusive, and should be interpreted in the light of neurologic and psychiatric assessment. Reuber's group in Sheffield have used a highly detailed conversational analysis technique that they first promoted in the study of dissociative seizures to look at the different patterns of clinical interaction between patients with dementia and patients with functional memory disorders). They (Jones et al., 2015) found five key factors which they argued might suggest functional origin: (1) whether the individual can answer questions about personal facts/information, with dementia patients being unable to say how old they are or where they live; (2) dementia patients were also unable to remember details of their memory lapses – this may be judged based on interaction with clinician; (3) to answer questions with multiple components; (4) dementia patients tended to delay before answering questions; and (5) they were unlikely to give spontaneous elaboration of detail in answers to questions.

Table 35.1

A range of factors indicating which memory problems are more likely to be functional than neurologic in nature (adapted from Stone et al., 2015)

Functional	Neurologic diseases
Young	Older
Attends alone	Attends with someone
Patient more aware of the problem than others	Others more aware of the problem than patient
Able to detail list of drugs, previous interactions with doctors	Less able
Watches TV dramas	Stops following drama
Marked variability	Less variability
Types of memory symptoms are usually within most people's normal experience	Types of memory symptoms are often out with normal experiences
"I used to have a brilliant memory"	Does not highlight previous "brilliant memory"
Can answer questions about personal facts/information	Unable to say how old they are or where they live
Can answer questions with multiple components	Can only manage single-component questions
Answering questions with normal flow	Tend to delay before answering questions
Frequently offers elaboration and detail	Unlikely to give spontaneous elaboration of detail
Confident in their interacting with the doctor	Lack confidence in their interactions
Answers questions in a way that suggests correct answer is known at some level, e.g., 50:50 questions at considerably less than chance or questions with answers that are always out by same small margin	Failures demonstrate a lack of knowledge of correct answer

In a further report, Elsey et al. (2015) found patients with "functional memory problems" were more likely to attend clinic alone, much less likely to look for any companion's help in answering questions, more likely to provide detail in answers to questions, were confident in their interaction with the doctor, and tended to give extended and detailed answers of memory lapses. By contrast, the dementia patients tended to look for assistance from their companion with questions, were much less confident, often unable to give structured answers, frequently answered "I don't know," and generally struggled to communicate meaningfully.

Andrew Larner has also examined some of these interactions systematically and had broadly similar, although less detailed, findings. In his clinic all patients are instructed in their booking letter to attend with a relative. Larner (2005) found that whether or not this instruction was actually obeyed had reasonable predictive validity for the presence or absence of dementia. They concluded that if attending the clinic with a relative, friend, or carer (that is, following the instructions given in the appointment letter) was considered a diagnostic test for dementia, it would have a sensitivity of 100% (95% confidence interval (CI) 96–100%, Wilson method), specificity of 35% (95% CI 26–46%), and positive and negative predictive values of 60% (95% CI 52–67%) and 100% (95% CI 90–100%), respectively. Positive likelihood ratio was 1.55 (95% CI 1.33–1.80, log method), judged unimportant, but negative likelihood ratio (0) was large. This supports the belief that attending the neurology clinic alone despite written instructions to the contrary is a robust sign of the absence of dementia.

NHS Evidence Clinical Knowledge Summary advises that the diagnosis of dementia be suspected "if, when you ask the person a simple question, they immediately turn to their partner — the so-called head-turning sign (HTS)." Larner (2012) tested this in a mixed cohort of 207 memory clinic attenders. For the whole cohort, 52 (25.1%) were HTS+ and 155 (74.9%) were HTS−. HTS+ was found to be very specific for the presence of cognitive impairment (0.98), but not very sensitive (0.60), with correspondingly excellent positive predictive value (0.94).

Schmidtke and colleagues (2008) argued that previous dissociative lapses may also indicate psychologic or functional problems. They proposed a Functional Memory Disorders Inventory of items, which they suggested may indicate psychologic causation (Table 35.2). Whilst this technique may heighten awareness of psychologic causation, we suggest caution and that it should not be used as a diagnostic indicator in its own right.

Cognitive testing may be normal, which may provide evidence to patients that their memory is not as bad as they thought. More commonly, though, formal testing may produce a range of minor abnormalities or low scores that must be interpreted with caution, considering both anxiety and also the possibility of suboptimal effort or exaggeration. Executive, attention, and memory difficulties are common, but there may be evidence of internal inconsistency mirroring that seen during the consultation. For example, patients may do much worse on simple tests of recall than they do on more complex delayed recall tests.

Pennington et al. (2015) described their experience of 196 patients attending their memory clinic, of whom 23 were diagnosed with so-called functional cognitive disorder (note that "cognitive" is a much broader concept than "memory," and should not be used interchangeably). On neuropsychologic testing, roughly half had

Table 35.2

The Functional Memory Disorders Inventory

Items related to a deficit of working memory and concentration	Do your forget errands on the way to their execution? Do you rapidly forget essential parts of a personal or telephone conversation? Do you experience disruptions of the thread of thoughts in conversations? Do you experience absent-mindedness and day dreaming during conversations?
Items related to a deficit of the registration of new contents	Do you forget important contents of conversations, appointments, and errands (timescale of days)? Do you experience difficulties understanding and registering the contents of news, reading, and lectures?
Items related to a deficit of retrieval	Do you experience blocks of retrieval of well-known names, phone numbers, PIN codes, etc. (but typically recall them later)? Do you commit errors, or experience "blackouts" during routine activities at work, at home, while driving, etc.? Do you experience difficulties finding words?
Item related to the variability of symptom severity	Is your memory impairment subject to variations, namely less marked during times of relaxation?

Reproduced from Schmidtke et al. (2008).

an invalid pattern of results, or failed tests of performance validity. Of those with valid neuropsychologic results, 80% scored in the normal range. Depression and anxiety were common but did not appear to be the primary cause of cognitive symptoms. Particular characteristics seen were excessively low self-rating of memory ability, and discrepancies between perceived and actual cognitive performance. The rate of unemployment was high, often due to the cognitive symptomatology.

A major factor in delineating the appropriate diagnosis is ensuring there is not another diagnosis that provides a better explanation of the presenting problem. Assessment of patients with unexplained memory problems may need to be multidisciplinary and to be undertaken at regular intervals not only to consider the possibility in some patients of developing dementia but also to undertake treatment of patients with psychogenic/functional memory disorders. We reiterate that crucial to any diagnosis is taking a good medical and psychiatric history, neurologic examination, medical state assessment, seeing an informant, and neuropsychologic assessment.

APPROACHES TO TREATMENT

If assessment leads to a confident diagnosis of an underlying psychologically based memory problem, some approaches to treatment have been suggested. As Stone and colleagues (2015) have noted, it is vital that patients understand and have some confidence in their diagnosis in order for therapeutic approaches to work. This in turn requires a clinician to be able to have confidence in the diagnosis and to deliver a clear explanation. The principles of communicating the diagnosis of functional or psychologic disorders are described in Chapter 44 and in Carson et al. (2016).

Some of the above diagnoses of a memory disorder have underlying etiologies for which pharmacologic and other treatments are available. This is true for depression and anxiety as well as stress- and/or trauma-related dissociative amnesia. If memory problems are due to depression or anxiety (including health anxiety or increased attention on memory problems), then attempting to treat this may lead to a substantial reduction in memory problems, and may even reverse them (Hejl et al., 2002; Koepsell and Monsell, 2012; Cassell and Humphreys, 2015). Cognitive-behavioral therapy is the most common technique, as it has been shown to be very useful and successful in depression and anxiety (Taylor and Asmundson, 2004; Butler et al., 2006; Marcus et al., 2007). Consistent with the necessity for individuals to understand their functional diagnosis, psychoeducational approaches towards treating depression and anxiety may also reduce memory problems (Donker et al., 2009). Finally, an intervention (MEmory Specificity Training, MEST) targeting to increase specificity of memories in depression has been shown to successfully increase specificity of autobiographic memory retrieval (Raes et al., 2009), so incorporating this into therapeutic techniques may be promising.

More recently, the use of other cognitive techniques has increased. Specifically, cognitive rehabilitation has been proposed to be helpful with functional memory problems but needs to be properly tested (Kapur et al., 2002; Migo et al., 2014). This may include errorless learning, the method of vanishing cues, the provision of and advice about the use of memory aids, and addressing beliefs about memory. Ideally, attempting to teach individuals to "reutilize" their memory may be useful, as they tend to associate their memory with failure and so functionally block the use of their memory. Psychogenic retrograde amnesia may be successfully targeted with various psychologic therapies, including those typically used in trauma-focused therapy (McKay and Kopelman, 2009; Cassell and Humphreys, 2015).

As discussed above, specialist memory clinics are not only tasked to assess memory problems, but also to maintain the adequate management and treatment of memory problems, and an important component of this is the continuous screening and monitoring of memory problems. It may become evident that an individual is in fact developing dementia if s/he is not responding to the various approaches to treating functional memory symptoms. Overall, treatment is essential, especially in those cases where it can stabilize or even reverse memory problems (Hejl et al., 2002).

CONCLUSION AND FUTURE DIRECTIONS

In conclusion, this chapter has given a brief insight into the current state of research into psychologic forms of memory disorders. Although there has been advocacy for the increasing availability and accessibility of memory services, they are still somewhat focused on the over-65 age group and are often specialized in assessing and managing dementia. Although this is a gain in our aging society, other memory problems are often neglected – both in research and in clinic. It has become clear that multispecialist and multidisciplinary input is required at all stages, and one might suggest that further research into these symptoms may increase both awareness and understanding. Through further national healthcare programs, this may then be passed down to individual professionals in various specialist memory clinics, in order to not only successfully identify and treat individuals with dementia, but also to support individuals with various other memory complaints. Future progress may require both increasing the accessibility to specialized memory clinics for assessment and treatment, and also increasing the diagnostic acumen of clinicians in cognitive disorders.

Further research will also facilitate the understanding of complex memory problems at all levels (symptoms, assessment, diagnosis, and treatment) as well as producing improved awareness of these problems in memory clinics. Individuals with subjective memory problems should no longer be diagnosed as "memory complainers," and even if their memory is assessed to be normal, they should receive an explanation as to how and why this is the case. Specialist services (including multidisciplinary teams) and enhanced training are required in order to serve these patients better and to improve their wellbeing and quality of life, as well as to reduce the impact on social and occupational functioning.

References

American Psychiatric Association (2013). Diagnostic and Statistical Manual of Mental Disorders, 5th edn. American Psychiatric Association, Washington, DC.

Anderson MC, Ochsner KN, Kuhl B et al. (2004). Neural systems underlying the suppression of unwanted memories. Science 303: 232–235.

Balash Y, Mordechovich M, Shabtai H et al. (2013). Subjective memory complaints in elders: depression, anxiety, or cognitive decline? Acta Neurol Scand 127 (5): 344–350.

Banerjee S, Willis R, Matthews D et al. (2007). Improving the quality of care for mild to moderate dementia: an evaluation of the Croydon Memory Service Model. Int J Geriatr Psychiatry 22 (8): 782–788.

Becker S, Wojtowicz JM (2007). A model of hippocampal neurogenesis in memory and mood disorders. Trends Cogn Sci 11 (2): 70–76.

Blackburn DJ, Shanks MF, Harkness KA et al. (2013). Political drive to screen for pre-dementia: not evidence based and ignores the harms of diagnosis. BMJ 347: f5125.

Burt DB, Zembar MJ, Niederehe G (1995). Depression and memory impairment: a meta-analysis of the association, its pattern, and specificity. Psychol Bull 117 (2): 285.

Butler AC, Chapman JE, Forman EM et al. (2006). The empirical status of cognitive-behavioural therapy: a review of meta-analyses. Clin Psychol Rev 26 (1): 17–31.

Carson A, Lehn A, Ludwig L et al. (2016). Explaining functional disorders in the neurology clinic: a photo story. Pract Neurol 16 (1): 56–61.

Cassell A, Humphreys K (2015). Psychological therapy for psychogenic amnesia: successful treatment in a single case study. Neuropsychol Rehabil: 1–16.

Commissaris CJAM, Ponds RWHM, Jolles J (1998). Subjective forgetfulness in a normal Dutch population: possibilities for health education and other interventions. Patient Educ Couns 34 (1): 25–32.

Doncaster E, McGeorge M, Orrell M (2011). Developing and implementing quality standards for memory services: The Memory Services National Accreditation Programme (MSNAP). Aging Ment Health 15: 23–33.

Donker T, Griffiths KM, Cuijpers P et al. (2009). Psychoeducation for depression, anxiety and psychological distress: a meta-analysis. BMC Med 7 (79).

Edwards MJ, Adams RA, Brown H et al. (2012). A Bayesian account of 'hysteria'. Brain 135 (11): 3495–3512.

Elsey C, Drew P, Jones D et al. (2015). Towards diagnostic conversational profiles of patients presenting with dementia or functional memory disorders to memory clinics. Patient Educ Couns 98: 1071–1077.

Fischer C, Schweizer TA, Atkins JA et al. (2008). Neurocognitive profiles in older adults with and without major depression. Int J Geriatr Psychiatry 23 (8): 851–856.

Grace GM, Nielson WR, Hopkins M et al. (1999). Concentration and memory deficits in patients with fibromyalgia syndrome. J Clin Exp Neuropsychol 21 (4): 477–487.

Hejl A, Høgh P, Waldemar G (2002). Potentially reversible conditions in 1000 consecutive memory clinic patients. J Neurol Neurosurg Psychiatry 73: 390–394.

Jones D, Drew P, Elsey C et al. (2015). Conversational assessment in memory clinic encounters: interactional profiling for differentiating dementia from functional memory disorders. Aging Ment Health 1–10.

Kapur N, Gilsky EL, Wilson BA (2002). External memory aids and computers in memory rehabilitation. 2004, In: AD Baddeley, MD Kopelman, BA Wilson (Eds.), The Essential Handbook of Memory Disorders for Clinicians, John Wiley, Chichester.

Kikuchi H, Fujii T, Abe N et al. (2009). Memory repression: brain mechanisms underlying dissociative amnesia. J Cogn Neurosci 22 (3): 602–613.

Koepsell TD, Monsell SE (2012). Reversion from mild cognitive impairment to normal or near-normal cognition: Risk factors and prognosis. Neurology 79 (15): 1591–1598.

Kopelman M (1987). Amnesia: organic and psychogenic. Br J Psychiatry 150: 428–442.

Kopelman M (1994). Structured psychiatric interview: psychiatric history and assessment of the mental state. Br J Hosp Med 52 (2/3): 93–99.

Kopelman M (2002). Disorders of memory. Brain 125: 2152–2190.

Kopelman M, Crawford S (1996). Not all memory clinics are dementia clinics. Neuropsychol Rehabil 6 (3): 187–202.

Larner AJ (2005). 'Who came with you?' A diagnostic observation in patients with memory problems? J Neurol Neurosurg Psychiatry 76: 1739.

Larner AJ (2012). Head turning sign: pragmatic utility in clinical diagnosis of cognitive impairment. J Neurol Neurosurg Psychiatry 83: 852–853.

Lindesay J, Marudkar M, van Diepen E et al. (2002). The second survey of memory clinics in the British Isles. Int J Geriatr Psychiatry 17 (1): 41–47.

Luce A, McKeith I, Swann A et al. (2001). How do memory clinics compare with traditional old age psychiatry services? Int J Geriatr Psychiatry 16 (9): 837–845.

MacQueen GM (2009). A meta-analysis examining clinical predictors of hippocampal volume in patients with major depressive disorder. J Psychiatr Neurosci: JPN 34 (1): 41.

MacQueen GM, Campbell S, McEwen BS et al. (2003). Course of illness, hippocampal function, and hippocampal volume in major depression. Proc Natl Acad Sci 100 (3): 1387–1392.

Marazziti D, Consoli G, Picchetti M et al. (2010). Cognitive impairment in major depression. Eur J Pharmacol 626 (1): 83–86.

Marcus DK, Gurley JR, Marchi MM et al. (2007). Cognitive and perceptual variables in hypochondriasis and health anxiety: a systematic review. Clin Psychol Rev 27 (2): 127–139.

McCaffrey RJ, Palav AA, O'Bryant S et al. (Eds.), (2003). Practitioner's Guide to Symptom Base Rates in Clinical Neuropsychology, Springer Verlag, New York.

McCaffrey RJ, Bauer L, Palav AA et al. (Eds.), (2006). Practitioner's Guide to Symptom Base Rates in the General Population, Springer Verlag, New York.

McKay GCM, Kopelman MD (2009). Psychogenic amnesia: when memory complaints are medically unexplained. Adv Psychiatr Treat 15 (2): 152–158.

Menon R, Larner AJ (2010). Use of cognitive screening instruments in primary care: the impact of national dementia directives (NICE/SCIE, National Dementia Strategy). Fam Pract: 1–5.

Merema MR, Speelman CP, Foster JK et al. (2013). Neuroticism (not depressive symptoms) predicts memory complaints in some community-dwelling older adults. Am J Geriatr Psychiatry 21 (8): 729–736.

Merten T, Merckelbach H (2013). Symptom validity testing in somatoform and dissociative disorders: a critical review. Psychol Inj Law 6 (1).

Migo EM, Haynnes BI, Harris L et al. (2014). Health and memory aids: levels of smartphone ownership in patients. J Ment Health 24 (5).

Montejo P, Montenegro M, Fernandez MA et al. (2011). Subjective memory complaints in the elderly: prevalence and influence of temporal orientation, depression and quality of life in a population-based stud in the city of Madrid. Aging Ment Health 15 (1): 85–96.

Nandrino J-L, Pezard L, Posté A et al. (2002). Autobiographical memory in major depression: a comparison between first-episode and recurrent patients. Psychopathology 35 (6): 335–340.

Nestler EJ, Barrot M, DiLeone RJ et al. (2002). Neurobiology of depression. Neuron 34 (1): 13–25.

Passmore AP, Craig DA (2004). The future of memory clinics. The Royal College of Psychiatrists 28 (10): 375–377.

Pennington C, Hayre A, Newson M et al. (2015). Functional cognitive disorder: a common cause of subjective cognitive symptoms. J Alzheimer's Dis 48: S19–S24.

Raes F, Williams JMG, Hermans D (2009). Reducing cognitive vulnerability to depression: a preliminary investigation of MEST in inpatients with depressive symptomology. J Behav Ther Exp Psychiatry 40 (1): 24–38.

Reuber M, Howlett S, Khan A et al. (2007). Non-epileptic seizures and other functional neurological symptoms: predisposing, precipitating, and perpetuating factors. Psychosomatics 48 (3): 230–238.

Royal College of Psychiatrists (2014). Report of Working Party on Alcohol-related Brain Damage. Royal College of Psychiatrists, London.

Schacter DL, Wang PL, Tulving E et al. (1982). Functional retrograde amnesia: a quantitative case study. Neuropsychologia 20 (5): 523–532.

Schmidtke K, Pohlmann S, Metternich B (2008). The syndrome of functional memory disorder: definition, etiology and natural course. Am J of Geriatr Psychiatry 16 (12): 981–988.

Silver JM (2012). Effort, exaggeration and malingering after concussion. J Neurol Neurosurg Psychiatry 83 (8): 836–841.

Stone J, Suvankar P, Blackburn D et al. (2015). Functional (psychogenic) cognitive disorders: a perspective from the neurology clinic. J Alzheimers Dis 48 (s1): s5–s17.

Taylor S, Asmundson GJG (2004). Treating Health Anxiety: A Cognitive-Behavioural Approach. Guilford Press, New York.

Vaccarino AL, Sills TL, Evans KR et al. (2008). Prevalence and association of somatic symptoms in patients with major depressive disorder. J Affect Disord 110 (3): 270–276.

Videbech P, Ravnkilde B (2004). Hippocampal volume and depression: a meta-analysis of MRI studies. Am J Psychiatry 161: 1957–1966.

World Health Organization (2010). The ICD-10 classification of mental and behavioural disorders: clinical descriptions and diagnostic guidelines, World Health Organization, Geneva.

Handbook of Clinical Neurology, Vol. 139 (3rd series)
Functional Neurologic Disorders
M. Hallett, J. Stone, and A. Carson, Editors
http://dx.doi.org/10.1016/B978-0-12-801772-2.00036-9

Chapter 36

Functional (dissociative) retrograde amnesia

H.J. MARKOWITSCH[1]* AND A. STANILOIU[1,2]

[1]*Department of Physiological Psychology, University of Bielefeld, Bielefeld, Germany*

[2]*Department of Psychiatry, Sunnybrook Hospital, Toronto, ON, Canada*

Abstract

Retrograde amnesia is described as condition which can occur after direct brain damage, but which occurs more frequently as a result of a psychiatric illness. In order to understand the amnesic condition, content-based divisions of memory are defined. The measurement of retrograde memory is discussed and the dichotomy between "organic" and "psychogenic" retrograde amnesia is questioned. Briefly, brain damage-related etiologies of retrograde amnesia are mentioned. The major portion of the review is devoted to dissociative amnesia (also named psychogenic or functional amnesia) and to the discussion of an overlap between psychogenic and "brain organic" forms of amnesia. The "inability of access hypothesis" is proposed to account for most of both the organic and psychogenic (dissociative) patients with primarily retrograde amnesia. Questions such as why recovery from retrograde amnesia can occur in retrograde (dissociative) amnesia, and why long-term new learning of episodic-autobiographic episodes is possible, are addressed. It is concluded that research on retrograde amnesia research is still in its infancy, as the neural correlates of memory storage are still unknown. It is argued that the recollection of episodic-autobiographic episodes most likely involves frontotemporal regions of the right hemisphere, a region which appears to be hypometabolic in patients with dissociative amnesia.

INTRODUCTION

The Greek/Latin word *hysteria* refers to suffering in the uterus. It was used to describe women who had excessive emotional reactions of fear or panic without a direct organic basis. Patients with a condition of hysteria usually became unconscious or semiconscious in anxiety-provoking situations and later lacked remembrances related to the circumstances of the hysteric attack – that is, they were retrogradely amnesic (Fig. 36.1).

Jean-Martin Charcot at the Salpêtrière Hospital in Paris studied and described patients with hysteria in the second half of the 19th century (see the review of Bogousslavsky, 2011). The concept became very prominent at the beginning of the 20th century, popularized not only by French authors, but also, for example, by Sigmund Freud, who had studied this condition at the Salpêtrière (e.g., Breuer and Freud, 1895; for reviews see Markowitsch, 1992a; Markowitsch and Staniloiu, in press). During the First World War hysteria was described in soldiers ("war trembler," "*Kriegszitterer*") and consequently lost its connotation as a "female" disease (Peckl, 2007). The name hysteria has nevertheless not only remained prominent in everyday language, but also in scientific communications up to today (e.g., Stone et al., 2006; Bell et al., 2011). It was listed as a disease category only in the early editions of the *Diagnostic and Statistical Manual* (DSM-II: American Psychiatric Association, 1968) and is used in association with (retrograde) amnesia up to today (e.g., Iglesias and Iglesias, 2009; Thomas-Antérion et al., 2010).

More recent versions of the DSM, including the present one (DSM-5: American Psychiatric Association, 2013), replaced the term and introduced (among others) the term "dissociative amnesia" (cf. Spiegel et al., 2011, who also criticize differences between DSM and the

*Correspondence to: Hans J. Markowitsch, Physiological Psychology, University of Bielefeld, POB 100131, 33501 Bielefeld, Germany. E-mail: hjmarkowitsch@uni-bielefeld.de

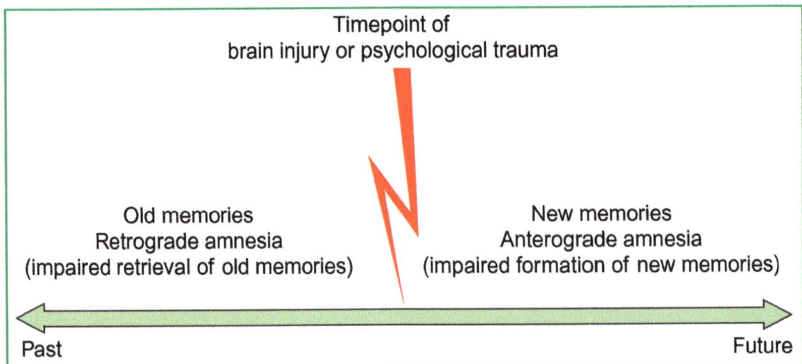

Fig. 36.1. After brain injury or a psychotraumatic event, memory may be impaired with respect to the remembering of old information (which was stored prior to the injury or the event), or with respect to the long-term acquisition of information with which the individual was confronted after the event or injury. The flash symbolizes the event or injury. Already Ribot (1882) noted that there is a gradient in retrograde amnesia: information dating back a long time is better preserved (can be retrieved more easily) than recently acquired information ("Ribot's law" or "law of regression"). (Reproduced from Staniloiu and Markowitsch, 2014.)

International Classification of Diseases, 10th edition (ICD-10: World Health Organization, 1992), and the lack of a proper definition of dissociative disorders). Spiegel et al. definite dissociation on p. 826 as:

> *a disruption of and/or discontinuity in the normal, subjective integration of one or more aspects of psychological functioning, including – but not limited to – memory, identity, consciousness, perception, and motor control. In essence, aspects of psychobiological functioning that should be associated, coordinated, and/or linked are not.*

"Dissociative amnesia" is seen as that subcategory of dissociative disorders in which memory and identity problems are pre-eminent. In a review we defined "dissociative amnesia" as an "inability to consciously recall autobiographical information in the absence of significant brain damage (as detectable by conventional structural neuroimaging)" (Staniloiu and Markowitsch, 2014, Panel 1, p. 2). The term is *a priori* theoretically loaded, since it assumes dissociation to be the primary or only pathogenetic mechanism. To avoid this, or to suggest alternative connotations, a number of additional terms are still widely used (cf. Panel 1 in Staniloiu and Markowitsch, 2014); among them are psychogenic amnesia, which of course emphasizes the psychic nature and origin of the amnesia and distinguishes it from "organic amnesia"; functional amnesia, which suggests that the amnesia serves a function for the affected individual; and mnestic block syndrome, which implies that the amnesia is potentially reversible (Markowitsch, 2002).

As dissociative amnesia can be seen in the tradition of the work of Charcot (1892), Janet (1893), Souques (1892), and other workers (see Markowitsch and Staniloiu, in press) of the 19th century, it can be regarded as more intensely studied than organic amnesic conditions prominent in this epoch (e.g., Korsakoff's disease: Markowitsch, 2010). In spite of its long tradition, dissociative amnesia remains an enigma, as it demonstrates that a primarily psychic condition – (most likely) induced by an adverse environment – can have effects on memory which outweigh those of severe brain injuries.

Before discussing dissociative amnesia in more detail, we will briefly introduce memory divisions as they are relevant for dissociative amnesia (having already defined that dissociative amnesia affects the autobiographic memory domain).

CONTENT-BASED MEMORY SYSTEMS

That memory is not a unity can best be inferred from clinical cases with disorders of memory and was consequently already investigated and described more than a century ago (Ribot, 1882; Markowitsch, 1992a; Markowitsch and Staniloiu, in press). In 1882 Ribot introduced and specified the distinction between anterograde and retrograde amnesia (Fig. 36.1). After some forms of brain damage or psychiatric disease, memory formation or memory retrieval may be impaired. A central question is whether this impairment is permanent, as is the anterograde memory impairment after certain kinds of brain damage (e.g., bilateral medial thalamic or hippocampal damage; cf. Markowitsch, 2008; Markowitsch and Staniloiu, 2012a), or whether it may be better seen as a time-limited blockade of retrieval (Markowitsch, 2002) which can be treated therapeutically.

Retrograde amnesia in principle has to be differentiated from forgetting, which occurs in everyday life situations and is therefore not a pathologic process (Markowitsch and Brand, 2010; Roediger et al., 2010); there is, however, an overlap between nonpathologic and pathologic forms of forgetting (Harris et al., 2010) and – as Sigmund Freud wrote already in 1901 – we never have a guarantee that our memories are correct (Freud, 1901a). In fact, false memories and memory distortions are more common than generally assumed (Loftus, 2006; Kühnel et al., 2008; Risius et al., 2013), and may play a role especially in forensic situations (Markowitsch and Staniloiu, 2011c).

Though predecessors existed 100 years ago (cf. Markowitsch, 1992a), the content-based division of memory, as used herein, distinguishes between a short-term and five long-term memory systems (Fig. 36.2). Of the five long-term memory systems shown in Figure 36.2, the first two (procedural memory, priming) are considered to be anoetic – that is, they lack or do not require conscious processing; the third and fourth memory systems (perceptual memory, semantic memory) are termed noetic – that is, they require conscious reflection, and the last memory system – the episodic-autobiographic one – is named autonoetic, which means that it requires self-reflection, self-awareness, and reconstructive processes. Interestingly, most neurologic and psychiatric patients manifest impairments principally in the episodic-autobiographic memory system, which indicates that this system requires a complex synchrony of neuronal assemblies (e.g., circuits for emotion and cognition) in order to function properly (cf. Figure 8 in Markowitsch, 2013, and the accompanying description).

MEASUREMENT PROBLEMS OF RETROGRADE AMNESIA

It is still much easier and much more valid to measure anterograde than retrograde memory functions (Markowitsch, 1992c). This problem is inherent in the deficit structure: It is always possible to apply stimulus material which is unknown to the patient, ask the patient to learn it, and measure learning progress. It is, however, much less reliable and valid to assess information which might or might not have been acquired properly or which might have got lost, or been suppressed or repressed with passing time. All patients have a very individual background determining what they learned, paid attention to, or neglected. Aside from a few stereotypically learned facts (own birthday, own name, names of parents, place of birth, and the like), knowledge depends on personal interests and intellectual background. Furthermore, episodic-autobiographic retrieval usually is accompanied by the feeling of autonoesis – of self-experience and emotional colorization (Staniloiu et al., 2010; Markowitsch and Staniloiu, 2011a, 2012a, b, 2013;

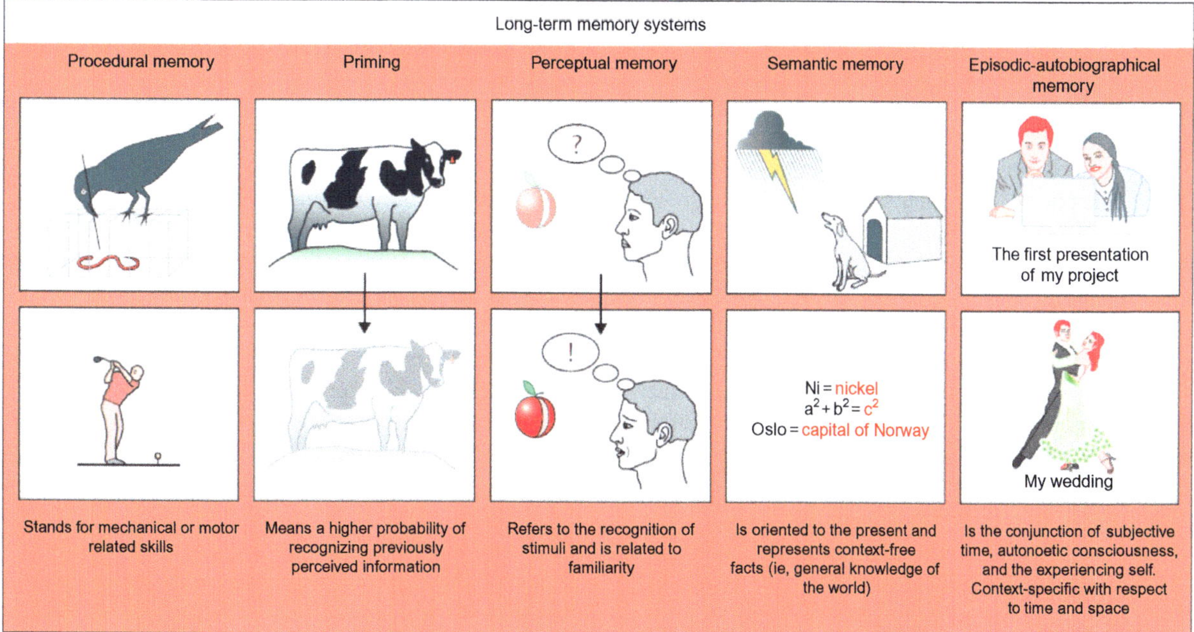

Fig. 36.2. The five long-term memory systems, based on Tulving's terminology and ideas (e.g., Tulving, 2005). These systems are assumed to develop from simple to complex (from left to right). Therefore, the simple systems, such as procedural memory and priming, exist in human beings from early childhood onward and in simple forms of animals, while the complex ones are only available in older children or in more advanced species. Tulving and others postulate that the episodic-autobiographic memory system exists in its full form only in (healthy) human beings. Also based on Tulving's work is the "remember–know" distinction: remembering occurs with a context and with conscious reflection ("reliving the event") and therefore refers to the episodic-autobiographic memory system, while knowing simply refers to yes or no distinctions without further connotations. (Reproduced from Staniloiu and Markowitsch, 2014, with permission from Elsevier).

Staniloiu and Markowitsch, 2012a, b, 2015; Markowitsch, 2013). For patients with dominant retrograde amnesia there is always the possibility that they relearned information about themselves which then is processed similarly to information learned about a third (unknown) person (Markowitsch et al., 1997b; Staniloiu and Markowitsch, 2012c; Markowitsch, 2013).

If a patient denies remembering anything from his or her personal past, one either can believe that, and not apply any autobiographic retrograde memory tests (cf., e.g., Fujiwara et al., 2008 or Markowitsch and Staniloiu, 2013 for descriptions), or try to apply symptom validity tests which again are not central, as they tap on anterograde memory abilities. Furthermore, the patient may still have stored his or her personal past, but is not aware of that (Mayes, 1988; Prigatano and Schacter, 1991; Schacter and Prigatano, 1991). This in fact may be the case in most patients with idiopathic amnesia, that is, amnesia of an unknown or uncertain cause (Markowitsch, 2002; see Panel 1 of Staniloiu and Markowitsch, 2014), or with so-called focal (as opposed to widespread cerebral) brain damage. For these cases indirect measures such as priming tasks (Damasio and Tranel, 1990; von Cramon et al., 1993) or application of galvanic skin response measures (Tranel and Damasio, 1985; Markowitsch et al., 1986; Damasio et al., 1991) might be used. Other problems are the possibility of increased emotional bluntness, especially after right-hemispheric lesions (Cimino et al., 1991; Schore, 2002; Moriguchi et al., 2006; Seidl et al., 2006; Anderson et al., 2011; cf. also Kihlstrom et al., 2013, who suggested that hypnosis might be mediated by the right hemisphere alone, and Quirin et al., 2013, who found electrophysiologically that emotions such as love are related to the right hemisphere). If there are psychiatric concomitants, a so-called overgeneral memory effect may be found; that is, the patients provide only very general information about their past life events and fail to show adequate emotional engagement (Williams et al., 1996; Watkins et al., 2000; Valentino et al., 2009). That variables such as vividness, contents, detail, and emotional colorization affect individual memories, especially if they stem from different time periods of the patient's life, was remarked already several decades ago (Squire and Cohen, 1982).

RETROGRADE AMNESIA: ORGANIC OR PSYCHOGENIC?

Since the early times of clinical brain research, relations between certain forms of brain damage and memory disturbances have been discussed. Interestingly, this research seemed to be more fruitful for anterograde than for retrograde memory, since for patients with anterograde amnesia distinct forms of brain damage were found (Markowitsch, 2008; Markowitsch and Staniloiu, 2012a). First two, and later three, types of brain damage leading to anterograde amnesia (with in part differing concomitant behavioral deficits) were established – medial temporal-lobe amnesia, diencephalic amnesia, and basal forebrain amnesia (cf. Table 1 in Markowitsch and Staniloiu, 2012a). It also was found that left-hemispheric damage leads to more severe deficits in the verbal, and right-hemispheric damage in the nonverbal, domains (Jokeit et al., 1997).

For retrograde amnesia such clearcut relations were much less obvious initially. Instead, especially patients with traumatic brain injury (TBI) were found to suffer from long-standing memory loss (Schlesinger, 1916; Russell and Nathan, 1946; Deelman et al., 1990; Rees, 2003; Anderson, 2004). Diffuse brain injury, including white-matter damage (Gale et al., 1995), and coma duration were seen as predictors of memory disturbances in the retrograde direction (Stuss and Richard, 1982; Markowitsch, 1999a). Already in 1899 Paul stated that "the degree or extent of amnesia is to a certain degree proportional to the duration of coma" (p. 264).

By far most cases with retrograde amnesia were, however, initially attributed to be of hysteric nature (Markowitsch, 1990a, b, 1992a). As mentioned above, hysteria was a very popular concept at the turn of the 20th century and was fostered from psychodynamic as well from other schools (Charcot, 1892; Breuer and Freud, 1895; Ganser, 1898, 1904; Janet, 1907; Matthies, 1908). Hysteria in those days meant emotional changes that lead to symptoms in sensory, motor, or mental domains. Aside from psychogenic blindness or paralysis, amnesia was especially often diagnosed and interpreted as a mechanism of protection against an adverse environment. As hysteria was considered to be a psychogenic illness, no underlying organic changes were assumed to exist. However, already in the 19th century Bennett (1878) had published a "case of cerebral tumour-symptoms simulating hysteria" and had questioned the dichotomy between organic and psychogenic illnesses. On page 120 he wrote about "Miss A., a young lady aged 16" (p. 114):

> *In conclusion, there appear to me to be at least two points of interest in this case: 1st, the anomalous symptoms of pressure caused by the tumour; and 2nd, that symptoms of what is called hysteria may co-exist with organic disease of the brain – whether independent of it or the result, being in this patient doubtful. Under any circumstances it serves to indicate what caution should be exercised in diagnosing, and more especially in treating, as hysteria, any nervous affection in women which may appear indefinite or mysterious.*

(A case with related symptomatology after brain disease was reported by Savage in the same year and in the same journal.)

While in later times many case reports appeared showing intermingling of brain disease or damage and psychic disturbances such as posttraumatic stress disorder or dissociative amnesia (Osnato, 1930; Silver et al., 1997; Joseph and Masterson, 1999; O'Neill of Tyrone and Fernandez, 2000; Kim et al., 2007; Mishra et al., 2011; Sehm et al., 2011; Pommerenke et al., 2012; Staniloiu and Markowitsch, 2014; Toussi et al., 2014), as long ago as 1870 a well-known medical doctor, Henry Maudsley (after whom a London hospital was named), wrote "Mental disorders are neither more nor less than nervous diseases in which mental symptoms predominate, and their entire separation from other nervous diseases has been a sad hindrance to progress" (p. 41). Maudsley's statement is remarkable particularly in light of the fact that neuropsychiatric societies were established only in the 1980s and 1990s.

The discussion on brain correlates of psychiatric diseases is, of course, continuing (cf. Pietrini, 2003) and – as Pietrini (2003) remarked – there is evidence for changes in glucose metabolism, in volume of limbic structures, and in white-matter changes in patients with dissociative disorders (Markowitsch et al., 2000a; Vermetten et al., 2006; Tramoni et al., 2009). Nevertheless, it should be emphasized again that extensive retrograde amnesia – aside from in patients with severe dementia (Piolino et al., 2003; Jetten et al., 2010) – seems more frequently to be a psychiatric than a neurologic disease. Already in 1911, Heine reviewed possible amnesic states and listed many with a psychologic background (Table 36.1). Similarly, a few years later, Schneider in 1928 formulated on p. 520 that there is evidence against a sharp distinction of organic and functional amnesic states.

In 2014 we reviewed the current understanding of dissociative amnesia, its epidemiology, clinical and psychologic features, and hypotheses for its occurrence. We view dissociative amnesia as a condition which is (in most cases) stress-related and is based on negative past experiences with which the patient could not cope adequately (Staniloiu and Markowitsch, 2014; Table 36.2). Patients with dissociative amnesia usually either had experienced a major negative event (such as in a life-threatening war situation), or, much more frequently, a number of negative events, the last of which led to dissociative amnesia (e.g., Markowitsch et al., 1999c). Because of this, we proposed the "two-hit hypothesis" as a likely cause for its occurrence, with two hits meaning "an additive or synergistic interaction between psychological and physical incidents" (p. 231) of a negative, adverse nature (see also Roberts et al., 2013).

Table 36.1

Conditions leading to memory disturbances according to Heine (1911, p. 55f)

1. Epileptic somnolence
2. Hysteric somnolence
3. States of unconsciousness and of mnestic activity after traumatic damage of the brain:
   1. Commotio cerebri
   2. Attempt to hang oneself
   3. Reanimation after hanging
4. States of somnolence with a relation to physiologic sleep
5. Hypnotic states
6. Migraine-based somnolence
7. Affect-based somnolence
8. Toxic somnolence, or disturbance of mind:
   1. Complicated states after intoxication
   2. Disease of the mind after carbon monoxide inhalation
9. Vasomotoric states of somnolence:
   1. Congestive (transitory mania)
   2. Angiospastic (raptus melancholicus)
10. Transitory disturbances of mind after infectious diseases
11. Paralytic attacks
12. Retrograde amnesia without previous disturbances of consciousness
13. Korsakoff's psychosis

SHORT REVIEW OF RETROGRADE AMNESIA AFTER STRUCTURAL BRAIN DAMAGE

As the topic here is functional retrograde amnesia, directly organic-based retrograde amnesia will only be briefly summarized. Etiologies for cases with predominant retrograde amnesia after brain diseases or brain injuries are: (1) TBI/minor brain injury; (2) viral infections such as herpes encephalitis; (3) degenerative brain diseases (e.g., Alzheimer's disease); (4) brain infarcts; (5) severe hypoxia (e.g., carbon monoxide poisoning, attempted hanging); and (6) Korsakoff's syndrome. Usually milder forms of retrograde amnesia are found in patients with transient epileptic amnesia and in transient global amnesia (TGA), in which it lasts by definition less than 24 hours. (TGA refers to an amnesic condition of sudden onset, usually affecting old people. It is triggered by sudden physical or psychic changes (e.g., considerable temperature change, unusual physical exercise, or an unexpected psychologic stress situation) and results in usually complete anterograde and partial retrograde amnesia in the episodic-autobiographic domain. It passes away within 24 hours.)

Brain infarcts and vascular brain damage

Brain infarcts usually lead to a combination of anterograde and retrograde memory disturbances with a higher

Table 36.2

Sequence of possible changes in brain–behavior interrelations induced by stress-conditions

Psychological or biological stress or trauma situations, especially in childhood
↓
Biological priming
Change in receptor structure
↓
Supersensitivity for excitatory neurotransmitters
↓
Latency phase
↓
(Re-)activation
via
Psychological mechanisms or biological events
(e.g., conflict, deprivation, accident, infection)
↓
Absence of adequate emotional-cognitive processing
↓
Second latency phase
↓
Dissociation between cognition and emotion
Psychobiologic stress reaction
↓
Depressive tendencies
↓
Dissociative amnesia / mnestic block syndrome

After Aldenhoff (1997) and Markowitsch (2000).

proportion of anterograde deficits (Markowitsch, 1988, 2008). Nevertheless there are case descriptions of severe and lasting retrograde amnesia also after damage to very focal regions such as the medial diencephalon (Hodges and McCarthy, 1993; Markowitsch et al., 1993b; for reviews, see: van der Werf et al., 2000; Carlesimo et al., 2011). In most of these patients retrograde amnesia follows Ribot's law, which states that old memories from childhood and youth are better preserved than recent memories from the last years (Ribot, 1882). (e.g., Markowitsch et al., 1993b). This clearly distinguishes brain-damaged patients from those with a dissociative amnesic condition where such a gradient is absent. It indeed seems that more widespread brain damage or a long-standing disease condition such as epilepsy can lead to more extensive retrograde amnesia, while restricted hippocampal damage may lead to more time-limited episodic-autobiographic memory loss (or inaccessibility). However, it needs to be emphasized that there may frequently be a difference between visible brain damage and existing brain damage, as was demonstrated, for example, for brain damage after heart attack (Markowitsch et al., 1997d).

Degenerative and metabolic brain diseases

Generally, most of the classic forms of dementia are subsumed under degenerative diseases. However, also metabolic, toxic, and viral diseases and continuing epilepsy-caused neural hyperactivity (excitotoxicity) may lead to brain degeneration. Therefore we will subsume Korsakoff's disease and herpes simplex encephalitis under this heading (even tuberculous meningitis might be added here, as Kapur mentioned in 1993).

Many of the group of dementia diseases lead in their more advanced stages to retrograde amnesia. This is due to a disintegration of cerebral networks involved in the storage of memories (Markowitsch, 2013). Seidl et al. (2006), for example, found that the more the condition of Alzheimer's disease progresses, the less detailed, less complete, and less comprehensive were reports of patients about their past. Furthermore, the number of reported events shrank with advancing disease. As an exception to the usual temporal gradient (Ribot's law) in dementias, in semantic dementia a reversed gradient seems to exist. Possible reasons for this were given by Kopelman (2002).

Korsakoff's disease is a thiamine deficiency-related degeneration of medial diencephalic nuclei, nowadays affecting mainly patients with severe alcohol abuse. Korsakoff's patients probably have been studied the longest among groups with different etiologies (Markowitsch, 1992a, 2010). Already in 1852 Huss wrote a book of roughly 600 pages on *Chronische Alkoholskrankheit oder Alcoholismus chronicus* [*Chronic Alcohol Disease or Alcoholismus chronicus*], in which he emphasized its negative effects on mental capacities, stating that memory becomes weak (p. 356). Markowitsch (2010) concluded from reviewing the available data on patients with Korsakoff's symptomatology that their memory deficits are principally "in the domain of (anterograde) episodic-autobiographic memories, and much less so in the domains of the other memory systems currently defined. With respect to semantic retrograde memories, the deficit is less pronounced, as can be inferred from a superior retrieval capacity under conditions of recognition compared to free recall." (p. 133). (cf. Markowitsch et al., 1984, 1986).

Epilepsy-related amnesic conditions are even found in patients with transient epileptic amnesia (Milton et al., 2010; Butler and Zeman, 2011; Soper et al., 2011) and are usually of anterograde nature (Bartsch and Butler, 2013). Long-lasting epilepsy may be accompanied by remote memory problems (Viskontas et al., 2000, 2002; Lah et al., 2006, 2008). Whether temporal extent and content-based broadness of retrograde amnesia vary with the extent of temporal-lobe damage still seems uncertain (Gold and Squire, 2006; Noulhiane et al., 2007; Insausti et al., 2013; Gregory et al., 2014).

Hypoxia

Hypoxic-ischemic brain lesions regularly result in cognitive disturbances (Anderson and Arciniegas, 2010). It is known that severe hypoxic conditions can lead to retrograde amnesia, probably due to reduced hippocampal volumes (Allen et al., 2006) or due to volume reductions in other brain regions (Hokkanen et al., 1995, 1996a, b; Markowitsch et al., 1997b; Kopelman et al., 2003). Especially cases with developmental amnesia demonstrate that hypoxia at birth may lead to medial temporal-lobe degeneration (reduced hippocampal volumes) and severe retrograde amnesia for the episodic-autobiographic domain (Staniloiu et al., 2013). For one of those patients it was detected that he had congenital absence of the mammillary bodies (Rosenbaum et al., 2014). These patients, however, constitute an exception within the category of patients with hypoxic-ischemic brain damage, as they probably were unable from early life on to consolidate episodic-autobiographic events. But also patients suffering from sudden hypoxia (e.g., after attempted hanging) (or even chronic hypoxia, as in sleep apnea patients) have long been found to suffer from partial (time-limited) retrograde amnesia (Boedeker, 1896; Markowitsch, 1992b; Reinhold et al., 2008).

A particularly interesting case with a background of hypoxia was published many decades ago by Grünthal and Störring. These authors investigated (1930) and followed up (Störring, 1931, 1936; Grünthal and Störring, 1933, 1956) a case of carbon monoxide intoxication with particular deficits in the anterograde memory range, but with massive retrograde amnesia as well. The patient's behavior with respect to memory performance, emotions, will, spontaneous activity, and ability to think and reflect consciously was documented over more than 120 pages in Störring's publication of 1931.

The patient's retrograde amnesia followed typically Ribot's law (the more recent the information is, the more likely it was lost, while, in contrast, the longer it had been stored, the more likely it was retained). He had a good ability to remember events from his youth, but practically no knowledge of his recent past. Grünthal and Störring (1930) speculated on the morphologic substrate of his amnesia and negated the existence of diffuse brain damage, but acknowledged the possibility "that the more refined physical-chemical processes of large brain areas might have suffered so differently in their dynamics or quality that especially the correlates of mnestic functions are affected" (p. 368). They preferred, however, to assume that distinct brain portions such as the mammillary bodies might have been damaged.

In 1933, the patient married his fiancée (who had already been mentioned in the 1930 report) and lived at home. He was still markedly amnesic and introduced his wife consistently as his fiancée. He was always happy to see her, as if he had just fallen in love. He showed appropriate behavioral stereotypes, such as taking off his hat when entering church or when being greeted, and was able to behave well during meals and to explain industrial drawings he had made about 10 years previously. But he used external help to memorize. For instance, he once explained that it must be Sunday because he was wearing a suit or that he would not be traveling on a train, as he was not dressed appropriately. He also assisted his wife in climbing a mountain as he remembered from the time before his accident that she had difficulties on such occasions.

It is interesting that, when asked about the present date, he always said "the last day of May, 1926," and in fact his accident had occurred on May 31 in 1926. His response resembles that of an amnesic patient who had had a stroke affecting the diencephalon and who always gave the year as 1981 – the year of his stroke – when asked in 1990 (Markowitsch et al., 1993b).

The case of Grünthal and Störring was revisited by Craver et al. (2014a). These authors discussed the pros and cons of the case with respect to being a true amnesic or a faker, citing also all the later work published on this case (e.g., Grünthal and Störring, 1954). A scientist, criticizing the description of Grünthal and Störring, also mentioned, according to Craver et al. (2014a), that the patient – Franz Breundl – at times gave implausible answers to questions, suggesting some kind of hysteric pseudodementia. If true, this might speak of features of Ganser's syndrome, a psychiatric disease characterized by *vorbeireden* (giving approximate answers, such as "3," in response to the question, "How many legs does a cat have?) and disturbed consciousness, and which for many years was subsumed under the category of psychogenic amnesic states (cf., e.g., the case given in Staniloiu et al., 2009).

Craver et al. (2014a) pointed out that philosophers might see in Breundl's case the continuity of personality in the absence of memory. One of us (H.J.M.) had a related case with carbon monoxide poisoning (due to a suicide attempt). This patient, however, seemed to have changed in personality due to his anterograde as well as retrograde memory loss. He usually appeared to be joyful and gregarious, demonstrating this also when he was invited to a TV talk show, where he immediately asked all women watching TV to make a date with him. From analyzing case descriptions of patients with retrograde dissociative amnesia, it seems that, though character traits may persist, a number of features of the self may be altered (Fradera and Kopelman, 2009; Rathbone et al., 2009, 2015; Staniloiu et al., 2010; Arzy et al., 2011; Markowitsch and Staniloiu, 2011a; Markowitsch, 2013).

Both the patient Breundl and this patient demonstrate that carbon monoxide poisoning as an etiology may be particularly prone to a mixture of organic (hippocampal degeneration) and psychogenic causes of retrograde as well as anterograde amnesia. (See also the descriptions of the anterograde psychogenic amnesic case Q. in Markowitsch and Staniloiu, 2013, of case T.A. in Markowitsch et al., 1999b, and of case F.L. in Smith et al., 2010.)

Traumatic brain injury/minor head trauma

TBI, accompanied by retrograde memory impairment, constitutes a very broad category ranging from minor head concussions to severe brain tissue damage (Russell, 1935, 1971; Russell and Nathan, 1946; Fisher, 1966; Lucchelli et al., 1995, 1998; Dean and Sterr, 2013). Temporary cardiac arrest may be added as related in its consequences to TBI. In war time, shot and shrapnel injuries were common (Kleist, 1934). Interestingly, the duration of retrograde amnesia varies considerably after TBI and is not always predictable from available variables (though coma duration is to some extent a predictor) (Markowitsch and Calabrese, 1996). Also a relation between posttraumatic amnesia duration and long-term cerebral atrophy was established (Wilde et al., 2006). Common to most forms of TBI is an inability to remember the immediate time period before and after the injury.

Another feature of patients with TBI is that TBI "seems to make patients particularly susceptible to depressive episodes, delusional disorder, and personal disturbances" (Koponen et al., 2002, p. 1315). (The same, at least with respect to depression and personal disturbances, holds true for patients with dissociative amnesia.) Such psychiatric changes may add to memory disturbances as it is known that there exists a strong relation between depression, personality disorders, and memory problems (Markowitsch et al., 1999c; Staniloiu and Markowitsch, 2014, 2015). A more refined analysis of the brain of TBI patients, for example, with diffusion tensor imaging or magnetization transfer ratio, may reveal microstructural changes that could account for continuing behavioral deficits (e.g., Back et al., 1998; Bendlin et al., 2008; Sidaros et al., 2008; cf. also Grafman et al., 1988; Markowitsch and Calabrese, 1996). Also the coma state may alter the usual biochemical inflow between neuronal assemblies representing stored information (Markowitsch, 1988). Prolonged disuse – also a consequence of coma and concussions – may enhance such detrimental effects.

Cases with severe amnesia after major TBI – relation to functional amnesia?

One of the best-known cases with both severe anterograde and retrograde amnesia is patient K.C., who had a motor cycle accident damaging several portions of his brain (Rosenbaum et al., 2005, 2009; Craver et al., 2014b).

Since the 1990s several papers, reporting complete or nearly complete retrograde amnesia in the episodic-autobiographic domain after combined temporopolar and frontal brain damage have been published (e.g., Kapur et al., 1992; Markowitsch et al., 1993a; Calabrese et al., 1996; Kroll et al., 1997; Markowitsch and Ewald, 1997; Levine et al., 1998) (Fig. 36.3). That is, such patients apparently had forgotten their whole life, and did not remember their partner or their profession. However, they could still read, write, and calculate or were able to relearn these skills quickly. Likewise, as our patient demonstrated, social skills, priming, and procedural memory were principally preserved (Markowitsch et al., 1993a). Similarly, case reports with mainly left-hemispheric cortical damage and severe retrograde amnesia in the semantic memory domain appeared from the late 1980s (De Renzi et al., 1987; Grossi et al., 1988; Markowitsch et al., 1999a). (The patient of De Renzi et al., however, did not have TBI, but herpes encephalitis; cf. also the encephalitis patient of Hokkanen et al., 1995, for whom the authors, however, excluded a psychogenic etiology.) These patients remembered their relatives, but were unable to recognize prominent politicians or actors.

It was assumed that the retrograde amnesia was "focal" or "isolated," that is, an isolated symptom that was the consequence of either the cortical damage or of some other mechanisms (e.g., Goldberg et al., 1982; Kapur et al.,

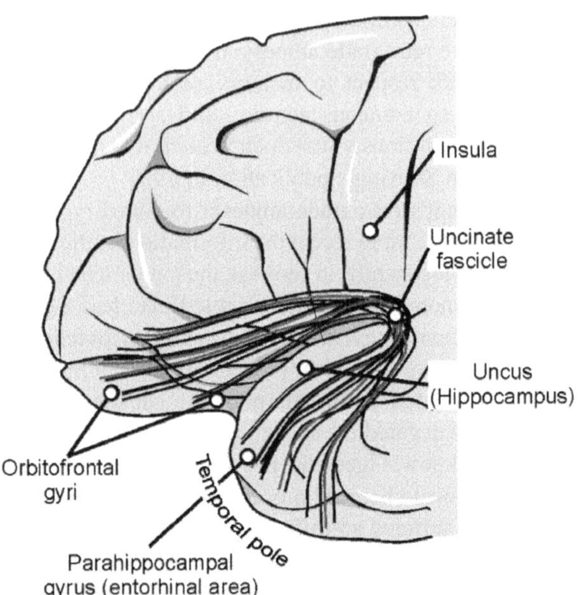

Fig. 36.3. The region of the temporofrontal cortex containing the uncinate fasciculus. It is assumed that this region is engaged in triggering the retrieval of consciously processed information – primarily semantic memory in the left hemisphere, and primarily episodic-autobiographic memory in the right hemisphere.

1989, 1992; Yoneda et al., 1992; Kapur, 1993; Hunkin et al., 1995; Hokkanen et al., 1995; Parkin, 1996; Levine et al., 1998, 2009; Fast and Fujiwara, 2001; Miller et al., 2001; Yamadori et al., 2001; Teramoto et al., 2005; Stracciari et al., 2008; Sehm et al., 2011). Sometimes also the expressions "disproportionate retrograde amnesia" (Kapur et al., 1996; Thomas-Antérion et al., 2014) or "permanent global amnesia" (Kritchevsky and Squire, 1993), or "pure retrograde amnesia" (Lucchelli et al., 1998) were used. This assumption was, however, questioned by Kopelman (2002), who also provided various different interpretations. As there were other – even earlier – cases with TBI (and other etiologies; e.g., Roman-Campos et al., 1980) and retrograde amnesia (e.g., Goldberg et al., 1981, 1982), the idea that at least some of the brain-damaged patients had dissociative amnesia or a combination of dissociative (psychogenic) and brain-organic amnesia was suggested (De Renzi et al., 1995, 1997; Markowitsch, 1996a, b) and the term "functional amnesia" was proposed for these cases (Lundholm, 1932; Schacter and Kihlstrom, 1989; De Renzi et al., 1997; Brandt and Van Gorp, 2006), implying that the amnesia served a function in their life. However, even in more recent times case reports appear which point to the "same faulty mechanism in the neural circuitry" (Ouellet et al., 2008, p. 27) in cases with brain damage (in the "organic" case of Ouellet et al., a wound in the right temporal lobe, caused by a nail gun) and after an intense emotional trauma in the other case of Ouellet et al. A similar view was already held by early researchers such as Syz (1937) and Maudsley (1870), and was also formulated in an editorial by Pietrini (2003) (see above).

DISSOCIATIVE AMNESIA WITH AND WITHOUT TBI

Nearly 150 years ago the first case reports of patients with so-called hysterical amnesia occurred and a number of them had a combination of minor TBI and a "hysterical amnesic state" (Markowitsch, 1992a). There is nearly always a problem when a minor head trauma leads to lasting retrograde amnesia (cf. Ruff and Jamora, 2009). If the patient is young and therefore probably of an immature personality structure, the likelihood for a psychiatric condition is even higher (Staniloiu and Markowitsch, 2014). While it is assumed that a long duration of the amnesia and the lack of compensation claims may speak for an organic origin (e.g., Hunkin et al., 1995), this cannot be seen as a rule. We have, for example, a patient whose variant of dissociative amnesia has lasted now for over 20 years – since 1994 (the case was first published in Markowitsch et al., 1999b).

There are a number of case descriptions of patients under 20 years of age, most of them still attending school (Reinhold and Markowitsch, 2007), who after minor accidents developed retrograde amnesia in the autobiographic domain. Lucchelli et al. (1998) described a 15-year-old boy who became retrogradely amnesic after a minor head bump; Markowitsch and Staniloiu (2013) described another one, who bumped against the opening door of a cigarette machine; Barbarotto et al. (1996) discussed a 38-year-old woman who slipped and fell in her office, resulting in pure retrograde amnesia, and a considerable number of patients were involved in motor vehicle accidents (De Renzi and Lucchelli, 1993; Stracciari et al., 1994; De Renzi et al., 1995, 1997; Mortati and Grant, 2012). For most of these patients, no brain injury could be detected on the basis of neuroimaging. In a few there was minor evidence for metabolic alterations, as inferred from single-photon emission computed tomography (SPECT) or positron emission tomography (PET) using radioactive water (Markowitsch et al., 1997b) or glucose (Markowitsch et al., 1998, 2000a; Brand et al., 2009; Thomas-Antérion et al., 2010, 2014). Some of the patients recovered from their amnesia after varying time periods (Lucchelli et al., 1998). Sometimes, it remained obscure whether any specific event had happened (Dalla Barba et al., 1997) and sometimes "purely" psychic conditions seemed likely (Kessler et al., 1997; Markowitsch et al., 1999c; Kritchevsky et al., 2004). A 9-year-old boy was diagnosed with TGA after suffering from retrograde and anterograde amnesia (Meijneke et al., 2014); there might have been a minor emotional trigger for his amnesia, as his new watch broke that day. As Bartsch and Deuschl (2010) remarked, an emotional – and therefore psychologic – trigger can be found in 30% of patients with TGA. While the authors did not consider a dissociative condition, there may in fact have been features of this, though the patient remembered facts like his name and address.

These and related cases (e.g., Reinhold and Markowitsch, 2009; Staniloiu and Markowitsch, 2012a, b, c; Markowitsch and Staniloiu, 2013) provoke the question on possible mechanisms of retrograde amnesia induction, maintenance, and resolution (Markowitsch and Staniloiu, 2012c). These will be discussed below.

THE PUZZLE OF RETROGRADE AMNESIA OCCURRENCE

The occurrence of retrograde amnesia is a puzzle, because, much more so than anterograde amnesia (Markowitsch, 2008; Markowitsch and Staniloiu, 2012a), it cannot be linked to a distinct neuropathology (cf. Kopelman, 2000). However, one of the distinct differences between patients with a clear organic cause and those with probable or likely psychogenic origin is the usually found gradient ("Ribot's law") in the organic, but not in the psychogenic, cases (Brown, 2002; Staniloiu and Markowitsch, 2012a–d, 2014, 2015). McKay and Kopelman (2009) even propose a reversed gradient for psychogenic amnesia. Furthermore, the cases with primarily psychogenic origin usually show some distinct personality features, namely a poor childhood or youth, an insecure personality profile as adults, a heightened vulnerability towards stress and stressful events, a lack of appropriate coping strategies against surprising or threatening situations, and a heightened susceptibility towards suggestions from others (Markowitsch, 2009).

In Tables 36.3 and 36.4 certain features accompanying severe and lasting retrograde amnesia of primarily organic and psychogenic origin are listed. For retrograde amnesia of direct organic origin, extent and locus of brain damage are considered to be responsible for the deficit. For retrograde amnesia with less obvious brain damage, as in mild head trauma and concussion, a number of factors were listed as possibly leading to a usually more transient or less severe retrograde amnesia. Among them are *contrecoup* damage, rotational forces leading to axonal and synaptic injury, gliosis, and biochemical changes at the microstructural level (Schoenfeld and Hamilton, 1977; Walker and Tesco, 2013). Demyelination and accompanying frontal-lobe dysfunctions have been added (Craver et al., 2014a), as well as intracranial microbleeding, hypoxia, and the formation of plaques with time.

Some of these aforementioned changes may more likely be seen with advanced neuroimaging techniques such as glucose PET, diffusion tensor imaging, magnetic resonance spectroscopy, or magnetization transfer imaging. This is clearly exemplified in a study of Ruff et al. (1994), who examined 9 patients suffering minor TBI with little or no evidence of computed tomography- or magnetic resonance imaging-proven brain damage, but with deficient neuropsychologic performance. PET examination on the other hand confirmed for all 9 patients the neuropsychologic evidence. On a similar line, Markowitsch and coworkers tried to prove an organic basis for primarily psychogenic forms of amnesia since 1997, mainly on the basis of PET investigations (Markowitsch, 1999d; Markowitsch et al., 1997a–c, 1998, 2000a; Brand et al., 2009). Other workers followed this line of research (Hennig-Fast et al., 2008; Stracciari et al., 2008; Tramoni et al., 2009), which revealed significant changes, most consistently in frontotemporal regions of the right hemisphere (Reinhold et al., 2006; Staniloiu and Markowitsch, 2010; Staniloiu et al., 2011). An overview of such studies is given in Table 4

Table 36.3

Distinct features of dissociative compared with direct organically based amnesias*

	Dissociative amnesias	Organically based amnesias (neurocognitive disorders)
Age at the time of diagnosis (years)	20–40	Variable
Course	Acute or chronic	Acute or chronic
Episodic-autobiographic anterograde amnesia	Less common	Most common
Episodic-autobiographic retrograde amnesia	Most common	Uncommon and rarely without anterograde amnesia
Loss of personal identity	Common	Uncommon
Preservation of learning of new facts	Usual, but not always	Rarely reported
Onset related to trauma or psychologic stress or conflicts	Common	Uncommon
Precipitants	Psychologic stress with or without physical events	Neural tissue damage (but also emotional precipitants in transient global amnesia)
Reversal of memory loss with hypnosis	Sometimes	No
Improvement with sedative hypnotics (e.g., pharmacologically facilitated interview)	Sometimes	No, or may worsen
Brain damage	In most cases not detectable by conventional neuroimaging techniques or postmortem	Usually structurally detectable or postmortem
Affected brain regions (metabolic or tissue damage)	Prefrontotemporal areas/limbic system	Variable, usually limbic areas

*Some criteria have been adapted from Table 4 of Spiegel and colleagues (2011).

Table 36.4

Similarities and differences between cases with retrograde amnesia due to organic or psychogenic causes

	Direct organic causation	Psychogenic causation
Initiating event	Traumatic brain injury, infarct, etc.	Psychic stress, mild head trauma*
Cognitive impairment beyond memory	Frequently and frequently severe	Usually limited, though existent
Factual self-knowledge	Usually preserved	Not preserved
Reversibility	Full reversibility infrequent	Full reversibility possible and sometimes quick
Gradient ("Ribot's law")	Usually existent	Nonexistent
Congruence of brain damage and degree of amnesia	Usually given	Usually not given
History of subtle personality disorder or premorbid psychiatric disease	Usually nonexistent	Usually more likely to exist

*It should be noted that, in transient global amnesia, about one-third of cases are triggered by an emotional stressor (Bartsch and Deuschl, 2010).
Partly after Reinhold and Markowitsch (2009).

of Staniloiu and Markowitsch (2014). Interestingly, while older studies emphasized the transience of dissociative amnesia, more recent work points to chronic conditions in a number of cases (Coons and Milstein, 1992; Markowitsch and Staniloiu, 2013; Staniloiu and Markowitsch, 2014).

On the other hand, visible and proven organic brain damage – contrary to classic descriptions – does not preclude the formation of dissociative amnesia (Lucchelli et al., 1995; Markowitsch, 1996a, b; Mishra et al., 2011; Pommerenke et al., 2012) (though this diagnosis is not always considered: see Wilson et al., 2015). The existence of cases with organic brain damage and dissociative amnesia indicates – similarly to TGA (Bartsch and Deuschl, 2010; Markowitsch and Staniloiu, 2012b) – that emotional stress as well as somatic-physical alterations may result in a similar symptomatology. Furthermore, in TGA the symptomatology is by definition transient and short, and in dissociative amnesia apparently rather complete recovery from the symptom of episodic-autobiographic amnesia has been found as well. While recovery seems always to be spontaneous in TGA, in dissociative amnesia it is more likely triggered by various mechanisms such as hypnosis, amytal injection, electric stimulation, drug medications, or – of course – conventional forms of psychotherapy (Naef, 1897; Bumke, 1924; Krarup, 1924; Schneider, 1928; Stuss and Guzman, 1988; Iglesias and Iglesias, 2009; Lee et al., 2011), though more or less spontaneous recovery has been reported as well (Lucchelli et al., 1995). Such findings encourage the postulation of an "inability of access" hypothesis for retrograde amnesia, thus leading to the idea that organic and psychogenic amnesia are similar insofar as both represent a frequently temporary (and partial or selective) memory loss, primarily affecting the episodic-autobiographic domain (Markowitsch, 1996a, b, 2002) (Fig. 36.2).

INABILITY OF ACCESS HYPOTHESIS

This hypothesis states that (episodic-autobiographic) memory still is stored in the brain, but that, due to an interruption in communication between brain network systems engaged in memory storage and in memory retrieval, a successful conscious recollection of episodes is blocked. Klein (2015) stated:

> *Recollection consists in two separate but interdependent parts. First, to count as an act of recollection (= memory) a mental state must be causally linked to an experience the individual formerly enjoyed. Second, memory is not simply* from *the past; it is a special way of being* about *the past ... To qualify as an act of memory, the content present in awareness must present itself as a re-experience of an experience previously had. This feeling of re-experiencing is directly given to consciousness, rather than the product of an act of inference or interpretation.*

There are two – at first glance – opposite ideas: one, that direct brain tissue damage is responsible for the blockage of old personal memories, and the other, that a psychic disturbance causes the observed retrograde amnesia (sometimes even just headache seems to result in persistent retrograde amnesia: Reinvang and Gjerstad, 1998). In fact, however, these two approaches are not mutually exclusive: they have a common denominator. Assuming that all psychic phenomena have an organic basis, the question is only how to measure the basis and how to find out about its plasticity (reversibility, stableness).

As mentioned before, the idea of "organicity" is not new (Maudsley, 1870; Flechsig, 1896a, b; Syz, 1937; Freud, 1954; Markowitsch, 1996a, b; Pietrini, 2003), though the separation between neurologic and psychiatric diseases seems to have even widened in the last decades (Markowitsch, 1999c). There are two prominent examples from the beginning of the 19th century, Freud and von Monakow. Freud started his career in neurology, publishing on fiber tracing and aphasia (see Markowitsch, 1992a) and worked from 1895 on an *Entwurf einer Psychologie* [Project of a Scientific Psychology], which was published only after his death (Freud, 1954; cf. Peper and Markowitsch, 2001). Freud was trained in neurobiologic subjects as a student of Ernst Brücke at the Physiological Institute of Vienna's University. Brücke was also a mentor to Exner, who took over Brücke's chair in 1891. Freud was consequently well acquainted with the work of Exner (1894), who was a pioneer in modeling brain circuits for affective and cognitive behavior (see Peper and Markowitsch, 2001). Freud (1954) assumed that ultimately a brain basis would be found for his psychoanalytic theories. He described psychologic phenomena as the routing of nervous energy in a neuron system and assumed that cerebral lesions and mental disorders have a common physiologic mechanism (cf. Jacobson, 1995).

A complementary approach came from von Monakow (1914) (see also Markowitsch and Pritzel, 1978; Engelhardt and da Mota Gomez, 2013). As explained in Markowitsch (1988), von Monakow divided shock into four types: (1) the shock of the surgeon (wound shock, traumatic shock); (2) psychic shock; (3) apoplectic shock (following a concussion of the brain); and (4) diaschisis (a usually sudden functional interruption in distinct, widely distributed central functional circuits). von Monakow in general favored a more holistic ("antilocalizationistic") approach in interpreting the consequences of brain damage. With his four forms of shock he acknowledged that both somatic-physiologic and psychic conditions can alter the functioning of the nervous system. And therefore he also at this early phase of brain research emphasized that intellectual functions can be suddenly disrupted by a variety of conditions.

Modern neuroimaging methods allow the investigation of structural as well as functional interruptions of the brain's circuitry and therefore narrow the gap between neurologic and psychiatric findings (Markowitsch, 1999c). The so-called trauma model seems to fit the findings best (Dalenberg et al., 2012; see also Vermetten et al., 2007; it is also in accordance with the writing of Freud, 1893, who considered hysteria to be caused by incompletely abreacted psychic traumata). Functional imaging findings in normal subjects attribute a role to the right-hemispheric anterior temporal lobes and the right inferolateral prefrontal cortex for triggering the recollection of episodic-autobiographic episodes (Fink et al., 1996). These regions furthermore contain emotion-processing structures such as the amygdala (Markowitsch and Staniloiu, 2011b) and are interconnected by various branches of the uncinate fascicle (Fig. 36.3), a fiber system which seems to be more expanded in the right hemisphere (Highley et al., 2002), and which seems to grow with advancing age of the individual (Lebel et al., 2008). Children reared in a deprived, neglectful environment show microstructural changes of the uncinate fascicle (Govindan et al., 2010) that may be accompanied by the so-called overgeneral memory effect, a phenomenon characterized by reduced specificity, detail, and emotional colorization of reported autobiographic episodes. A similar effect can be found in patients with Alzheimer's disease (Seidl et al., 2006). While normal individuals, requested to recollect autobiographic information from their past, demonstrate increased frontotemporal activity, particularly in the right hemisphere (Fink et al., 1996), patients with dissociative amnesia show a decreased activation in this area (Markowitsch et al., 1997b; Brand et al., 2009), or a very selective right anterior temporal increase only, which corresponds with reporting affect-related excitation towards past events which cannot be consciously narrated (Markowitsch et al., 1997c).

A major question is how the dysfunction of this combination of areas is initiated and maintained. As stress is acting, and has acted, nearly universally in patients with dissociative amnesia (Arrigo and Pezdek, 1997; Markowitsch, 1999b, 2006; Bremner, 2005, 2010; Igwe, 2013; Wabnitz et al., 2013; Magnin et al., 2014), an overflow of stress hormones (glucocorticoids; O'Brien, 1997; de Kloet et al., 2005a, b; Lupien et al., 2005, 2009; de Kloet and Rinne, 2007) and an altered activity of the hypothalamic–pituitary–adrenal axis (Heim et al., 2008) is postulated to occur, blocking the retrieval of stress-related memories and possibly also generalizing to other memories of an emotional nature (Markowitsch et al., 1999c; Markowitsch, 2002; Fujiwara and Markowitsch, 2006a; cf. Wolf, 2009; Brand and Markowitsch, 2010; O'Brien, 2011; Wingenfeld and Wolf, 2014; Staniloiu and Markowitsch, 2015). Stress, induced by traumatic events during childhood or youth, seems to result in a long-term change in the brain's response to further stress situations later in (adult) life (Markowitsch, 1999b, 2000; Spiegel et al., 2013).

Hippocampal formation and the amygdala play central roles in emotion-related memory processing (Heim et al., 2008; Lupien et al., 2011; Markowitsch and Staniloiu, 2011b; Markowitsch, 2013; cf. also the discussion between Anderson, 2004, and Rees, 2003, on the interaction between brain damage, stress, and cognitive consequences). Amygdala and hippocampal formation possess the highest density of stress hormones in the brain. Consequently, several studies reported damage to brain structures after stress and psychic trauma conditions (e.g., Sapolsky, 1996a, b, 2000; Bremner, 2005). Memory problems accompanying stress are consequently a common occurrence (Markowitsch, 1999b, 2006; Lupien and Maheu, 2000; Valentino et al., 2009; Quesada et al., 2012). And, as a number of studies found a functional lateralization, with the right hemisphere processing emotionally laden information and the left one neutral facts (Markowitsch et al., 1999a; Schore, 2002, 2005; Moriguchi et al., 2006; Gregory et al., 2014), it makes sense that functional imaging studies principally confirmed the idea of right-hemispheric episodic-autobiographic memory (see Fink et al., 1996; Markowitsch et al., 2000a, b; LaBar and Cabeza, 2006).

A relation to conscious memory suppression has been proposed as well (cf. Kikuchi et al., 2010; Staniloiu and Markowitsch, 2014). In a number of more recent articles, mechanisms of willful memory suppression were analyzed (e.g., Paz-Alonso et al., 2009, 2013; Benoit and Anderson, 2012; Detre et al., 2013; van Schie et al., 2013), a skill which might also be used to conceal guilty knowledge (e.g., Bergström et al., 2013) and which is related to prefrontal activation (Anderson et al., 2004). We have studied patients who first willfully pretended to be amnesic, but later apparently had dissociative amnesia which they no longer could control willfully. Such patients therefore demonstrate that there may be brain mechanisms which, as a consequence of stress, lead to a block of the possibility to retrieve subjectively problematic memories (cf. Fig. 15.2 of Fujiwara and Markowitsch, 2006a, and the corresponding explanation in the text). There also seems to be a relation between prefrontal activity and susceptibility to hypnosis and hysteria (Bell et al., 2011); posthypnotic amnesia has been discussed as a model for dissociative amnesia (Cox and Barnier, 2003).

The probable mechanism acting in dissociative amnesia may be comparable to when one is trying to reconstruct the contents of a dream after having been awake for some time: there may be very vague schemes, but it is not possible to arrange a united scene which includes a "what, where, when" trilogy and a first-person perspective (Markowitsch and Staniloiu, 2013). This idea has similarities to the index theory of memory (Teyler and Rudy, 2007), which assumes that there has to be an interaction between limbic regions – such as the hippocampus – and neocortical ones for conscious retrieval of information (Llewellyn, 2013). Similarly, the lack of identity feelings has parallels to sleep conditions or to conditions of dementia (Jetten et al., 2010; Stickgold and Walker, 2013), where the corticolimbic network is so broken and unstable that a coherent resonance pattern, creating identity, cannot be established. Both the unstable identity and memory conditions are preserved as long as under conditions of psychic effort stress hormones are released and block retrieval. There may be a process of prolonged continuity which then leads to alterations in the neuronal network so that with time also the connectivity between brain structures becomes damaged so that the ability to re-establish a united self (Staniloiu et al., 2010; Markowitsch and Staniloiu, 2011a; Markowitsch, 2013) and access to the personal past remains chronically impaired.

Such a condition may also follow or be strengthened by direct tissue damage in regions which usually are involved in accessing stored episodes and in preparing them for conscious reconstruction. For instance, brain damage that includes frontotemporal regions of primarily the right hemisphere can trigger the blockade of retrieving episodic-autobiographic episodes (Calabrese et al., 1996; Kroll et al., 1997). Of special interest, and somewhat puzzling, is why at least some patients with organic brain damage and retrograde amnesia are able to acquire new episodic-autobiographic information long-term, while they remain unable to retrieve old information. This issue was discussed in Kroll et al. (1997); alternative retrieval paths were suggested for the newly acquired episodes or the possibility

> *that the storage of memory content is composed according to landmarks (e.g. around an important event such as the Second World War). This could then result in the inability to recall events which occurred prior to the landmark of the brain damage, while not affecting those stored thereafter (Treadway et al., 1992; Hodges and McCarthy, 1993) (Kroll et al., 1997, p. 1396).*

It was also referred to Wolpaw's (1971) hypothesis "that brain damage which is especially traumatic … may disrupt the association between memories due to the 'missing link' (temporofrontal junction area) which is necessary for the organized triggering of (frontal portion) and access to (temporal portion) the engrams" (Kroll et al., 1997, p. 1396). A related hypothesis was put forward by Lucchelli et al. (1995), who suggested the existence of a reversible distortion of "neuronal pattern matrices." And, finally, one can mention the work of Mace, who argued for involuntary memory chaining in autobiographic memory recall and that events always consolidate in the same conceptual class or network (Mace et al., 2010, 2013; Mace, 2014). His ideas imply that memories may be consciously activated via spreading activations. In contrast, this could mean that, if one or a few critical mnemonic events are suppressed, this can in principle spread to all mnemonic events.

HOW CAN RECOVERY OCCUR?

Even in cases with direct organic amnesia (thalamic stroke), sudden recovery may occur (Lucchelli et al., 1995). In case G.R. of Lucchelli et al. (1995), this occurred when he was in a special, somewhat uncomfortable and unusual situation – similar to a very related one that had occurred some 25 years before. The second case of Lucchelli et al. (1995) – patient M.M., who had had a car accident, but no visible structural brain damage – recovered from his severe autobiographic retrograde amnesia 1 month after the accident, triggered by the fact that he had made the same error while playing tennis as he had done years before. One of our patients (patient D.F.) showed partial memory recovery after being confronted with a slaughter scene 10 months after the onset of her amnesia (Reinhold and Markowitsch, 2009). This slaughter scene involved putting her hands in pig blood; it triggered an event of homicide in China after which she had become amnesic. She still felt guilty that she did not intervene or help and this negative feeling may have prolonged her partial autobiographic amnesia. One of our dissociative amnesic patients was extensively documented in a book entitled *Der Mann, der sein Gedächtnis verlor* [*The Man, who Lost his Memory*] (Kruse, 2010). The journalist Kuno Kruse, who followed his life for more than 5 years, found that certain confrontations with emotion-laden loci and comrades from his past triggered a few memories of his childhood, while others – for an outsider, similar situations – failed to do so. Also listening to music or playing the piano (which the patient had done in childhood) evoked a few broken memories.

These cases demonstrate the importance of the concept of state dependency of memory, originally proposed by Semon in 1904 – together with the concept of "ecphory" (Markowitsch and Staniloiu, in press). Tulving in 1983 reintroduced both concepts and brought them to general attention. Semon also stated in his 1904 monograph that engrams are rarely lost after brain damage – there is just an inability to access (to ecphorize) still fully intact memories. Tulving described ecphory as the process by which retrieval cues interact with stored information so that an image or a representation of the information in question appears. Retrieval cues may occur as other thought associations or as cues from the environment. If the retrieval cues are very different from those existing during encoding, distortions in remembrance may occur – a phenomenon taken up by Sigmund Freud in a number of variations (Breuer and Freud, 1895; Freud, 1901a, b, 1910), and named "encoding specificity principle" in modern literature (Tulving and Thompson, 1973).

Though the encoding specificity principle is in general considered a valid hypothesis, Naime (2002) opposes it in his critique. Naime assumes that it is not so much the match between states of encoding and of retrieval, but cue distinctiveness. He proposes that retrieval is successful if there is a highly distinctive (though possibly only minimal) overlap between the encoding and retrieval conditions ("relative diagnostic match"). Memory is characterized by him as an active process of discrimination. A more recent study by Goh and Lu (2012) tested and supported Naime's proposal. Also Naime's ideas could explain the retrieval impairment of patients with retrograde episodic-autobiographic amnesia: Such patients cannot recognize and discriminate proper cues that would trigger the respective memories. An analogy to this hypothesis might be when a certain word or scene occurring during the daytime triggers the remembrance of a dreamwhich otherwise would have been "forgotten" (or inaccessible).

It seems that only a kind of reconnection between new events similar to the blocked ones triggers memory recovery – by unblocking the pathways to the autobiographic engrams. This phenomenon can be found in very old anecdotic texts in which it is stated that one should cure a shock condition by introducing a similar shock. Some of the present therapeutic approaches for patients with dissociative amnesia may have a related rationale for unblocking memories, namely hypnosis or the sodium amytal abreaction procedure ("truth drug").

WHY IS ANTEROGRADE LEARNING OF AUTOBIOGRAPHIC EPISODES USUALLY UNIMPAIRED OR MUCH LESS IMPAIRED THAN RETROGRADE MEMORY?

After onset of a memory-blocking event patients are in a different setting, compared to their life before – their life is split into an inaccessible personal past and a new, accessible present. There is frequently the observation that the new present differs emotionally from the past. Many patients – whether with structural brain damage or with dissociative amnesia – live in a very different emotional condition compared to that prior to the amnesia-triggering event (Reinhold and Markowitsch, 2009; Staniloiu et al., 2010; Staniloiu and Markowitsch, 2012a–c). Already before the turn of the 20th century, Janet (1893) and then Breuer and Freud (1895) named one of these altered conditions "*la belle indifférence*"; it describes a flattening of emotions. In a survey based on 11 reports, Stone et al. (2006) found that only 21% of patients with conversion disorder and 29% with organic disease showed *la belle indifférence*. However, there was a considerable variance between studies (0–54% in 356 patients with conversion disorder and 0–60% in 157 patients with organic disease). Whether *la belle indifférence* is indeed rarer than noted in the literature (e.g., Kleist, 1918; Kiersch, 1962; Reinhold and Markowitsch, 2007, 2009; Serra et al., 2007; Pommerenke et al., 2012) is a still open issue. Staniloiu and Markowitsch (2014) wrote that many patients with dissociative amnesia "report feeling distressed by their amnesic syndromes" (p. 229). An observation we made is that patients with retrograde amnesia encode new information likely in an emotionally flat manner (Markowitsch et al., 1993a; Reinhold and Markowitsch, 2007, 2009; Staniloiu and Markowitsch, 2012b; Markowitsch and Staniloiu, 2013) and may show impaired somatic responses to emotional stimuli (Reinhold and Markowitsch, 2009; Tramoni et al., 2009). In patients with dissociative (conversion) amnesia heart rate variability is lower than in healthy participants (Tramoni et al., 2009; van der Kruijs et al., 2014). Furthermore, patients with dissociative amnesia frequently show signs of depression and alexithymia (Markowitsch et al., 1998, 1999c, 2000b; Maldano and Spiegel, 2008; Moriguchi et al., 2009; Staniloiu et al., 2010). All this impairs theory of mind functions and foresight, and reduces the patient to an extended noetic present (Suddendorf et al., 2009) with resignation and lack of concern. And in fact, this is a not uncommon observation in patients with retrograde amnesia: they can and do learn new information, but they do this in a neutral, unengaged manner – they are unable to resonate with their social and biologic environment (Markowitsch, 1998).

It is obvious that there are also patients pretending to be amnesic or exaggerating their deficit – for example, in legal or forensic situations – and that proper assessment has to be performed in order to preclude faking in such cases (Bass and Halligan, 2007; Jenkins et al., 2009; Markowitsch and Staniloiu, 2011c; Boone, 2013). Already in 1943 Lennox wrote that feigned amnesia may accompany both organic and psychogenic amnesia. He suggested that some patients may manifest a combination of three types of amnesia ("pathological" [organic], "psychological," and "feigned"; Lennox, 1943, p. 741). Similarly, Barbarotto et al. later (1996) described a case under the heading "A case of simulated, psychogenic or focal pure retrograde amnesia: Did an entire life become unconscious?" (A similar case with a similar title was published by Weusten et al., 2013.) We had several patients who started with conscious memory suppression or faking of amnesia and apparently ended with true dissociative amnesia. Changes in the brain's circuitry therefore may occur as a consequence of certain patterns of thinking and acting – a phenomenon that may have relations to the concepts of embodiment (Pfeifer and Bongard, 2007; Campbell and Garcia, 2009; Dove, 2011) and extended mind (Clark and Chalmers, 1998; Clark, 2008).

CONCLUSIONS

Aside from cases with major cortical degeneration such as in most forms of dementia, the brain correlates of retrograde amnesia are still unclear. Reasons for this most likely have to do with the uncertainty about how memories – especially episodic-autobiographic episodes – are stored (and retrieved) in the brain. For memory storage, ideas exist which assume distinct storage places, based on findings that some patients showed an inability to retrieve specific categories of information after circumscribed brain damage (e.g., Warrington and Shallice, 1984; Damasio, 1990; De Renzi and Lucchelli, 1994), gnostic units (John, 1975; Quiroga, 2013), grandmother (Gross, 2002), and concept cells (Quiroga et al., 2005, 2008; Quiroga, 2012), statistically distributed (John, 1972), and holistic representations (Pribram, 1971; Deacon, 1989), or a compromise between such ideas (Markowitsch, 1985, 2013; Mesulam, 1990, 2000). This variety of approaches demonstrates an *ignoramus* – we do not know. Similarly, there are at present only speculations on how stored memories are accessed and how access is blocked. This is a continuing issue, especially for dissociative or psychogenic amnesia, though the expression "psychogenic amnesia" can already be found as the headline of a commentary in the *Lancet* in 1935 in which the writer warns of the "incompleteness of purely psychological explanations of amnesia, and the occasional practical risks of accepting them as final" (Anonymous, 1935).

Regions of the frontotemporal cortex have, however, frequently been associated with retrograde amnesia. They are also most commonly affected in TBI, the etiology most closely associated with retrograde amnesia. Damage to these regions – in addition to memory – also affects social-emotional processing, inhibitory processes, attention, and consciousness (e.g., Feuchtwanger, 1923; Damasio, 1999; Eluvathingal et al., 2006; Fujiwara and Markowitsch, 2006b; LaBar and Cabeza, 2006; Sturm et al., 2006; Schulte-Rüther et al., 2007, 2011; Marinkovic et al., 2011; Vandekerckhove et al., 2014). Furthermore, they are intimately interconnected (e.g., Horel, 1978; Sarter and Markowitsch, 1984; Ebeling and von Cramon, 1992; Kier et al., 2004; Eluvathingal et al., 2006; Diehl et al., 2008; Phan Luan et al., 2009; Staniloiu and Markowitsch, 2012e). It is therefore likely that the complex network of emotion-embedded memory functions and autonoetic consciousness becomes disturbed both after direct brain damage and after major biochemical alterations (Markowitsch, 1996a, b, 1998; O'Brien, 1997; Lupien et al., 2005, 2009). Attentional dysfunctions and processes of increased inhibition may strengthen and maintain the block of information retrieval (or, more generally, of consciously forming representations of events), as delineated in the model depicted in Figure 15.2 of Fujiwara and Markowitsch (2006a).

Another, related model was proposed by R.J. Brown (2004) to account for medically unexplained symptoms. It proposes body-focused attention as psychologic defense. The model assumes "that traumatic events such as physical, sexual, and emotional abuse often lead to the use of body-focused attention as a means of avoiding the affect and cognitive activity associated with experiences of this sort" (p. 806). Also Chadda and Raheja (2002) argue with a narrowed attention in patients with dissociative amnesia. Support for such ideas comes from findings showing a forgetting-related downregulation of neural synchrony mediated by the prefrontal cortex (Hanslmeyer et al., 2012) and from the study of Brand et al. (2009). These authors combined brain glucose PET data from 14 patients with dissociative amnesia in order to detect brain regions with changed activity patterns. They found a significant metabolic reduction in the right ventromedial prefrontal cortex, extending in principle to the right anterior temporal cortex (Fig. 36.4). Their data are in agreement with previous findings demonstrating increased PET activation (radioactive water PET) in individuals retrieving autobiographic episodes from their past (Fink et al., 1996) and with data from patients with damage to the right frontotemporal brain failing to retrieve memories from their personal past (Markowitsch et al., 1993a; Kroll et al., 1997; Levine et al., 1998, 2009).

Further support for the involvement of the prefrontal cortex in memory retrieval comes from a study of Kunii et al. (2012). These authors conducted a sequential cerebral blood flow (CBF) study with SPECT in an ex-convict with dissociative amnesia. They carried out CBF-SPECT measurement during memory retrieval 10, 50, 86, 114, and 146 days after admission, while the patient gradually recovered from his amnesia during this time period. A regions-of-interest analysis revealed a continuous increase in frontal cortex regional CBF during the process of recovery (increased retrieval) and suggested, in the eyes of the authors, that the frontal cortex might be inhibited (less active) during dissociative amnesia. Alternatively, or in addition to this function, a heightened activation could reflect "an active mental defense against unwanted memories of which the patient was not aware due to strong repression" (p. 624). This last remark they made with reference to the findings of Anderson et al. (2004) on neural systems underlying the suppression of unwanted memories.

So, at least with respect to recollecting past personal episodes, it seems that there is evidence for a crucial involvement of the right temporofrontal cortex. What, however, remains to be unraveled are especially the conditions for recovery from retrograde episodic-autobiographic amnesia. From the sparse results available (see above), it seems that even full recovery can occur in less severely brain-damaged patients and in principle in most patients with dissociative amnesia. Supportive or triggering factors for recovery have to be established, especially for more severe cases, in addition to the conventional forms of therapy (McKay and Kopelman, 2009; Staniloiu and Markowitsch, 2014). The neuropathology of retrograde amnesia is still much more a riddle than that of anterograde amnesia. Probably, more subtle forms of brain damage, occurring in a considerable proportion of patients with retrograde compared to anterograde amnesia, have to be investigated (changes in biochemistry, in the neuropil) (Markowitsch and Staniloiu, 2012a). Findings of electric brain stimulation (Doty, 1970; Bancaud et al., 1994) and electroconvulsive therapy (Hihn et al., 2006; Sackeim et al., 2007; Fraser et al., 2008) point in the direction that circuits and association fibers seem to play a particular role in evoking conscious memories.

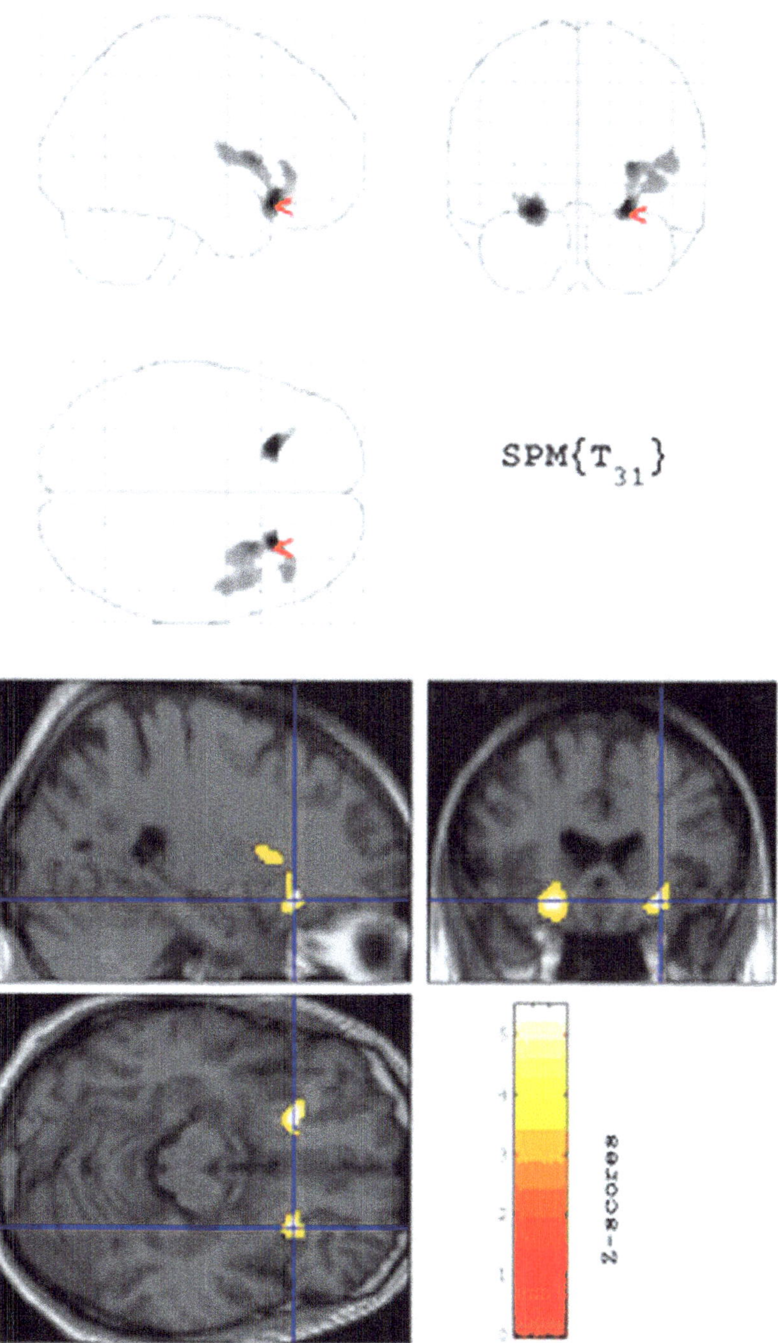

Fig. 36.4. Relative decreases in regional cerebral glucose metabolism in 14 patients with dissociative amnesia relative to 19 control individuals (sagittal, frontal, and horizontal views as "glass brains" and superimposed on magnetic resonance imaging (MRI) sections: MRI template). The blue cross indicates the locus of the only significantly deactivated spot in the right inferolateral prefrontal cortex ($p_{corrected} < 0.001$, $x = 26$ mm, $y = 24$ mm, $z = -14$ mm). The homologous hypometabolic region within the left inferolateral prefrontal cortex failed to reach significance ($p_{corrected} < 0.083$, $x = 22$ mm, $y = 24$ mm, $z = -14$ mm). (Reproduced from Brand et al. (2009), Figure 1, with permission of Elsevier.)

References

Aldenhoff J (1997). Überlegungen zur Psychobiologie der Depression. Nervenarzt 68: 379–389.

Allen JS, Tranel D, Bruss J et al. (2006). Correlations between regional brain volumes and memory performance in anoxia. J Clin Exp Neuropsychol 28: 457–476.

American Psychiatric Association (1968). Diagnostic and Statistical Manual of Mental Disorders (2nd ed): DSM-II, American Psychiatric Association, Washington, DC, USA.

American Psychiatric Association (2013). Diagnostic and Statistical Manual of Mental Disorders—Fifth Edition: DSM-5, American Psychiatric Publishing, Washington, DC, USA.

Anderson SD (2004). Mild traumatic brain injury and memory impairment. Arch Phys Med Rehabil 85: 862.

Anderson CA, Arciniegas DB (2010). Cognitive sequelae of hypoxic-ischemic brain injury: a review. NeuroRehab 26: 47–63.

Anderson MC, Ochsner KN, Kuhl B et al. (2004). Neural systems underlying the suppression of unwanted memories. Science 303: 232–235.

Anderson ND, Davidson PSR, Mason WP et al. (2011). Right frontal lobe mediation of recollection- and familiarity-based verbal recognition memory: evidence from patients with tumor resections. J Cogn Neurosci 23: 3804–3816.

Anonymous (1935). Psychogenic amnesia. Lancet 26: 953.

Arrigo JM, Pezdek K (1997). Lessons from the study of psychogenic amnesia. Curr Direct Psychol Sci 6: 148–152.

Arzy S, Collette S, Wissmeyer M et al. (2011). Psychogenic amnesia and self-identity: a multimodal functional investigation. Eur J Neurol 18: 1422–1425.

Back T, Haag C, Buchberger A et al. (1998). Diffusionsgewichtetes MR–Imaging bei einem Fall von dissoziativer Amnesie. Nervenarzt 69: 909–912.

Bancaud J, Brunet-Bourgin F, Chauvel P et al. (1994). Anatomical origin of déjà vu and vivid 'memories' in human temporal lobe epilepsy. Brain 117: 71–90.

Barbarotto R, Laiacona M, Cocchini G (1996). A case of simulated, psychogenic or focal pure retrograde amnesia: did an entire life become unconscious? Neuropsychologia 34: 575–585.

Bartsch T, Butler C (2013). Transient amnesic syndromes. Nat Rev Neurol 9: 86–97.

Bartsch T, Deuschl G (2010). Transient global amnesia: functional anatomy and clinical implications. Lancet Neurol 9: 205–214.

Bass C, Halligan PW (2007). Illness related deception: social or psychiatric problem? J Roy Soc Med 100: 81–84.

Bell V, Oakley DA, Halligan PW et al. (2011). Dissociation in hysteria and hypnosis: evidence from cognitive neuroscience. J Neurol Neurosurg Psychiatry 82: 332–339.

Bendlin BB, Ries ML, Lazar M et al. (2008). Longitudinal changes in patients with traumatic brain injury assessed with diffusion-tensor and volumetric imaging. Neuroimage 42: 503–514.

Bennett AH (1878). Case of cerebral tumour-symptoms simulating hysteria. Brain 1: 114–120.

Benoit RG, Anderson MC (2012). Opposing mechanisms support the voluntary forgetting of unwanted memories. Neuron 76: 450–460.

Bergström ZM, Anderson MC, Buda M et al. (2013). Intentional retrieval suppression can conceal guilty knowledge in ERP memory detection tests. Biol Psychiatry 94: 1–11.

Boedeker J (1896). Ueber einen Fall von retro- und anterograder Amnesie nach Erhängungsversuch. Arch Psychiatr Nervenkrankht 29: 647–650.

Bogousslavsky J (2011). Hysteria after Charcot; Back to the future. Front Neurol Neurosci 29: 137–161.

Boone KB (2013). Clinical Practice of Forensic Neuropsychology, Guilford Press, New York.

Brand M, Markowitsch HJ (2010). Aspects of forgetting in psychogenic amnesia. In: S Della Sala (Ed.), Forgetting, Psychology Press, Hove, East Sussex, pp. 239–251.

Brand M, Eggers C, Reinhold N et al. (2009). Functional brain imaging in fourteen patients with dissociative amnesia reveals right inferolateral prefrontal hypometabolism. Psychiatr Res Neuroimag Sect 174: 32–39.

Brandt J, Van Gorp WG (2006). Functional ("psychogenic") amnesia. Semin Neurol 26: 331–340.

Bremner JD (2005). Effects of traumatic stress on brain structure and functions: relevance to early responses to trauma. J Trauma Dissoc 6: 51–68.

Bremner JD (2010). Cognitive processes in dissociation: Comment on Giesbrecht et al. (2008). Psychol Bull 136: 1–6.

Breuer J, Freud S (1895). Studien über Hysterie. Deuticke, Vienna.

Brown AS (2002). Consolidation theory and retrograde amnesia in humans. Psychonom Bull Rev 9: 403–425.

Brown RJ (2004). Psychological mechanisms of medically unexplained symptoms: an integrative conceptual model. Psychol Bull 130: 793–812.

Bumke O (1924). Lehrbuch der Geisteskrankheiten, JF Bergmann, Munich.

Butler CR, Zeman A (2011). The causes and consequences of transient epileptic amnesia. Behav Neurol 24: 299–305.

Calabrese P, Markowitsch HJ, Durwen HF et al. (1996). Right temporofrontal cortex as critical locus for the ecphory of old episodic memories. J Neurol Neurosurg Psychiatry 61: 304–310.

Campbell BC, Garcia JR (2009). Neuroanthropology: evolation and emotional embodiment. Front Evolut Neurosci 1: 1–6. Art. 4.

Carlesimo GA, Lombardi MG, Caltagirone C (2011). Vascular thalamic amnesia: a reappraisal. Neuropsychologia 49: 777–789.

Chadda RK, Raheja D (2002). Amnesia for autobiographical memory: a case series. Indian J Psychiatr 44: 283–288.

Charcot JM (1892). Sur un cas d'amnésie retro-anterograde. Rev Med 12: 81–96.

Cimino CR, Verfaellie M, Bowers D et al. (1991). Autobiographical memory: influence of right hemisphere damage on emotionality and specificity. Brain Cognit 15: 106–118.

Clark A (2008). Supersizing the mind: Embodiment, Action, and the Cognitive Extension, Oxford University Press, London.

Clark A, Chalmers DJ (1998). The extended mind. Analysis 58: 10–23.

Coons PM, Milstein V (1992). Psychogenic amnesia: a clinical investigation of 25 Cases. Dissociation 5: 73–79.

Cox RE, Barnier AJ (2003). Posthypnotic amnesia for a first romantic relationship: forgetting the entire relationship versus forgetting selected events. Memory 11: 307–318.

Craver CF, Graham B, Rosenbaum RS (2014a). Remembering Mr. B. Cortex 59: 153–184.

Craver CF, Kwan D, Steindam C et al. (2014b). Individuals with episodic amnesia are not stuck in time. Neuropsychologia 57: 181–195.

Dalenberg CJ, Brand BL, Gleaves DH et al. (2012). Evaluation of the evidence for the trauma and fantasy models of dissociation. Psychol Bull 138: 150–188.

Dalla Barba G, Mantovan MC, Ferruzza E et al. (1997). Remembering and knowing the past: a case study of isolated retrograde amnesia. Cortex 33: 143–154.

Damasio AR (1990). Category-related recognition defects as a clue to the neural substrates of knowledge. Trends Neurosci 13: 95–98.

Damasio AR (1999). The feeling of what happens. Body and emotion in the making of consciousness. Harcourt, San Diego.

Damasio AR, Tranel D (1990). Knowing that 'Colorado' goes with 'Denver' does not imply knowledge that 'Denver' is in 'Colorado'. Behav Brain Res 40: 193–200.

Damasio AR, Tranel D, Damasio HC (1991). Somatic markers and the guidance of behavior: Theory and preliminary testing. In: HS Levin, HM Eisenberg, AL Benton (Eds.), Frontal Lobe Function and Dysfunction, Oxford University Press, New York, pp. 217–229.

de Kloet ER, Rinne T (2007). Neuroendocrine markers of early trauma. In: E Vermetten, MJ Dorahy, D Spiegel (Eds.), Traumatic Dissociation. Neurobiology and Treatment, American Psychiatric Publishing, Arlington, VA, pp. 139–156.

de Kloet R, Joels M, Holsboer F (2005a). Stress and the brain: from adaptation to disease. Nat Rev Neurosci 6: 463–475.

de Kloet ER, Sibug RM, Helmerhorst FM et al. (2005b). Stress, genes and the mechanism of programming the brain for later life. Neurosci Biobehav Rev 29: 271–281.

De Renzi E, Lucchelli F (1993). Dense retrograde amnesia, intact learning capability and abnormal forgetting rate: a consolidation deficit? Cortex 29: 449–466.

De Renzi E, Lucchelli F (1994). Are semantic systems separately represented in the brain? The case of living category impairment. Cortex 30: 3–25.

De Renzi E, Liotti M, Nichelli P (1987). Semantic amnesia with preservation of autobiographic memory. A case report. Cortex 23: 575–597.

De Renzi E, Lucchelli F, Muggia S et al. (1995). Persistent retrograde amnesia following a minor head trauma. Cortex 31: 531–542.

De Renzi E, Lucchelli F, Muggia S et al. (1997). Is memory without anatomical damage tantamount to a psychogenic deficit? The case of pure retrograde amnesia. Neuropsychologia 35: 781–794.

Deacon TW (1989). Holism and associationism in neuropsychology: An anatomical synthesis. In: E Perecman (Ed.), Integrating Theory and Practice in Clinical Neuropsychology, LEA, Hillsdale, NJ, pp. 1–47.

Dean PJA, Sterr A (2013). Long-term effects of mild traumatic brain injury on cognitive performance. Front Hum Neurosci 7. Art. 30.

Deelman BG, Saan RJ, Van Zomeren AH (1990). Traumatic Brain Injury; Clinical, Social, and Rehabilitational Aspects. Swets & Zeitlinger, Lisse.

Detre GJ, Natarajan A, Gershman SJ et al. (2013). Moderate levels of activation lead to forgetting in the think/no-think paradigm. Neuropsychologia 51: 2371–2388.

Diehl B, Busch RM, Duncan JS et al. (2008). Abnormalities in diffusion tensor imaging of the uncinate fasciculus relate to reduced memory in temporal lobe epilepsy. Epilepsia 49: 1409–1418.

Doty RW (1970). On butterflies in the brain. In: VS Rusinov (Ed.), Electrophysiology of the Central Nervous System, Plenum Press, New York, pp. 97–106.

Dove G (2011). On the need for embodied and dis-embodied cognition. Front Psychol 1: 1–13 Art. 242.

Ebeling U, von Cramon D (1992). Topography of the uncinate fascicle and adjacent temporal fiber tracts. Acta Neurochir (Vienna) 115: 143–148.

Eluvathingal TJ, Chugani HT, Behen ME et al. (2006). Abnormal brain connectivity in children after early severe socioemotional deprivation: a diffusion tensor imaging study. Pediatrics 117: 2093–2100.

Engelhardt E, da Mota Gomez M (2013). Shock, diaschisis and von Monakow. Arq Neuropsiquiatr 71: 487–489.

Exner S (1894). Entwurf zu einer physiologischen Erklärung der psychischen Erscheinungen. Franz Deuticke, Leipzig.

Fast K, Fujiwara E (2001). Isolated retrograde amnesia. Neurocase 7: 269–282.

Feuchtwanger E (1923). Die Funktionen des Stirnhirns, Springer, Berlin.

Fink GR, Markowitsch HJ, Reinkemeier M et al. (1996). Cerebral representation of one's own past: neural networks involved in autobiographical memory. J Neurosci 16: 4275–4282.

Fisher CM (1966). Concussion amnesia. Neurology 16: 826–830.

Flechsig P (1896a). Die Lokalisation der geistigen Vorgänge, insbesondere der Sinnesempfindungen des Menschen. Veit, Leipzig.

Flechsig P (1896b). Gehirn und Seele, Veit, Leipzig.

Fradera A, Kopelman MD (2009). Memory disorders. In: LR Squire (Ed.), Encyclopedia of Neuroscience, Vol. 5. Academic Press, Oxford, pp. 751–760.

Fraser LM, O'Caroll RE, Ebmeier KP (2008). The effect of electroconvulsive therapy on autobiographic memory: a systematic review. J ECT 24: 10–17.

Freud S (1893). Über den psychischen Mechanismus hysterischer Phänomene. Wien Med Presse 34: 121–126 and 165–167.

Freud S (1901a). Zum psychischen Mechanismus der Vergesslichkeit. Monatsschr Psychiatr Neurol 4 (5): 436–443.

Freud S (1901b). Zur Psychopathologie des Alltagslebens (Vergessen, Versprechen, Vergreifen) nebst Bemerkungen über eine Wurzel des Aberglaubens. Monatsschr Psychiatr Neurol 10: 1–32 and 95–143.

Freud S (1910). Über Psychoanalyse. Fünf Vorlesungen gehalten zur 20jährigen Gründungsfeier der Clark University in Worcester Mass. September 1909, F. Deuticke, Leipzig.

Freud S (1954). Project for a scientific psychology. In: M Bonaparte, A Freud, E Kris (Eds.), The Origins of Psychoanalysis, Letters to Wilhelm Fliess, Drafts and Notes, Basic Books, New York, pp. 1887–1902.

Fujiwara E, Markowitsch HJ (2006a). Brain correlates of binding processes of emotion and memory. In: H Zimmer, AM Mecklinger, U Lindenberger (Eds.), Binding in Human Memory – A Neurocognitive Perspective, Oxford University Press, Oxford, UK, pp. 379–410.

Fujiwara E, Markowitsch HJ (2006b). Das mnestische Blockadesyndrom: Hirnorganische Korrelate von Angst und Stress. In: G Schiepek (Ed.), Neurobiologische Korrelate der Psychotherapie, Schattauer, Stuttgart, pp. 186–212.

Fujiwara E, Brand M, Kracht L et al. (2008). Functional retrograde amnesia: a multiple case study. Cortex 44: 29–45.

Gale SD, Johnson SC, Bigler ED et al. (1995). Nonspecific white matter degeneration following traumatic brain injury. J Int Neuropsychol Soc 1: 17–28.

Ganser SJ (1898). Ueber einen eigenartigen hysterischen Dämmerzustand. Arch Psychiatr Nervenkrankht 30: 633–640.

Ganser SJ (1904). Zur Lehre vom hysterischen Dämmerzustande. Arch Psychiatr Nervenkrankht 38: 34–46.

Goh WD, Lu SHX (2012). Testing the myth of the encoding–retrieval match. Mem Cogn 40: 28–39.

Gold JJ, Squire LR (2006). The anatomy of amnesia: Neurohistological analysis of three new cases. Learn Mem 13: 699–710.

Goldberg E, Antin SP, Bilder Jr RM et al. (1981). Retrograde amnesia: possible role of mesencephalic reticular activation on long-term memory. Science 213: 1392–1394.

Goldberg E, Hughes JEO, Mattis S et al. (1982). Isolated retrograde amnesia: different etiologies, same mechanisms? Cortex 18: 459–462.

Govindan RM, Behen ME, Helder E et al. (2010). Altered water diffusivity in cortical association tracts in children with early deprivation identified with tract-based spatial statistics. Cerebr Cort 20: 561–569.

Grafman J, Jonas BS, Martin A et al. (1988). Intellectual function following penetrating head injury in Vietnam veterans. Brain 111: 169–184.

Gregory E, McCloskey M, Landau B (2014). Profound loss of general knowledge in retrograde amnesia: evidence form an amnesic artist. Front Hum Neurosci 8: 1–10 Art. 287.

Gross CG (2002). Genealogy of the "grandmother cell". Neuroscientist 8: 512–518.

Grossi D, Trojano L, Grasso A et al. (1988). Selective "semantic amnesia" after closed-head injury. A case report. Cortex 24: 457–464.

Grünthal E, Störring GE (1930). Über das Verhalten bei umschriebener, völliger Merkunfähigkeit. Monatsschr Psychiatr Neurol 74: 354–369.

Grünthal E, Störring GE (1933). Ergänzende Beobachtungen und Bemerkungen zu dem in Band 74 (1930) dieser Zeitschrift beschriebenen Fall mit reiner Merkunfähigkeit. Monatsschr Psychiatr Neurol 77: 374–382.

Grünthal E, Störring GE (1954). Einige Bemerkungen zu dem Aufsatz von F. Lotmar: Zur psychophysiologischen Deutung 'isolierten' dauernden Merkfähigkeitsverlustes von extremem Grade nach initialer Kohlenmonoxydschädigung eines Unfallversicherten. Schweiz Arch Neurol Psychiatrie 74: 179.

Grünthal E, Störring GE (1956). Abschließende Stellungnahme zu der vorstehenden Arbeit von H. Völkel und R. Stolze über den Fall B. Monatsschr Neurol Psychiatr 132: 309–311.

Hanslmeyer S, Volberg G, Wimber M et al. (2012). Prefrontally driven downregulation of neural synchrony mediated goal-directed forgetting. J Neurosci 32: 14742–14751.

Harris CB, Sutton J, Barnier AJ (2010). Autobiographical forgetting, social forgetting, and situated forgetting. In: S Della Sala (Ed.), Forgetting, Psychology Press, Hove, East Sussex, pp. 253–284.

Heim C, Mletzko T, Purselle D et al. (2008). The dexamethasone/corticotropin-releasing factor test in men with major depression: role of childhood trauma. Biol Psychiatry 63: 398–405.

Heine R (1911). Die forensische Bedeutung der Amnesie [The forensic significance of amnesia]. Vierteljahresschr gerichtl Med (3 Folge) 42: 51–93.

Hennig-Fast K, Meister F, Frödl T et al. (2008). A case of persistent retrograde amnesia following a dissociative fugue: neuropsychological and neurofunctional underpinnings of loss of autobiographical memory and self-awareness. Neuropsychologia 46: 2993–3005.

Highley JR, Walker MA, Esiri MM et al. (2002). Asymmetry of the uncinate fasciculus: a post-mortem study of normal subjects and patients with shizophrenia. Cerebr Cort 12: 1218–1224.

Hihn H, Baune BT, Michael N et al. (2006). Memory performance in severely depressed patients treated by electroconvulsive therapy. J ECT 22: 189–195.

Hodges JR, McCarthy RA (1993). Autobiographical amnesia resulting from bilateral paramedian thalamic infarction. Brain 116: 921–940.

Hokkanen L, Launes J, Vataja R et al. (1995). Isolated retrograde amnesia for autobiographical material associated with acute left temporal lobe encephalitis. Psychol Med 25: 203–208.

Hokkanen L, Phil L, Salonen O et al. (1996a). Amnesia in acute herpetic and nonherpetic encephalitis. Arch Neurol 53: 972–978.

Hokkanen L, Poutiainen E, Valanne L et al. (1996b). Cognitive impairment after acute encephalitis: comparison of herpes simplex and other aetiologies. J Neurol Neurosurg Psychiatry 61: 478–484.

Horel JA (1978). The neuroanatomy of amnesia. A critique of the hippocampal memory hypothesis. Brain 101: 403–445.

Hunkin NM, Parkin AJ, Bradley VA et al. (1995). Focal retrograde amnesia following closed head injury: a case study and theoretical account. Neuropsychologia 33: 509–523.

Huss M (1852). Chronische Alkoholskrankheit oder Alcolismus chronicus – Ein Beitrag zur Kenntniss der Vergiftungs-Krankheiten, nach eigener und anderer Erfahrung, C.E. Fritze, Stockholm.

Iglesias A, Iglesias A (2009). Diagnosis and hypnotic treatment of an unusual case of hysterical amnesia. Am J Clin Hypnosis 52: 123–131.

Igwe MN (2013). Dissociative fugue symptoms in a 28-year-old male Nigerian medical student: a case report. J Med Case Rep 7: 143.

Insausti R, Annese J, Amaral DG et al. (2013). Human amnesia and the medial temporal lobe illuminated by neuropsychological and neurohistological findings for patient E.P. Proc Natl Acad Sci U S A 110: E1953–E1962.

Jacobson M (1995). Foundations of Neuroscience, Plenum Press, New York.

Janet P (1893). L'amnésie continue. Rev Gen Sci 4: 167–179.

Janet P (1907). The Major Symptoms of Hysteria, Macmillan, New York.

Jenkins KG, Kapur N, Kopelman MD (2009). Retrograde amnesia and malingering. Curr Opin Neurol 22: 601–605.

Jetten J, Haslam C, Pugliese C et al. (2010). Declining autobiographical memory and the loss of identity; Effects on well-being. J Clin Exp Neuropsychol 32: 408–416.

John ER (1972). Switchboard versus statistical theories of learning and memory. Science 177: 850–864.

John ER (1975). Konorski's concept of gnostic areas and units: some electrophysiological considerations. Acta Neurobiol Exp (Wars) 35: 417–429.

Jokeit H, Ebner A, Holthausen H et al. (1997). Individual prediction of change in delayed recall of prose passages after left-sided anterior temporal lobectomy. Neurology 49: 481–487.

Joseph S, Masterson J (1999). Posttraumatic stress disorder and traumatic brain injury: are they mutually exclusive? J Traumat Stress 12: 437–453.

Kapur N (1993). Focal retrograde amnesia in neurological disease: a critical review. Cortex 29: 217–234.

Kapur N, Young A, Bateman D et al. (1989). Focal retrograde amnesia: a long term clinical and neuropsychological follow-up. Cortex 25: 387–402.

Kapur N, Ellison D, Smith MP et al. (1992). Focal retrograde amnesia following bilateral temporal lobe pathology. Brain 115: 73–85.

Kapur N, Scholey K, Moore E et al. (1996). Long-term retention deficits in two cases of disproportionate retrograde amnesia. J Cognit Neurosci 8: 416–434.

Kessler J, Markowitsch HJ, Huber R et al. (1997). Massive and persistent anterograde amnesia in the absence of detectable brain damage – anterograde psychogenic amnesia or gross reduction in sustained effort? J Clin Exp Neuropsychol 19: 604–614.

Kier EL, Staib LH, Davis LM et al. (2004). MR Imaging of the temporal stem: anatomic dissection tractography of the uncinate fasciculus, inferior occipitofrontal fasciculus, and Meyer's loop of the optic radiation. Am J Neuroradiol 25: 677–691.

Kiersch TA (1962). Amnesia: a clinical study of ninety-eight cases. Am J Psychiatry 119: 57–60.

Kihlstrom JF, Glisky ML, McGovern S et al. (2013). Hypnosis in the right hemisphere. Cortex 49: 393–399.

Kikuchi H, Fujii T, Abe N et al. (2010). Memory repression: brain mechanisms underlying dissociative amnesia. J Cogn Neurosci 22: 602–613.

Kim E, Lauterbach EC, Reeve A et al. (2007). Neuropsychiatric complications of traumatic brain injury: a critical review of the literature (A report by the ANPA Committee on Research). J Neuropsychiatr Clin Neurosci 19: 106–127.

Klein S (2015). What memory is. WIREs Cogn Sci 6: 1–38.

Kleist K (1918). Schreckpsychosen. Zeitschr Psychiatr Psychgerichtl Med 74: 432–510.

Kleist K (1934). Gehirnpathologie, Barth, Leipzig.

Kopelman MD (2000). Focal retrograde amnesia and the attribution of causality: an exceptionally critical review. Cogn Neuropsychol 17: 585–621.

Kopelman MD (2002). Disorders of memory. Brain 125: 2152–2190.

Kopelman MD, Lasserson D, Kingsley DR et al. (2003). Retrograde amnesia and the volume of critical brain structures. Hippocampus 13: 879–891 [See comment in PubMed Commons below.].

Koponen S, Taiminen T, Portin R et al. (2002). Axis I and axis II psychiatric disorders after traumatic brain injury: a 30-year follow-up study. Am J Psychiatry 159: 1315–1321.

Krarup F (1924). Hypnoide Handlungen, Amnesie, Wiedererinnerung durch Hypnose. Z Ges Neurol Psychiat 90: 638–645.

Kritchevsky M, Squire LR (1993). Permanent global amnesia with unknown etiology. Neurology 43: 326–332.

Kritchevsky M, Chang J, Squire LR (2004). Functional amnesia: clinical description and neuropsychological profile of 10 cases. Learn Mem 11: 213–226.

Kroll N, Markowitsch HJ, Knight R et al. (1997). Retrieval of old memories – the temporo-frontal hypothesis. Brain 120: 1377–1399.

Kruse K (2010). Der Mann, der sein Gedächtnis verlor. Hoffmann and Campe, Hamburg.

Kühnel S, Woermann FG, Mertens M et al. (2008). Involvement of the orbitofrontal cortex during correct and false recognitions of visual stimuli. Implications for eyewitness decisions on an fMRI study using a film paradigm. Brain Imag Behav 2: 163–176.

Kunii Y, Okano T, Mashiko H et al. (2012). Serial changes in cerebral blood flow single photon emission computed tomography findings during memory retrieval in a case of psychogenic amnesia. Psychiatr Clin Neurosci 66: 623–624.

LaBar KS, Cabeza R (2006). Cognitive neuroscience of emotional memory. Nat Rev Neurosci 7: 54–64.

Lah S, Lee T, Grayson S et al. (2006). Effects of temporal lobe epilepsy on retrograde memory. Epilepsia 47: 615–625.

Lah S, Lee T, Grayson S et al. (2008). Changes in retrograde memory following temporal lobectomy. Epilepsy Behav 13: 391–396.

Lebel CW, Leemans L, Phillips L et al. (2008). Microstructural maturation of the human brain from childhood to adulthood. Neuroimage 40: 1044–1055.

Lee S-S, Park S, Park S-S (2011). Use of Lorazepan in drug-assisted interviews: two cases of dissociative amnesia. Psychiatry Investig 8: 377–380.

Lennox WG (1943). Amnesia, real and feigned. Am J Psychiatry 99: 732–743.

Levine B, Black SE, Cabeza R et al. (1998). Episodic memory and the self in a case of isolated retrograde amnesia. Brain 121: 1951–1973.

Levine B, Svoboda E, Turner GR et al. (2009). Behavioral and functional neuroanatomical correlates of anterograde autobiographical memory in isolated retrograde amnesic patient M.L. Neuropsychologia 47: 2188–2196.

Llewellyn S (2013). Such stuff as dreams are made on? Elaborative encoding, the ancient art of memory, and the hippocampus. Behav Brain Sci 36: 589–659.

Loftus EF (2006). Recovered memories. Annu Rev Clin Psychol 2: 469–508.

Lucchelli F, Muggia S, Spinnler H (1995). The 'Petit Madelaines' phenomenon in two amnesic patients. Sudden recovery of forgotten memories. Brain 118: 167–183.

Lucchelli F, Muggia S, Spinnler H (1998). The syndrome of pure retrograde amnesia. Cogn Neuropsychiatry 3: 91–118.

Lundholm H (1932). The riddle of functional amnesia. J Abnorm Soc Psychol 26: 355–366.

Lupien SJ, Maheu FS (2000). Memory and stress. In: H Fink (Ed.), 2nd ed. Encyclopedia of Stress, Vol. 2 F-N. Elsevier, Amsterdam, pp. 693–699.

Lupien SJ, Fiocco A, Wan N et al. (2005). Stress hormones and human memory function across the lifespan. Psychoneuroendocrinol 30: 225–242.

Lupien SJ, McEwen BS, Gunnar MR et al. (2009). Effects of stress throughout the lifespan on the brain, behavior and cognition. Nat Revs Neurosci 10: 434–445.

Lupien SJ, Parent S, Evans AC et al. (2011). Larger amygdala but no chance in hippocampal volume in 10-year-old children exposed to maternal depressive symptomatology since birth. Proc Natl Acad Sci U S A 108: 14324–14329.

Mace JH (2014). Involuntary autobiographical memory chains: implications for autobiographical memory organization. Front Psychiatr 5. Art. 193.

Mace JH, Clevinger AM, Martin C (2010). Involuntary memory chaining versus event cuing: which is a better indicator for autobiographical memory organization. Memory 18: 845–854.

Mace JH, Clevinger AM, Bernas RS (2013). Involuntary memory chains: what do they tell us about autobiographical memory organization? Memory 21: 324–335.

Magnin E, Thomas-Anterion C, Sylvestre G et al. (2014). Conversion, dissociative amnesia, and Ganser syndrome in a case of "chameleon" syndrome: anatomo–functional findings. Neurocase 20: 27–36.

Maldano JR, Spiegel D (2008). Dissociative disorders. In: RE Hales, SC Yudofsky, GO Gabbard (Eds.), The American Psychiatric Publishing Textbook of Psychiatry, American Psychiatric Publishing, Washington, DC, pp. 665–710.

Marinkovic K, Baldwin S, Courtney MG et al. (2011). Right hemisphere has the last laugh: neural mechanisms of joke appreciation. Cogn Affect Behav Neurosci 11: 113–130.

Markowitsch HJ (1985). Hypotheses on mnemonic information processing by the brain. Internat J Neurosci 27: 191–227.

Markowitsch HJ (1988). Individual differences in memory performance and the brain. In: HJ Markowitsch (Ed.), Information Processing by the Brain, Huber, Toronto, pp. 125–148.

Markowitsch HJ (1990a). Early concepts of transient disorders with symptoms of amnesia. In: HJ Markowitsch (Ed.), Transient Global Amnesia and Related Disorders, Hogrefe & Huber, Toronto, pp. 4–14.

Markowitsch HJ (1990b). Transient psychogenic amnesic states. In: HJ Markowitsch (Ed.), Transient Global Amnesia and Related Disorders. Hogrefe & Huber, Toronto, pp. 181–190.

Markowitsch HJ (1992a). Intellectual Functions and the Brain. An Historical Perspective, Hogrefe & Huber, Toronto.

Markowitsch HJ (1992b). The neuropsychology of hanging – an historical perspective. J Neurol Neurosurg Psychiatry 55: 507.

Markowitsch HJ (1992c). Das gestörte Altgedächtnis: Diagnoseverfahren bei Hirngeschädigten. Rehabilitation 31: 11–19.

Markowitsch HJ (1996a). Organic and psychogenic retrograde amnesia: two sides of the same coin? Neurocase 2: 357–371.

Markowitsch HJ (1996b). Retrograde amnesia: similarities between organic and psychogenic forms. Neurol Psychiatr Brain Res 4: 1–8.

Markowitsch HJ (1998). The mnestic block syndrome: environmentally induced amnesia. Neurol Psychiatr Brain Res 6: 73–80.

Markowitsch HJ (1999a). Koma und Hirntod: Funktionelle Anatomie von Bewußtsein und Bewußtseinsstörungen. In: HC Hopf, G Deuschl, HC Diener et al. (Eds.), Neurologie in Praxis und Klinik, Vol. 1. Thieme, Stuttgart, pp. 60–65.

Markowitsch HJ (1999b). Stress-related memory disorders. In: L-G Nilsson, HJ Markowitsch (Eds.), Cognitive Neuroscience of Memory, Hogrefe, Göttingen, pp. 193–211.

Markowitsch HJ (1999c). Neuroimaging and mechanisms of brain function in psychiatric disorders. Curr Opin Psychiatry 12: 331–337.

Markowitsch HJ (1999d). Functional neuroimaging correlates of functional amnesia. Memory 7: 561–583.

Markowitsch HJ (2000). Repressed memories. In: E Tulving (Ed.), Memory, consciousness, and the brain: The

Tallinn conference, Psychology Press, Philadelphia, PA, pp. 319–330.
Markowitsch HJ (2002). Functional retrograde amnesia – mnestic block syndrome. Cortex 38: 651–654.
Markowitsch HJ (2006). Brain imaging correlates of stress-related memory disorders in younger adults. Biol Psychiatr Psychopharmacol 8: 50–53.
Markowitsch HJ (2008). Anterograde amnesia. In: G Goldenberg, BL Miller (Eds.), Handbook of Clinical Neurology, 3rd Series, Vol. 88: Neuropsychology and Behavioral Neurology, Elsevier, New York, pp. 155–183.
Markowitsch HJ (2009). Stressbedingte Erinnerungsblockaden. Neuropsychologie und Hirnbildgebung. Psychoanalyse 13: 246–255.
Markowitsch HJ (2010). Korsakoff's syndrome. In: GF Koob, M Le Moal, RF Thompson (Eds.), Encyclopedia of Behavioral Neuroscience, Vol. 2. Academic Press, Oxford, pp. 131–136.
Markowitsch HJ (2013). Memory and self – neuroscientific landscapes. ISRN Neurosci. Art. ID 176027.
Markowitsch HJ, Brand M (2010). Forgetting: A historical perspective. In: S Della Sala (Ed.), Forgetting, Psychology Press, Hove, East Sussex, pp. 22–34.
Markowitsch HJ, Calabrese P (1996). Commonalities and discrepancies in the relationship between behavioural outcome and the results of neuroimaging in brain-damaged patients. Behav Neurol 9: 45–55.
Markowitsch HJ, Ewald K (1997). Right-hemispheric fronto-temporal injury leading to severe autobiographical retrograde and moderate anterograde episodic amnesia. Neurol Psychiatr Brain Sci 5: 71–78.
Markowitsch HJ, Pritzel M (1978). Von Monakow's diaschisis concept: Comments on West et al. (1976). Behav Biol 22: 411–412.
Markowitsch HJ, Staniloiu A (2011a). Memory, autonoetic consciousness, and the self. Consciousn Cognit 20: 16–39.
Markowitsch HJ, Staniloiu A (2011b). Amygdala in action: relaying biological and social significance to autobiographic memory. Neuropsychologia 49: 718–733.
Markowitsch HJ, Staniloiu S (2011c). Neuroscience and the law. Cortex 47: 1248–1251.
Markowitsch HJ, Staniloiu S (2012a). Amnesic disorders. Lancet 380: 1429–1440.
Markowitsch HJ, Staniloiu A (2012b). A rapprochement between emotion and cognition: amygdala, emotion and self relevance in episodic-autobiographical memory. Behav Brain Sci 35: 164–166.
Markowitsch HJ, Staniloiu A (2012c). Towards a re-conceptualizing of brain injury: the case of dissociative disorders and transient global amnesia. Brain Inj 26: 198–199.
Markowitsch HJ, Staniloiu A (2013). The impairment of recollection in functional amnesic states. Cortex 49: 1494–1510.
Markowitsch HJ, Staniloiu A (in press). History of memory. In: W Barr, LA Bielauslas (Eds.), Oxford Handbook of the History of Clinical Neuropsychology. Oxford University Press, Oxford.
Markowitsch HJ, Kessler J, Bast-Kessler C et al. (1984). Different emotional tones significantly affect recognition performance in patients with Korsakoff psychosis. Internat J Neurosci 25: 145–159.
Markowitsch HJ, Kessler J, Denzler P (1986). Recognition memory and psychophysiological responses towards stimuli with neutral and emotional content. A study of Korsakoff patients and recently detoxified and longterm abstinent alcoholics. Internat J Neurosci 29: 1–35.
Markowitsch HJ, Calabrese P, Liess J et al. (1993a). Retrograde amnesia after traumatic injury of the temporo-frontal cortex. J Neurol Neurosurg Psychiatry 56: 988–992.
Markowitsch HJ, von Cramon DY, Schuri U (1993b). Mnestic performance profile of a bilateral diencephalic infarct patient with preserved intelligence and severe amnesic disturbances. J Clin Exp Neuropsychol 15: 627–652.
Markowitsch HJ, Calabrese P, Fink GR et al. (1997a). Impaired episodic memory retrieval in a case of probable psychogenic amnesia. Psychiatr Res Neuroimag Sect 74: 119–126.
Markowitsch HJ, Fink GR, Thöne AIM et al. (1997b). Persistent psychogenic amnesia with a PET-proven organic basis. Cogn Neuropsychiatry 2: 135–158.
Markowitsch HJ, Thiel A, Kessler J et al. (1997c). Ecphorizing semi-conscious episodic information via the right temporopolar cortex – a PET study. Neurocase 3: 445–449.
Markowitsch HJ, Weber-Luxenburger G, Ewald K et al. (1997d). Patients with heart attacks are not valid models for medial temporal lobe amnesia. A neuropsychological and FDG-PET study with consequences for memory research. Eur J Neurol 4: 178–184.
Markowitsch HJ, Kessler J, Van der Ven C et al. (1998). Psychic trauma causing grossly reduced brain metabolism and cognitive deterioration. Neuropsychologia 36: 77–82.
Markowitsch HJ, Calabrese P, Neufeld H et al. (1999a). Retrograde amnesia for world knowledge and preserved memory for autobiographic events. A case report. Cortex 35: 243–252.
Markowitsch HJ, Kessler J, Kalbe E et al. (1999b). Functional amnesia and memory consolidation. A case of persistent anterograde amnesia with rapid forgetting following whiplash injury. Neurocase 5: 189–200.
Markowitsch HJ, Kessler J, Russ MO et al. (1999c). Mnestic block syndrome. Cortex 35: 219–230.
Markowitsch HJ, Kessler J, Weber-Luxenburger G et al. (2000a). Neuroimaging and behavioral correlates of recovery from mnestic block syndrome and other cognitive deteriorations. Neuropsychiatry Neuropsychol Behav Neurol 13: 60–66.
Markowitsch HJ, Thiel A, Reinkemeier M et al. (2000b). Right amygdalar and temporofrontal activation during autobiographic, but not during fictitious memory retrieval. Behav Neurol 12: 181–190.
Matthies (1908). Über einen Fall von hysterischem Dämmerzustand mit retrograder Amnesie. Allgemeine Zeitschr Psychiatr Grenzgeb 65: 188–206.

Maudsley H (1870). Body and Mind: An inquiry into their connection and mutual influence, specially in reference to mental disorders, Macmillan, London.

Mayes AR (1988). Human Organic Memory Disorders, Cambridge University Press, Cambridge, UK.

McKay GCM, Kopelman MD (2009). Psychogenic amnesia: when memory complaints are medically unexplained. Adv Psychiatr Treatment 15: 152–158.

Meijneke RWH, van de Ven EA, Schippers HM (2014). Een 9-jarige jongen met plotselig geheugenverlies. Ned Tijdschr Geneeskd 158: A6962.

Mesulam M-M (1990). Large-scale neurocognitive networks and distributed processing for attention, language, and memory. Ann Neurol 28: 597–613.

Mesulam M-M (2000). Behavioral neuroanatomy: Large-scale networks, association cortex, frontal syndromes, the limbic system, and hemispheric specializations. In: M-M Mesulam (Ed.), Principles of Behavioral and Cognitive Neurology, 2nd ed. Oxford University Press, New York, pp. 1–120.

Miller LA, Caine D, Harding A et al. (2001). Right medial thalamic lesion causes isolated retrograde amnesia. Neuropsychologia 39: 1037–1046.

Milton F, Muhlert N, Pindus DM et al. (2010). Remote memory deficits in transient epileptic amnesia. Brain 133: 1368–1379.

Mishra NK, Russmann H, Granziera C et al. (2011). Mutism and amnesia following high-voltage electrical injury: psychogenic symptomatology triggered by organic dysfunction? Eur Neurol 66: 229–234.

Moriguchi Y, Ohnishi T, Lane RD et al. (2006). Impaired self-awareness and theory of mind: an fMRI study of mentalizing in alexithymia. Neuroimage 32: 1472–1482.

Moriguchi Y, Ohnishi T, Decety J et al. (2009). The human mirror neuron system in a population with deficient self-awareness: an fMRI study in alexithymia. Hum Brain Mapp 30: 2063–2076.

Mortati K, Grant AC (2012). A patient with distinct dissociative and hallucinatory fugues. BMJ Case Rep. http://dx.doi.org/10.1136/bcr.11.2011.5078.

Naef M (1897). Ein Fall von temporärer, totaler, theilweise retrograder Amnesie (durch Suggestion geheilt). Zeitschr Hypnotismus 6: 321–355.

Naime JS (2002). The myth of the encoding-retrieval match. Memory 10: 389–395.

Noulhiane M, Piolino P, Hasboun D et al. (2007). Autobiographical memory after temporal lobe resection: neuropsychological and MRI volumetric findings. Brain 130: 3184–3199.

O'Brien JT (1997). The 'glucocorticoid cascade' hypothesis in man. Br J Psychiatry 170: 199–201.

O'Brien DJ (2011). Unconscious by any other name. Nature Rev Neurosci 12: 302.

O'Neill of Tyrone A, Fernandez JM (2000). Dissociative disorder associated with a colloid cyst of the third ventricle: organic or psychogenic amnesia? Psychother Psychosom 69: 108–109.

Osnato M (1930). The rôle of trauma in various neuropsychiatric conditions. Am J Psychiatry 86: 643–660.

Ouellet J, Rouleau I, Labrecque R et al. (2008). Two routes to losing one's past life: a brain trauma, an emotional trauma. Behav Neurol 20: 27–38.

Parkin AJ (1996). Focal retrograde amnesia: a multi-faceted disorder? Acta Neurol Belg 96: 43–50.

Paul M (1899). Beiträge zur Frage der retrograden Amnesie. Arch Psychiatr Nervenkrankht 32: 251–282.

Paz-Alonso PM, Ghetti S, Matlen BJ et al. (2009). Memory suppression is an active process that improves over childhood. Front Hum Neurosci 3. Art. 24.

Paz-Alonso PM, Bunge SA, Anderson MC et al. (2013). Strength of coupling within a mnemonic control network differentiates those who can and cannot suppress memory retrieval. J Neurosci 33: 5017–5026.

Peckl P (2007). "Patient will früher immer gesund gewesen sein" - der "Kriegszitterer" im Spiegel der Lazarettkrankenakten deutscher Soldaten im Ersten Weltkrieg Praxis. Praxis 96: 2075–2079.

Peper M, Markowitsch HJ (2001). Pioneers of affective neuroscience and early conceptions of the emotional brain. J Hist Neurosci 10: 58–66.

Pfeifer R, Bongard J (2007). How the Body Shapes the Way we Think. MIT Press, Cambridge, MA.

Phan Luan K, Orlichenko A, Boyd E et al. (2009). Preliminary evidence of white matter abnormality in the uncinate fasciculus in generalized social anxiety disorder. Biol Psychiatry 66: 691–694.

Pietrini P (2003). Toward a biochemistry of mind? Am J Psychiary 160: 1907–1908.

Piolino P, Desgranges B, Belliard S et al. (2003). Autobiographical memory and autonoetic consciousness: triple dissociation. Brain 126: 2203–2219.

Pommerenke K, Staniloiu A, Markowitsch HJ et al. (2012). Ein Fall von retrograder Amnesie nach Resektion eines Medullablastoms – psychogen/funktionell oder organisch? Neurol Rehab 18: 106–116.

Pribram KH (1971). Languages of the Brain. Experimental Paradoxes and Principles in Neuropsychology, Prentice-Hall, Englewood Cliffs, NJ.

Prigatano GP, Schacter DL (Eds.), (1991). Awareness of Deficit after Brain Injury. Clinical and Theoretical Issues, Oxford University Press, New York.

Quesada AA, Wiemers US, Schoofs D et al. (2012). Psychosocial stress exposure impairs memory retrieval in children. Psychoneuroendocrinology 37: 125–136.

Quirin M, Gruber T, Kuhl J et al. (2013). Is love right? Prefrontal resting brain asymmetry is related to the affiliation motive. Front Hum Neurosci 7. http://dx.doi.org/10.3389/fnhum.2013.00902. Art. 902.

Quiroga R (2012). Concept cells: the building blocks of declarative memory functions. Nat Rev Neurosci 13: 587–597.

Quiroga R (2013). Gnostic cells in the 21st century. Acta Neurobiol Exp (Wars) 73: 463–471.

Quiroga R, Reddy L, Kreiman G et al. (2005). Invariant visual representation by single neurons in the human brain. Nature 435: 1102–1107.

Quiroga R, Kreiman G, Koch C et al. (2008). Sparse but not "Grandmother-cell" coding in the medial temporal lobe. Trends Cognit Sci 12: 88–91.

Rathbone C, Moulin CJA, Conway MA (2009). Autobiographical memory and amnesia: using conceptual knowledge to ground the self. Neurocase 15: 405–418.

Rathbone C, Ellis J, Baker I et al. (2015). Self, memory, and imaging the future in a case of psychogenic amnesia. Neurocase 21: 727–737.

Rees PM (2003). Contemporary issues in mild traumatic brain injury. Arch Phys Med Rehabil 84: 1885–1894.

Reinhold N, Markowitsch HJ (2007). Emotion and consciousness in adolescent psychogenic amnesia. J Neuropsychol 1: 53–64.

Reinhold N, Markowitsch HJ (2009). Retrograde episodic memory and emotion: a perspective from patients with dissociative amnesia. Neuropsychologia 47: 2197–2206.

Reinhold N, Kühnel S, Brand M et al. (2006). Functional neuroimaging in memory and memory disturbances. Curr Med Imag Rev 2: 35–57.

Reinhold N, Clarenbach P, Markowitsch HJ (2008). Kognition und Gedächtnis bei Patienten mit schlafbezogenen Atmungsstörungen - Verlaufsuntersuchung über eine dreimonatige nCPAP-Therapie. Zeitschr Neuropsychol/J Neuropsychol 19: 15–22.

Reinvang I, Gjerstad L (1998). Focal retrograde amnesia associated with vascular headache. Neuropsychologia 36: 1335–1341.

Ribot T (1882). Diseases of Memory, D Appleton, New York.

Risius U-M, Staniloiu A, Piefke M et al. (2013). Retrieval, monitoring and control processes: A 7 Tesla fMRI approach to memory accuracy. Front Behav Neurosci 7: 1–21. Art. 24.

Roberts I, Gluck N, Smith MS et al. (2013). Postanesthesia persistent amnesia in a patient with a prior history of dissociative fugue state : the case for the two-hit hypothesis. Am J Psychiatry 170: 1398–1400.

Roediger III HL, Weinstein Y, Agarwal PK (2010). Forgetting. Prelminary considerations. In: S Della Sala (Ed.), Forgetting, Psychology Press, Hove, East Sussex, pp. 1–22.

Roman-Campos G, Poser CM, Wood FB (1980). Persistent retrograde memory deficit after transient global amnesia. Cortex 16: 509–518.

Rosenbaum RS, Köhler S, Schacter DL et al. (2005). The case of K.C.: contributions of a memory-impaired person to memory theory. Neuropsychologia 43: 989–1021.

Rosenbaum RS, Gilboa A, Levine B et al. (2009). Amnesia as an impairment of detail generation and binding: evidence from personal, fictional, and semantic narratives in K.C. Neuropsychologia 47: 2181–2187.

Rosenbaum RS, Gao F, Honjo K et al. (2014). Congenital absence of the mammillary bodies: a novel finding in a well-studied case of developmental amnesia. Neuropsychologia 65: 82–87.

Ruff RM, Jamora CW (2009). Myths and mild traumatic brain injury. Psychol Inj Law 2: 34–42.

Ruff RM, Crouch JA, Troster AI et al. (1994). Selected cases of poor outcome following a minor brain trauma: comparing neuropsychological and positron emission tomography assessment. Brain Inj 8: 297–308.

Russell WR (1935). Amnesia following head injuries. Lancet 2: 762–763.

Russell WR (1971). The Traumatic Amnesias, Oxford University Press, London.

Russell WR, Nathan PW (1946). Traumatic amnesia. Brain 69: 280–300.

Sackeim HA, Prudic J, Fuller R et al. (2007). The cognitive effects of electroconvulsive therapy in community settings. Neuropsychopharm 32: 244–254.

Sapolsky RM (1996a). Why stress is bad for your brain. Science 273: 749–750.

Sapolsky RM (1996b). Stress, glucocorticoids, and damage to the nervous system: the current state of confusion. Stress 1: 1–19.

Sapolsky RM (2000). Glucocorticoids and hippocampal atrophy in neuropsychiatric disorders. Arch Gen Psychiatry 57: 925–935.

Sarter M, Markowitsch HJ (1984). Collateral innervation of the medial and lateral prefrontal cortex by amygdaloid, thalamic, and brain stem neurons. J Comp Neurol 224: 445–460.

Savage GH (1878). Acute mania associated with abscess of the brain. Brain 1: 265–269.

Schacter DL, Kihlstrom JF (1989). Functional amnesia. In: F Boller, J Grafman (Eds.), Handbook of Neuropsychology, Vol. 3. Elsevier, Amsterdam, pp. 209–231.

Schacter DL, Prigatano GP (1991). Forms of unawareness. In: GP Prigatano, DL Schacter (Eds.), Awareness of Deficit after Brain Injury. Clinical and Theoretical Issues, Oxford University Press, New York, pp. 258–262.

Schlesinger H (1916). Hochgradige retrograde Amnesie nach Gehirnverletzung. Muenchner med Wochenschr Nr 1: 18.

Schneider K (1928). Die Störungen des Gedächtnisses. In: P Bumke (Ed.), Handbuch der Geisteskrankheiten, Vol. 1. Springer, Berlin, pp. 508–529.

Schoenfeld TA, Hamilton LW (1977). Secondary brain changes following lesions: a new paradigm for lesion experimentation. Physiol Behav 18: 951–967.

Schore AN (2002). Dysregulation of the right brain: a fundamental mechanism of traumatic attachment and the psychopathogenesis of posttraumatic stress disorder. Austral New Zealand J Psychiatry 36: 9–30.

Schore AN (2005). Back to basics: attachment, affect regulation, and the developing right brain: linking developmental neuroscience to pediatrics. Pediatr Rev 26: 204–217.

Schulte-Rüther M, Markowitsch HJ, Fink GR et al. (2007). Mirror neuron and theory of mind mechanisms involved in face-to-face interactions: an fMRI approach to empathy. J Cogn Neurosci 19: 1354–1372.

Schulte-Rüther M, Greimell E, Markowitsch HJ et al. (2011). Dysfunctional Brain Networks Supporting Empathy in Adults with Autism Spectrum Disorder: an fMRI Study. Soc Neurosci 6: 1–21.

Sehm B, Frisch S, Thöne-Otto A et al. (2011). Focal retrograde amnesia: voxel-based morphometry findings in a case without MRI lesions. PLoS One 6: e26538.

Seidl U, Markowitsch HJ, Schröder J (2006). Die verlorene Erinnerung. Störungen des autobiographischen Gedächtnisses bei leichter kognitiver Beeinträchtigung und Alzheimer-Demenz. In: H Welzer, HJ Markowitsch (Eds.), Warum Menschen sich erinnern können. Fortschritte der interdisziplinären Gedächtnisforschung, Klett, Stuttgart, pp. 286–302.

Semon R (1904). Die Mneme als erhaltendes Prinzip im Wechsel des organischen Geschehens, Wilhelm Engelmann, Leipzig.

Serra L, Fadda L, Buccione I et al. (2007). Psychogenic and organic amnesia: a multidimensional assessment of clinical, neuroradiological, neuropsychological and psychopathological features. Behav Neurol 18: 53–64.

Sidaros A, Engberg AW, Sidaros K et al. (2008). Diffusion tensor imaging during recovery from severe traumatic brain injury and relation to clinical outcome: a longitudinal study. Brain 131: 559–572.

Silver JM, Rattok J, Anderson K (1997). Post-traumatic stress disorder and traumatic brain injury. Neurocase 3: 151–157.

Smith CN, Frascino JC, Kripke DL et al. (2010). Losing memories overnight: a unique form of human amnesia. Neuropsychologia 38: 2833–2840.

Soper AC, Wagner MT, Edwards JC et al. (2011). Transient epileptic amnesia: a neurosurgical case report. Epilepsy Behav 20: 709–713.

Souques A (1892). Essai sur l'amnesie retro-anterograde dans l'hysterie, les traumatismes cerebraux et l'alcoolisme chronique [Essay about retrograde-anterograde amnesia in hysteria, cerebral trauma and chronic alcoholism]. Revue de Medicine 13: 367–401.

Spiegel D, Loewenstein RJ, Lewis-Fernandet R et al. (2011). Dissociative disorders in DSM-5. Depress Anxiety 28: 824–852.

Spiegel D, Lewis-Fernández R, Lanius R et al. (2013). Dissociative disorders in DSM-5. Annu Rev Clin Psychol 9: 299–326.

Squire LR, Cohen NJ (1982). Remote memory, retrograde amnesia, and the neuropsychology of memory. In: LS Cermak (Ed.), Human Memory and Amnesia, LEA, Hillsdale, NJ, pp. 275–303.

Staniloiu A, Markowitsch HJ (2010). Searching for the anatomy of dissociative amnesia. J Psychol 218: 96–108.

Staniloiu A, Markowitsch HJ (2012a). Towards solving the riddle of forgetting in functional amnesia: recent advances and current opinions. Front Psychol 3. Article 403.

Staniloiu A, Markowitsch HJ (2012b). The remains of the day in dissociative amnesia. Brain Sci 2: 101–129.

Staniloiu A, Markowitsch HJ (2012c). Dissociation, memory, and trauma narrative. J Lit Theory 6: 103–130.

Staniloiu A, Markowitsch HJ (2012d). Functional amnesia: Definition, types, challenges and future directions. In: E Abdel-Rahman, RA Balogun (Eds.), Functional Impairment: Management, Types and Challenges, Nova Science Publishers, Hauppauge, NY, pp. 87–123.

Staniloiu A, Markowitsch HJ (2012e). The splitting of the brain: A reorientation towards fiber tracts damage in amnesia. In: AJ Schäfer, J Müller (Eds.), Brain Damage: Causes, Management, and Prognosis, Nova Science Publishers, Hauppauge, NY, pp. 41–70.

Staniloiu A, Markowitsch HJ (2014). Dissociative amnesia. Lancet Psychiatry 1: 226–241.

Staniloiu A, Markowitsch HJ (2015). Amnesia, psychogenic. In: JD Wright (Ed.), International Encyclopedia of the Social and Behavioral Sciences, Vol. 1. Elsevier Science, Oxford, pp. 651–658.

Staniloiu A, Bender A, Smolewska K et al. (2009). Ganser syndrome with work–related onset in a patient with a background of immigration. Cogn Neuropsychiatry 14: 180–198.

Staniloiu A, Markowitsch HJ, Brand M (2010). Psychogenic amnesia – A malady of the constricted self. Consciousn Cognit 19: 778–801.

Staniloiu A, Vitcu I, Markowitsch HJ (2011). Neuroimaging and dissociative disorders. In: V Chaudhary (Ed.), Advances in Brain Imaging, INTECH – Open Access Publishing, Rijecka, Croatia, pp. 11–34.

Staniloiu A, Borsutzky S, Woermann F et al. (2013). Social cognition in a case of amnesia with neurodevelopmental mechanisms. Front Cognit 4: 1–28. Art. 342.

Stickgold T, Walker MP (2013). Sleep-dependent memory triage: evolving generalization through selective processing. Nat Neurosci 16: 139–145.

Stone J, Smyth R, Carson A et al. (2006). La belle indifference in conversion symptoms and hysteria: systematic review. Br J Psychiatr 188: 204–209.

Störring GE (1931). Über den ersten reinen Fall eines Menschen mit völligem, isoliertem Verlust der Merkfähigkeit. (Gleichzeitig ein Beitrag zur Gefühls-, Willens- und Handlungspsychologie). Arch ges Psychol 81: 257–384.

Störring GE (1936). Gedächtnisverlust durch Gasvergiftung: Ein Mensch ohne Zeitgedächtnis. Arch gesamt Psychol 96: 436–511.

Stracciari A, Ghidoni E, Guarino M et al. (1994). Post-traumatic retrograde amnesia with selective impairment of autobiographical memory. Cortex 30: 459–468.

Stracciari A, Fonti C, Guarino M (2008). When the past is lost: Focal retrograde amnesia. Focus on the "functional" form. Behav Neurol 20: 113–125.

Sturm VE, Rosen HJ, Allison S et al. (2006). Self-conscious emotion deficits in frontotemporal lobar degeneration. Brain 129: 2508–2516.

Stuss DT, Guzman DA (1988). Severe remote memory loss with minimal anterograde amnesia: a clinical note. Brain Cogn 8: 21–30.

Stuss DT, Richard MT (1982). Neuropsychological sequelae of coma after head injury. In: LP Ivan, DA Bruce (Eds.), Coma, Physiopathology, Diagnosis and Management, Springfield, IL, Charles C Thomas, pp. 193–210.

Suddendorf T, Addis DR, Corballis MC (2009). Mental time travel and the shaping of the human mind. Phil Trans Roy Soc Lond B 364: 1317–1324.

Syz H (1937). Recovery from loss of mnemonic retention after head trauma. J Gen Psychol 17: 355–387.

Teramoto S, Uchiyama M, Higurashi N et al. (2005). A case of isolated retrograde amnesia following brain concussion. Pediatr Int 47: 469–472.

Teyler TJ, Rudy JW (2007). The hippocampal indexing theory and episodic memory: updating the index. Hippocampus 17: 1158–1169.

Thomas-Antérion C, Guedj E, Decousus M et al. (2010). Can we see personal identity loss? A functional imaging study of typical 'hysterical amnesia'. J Neurol Neurosurg Psychiatry 81: 468–469.

Thomas-Antérion C, Dubas F, Decousus M et al. (2014). Clinical characteristics and brain PET findings in 3 cases of dissociative amnesia: disproportionate retrograde deficit and posterior middle temporal gyrus hypometabolism. Neurophysiol Clin 44: 355–362.

Toussi A, Bryk J, Alam A (2014). Forgetting heart break: a fascinating case of transient left ventricular apical ballooning syndrome associated with dissociative amnesia. Gen Hosp Psychiatry 36: 225–227.

Tramoni E, Aubert-Khalfa S, Guye M et al. (2009). Hypo–retrieval and hyper–suppression mechanisms in functional amnesia. Neuropsychologia 47: 611–624.

Tranel D, Damasio AR (1985). Knowledge without awareness: an autonomic index of facial recognition by prosopagnosics. Science 228: 1453–1454.

Treadway M, McCloskey M, Gordon B et al. (1992). Landmark life events and the organization of memory: Evidence from functional retrograde amnesia. In: S-A Christianson (Ed.), The Handbook of Emotion and Memory. Research and Theory, LEA, Hillsdale, NJ, pp. 389–410.

Tulving E (1983). Elements of Episodic Memory, Clarendon Press, Oxford.

Tulving E (2005). Episodic memory and autonoesis: uniquely human? In: H Terrace, J Metcalfe (Eds.), The missing link in cognition: evolution of self-kmowing consciousness, Oxford University Press, New York, pp. 3–56.

Tulving E, Thompson D (1973). Encoding specificity and retrieval processes in episodic memory. Psychol Rev 80: 352–373.

Valentino K, Toth SL, Cicchetti D (2009). Autobiographical memory functioning among abused, neglected, and nonmaltreated children: the overgeneral memory effect. J Child Psychol Psychiatry 50: 1029–1038.

van der Kruijs SJ, Bodde NM, Carrette E et al. (2014). Neurophysiological correlates of dissociative symptoms. J Neurol Neurosurg Psychiatry 85: 174–179.

van der Werf YD, Witter MP, Uylings HBM et al. (2000). Neuropsychology of infarctions in the thalamus: a review. Neuropsychologia 38: 613–627.

van Schie K, Geraerts E, Anderson MC (2013). Emotional and non-emotional memories are suppressible under direct suppression instructions. Cogn Emot 27: 1122–1131.

Vandekerckhove M, Plessers M, Van Mieghem A et al. (2014). Impaired facial emotion recognition in patients with ventromedial prefrontal hypoperfusion. Neuropsychology 28: 605–612.

Vermetten E, Schmahl C, Lindner S et al. (2006). Hippocampal and amygdalar volumes in dissociative identity disorder. Am J Psychiatry 163: 630–636.

Vermetten E, Dorahy MJ, Spiegel D (Eds.), (2007). Traumatic Dissociation. Neurobiology and Treatment. American Psychiatric Publishing, Arlington, VA.

Viskontas IV, McAndrews MP, Moscovitch M (2000). Remote episodic memory deficits in patients with unilateral temporal lobe epilepsy and excisions. J Neurosci 20: 5853–5857.

Viskontas IV, McAndrews MP, Moscovitch M (2002). Memory for famous people in patients with unilateral temporal lobe epilepsy and excisions. Neuropsychology 16: 472–480.

von Cramon DY, Markowitsch HJ, Schuri U (1993). The possible contribution of the septal region to memory. Neuropsychologia 31: 1159–1180.

Von Monakow C (1914). Die Lokalisation im Grosshirn und der Abbau der Funktion durch kortikale Herde, Bergmann, Wiesbaden.

Wabnitz P, Gast U, Catani C (2013). Differences in trauma history and psychopathology between PTSD patients with and without co-occurring dissociative disorders. Eur J Psychotraumatol 4: 21452.

Walker KR, Tesco G (2013). Molecular mechanisms of cognitive dysfunction following traumatic brain injury. Front Aging Neurosci 5: 1–25. Art. 29.

Warrington EK, Shallice T (1984). Category specific semantic impairments. Brain 107: 829–854.

Watkins E, Teasdale JD, Williams RM (2000). Decentring and distraction reduce overgeneral autobiographical memory in depression. Psychol Med 30: 911–920.

Weusten LH, Severeijns R, Leue C (2013). Een omvangrijke retrograde amnesie van bijna 30 jaar en de rol van organische, intentionele en psychogene factoren. Tijdschr Psychiatrie 55: 281–285.

Wilde EA, Bigler ED, Pedroza C et al. (2006). Post-traumatic amnesia predicts long-term cerebral atrophy in traumatic brain injury. Brain Inj 20: 695–699.

Williams JM, Ellis NC, Tyers C et al. (1996). The specificity of autobiographical memory and imageability of the future. Mem Cogn 24: 116–125.

Wilson BA, Robertson C, Ashworth F (2015). Identity Unknown, Psychology Press, Hove, East Sussex.

Wingenfeld K, Wolf OT (2014). Stress, memory, and the hippocampus. In: K Szabo, MG Hennerici (Eds.), The Hippocampus in Clinical Neuroscience, Karger, Basel, pp. 1–12.

Wolf OT (2009). Stress and memory in humans: Twelve years of progress? Brain Res 293: 142–154.

Wolpaw JR (1971). The aetiology of retrograde amnesia. Lancet 2: 356–358.

World Health Organization (1992). Classification of Mental and Behavioral Disorders: Clinical Descriptions and Diagnostic Guidelines: ICD-10, World Health Organization, Geneva.

Yamadori A, Suzuki K, Shimada M et al. (2001). Isolated and focal retrograde amnesia: a hiatus in the past. Tohoku J Exp Med 193: 57–65.

Yoneda Y, Yamadori A, Mori E et al. (1992). Isolated prolonged retrograde amnesia. Eur Neurol 32: 340–342.

Handbook of Clinical Neurology, Vol. 139 (3rd series)
Functional Neurologic Disorders
M. Hallett, J. Stone, and A. Carson, Editors
http://dx.doi.org/10.1016/B978-0-12-801772-2.00037-0

Chapter 37

Functional (psychogenic) dizziness

M. DIETERICH[1,2]*, J.P. STAAB[3], AND T. BRANDT[2]

[1]*Department of Neurology, Ludwig-Maximilians-University Munich, Klinikum Grosshadern, Munich, Germany*

[2]*German Center for Vertigo and Balance Disorders, Ludwig-Maximilians-University Munich, Klinikum Grosshadern, Munich, Germany*

[3]*Department of Psychiatry and Psychology, Mayo Clinic, Rochester, MN, USA*

Abstract

Functional and psychiatric disorders that cause vestibular symptoms (i.e., vertigo, unsteadiness, and dizziness) are common. In fact, they are more common than many well-known structural vestibular disorders. Neurologists and otologists are more likely to encounter patients with vestibular symptoms due to persistent postural-perceptual dizziness or panic disorder than Ménière's disease or bilateral vestibular loss. Successful approaches to identifying functional and psychiatric causes of vestibular symptoms can be incorporated into existing practices without much difficulty. The greatest challenge is to set aside dichotomous thinking that strongly emphasizes investigations of structural diseases in favor of a three-pronged approach that assesses structural, functional, and psychiatric disorders simultaneously.

The pathophysiologic mechanisms underlying functional and psychiatric causes of vestibular symptoms are better understood than many clinicians realize. Research methods such as advanced posturographic analysis and functional brain imaging will push this knowledge further in the next few years. Treatment plans that include patient education, vestibular rehabilitation, cognitive and behavioral therapies, and medications substantially reduce morbidity and offer the potential for sustained remission when applied systematically. Diagnostic and therapeutic approaches are necessarily multidisciplinary in nature, but they are well within the purview of collaborative care teams or networks of clinicians coordinated with the neurologists and otologists whom patients consult first.

INTRODUCTION

This chapter reviews common functional and psychiatric disorders that cause vestibular symptoms, starting with a discussion of the definitions, differential diagnosis, putative pathophysiologic mechanisms, and treatment strategies of two functional vestibular disorders that are defined explicitly in the neuro-otologic literature, namely phobic postural vertigo (PPV) (Brandt and Dieterich, 1986) and chronic subjective dizziness (CSD) (Staab and Ruckenstein, 2007a). These disorders share many features, but also differ in important ways that have not yet been reconciled experimentally. The chapter then introduces persistent postural-perceptual dizziness (PPPD), a condition based on the common features of PPV and CSD, which was defined for the first time in the beta draft version of the *International Classification of Diseases*, 11th edition (ICD-11: WHO, 2015a). Less common functional vestibular presentations, which have been observed clinically but not studied formally, are discussed briefly. The chapter ends with a review of the clinical manifestations, differential diagnosis, and treatment of psychiatric disorders that cause vestibular symptoms. As a whole, the chapter offers guidance for efficiently and effectively identifying

*Correspondence to: Marianne Dieterich, MD, FANA, FEAN, Department of Neurology, Ludwig-Maximilians-University Munich, Klinikum Grosshadern, Marchioninistrasse 15, D-81377 Munich, Germany. Tel: +49-89-44007-2570, E-mail: Marianne.Dieterich@med.uni-muenchen.de

functional and psychiatric causes of vestibular symptoms based on pertinent positives in the clinical history plus supporting evidence from physical examinations and laboratory testing. None of these disorders has a pathognomonic symptom or sign, but they all have key features that suggest their presence whether or not other illnesses are active, too.

The term "vestibular symptoms" is used in this chapter to denote vertigo, unsteadiness, and dizziness, collectively, regardless of cause. This is in keeping with nomenclature proposed by the Committee for Classification of Vestibular Disorders of the Bárány Society (Bisdorff et al., 2009), which further defined vertigo as a false or distorted sensation of movement, unsteadiness as a feeling of rocking or swaying when upright, and dizziness as a nonmotion sensation of disordered spatial orientation. Functional and psychiatric disorders that cause vestibular symptoms are considered separately from one another and from structural vestibular diseases. That is because experimental data show that they occur independently (Brandt, 1996; Staab and Ruckenstein, 2003, 2007a; Eckhardt-Henn, et al., 2008). Their separate contributions to vestibular morbidity have to be recognized and their interactions with one another understood explicitly. Herein, functional vestibular disorders are defined positively (i.e., by the presence of identifiable and unique sets of symptoms) and not negatively (i.e., by the absence of structural deficits). Psychiatric disorders that cause vestibular symptoms are defined by their relevant diagnostic criteria in ICD-10 (WHO, 1993), and the *Diagnostic and Statistical Manual of Mental Disorders*, 5th edition (DSM-5: American Psychiatric Association, 2013).

Retrospective, cross-sectional, and prospective studies conducted over three decades suggest that 8–10% of patients with vestibular symptoms have an anxiety or depressive disorder as the primary cause of their illness (see Staab, 2013, for review). One in eight will develop a *de novo* anxiety or depressive disorder triggered by an acute vestibular disease (Godemann et al., 2006), and a total of 30–50% will manifest anxiety or depressive morbidity over the course of their vestibular illness (Eagger et al., 1992; Eckhardt-Henn et al., 2003; Kammerlind et al., 2005; Lahmann et al., 2015). Another 15–20% will primarily manifest the functional vestibular syndromes of PPV (Brandt et al., 2013) or CSD (Staab, 2012). Thus, functional and psychiatric disorders may be primary, secondary, or comorbid problems in many patients presenting for evaluation of vestibular symptoms. In other words, these conditions are common causes, consequences, and complications of vestibular symptoms. They are often responsible for the greatest portion of morbidity and disability, especially in patients with chronic complaints.

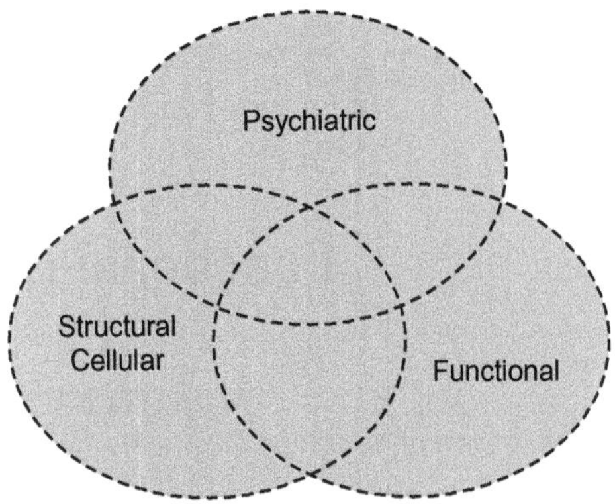

Fig. 37.1. General diagnostic classification of vestibular disorders. Structural/cellular, somatic/functional, and psychiatric disorders may independently cause vestibular symptoms. They also may coexist in any combination of primary, secondary, and coexisting conditions.

These data demonstrate that the traditional dichotomous classification of vestibular symptoms as "organic" or "psychogenic" is unworkable. Structural/cellular, functional, and psychiatric disorders manifest independently and in all possible combinations as primary and secondary conditions (Fig. 37.1). Therefore, it is inherently illogical to approach diagnostic assessments in a binary manner (Staab, 2013). The presence or absence of one group of illnesses (e.g., structural/cellular diseases) provides no definitive information about the presence or absence of the others. All must be considered independently and simultaneously to construct complete and accurate diagnostic formulations. Furthermore, the common hierarchic approach to diagnostic evaluations in which structural and cellular diagnoses are considered first, and then other illnesses are added to the differential diagnosis only when medical testing is negative, belies the epidemiologic evidence that functional and psychiatric disorders are among the most common causes of vestibular morbidity.

Before proceeding with a review of specific disorders, two commonly held beliefs about functional conditions merit discussion because they are not supported by recent evidence. Disability status, healthcare utilization, and patient dissatisfaction with medical care are generally thought to be greater among patients with functional disorders than among those with structural diseases. However, the results of clinical and population-based epidemiologic studies suggest otherwise. Adverse health outcomes were predicted not by the type or cause of physical symptoms, but by two other factors: the total number of physical symptoms from all causes (i.e., total symptom burden) (Tomenson et al., 2012, 2013) and the presence of coexisting anxiety or depressive disorders (Hanel et al., 2009). This general finding was recently confirmed in a study of patients with vestibular illnesses

(Lahmann et al., 2015). Those with functional or psychiatric disorders were no more impaired than those with structural illnesses. Earlier investigations that reported less impairment among patients with structural diseases (Furman and Jacob, 1997; Yardley and Redfern, 2001; Eckhardt-Henn et al., 2003) mixed functional and psychiatric conditions together, precluding evaluation of the independent effects of each.

The second belief is that experiences of psychologic traumatization and adverse life events differentially cause functional and psychiatric presentations of neurologic symptoms. These long-held theories were contradicted in a recent study of patients with vestibular symptoms (Radziej et al., 2015). Childhood and adulthood adversity was no more common among patients with functional or psychiatric versus structural causes of vestibular symptoms. A history of adversity was a risk factor for greater symptom severity and handicap regardless of the causes of illness. Thus, a history of adverse life events did not help with the differential diagnosis of vestibular symptoms. Rather, it increased the likelihood of poorer outcomes regardless of final diagnosis.

FUNCTIONAL CAUSES OF VESTIBULAR SYMPTOMS

Phobic postural vertigo

The functional vestibular syndrome of PPV is among the most common disorders encountered in neuro-otologic practice, although it is often not recognized. In a tertiary referral dizziness unit (the German Center for Vertigo and Balance Disorders), it was the second most common diagnosis, identified in 15% of 17 700 adult outpatients, behind only benign paroxysmal positional vertigo (Brandt et al., 2013). In another tertiary dizziness unit, 23% of 3113 patients suffered from PPV (Obermann et al., 2015). The frequency of this diagnosis in other centers and countries varied considerably, from 2.5% (Ketola et al., 2009) to 16% (Lopez-Gentili et al., 2003), possibly because of the sensitivity of diagnostic processes. In childhood and adolescence, functional and psychiatric causes of vestibular symptoms, including PPV, account for up to 21% of diagnoses. They are second in frequency to the migrainous syndrome of benign paroxysmal vertigo of childhood (39%) (Batu et al., 2015).

The cardinal symptoms and features of PPV include the following (Brandt and Dieterich, 1986; Brandt, 1996; Brandt et al., 2013):

1. Patients complain about postural dizziness and subjective stance and gait unsteadiness without this being evident to an observer; moreover, their findings in neuro-otologic tests are normal.
2. Dizziness is often described as light-headedness with varying degrees of unsteadiness of stance and gait, attack-like fear of falling without actually falling (Schlick et al., 2016), in part also unintentional body swaying of short duration.
3. The attacks often occur in typical situations known to be external triggers of other phobic syndromes (e.g., bridges, driving a car, empty rooms, long corridors, large crowds of people in a store or restaurant) or during visual stimulation (e.g., cinema, television, store).
4. Symptoms improve or resolve during sporting activities (cycling, tennis) and during more complicated balance conditions, whereas they reappear at rest or under simpler conditions (e.g., standing after cycling).
5. During the course of the illness, patients begin to generalize the symptoms and increasingly avoid the triggering stimuli. During or shortly after the attacks (frequently mentioned only when asked), patients report vegetative disturbances and anxiety; most also report attacks of vertigo/dizziness without anxiety.
6. If asked, patients usually report that their symptoms improve after imbibing a little alcohol.
7. Initially there is often a structural vestibular illness (e.g., vestibular neuritis or benign paroxysmal positional vertigo that resolves) (Huppert et al., 1995) or special psychosocial stress situations (Kapfhammer et al., 1997).
8. Patients with PPV often exhibit obsessive-compulsive and perfectionistic personality traits and reactive-depressive symptoms during the course of the disease.

The diagnosis of PPV depends on positively identifying these clinical features. It is not sufficient to simply exclude structural causes of vestibular symptoms. PPV is not a diagnosis of exclusion.

Clinical aspects and course of the illness

The combination of postural dizziness with subjective instability of stance and gait in patients with normal findings on otoneurologic examination and vestibular and balance tests (e.g., video-oculography, including caloric irrigation, neuroimaging), and the absence of other disorders that could explain the symptoms are characteristic. The monosymptomatic subjective disorder of balance is connected with standing or walking, and manifests with attack-like worsening that occurs with or without recognizable triggers and with or without accompanying anxiety. The absence of recognizable triggers or vertigo without accompanying anxiety causes many patients – and occasionally the doctor treating them – to doubt the diagnosis of a functional vestibular disorder.

Patients with PPV generally have a compulsive personality as their most pronounced personality trait, a tendency to intensified introspection, and a need to keep everything under control. They are more likely to be ambitious and place high demands on themselves, and are often easily irritated and fearful (Kapfhammer et al., 1997).

Such patients rarely go to a psychiatrist first; they tend to seek care of neurologists or otologists, the specialists associated with their primary physical symptoms. They consider themselves to have a physical (i.e., structural or cellular, not functional) illness. However, as PPV is not yet part of the diagnostic repertoire of most neurologists or ear, nose, and throat doctors, the illness often lasts quite a long time before a diagnosis is established (an average of 3 years for 154 patients with PPV: Huppert et al., 1995). The diagnosis is established only after a number of visits to different specialists, superfluous laboratory examinations, and erroneous classifications such as "cervicogenic vertigo" or "recurrent vertebrobasilar ischemia", with correspondingly unsuccessful treatment attempts.

PPV is the most frequent cause of dizziness or vertigo in younger adults. A follow-up study confirmed that PPV is a unique clinical entity, which can be clearly differentiated from psychiatric disorders such as panic disorder with or without agoraphobia (Kapfhammer et al., 1997). Another longitudinal follow-up study (5–16 years) on 106 patients showed that physical symptoms improved at a rate of 75%; the symptoms had fully resolved in 27% (Huppert et al., 2005). In none of these patients did the diagnosis have to be revised. PPV can manifest in adults of every age, but there is a bimodal distribution with a peak in the second and fifth decades (it is the most common form of vertigo in this age group), and it shows no sexual predominance. If PPV remains untreated, the symptoms worsen, a generalization of the precipitating stimuli develops, and avoidance behavior may increase until the patient is unable to leave his/her own apartment without help.

Differential diagnosis

The differential diagnosis of PPV includes structural vestibular disorders, other medical illnesses, and psychiatric syndromes.

The most important structural vestibular and medical illnesses include:

- vestibular migraine
- orthostatic dysregulation
- bilateral vestibulopathy
- neurodegenerative disorders (spinocerebellar ataxias, multisystem atrophy, dementia)
- episodic ataxia type 2
- primary orthostatic tremor with a pathognomonic frequency peak of 14–16 Hz in electromyography and posturography (Yarrow et al., 2001)
- vestibular paroxysmia
- perilymph fistula/superior canal dehiscence syndrome
- central vestibular syndromes
- posttraumatic otolith dizziness.

The most important functional and psychiatric syndromes include the following (Brandt et al., 2013):

- panic disorder with or without agoraphobia
- other psychiatric or medical disorders that cause panic attacks or chronic anxiety
- space phobia (Marks, 1981)
- visual vertigo (Bronstein, 1995, 2004)
- *mal de débarquement* syndrome (Murphy, 1993)

CSD (Staab, 2012), which will be discussed in the next section, has a broad overlap with PPV.

Despite the relatively long lists of diseases and disorders in the differential diagnosis of PPV, the combination of specific complaints, normal physical findings, and primary personality type is so characteristic that there is seldom any doubt as to the diagnosis after the first examination (Brandt, 1996; Kapfhammer et al., 1997).

Pathophysiologic mechanisms

To explain the illusory perception of postural vertigo and stance instability, Brandt and Dieterich hypothesized a disturbance of space constancy. This results from a partial decoupling of the actual reafference signal from the efference copy signal for active head and body movements (Brandt and Dieterich, 1986; Brandt, 1996). Under normal conditions, humans do not perceive slight, self-generated body sway or head movements as accelerations during upright stance. The environment also appears to be stationary during active movements, although there are shifts of retinal images caused by these relative movements. Space constancy seems to be maintained by the simultaneous occurrence of a voluntary impulse to initiate a movement and in parallel the delivery of adequate information to identify self-motion (Fig. 37.2). According to Von Holst and Mittelstaedt (1950), this efference copy may provide a sensory pattern of expectation based on earlier experience (internal model). The movement-triggered actual sensory information is then so interpreted that self-motion can be differentiated from the motion of the environment. If this efference copy is missing, e.g., if we move the eyeball with a finger on the eyelid, illusory movements of the environment occur, so-called oscillopsia. The sensation of vertigo described by these patients (involving

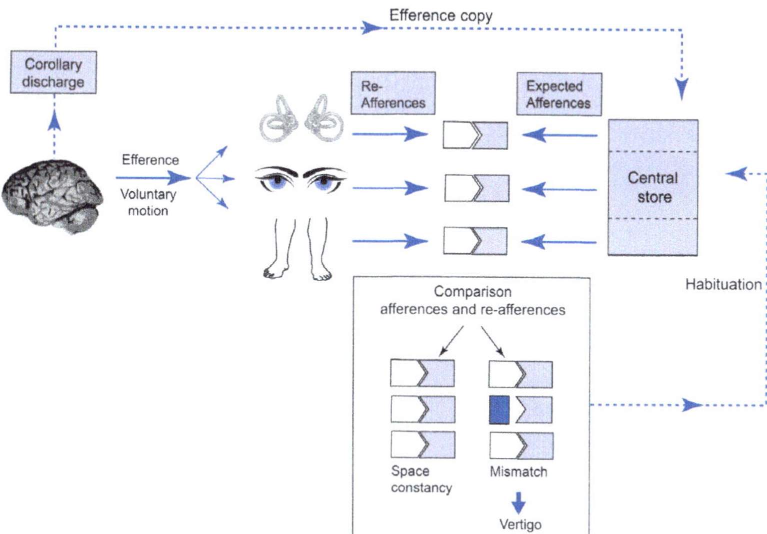

Fig. 37.2. Schematic drawing showing how vertigo/dizziness develops due to a disturbance of the space-constancy mechanism during active motion.

Voluntary head movements lead to stimulation of the vestibular, visual, and somatosensory sensory organs. Their messages are compared with a multisensory pattern of expectation provided by an internal model that was calibrated by earlier experience of motion. The expected pattern is prepared simultaneously by the efference-copy signal, which is sent in parallel with the voluntary movement impulse. If the concurrent sensory stimulation and the pattern of expectation are in agreement, the self-motion is perceived and "space constancy" is maintained. However, if there is an incongruence between the incoming and the expected pattern due to a partial "decoupling" of the efference-copy signal and the re-afference, a sensorimotor mismatch, then vertigo and imbalance develop. The subject no longer experiences a voluntary head movement in a stationary surrounding, but rather a threatening disorientation with exogenic head acceleration and a concurrent illusory movement of the surrounding. (Modified after Brandt, 1996.)

involuntary body sway and the occasional perception of individual head movements as disturbing external perturbations with simultaneous illusional movements of the surroundings) can be explained by a transient decoupling of efference copy and re-afference, i.e., a mismatch occurs between the anticipated and the actual motion (Brandt et al., 2013). Healthy people can experience similar mild sensations of vertigo without simultaneous anxiety during a state of total exhaustion, when the difference between voluntary head movements and involuntary sway becomes blurred. In patients with PPV, this partial decoupling may be caused by their constant preoccupation with anxious monitoring and checking of balance. This leads to the perception of sensorimotor adjustments that would otherwise be made unconsciously by means of learned (and reflex-like) muscle activation programs called up to maintain upright posture.

Precise posturographic analyses show that patients with PPV increase their postural sway during normal stance by co-contracting the flexor and extensor muscles of the foot (Brandt et al., 2012). This is evidently an expression of an unnecessary fearful strategy to control stance. Subjective imbalance in PPV is associated with characteristic changes in the coordination of open- and closed-loop mechanisms of postural control by which sensory feedback is used unnecessarily during simple, undisturbed stance (Wuehr et al., 2013) (Fig. 37.3). Healthy subjects use this strategy only when in real danger of falling. During difficult balancing tasks, such as tandem stance with eyes closed, the posturographic data of the patients with PPV do not differ from those of healthy subjects, i.e., the more difficult the demands of balance, the more the balance performance of the patients with PPV matches that of normal individuals (Querner et al., 2000; Fig. 37.4). Patients often report that unsteadiness especially increases when looking at moving visual scenes. However, when exposed to large-field visual motion stimulation in the roll plane, body sway did not exhibit a physiological visually increased body sway that could increase risk of falling (Querner et al., 2002). This is compatible with a lower threshold for closed-loop postural control by a stiffening of the musculoskeletal system (Wuehr et al., 2013).

Co-contraction of the entire gravity muscles and altered interactions between open- and closed-loop postural control culminate in a circular cascade of symptoms or a so-called vicious circle of postural instability (Wuehr et al., 2013; Brandt et al., 2015a) (Fig. 37.3). This is very similar to postural control of subjects with fear of heights.

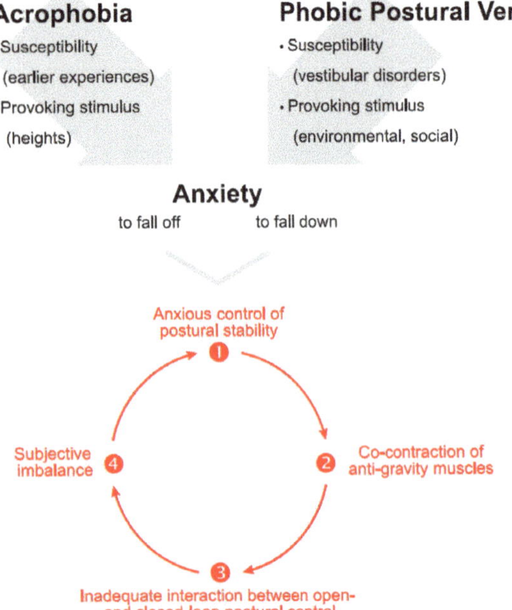

Fig. 37.3. Acrophobia and phobic postural vertigo are two different disorders that share anxiety of falling as a major symptom, although those afflicted do not fall. Both are characterized by an individual susceptibility to the condition. In acrophobia individuals often have had earlier experiences at heights, whereas in phobic postural vertigo the experiences are often initiated by a vestibular disorder. The provoking stimuli are disease-specific, but both end in a common circular cascade of symptoms, the so-called vicious circle (bottom). Anxious concentration on control of postural stability triggers co-contraction of the antigravity muscles, thereby causing an inadequate mode of interaction between open- and closed-loop mechanisms within the postural control systems. This leads to subjective imbalance, which in turn enhances anxious control of posture. (Modified after Brandt et al., 2015a.)

Both conditions – PPV and acrophobia – share two criteria: there is a dissociation between the subjective and objective risk of falling, and typically both conditions do not lead to an increased number of falls compared to normal controls (Brandt et al., 2015a; Schlick et al., 2016). Anxiety also affects ocular motor reflexes and gaze control (Staab, 2014). Acrophobic subjects tend to freeze their gaze to the horizon when exposed to heights (Kugler et al., 2014) (Fig. 37.5).

The use of automatized analysis of sway patterns in posturography under various conditions (e.g., with eyes open or closed, standing on firm ground or on foam rubber) together with a neuronal network allows in many cases a decision as to whether, for example, a PPV is present versus other conditions in the differential diagnosis (e.g., bilateral vestibulopathy, orthostatic tremor, or cerebellar syndrome) (Krafczyk et al., 2006; Brandt et al., 2012).

Pragmatic therapy

A doctor–patient consultation that provides a detailed explanation of the mechanism of the disease and of the necessity of self-controlled desensitization (i.e., the patient should consciously confront situations that induce dizziness) is essential for the therapy to succeed.

Treatment is based on three or four measures:

1. a thorough diagnostic evaluation to demonstrate to patients that their symptoms fit the definition of PPV and that they do not have an active structural disorder
2. education about the nature of the disorder
3. desensitization by self-exposure to triggers and regular exercise (physical therapy)
4. in case of relevant psychiatric comorbidity or if symptoms persist, cognitive-behavioral therapy with or without accompanying pharmacotherapy.

The most important therapeutic measure is to relieve patients of their fear of having a structural illness by careful examination and explanation of the functional mechanisms underlying the disorder (i.e., increased self-observation in the context of the corresponding primary personality structure). Desensitization by exposure to provoking situations should follow (i.e., the patient should not avoid such situations but, on the contrary, seek them out). At the same time, regular exercise has proven to be helpful to give patients confidence in their sense of balance. If explanation and self-desensitization do not result in sufficient improvement after a few weeks to months, then cognitive-behavioral therapy with or without drug therapy should be started. Selective serotonin reuptake inhibitors (e.g., paroxetine, citalopram, fluvoxamine, or sertraline) or tricyclic antidepressive agents may be used for 3–6 months. In a few patients it is necessary to initially combine these drugs with an anxiolytic drug (e.g., lorazepam), but only for a short time (for days to a few weeks) in order to avoid addiction to these drugs.

In a follow-up study (0.5–5.5 years after the initial diagnosis) involving 78 patients, 72% were free of symptoms or exhibited a clear improvement after this therapeutic strategy (Brandt et al., 1994). Fortunately, this long-term follow-up study showed no sign of an erroneous diagnosis. Identical results were also found in a longer-term follow-up study over 5–16 years (Huppert et al., 2005).

Cognitive-behavioral therapy in combination with vestibular rehabilitation was shown to significantly improve symptoms in controlled studies of small groups of patients with chronic nonspecific dizziness (Johansson et al., 2001; Andersson et al., 2006; Schmid et al., 2011). Holmberg and coworkers (2006) investigated the efficacy of cognitive-behavioral therapy

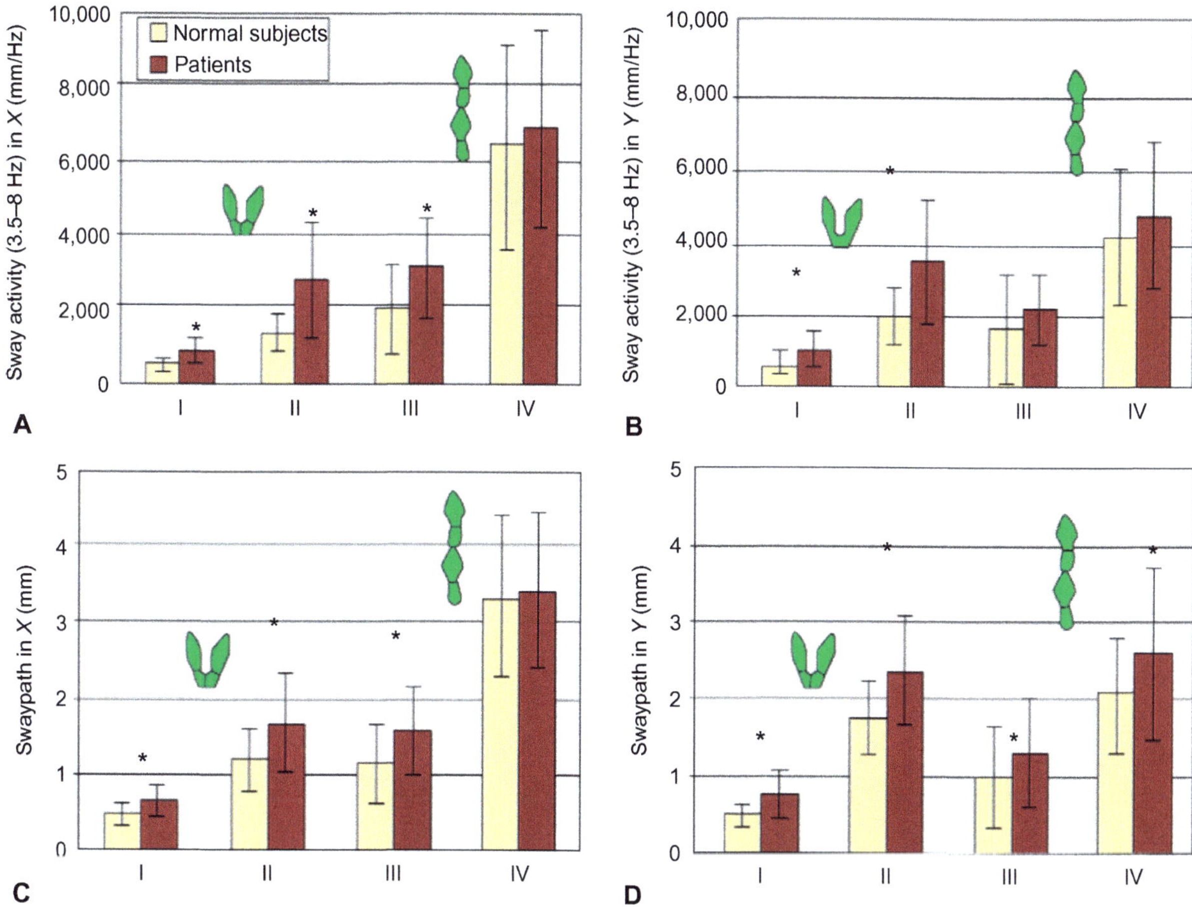

Fig. 37.4. Sway parameters revealed by a posturographic examination of healthy subjects and patients with phobic postural vertigo during different conditions of stance of increasing difficulty (I, normal stance with eyes open; II, normal stance with eyes closed; III, tandem stance with eyes open; IV, tandem stance with eyes closed). The more difficult the conditions, the more normal the performance of patients with phobic postural vertigo (*t*-test, $*p<0.05$; $**p<0.01$). (Modified after Querner et al., 2000.)

for PPV in a randomized trial of 31 patients. They found that 12 weeks of cognitive-behavioral therapy was superior to self-directed desensitization exercises when assessed at the end of treatment. However, a follow-up examination after 1 year determined that the positive effect was not maintained (Holmberg et al., 2007). It is possible that a combination of cognitive-behavioral therapy with psychoeducation, medication, and physiotherapy may be more suitable (pilot study: Tschan et al., 2012; Best et al., 2015).

The readiness of most of the patients, who experience much stress as a result of their suffering, to understand the functional mechanism of PPV and to overcome it by desensitization is a positive experience for both patients and clinicians.

Chronic subjective dizziness

Beginning in the early 2000s, Staab and colleagues (Staab et al., 2004; Staab and Ruckenstein, 2007a) began a series of investigations that led to the description of the syndrome of CSD. Inspired by the available literature on PPV, as well as studies of space motion discomfort (Jacob et al., 1993) and visual vertigo (Bronstein, 1995), they defined CSD as (Staab and Ruckenstein, 2007a):

1. persistent (duration $\geq$3 months) sensations of nonvertiginous dizziness, light-headedness, heavy-headedness, or subjective imbalance present on most days
2. chronic (duration $\geq$3 months) hypersensitivity to one's own motion, which is not direction-specific, and to the movements of objects in the environment
3. exacerbation of symptoms in settings with complex visual stimuli such as grocery stores or shopping malls or when performing precision visual tasks such as reading or using a computer
4. absence of currently active physical (i.e., structural or cellular) neuro-otologic illnesses, other

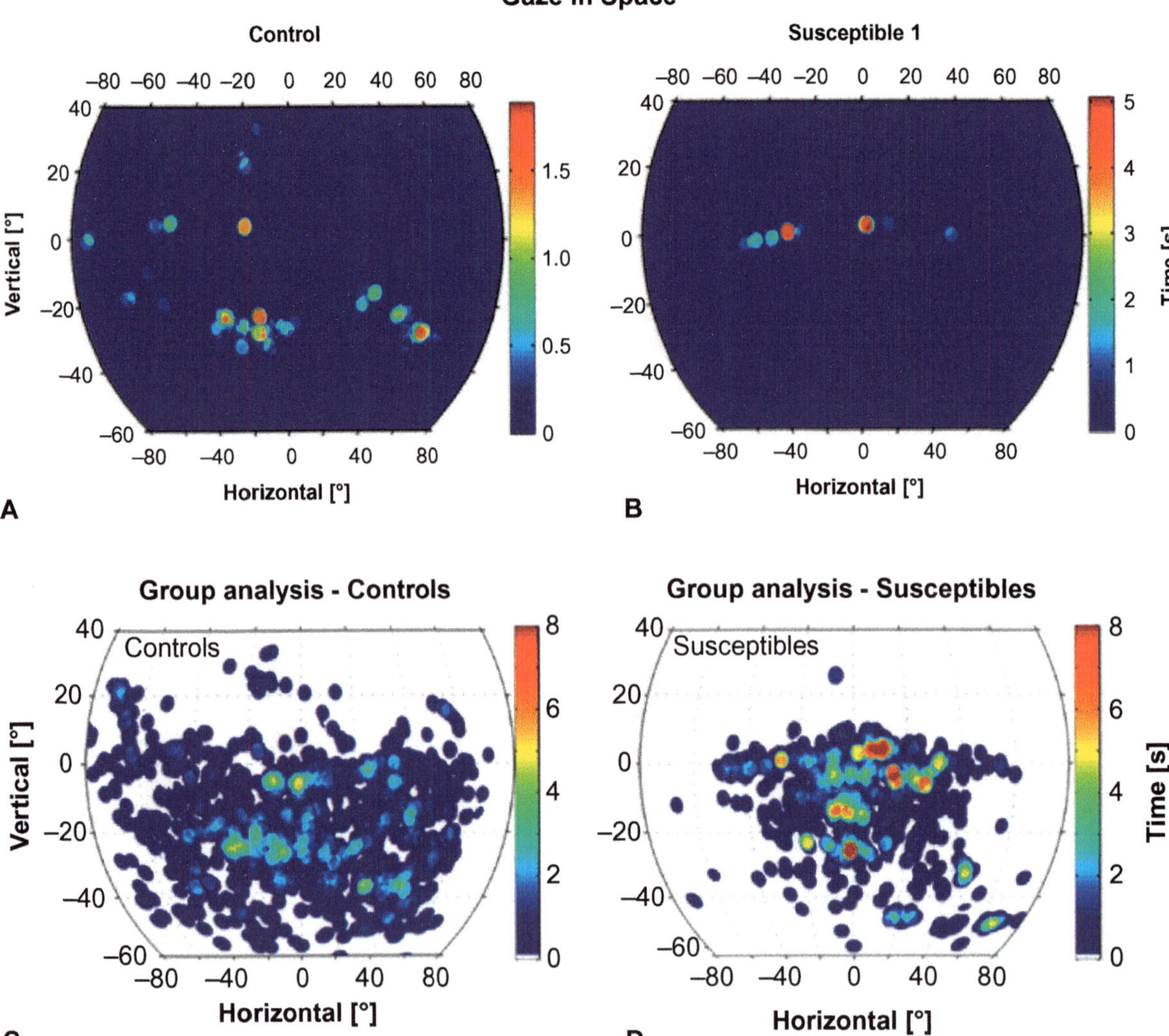

Fig. 37.5. Visual exploration behavior of subjects susceptible to fear of heights (right side) and of control subjects (left side) while standing on an emergency balcony 20 meters above ground level. Eye movements were measured by infrared eye-tracking goggles with inertial sensors for simultaneous recording of head movements. Gaze in space was calculated from eye-in-head and head movements. (**A**) The distributions of fixations in space during approximately 30 seconds are depicted for an individual control subject and for a susceptible subject. Note the preferred fixation along the horizon of the susceptible individual (top right). (**B**) Restricted visual exploration is also evident in the group analysis ($n = 16$): there is a tendency to freeze gaze to a small area straight ahead on the horizon or somewhat below it (bottom right). (Modified after Brandt et al., 2015a.)

definite medical conditions, or use of medications that may cause dizziness, or inability of such conditions to account for the full extent of dizziness or disability

5. results from radiographic imaging of the brain that exclude neuro-otologically significant anatomic lesions
6. findings from balance function tests that are in the reference range or are not indicative of a definitive structural vestibular deficit.

A later update of this definition (Staab, 2012) added a postural criterion similar to PPV (i.e., symptoms worse when in an upright posture) and refined the last three criteria to allow for the coexistence of CSD with other active vestibular disorders (i.e., positive findings on physical examination, balance function tests, or neuroimaging signified the presence of the comorbid condition rather than excluded CSD).

Comparing the definitions of CSD and PPV reveals several differences. The criteria for CSD emphasize persistent unsteadiness and dizziness. They do not include intermittent attacks of vestibular symptoms. They also focus more strongly on provocation of symptoms by visual stimuli than upright posture, even after the addition of the postural criterion. Psychologic elements such as obsessive personality traits, phobic behaviors, and mild anxiety and depressive symptoms were excluded, as these were considered to be risk factors or comorbid conditions, not core features of the disorder.

Research on CSD has included studies of its precipitants, clinical course, differential diagnosis, relationship to psychologic factors, treatment, and most recently, neurophysiologic and neuroimaging correlates (Staab and Ruckenstein, 2003, 2005, 2007a, b; Staab et al., 2010; Neff et al., 2012).

Clinical aspects and course of the illness

The largest study of CSD ($n = 345$) enumerated its precipitants (Staab and Ruckenstein, 2007a). These included acute or episodic vestibular syndromes such as vestibular neuritis or benign paroxysmal positional vertigo (25%), panic attacks, especially in young adults (15–20%), vestibular migraine (15–20%), generalized anxiety (15%), mild traumatic brain injury (concussion or whiplash), especially in young men (10–15%), and autonomic dysregulation (7%). A collection of other medical events (e.g., dysrhythmias, adverse drug reactions) that had the ability to produce dizziness or disrupt balance completed the list at 1–2% each. This list includes the types of triggering events described for PPV (Brandt and Dieterich, 1986; Brandt, 1996). The most common precipitants found for CSD were neurologic and otologic disorders. Psychosocial stressors were observed to exert their effects via panic attacks or generalized anxiety.

The clinical course of CSD was found to be influenced by pre-existing and coexisting conditions. In particular, patients with pre-existing anxiety diatheses in the form of personal or family histories of anxiety disorders had more chronic symptoms (Staab and Ruckenstein, 2003) and less robust responses to treatment with selective serotonin reuptake inhibitors (Staab and Ruckenstein, 2005). The duration of illness was measured in months to years, with an average duration of 4.5 years at the time of tertiary consultation (Staab and Ruckenstein, 2007a), due at least in part to the limited recognition of the disorder by neurologists and otologists previously described for PPV (Huppert et al., 1995).

Coexisting anxiety and depressive disorders are common, but not universal, in patients with CSD. In a diagnostic validation study of patients with CSD ($n = 107$), 60% had clinically significant anxiety symptoms and 45% had clinically significant depression symptoms, but, importantly, 25% had no problematic anxiety or mood symptoms on self-report measures, standardized clinician-administered psychiatric diagnostic screening, or psychosomatic examinations (Staab et al., 2010). Thus, CSD, like PPV, can exist apart from any psychiatric comorbidity.

Coexisting vestibular syndromes and other medical diseases also affect the course of illness for patients with CSD. Episodic conditions such as vestibular migraine or Ménière's disease create a clinical picture of recurrent attacks of vertigo and associated headache or hearing symptoms, respectively, superimposed on a baseline of persistent dizziness and unsteadiness due to CSD (Neff et al., 2012). Coexisting chronic medical conditions such as postural orthostatic tachycardia syndrome produce an intertwined set of persistent symptoms (Staab and Ruckenstein, 2007b).

Differential diagnosis

The differential diagnosis of CSD mirrors the list above for PPV. Assessment must be made of residua or recurrences of precipitating conditions (e.g., uncompensated peripheral vestibular deficits, recurrent attacks of vestibular migraine), coexisting disorders (e.g., postconcussive syndrome, generalized anxiety disorder), and illnesses that may partially mimic its symptoms (e.g., *mal de débarquement*, orthostatic tremor).

Pathophysiologic mechanisms

The pathophysiologic processes postulated for CSD are illustrated in Figure 37.6 (Staab, 2013). Starting at the left, precipitating events trigger a combination of physiologic and behavioral adaptations that are normally expected in response to acute vestibular syndromes or other conditions that disrupt balance function. These include a shift in sensory integration to favor visual or somatosensory inputs, increased attention to head and body motion, and increased caution with ambulation, all of which have been measured in normal individuals under postural threat (Brown et al., 2002; Gage et al., 2003). As acute events remit, however, the effects of predisposing anxiety-related personality traits and acutely anxious responses to the inciting events delay a return to normal postural and oculomotor control (middle of figure). This means that high-risk strategies, properly evoked by the original events, continue to be used to manage routine movements and responses to low-demand space and motion stimuli in the environment (right of figure). The unnatural quality of these circumstances perpetuates a misperception that high-risk strategies are still required, sustaining the condition over time. Additional psychiatric morbidity may or may not develop depending on the individual patient (top right of figure).

This hypothesis is compatible with the pathophysiologic mechanisms proposed by Brandt and Dieterich to explain PPV (Brandt and Dieterich, 1986; Brandt, 1996). In fact, it is conceivable that the failure to return to normal low-risk postural control depicted in

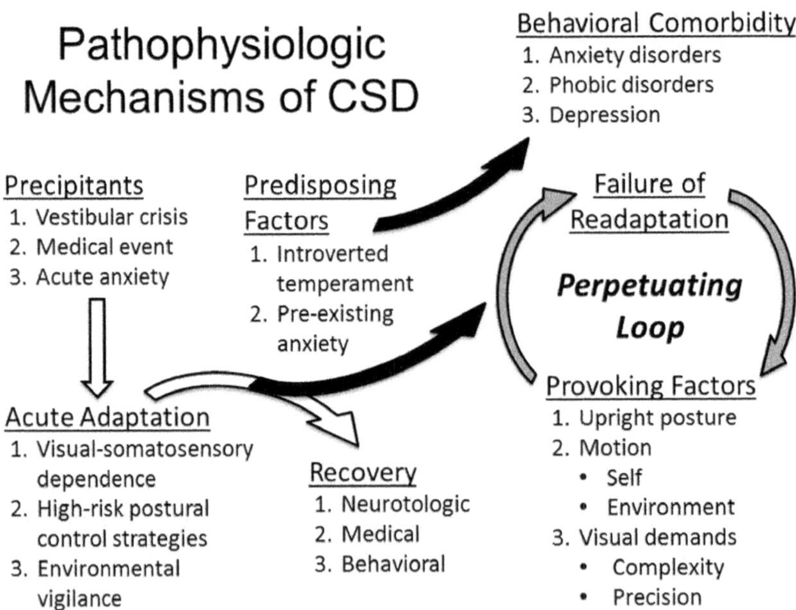

Fig. 37.6. Graphic depiction of putative pathophysiologic mechanisms in chronic subjective dizziness (CSD). The normal response to acute vestibular or balance symptoms includes a transient shift to high demand (stiffer) postural control and visual dependence (left of figure). A pre-existing anxiety diathesis and highly anxious response to acute physical symptoms increases the likelihood that this shift will persist and not revert back to normal (middle of figure). The result is maladaptive use of high-demand strategies, even for routine control of posture, gait, and gaze, with or without the development of psychiatric comorbidity (right of figure). (Reproduced from Staab (2013), with permission from Oxford University Press.)

Figure 37.6 may be related to different thresholds for the use of efference copy/re-afferent matching to drive postural feedback control in high- versus low-demand states. Anxiety-related perceptions of continued threat could extend the use of high-risk postural feedback control mechanisms such as co-contraction of leg musculature to the low-demand situations that normally re-emerge as acute precipitants resolve. However, there are two differences in the mechanisms proposed for PPV and CSD. The pathophysiologic processes of Figure 37.6 include greater specificity about anxiety-related personality traits and greater attention to shifts in multisensory integration toward visual dependence than the processes suggested for PPV, which emphasize abnormalities of postural control.

Concepts of anxiety-related personality traits have advanced since the inclusion of obsessive compulsive personality traits in the original description of phobic original postural vertigo in 1986 (Brandt and Dieterich, 1986). In particular, an anxious temperament (also called high trait anxiety) comprised of high levels of neuroticism and low levels of extraversion (high N, low E) has emerged as a risk factor for depressive and anxiety disorders, and increased morbidity in functional disorders (Bienvenu et al., 2007; Schrier et al., 2013; Torres et al., 2013). Neuroticism and extraversion, along with openness, agreeableness, and conscientiousness, are the five fundamental traits in contemporary models of human personality, which can be measured with the NEO Personality Inventory (Costa and McCrae, 1992). Staab et al. (2014) used the NEO to determine that patients with CSD were significantly more likely to possess a composite high-N, low-E temperament than a comparison group of patients with coexisting vestibular and anxiety disorders who had similar levels of dizziness, anxiety, and depression (67% vs. 25%, respectively, odds ratio = 6.0, $p < 0.05$).

These same traits may affect brain responses to vestibular stimulation. In a functional magnetic resonance imaging (fMRI) study of normal individuals (Indovina et al., 2014), higher levels of neuroticism were associated with greater activity in the brainstem, cerebellar fastigium, and visual cortex (V2) and reduced activity in the supramarginal gyrus in response to sound-evoked vestibular stimulation. Higher levels of neuroticism also were associated with greater connectivity between the amygdala and brainstem, amygdala and fastigium, inferior frontal gyrus and supramarginal gyrus, and inferior frontal gyrus and V2. Lower levels of extraversion were associated with greater activity of the amygdala and less connectivity between the amygdala and orbitofrontal areas that modulate its function. Separately, moderate versus low-trait anxiety was shown to reduce the threshold at which high-risk (stiffened) postural control strategies were employed in response to visual and cognitive demands on balance (Hainault et al., 2011). Thus, high neuroticism and low extraversion may increase the risk for development of CSD because they increase reactivity and connectivity of vestibular-visual and anxiety networks in the brain, and reduce the threshold for employing high-risk postural control processes. In contrast, the personality traits of resilience, optimism, and belief that the travails of life are manageable (essentially the opposite of high N, low E) were associated with less likelihood of developing persistent functional dizziness in the year after acute vestibular syndromes (Tschan et al., 2011).

Results of the first structural and functional imaging studies to investigate brain morphology, activity, and connectivity in patients with functional vestibular syndromes have recently been completed (Indovina et al., 2015; Zu Eulenburg et al., personal communication; Sohsten et al., personal communication). A structural and functional imaging investigation found links between physical and psychologic symptoms and regional gray-matter density in patients with PPV (Zu Eulenburg et al., personal communication) (Fig. 37.7). Specifically, patients with PPV versus normal control subjects had lower regional gray-matter density in the medial orbitofrontal cortex, which correlated with the duration of dizziness symptoms and reduced activation of that region in response to the motion aftereffect of vestibular stimulation. Furthermore, scores on the Beck Depression Inventory correlated negatively with gray-matter density in the caudal vermis and cerebellar tonsil.

In an fMRI study, brain activity and connectivity in frontal, vestibular, and visual cortical regions were found to differ between patients with CSD and normal individuals (Indovina et al., 2015; Fig. 37.8). Patients with CSD demonstrated reduced activity relative to controls in the parietoinsular vestibular cortex (PIVC), anterior insula, anterior cingulate cortex, inferior frontal gyrus, and hippocampus in response to sound-evoked vestibular stimulation (otolith activation by short tone bursts). Patients with CSD also showed negative connectivity between the anterior insula and PIVC, anterior insula and middle occipital cortex, hippocampus and PIVC, and anterior cingulate cortex and PIVC.

A second fMRI study using emotional pictures (non-motion stimuli) (Sohsten et al., personal communication) found reduced activation of the amygdala and anterior cingulate cortex in response to standardized, negatively valenced pictures in patients with PPPD versus individuals who had recovered well from the types of acute

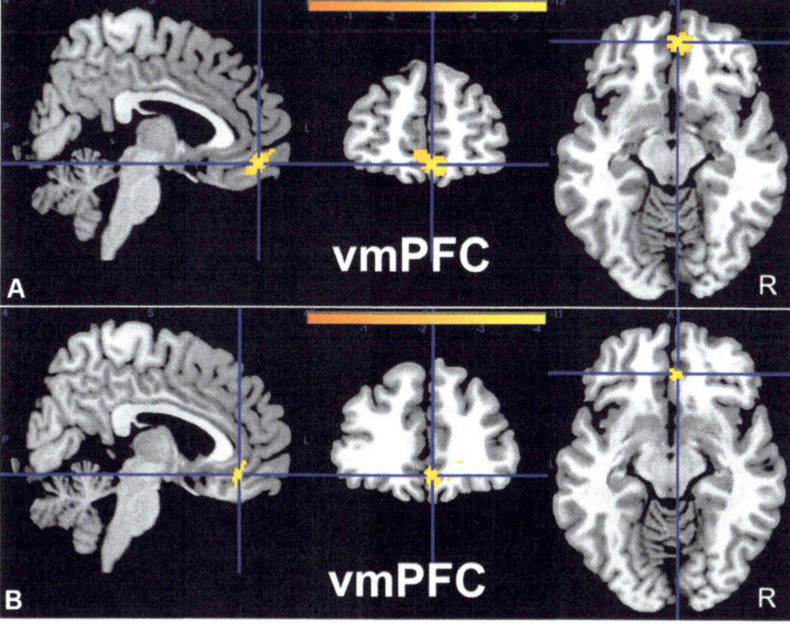

Fig. 37.7. Multimodal images of a cohort of patients with functional dizziness (phobic postural vertigo) derived from task-based functional magnetic resonance imaging to show neural responses (**A**) as well as voxel-based morphometry (VBM) to delineate structural changes (**B**). (**A**) Significantly stronger deactivation of the ventromedial prefrontal cortex (vmPFC) during the motion aftereffect following visual stimulation in patients with functional dizziness ($n=21$) compared to age- and gender-matched controls performing the same task ($p<0.05$ false discovery rate (FDR) cluster corrected). All scales reflect z-scores. The area vmPFC is known to play a significant role in fear extinction and self-value-based decision making. (**B**) Significantly lower gray-matter density information in the vmPFC of patients with functional dizziness ($n=38$), suggesting regional atrophy in comparison to an age-matched control group ($p<0.05$ FDR cluster corrected, VBM 12). Thus, converging multimodal evidence was found for the importance of vmPFC in functional dizziness. (Zu Eulenburg et al., personal communication.)

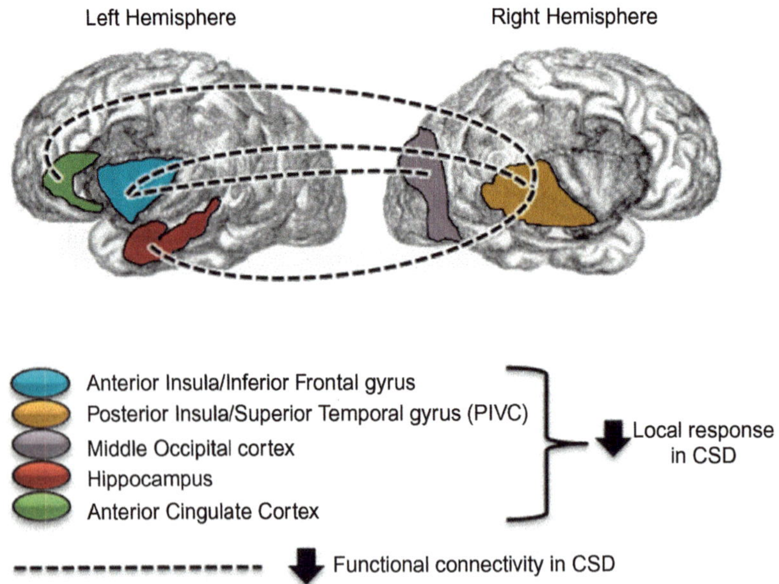

Fig. 37.8. Summary of regional activity and connectivity changes in patients with chronic subjective dizziness (CSD) versus healthy controls in response to a sound-evoked vestibular stimulus (otolith stimulation by a 10-ms, 500-Hz, 100-dB tone burst). Patients with CSD had reduced activation in the parietoinsular vestibular cortex (PIVC) (superior temporal gyrus/posterior insula), inferior frontal gyrus/anterior insula, hippocampus, and anterior cingulate cortex (downward arrows) and more negative functional connectivity between the PIVC and three other regions (anterior insula, anterior cingulate, and hippocampus), as well as between the anterior insula and middle occipital cortex (dashed lines). This suggests that CSD is associated with widespread changes in brain networks connecting regions responsible for processing space–motion information (PIVC, visual cortex, and hippocampus), body awareness (anterior insula), and contextual responses to noxious or threatening stimuli (hippocampus, anterior cingulate, anterior insula). (Reproduced from Indovina et al., 2015, with permission.)

vestibular symptoms that can trigger PPPD. Taken together, these early imaging results support models of the PPV and CSD (and, by extension, PPPD), which suggest that its pathophysiologic mechanisms involve widespread structural and functional alterations in sensory cortical areas (PIVC and visual cortices), regions involved in spatial information processing (hippocampus), postural control (cerebellar vermis), and threat assessment (amygdala), and the frontal/prefrontal regions that modulate their activity (orbitofrontal cortex, anterior insula, anterior cingulate). Future investigations are needed to extend these results and evaluate the effects of physical activity levels, mental state, pre-existing personality traits, and treatment.

The putative pathophysiologic mechanisms of CSD also suggest that increased sensitivity to visual motion stimuli, complex patterns in the environment, and performance of tasks requiring sustained visual focus result from increased visual dependence. This is the process thought to underlie visual vertigo (Bronstein, 1995, 2004). In a prospective study, patients with chronic nonvertiginous dizziness that persisted for 6 months or more after bouts of acute vestibular neuritis were significantly more likely to demonstrate visual dependence measured by the Rod and Disk Test than their counterparts who recovered without residual symptoms or normal control subjects (Cousins et al., 2014). The Rod and Disk Test measures the extent to which a rotating background of dots alters an individual's visual estimate of true vertical compared to a stationary background. That study was not designed to investigate CSD, but its methods have been extended to patients with CSD in an ongoing study.

Treatment

The efficacy of serotonergic antidepressants (Staab et al., 2004; Staab, 2011), vestibular habituation exercises (Thompson et al., 2015), and cognitive-behavioral therapy (Edelman et al., 2012; Mahoney et al., 2013) has been investigated in patients with CSD in open-label, retrospective follow-up, and randomized controlled trials, respectively. Additional studies of these treatments in cohorts of patients with chronic, but nonspecific, dizziness lend further support to their use (see Staab, 2012, for reviews).

The first treatment trial for CSD was a 16-week, prospective, open-label study of flexibly dosed sertraline (25–200 mg/day) in 20 patients (Staab et al., 2004). Fifteen patients completed the trial with a median endpoint dose of 100 mg/day; 11 (73%) had a positive response measured as a >50% reduction in scores on the Dizziness Handicap Inventory, including 6 (40%) who achieved complete remission. The other pharmacologic study that focused specifically on patients with CSD was a case series of venlafaxine treatment in 32 patients who also had vestibular migraine with ($n=20$) or without ($n=12$) a third diagnosis of an anxiety disorder. Patients with all three disorders were twice as likely to respond (65% vs. 33%) as those with CSD plus vestibular migraine, but no psychiatric morbidity. Response meant halving of both dizziness and headache severity.

Four more open-label studies and a case series have examined the efficacy of the other five selective serotonin reuptake inhibitors (Staab et al., 2002; Horii et al., 2004, 2007; Simon et al., 2005) and the serotonin norepinephrine reuptake inhibitor, milnacipran (Horii et al., 2008) in patients with chronic nonspecific dizziness. The entry criterion for these studies was not a diagnosis of CSD *per se*, but persistent dizziness in the absence of structural vestibular disorders. Collectively, 66–84% of patients had positive responses and most tolerated the medications well, in keeping with the results of the studies of patients with CSD.

Vestibular habituation is a well-established physiotherapy treatment for patients with vestibular symptoms, though its pivotal trials were conducted in cohorts of patients with mixed, often undefined, causes of chronic dizziness (Telian et al., 1990; Shepard et al., 1993; Yardley et al., 1998, 2004). Clinically, vestibular habituation has been used for more than a decade to treat patients with CSD, though its efficacy was not investigated until a just-published telephone follow-up of patients identified by retrospective chart review showed that almost all patients found consultation with a physical therapist to be helpful and more than half (14/26) obtained significant relief from sensitivity to head/body movement and visual motion stimuli (Thompson et al., 2015).

One randomized controlled trial of cognitive-behavioral therapy (Edelman et al., 2012) with 6-month follow-up (Mahoney et al., 2013) has been completed in patients with CSD. This intervention targeted dizziness, body vigilance, and perceptions of dizziness-related handicaps. Forty-four patients were randomly assigned to three sessions of cognitive-behavioral therapy or a wait-list control. Patients who received active treatment showed large reductions in dizziness and dizziness-related handicaps at the end of treatment (Edelman et al., 2012), benefits that were sustained at 6-month re-evaluation (Mahoney et al., 2013). The major difference between these studies and the earlier investigations of Holmberg and coworkers (2006, 2007), that showed no lasting benefits of cognitive behavior therapy for patients with PPV, is that patients with CSD were treated early. In fact, they were enrolled in treatment within 8 weeks of triggering events as the disorder was emerging, but not fully established, whereas patients in the studies of PPV had long-standing symptoms. This suggests that cognitive-behavioral therapy may prevent the development of CSD, if administered early, whereas it may have less benefit for patients with lengthy illnesses.

Persistent postural-perceptual dizziness

In 2010, the Committee for Classification of Vestibular Disorders of the Bárány Society (Bisdorff et al., 2013) commissioned a Behavioral Subcommittee to examine the extant literature on PPV and CSD as well as space motion discomfort (Jacob et al., 1993, 2009) and visual vertigo (Bronstein, 1995, 2004), to determine if published data suggested the presence of one or more unique clinical conditions. Space motion discomfort is a combination of uneasiness about spatial orientation and balance, feelings of swaying or rocking when still, and increased awareness of motion stimuli that can be exacerbated by a person's own movement or exposure to moving or patterned objects in the environment (Jacob et al., 1993). Visual vertigo, now called visually induced dizziness, is a sensation of unsteadiness or dizziness that occurs on exposure to complex or moving visual stimuli and develops in a portion of patients following bouts of acute peripheral or central vestibular losses (Bronstein, 1995, 2004). Members of the subcommittee reached consensus about the presence of one distinctly definable disorder, which they termed PPPD, in keeping with the nomenclature of the Bárány Society's classification project (Bisdorff et al., 2009). The subcommittee prepared a 100-word narrative description of PPPD that was included in the Bárány Society's recommendations to the World Health Organization for updates to the ICD. The WHO has added this definition to the beta draft version of ICD-11:

> *Persistent non-vertiginous dizziness, unsteadiness, or both lasting three months or more. Symptoms are present most days, often increasing throughout the day, but may wax and wane. Momentary flares may occur spontaneously or with sudden movement. Affected individuals feel worst when upright, exposed to moving or complex visual stimuli, and during active or passive head motion. These situations may not be equally provocative. Typically, the disorder follows occurrences of acute or episodic vestibular or balance-related problems. Symptoms may begin intermittently, and then consolidate. Gradual onset is uncommon (WHO, 2015a).*

This definition was drawn primarily from key features shared by PPV and CSD. As such, much of the research on those two disorders is expected to be applicable to PPPD. For example, Thompson et al. (2015) applied the criteria of PPPD retrospectively to patients enrolled in their study of vestibular habituation for CSD and found that the results held. Nonetheless, validation of the diagnostic criteria for the new disorder, assessment of possible variations or subtypes (e.g., a predominantly postural subtype akin to PPV or a predominantly visual subtype like CSD), understanding of its pathophysiologic mechanisms, and best strategies for treatment await future investigations.

Additional functional vestibular presentations

The vestibular symptoms caused by PPV and CSD are not the only persistent functional vestibular symptoms encountered in clinical practice. Some patients describe unrelenting and unchanging vestibular symptoms that lack any identifiable pattern of provoking or mitigating factors yet are highly distressing and debilitating. Their continuous nature, unwavering quality in the face of typical motion provocations, abnormal complexity, and high level of resulting burden distinguish them from the more common episodic or fluctuating symptoms reported by patients with structural vestibular disorders, PPV, CSD, and well-defined psychiatric causes of vestibular symptoms (see next section). In many patients, these constant vestibular symptoms are accompanied by other chronic complaints such as fatigue and pain. This raises the possibility that patients with these symptoms are suffering from a somatic symptom disorder (DSM-5: American Psychiatric Association, 2013) or bodily distress disorder (ICD-11 beta draft: WHO, 2015b). Future investigations will have to examine this prospect.

PSYCHIATRIC CAUSES OF VESTIBULAR SYMPTOMS

Psychiatric disorders may be the primary causes or secondary complications of vestibular syndromes. Primary psychiatric disorders occur without other preceding vestibular syndromes. Secondary psychiatric disorders develop after the onset of primary vestibular disorders and often outlast their remission (Huppert et al., 1995; Staab and Ruckenstein, 2003; Dieterich and Eckhardt-Henn, 2006; Eckhardt-Henn et al., 2008) (Fig. 37.9). In some cases, psychiatric disorders occur first, but do not manifest vertigo, unsteadiness, or dizziness. Then, with the onset of a vestibular disorder, they increase in severity and contribute to overall morbidity in an interactive manner (Staab and Ruckenstein, 2003). Psychiatric disorders also may trigger functional vestibular syndromes such as PPV or CSD (Fig. 37.9).

Psychiatric disorders that may cause or contribute to vestibular symptoms, ranked by likelihood of doing so, are:

1. anxiety and phobic disorders
2. traumatic stress and obsessive-compulsive disorders (via associated panic attacks and chronic anxiety)
3. depressive disorders
4. somatic symptom disorder/bodily distress disorder (mentioned above)
5. dissociative disorders (including depersonalization/derealization syndromes).

The prevalence of these disorders as primary causes of vestibular symptoms has been estimated at about 8–10% among all patients in specialty neuro-otology centers (Staab, 2013), most of that due to disorders that produce

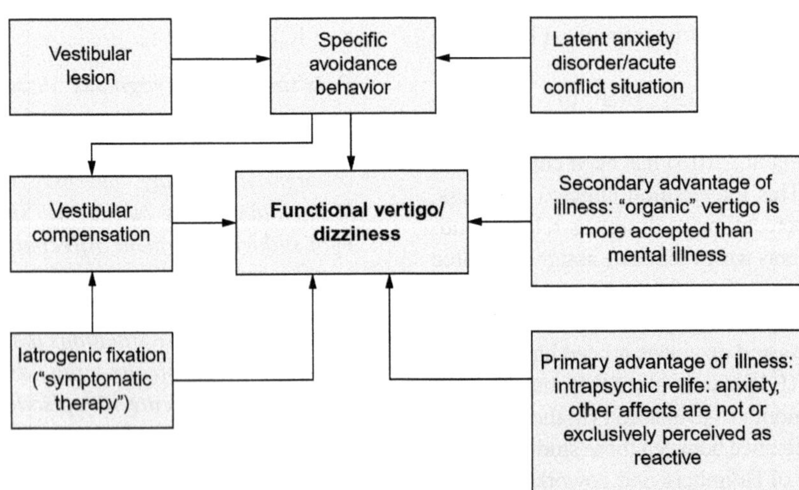

Fig. 37.9. Pathogenetic model of phobic postural vertigo: secondary functional or psychiatric vertigo/dizziness, triggered by organic vertigo/dizziness. (Modified after Dieterich and Eckhardt-Henn, 2006, a pathogenetic model for somatoform vertigo and dizziness.)

dizziness during panic attacks or flares of chronic anxiety or depression. Rates of psychiatric comorbidity in patients with structural or functional vestibular syndromes are much higher. In a cross-sectional diagnostic study of 547 patients recruited from a specialized interdisciplinary treatment center for vertigo/dizziness, nearly 50% of all patients had an active psychiatric disorder detected by standardized, clinician-administered, psychiatric diagnostic interviews (the Structured Clinical Interview for DSM-IV Axis I Disorders: SCID-I) (Best et al., 2009a; Hanel et al., 2009; Lahmann et al., 2015). However, the prevalence of psychiatric comorbidity was not uniform across all structural vestibular disorders. The highest rates were found in patients suffering from vestibular migraine (49%) and vestibular paroxysmia (51%). Lower rates were seen in vestibular neuritis (37%) and bilateral vestibular failure (24%). These results were in agreement with an earlier study that used both structured interviews and psychometric tests and found a high point prevalence of psychiatric comorbidity in patients with vestibular migraine (65%) and Ménière's disease (57%) versus much lower rates in patients with vestibular neuritis (22%) and benign paroxysmal positional vertigo (15%) (Eckhardt-Henn et al., 2008). By comparison, the prevalence of psychiatric morbidity in the general population is about 20% (Kessler et al., 2005). Patients with active psychiatric disorders had more vertigo-related handicaps, more physical and psychologic symptoms, and a lower psychologic quality of life than their counterparts without psychiatric comorbidity (Best et al., 2009b; Lahmann et al., 2015).

Prospective reports have offered additional details. In a study that followed patients with various causes of vertigo for 1 year (Best et al., 2009a), patients with vestibular migraine had sustained elevations in rates of psychiatric morbidity, whereas those with Ménière's disease, vestibular neuritis, and benign paroxysmal positional vertigo exhibited normal or normalizing values over time (Fig. 37.10). Patients with vestibular migraine reported stronger vestibular symptoms, felt themselves more hindered in their daily life by dizziness, and had more anxiety than patients with other vestibular disorders (Tschan et al., 2008, 2011; Best et al., 2009b). Interestingly, patients with vestibular migraine also may have increased susceptibility to functional vestibular comorbidity. In one study, the rate of coexisting CSD was 31% for subjects with vestibular migraine versus 5.5% for individuals with Ménière's disease (Neff et al., 2012). The development of secondary morbidity may be predicated most strongly on patients' initial reactions to acute vestibular events. Several studies have shown that it is not the extent of structural deficits that predict long-term morbidity (Best et al., 2006, 2009a; Cousins et al., 2014), but the level of anxiety and vigilance about vertigo and dizziness during and after acute vestibular syndromes (Godemann et al., 2006; Heinrichs et al., 2007).

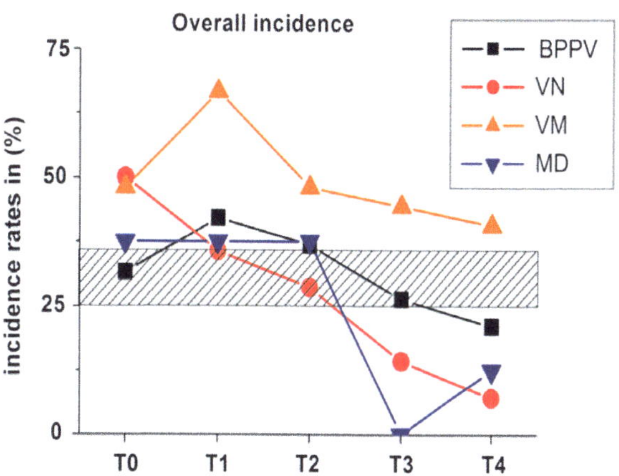

Fig. 37.10. Prospective longitudinal analysis of the incidence (in %) of the development of a functional/psychiatric disorder in the course of illness in patients with various vestibular vertigo syndromes. Patients with vestibular migraine develop a secondary functional disorder conspicuously more often. BPPV, benign peripheral paroxysmal positioning vertigo; VN, vestibular neuritis; VM, vestibular migraine; MD, Ménière's disease; T0, time of the diagnosis of the illness; T1, 6 weeks; T2, 3 months; T3, 6 months; T4, 1 year. (Modified after Best et al., 2009a with permission from Springer Science and Business Media.)

Patients with functional vestibular disorders also have high rates of psychiatric comorbidity. Cross-sectional and follow-up studies of patients with PPV (Kapfhammer et al., 1997; Holmberg et al., 2005) and CSD (Staab and Ruckenstein, 2007a; Staab et al., 2010) found the prevalence of anxiety and depressive disorders to be about 75% for patients with long-term illness. Patients with one psychiatric disorder that generates vestibular morbidity may be prone to additional psychiatric problems. For example, individuals with a susceptibility to visual height intolerance and those with the psychiatric diagnosis of acrophobia (specific phobia of heights) also exhibited comorbid anxiety and depressive disorders (Kapfhammer et al., 2015).

Detecting functional and psychiatric disorders – importance of patient history

The large number of possible combinations of primary and secondary structural, functional, and psychiatric disorders (Fig. 37.1) may make the complete assessment of vestibular symptoms seem an impossibly daunting task, but it is not. Recognition of functional and psychiatric diagnoses is mainly based on patients' descriptions of their symptoms and associated behavioral changes. Years ago, Trimble wrote in 1984 that:

Assessment of etiology, particularly where objectively determined neurological accompanying signs are minimal or absent [or cannot explain the full extent of illness], will depend therefore on an understanding of the patient in whom the symptom is arising, his [or her] background quality of interpersonal relationships, and the life situation in which the symptoms have arisen (text in brackets added from Staab, 2013).

In practice, the task is simpler than that, as diagnostic methods have improved dramatically since Trimble wrote these words.

The clinical history is paramount because functional and psychiatric vestibular disorders are diagnosed by history (Fig. 37.11). There are no single pathognomonic symptoms for these illnesses, but key elements of clinical history are more common in structural versus functional versus psychiatric syndromes (Brandt, 1999; Staab, 2013; Brandt et al., 2015b). Combinations of symptoms and their temporal associations are keys to properly making (i.e., ruling in) diagnoses (Table 37.1). Importantly, however, the existence of features in one category does not exclude disorders in other categories from consideration. High rates of comorbidity make it impossible to use the presence of one set of features to eliminate (i.e., rule out) other illnesses.

For example, a patient with episodic vertigo accompanied by nausea, vomiting, and ataxia is most likely to have a peripheral or central structural abnormality (e.g., benign paroxysmal positional vertigo, brainstem stroke), whereas an individual with episodic dizziness accompanied by palpitations, dyspnea, tremulousness, paresthesias, and fear of becoming incapacitated is most likely to have a psychiatric disorder (e.g., an anxiety disorder with panic attacks). Structural disorders such as benign paroxysmal positional vertigo may produce unsteadiness rather than vertigo and psychiatric

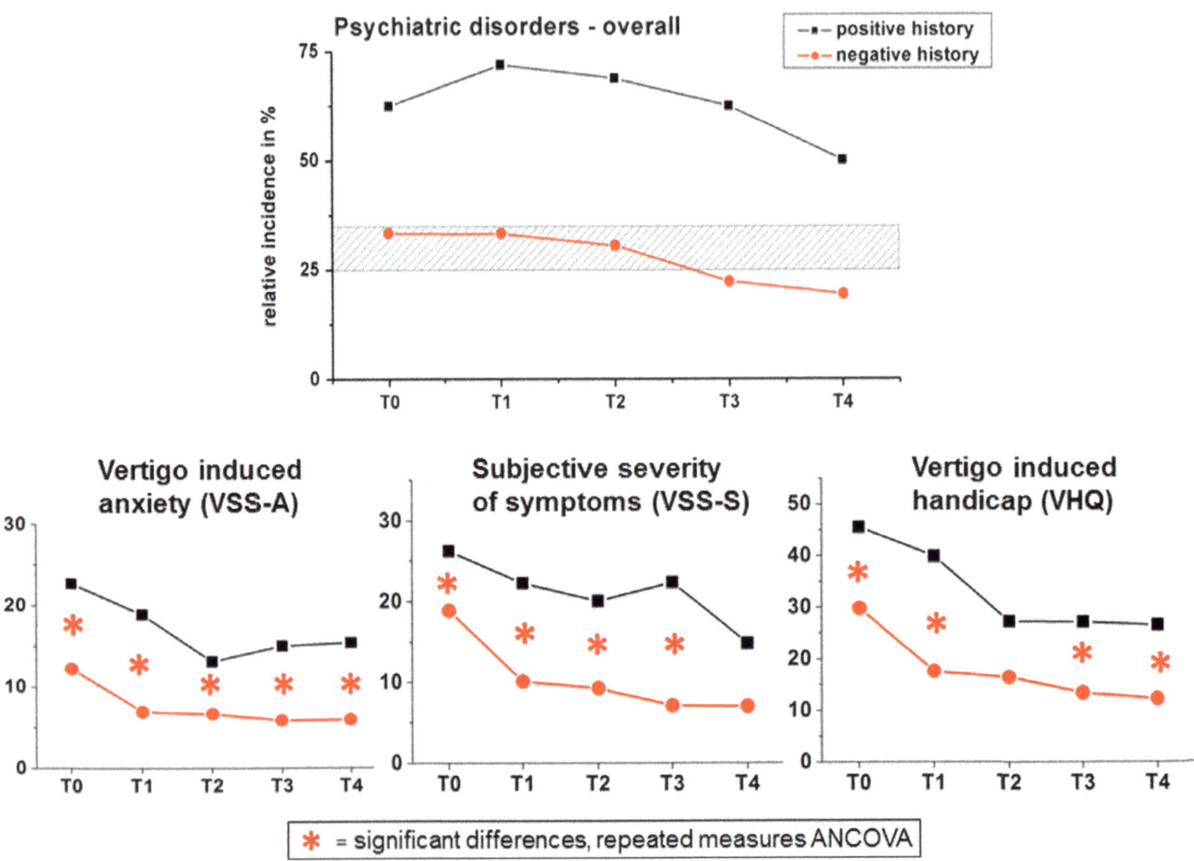

Fig. 37.11. Prospective study of patients with acute vestibular disorders during a follow-up over 1 year (T0–T4). Relative incidence (in %) of a patient becoming ill with a functional or psychiatric disorder within 6 months after having an acute vestibular syndrome (such as benign peripheral paroxysmal positioning vertigo, vestibular neuritis, vestibular migraine, Ménière's disease) dependent on his/her history of pre-existing psychiatric illness (top: negative history in red, positive history in black). Vertigo-induced anxiety (VSS-A), subjective severity of symptoms (VSS-S), and vertigo-induced handicap (VHQ) of the same patients (bottom). T0, time of the diagnosis of the illness; T1, 6 weeks; T2, 3 months; T3, 6 months; T4, 1 year. Modified after Best et al., 2009a, b.)

Table 37.1

Signs and symptoms in acute and chronic syndromes of structural, functional, and psychiatric vestibular disorders

		Structural disorders	Functional disorders	Psychiatric disorders
Acute or episodic syndromes	Vestibular symptoms	Vertigo attacks		Dizziness Unsteadiness
	Motion sensitivity	Vertigo in specific positions Vertigo with rapid head tilts or turns		Fear of provocative motion
	Aural symptoms	Fluctuating hearing loss Unilateral tinnitus		
	Autonomic and vegetative symptoms	Nausea Emesis	Mild queasiness without emesis Mild diaphoresis, tremulousness	Chest pain, palpitations, dyspnea, tremulousness, paresthesias
	Posture and gait abnormalities	Direction-specific pulsion or falls Drop attacks Ataxia	Variable gait and stance deficits Excessive upper-body motion	Excessive caution
	Emotional symptoms			Fear of falling or heights Fear of becoming incapacitated or accidentally harming others
Chronic syndromes	Vestibular symptoms	Unsteadiness Dizziness	Unsteadiness Dizziness	Unsteadiness Dizziness
	Motion sensitivity	Vertigo, unsteadiness, or oscillopsia with rapid head movements	Unsteadiness or dizziness with motion of self in any direction or movement in the environment	Avoidance of provocative motion environments
	Aural symptoms	Progressive hearing loss Unilateral tinnitus		Variable tinnitus
	Autonomic and vegetative symptoms		Chronic fatigue	Tension, restlessness, insomnia, fatigue, weight change Cognitive complaints
	Postural and gait abnormalities	Progressive decline in gait speed or fluidity Gradually increasing frequency of falls	Postural unsteadiness or dizziness Variable sensations of impending falls, toppling over, or floating off the ground	Excessive caution Unnecessary use of gait aids
	Emotional symptoms			Catastrophic worries about consequences of symptoms Demoralization or sadness Pessimism or hopelessness

disorders may generate panic attacks with minor vertiginous sensations; however, associated symptoms still elucidate the diagnosis. Coexisting illnesses may be detected in a similar manner. A patient with episodes of vertigo, unilateral tinnitus, and fluctuating hearing plus complete avoidance of driving lest an attack incapacitate him resulting in a crash most likely has Ménière's disease plus a specific phobia of vertigo. Reduction of vertigo attacks by adequate treatment of Ménière's disease alone may not eliminate his phobic beliefs and behaviors. Simultaneous treatment of the phobic disorder conditions is likely to be needed.

Patients' dominant symptoms may change over time as one disorder begets another, so it is important to follow the temporal evolution of their illnesses. Misattribution of all symptoms to the initial illnesses may incorrectly keep the focus of diagnostic evaluations and treatment on those conditions, even if they have remitted. Here too, Table 37.1 offers helpful guidance for establishing the diagnosis, as illustrated in these case vignettes.

CASE HISTORY 37.1

One year before presenting for evaluation, a 48-year-old woman experienced an acute vestibular syndrome of vertigo, nausea, vomiting, and gait instability that resolved over a 3-week period. However, she developed daily nonvertiginous dizziness that was worse when standing than when lying down. Symptoms were better when she walked at a modest pace than when she stood still. She experienced momentary bouts of unsteadiness that provoked mild anxiety, but not panic attacks. She was a perfectionist by nature. Diagnosis: This patient had a primary structural disorder (vestibular neuritis) that triggered a secondary functional disorder (PPV).

CASE HISTORY 37.2

A man presented with a 2-year history of abnormal gait and recurrent attacks of vertigo, unsteadiness, and dizziness. He walked down the hall to the exam room with a very slow gait that had a markedly prolonged stance phase, such that he balanced motionless on each foot for 1–2 seconds between steps. His illness began when he was serving in the military in a transportation company. His vehicle was attacked with a roadside bomb. He was knocked unconscious and then awoke with acute vertigo and unilateral hearing loss. Vertigo resolved with 8 weeks of physical therapy and hearing loss gradually improved. Two months later he began to have recurrent attacks of positional vertigo lasting 1–2 minutes. He also had frequent nightmares, insomnia, heightened startle, and daytime panic attacks that produced intense feelings of dizziness and unsteadiness. In response to these two sets of recurrent vestibular symptoms, he became more and more cautious with his gait. He was successfully taught to treat his positional vertigo with canalith repositioning maneuvers and he received psychotherapy for his traumatic stress symptoms, but his gait disturbance remained. Diagnosis: This patient had a primary structural disorder (labyrinthine concussion) leading to a secondary structural disorder (posttraumatic benign paroxysmal positional vertigo). He also had a coexisting primary psychiatric disorder (posttraumatic stress disorder) that manifested with recurrent vestibular symptoms. Together, these three illnesses induced a secondary functional gait disorder.

Although the last case involved psychologic trauma, it illustrates an important general concept. A history of psychosocial stressors or adverse life events, even if temporally connected to the course of vestibular symptoms, is an unreliable indicator of functional or psychiatric vestibular diagnosis. Childhood and adulthood adversity is equally prevalent in patients with structural versus functional/psychiatric causes of vestibular symptoms (Radziej et al., 2015).

Validated self-reports can aid in the detection of psychiatric morbidity. These require just a few minutes of time and can be administered in the office, clinic, or hospital (Staab, 2013). Two questionnaires that are short and easy to use are the Patient Health Questionnaire for depression (PHQ-9: Spitzer et al., 1999) and the Generalized Anxiety Disorder Scale for anxiety symptoms (GAD-7: Spitzer et al., 2006). Both are available in multiple languages and can be downloaded free of charge from the website phqscreeners.com. They have been validated in neuro-otologic patients (Persoons et al., 2003).

Treatment of psychiatric vestibular disorders

The treatment of psychiatric disorders that cause vestibular symptoms depends on several factors, including the specific psychiatric diagnosis, whether the psychiatric conditions are the only active diagnoses or coexist with structural or functional illnesses, patients' psychosocial circumstances, and patients' preferences for treatment. Major clinical trials of pharmacologic and psychotherapeutic treatments for anxiety and mood disorders conducted within the field of psychiatry over the last several decades have not separated patients by specific physical symptoms (e.g., chest pain versus dizziness). There has not been any indication of a differential effect on physical symptoms, though that has not been systematically sought. Therefore, treatment choices for psychiatric disorders that manifest vestibular symptoms currently follow the established therapies for those disorders in general. In the absence of explicit testing of these treatments in patients with predominantly vestibular symptoms, three considerations may improve therapeutic outcomes:

1. The first consideration is that vestibular rehabilitation can be quite effective in reducing anxiety and depressive symptoms even in the absence of other psychiatric or psychologic interventions (Meli et al., 2007). Many psychiatrists and psychotherapists are unfamiliar with this procedure, so a collaborative recommendation for physical therapy may add a useful intervention to patients' treatment plans.
2. The second consideration is the need to coordinate medications when structural and functional disorders coexist with psychiatric conditions. There are opportunities for parsimonious overlaps in medication management, but also for duplicative therapies, adverse interactions, and a few contraindicated combinations. The large number of potential medication choices precludes review here. However, establishing a plan for collaboration among prescribing clinicians and regular checks of drug interaction databases can minimize potential missteps.
3. The third consideration is proper recognition of specific therapies for the functional vestibular syndromes of PPV and CSD that were reviewed above. Adaptations of existing and new medication and nonmedication therapies from neuro-otology and psychiatry will continue and will be guided by emerging mechanistic research.

Several small and pilot studies have investigated multimodality interventions for patients with chronic dizziness. These have not been diagnosis-specific. Older investigations targeted patients with chronic nonspecific dizziness (e.g., Jacob et al., 2001; Johansson et al., 2001). More recent interventions addressed dysfunctional illness beliefs and behaviors in patients with chronic vestibular morbidity. A pilot study suggested that a combined approach using psychoeducation, cognitive-behavioral therapy, physical therapy, and antidepressant drugs, when needed, may reduce dysfunctional illness behaviors and dizziness (Tschan et al., 2012). This combined approach improved not only the dizziness symptoms but also the postural strategy (Best et al., 2015). After a time period of at least 1 year (average 32 months) with this flexible treatment, 78% of patients reported a sustained reduction of dizziness symptoms (Schaaf and Hesse, 2015). This study offers three important lessons. First, individualized use of currently available therapies offers significant benefits when patients receive diagnostic evaluations that are thorough enough to guide multidisciplinary treatment plans. Second, a systematic approach to treatment over several weeks to months may be needed to achieve favorable outcomes. Third, treatment gains can be sustained.

References

American Psychiatric Association (2013). Diagnostic and Statistical Manual of Mental Disorders, 5th edn. American Psychiatric Press, Washington, DC.

Andersson G, Asmundson GJ, Denev J et al. (2006). A controlled trial of cognitive behavior therapy combined with vestibular rehabilitation in the treatment of dizziness. Behav Res Ther 44: 1265–1273.

Batu ED, Anlar B, Topcu M et al. (2015). Vertigo in childhood: a retrospective series of 100 children. Eur J Paed Neurol 19: 226–232.

Best C, Eckhardt-Henn A, Diener G et al. (2006). Interaction of somatoform and vestibular disorders. J Neurol Neurosurg Psychiatry 77: 658–664.

Best C, Eckhardt-Henn A, Tschan R et al. (2009a). Psychiatric morbidity and comorbidity in different vestibular vertigo syndrome: results of a prospective longitudinal study over one year. J Neurol 256: 58–65.

Best C, Eckhardt-Henn A, Tschan R et al. (2009b). Who is a risk for psychiatric distressed after vestibular disorder? Results from a prospective one-year follow-up. Neuroscience 164: 1579–1587.

Best C, Tschan R, Stieber N et al. (2015). STEADFAST: Psychotherapeutic intervention improves postural strategy of somatoform vertigo and dizziness (SVD). Behav Neurol 2015: 456850. http://dx.doi.org/10.1155/2015/456850.

Bienvenu OJ, Hettema JM, Neale MC et al. (2007). Low extraversion and high neuroticism as indices of genetic and environmental risk for social phobia, agoraphobia, and animal phobia. Am J Psychiatry 164 (11): 1714–1721.

Bisdorff A, von Brevern M, Lempert T et al. (2009). Classification of vestibular symptoms: towards an international classification of vestibular disorders. J Vestib Res 19 (1-2): 1–13.

Bisdorff AR, Staab JP, Newman-Toker DE (2013). Vestibular symptoms, balance, and their disorders: How will we classify them? In: AM Bronstein (Ed.), Oxford Textbook of Vertigo and Imbalance, Oxford University Press, Oxford, UK, pp. 171–178.

Brandt T (1996). Phobic postural vertigo. Neurology 46: 1515–1519.

Brandt T (1999). Vertigo, its multisensory syndromes, 2nd edn. Springer, Heidelberg.

Brandt T, Dieterich M (1986). Phobischer Attacken-Schwankschwindel, ein neues Syndrom. Munch Med Wochenschr 128: 247–250.

Brandt T, Huppert D, Dieterich M (1994). Phobic postural vertigo: a first follow-up. J Neurol 241: 191–195.

Brandt T, Strupp M, Novozhilov S et al. (2012). Artificial neural network posturography detects the transition of vestibular neuritis to phobic postural vertigo. J Neurol 259: 182–184.

Brandt T, Dieterich M, Strupp M (2013). Vertigo and Dizziness: Common Complaints, 2nd edn. Springer, London.

Brandt T, Kugler G, Schniepp R et al. (2015a). Acrophobia impairs visual exploration and balance during standing and walking. Ann N Y Acad Sci 1343: 37–48.

Brandt T, Strupp M, Dieterich M (2015b). Functional dizziness: diagnostic keys and differential diagnosis. J Neurol 262: 1977–1980.

Bronstein AM (1995). The visual vertigo syndrome. Acta Otolaryngol (Stockh) 520: 45–48.

Bronstein AM (2004). Vision and vertigo: some visual aspects of vestibular disorders. J Neurol 251: 381–387.

Brown LA, Gage WH, Polych MA et al. (2002). Central set influences on gait. Age-dependent effects of postural threat. Exp Brain Res 145: 286–296.

Costa PT, McCrae RR (1992). NEO Personality Inventory Revised (NEO-PI-R™), Psychological Assessments Resources, Lutz, FL, USA.

Cousins S, Cutfield NJ, Kaski D et al. (2014). Visual dependency and dizziness after vestibular neuritis. PLoS One 9 (9): e105426.

Dieterich M, Eckhardt-Henn A (2006). Neurological and somatoform vertigo syndromes. In: P Henningsen, H Gündel, A Ceballos-Baumann (Eds.), Neuro-Psychosomatik. Grundlagen und Klinik neurologischer Psychosomatik. Schattauer, Stuttgart, pp. 253–265.

Eagger S, Luxon LM, Davies RA et al. (1992). Psychiatric morbidity in patients with peripheral vestibular disorder: a clinical and neuro-otological study. J Neurol Neurosurg Psychiatry 55: 383–387.

Eckhardt-Henn A, Breuer P, Thomalske C et al. (2003). Anxiety disorders and other psychiatric subgroups in patients complaining of dizziness. J Anxiety Disord 431: 1–20.

Eckhardt-Henn A, Best C, Bense S et al. (2008). Psychiatric comorbidity in different organic vertigo syndromes. J Neurol 255: 420–428.

Edelman S, Mahoney AE, Cremer PD (2012). Cognitive behavior therapy for chronic subjective dizziness: a randomized, controlled trial. Am J Otolaryngol 33: 395–401.

Furman JM, Jacob RG (1997). Psychiatric dizziness. Neurology 48: 1161–1166.

Gage WH, Sleik RJ, Polych MA et al. (2003). The allocation of attention during locomotion is altered by anxiety. Exp Brain Res 150: 385–394.

Godemann F, Schabowska A, Naetebusch B et al. (2006). The impact of cognitions on the development of panic and somatoform disorders: a prospective study in patients with vestibular neuritis. Psychol Med 36: 99–108.

Hainault JP, Caillet G, Lestienne FG et al. (2011). The role of trait anxiety on static balance performance in control and anxiogenic situations. Gait Posture 33: 604–608.

Hanel G, Henningsen P, Herzog W et al. (2009). Depression, anxiety, and somatoform disorders: Vague or distinct categories in primary care? Results from a large cross-sectional study. J Psychosom Res 67: 189–197.

Heinrichs N, Edler C, Eskens S et al. (2007). Predicting continued dizziness after an acute peripheral vestibular disorder. Psychosom Med 69: 700–707.

Holmberg J, Karlberg M, Harlacher U et al. (2005). Experience of handicap and anxiety in phobic postural vertigo. Acta Otolaryngol 125 (3): 270–275.

Holmberg J, Karlberg M, Harlacher U et al. (2006). Treatment of phobic postural vertigo. A controlled study of cognitive-behavioral therapy and self-controlled desensitization. J Neurol 253: 500–506.

Holmberg J, Karlberg M, Harlacher U et al. (2007). One-year follow-up of cognitive behavioral therapy for phobic postural vertigo. J Neurol 254: 1189–1192.

Horii A, Mitani K, Kitahara T et al. (2004). Paroxetine, a selective serotonin reuptake inhibitor, reduces depressive symptoms and subjective handicaps in patients with dizziness. Otol Neurotol 25: 536–543.

Horii A, Uno A, Kitahara T et al. (2007). Effects of fluvoxamine on anxiety, depression, and subjective handicaps of chronic dizziness patients with or without neuro-otologic diseases. J Vestib Res 17: 1–8.

Horii A, Kitahara T, Masumura C et al. (2008). Effects of milnacipran, a serotonin noradrenaline reuptake inhibitor (SNRI) on subjective handicaps and posturography in dizzy patients. Available online at Abstracts from the XXVth Congress of the Barany Society, Kyoto, Japan. http://www.acplan.jp/barany2008/. (accessed 9 July 2011).

Huppert D, Kunihiro T, Brandt T (1995). Phobic postural vertigo (154 patients): its association with vestibular disorders. J Audiol 4: 97–103.

Huppert D, Strupp M, Rettinger N et al. (2005). Phobic postural vertigo – a long-term follow-up (5 to 15 years) of 106 patients. J Neurol 252: 564–569.

Indovina I, Ricelli R, Staab JP et al. (2014). Personality traits modulate subcortical and cortical vestibular and anxiety responses to sound-evoked otolithic receptor stimulation. J Psychosom Res 77 (5): 391–400.

Indovina I, Riccelli R, Chiarella G et al. (2015). Role of the insula and vestibular system in patients with chronic subjective dizziness: an fMRI study using sound-evoked vestibular stimulation. Front Behav Neurosci 9: 334.

Jacob RG, Woody SR, Clark DB et al. (1993). Discomfort with space and motion: a possible marker of vestibular dysfunction assessed by the Situational Characteristics Questionnaire. J Psychopathol Behav Assess 15: 299–324.

Jacob RG, Whitney SL, Detweiler-Shostak G et al. (2001). Vestibular rehabilitation for patients with agoraphobia and vestibular dysfunction: a pilot study. J Anxiety Disord 15: 131–146.

Jacob RG, Redfern MS, Furman JM (2009). Space and motion discomfort and abnormal balance control in patients with anxiety disorders. J Neurol Neurosurg Psychiatry 80: 74–78.

Johansson M, Akerlund D, Larsen HC et al. (2001). Randomized controlled trial of vestibular rehabilitation combined with cognitive-behavioral therapy for dizziness in older people. Otolaryngol Head Neck Surg 125: 151–156.

Kammerlind AS, Ledin TE, Skargren EI et al. (2005). Long-term follow-up after acute unilateral vestibular loss and comparison between subjects with and without remaining symptoms. Acta Otolaryngol (Stockh) 125: 946–953.

Kapfhammer HP, Mayer C, Hock U et al. (1997). Course of illness in phobic postural vertigo. Acta Neurol Scand 95: 23–28.

Kapfhammer HP, Huppert D, Grill E et al. (2015). Visual height intolerance and acrophobia: clinical characteristics and comorbidity patterns. Eur Arch Psychiatry Clin Neurosci 265 (5): 375–385.

Kessler RC, Chiu WT, Demler O et al. (2005). Prevalence, severity, and comorbidity of 12-month DSM-IV disorders in the National Comorbidity Survey Replication. Arch Gen Psychiatry 62: 617–627.

Ketola S, Niemensivu R, Henttonen A et al. (2009). Somatoform disorders in vertiginous children and adolescents. Int J Pediatr Otorhinolaryngol 73 (7): 933–936.

Krafczyk S, Tietze S, Swoboda W et al. (2006). Artificial neural network: a new diagnostic posturographic tool for disorders of stance. Clin Neurophysiol 117: 1692–1698.

Kugler G, Huppert D, Schneider E et al. (2014). Fear of heights freezes gaze to the horizon. J Vest Res 24 (5-6): 433–441.

Lahmann C, Henningsen P, Brandt T et al. (2015). Psychiatric comorbidity and psychosocial impairment among patients with vertigo and dizziness. J Neurol Neurosurg Psychiatry 86: 302–308.

Lopez-Gentili LI, Kremenchutzky M, Salgado P (2003). A statistical analysis of 1300 patients with dizziness-vertigo. Its most frequent cases. Rev Neurol 36 (5): 417–429.

Mahoney AEJ, Edelman S, Cremer PD (2013). Cognitive behavior therapy for chronic subjective dizziness: longer-term gains and predictors of disability. Am J Otolaryngol 34: 115–120.

Marks JM (1981). Space "phobia": a pseudo-agoraphobic syndrome. J Neurol Neurosurg Psychiatry 48: 729–735.

Meli A, Zimatore G, Badaracco C et al. (2007). Effects of vestibular rehabilitation therapy on emotional aspects in chronic vestibular patients. J Psychosom Res 63: 185–190.

Murphy TP (1993). Mal de debarquement syndrome: a forgotten entity? Otolaryngol Head Neck Surg 109: 10–13.

Neff BA, Staab JP, Eggers SD et al. (2012). Auditory and vestibular symptoms and chronic subjective dizziness in patients with Meniere's disease, vestibular migraine, and Meniere's disease with concomitant vestibular migraine. Otol Neurotol 33 (7): 1235–1244.

Obermann M, Bock E, Sabev N et al. (2015). Long-term outcome of vertigo and dizziness associated disorders following treatment in specialized tertiary care: the Dizziness and Vertigo Registry (DiVeR) Study. J Neurol 262 (9): 2083–2091.

Persoons P, Luyckx K, Desloovere C et al. (2003). Anxiety and mood disorders in otorhinolaryngology outpatients presenting with dizziness: validation of the self-administered PRIME- MD Patient Health Questionnaire and epidemiology. Gen Hosp Psychiatry 25: 316–323.

Querner V, Krafczyk S, Dieterich M et al. (2000). Patients with somatoform phobic postural vertigo: the more difficult the balance task, the better the balance performance. Neurosci Lett 285: 21–24.

Querner V, Krafczyk S, Dieterich M et al. (2002). Somatoform phobic postural vertigo: body sway during optokinetically induced roll vection. Exp Brain Res 143: 269–275.

Radziej K, Schmid G, Dinkel A et al. (2015). Psychological traumatization and adverse life events in patients with organic and functional vestibular symptoms. J Psychosom Res 79 (2): 123–129.

Schaaf H, Hesse G (2015). Patients with long-lasting dizziness: a follow-up after neurotological and psychotherapeutic inpatient treatment after a period of at least 1 year. Eur Arch Otorhinolaryngol 272 (6): 1529–1535.

Schlick C, Schniepp R, Loidl V et al. (2016). Falls and fear of falling in vertigo and balance disorders: a controlled cross sectional study. J Vestib Res 25 (5-6): 241–251.

Schmid G, Henningsen P, Dieterich M et al. (2011). Psychotherapy in vertigo – a systematic review. J Neurol Neurosurg Psych 82 (6): 601–606.

Schrier AC, de Wit MA, Krol A et al. (2013). Similar associations between personality dimensions and anxiety or depressive disorders in a population study of Turkish-Dutch, Moroccan-Dutch, and native Dutch subjects. J Nerv Ment Dis 201 (5): 421–428.

Shepard NT, Telian SA, Smith-Wheelock M et al. (1993). Vestibular and balance rehabilitation therapy. Ann Otol Rhinol Laryngol 102 (3 Pt 1): 198–205.

Simon NM, Parker SW, Wernick-Robinson M et al. (2005). Fluoxetine for vestibular dysfunction and anxiety: a prospective pilot study. Psychosomatics 46: 334–339.

Spitzer RL, Kroenke K, Williams JBW (1999). Validation and utility of a self-report version of PRIME- MD – The PHQ primary care study. JAMA 282: 1737–1744.

Spitzer RL, Kroenke K, Williams JBW et al. (2006). A brief measure for assessing generalized anxiety disorder – The GAD-7. Arch Intern Med 166: 1092–1097.

Staab JP (2011). Clinical clues to a dizzying headache. J Vestib Res 21 (6): 331–340.

Staab JP (2012). Chronic subjective dizziness. Continuum (Minneap Minn) 18: 1118–1141.

Staab JP (2013). Behavioural neuro-otology. In: AM Bronstein (Ed.), Oxford Textbook of Vertigo and Imbalance, Oxford University Press, Oxford, UK, pp. 333–346.

Staab JP (2014). The influence of anxiety on ocular motor control and gaze. Curr Opin Neurol 27: 118–124.

Staab JP, Ruckenstein MJ (2003). Which comes first? Psychogenic dizziness versus otogenic anxiety. Laryngoscope 113: 1714–1718.

Staab JP, Ruckenstein MJ (2005). Chronic dizziness and anxiety: effect of course of illness on treatment outcome. Arch Otolaryngol Head Neck Surg 131: 675–679.

Staab JP, Ruckenstein MJ (2007a). Expanding the differential diagnosis of dizziness. Arch Otolaryngol Head Neck Surg 13: 170–176.

Staab JP, Ruckenstein MJ (2007b). Autonomic nervous system function in chronic dizziness. Otol Neurotol 28 (6): 854–859.

Staab JP, Ruckenstein MJ, Solomon D et al. (2002). Serotonin reuptake inhibitors for dizziness with psychiatric symptoms. Arch Otolaryngol Head Neck Surg 128: 554–560.

Staab JP, Ruckenstein MJ, Amsterdam JD (2004). A prospective trial of sertraline for chronic subjective dizziness. Laryngoscope 114: 1637–1641.

Staab J, Eggers S, Neff B et al. (2010). Validation of a clinical syndrome of persistent dizziness and unsteadiness. J Vestib Res 12: 149–268.

Staab JP, Rohe DE, Eggers SD et al. (2014). Anxious, introverted personality traits in patients with chronic subjective dizziness. J Psychosom Res 76 (1): 80–83.

Telian SA, Shepard NT, Smith-Wheelock M et al. (1990). Habituation therapy for chronic vestibular dysfunction: preliminary results. Otolaryngol Head Neck Surg 103 (1): 89–95.

Thompson KJ, Goetting JC, Staab JP et al. (2015). Retrospective review and telephone follow-up to evaluate a physical therapy protocol for treating persistent postural-perceptual dizziness: a pilot study. J Vestib Res 25: 97–104.

Tomenson B, McBeth J, Chew-Graham CA et al. (2012). Somatization and health anxiety as predictors of health care use. Psychosom Med 74 (6): 656–664.

Tomenson B, Essau C, Jacobi F et al. (2013). Total somatic symptom score as a predictor of health outcome in somatic symptom disorders. Br J Psychiatry 203 (5): 373–380.

Torres X, Bailles E, Valdes M et al. (2013). Personality does not distinguish people with fibromyalgia but identifies subgroups of patients. Gen Hosp Psychiatry 35 (6): 640–648.

Trimble MR (1984). Psychiatric aspects of vertigo. In: MR Dix, DD Hood (Eds.), Vertigo, Wiley, Chichester, pp. 345–358.

Tschan R, Wiltink J, Best C et al. (2008). Validation of the German version of the vertigo symptom scale (VSS) in patients with organic of somatoform dizziness and healthy controls. J Neurol 255 (8): 1168–1175.

Tschan R, Best C, Beutel M et al. (2011). Patients' psychological well-being and resilient coping protect from secondary somatoform vertigo and dizziness (SVD) one year after vestibular disease. J Neurol 258: 104–112.

Tschan R, Eckhardt-Henn A, Scheurich V et al. (2012). Steadfast-effectiveness of a cognitive behavioral self-management program of patients with somatoform vertigo and dizziness. Psychother Psychosom Med Psychol 62 (3-4): 111–119.

Von Holst E, Mittelstaedt H (1950). Das Reafferenzierungsprinzip (Wechselwirkungen zwischen Zentralnervensystem und Peripherie). Naturwissenschaften 37: 461–476.

WHO (1993). The ICD-10 Classification of Mental and Behavioral Disorders, Clinical Description and Diagnostic Guidelines, WHO, Geneva.

WHO (2015a). International Classification of Diseases, 11th edition, beta draft, Persistent postural-perceptual dizziness. Available online at http://id.who.int/icd/entity/2005792829(accessed 19 September 2015).

WHO (2015b). International Classification of Diseases, 11th edition, beta draft, Bodily distress disorder. Available online at http://id.who.int/icd/entity/767044268 (accessed 19 September 2015).

Wuehr M, Pradhan C, Novozhilov S et al. (2013). Inadequate interaction between open- and closed-loop postural control in phobic postural vertigo. J Neurol 260 (5): 1314–1323.

Yardley L, Redfern MS (2001). Psychological factors influencing recovery from balance disorders. J Anxiety Disord 15: 107–119.

Yardley L, Beech S, Zander L et al. (1998). A randomized controlled trial of exercise therapy for dizziness and vertigo in primary care. Br J Gen Pract 48 (429): 1136–1140.

Yardley L, Donovan-Hall M, Smith HE et al. (2004). Effectiveness of primary care–based vestibular rehabilitation for chronic dizziness. Ann Intern Med 141: 598–605.

Yarrow K, Brown P, Gresty MA et al. (2001). Force platform recordings in the diagnosis of primary orthostatic tremor. Gait Posture 13: 27–34.

Handbook of Clinical Neurology, Vol. 139 (3rd series)
Functional Neurologic Disorders
M. Hallett, J. Stone, and A. Carson, Editors
http://dx.doi.org/10.1016/B978-0-12-801772-2.00038-2

Chapter 38

Urologic symptoms and functional neurologic disorders

I. HOERITZAUER[1], V. PHÉ[2], AND J.N. PANICKER[3]*

[1]*Centre for Clinical Brain Sciences, University of Edinburgh, UK*

[2]*Department of Uro-Neurology, The National Hospital for Neurology and Neurosurgery, London, UK and Department of Urology, Pitié-Salpêtrière Academic Hospital, Paris, France*

[3]*Department of Uro-Neurology, The National Hospital for Neurology and Neurosurgery and UCL Institute of Neurology, Queen Square, London*

Abstract

The term functional urologic disorders covers a wide range of conditions related broadly to altered function rather than structure of the lower urinary tract, mainly of impaired urine voiding or storage. Confusingly, for a neurologic readership, these disorders of function may often be due to a urologic, gynecologic, or neurologic cause. However, there is a subset of functional urologic disorders where the cause remains uncertain and, in this chapter, we describe the clinical features of these disorders in turn: psychogenic urinary retention; Fowler's syndrome; paruresis (shy-bladder syndrome); dysfunctional voiding; idiopathic overactive bladder, and interstitial cystitis/bladder pain syndrome. Some of these overlap in terms of symptoms, but have become historically separated. Psychogenic urinary retention in particular has now largely been abandoned as a concept, in part because of the finding of specific urethral electromyogram findings in patients with this symptom now described as having Fowler's syndrome, and their successful treatment with sacral neurostimulation.

In this chapter we review the poorly researched interface between these "idiopathic" functional urologic disorders and other functional disorders (e.g., irritable-bowel syndrome, fibromyalgia) as well as specifically functional neurologic disorders. We conclude that there may be a relationship and overlap between them and that this requires further research, especially in those idiopathic functional urologic disorders which involve disorders of the urethral sphincter (i.e., voluntary muscle).

INTRODUCTION

Functional neurologic disorders, such as functional tremor or functional limb weakness, are diagnosed based on positive signs, such as entrainment of functional tremor or Hoover's sign of functional leg weakness, which demonstrate an underlying intact structure to the nervous system. Confusingly, for a neurologic readership, there is much less of a dichotomy in the urologic literature between functional and structural disorders. The term functional urologic disorders covers a wide range of disorders in which abnormal functioning of the lower urinary tract (LUT) causes urologic symptoms. Most functional urologic symptoms have a clear organic pathology (e.g., urologic, gynecologic, or neurologic) that is uncovered during clinical assessment or investigation. There are, however, some functional urologic disorders where the LUT dysfunction is evident through investigations, but the etiology is unclear.

Functional disorders of the LUT manifest as voiding dysfunction, storage dysfunction, or both. The symptoms of storage dysfunction include urinary urgency, daytime frequency, nighttime frequency, nocturia, and/or urge urinary incontinence (Abrams et al., 2002; Hayllen et al., 2010). Voiding dysfunction manifests with

*Correspondence to: Jalesh N. Panicker, Department of Uro-Neurology, The National Hospital for Neurology and Neurosurgery and UCL Institute of Neurology, Queen Square, London WC1N 3BG, UK. E-mail: j.panicker@ucl.ac.uk

symptoms of urinary hesitancy, intermittent flow and slow stream, straining to void, a sensation of incomplete bladder emptying after voiding and double voiding, characterized by the need to urinate again soon after voiding (Abrams et al., 2002). In the most severe case, patients may even be in urinary retention.

We start this chapter with a description of LUT function in health and a summary of what is known about the brain–bladder axis. We then focus on the following presentations where there is no clear cause for dysfunction: psychogenic urinary retention; Fowler's syndrome; paruresis (shy-bladder syndrome); dysfunctional voiding; interstitial cystitis/bladder pain syndrome, and overactive bladder (OAB). Some of these overlap in terms of symptoms, but have become historically separated.

We then discuss what evidence there is for an overlap between these disorders and functional somatic disorders such as fibromyalgia (FM) and irritable bowel as well as functional neurologic disorders such as functional movement disorders or dissociative (nonepileptic) seizures. Functional somatic disorders have been recognized in patients with idiopathic functional urologic disorders, and LUT dysfunction has also been documented in patients with a range of functional somatic disorders. The nature of the association, however, is uncertain and whether these are the manifestations of a common underlying abnormal working of the nervous system, or merely represent the coincidental existence of two independent processes, is yet to be systematically explored.

LOWER URINARY TRACT FUNCTIONS IN HEALTH

In health, the LUT remains in the storage phase, acting as a low-capacity reservoir of urine, 99% of the time. Storage is dependent on sympathetic and somatic-mediated contraction of the internal and external urethral sphincters, respectively, and sympathetic-mediated inhibition of the detrusor. During the storage phase, the pontine micturition center (PMC) is tonically inhibited by activity from cortical and subcortical centers, such as the prefrontal cortex, anterior cingulate gyrus, and insula (de Groat et al., 2015). Increasingly stronger signals through the sacral afferents during the storage phase are primarily responsible for initiating a switch to the voiding phase (Valentino et al., 2011). When deemed socially appropriate and safe, tonic inhibition of the PMC from the periaqueductal gray (PAG) is released, resulting in relaxation of the urethral sphincters and pelvic floor, and parasympathetic-mediated activation of the detrusor, voiding ensues (Panicker and Fowler, 2010).

CURRENT MODELS OF THE BRAIN–BLADDER AXIS

A more indepth review of the complex higher cortical pathways is useful to gain a better understanding of the bladder–brain axis and explore the association between functional disorders and LUT symptoms. Current understanding of LUT regulation suggests connection between the LUT and higher centers, including emotion, arousal, and motivation. Additionally, three circuits of micturition are postulated (Griffiths, 2015). The micturition system works largely unconsciously via PAG and parahippocampal regions of the temporal cortex to monitor the slowly filling bladder (Kavia et al., 2010; Tadic et al., 2013). Once it is socially appropriate and safe to void, activation of the medial prefrontal cortex triggers the PAG to activate the PMC. This circuit is hypothesized to be closely linked not only anatomically to the amygdala, but also emotionally linked to the crucial aspect of safety required for voiding.

In patients who experience the threat of involuntary leakage with or without the sense of urgency, two other circuits are activated. One involves the insula and prefrontal cortex. The insula is known to receive homeostatic information from the whole body, with increasing activation as the bladder progressively fills. The prefrontal cortex has connections to the limbic system, associated with emotional and social contextualized decision making and involved in working memory. In response to the threat of involuntary voiding, the medial prefrontal cortex is inhibited by activity from the insula and lateral prefrontal cortex. Reduced medial prefrontal cortex activation inhibits PAG activation and raises the threshold micturition level (Tadic et al., 2011).

The anterior cingulate gyrus is responsible for motivation and adjustments of bodily arousal states in response to mental stress. It is coactivated with the supplementary motor area, which controls striated muscles such as those in the pelvic floor and external urethral sphincter (Critchley, 2003). In response to the threat of involuntary voiding and the sensation of urge, activation of both the supplementary motor cortex and the dorsal anterior cingulate gyrus occurs. These two areas are thought to be responsible for simultaneous pelvic floor and urethral sphincter contraction and the anterior cingulate gyrus is thought to create the motivation to visit a toilet (Schrum et al., 2011).

The PAG is thought to play a significant role linking between higher centers and the LUT, with projections to the thalamus, hypothalamus, and amygdala, while also receiving information from the bladder (Griffiths and Fowler, 2013; Griffiths, 2015). The PAG modulates the voiding threshold using the information received from the higher centers. If it is unsafe or socially inappropriate to void, the micturition threshold will be increased and the need to void reduced until there are higher bladder volumes. Brainstem nuclei such as the locus coeruleus modulate behaviors related to LUT function. The locus coeruleus system initiates and maintains arousal and facilitates shifts between focused attention and scanning attentiveness (Berridge and Waterhouse, 2003). Activation of the PMC and hence the locus coeruleus results in a switch from nonvoiding to voiding-related behaviour. Experiments in rodent models have shown that the expected pattern of increased activity from the locus coeruleus with increasing bladder pressure is lost 2 weeks after partial bladder outlet obstruction, even when bladder pressure increased to the micturition threshold (Rickenbacher et al., 2008). This may be relevant in understanding why some individuals with chronic urinary retention may have high volume retention without a sensation of urge or bladder fullness. It also suggests that persistent outlet obstruction leads to a loss of central regulation of LUT function.

As well as the loss of sensitivity to increases in bladder pressure, the locus coeruleus neurons also showed increased basal activity of 40% compared with sham rats (Rickenbacher et al., 2008). This elevated basal activity is associated with hyperarousal, difficulty focusing on an ongoing task, and neurobehavioral impairments such as anxiety and sleep impairment. Theta oscillations were prominent on electroencephalogram, which ties in with loss of ability to differentiate between differing bladder pressures. Theta oscillations play a role in sensorimotor integration by coordinating activity in various brain regions on the basis of sensory input to update motor plans (Caplan et al., 2003). The presence of these may also cause difficulty with nonbladder sensorimotor processing.

ASSESSMENT OF FUNCTIONAL UROLOGIC DISORDERS

History and examination are essential to consider potential urologic and gynecologic pathologies such as prostate enlargement, pelvic organ prolapse, tumors, or neurologic disorders such as multiple sclerosis, spinal pathology, or Parkinson's disease. A bladder diary aids with assessment of the functional bladder capacity, urinary frequency, and the number of leakage or urgency episodes. Noninvasive investigations such as uroflowmetry and measurement of the postvoid residual by ultrasound or in–out catheterization help to uncover voiding dysfunction and incomplete bladder emptying. Urodynamics helps to identify the pattern of LUT dysfunction, such as detrusor instability or voiding dysfunction, but does not necessarily inform the etiology. Although the majority of patients presenting with "functional" problems with their bladder will have a cause identified during the course of investigations, many will not, and these are the disorders we consider in this chapter.

PSYCHOGENIC URINARY RETENTION

There are numerous causes for urinary retention; most commonly this arises in the setting of structural urologic lesions or an established neurologic disorder (Panicker et al., 2010; Smith et al., 2013). Reports of an association between psychologic factors and urinary retention began to appear in the 1800s, under the term "hysterical ischuria" (Charcot, 1877; Dejerine and Gauckler, 1913). We have found reports of 109 patients with a diagnosis of "psychogenic urinary retention," with the majority ($n = 84$) reported prior to 1985. The diagnosis was made after medical investigations to exclude urologic, gynecologic, or neurologic causes (Margolis, 1965; Bridges et al., 1966; Blaivas et al., 1977; Barrett, 1978; Korzets et al., 1985; Nicolau et al., and 1991; Bilanakis, 2006). Triggering events and secondary gain were typically then sought and urologists were urged to look for recent life stressors and positive psychologic features to make the diagnosis (Wahl and Golden, 1963).

Psychogenic urinary retention was reported most commonly in young women, with an average age of onset of 29 years based on a review of 15 papers. Emotional deprivation during childhood seemed to be a predisposing factor in many cases (Wahl and Golden, 1963; Montague and Jones, 1979), and there were several reports of patients having nocturnal enuresis and urinary tract infections (UTIs) (Wahl and Golden, 1963; Lamontagne and Marks, 1973; Christmas et al., 1991).

The literature is replete with predisposing and precipitating factors, including perceived stress, such as unhappy marriage or home life (Montague and Jones, 1979; Korzets et al., 1985), feelings of guilt or fear of punishment, often for promiscuous sexual activity (Wahl and Golden, 1963; Montague and Jones, 1979), and depression and anxiety (Blaivas et al., 1977; Montague and Jones, 1979). Patients' unhelpful thoughts about genitourinary sensations as being "dirty" (Williams and Johnson, 1956) and "tense and unassertive" (Lamontagne and Marks, 1973) or "emotionally overcontrolled" (Montague and Jones, 1979) personalities were also felt to predispose to abnormal bladder functions. In several patients, urinary retention was precipitated by physical triggers such as UTI, road traffic accident, surgery, or childbirth (Cardenas et al., 1986).

Modeling from parents with genitourinary problems, sudden death of a friend or colleague from renal disease, iatrogenesis due to recurrent questions about urinary dysfunction, or minor symptoms which escalated with frequent medical reviews were also reported (Norden and Friedman, 1961; Wahl and Golden, 1963). Rape (Williams and Johnson, 1956; Montague and Jones, 1979) and murderous rage (Williams and Johnson, 1956) were reported in only 2 patients, but are often quoted in case series introductions or discussions as potential precipitating factors.

Many patients reported unexplained sensory symptoms or pain and headaches (Williams and Johnson, 1956; Lamontagne and Marks, 1973; Montague and Jones, 1979). These symptoms improved with improving urinary symptoms. Psychogenic urinary retention was only associated with renal dysfunction in 2 cases (Knox, 1960; Korzets et al., 1985). Perceived benefits included freedom from unhappy home or sexual situations, the ability to exert control in situations in which the patient was being exploited, and being unburdened from many household duties expected of a woman at that time (Wahl and Golden, 1963; Montague and Jones, 1979).

Treatment outcomes were generally only published in patients who significantly improved. However, many patients underwent unnecessary surgery, such as urethral dilatation, urethral elongation, and hysterectomy before a diagnosis of psychogenic urinary retention was made and specific treatment commenced (Montague and Jones, 1979; Cardenas et al., 1986). It is unclear, however, what proportion of patients diagnosed with psychogenic urinary retention were left with a permanent indwelling catheter or escalating surgical options for long-term treatment (Blaivas et al., 1977). Treatment was initially described with psychoanalysis, but in more recent literature, studies of systematic desensitization with relaxation training and biofeedback-monitored relaxation training were described (Lamontagne and Marks, 1973; Montague and Jones, 1979; Nicolau et al., 1991).

Reviewing the literature, there are also case reports of psychogenic urinary retention, which in hindsight clearly had a nonpsychogenic cause. For example, a case was reported in 1891 of a young woman developing urinary retention and this was attributed to her being frightened by a man with a traveling bear. However, there was also mention of abnormal sensations of tight rings around her lower thighs, reduced sensation and power in her legs, and bowel disturbance, which gradually improved over 6 months (Little, 1891). It seems possible that this was due to an inflammatory conus lesion which would not have been diagnosed with the investigations at the time. The danger of making a diagnosis of psychogenic or functional neurologic disorder in the absence of positive signs, such as Hoover's sign of functional weakness, is highlighted by this case and caution should therefore be exercised when exploring this area. Although urinary retention was included in the *Diagnostic and Statistical Manual of Mental Disorders* (DSM-IV) (American Psychiatric Association, 2000) as one of the symptoms of somatization disorder, there are few studies which refer to this condition in the recent literature.

FOWLERS SYNDROME

At a time when several of the cases of unexplained urinary retention were being labeled as "psychogenic," Clare Fowler and colleagues investigated the electromyogram (EMG) activity of the striated urethral sphincter and reported abnormal findings in 72% of the 48 women they examined (Fowler and Kirby, 1986). The findings they reported were complex repetitive discharges (CRDs) and decelerating bursts (DB), and this abnormal EMG activity suggested a biologic basis for urinary retention in young women who hitherto were told they had psychogenic urinary retention. Further investigation of this patient subgroup found that they were young women with an average age of 27 years, who, despite retaining urine, typically more than 1 liter, did not report urgency. They often reported an unpleasant sensation of "something gripping" during catheter withdrawal (and insertion), which was so severe that 28% of the original cohort received suprapubic catheters (Swinn and Fowler, 2001). Two-thirds of patients reported a triggering event at the onset of retention, most commonly surgery but also childbirth, UTI, or an acute medical condition. Many women note a long history of voiding difficulty prior to their initial episode of urinary retention (Swinn and Fowler, 2001). Subsequent investigations showed that women with an abnormal EMG often had a high urethral pressure profile and sphincter volume (Wiseman et al., 2002). The abnormality is thought to be a nonrelaxing striated urethral sphincter, which causes abnormally high urethral pressures and impaired voiding. Activation of sphincter afferents is likely to be having a reflex inhibitory effect on detrusor afferent and efferent activity, resulting in complete urinary retention and poor sensations of bladder fullness (Ramm et al., 2012). Our current understanding of the etiology of Fowler's syndrome is that it likely occurs due to upregulation of spinal enkephalins (Panicker et al., 2012), naturally occurring opiates, which reduce bladder sensation and negatively feed back to the sacral nerve roots, so that urethral sphincter sympathetic tone remains elevated and the PAG and PMC are not activated, even with large-volume bladder filling. The effect of upregulated spinal enkephalins is likely to be exacerbated by exogenous opiates.

The diagnosis is often difficult to establish and women with Fowler's syndrome see on average three consultants before their diagnosis is reached (Kavia et al., 2006). Although the urethral sphincter EMG findings are characteristic for this condition, in recent years two papers and two abstracts, one of which was a 10-year follow-up of the first, reported that these findings may be seen in the external urethral sphincter of apparently healthy women (Kujawa et al., 2001; Ramm et al., 2012; Tawadros et al., 2015). The number of participants in these studies were small, but they do raise some interesting questions about the specificity of these EMG findings to Fowler's syndrome, and also the effects of the menstrual cycle on EMG changes. The finding of CRDs and DBs in apparently asymptomatic young women suggests that only when the inhibitory signal is sufficiently strong will urinary retention occur. The EMG changes should therefore be considered with the clinical features before making a diagnosis of Fowler's syndrome. The finding of an elevated urethral pressure profile (>92 – age cm water) or urethral sphincter volume (>1.8 cm^3) aids the diagnosis (Wiseman et al., 2002). The finding of CRDs and DBs, however, remains prognostically useful as patients with these changes have improved outcomes following sacral neuromodulation (De Ridder et al., 2007).

The only currently useful long-term treatment for Fowler's syndrome is sacral neuromodulation, which has successful outcomes, with up to 70% of patients regaining the ability to void normally with postvoid residuals of ≤100 mL, on follow-up of up to 10 years (De Ridder et al., 2007; Elneil, 2010). Sacral neuromodulation appears to work by overriding the negative feedback from the sacral nerves. On imaging studies of 6 women with sacral neuromodulation, the previously reduced activity in the PAG and other higher brain centers shows restoration of normal or near normal activity after sacral neuromodulation insertion (Kavia et al., 2010). A recent open-label pilot study of 10 women demonstrated that urethral sphincter injection of botulinum toxin was associated with improvement in their urinary symptoms and objective improvements on urodynamic testing, and this potentially represents a less invasive option with few side-effects (Panicker et al., 2016).

Somatic comorbidities have been reported in women with Fowler's syndrome. A retrospective study of the hospital records of 62 women with Fowler's syndrome found that almost a quarter of patients (24%) with Fowler's syndrome had functional neurologic symptoms, including loss of consciousness, limb weakness, sensory disturbance, and memory impairment (Hoeritzauer et al., 2016). There are no comparison data in patients with other urologic or uro-neurologic disorders; however, based upon population prevalence of 2–33 per 100 000 for dissociative seizure (Reuber, 2008) or 1.7% of the population for patients with multiple idiopathic symptoms (Engel et al., 2002), this represents a high degree of comorbidity burden. Further studies are required to explore the reasons for this, whether due to a long diagnostic limbo prior to diagnosis or possibly because patients with Fowler's syndrome are more likely to have functional somatic comorbidities. Patients with Fowler's syndrome may be missing a useful opportunity to treat their disorder in the context of other relevant comorbidities. In a separate prospective series of 62 patients treated with sacral neuromodulation, 26.6% of patients with Fowler's syndrome and 44% of patients with chronic idiopathic urinary retention screened with the Patient Health Questionnaire were defined as being at risk for somatization based upon their scores (De Ridder et al., 2007).

Fifty percent of patients with Fowler's syndrome suffered from unexplained chronic abdominopelvic, back, leg, or widespread pain (Hoeritzauer et al., 2016). A recent study of gynecologic pathology in patients with Fowler's syndrome found rates similar to that expected in the general population, so it is unlikely that these chronic pain syndromes were caused by an underlying undiagnosed pelvic pathology (Karmarkar et al., 2015).

PARURESIS

Paruresis, also called "shy" or "bashful" bladder syndrome, is defined by DSM-5 (DSM-5 300.23: American Psychiatric Association, 2000) as a social anxiety disorder (social phobia) characterized by fear and avoidance of urinating in public toilets when other individuals are present. It is characterized by a situation-specific voiding dysfunction which usually occurs in adolescence following an unpleasant experience such as being rushed to urinate or being teased or harassed (Hammelstein et al., 2005; Soifer et al., 2010). Awareness of others waiting for the toilet often further exacerbates symptoms. Paruresis is not associated with the fear of contamination (Vythilingum et al., 2002), and 20% of patients report no anxiety, but merely the inability to void in public toilets. Despite the subgroup with no anxiety, rates of psychologic comorbidity are quite high in the general paruresis population. Social anxiety disorders (29%), a major depressive episode (22%), alcohol abuse (14%), preparuresis obsessive compulsive disorder or significant problematic embarrassment all occur and should be sought (Vythilingum et al., 2002; Kaufman, 2005).

Paruresis is seldom investigated, and there is poor knowledge about the disorder in medical circles. However, it is associated with significant morbidity and patients report high levels of shame, limitations to activities such as traveling or dating, and professional work (Vythilingum et al., 2002). The prevalence and gender ratios are uncertain; however, men are more likely to seek treatment and respond to questionnaires. Prevalence varies depending on how the question is phrased, as many as 6% of the population are fearful of using a public toilet (Ruscio and Brown, 2008), but situational inability to void seems to occur in only about 3% of the population (Hammelstein et al., 2005). Perhaps because of its low profile or the embarrassment associated with the condition, only about 30% of individuals seek treatment. Paruresis is often triggered by the triad of close physical or psychologic proximity with the individual, the presence of either familiar persons or the presence of strangers in the toilet, and temporary psychologic states, especially anxiety. Cognitive behavioral therapy with graded exposure techniques and biofeedback is the treatment offered for this condition (Rogers, 2003; Boschen, 2008; Soifer et al., 2010).

DYSFUNCTIONAL VOIDING AND HINMAN–ALLEN SYNDROME

Dysfunctional voiding is characterized by an intermittent or fluctuating urinary flow which occurs due to involuntary intermittent contractions of the striated urethral sphincter and/or levator muscles during voiding in otherwise neurologically intact individuals (Jeong et al., 2014; King and Goldman, 2014).

Despite this being primarily a problem of voiding, individuals with dysfunctional voiding, who are most often females, commonly present with symptoms of urgency and frequency. Incomplete bladder emptying is common, resulting in recurrent UTIs. Most patients have symptom onset from childhood.

The etiology is unclear; however, it is currently thought that dysfunctional voiding is a learned behavior in response to infection, trauma, detrusor overactivity causing stress incontinence, or psychologic factors (Karmakar and Sharma, 2014). Rates of depression and anxiety are greater than in asymptomatic controls (Fan et al., 2008) and dysfunctional voiding is more common in individuals with a history of sexual abuse (Ellsworth et al., 1995; Davila et al., 2003). Dysfunctional voiding is found in 2% of adults referred for urodynamic assessment, and the most common finding is a specific staccato pattern and dilated proximal urethra seen on voiding cystourethrogram (Glassberg and Combs, 2014). Treatment is primarily with biofeedback, which is thought to be successful in 60–90% of patients (Chin-Peuckert and Salle, 2001). However, a recent meta-analysis of all randomized studies of biofeedback ($n=5$) for dysfunctional voiding in children has shown no benefit over controls (Fazeli et al., 2015). This may be due to poor trial data and the heterogeneity within the dysfunctional voiding group. Biofeedback is thought to be much more successful in patients with involuntary intermittent contraction of the levator muscles.

A severe form of dysfunctional voiding, known as Hinman–Allen syndrome or nonneurogenic neurogenic bladder, is characterized by external urethral sphincter dysfunction, recurrent UTIs, and damage to the upper urinary tracts (Phillips and Uehling, 1993; Hinman, 1994). Hinman–Allen syndrome has been attributed to primarily psychologic causes since its inception. Children were described as having “failed personalities,” and parental divorce and “family disarray” were felt to be contributing factors (Hinman and Baumann, 2002). Up to 40% of patients have severe urinary tract morbidity, resulting in chronic renal failure (Yang and Mayo, 1997; Silay et al., 2011). The focus on psychologic etiology has been questioned with the publication of 9 cases of babies under 30 months having features of severe dysfunctional voiding (Jayanthi et al., 1997; Al Mosawi, 2007; Chaichanamongkol et al., 2008). There are moves towards allying this condition more closely to syndromes of elimination disorders such as urofacial syndrome (Ochoa syndrome or hydronephrosis with peculiar facial expression) (Ochoa, 2004; Roberts et al., 2014). Urofacial syndrome is a genetic disorder with similar findings on investigation to Hinman–Allen syndrome, but additionally patients have a characteristic facies on smiling, akin to crying (Ochoa, 2004; Roberts et al., 2014; Tu et al., 2014). It occurs due to an abnormality on chromosome 10 in the region of 10q23-q24 which codes for the genes *HSPE2* or *LRIG2* (Ochoa, 2004; Roberts et al., 2014). Only a small genetic study of 22 patients with Hinman–Allen syndrome has been performed and no abnormalities were detected; however, further studies are required (Bulum et al., 2015).

OVERACTIVE BLADDER

OAB is a syndrome defined by the International Continence Society as “urinary urgency, usually accompanied by frequency and nocturia, with or without urgency urinary incontinence in the absence of UTI or other obvious pathology” (Abrams et al., 2002). The diagnosis is made based upon the patient’s self-reported symptoms of urinary urgency, frequency, nocturia, and/or urgency urinary incontinence. Whilst urgency is difficult to measure clinically, urinary frequency is defined as voiding more than eight times per day, nocturia in OAB as passing small amounts of urine several times overnight, and urgency urinary incontinence can be recorded using a diary (Gormley et al., 2015). There are several conditions that may result in these symptoms; however, in a subset of individuals with “idiopathic” OAB, the cause remains obscure despite extensive investigations.

Patients with OAB report considerable morbidity. They have significantly worse health-related quality of life, are less likely than individuals without OAB to be employed, and may report sexual dysfunction (Ergenoglu et al., 2013; Tang et al., 2014). Patients with urinary incontinence (wet OAB) are more severely affected than those without incontinence (dry OAB). Disease-specific and global quality-of-life scores are lower and patients are less productive, and have greater health resource allocation (Tang et al., 2014). OAB is a long-term problem for the majority of patients and is underreported and undertreated (Getsios et al., 2005; Ergenoglu et al., 2013).

OAB is associated with high levels of anxiety and depression (Matsuzaki et al., 2012; Matsumoto et al., 2013; Vrijens et al., 2015). A recent systematic review reported a positive association between depression and OAB in 26/35 studies, and between anxiety and OAB in 6/9 studies. There was strong evidence of OAB developing in patients who had depression, with an odds ratio 1.15–5.78, although it was not possible to assess causality (Vrijens et al., 2015). The occurrence of OAB symptoms is associated with worse quality-of-life scores, embarrassment, and social isolation (Wagg et al., 2007; Tang et al., 2014).

Anxiety in healthy individuals can cause increased urinary frequency and urgency. Charcot and contemporaries used the term "pollakiuria" to describe "frequent and repeated micturition which one experiences under the stress of an emotion" (Dejerine and Gauckler, 1913). Animal studies suggested that chronic stress in anxiety-prone animals resulted in bladder hyperalgesia, which may contribute to the pathogenesis of LUT symptoms in affective disorders (Lee et al., 2015).

There is limited literature exploring LUT symptoms in patients with pathologic anxiety disorders. In one longitudinal community study, anxiety appeared to have a causative role in the occurrence of urge incontinence (Perry et al., 2006). Females aged over 40 years old were asked through a community postal survey about anxiety and depression using the Hospital Anxiety and Depression scale, and urinary symptoms, and followed up for a year. It was observed that the presence of urge incontinence and urinary frequency predicted the development of anxiety and depression. Moreover, anxiety predicted urge incontinence, whereas depression did not. In contrast, stress incontinence did not predict either anxiety or depression (Perry et al., 2006).

Four randomized controlled trials demonstrated that successful treatment of OAB resulted in a significant improvement in patients' affective symptoms (Vrijens et al., 2015). The relationship between depression, anxiety, and OAB is postulated to be due to altered serotonin and norepinephrine levels causing OAB. This is on the basis of animal models demonstrating that serotonin and norepinephrine have a modulatory effect on Onuf's nucleus, which prevents accidental voiding when abdominal pressure increases, that serotonin inhibits the parasympathetic voiding activity and stimulates sympathetic activity, and that frequency is reduced after administration of selective serotonin reuptake inhibitors (Redaelli et al., 2015).

An alternative mechanism is through the central effect of increased corticotropin-releasing factor, released due to dysregulation of the hypothalamic–pituitary–adrenal axis, causing both bladder and mood symptoms, as seen in rodent models (Wood et al., 2013).

Recently three studies investigated functional somatic syndrome comorbidities in OAB and found irritable-bowel syndrome (IBS) occurring in up to one-third of patients with OAB, with a background population rate of 20% (Matsumoto et al., 2013). Patients with fibromyalgia (FM) were significantly more likely to have OAB and more severe OAB symptoms correlated to more severe FM symptoms. There was a significant overlap between OAB and functional dyspepsia in population-based studies (Persson et al., 2015). A history of sexual abuse was found to be associated with urinary frequency, urgency, and nocturia in at least three studies (Davila et al., 2003; Fitzgerald et al., 2007; Link et al., 2007). Among these studies, one fulfilled the Bradford Hill criteria for causality (Link et al., 2007).

INTERSTITIAL CYSTITIS/BLADDER PAIN SYNDROME AND FUNCTIONAL SOMATIC SYNDROMES

Interstitial cystitis/bladder pain syndrome (IC/BPS) is defined by the Society for Urodynamics and Female Urology as "an unpleasant sensation (pain, pressure, discomfort) perceived to be related to the urinary bladder, associated with lower urinary tract symptoms of more than six weeks duration, in the absence of infection or other identifiable cause" (Hanno et al., 2011). Voiding helps to reduce pain (Hanno et al., 2011). Patients with IC/BPS have a worse quality of life compared to healthy individuals, as well as to patients with OAB, due to effects on emotion, social limitations, and personal relationships (Kim and Oh, 2010).

Several studies have shown that patients with IC/BPS report comorbidities with functional somatic disorders such as IBS, FM, chronic fatigue syndrome (CFS), and vulvodynia (Aaron and Buchwald, 2001; Buffington, 2004; Rodríguez et al., 2009). Moreover, patients reporting an increasing number of functional somatic syndromes, particularly FM, CFS, and IBS, have a greater risk for IC/BPS (Warren et al., 2011). In a systematic review, 16 of 25 publications found overlap between painful urologic pelvic pain syndromes and nonurologic syndromes (Rodríguez et al., 2009). Four studies were of patients with IC, and these showed higher rates of IBS (22.5% vs. 7% of controls), higher rates of backache, dizziness, arthralgia, abdominal cramps, and headache than controls, generalized pain in 27% vs. 7% of controls, and the women with IC were 11 times more likely to be diagnosed with IBS compared with controls. In patients who had FM, 12% of patients met the criteria for IC, and in patients with chronic pelvic pain, IBS was found in 22.4% of patients, 40% of whom had IC. Twin studies found that twins with fatigue were 2–20 times more likely to have IC than twins without fatigue (Rodríguez et al., 2009). Most of the studies exploring the association of LUT symptoms and functional somatic syndromes have focused on pain disorders and therefore the association of IC/BPS and functional somatic symptoms may be overrepresented in the literature.

There is also evidence for disproportionate levels of sexual abuse, high levels of depression, and panic disorder in patients with IC/BPS (Peters et al., 2007; Clemens et al., 2008). Several studies have investigated the association between abuse and IC/BPS. Physical, mental, or sexual abuse was found in 37% of patients with IC vs. 24% of symptom-free controls, and sexual abuse occurred in 18 vs. 8% in a population responding to a survey ($n = 215$ vs. $n = 464$ symptom-free controls) and 25/76 women (33%) seen in clinic (Peters et al., 2007).

There is no definitive treatment for IC/BPS. Treatment is tailored to the individual patient, with holistic multimodal multidisciplinary input to maximize efficacy. First-line treatments include stress reduction, patient education, use of nonprescription analgesics, pelvic floor relaxation, and dietary manipulation (De Bock et al., 2011).

Oral medications are generally the first-line treatment therapy, including antiallergics, amitriptyline, pentosan polysulfate sodium (Elmiron) and immunosuppressants. The choice of analgesic should be made in collaboration with a specialist pain management team. In case of failure of oral therapy, intravesical drugs (local anesthetics, hyaluronic acid, heparin) are administered; the intravesical route improves drug bioavailability, establishing high drug concentrations at the target, and is associated with fewer systemic side-effects. Disadvantages include the need for intermittent catheterization, which can be painful in BPS patients, cost, and risk of infection. Although bladder hydrodistension is a common treatment for BPS, the scientific justification is scanty. It can be a part of the diagnostic evaluation, but has a limited therapeutic role. Botulinum toxin A may have an antinociceptive effect through bladder afferent pathways, producing symptomatic and urodynamic improvement (Engeler et al., 2015). Sacral neuromodulation is associated with improvements in the symptoms of refractory BPS, with good long-term success seen in 72% (Engeler et al., 2015). Endourologic destruction of bladder tissue aims to eliminate urothelial lesions, mostly Hunner's ulcers, and can be helpful in the relief of pain and urgency. Ablative organ surgery should be a last resort and should be performed only by surgeons knowledgeable about BPS. Unfortunately, no single treatment seems to work for patients over a prolonged period of time (Hanno et al., 2011).

The etiology of IC/BPS is unclear and, whilst many studies have investigated association, causality remains elusive. Discussion of etiology involves physiologic and psychologic hypotheses (Aaron and Buchwald, 2001; Warren, 2014). The current favored hypothesis is that central brain processing of pain is different in patients with IC than in healthy controls. A recent imaging study using voxel-based morphometry of 33 patients with IC and no other comorbidities showed increased gray matter in the supplementary motor area, the superior parietal lobule/precuneus bilaterally, and the right primary somatosensory cortex. In the right primary somatosensory cortex volume changes also correlated with clinical measurement of pain, anxiety, and urologic symptoms (Kairys et al., 2015). It was suggested by the authors that increased gray matter in the precuneus might be caused by alterations in the higher pain connections in a similar manner to those seen in FM. Alternatively, the increases could be due to bottom-up changes to the higher-center connections caused by prolonged severe pain.

FREQUENCY OF UROLOGIC SYMPTOMS IN FUNCTIONAL/PSYCHOGENIC DISORDERS

Although rarely reported in the literature, LUT symptoms have been observed in patients with functional neurologic disorders. The only study of LUT dysfunction in patients with functional neurologic disorders is a retrospective review of 150 patients diagnosed with definite or probable functional movement disorders between 2006 and 2014 from the National Hospital for Neurology and Neurosurgery in London (Batla et al., 2016). Patient notes were screened retrospectively and patients with LUT symptoms were administered questionnaires for urinary symptoms and LUT-related quality of life. Thirty of the 150 patients with functional movement disorders had LUT symptoms; 20 of the 49 (41%) patients with fixed dystonia, 8 of the 57 (14%) patients with tremor, and 2 of the 14 (14%) patients with mixed movement disorders. LUT questionnaires were completed by 22 of the 30 patients, all of whom were female, the majority of whom had symptoms of OAB ($n = 14$). The remaining patients complained of stress urinary incontinence ($n = 5$) and low stream ($n = 3$). Opiate use was correlated with low stream ($p = 0.02$). The 5 most severely affected patients, 3 of whom had urinary retention and recurrent UTIs, and all of whom were using opiates, underwent urodynamic evaluation. No clear pattern of abnormality was evident and no neurologic or urologic cause was found. The 3 patients with urinary retention were initially managed with suprapubic catheterization and then had successful outcomes with sacral neuromodulation. Patients with fixed dystonia had the most severe symptoms, but the quality of life for all patients was negatively affected. LUT symptoms in other neurologic disorders are known to negatively affect quality of life; further studies in patients with functional neurologic disorders are required (Panicker and Fowler, 2015).

OPIATE USE AND LUT DYSFUNCTION

Pain is a well-known comorbidity in many functional conditions and high rates of prescription opiate use have been described (Pearson et al., 2014). The association between opiate use and LUT dysfunction is less well known amongst general physicians and patients, and could be contributing to LUT dysfunction in patients with neurologic and urologic disorders (Elneil, 2010; Panicker et al., 2012). In a study of 61 consecutive female patients reviewed at Queen's Square with unexplained urinary retention, 24 patients were taking regular opiates, 3 of whom were taking more than one opiate. Five of these patients were diagnosed with Fowler's syndrome, but 13 of the patients had no known cause for their voiding dysfunction. Patients had been prescribed opiates for unexplained predominantly abdominopelvic, musculoskeletal, or mechanical pain syndromes (Panicker et al., 2012). On discontinuing opiates, 2 of the 24 patients reported improvement in LUT symptoms. Intravenous ($n = 72$) (Malinovsky et al., 1998) and intrathecal ($n = 45$) (Kuipers et al., 2004) opiates have been shown to reduce bladder sensation, increase residual volume, and affect the urge to void and the ability to micturite in some patients, with dose-dependent effects (Kuipers et al., 2004). Opiates are thought to affect the bladder peripherally by increasing parasympathetic tone and centrally acting on spinal enkephalins and mu receptors in the PAG (Matsumoto et al., 2004).

IS THERE AN ASSOCIATION BETWEEN LUT DYSFUNCTION AND FUNCTIONAL DISORDERS?

The term "functional disorders" encompasses overlapping syndromes including CFS, FM, IBS, myofascial pain, and temporomandibular joint disease (Clauw, 2010). The overlap of symptoms is well documented (Wessely et al., 1999; Clauw and Crofford, 2003; Wessely and White, 2013). The way in which these conditions overlap with functional disorders seen in neurologic practice, such as functional movement disorder and dissociative (nonepileptic) attacks, is also now well documented.

Reflecting on the LUT dysfunction discussed in this chapter and its relationship with functional disorders, the initial problem is the dearth of studies that have attempted to specifically answer the question as to whether functional urologic disorders could share an etiology with functional neurologic and somatic disorders.

It is known that the LUT is regulated by a complex interconnected network of higher centers involved in arousal, focus, understanding of safety and social propriety, emotion and motor activity. This system is informed by afferent signals from the LUT via the spinal cord, and the PAG and PMC are important brainstem centers involved in the coordination of urethral, pelvic floor, and detrusor contractions. There are many points at which this network can go wrong, yet present with a limited repertoire of LUT symptoms. Understanding of the bladder–brain axis is exponentially increasing through basic, clinical, and imaging science. Increasing knowledge of neural networks has changed the understanding of disease from simply biologic or psychologic processes to an awareness of disease as something spanning both, and affected by environment and beliefs, as well as genes, which all come together to create the patient's disease phenotype. In functional neurologic disorders, the field is moving away from the dualistic understanding of psychogenic versus organic etiology. This allows a functional model to emerge that comfortably incorporates psychologic and physiologic disturbances.

Considering whether these disorders have features which overlap with functional somatic syndromes, such as IBS, FM, or hyperventilation syndrome, the criteria from Wessely et al. (1999) will be used.

Patients with one functional syndrome frequently meet diagnostic criteria for other syndromes

The prevalence of other functional disorders in patients with OAB, IC, paruresis, and Fowler's syndrome has been discussed above.

Sex

IC, idiopathic OAB syndrome, Fowler's syndrome, and dysfunctional voiding affect predominantly women, whereas paruresis is likely to affect men more often. Some functional neurologic disorders such as functional propriospinal myoclonus have a male preponderance (van der Salm et al., 2014).

Emotional problems

Depression and anxiety are reported more in patients with idiopathic OAB, IC, paruresis, dysfunctional voiding, and Fowler's syndrome compared to healthy controls. However, the impact of a chronic LUT disorder on mood requires further study before attempting to make an association between psychologic comorbidities and urologic disorders.

Physiology

Much of the current research of IC, idiopathic OAB, and Fowler's syndrome hypothesizes that there is a central mechanism (brain $\pm$ spinal cord) causing the disorder rather than an abnormality which is solely bladder-based (Kavia et al., 2010; Tadic et al., 2011; Kairys et al., 2015). Paruresis is treated with cognitive-behavioral therapy, recognizing that a central mechanism of inhibition exists that must be unlearned.

History of childhood abuse or neglect

While this is frequently referenced in older psychogenic urinary retention literature, there are few studies which explore this, except in the IC and dysfunctional voiding literature (Ellsworth et al., 1995; Davila et al., 2003; Mayson and Teichman, 2009). In the Boston Area Community Health study ($n = 5506$), sexual and physical abuse and the prevalence of urinary frequency, urgency, and nocturia met the Bradford Hill criteria to suggest causality (Link et al., 2007). Given the frequency of these urinary symptoms in the population, background rates of childhood and adult adversity and potential pathophysiologic mechanisms should be investigated in a range of neurologic, gynecologic, and functional urologic conditions.

Many patients with idiopathic functional urologic disorders share similar characteristics with patients who have functional somatic disorders. The LUT is unique amongst visceral organs because of the highly organized central neural network that regulates its functions and affords higher-level voluntary input, and therefore it is likely that there exists an association between LUT dysfunction and functional syndromes. Though tests such as urodynamics help to uncover the pathophysiologic correlate of LUT symptoms, the test is unable to provide information about the etiology or behavioral underpinnings responsible for the LUT dysfunction. Studies are therefore required that are designed to specifically evaluate the nature of the association between LUT dysfunction and functional syndromes and explore causality. Recognizing the interface between emotion, motivation, memory, and LUT functions would allow for a more comprehensive approach to patients presenting with functional disorders.

ACKNOWLEDGMENTS

JNP undertook this work at UCLH/UCL Institute of Neurology and is supported in part by funding from the UK Department of Health NIHR Biomedical Research Centres funding scheme. IH is funded by an ABN/Patrick Berthoud Clinical Research Training Fellowship. VP was supported by the European Urological Scholarship Programme.

References

Aaron L, Buchwald D (2001). A review of the evidence for overlap among unexplained clinical conditions. Ann Intern Med 134: 868–881.

Abrams P, Cardozo L, Fall M et al. (2002). The standardisation of terminology in lower urinary tract function: report from the standardisation sub-committee of the International Continence Society. Urology 21: 167–178.

Al Mosawi AJ (2007). Identification of nonneurogenic neurogenic bladder in infants. Urology 70 (2): 355–356. discussion 356–7.

American Psychiatric Association (2000). Diagnostic and statistical manual of mental disorders, 4th ed., text rev. Washington, DC.

Barrett DM (1978). Evaluation of psychogenic urinary retention. J Urol 120 (2): 191–192.

Batla A, Pareés I, Edwards MJ et al. (2016). Lower urinary tract dysfunction in patients with functional movement disorders. J Neurol Sci 361: 192–194.

Berridge CW, Waterhouse BD (2003). The locus coeruleus-noradrenergic system: modulation of behavioral state and state-dependent cognitive processes. Brain Res Rev 42 (1): 33–84.

Bilanakis N (2006). Psychogenic urinary retention. Gen Hosp Psychiatry 28: 259–261.

Blaivas G, Labib B, Medical TE (1977). Acute urinary retention in women. Complete urodynamic evaluation. Urology X (4): 383–389.

Boschen MJ (2008). Paruresis (psychogenic inhibition of micturation): cognitive behavioral formulation and treatment. Depress Anxiety 25 (11): 903–912.

Bridges PK, Koller KM, Wheeler TK (1966). Psychiatric referrals in a general hospital. Acta Psychiatr Scand 42: 171–182.

Buffington CA (2004). Comorbidity of interstitial cystitis with other unexplained clinical conditions. J Urol 172 (October): 1242–1248.

Bulum B, Ozcakar ZB, Duman D et al. (2015). HPSE2 mutations in urofacial syndrome, non-neurogenic neurogenic bladder and lower urinary tract dysfunction. Nephron 130 (1): 54–58.

Caplan JB, Madsen JR, Schulze-Bonhage A et al. (2003). Human theta oscillations related to sensorimotor integration and spatial learning. J Neurosci 23 (11): 4726–4736.

Cardenas DD, Larson J, Egan KJ (1986). Hysterical paralysis in the upper extremity of chronic pain patients. Arch Phys Med Rehabil 67: 190–193.

Chaichanamongkol V, Ikeda M, Ishikura K et al. (2008). An infantile case of Hinman syndrome with severe acute renal failure. Clin Exp Nephrol 12 (4): 309–311.

Charcot JM (1877). Lectures on the Disease of The Nervous System, J.E. Adlard, plate V, London, pp. 225–245.

Chin-Peuckert L, Salle JL (2001). A modified biofeedback program for children with detrusor-sphincter dyssynergia: 5-year experience. J Urol 166 (4): 1470–1475.

Christmas TJ, Noble JG, Watson JM et al. (1991). Use of biofeedback in treatment of psychogenic voiding dysfunction. Urology 37 (1): 43–45.

Clauw DJ (2010). Perspectives on fatigue from the study of chronic fatigue syndrome and related conditions. PM and R 2 (5): 414–430.

Clauw DJ, Crofford LJ (2003). Chronic widespread pain and fibromyalgia: what we know, and what we need to know. Best practice and research. Clin Rheumatol 17 (4): 685–701.

Clemens JQ, Brown SO, Calhoun E (2008). Mental health diagnoses in patients with interstitial cystitis/painful bladder syndrome and chronic prostatitis/chronic pelvic pain syndrome: a case/control study. J Urol 180 (October): 1378–1382.

Critchley HD (2003). Human cingulate cortex and autonomic control: converging neuroimaging and clinical evidence. Brain 126 (10): 2139–2152.

Davila GW, Bernier F, Franco J et al. (2003). Bladder dysfunction in sexual abuse survivors. J Urol 170 (2 Pt 1): 476–479.

De Bock F, Dirckx J, Wyndaele J-J (2011). How are we going to make progress treating bladder pain syndrome? ICI-RS 2013. Neurourol Urodyn 30: 169–173.

de Groat WC, Griffiths D, Yosimura N (2015). Neural control of the lower urinary tract. Compr Physiol 5 (1): 327–396.

De Ridder D, Ost D, Bruyninckx F (2007). The presence of Fowler's syndrome predicts successful long-term outcome of sacral nerve stimulation in women with urinary retention. Eur Urol 51 (1): 229–233. discussion 233–4.

Dejerine J, Gauckler E (1913). The Psychoneuroses and their Treatment By Psychotherapy, J B Lippincott, Philadelphia, 52.

Ellsworth PI, Merguerian PA, Copening ME (1995). Sexual abuse: another causative factor in dysfunctional voiding. J Urol 153 (3 Pt 1): 773–776.

Elneil S (2010). Urinary retention in women and sacral neuromodulation. Int Urogynecol J Pelvic Floor Dysfunct 21 (October): 475–483.

Engel CC, Liu X, Hoge C et al. (2002). Multiple idiopathic physical symptoms in the ECA study: competing-risks analysis of 1-year incidence, mortality, and resolution. Am J Psychiatry 159 (June): 998–1004.

Engeler D, Baranowski AP, Borovicka J et al. (2015). Guidelines on chronic pelvic pain, European Association of Urology, pp. 30–32. Available at: http://uroweb.org/wp-content/uploads/25-Chronic-Pelvic-Pain_LR_full.pdf.

Ergenoglu AM, Yeniel AO, Itil IM et al. (2013). Overactive bladder and its effects on sexual dysfunction among women. Acta Obstet Gynecol Scand 92: 1202–1207.

Fan Y-H, Lin AT, Wu HM et al. (2008). Psychological profile of female patients with dysfunctional voiding. Urology 71 (4): 625–629.

Fazeli MS, Lin Y, Nikoo N et al. (2015). Biofeedback for nonneuropathic daytime voiding disorders in children: a systematic review and meta-analysis of randomized controlled trials. J Urol 193 (1): 274–280.

Fitzgerald MP, Link CL, Litman HJ et al. (2007). Beyond the lower urinary tract: the association of urologic and sexual symptoms with common illnesses. Eur Urol 52: 407–415.

Fowler C, Kirby R (1986). Electromyography of urethral sphincter in women with urinary retention. The Lancet 1455–1457. June.

Getsios D, El-Hadi W, Caro I et al. (2005). Pharmacological management of overactive bladder. Pharmacoeconomics 23 (5): 995–1006.

Glassberg KI, Combs AJ (2014). Lower urinary tract dysfunction in childhood: what's really wrong with these children? Curr Bladder Dysfunct Rep 9 (4): 389–400.

Gormley EA, Lightner DJ, Faraday M et al. (2015). Diagnosis and treatment of overactive bladder (non-neurogenic) in adults: AUA/SUFU guideline amendment. J Urol: 1–9 (January).

Griffiths D (2015). Functional imaging of structures involved in neural control of the lower urinary tract. Neurology of Sexual and Bladder Disorders: Handbook Of Clinical Neurology, 130: Elsevier, Amsterdam, pp. 121–133.

Griffiths DJ, Fowler CJ (2013). The micturition switch and its forebrain influences. Acta Physiol 207 (1): 93–109.

Hammelstein P, Pietrowsky R, Merbach M et al. (2005). Psychogenic urinary retention ('paruresis'): diagnosis and epidemiology in a representative male sample. Psychother Psychosom 74 (5): 308–314.

Hanno PM, Burks DA, Clemens JO et al. (2011). Infection/inflammation AUA guideline for the diagnosis and treatment of interstitial cystitis/bladder pain syndrome. J Urol 185: 2162–2170.

Hayllen B, Maher CF, Barber MD et al. (2010). An International Urogynaecological Association (IUGA)/International Continence Society (ICS) joint report on the terminology for female pelvic floor dysfunction. Neurourol Urodyn 29: 4–20.

Hinman F, Lear EA (1994). A no-nonsense reply. Urology 43 (6): 763–764.

Hinman F, Baumann FW (2002). Vesical and ureteral damage from voiding dysfunction in boys without neurologic or obstructive disease. J Urol 167 (2 Pt 2): 1069–1073.

Hoeritzauer I, Stone J, Fowler C et al. (2016). Fowler's syndrome of urinary retention: a retrospective study of co-morbidity. Neurourology and Urodynamics 35: 601–603.

Jayanthi VR, Khoury AC, McLorie GA et al. (1997). The nonneurogenic neurogenic bladder of early infancy. J Urol 158 (3 Pt 2): 1281–1285.

Jeong SJ, Yeon JS, Lee JK et al. (2014). Chronic lower urinary tract symptoms in young men without symptoms of chronic prostatitis: Urodynamic analyses in 308 men aged 50 years or younger. Korean J Urol 55: 341–348.

Kairys AE, Schmidt-Wijcke T, Pulu T et al. (2015). Increased brain gray matter in the primary somatosensory cortex is associated with increased pain and mood disturbance in patients with interstitial cystitis/painful bladder syndrome. J Urology 193 (1): 131–137.

Karmakar D, Sharma J (2014). Current concepts in voiding dysfunction and dysfunctional voiding: A review from a urogynaecologist's perspective. J Mid-Life Health 5 (3): 104.

Karmarkar R, Abtahi B, Saber-Khalaf M et al. (2015). Gynaecological pathology in women with Fowler's syndrome. Eur J Obstet Gynecol 194: 54–57.

Kaufman KR (2005). Monotherapy treatment of paruresis with gabapentin. Int Clin Psychopharmacol 20 (1): 53–55.

Kavia RBC, Datta SN, Dasgupta R et al. (2006). Urinary retention in women: its causes and management. BJU Int 97 (2): 281–287.

Kavia R, Dasgupta R, Critchley H et al. (2010). A functional magnetic resonance imaging study of the effect of sacral neuromodulation on brain responses in women with Fowler's syndrome. BJU Int 105 (3): 366–372.

Kim SH, Oh SJ (2010). Comparison of voiding questionnaires between female interstitial cystitis and female idiopathic overactive bladder. Int Neurourol J 14: 86–92.

King AB, Goldman HB (2014). Bladder outlet obstruction in women : functional causes. Curr Urol Rep 15 (436): 1–9.

Knox SJ (1960). Psychogenic urinary retention after parturition, resulting in hydronephrosis. Br Med J 12: 1422–1424.

Korzets Z, Garb R, Lewis S et al. (1985). Reversible renal failure due to psychogenic urinary retention. Postgrad Med J 61: 465–468.

Kuipers PW, Kamphuis ET, van Venrooij GE et al. (2004). Intrathecal opioids and lower urinary tract function: a urodynamic evaluation. Anesthesiology 100 (6): 1497–1503.

Kujawa M, Reid F, Ellis A et al. (2001). Are "whaling" women normal? Br J Urol 41 (s1): p.P162.

Lamontagne Y, Marks IM (1973). Psychogenic urinary retention: treatment by prolonged exposure. Behav Ther 4: 581–585.

Lee UJ, Ackerman AL, Wu A et al. (2015). Chronic psychological stress in high-anxiety rats induces sustained bladder hyperalgesia. Physiol Behav 139: 541–548.

Link CLC, Luffey KE, Steers WD et al. (2007). Is abuse causally related to urologic symptoms? Results from the Boston Area Community Health (BACH) Survey. Eur Urol 52 (2): 397–406.

Little J (1891). Hysterical ischuria. The Lancet 4: 12.

Malinovsky JM, Le Normand L, Lepage JY et al. (1998). The urodynamic effects of intravenous opioids and ketoprofen in humans. Anesth Analg 87 (2): 456–461.

Margolis GJ (1965). A review of literature on psychogenic urinary retention. J Urol 94 (3): 257–258.

Matsumoto S, Levendusky MC, Longhurst PA et al. (2004). Activation of mu opioid receptors in the ventrolateral periaqueductal gray inhibits reflex micturition in anesthetized rats. Neurosci Lett 363 (2): 116–119.

Matsumoto S, Hashizume K, Wada N et al. (2013). Relationship between overactive bladder and irritable bowel syndrome: a large-scale internet survey in Japan using the overactive bladder symptom score and Rome III criteria. BJU Int 111: 647–652.

Matsuzaki J, Suzuki H, Fukushima Y et al. (2012). High frequency of overlap between functional dyspepsia and overactive bladder. Neurogastroenterol Motil 24: 821–827.

Mayson BE, Teichman JMH (2009). The relationship between sexual abuse and interstitial cystitis/painful bladder syndrome. Curr Urol Rep 10 (6): 441–447.

Montague D, Jones RL (1979). Psychogenic urinary retention. Urology XIII (1): 30–35.

Nicolau R, Toro J, Prado CP (1991). Behavioral treatment of a case of psychogenic urinary retention. J Behav Ther Exp Psychiatry 22 (1): 63–68.

Norden C, Friedman E (1961). Psychogenic urinary retention. Report of two cases. New Engl J Med 264 (21): 1096–1097.

Ochoa B (2004). Can a congenital dysfunctional bladder be diagnosed from a smile? The Ochoa syndrome updated. Pediatr Nephrol 19 (1): 6–12.

Panicker JN, Fowler CJ (2010). The bare essentials: uro-neurology. Pract Neurol 10 (3): 178–185.

Panicker JN, Fowler CJ (2015). Lower urinary tract dysfunction in patients with multiple sclerosis. In: DB Vodušek, F Boller (Eds.), Handbook of Clinical Neurology, Elsevier, Amsterdam, pp. 371–381.

Panicker JN, DasGupta R, Elneil S et al. (2010). Urinary retention. In Pelvic Organ Dysfunction in Neurological Disease: Clinical Management and Rehabilitation, Cambridge University Press, Cambridge, pp. 293–306.

Panicker JN, Game X, Khan S et al. (2012). The possible role of opiates in women with chronic urinary retention: observations from a prospective clinical study. J Urol 188 (2): 480–484.

Panicker JN, Seth JH, Khan S et al. (2016). Open-label study evaluating outpatient urethral sphincter injections of onabotulinumtoxinA to treat women with urinary retention due to a primary disorder of sphincter relaxation (Fowler's syndrome). BJU Int 117: 809–813.

Pearson JS, Pollard C, Whorwell PJ (2014). Avoiding analgesic escalation and excessive healthcare utilization in severe irritable bowel syndrome: a role for intramuscular anticholinergics? Ther Adv Gastroenterol 7 (6): 232–237.

Perry S, McGrother CW, Turner K (2006). An investigation of the relationship between anxiety and depression and urge incontinence in women: development of a psychological model. Br J Health Psychol 11: 463–482.

Persson R, Wensaas KA, Hanevik K et al. (2015). The relationship between irritable bowel syndrome, functional dyspepsia, chronic fatigue and overactive bladder syndrome: a controlled study 6 years after acute gastrointestinal infection. BMC Gastroenterol 15 (1): 66.

Peters KM, Kalinowski SE, Carrico DJ et al. (2007). Fact or fiction – is abuse prevalent in patients with interstitial cystitis? Results from a community survey and clinic population. J Urol 178 (September): 891–895.

Phillips E, Uehling D (1993). Hinman syndrome: a vicious cycle. Pediatr Urol 42 (3): 317–319.

Ramm O, Mueller ER, Brubaker L et al. (2012). Complex repetitive discharges – a feature of the urethral continence mechanism or a pathological finding? J Urol 187 (6): 2140–2143.

Redaelli M, Ricatti MJ, Simonetto M et al. (2015). Serotonin and noradrenaline reuptake inhibitors improve micturition control in mice. PLoS One 10 (3): p.e0121883.

Reuber M (2008). Psychogenic nonepileptic seizures: answers and questions. Epilepsy Behav 12: 622–635.

Rickenbacher E, Baez MA, Hale L et al. (2008). Impact of overactive bladder on the brain: central sequelae of a visceral pathology. Proc Natl Acad Sci U S A 105 (30): 10589–10594.

Roberts NA, Woolf AS, Stuart HM et al. (2014). Heparanase 2, mutated in urofacial syndrome, mediates peripheral neural development in *Xenopus*. Hum Mol Genet 23 (16): 4302–4314.

Rodríguez MÁB, Afari N, Buchwald DS (2009). Evidence for overlap between urological and nonurological unexplained clinical conditions. J Urol 182 (5): 2123–2131.

Rogers G (2003). Treatment of paruresis in the context of benign prostatic hyperplasia: a case report. Cogn Behav Pract 1985: 168–177.

Ruscio A, Brown T (2008). Social fears and social phobia in the USA: results from the National Comorbidity Survey Replication. Psychol Med 38 (1): 15–28.

Schrum A, Wolff S, van der Horst C et al. (2011). Motor cortical representation of the pelvic floor muscles. J Urol 186 (1): 185–190.

Silay MS, Tanriverdi O, Karatag T et al. (2011). Twelve-year experience with Hinman-Allen syndrome at a single center. Urology 78 (6): 1397–1401.

Smith MD, Seth JH, Fowler CJ et al. (2013). Urinary retention for the neurologist. Pract Neurol 13 (5): 288–291.

Soifer S, Himle J, Walsh K (2010). Paruresis (shy bladder syndrome): a cognitive-behavioral treatment approach. Soc Work Health Care 49 (5): 494–507.

Swinn M, Fowler C (2001). Isolated urinary retention in young women, or Fowler's syndrome. Clin Auton Res 11 (5): 309–311.

Tadic S, Griffiths D, Schaefer W et al. (2011). Brain activity underlying impaired continence control in older women with overactive bladder. Neurourol Urodyn 31: 652–658.

Tadic S, Tannenbaum C, Resnick SM et al. (2013). Brain responses to bladder filling in older women without urgency incontinence. Neurourol Urodyn 32: 435–440.

Tang DH, Colayco DC, Khalaf KM et al. (2014). Impact of urinary incontinence on healthcare resource utilization, health-related quality of life and productivity in patients with overactive bladder. BJU Int 113: 484–491.

Tawadros C, Burnett K, Derbyshire LF et al. (2015). External urethral sphincter electromyography in asymptomatic women and the influence of the menstrual cycle. BJU Int 116 (3): 423–431.

Tu Y, Yang P, Yang J et al. (2014). Clinical and genetic characteristics for the urofacial syndrome (UFS). Int J Clin Exp Pathol 7 (5): 1842–1848.

Valentino RJ, Wood SK, Wein SJ et al. (2011). The bladder–brain connection: putative role of corticotropin-releasing factor. Nat Rev Urol 8 (1): 19–28.

van der Salm SMA, Erro R, Cordivari C et al. (2014). Propriospinal myoclonus: clinical reappraisal and review of literature. Neurology 83: 1862–1870.

Vrijens D, Drossaerts J, van Koeveringe G et al. (2015). Affective symptoms and the overactive bladder – A systematic review. J Psychosom Res 78: 95–108.

Vythilingum B, Stein DJ, Soifer S (2002). Is "shy bladder syndrome" a subtype of social anxiety disorder? A survey of people with paruresis. Depress Anxiety 16 (2): 84–87.

Wagg AS, Cardozo L, Chapple C et al. (2007). Overactive bladder syndrome in older people. BJU Int 99: 502–509.

Wahl CW, Golden JS (1963). Psychogenic urinary retention. Psychosom Med xxv (6): 543–555.

Warren JW (2014). Bladder pain syndrome/interstitial cystitis as a functional somatic syndrome. J Psychosom Res 77 (6): 510–515.

Warren JW, Van De Merwe JP, Nickel JC (2011). Interstitial cystitis/bladder pain syndrome and nonbladder syndromes: Facts and hypotheses. Urology 78 (4): 727–732.

Wessely S, White PD (2013). There is only one functional somatic syndrome. Br J Psychiatr 185: 95–96.

Wessely S, Nimnuan C, Sharpe M (1999). Functional somatic syndromes: one or many? Lancet 354: 936–939.

Williams G, Johnson A (1956). Recurrent urinary retention due to emotional factors; report of a case. Psychosom Med 18 (1): 77–80.

Wiseman O, Swinn MJ, Brady CM et al. (2002). Maximum urethral closure pressure and sphincter volume in women with urinary retention. J Urol 167 (March): 1348–1352.

Wood SK, McFadden K, Griffin T et al. (2013). A corticotropin-releasing factor receptor antagonist improves urodynamic dysfunction produced by social stress or partial bladder outlet obstruction in male rats. Am J Physiol 304 (11): R940–R950.

Yang C, Mayo E (1997). Morbidity of dysfunctional voiding syndrome. Pediatr Urol 49 (3): 445–448.

Handbook of Clinical Neurology, Vol. 139 (3rd series)
Functional Neurologic Disorders
M. Hallett, J. Stone, and A. Carson, Editors
http://dx.doi.org/10.1016/B978-0-12-801772-2.00039-4

Chapter 39

Functional disorders of swallowing

A. BAUMANN[1] AND P.O. KATZ[2]*

[1]*Department of Internal Medicine, Albert Einstein Medical Center, Philadelphia, PA, USA*

[2]*Division of Gastroenterology, Albert Einstein Medical Center, Philadelphia, PA, USA*

Abstract

Swallowing involves complex coordination of the neuromuscular anatomy and physiology of the oropharynx and esophagus, controlled by the enteric and central nervous systems. Dysphagia is classified as either oropharyngeal or esophageal and results from mechanical or structural disturbances. Videofluoroscopy, fiberoptic endoscopic evaluation of swallowing, barium swallow, manometry, and endoscopy are common modalities utilized in diagnosis, but none is as important as a patient's history. Functional dysphagia is a diagnosis of exclusion and is based on Rome criteria. Its mechanism is unknown but potentially related to visceral hypersensitivity, inappropriate pain perception, or unidentified contraction abnormalities. Its management is mainly supportive; however, there is literature to suggest, but not confirm, benefit with the use of antidepressants. Continued understanding of functional dysphagia and other functional esophageal disorders, including globus sensation, will require further investigation into diagnostic algorithms and finding treatment methods.

INTRODUCTION

Swallowing is a natural yet complex process that is taken for granted every day. When structural anatomy or neurophysiology is disturbed, this process becomes dysfunctional. In addition to a thorough history, diagnostic testing is available which helps to classify and understand the etiology of the dysphagia, allowing for appropriate treatment. Functional dysphagia, on the other hand, is a diagnosis of exclusion and its management remains unproven. This chapter will discuss the basic anatomy and physiology of swallowing and the classification and diagnosis of dysphagia, but focus mainly on the current understanding of functional dysphagia and its management. Lastly, it will touch briefly on the functional esophageal disorder globus sensation.

SWALLOWING

Anatomy

A normal swallow relies on structural support from bones and cartilage as well as coordination of several muscles, controlled by cranial and peripheral nerves. The tongue consists of four intrinsic and four extrinsic muscles. The pharynx relies on three constrictor muscles, and the esophagus has two layers of muscle fibers, one circular and one longitudinal in orientation. The tongue, oropharynx, upper esophageal sphincter (UES), and proximal esophageal body are composed of striated muscle. The distal esophageal body and lower esophageal sphincter (LES) are composed of smooth muscle. The remaining esophagus is a transition zone composed of both muscle types (Lind, 2003).

There is a switch in neural control that governs the muscle movements of a swallow. Striated muscle motor endplates are directly innervated by cranial nerves V, VII, IX, X, and XII originating from cell bodies within the nucleus ambiguus of the brainstem, while smooth muscle is innervated by the myenteric plexus, which communicates with the vagus nerve originating from cell bodies within the dorsal motor nucleus. These neurons may be inhibitory or stimulatory to the smooth muscle (Dodds, 1989; Lind, 2003).

*Correspondence to: Philip O. Katz, MD, FACG, Division of Gastroenterology, Albert Einstein Medical Center, 5401 Old York Road, Klein 363, Philadelphia PA 19141, USA. Tel: +1-215-456-8217, E-mail: katzp@einstein.edu

Physiology

There are three phases of swallowing: oral phase, pharyngeal phase, and esophageal phase. The oral phase is voluntary; however, both peripheral sensory input from the oral cavity as well as central nervous system (CNS) control are required to initiate this phase (Cook and Kahrilas, 1999). The oral phase can be further divided into two phases: (1) the oral preparatory phase, when mastication and food bolus formation occur; and (2) the oral transport phase, when the tongue pushes the food bolus against the palate and moves it toward the pharynx.

The pharyngeal phase is an involuntary reflex that moves the bolus from the pharynx to the proximal portion of the esophagus. This phase occurs within 1 second and coordinates: (1) soft-palate elevation and nasopharynx closure; (2) UES relaxation and opening; (3) laryngeal vestibule closure; (4) bolus loading on the tongue; (5) tongue propulsion of the bolus; and (6) pharyngeal evacuation of debris by pharyngeal constrictor contraction (Cook and Kahrilas, 1999). The pharyngeal phase is thus responsible for preventing the bolus from entering the nasal cavity or larynx. The pharyngeal upper, middle, and lower constrictors contract in a slow wave preceded by a rapid relaxation wave, allowing for accommodation of the bolus (Dodds, 1989).

The esophageal phase is also involuntary and moves the bolus distally to the stomach via peristalsis. Primary peristalsis within the esophagus is initiated by the swallow and accompanied by LES relaxation. Secondary peristalsis creates a wave triggered by esophageal distension (Lind, 2003). Secondary peristalsis has lower-amplitude contractions on manometry than primary (Paterson et al., 1991). During peristalsis, the circular muscle layer contracts, generating localized pressure by closing the lumen at progressive intervals along the esophagus. This peristaltic force is theoretically amplified by longitudinal muscle contractions that shorten the contracting segments and lower the degree of force required to move the bolus (Brasseur et al., 2007). Esophageal smooth muscle causes peristalsis similar to pharyngeal constrictors with a rapid relaxation wave followed by a slow contraction wave; however, within the distal esophagus striated muscle creates and modifies peristalsis based on peripheral sensory input (Dodds, 1989). Potentially due to the switch in neural control, there appear to be two contraction waves that form during peristalsis, one above the transition zone of striated and smooth muscle and one below. Manometry and fluoroscopy studies have demonstrated a spatial jump of approximately 3.32 cm across this zone and between the two contraction waves. This area remains susceptible to bolus retention (Ghosh et al., 2006).

DYSPHAGIA

Etiology

Dysphagia is a feeling of abnormal food transit upon swallowing. It typically occurs secondary to abnormal anatomy or physiology and is classified as oropharyngeal or esophageal dysphagia based on its origin.

Oropharyngeal dysphagia is impaired transfer of a bolus from the mouth to the esophagus and can be described as a difficulty with swallow initiation. It is often accompanied by coughing, choking, recurrent aspiration, and subsequent regurgitation upon swallowing. It may originate from a motor neuron disorder, a CNS disorder (e.g., cerebral vascular accident and multiple sclerosis), a neuromuscular junction disorder (e.g., myasthenia gravis), or a striated muscle disorder (e.g., muscular dystrophy) (Lind, 2003). However, other functional and structural causes exist, and include cricopharyngeal dysfunction (UES relaxation dysfunction), malignancy, and even prolonged endotracheal intubation.

Esophageal dysphagia is a difficulty in movement of a bolus from the upper esophagus to the stomach. It is frequently described as a sensation of food lodging or feeling stuck in the chest. Etiologies are typically either structural or motility-related. Structural and mucosal lesions include esophageal strictures, rings and webs, esophagitis (eosinophilic, infectious, or erosive), and malignancy (intrinsic or extrinsic) (Kahrilas and Smout, 2010). Motility disorders can originate from a smooth-muscle disorder (e.g., scleroderma), a myenteric plexus disturbance (e.g., achalasia), or the less understood (e.g., distal esophageal spasm, ineffective esophageal motility, hypertensive LES, and nutcracker esophagus) (Lind, 2003).

Diagnosis

Diagnosis of dysphagia is reliant on a detailed history, which can often delineate oropharyngeal from esophageal causes as well as anatomic from motor causes. For instance, neurologic symptoms often are clues to oropharyngeal dysphagia since it originates mainly from CNS and neuromuscular disorders. In addition, dysphagia to solids and liquids typically reflects an esophageal motility disorder, whereas progressive dysphagia to solids reflects a structural disorder. Various diagnostic testing is subsequently available to confirm the cause.

Videofluoroscopy, transnasal endoscopy, manometry, and fiberoptic endoscopic evaluation of swallowing are used in the diagnosis of oropharyngeal dysphagia. Real-time magnetic resonance imaging is a newer modality that may provide a more comprehensive evaluation of swallowing, and therefore better illustrate where the oropharyngeal dysfunction occurs (Olthoff et al., 2014).

Esophagogastroduodenoscopy (EGD) and barium swallow are traditionally used in the initial diagnosis of esophageal dysphagia, evaluating mainly for structural lesions. In addition, barium swallow as well as esophageal intraluminal impedance testing and radionuclide transit studies provide information about esophageal transit and limited data regarding motility. Esophageal manometry has been the gold standard for evaluation of motility disorders. The recent development of high-resolution manometry has offered potential for greater diagnostic yield (Gyawali et al., 2013).

FUNCTIONAL DYSPHAGIA

Definition

Dysphagia may exist without an identifiable cause. The Rome diagnostic criteria are available for all functional gastrointestinal disorders. Rome III diagnostic criteria define functional dysphagia as three criteria present for the prior 3 months with onset of symptoms at least 6 months before the diagnosis. The three criteria include: a sense of food sticking or passing with difficulty through the esophagus, an absence of objective evidence of gastroesophageal reflux disease (GERD), and an absence of histopathology-based evidence of an esophageal motility disorder (Galmiche et al., 2006).

Diagnosis

Functional dysphagia is a diagnosis of exclusion. An algorithmic approach (Fig. 39.1) should be used to exclude other diagnoses, including performance of an EGD, barium swallow, proton pump inhibitor (PPI) trial, and manometry. EGD with biopsy is performed first to exclude mucosal or structural lesions. If nothing is discovered, then barium swallow should be done to confirm, which may also give insight into possible motility disorders. If reflux symptoms are present, a trial of PPI therapy can be initiated. Response may indicate GERD as the true etiology; however, objective evidence of GERD should be excluded by EGD or pH testing. Then manometry should be preformed to rule out motility disorders. If dysphagia is felt to be cervical, a videofluoroscopic swallowing study is appropriate to evaluate for oropharyngeal disorders. If all of these studies result in no diagnosis, then functional dysphagia is the diagnosis (Kahrilas and Smout, 2010).

Pathophysiology

The pathophysiology of functional dysphagia is poorly understood, and one encompassing mechanism is not defined. This ambiguity may be secondary to the complexity of esophageal neurophysiology. For instance, esophageal pain is thought to be influenced by the hypothalamic–pituitary–adrenal axis and the autonomic nervous system (ANS) through a stress-responsive system; however, this bidirectional brain–gut interaction is not well understood. The enteric nervous system, a division of the ANS, is involved in esophageal motility and sensation, but its roles are also not completely known (Woodland et al., 2013).

Visceral hypersensitivity is thought to be a potential cause of many functional gastrointestinal disorders.

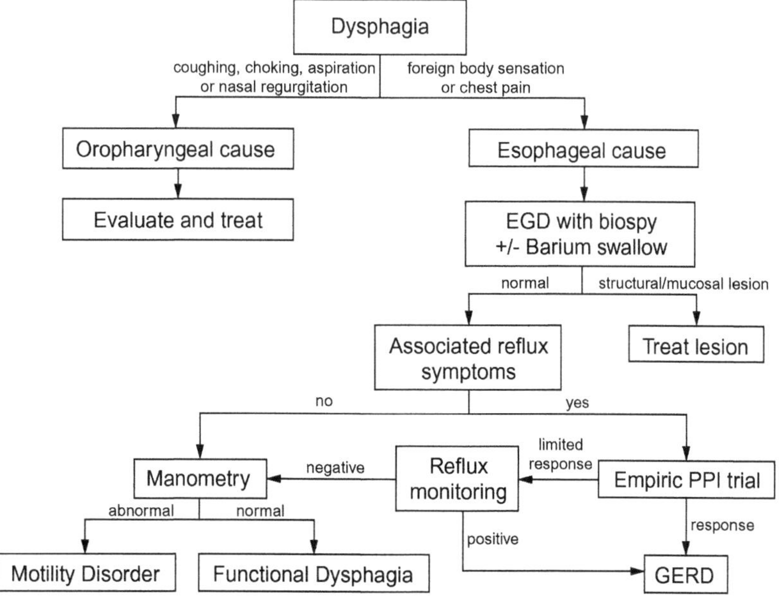

Fig. 39.1. Diagnostic algorithm for dysphagia. EGD, esophagogastroduodenoscopy; PPI, proton pump inhibitor; GERD, gastroesophageal reflux disorder.

For instance, studies have demonstrated heightened sensitivity of the esophagus to balloon distension in patients with functional chest pain (Barish et al., 1986; Richter et al., 1986). It is thought that mechanical stimuli are inappropriately interpreted as painful due to disturbance in the brain–gut axis causing sensory input upregulation. This may occur due to variations in: (1) mechanoreceptor activation within the gut, involving the ENS; (2) sensory conduction along the spinal column; or (3) sensory processing within the brainstem (Sarnelli et al., 2004). These alterations lead to peripheral or central sensitization. Peripheral sensitization is thought to potentially be caused by mucosal inflammation within the gut facilitating stimulatory access to nociceptors and sensitizing afferents to increasing amounts of noxious stimuli (Woodland et al., 2013).

Functional dysphagia has also been proposed to be secondary to motility disturbances causing abnormal transit. Patients with nonobstructive dysphagia, but not normal individuals, have demonstrated symptoms in association with repetitive, simultaneous contractions distal to an inflated intraesophageal balloon during a manometry study. This may demonstrate that spasms distal to a food bolus cause functional resistance to bolus transit, and therefore, a sensation of dysphagia (Deschner et al., 1989).

Thus, balloon distension, and in theory a food bolus, could cause esophageal symptoms either via inappropriate sensory perception or abnormal transit resulting from uncoordinated contractions. Further study has demonstrated that esophageal sensory and motor abnormalities may occur through different mechanisms in patients with functional esophageal disorders while both contributing to patient symptoms. This would support both theories; however, functional dysphagia has been more specifically linked to sensory disturbance independently of manometry findings (Clouse et al., 1991).

Treatment

Treatment of functional dysphagia is mainly supportive, including reassurance, avoidance of precipitating foods, and proper mastication (Galmiche et al., 2006). Reassurance benefits many patients with functional gastrointestinal disorders by emphasizing the benign nature of their disease. Medical and endoscopic treatments are available, but not validated in functional dysphagia patients. No randomized controlled trials exist for the treatment of functional dysphagia. The tetracyclic antidepressant, trazodone, tricyclic antidepressants, and selective serotonin reuptake inhibitors have been studied as potential treatment options in functional esophageal disorders, because these disorders are thought to be related to esophageal hypersensitivity. For instance, trazodone modified symptoms in patients with esophageal contraction abnormalities in a small controlled trial (Clouse et al., 1987). Imipramine has been shown to decrease pain in healthy males and noncardiac chest pain patients (Cannon et al., 1994; Peghini et al., 1998). Citalopram has been shown to raise stimuli thresholds and benefit patients with esophageal hypersensitivity and functional heartburn (Broekaert et al., 2006; Viazis et al., 2012). Although psychiatric comorbidities are common in these patients, the effects of these drugs appear to be independent of psychiatric effects and do not appear to affect esophageal motility (Clouse et al., 1987; Cannon et al., 1994). A recent systematic review including randomized controlled trials showed that antidepressants cause visceral analgesia in functional esophageal disorders; however, none of these trials included functional dysphagia (Weijenborg et al., 2015). There is hope to extrapolate available data to functional dysphagia patients but caution is needed.

Empiric dilation of the esophagus is another treatment modality, but available studies show conflicting data. One randomized study showed no benefit of empiric dilation with an 18-mm balloon over a matched sham group in patients with dysphagia lacking endoscopic evidence of an etiology (Scolapio et al., 2001). Another randomized study in patients with non-obstructive dysphagia compared 26 F and 50 F Maloney dilators. Both dilators showed insignificant improvement in frequency of dysphagia, but the larger dilator showed significant improvement in the variety of foods causing dysphagia (e.g., diet score). Of note, 43.4% of participants had nonspecific motility disorders (Colon et al., 2000).

GLOBUS SENSATION

Globus sensation is another functional esophageal disorder that should be distinguished from dysphagia. The Rome III diagnostic criteria define it as a nonpainful feeling of a lump in the throat, which occurs between meals and in the absence of dysphagia, odynophagia, GERD, or a histopathology-based esophageal motility disorder. These criteria must exist for at least 3 months with onset 6 months before diagnosis (Galmiche et al., 2006). Globus sensation is also a diagnosis of exclusion and diagnostic testing is usually governed by history and may include an otolaryngologic specialty evaluation, EGD, PPI trial, manometry or pH-impedance monitoring. The Rome criteria define globus as a single diagnosis rather than as a part of a syndrome; thus, if dysphagia or GERD coexists, then evaluation of these diagnoses should precede workup for globus sensation (Galmiche et al., 2006; Kahrilas and Smout, 2010; Selleslagh et al., 2014). Although psychiatric disorders like anxiety and depression have been shown to coexist with functional gastrointestinal disorders, it is unclear which comes first. Having a diagnosis of exclusion can make a patient feel misunderstood and unhopeful (Selleslagh et al., 2014).

The etiology of globus sensation is undefined, as the current literature includes weak methodology. Similar to functional dysphagia, oropharyngeal structural lesions, hypertensive UES, GERD, esophageal dysmotility, and psychiatric disorders have been investigated as associations. The results of these studies are conflicting, with no true consensus. Akin to other functional gastrointestinal disorders, visceral hypersensitivity is a probable underlying component. Globus sensation is unlikely to be defined by one unifying pathology but rather varies amongst individuals and/or is multifactorial (Selleslagh et al., 2014).

After exhaustive investigation, including PPI trial, treatment is mainly reassurance and supportive care, as globus sensation often resolves on its own (Galmiche et al., 2006; Kahrilas and Smout, 2010; Selleslagh et al., 2014). However, speech therapy was successful in one small controlled trial (Khalil et al., 2003), but further research is needed. Additionally, antidepressants and cognitive-behavioral therapy may be considered in the presence of coexisting diagnosed psychiatric disorders (Lee and Kim, 2012).

CONCLUSION

Functional dysphagia is a diagnosis of exclusion, without a complete understanding of pathophysiology or proven treatment modalities. Treatment is anecdotal and based on studies done in other functional esophageal disorders. Currently each case should be individualized with attention to cost versus benefit before starting any treatment. Reassurance of the benign nature of the symptoms, appropriate use of antidepressant medications, and dietary modifications are the mainstay of treatment. In appropriate patients empiric esophageal dilation may be considered. Future research should focus on assessing quality of life and symptom burden in this population in hopes of improving patient outcomes.

Globus sensation should not be confused with dysphagia; however, like functional dysphagia, it is a diagnosis of exclusion without a unifying etiology. It often resolves on its own with reassurance. Clinically, physicians should focus on coordination of patient care via communication between otolaryngologic specialists, gastroenterologists, psychiatrists, and primary care physicians.

References

Barish CF, Castell DO, Richter JE (1986). Graded esophageal balloon distension: a new provocative test for noncardiac chest pain. Dig Dis Sci 31: 1292–1298.

Brasseur JG, Nicosia MA, Pal A et al. (2007). Function of longitudinal vs. circular muscle fibers in esophageal peristalsis, deduced with mathematical modeling. World J Gastroenterol 13: 1335–1346.

Broekaert D, Fischler B, Sifrim D et al. (2006). Influence of citalopram, a selective serotonin reuptake inhibitor, on oesophageal hypersensitivity: a double-blind, placebo-controlled study. Aliment Pharmacol Ther 23: 365–370.

Cannon RO, Quyyumi AA, Mincemoyer R et al. (1994). Imipramine in patients with chest pain despite normal coronary angiograms. N Engl J Med 330: 1411–1417.

Clouse RE, Lustman PJ, Eckert TC et al. (1987). Low-dose trazodone for symptomatic patients with esophageal contraction abnormalities. A double-blind, placebo-controlled trial. Gastroenterology 92: 1027–1036.

Clouse RE, McCord GS, Lustman PJ et al. (1991). Clinical correlates of abnormal sensitivity to intraesophageal balloon distension. Dig Dis Sci 36: 1040–1045.

Colon VJ, Young MA, Ramirez FC (2000). The short- and long-term efficacy of empirical esophageal dilation in patients with nonobstructive dysphagia: a prospective, randomized study. Am J Gastroenterol 95: 910–913.

Cook IJ, Kahrilas PJ (1999). AGA technical review on management of oropharyngeal dysphagia. Gastroenterology 116: 455–478.

Deschner WK, Maher KA, Cattau EL et al. (1989). Manometric responses to balloon distention in patients with nonobstructive dysphagia. Gastroenterology 97: 1181–1185.

Dodds WJ (1989). The physiology of swallowing. Dysphagia 3: 171–176.

Galmiche JP, Clouse RE, Balint A et al. (2006). Functional esophageal disorders. Gastroenterology 130: 1459–1465.

Ghosh SK, Janiak P, Schwizer W et al. (2006). Physiology of the esophageal pressure transition zone: separate contraction waves above and below. Am J Physiol Gastrointest Liver Physiol 290: G568–G576.

Gyawali CP, Bredenoord AJ, Conklin JL et al. (2013). Evaluation of esophageal motor function in clinical practice. Neurogastroenterol Motil 25: 99–133.

Kahrilas PJ, Smout AJ (2010). Esophageal disorders. Am J Gastroenterol 105: 747–756.

Khalil HS, Bridger MW, Hilton-Pierce M et al. (2003). The use of speech therapy in the treatment of globus pharyngeus patients. A randomized controlled trial. Rev Laryngol Otol Rhinol 124: 187–190.

Lee BE, Kim GH (2012). Globus pharyngeus: a review of its etiology, diagnosis and treatment. World J Gastroenterol 18: 2462–2471.

Lind CD (2003). Dysphagia: evaluation and treatment. Gastroenterol Clin N Am 32: 553–575.

Olthoff A, Zhang S, Schweizer R et al. (2014). On the physiology of normal swallowing as revealed by magnetic resonance imaging in real time. Gastroenterol Res Pract 2014: 493174.

Paterson WG, Hynna-Liepert TT, Selucky M (1991). Comparison of primary and secondary esophageal peristalsis in humans: effect of atropine. Am J Physiol 260: G52–G57.

Peghini PL, Katz PO, Castell DO (1998). Imipramine decreases oesophageal pain perception in human male volunteers. Gut 42: 807–813.

Richter JE, Barish CF, Castell DO (1986). Abnormal sensory perception in patients with esophageal chest pain. Gastroenterology 91: 845–852.

Sarnelli G, Vandenberghe J, Tack J (2004). Visceral hypersensitivity in functional disorders of the upper gastrointestinal tract. Dig Liver Dis 36: 371–376.

Scolapio JS, Gostout CJ, Schroeder KW et al. (2001). Dysphagia without endoscopically evident disease: to dilate or not. Am J Gastroenterol 96: 327–330.

Selleslagh M, van Oudenhove L, Pauwels A et al. (2014). The complexity of globus: a multidisciplinary perspective. Nat Rev Gastroenterol Hepatol 11: 220–233.

Viazis N, Keyogiou A, Kanellopoulos AK et al. (2012). Selective serotonin reuptake inhibitors for the treatment of hypersensitive esophagus: a randomized, double-blind, placebo-controlled study. Am J Gastroenterol 107: 1662–1667.

Weijenborg PW, de Schepper HS, Smout AJ et al. (2015). Effects of antidepressants in patients with functional esophageal disorders or gastroesophageal reflux disease: a systematic review. Clin Gastroenterol Hepatol 13: 251–259. e1.

Woodland P, Sifrim D, Krarup AL et al. (2013). The neurophysiology of the esophagus. Ann N Y Acad Sci 1300: 53–70.

Handbook of Clinical Neurology, Vol. 139 (3rd series)
Functional Neurologic Disorders
M. Hallett, J. Stone, and A. Carson, Editors
http://dx.doi.org/10.1016/B978-0-12-801772-2.00040-0

Chapter 40

Pediatric functional neurologic symptoms

P.J. GRATTAN-SMITH* AND R.C. DALE
Department of Neurology, Westmead Children's Hospital, Sydney, Australia

Abstract

Functional neurologic disorders (FND) of children have many similarities to those of adults, and there is a potential to learn much from the study of FND in children. In this chapter we discuss multiple aspects of pediatric FND. These include their frequency, historic features, the diagnosis, and controversies over the nature of FND and the "correct" name that should be used. We also discuss methods of informing the child and family of the diagnosis, treatment, and prognosis. FND of children typically affect girls in the 10–14-years age range. The presentation is often polysymptomatic, with pain and lethargy accompanying loss of motor function. A common situation is a perfectionistic child who has taken on too much in her academic, sporting, cultural, and social life. Some children respond readily to treatment, but others have a prolonged illness.

PEDIATRIC FUNCTIONAL NEUROLOGIC SYMPTOMS

Functional neurologic disorders (FND) of children have many similarities to those of adults, and in this chapter there will be overlap with other parts of the book. However, there is a potential to learn much from the study of FND in children. The naïve simplicity of FND in the young child may give us clues to the nature of FND in older children and adults. There is also a long-standing belief that FND in adults can result from the persisting aftereffects of childhood trauma, and adults with FND may have first developed their symptoms in childhood.

The first great difficulty when approaching FND at all ages is the choice of a name that is acceptable to both the patient and the doctors who make the diagnosis. Throughout this chapter we will use the term "functional." However, we have misgivings about this word, which will be discussed later. In quoting various authors we will use the term they employed, realizing that, for example, "hysteria" is generally not now regarded as an acceptable term. "Functional," "hysteria," "conversion disorder," "psychogenic," "symptoms unexplained by organic disease," or "medically unexplained illness" will be taken to have essentially the same meaning.

HOW COMMON ARE PEDIATRIC FUNCTIONAL NEUROLOGIC SYMPTOMS?

Taylor observed: "Hysteria, the laying claim to sickness for which there is no objective evidence, is a commonplace reaction, and those who become dignified by a formal diagnosis are a severe, extreme or fortuitous selection" (Taylor, 1986).

There have been two recent surveillance reports of the incidence of conversion disorder in childhood. In the study of Ani et al. (2013), over a 15-month surveillance period there were 204 confirmed cases in the UK and Ireland, giving an estimated 12-month incidence of 1.30/100 000. When looked at in terms of age, the incidence was 0.26/100 000 among children younger than 10 years and 3.04/100 000 for children 10–15 years old.

Koslowska et al. (2007), in a surveillance study of Australian children under 16 years of age, found an annual incidence of conversion disorder of 2.3/100 000. In children younger than 10 years of age, the incidence was 0.8/100 000. However, in New South Wales, the overall incidence was 4.2/100 000, perhaps due to more diligent reporting.

*Correspondence to: P.J. Grattan-Smith, Department of Neurology, Westmead Children's Hospital, Westmead 2145, Sydney, NSW, Australia. Tel: +61-414-765-835, E-mail: pgrattan-smith@iinet.net.au

HOW DO CHILDREN WITH FUNCTIONAL NEUROLOGIC DISORDERS PRESENT?

In the study by Ani et al. (2013), the age range was 7–15 years, with a median age of 12.5 years. Three-fourths were females, and the female predominance was retained in younger children, being 76% of those under 10 years. No child was seen younger than 7 years of age. The core symptoms were: motor weakness (63%), abnormal movements (43%), nonepileptic seizures (40%), anesthesia/paresthesia (32%), diminished consciousness (29%), visual loss (23%), limb paralysis (22%), loss of speech (19%), and hearing loss (8%). In 69% of the children there was more than one core symptom. Associated symptoms include pain (55%) and fatigue (34%).

In the study by Koslowska et al. (2007), the average age was 11.8 years and 71% were female. Multiple symptoms were again seen, with 64% having more than one symptom and 15% three or more symptoms. Disturbance of voluntary motor function was present in 63%, with 37% having paresis and 33% an abnormal gait. Abnormal movements were seen in 17% and nonepileptic seizures in 23%. There was an almost identical incidence of pain and fatigue, with pain present in 56% and fatigue in 34%.

From these two studies from different ends of the earth, it can be seen that, when doctors diagnose conversion disorder in childhood, there is a typical profile. The child is most commonly between 10 and 14 years of age, is female, has multiple symptoms and, as well as loss of function, often also has sensory disturbance and fatigue. A surveillance study, of course, has significant limitations.

In a case review done 20–25 years earlier, the clinical features of 52 children admitted to hospital with conversion disorder over a 10-year period were reviewed (Grattan-Smith et al., 1988). Although this was a chart review study, the findings were almost identical to the two surveys. Seventy-five percent of the children were female and 62% were between the age of 10 and 12 years. There were three children under the age of 8. An abnormal gait was present in 66%. Of those with an abnormal gait, 44% could not move at all with leg pain and most of the remainder had classic presentations such as monoparesis, paraplegia, hemiparesis, and ataxia. In two children walking was impeded by a generalized tremor, and two had a "parkinsonian" gait. Other presentations included nonepileptic seizures, sneezing, stridor, aphasia, and globus hystericus. Overall, 77% complained of pain, paresthesia, or anesthesia.

There have been multiple studies with similar findings and it is clear that the presentation of FND in children has a remarkable similarity over time and place.

HISTORIC FEATURES

The history of FND probably stretches back to the beginning of time, or at least to the ancient Egyptians. Both Mayer (1899) and Hecht (1907) believed that it was Briquet who was the person most responsible for the realization that FND occurred not only in women and men, but also in children. Hecht comments:

> *It was reserved for Briquet in 1859, to correlate facts from his vast material that have given unqualified support from that day to this of the occurrence of juvenile hysteria as a common affection. His apparently extravagant claim that one-fifth of all cases of hysteria are developed before the twelfth year and that about 5 percent of the patients are males has found reiteration in the most recent figures by Bruns, who states that the ratios established "are not excessive, but less than the actual truth."*

In the controversies and heated debates that have characterized the last 100 or more years of thought about FND, a criticism that is frequently leveled at opponents is the view that they are out of date and do not have a grasp of modern thought on the topic. However, as the philosopher Santayana observed: "Those who cannot remember the past are condemned to repeat it." Between 1897 and 1907 in the *Journal of the American Medical Association* there were four articles published with the identical title, "Hysteria in children" (Burr, 1897; Biller, 1898; Mayer, 1899; Hecht, 1907). A quick review of these articles shows us that, although there has been much name changing and name calling in the last 100 years, doctors of that time faced the exact same problems with diagnosis and treatment of FND that we do. To illustrate this, brief extracts from these articles are listed below.

Epidemiology

Holt's view that hysteria is "very rare before the seventh or eighth year, occurring most often in children after the age of 10" is cited. Hecht adds: "The average sex ratio between children is 2 to 1 in favour of the female, but with approaching puberty the tendency is for female types to increase and male types to decrease."

The predicament of the child

Mayer:

> *Often the cause of the child's hysteria is fright caused by a drunken father nightly beating mother and child, or fear of a whipping by a stern teacher.*

Biller:

[children with hysteria] suffer greatly from competitive examinations at school, and from the extra work that is often imposed upon them in preparing for school entertainments – especially in preparing for public recitations.

The provocation of an FND by minor injury or illness

Hecht:

That hysterical symptoms are frequently engrafted on symptoms of organic disease and long outlast the latter, is, of course, not to be lost sight of ... Slight cause, then, and grave consequence should arouse immediately a suspicion of hysteria.

Controversies over the cause

Mayer:

Before proceeding further let us see what the basis of hysteria is. It is a question often asked, but never answered. Still, there is an underlying groundwork to every case. We do not refer to hypotheses. Many of these have been advanced, as that of Janet, that hysteria is due to a weakening of the psychologic synthesis; of Myers, that it is due to a disease of the hypnoid stratum, and of Liebermeister that it is a subcortical disturbance.

The difficulty in separating organic disease from FND

Hecht:

The greatest difficulty lies not so much in mistaking organic disease for hysteria, and vice versa, as in failing to appreciate that organic disease may be and frequently is complicated by hysteria.

Malingering

Mayer:

Just as hard as it is to diagnose the hysteric or organic nature of an affection in some cases, is it to distinguish simulation from hysteria.

Treatment of the symptom or the underlying cause?

Burr:

I have used the word cure several times. I wish it to be understood to refer only to the specific attack and not to the inherited predisposition. We usually cure not the hysteria but the attack ... These children need not only treatment for the attack, but most careful education of the will and the emotions, to save them in the future from suffering from hysteria.

Treatment difficulties and the tendency of families to seek alternative methods

Biller:

the patient becomes dissatisfied and passes, frequently, into the hands of some quack or charlatan, who thrives by accidentally – and probably unconsciously – knowing how to take advantage of some of the tricks of this powerful but susceptible enemy of the human family.

Prognosis

Hecht:

Just a word in reference to the prognosis, which in children is infinitely better than adults.

This brief review reminds us that in discussing FND we need to retain a sense of humility as, rather than standing on the shoulders of giants, we may be blindly stumbling along a well-worn path.

DIAGNOSIS OF FUNCTIONAL NEUROLOGICAL DISORDERS

In thinking about the signs that alert us that a child may have a FND, a historic perspective is helpful. Charcot, who believed hysteria was a functional (in the sense of organic) disorder identified stigmata of the disease, including hemianesthesia, the provocation of hysteric attacks by ovarian irritation, their cessation by ovarian pressure, and the presence of hysterogenic zones. (For a detailed description, see Gamgee (1878) and Jane Avril's recollections of her time at the Salpêtrière (Bonduelle and Gelfand, 1999). From these accounts it is clear that at that time the Salpêtrière itself had become a hysterogenic zone.)

In 1922 Henry Head described the positive signs of hysteria:psychogenic

These physical signs are as definite and specific as those of any other disease. Hysteria is sometimes said to "imitate" organic affections; but this is a highly misleading statement. The mimicry can only deceive an observer ignorant of the signs of hysteria or content with perfunctory examination.

Many subsequent multiedition neurologic textbooks such as those of Walshe and de Jong gave detailed descriptions of how to recognize FND.

In 1965 Eliot Slater attacked the existence of hysteria and took particular exception to Head's paper:

> *What are the positive signs of "hysteria"? Unfortunately Head could not describe any common characteristic by which these signs could be recognized, and he dealt with them by enumeration... What is given is a list, which might be enlarged without limit... The only thing that "hysterical" patients can be shown to have in common is that they are all patients.*

For the next 30 years doctors dealing with both adults and children either did not make the diagnosis of FND, or when they made it, were reminded they were likely to be misdiagnosing a substantial proportion of their patients, who in fact had an organic disease. Goodyer (1986) said of the diagnosis of hysteria in children: "Somewhere between 25–30% of children who receive this diagnosis will be shown to have an organic illness likely to have caused the presenting symptoms."

In 1998, a paper was published by Crimlisk et al., entitled "Slater revisited." The authors reported 64 patients with "medically unexplained motor symptoms," and at follow-up only 3 had developed an organic illness that fully or partly explained their psychiatric presentation. In 2009 Stone et al. published a multinational paper of patients with "symptoms unexplained by organic disease," where at 18-month follow-up "only 4 out of 1030 patients (0.4%) had acquired an organic disease diagnosis that was unexpected at initial assessment and plausibly the cause of the patients' original symptoms." Multiple papers have come to a similar conclusion. The tide has turned and the general view is that organic disease and FND are most often clearly separable.

In 2012 Edwards and Bhatia, in discussing functional movement disorders (FMD), observed:

> *The key clinical feature that separates patients with FMD from those with organic movement disorders is that the movements have features that one would usually associate with voluntary movement (distractibility, resolution with placebo, and presence of pre-movement potentials), but patients report them as being involuntary and not under their control. There seem to be just two logical explanations for this feature: either movements are deliberately feigned or there must be a brain mechanism that allows voluntary movement to occur but to be experienced subjectively as involuntary.*

Edwards and Bhatia believe the second alternative applies. In framing their argument in such a black-and-white fashion, they are at the same time promoting it. The concept that symptoms could be deliberately feigned introduces a harsh moral judgment that would be unacceptable to almost all patients with FND, and most doctors who treat them.

Nevertheless, we believe this is an extremely important statement. The "apparently voluntary" impression provides a unifying principle in the detection of FND. It can be applied to its kaleidoscope of manifestations and is a guiding principle for the "lists" of signs of FND. It explains how for so long neurologists have been able to make the diagnosis of an FND without relying on the psychiatric history. Walshe (1952) at least hinted at the same conclusion:

> *Current theories of the genesis of the psychoneuroses require that the psychological processes underlying them should be below the threshold of consciousness, and the clear evidence to the contrary sometimes provided by clinical experience has been ignored or suppressed in the interests of theory.*

Brain (1955) in discussing the symptoms observed:

> *it follows that the hysterical symptom is always the expression of an idea in the patient's mind. Thus hysterical aphonia expresses the idea "I have lost my voice," hysterical paralysis the idea "I cannot move my limb" and so on. This fact is of great diagnostic importance, for it is impossible that the patient's idea of a symptom should correspond with a similar symptom produced by organic disease, and the resulting discrepancy renders possible the diagnosis of the one from the other.*

There is insufficient space to systematically go through all the signs that can be seen in children with FND. They are substantially the same as those that occur in adults and have been recognized for more than 100 years. The diagnosis is usually easy in the young child. The following examples seen by the authors reflect the broad variety of presentations.

1. A child complaining of anesthesia is asked to close her eyes and to say "yes" if she can feel the subtle touch of cotton wool and "no" if she can't feel it. Every time she is touched she says "no."
2. A child is unable to walk but can lift his legs against gravity when lying on a bed. His tone, reflexes and Babinski sign are normal. When held upright his legs are retracted tightly up against his abdomen and held there, making it impossible for him to walk.

3. A child complains of hemianesthesia. During the history, when asked if stress could have a role in her symptoms, she replies politely "it is not possible, doctor!" Examination reveals total hemianesthesia to all sensory modalities. This operates at the exact midline. When a vibration fork is placed on her forehead 1 cm from the dividing line on the "normal" side, she accurately experiences vibration and can appreciate the cold metal. When it is placed 1 cm on the "abnormal" side, she can feel nothing at all.
4. A child complains of double vision which persists when one eye is closed. A pen is held 1 meter from her nose and then as it moved towards her nose she is asked to say how many pens she can see. She replies "2," "3," "4," and then "lots" just as it reaches her nose.

In the young child there can be an almost comical aspect to the symptoms. This usually evokes a strong care-giving approach from the parents, and at the same time they are usually content that there is no serious underlying disease. In older children, especially when the problem has been of long standing and many doctors have been involved, diagnosis and management can be extremely difficult. There are often multiple symptoms, combined with extreme anxiety and distress, which reverberate back and forth between the child and the parents. If, for example, the presentation is with an immobile and painful limb that is cold and wasted, it is much more difficult to be sure the problem is functional. Although the signs of FND are reliable, it is by no means always easy to decide they are present. When there are a large number of symptoms and signs in someone who is otherwise well ("too much smoke and not enough fire") or there is a steady accumulation of clinical improbabilities, the diagnosis of FND is considered, but it can take quite some time to convince yourself of this, let alone the child and family.

As well as the sense of a movement appearing voluntary, we would add that if there is a feeling of move and countermove, then this is highly suggestive of an FND. For example, an intelligent older child with a tremor who is asked to do "serial sevens" may give hopelessly incorrect answers, defeating the purpose of the examiner in asking this. Fahn and Jankovic (2007), in discussing the role of distraction in diagnosing psychogenic tremor in adults, observe: "many patients are too aware to distract easily." In the motor examination Head (1922) described "an instinctive opposition to external commands." Walshe (1952) wrote of "The Law of Antagonistic Effort: ... another feature of hysterical weakness is the tendency to perform a movement opposite to that demanded." The impression of a mind actively at work is an important clue.

ARE FUNCTIONAL NEUROLOGIC DISORDERS PSYCHOGENIC?

There is a current controversy about whether the term "psychogenic" movement disorders should be replaced by "functional" movement disorders. Edwards et al. (2014a) believe we should stop using "psychogenic," "a term that defines the disorder with regard to a proposed aetiology, which is poorly defined and is not supported by current evidence..."

What is the evidence for psychologic disturbance in children diagnosed as having FND? In the two recent surveys of FND, antecedent stressors were reported, in 62% of children by Koslowska et al. (2007), and 81% by Ani et al. (2013). In the paper of Ani et al., the most common antecedent stressor was bullying at school. How do we assess the significance of such stressors? Slater (1965) correctly asserted: "trouble, discord, anxiety and frustration are so prevalent at all stages of life that their mere occurrence near to the time of onset of an illness does not mean very much." What about the psychologic state of the children? In the study of Ani et al., 78% (160/204) of children where a psychiatric history was available had had no known mental disorder prior to the episode of conversion disorder. Of those with a premorbid psychiatric diagnosis, anxiety disorder was reported in 21/200 (11%) and depressive disorder in 10/194 (5%). This supports the proposition that most children with FND appear "normal" psychologically before the onset of FND.

The difficulty here is: how do you assess psychologic health? In the Freudian era therapists could see problems everywhere:

> *jealousies between brothers and sisters, a scolding nurse, a tyrannous father, or a spoiling mother. However, there is no need whatever to stop at this point, for any logical and sufficiently persistent search for the "cause" will recognise the importance of the breast as being the causal centre of all subsequent disasters, in that it was administered, whether injudiciously or not, by the mother. And why stop here, for there is the awful event of the birth trauma itself (Howe, 1934).*

The psychiatry pendulum has now swung far in the direction of a "biologic" approach. Shorvon (2007), in discussing the battles of Freud and his followers, observed:

> *All this seems faintly ridiculous to contemporary psychiatric theory, bound up as it is in receptor*

> *chemistry and functional neuroimaging (contemplate the mockery of this in future generations) – but it was a battle of ferocious intensity and importance at the time.*

It is a not uncommon experience to see a child who seems clearly to have an FND and an identifiable cause such as too much pressure to succeed, and be told that a psychologist has given the child the "all clear." In a sense, this is correct, in that the child has not suffered a severe trauma such as sexual abuse (a concern from the time of Freud but identified as a possible cause in only 4% of the children in the Koslowska et al. (2007) study).

We have found Taylor's writings helpful in understanding the genesis of FND (Taylor, 1986). He notes: "there is little evidence to support the idea of psychopathology in children with hysterical symptoms." Taylor believes FND "are generated as a defence mechanism" and children "exhibit distress through whatever scope is left to them. The body speaks what the tongue cannot utter." Taylor describes the elements of pediatric FND. The first requirement is the child is in a "predicament" where all apparent solutions are blocked. The second is an "ally" who helps to "promote the sickness." The ally acts "like a manager and will vigorously defend the 'right to be sick' and pursue disease explanations relentlessly." The third component is a "model of the sickness." The model can appear in many ways. There may be a family member with Parkinson's disease or the child may have seen a television program about Lyme disease.

In Taylor's formulation, doctors can be a particular problem:

> *Doctors in particular, and other health care workers to some extent, can provide well for all these elements. They can block alternative explanations by patients, or by failing to take an adequate history of their predicament fail totally to discern it. They are powerful allies in sickness promotion, and can be sucked into the system quite unwittingly, especially if they have an investment in a biomedical diagnosis. They provide a variety of models and can offer suggestions which improve the credibility of the sickness.*

A common predicament currently encountered is the girl who is simply doing too much. She may be the best student in the class, the class captain, may excel at multiple sports, do dancing or gymnastics, drama or debating, and play one or more musical instruments. Often she has taken all this on willingly, and it is not due to parental pressure. When asked, how much time do you spend per week doing absolutely nothing? she will look back incredulously. Over time, the need for perfection in so many areas is too much and sickness is the only defense. These children can exhibit the same determination and persistence in being sick as they do in all other areas of their life. Grattan-Smith et al. (1988) (looking at children mainly from the 1970s, when life seemed a lot easier) called them the "difficult" group, as they presented particular problems in both diagnosis and management. "They were generally 'good' children, serious minded, compliant and perfectionistic, who came from families with high expectations of them and were anxious about illness." There are, of course, many other predicaments, including physical or sexual abuse, but these seem to be a relatively uncommon cause in recent reports of FND.

INFORMING THE CHILD AND FAMILY OF THE DIAGNOSIS

Neurologists are rarely involved in the treatment of FND but have a crucial role in informing the child and family of the diagnosis. Part of the argument for "functional" is that it is a word that is more acceptable to patients. However, rather than the word, it is the diagnosis of the child having a psychologic problem that is unacceptable to many patients and families (and doctors). Paget wrote in 1873: "To call a patient hysterical is taken by many people as meaning that she is silly, or shamming, or could get well if she pleased." This remains a common reaction. It is therefore of extreme importance that the discussion of the diagnosis of pediatric FND is done in a careful and sensitive manner and with plenty of time available. The first step is countering the suspicion that, cloaked in medical professionalism, you are accusing the child of "faking it."

There are many ways to have this discussion and each of us has to find a way that feels natural and is effective. The following approach is simply one example. We prefer the term "stress-related" to "functional" or "psychogenic." The discussion takes place once it is clear that organic disease has been excluded as far as can be done reasonably. Often this is after blood tests and magnetic resonance imaging (MRI) scans have been performed. These tests have an important role in persuading the child and the family that the symptoms are being taken seriously, and the child does not have a brain tumor or multiple sclerosis. Investigations should be done as soon as possible and not strung out over weeks, if at all possible. At the time of ordering the tests the child and family should be told that a stress-related problem seems highly likely, but we want to be careful.

The child is seen with the parents and, given that most often the child is 10 years or older, the discussion is directed towards the child with the parents listening and free to ask questions as the discussion proceeds. It follows these broad lines:

As I have previously suggested, your problems are very likely to be stress-related. For more than a hundred years doctors have recognized that the signs and symptoms you have indicate that you are under stress. This is good news. There are many diseases that leave children severely disabled or that are fatal, and here there can be a complete recovery.

I commonly see children with such reactions. From my own experience and many articles written by doctors, it is clear that children with these reactions are not disturbed or "crazy" and are not being abused at home. Rather, they are usually high-achieving kids who are very thoughtful and considerate towards other people. At the same time they tend to want to keep their feelings to themselves so as not to worry others, especially their parents.

Over a period of time the child comes under the pressure of multiple stressful events. Each one by itself is manageable but they build up and act all together. The child tries to ignore them and keep them out of the conscious mind but they are there. There is then often an injury or illness that would usually cause a problem that would only last a few days. However, the stress then takes over. The symptoms then last much longer and are much more severe than they otherwise would have been. It can take some time to get back to normal, but full recovery is expected.

One way of looking at this is that the body knows it is under pressure and as a defense against stress "shuts down" to bring a change in the situation.

The discussion usually includes many questions from the parents (and child), often initially with complete disbelief that a child previously so high-functioning could be brought down by stress. At that time historic examples such as Horatio Nelson and Florence Nightingale can be discussed as people who were very high achievers despite being subject to stress. The concept of the necessity of stress for peak performance is also covered, accompanied with the advice that stress is "a good servant but a poor master." What is needed is some finetuning, not a drastic change. The child is told that it is important to always put in a full effort, but it is impossible to be perfect at all times. Depending on how the meeting is going, giants of the past can be cited, such as, "perfect is the enemy of good" (Voltaire) or "better a diamond with a flaw than a pebble without" (Confucius).

Although in FMD the apparently voluntary nature of the signs is important in making the diagnosis, a discussion with the child and family of whether or not the signs could be deliberately feigned is recipe for certain disaster. We believe this is not the place for the moral judgments implicit in psychiatric terms such as unconscious, conscious, factitious, and malingering. It is far better to consider the signs neutrally, as a signal of distress, and make plans for the best way to deal with them.

This discussion is aimed at putting the concept of external stresses being brought to bear on a sensitive child before the child and family. There is no need to try to win every point in the discussion. Nor should it be expected that the child and family will agree with you immediately. Some families seem never to agree, but in the study of Ani et al. (2013), "over 90% of families had some level of acceptance for a nonorganic explanation." Depending on how unwell the child is, and the response to these suggestions, plans can then be made for future management.

TREATMENT OF FUNCTIONAL NEUROLOGIC DISORDERS

After being told their problems are likely to be the result of stress combined with suggestions of how to best reduce this, some children readily accept the concept and the symptoms settle quickly. Others have prolonged illnesses. These children require psychiatric evaluation and often admission to hospital. Here the treatment is usually multidisciplinary and may include family therapy, individual psychotherapy, medication for comorbid anxiety and depression, physiotherapy, and occupational therapy (Calvert and Jureidini, 2003; Koslowska et al., 2012). The stay is usually not short: "admissions typically last two weeks" (Koslowska et al., 2012). Helping these children involves intensive and persistent effort from many people. Emphasis is placed on the physical signs; for example, the child may be given a program of walking progressively longer distances each day or two, e.g., walk 10 metres (Monday/Tuesday), 25 metres (Wednesday/Thursday), 20 metres twice (Friday/Saturday), and 50 metres (Sunday/Monday) (Calvert and Jureidini, 2003).

In terms of the concept of the child's predicament and models, it is interesting to see that part of the program of Koslowska et al. (2007) involves a limitation of parental visiting hours. These are restricted to 2–3 hours at the end of the day. They note: "We have retained this component of treatment because we have found that when parents remain on the ward at all times, the rehabilitation admissions have not been successful." Part of the reason for this is:

the parents' concern for the child is often expressed in strong non-verbal communications of anxiety, solicitous questions about the child's symptoms, and caregiving responses to alleviate or manage the symptoms. Unfortunately, these "caring" behaviors often trigger and intensify the child's symptoms.

This requirement of reduction of parental contact was the advice given more than 100 years ago, although with greater severity. From Mayer:

Unfortunately, it is just in these cases that the parents are unable to treat their children as desired. For this reason, isolation is necessary. The child, brought to a hospital, realizes itself alone; it cannot call on weak parents to act against the injunctions of the physician ... Stop all visits, even letters.

From Hecht:

When one is denied the intelligent and obedient cooperation of parents, and this is only too often the case, isolation becomes an imperative measure. Isolation to be complete and effective means no visitors, no letters, no messages; in short, no reminders of the past.

It seems likely that intensive inpatient programs work by enabling the child to rest and get better slowly without loss of dignity while psychologic and family problems are addressed. It is of vital importance to avoid a contest of wills, which is highly likely to degenerate into a lose–lose situation. Children in the 10–14-years age group can be extraordinarily strong-willed. The story of the 12-year-old "Welsh fasting girl" Sarah Jacobs is an extreme example. She and her parents claimed that she had not eaten for 2 years. According to the *Spectator* (1869), Sarah was "a pretty little creature, [she] was exhibited to all comers lying in bed, attired as a bride, and the fame of her went abroad over all England." A team of "watchers" came from Guy's Hospital to ensure she was not surreptitiously receiving food. Refusing to eat or drink despite only having to ask for it, she died 8 days later. Again from the *Spectator*: "The girl, however, either from pride, or obstinacy, or ignorance of her danger – held out." (The parents and medical committee were subsequently charged with "killing and slaying" the poor girl (*Lancet*, 1870).)

It is easy to criticize the amount of time and effort and the long hospital stays needed to help some of these children, but many are very ill. Trying to "force them" to get better sooner can result in an escalation of symptoms and an even more prolonged illness.

PROGNOSIS

The impression going back to Hecht is that most children with FND do well. Goodyer's impression is that:

Many of the children appear to be free from psychiatric disturbance and the outcome in terms of the presenting symptoms is generally good, with most of the children at follow-up one to ten years later free of psychiatric, social or educational difficulties. However, for a small percentage the outcome is poor (Goodyer, 1986).

In the study of Grattan-Smith et al. (1988), 44% were symptomfree at discharge from hospital and another 17% were markedly improved. In the study of Ani et al. (2013), at 1 year, of those who could be followed, around 90% showed an improvement in neurologic symptom. In addition, 28% had been diagnosed with a new psychiatric disorder, including anxiety disorder (14%), depressive disorder (13%), and school phobia (9%). Long-term follow-up studies of children with FND have proven difficult to implement, and the full picture might not be seen until 30–40 years after presentation.

FUNCTIONAL OR PSYCHOGENIC?

As discussed above, there is currently intense controversy over whether "functional" or "psychogenic" is a better term (Edwards et al., 2014a, b; Fahn and Olanow, 2014; Ganos et al., 2014; Jankovic, 2014; La Faver and Hallett, 2014). This is likely to be covered in detail in other parts of the book and we will only discuss it briefly. We believe psychogenic is a better word than functional. It is straightforward and makes clear what is meant. We believe functional is not a good word in this setting as it lacks clarity. For example, where does it sit with functional imaging, functional MRI, and functional neuroanatomy? Reflecting this, there are also practical consequences. In December 2014 a PubMed search for "psychogenic movement disorders in children" resulted in 81 hits. For "functional movement disorders in children," the number was 888, with most not relevant to the purpose of the search. When the search was repeated with "in children" deleted, "psychogenic" produced 495 hits and "functional," 10 934.

In a recent review of the use of the word, the conclusion was that "functional" is "a simplifying euphemism allowing neurologists to use one term to mean one thing to colleagues and another to patients" (Kanaan et al., 2012). It seems that the proponents of "functional" are, in reality, more opponents of "psychogenic" as they do not believe the underlying cause is psychologic disturbance. In the search for a better word, Babinski suggested "pithiatism," meaning curable by persuasion, but this did not catch on in the English literature (Derouesné, 2009). More recently, terms such as "symptoms unexplained by organic disease" and "medically unexplained illness" were tried, but their limitations are so obvious that the ambiguous "functional" has now been resurrected. If the child's problems are not the result of mental suffering, what hypothesis do we employ to explain the symptoms? How do we reconcile saying to the child and family, "there is a functional disturbance of the brain," followed by "I believe we need the help of a psychiatrist." (There have been suggestions that psychiatrists have no value in the treatment of FND, but this is not our position.)

The opponents of "psychogenic" also see it as promoting dualism, the concept that the mind and brain are distinct entities that can interact with each other. Opposition to dualism is a strong current theme among some neuroscientists, with Mudrik and Maoz (2014) urging their colleagues to root out "closet dualism." The problem is that many people, and, in particular, children, perceive the mind and body as separate entities. If even neuroscientists are prone to disciplinary lapses, the avoidance of dualism, rather than adding scientific rigor, seems more of a distraction from the prime purpose of helping the child and family.

We certainly agree that "psychogenic" is not without its problems. As outlined above, in discussions with the child and family we often use the term "stress-related" in the sense of a sensitive child subject to powerful external forces, rather than "psychogenic," which could be seen as implying intrinsic flaws and weaknesses in the child. Far more important than the term used is the attitude of the person using the term, and what the child and family understand is being said.

References

Ani C, Reading R, Lynn R et al. (2013). Incidence and 12-month outcome of non-transient childhood conversion disorder in the UK and Ireland. Br J Psychiatry 202: 413–418.

Biller JG (1898). Hysteria in Children. JAMA XXXI: 1338–1340.

Bonduelle M, Gelfand T (1999). Hysteria behind the scenes: Jane Avril at the Salpêtrière. J Hist Neurosc 8: 35–42.

Brain R (1955). Diseases of the Nervous System, 5th edn. Oxford University Press, London, pp. 969–972.

Burr CW (1897). Hysteria in Children. JAMA XXIX: 1151–1152.

Calvert P, Jureidini J (2003). Restrained rehabilitation: an approach to children and adolescents with unexplained signs and symptoms. Arch Dis Child 88: 399–402.

Crimlisk HL, Bhatia K, Cope H et al. (1998). Slater revisited: 6 year follow up study of patients with medically unexplained motor symptoms. BMJ 316: 582–586.

Derouesné C (2009). Pithiatism versus hysteria. In: J Philippon, J Poirier (Eds.), Joseph Babinski. A Biography, Oxford University Press, Oxford, pp. 297–320.

Edwards MJ, Bhatia KP (2012). Functional (psychogenic) movement disorders: merging mind and brain. Lancet Neurol 11: 250–260.

Edwards MJ, Stone J, Lang AE (2014a). From psychogenic movement disorder to functional movement disorder: it's time to change the name. Mov Disord 29: 849–852.

Edwards MJ, Stone J, Lang AE (2014b). Functional/psychogenic movement disorders: do we know what they are? Mov Disord 29: 1696–1697.

Fahn S, Jankovic J (2007). Principles and Practice of Movement Disorders, Churchill Livingstone, Philadelphia, PA, pp. 597–613.

Fahn S, Olanow CW (2014). "Psychogenic movement disorders": they are what they are. Mov Disord 29: 853–856.

Gamgee A (1878). An account of a demonstration on the phenomena of hystero-epilepsy: and on the modification which they undergo under the influence of magnets and solenoids; given by Professor Charcot at the Salpêtrière. BMJ 2: 545–548.

Ganos C, Erro R, Bhatia KP et al. (2014). Comment on psychogenic versus functional movement disorders. Mov Disord 29: 1696.

Goodyer IM (1986). Monosymptomatic hysteria in childhood, family and professional systems involvement. J Fam Ther 8: 253–266.

Grattan-Smith P, Fairley M, Procopis P (1988). Clinical features of conversion disorder. Arch Dis Child 63: 408–414.

Head H (1922). An address on the diagnosis of hysteria. BMJ 1: 827–829.

Hecht D (1907). Hysteria in children. JAMA XLVIII: 670–677.

Howe EG (1934). The causal fallacy. Lancet 1: 611–615.

Jankovic J (2014). "Psychogenic" versus "functional" movement disorders? That is the question. Mov Disord 29: 1697–1698.

Kanaan RA, Armstrong D, Wessely SC (2012). The function of 'functional': a mixed methods investigation. JNNP 83: 248–250.

Koslowska K, Nunn K, Rose D et al. (2007). Conversion disorder in Australian paediatric practice. J Am Acad Child Adolesc Psychiatry 46: 168–175.

Koslowska K, English M, Savage B et al. (2012). Multimodal rehabilitation: a mind–body, family-based intervention for children and adolescents impaired by medically unexplained symptoms. Part 1: The Program. Am J Fam Ther 40: 399–419.

Lancet (1870). The Welsh fasting girl and the medical committee. Lancet 95 (1): 360–361.

La Faver K, Hallett M (2014). Functional or psychogenic: what's the better name? Mov Disord 29: 1698–1699.

Mayer EE (1899). Hysteria in children. JAMA XXXIII: 945–949.

Mudrik L, Maoz U (2014). "Me and my brain": exposing neuroscience's closet dualism. J Cogn Neurosci 27 (2): 211–221.

Paget J (1873). Clinical lectures on the nervous mimicry of organic diseases. Lancet 2: 511–513.

Shorvon S (2007). Fashion and cult in neuroscience – the case of hysteria. Brain 130: 3342–3348.

Slater E (1965). Diagnosis of "hysteria". BMJ 1: 1395–1399.

Spectator (1869). 25 December, p 9.

Stone J, Carson A, Duncan R (2009). Symptoms "unexplained by organic disease" in 1144 new neurology outpatients: how often does the diagnosis change at follow-up? Brain 132: 2878–2888.

Taylor DC (1986). Hysteria, play-acting and courage. Br J Psychol 149: 37–41.

Walshe FMR (1952). Diseases of the Nervous System, 7th edn. E&S Livingston, Edinburgh, pp. 338–347.

Handbook of Clinical Neurology, Vol. 139 (3rd series)
Functional Neurologic Disorders
M. Hallett, J. Stone, and A. Carson, Editors
http://dx.doi.org/10.1016/B978-0-12-801772-2.00041-2

Chapter 41

Posttraumatic functional movement disorders

C. GANOS[1,2], M.J. EDWARDS[3], AND K.P. BHATIA[1]*

[1]*Sobell Department of Motor Neuroscience and Movement Disorders, National Hospital for Neurology and Neurosurgery, Queen Square, London, UK*

[2]*Department of Neurology, University Medical Center Hamburg-Eppendorf (UKE), Hamburg, Germany*

[3]*Department of Molecular and Clinical Sciences, St George's University of London and Atkinson Morley Regional Neuroscience Centre, St George's University Hospitals NHS Foundation Trust, London, UK*

Abstract

Traumatic injury to the nervous system may account for a range of neurologic symptoms. Trauma location and severity are important determinants of the resulting symptoms. In severe head injury with structural brain abnormalities, the occurrence of trauma-induced movement disorders, most commonly hyperkinesias such as tremor and dystonia, is well recognized and its diagnosis straightforward. However, the association of minor traumatic events, which do not lead to significant persistent structural brain damage, with the onset of movement disorders is more contentious. The lack of clear clinical-neuroanatomic (or symptom lesion) correlations in these cases, the variable timing between traumatic event and symptom onset, but also the presence of unusual clinical features in a number of such patients, which overlap with signs encountered in patients with functional neurologic disorders, contribute to this controversy. The purpose of this chapter is to provide an overview of the movement disorders, most notably dystonia, that have been associated with peripheral trauma and focus on their unusual characteristics, as well as their overlap with functional neurologic disorders. We will then provide details on pathophysiologic views that relate minor peripheral injuries to the development of movement disorders and compare them to knowledge from primary organic and functional movement disorders. Finally, we will comment on the appropriate management of these disorders.

PERIPHERAL TRAUMA AND MOVEMENT DISORDERS – EVOLUTION OF A CONCEPT

One of the earliest accounts on peripheral trauma-induced movement disorders (PTMD) in the English language was provided by Gowers, who described the development of "writing spasm" in a naval officer, following a minor thumb injury (Gowers, 1888). A few years earlier, Charcot had already described several cases with abnormal limb posturing to contractures following minor peripheral injury and argued in favor of hysteria as the underlying diagnosis (Charcot, 1877). There continued to be reports of physical trauma (or proposed physical trauma) associated with the development of neurologic and other symptoms, including "railway spine," where the vibration of train carriages was held responsible for a variety of different ailments (Trimble, 1981).

In more recent times, Sheehy and Marsden (1980) argued on a presumable association between neck trauma and onset of cervical dystonia, and Schott (1981) provided a detailed clinical account of 5 cases of painful-legs/moving-toes syndrome following peripheral injury. Only 3 years later, Marsden and colleagues (1984) described 4 unusual cases of tonic spasms and clonic limb jerking following minor peripheral injury, further sparking interest in PTMD. The main and distinct features of these cases were not only the largely tonic character of the abnormal movements associated with peripheral trauma, but also that all 4 patients developed severe pain and trophic changes of the skin and/or bones related to, what was at the time labeled as, sympathetic algodystrophy or Sudeck's atrophy.

*Correspondence to: Kailash P. Bhatia, Clinical Movement Disorders Group, Sobell Department of Motor Neuroscience and Movement Disorders, UCL Institute of Neurology, Queen Square, London, UK. E-mail: k.bhatia@ucl.ac.uk

Subsequently, Scherokman et al. (1986) reported 4 cases of adult-onset focal hand dystonia with largely task-induced dystonic posturing of one hand with concomitant or subsequent development of peripheral neuropathy in the same hand and emphasized the potential pathophysiologic link between peripheral nerve injury and (secondary) focal dystonia.

Following these reports, larger case series provided detailed accounts of adult patients who suffered minor peripheral injuries and developed sustained abnormal limb and/or neck postures, spasms, and/or tremor, corroborating the association of movement disorders with disabling pain and trophic skin changes (Schott, 1986; Jankovic and Van der Linden, 1988; Schwartzman and Kerrigan, 1990; Bhatia et al., 1993).

While all descriptions essentially described the same characteristic syndrome, different weight was given by each author to different clinical aspects. Schott (1986), for example, emphasized the association of abnormal movements with causalgia (a term analogous to Sudeck's atrophy, which was first coined by Dunglinson in 1867 to describe the disabling pain following peripheral nerve injury, as in the traumatic war cases described by Mitchel in 1864 (Headley, 1987)). Jankovic and van der Linden (1988) highlighted the role of peripheral trauma as a rare cause of movement disorders, whereas Schwartzman and Kerrigan (1990) focused on the varied phenotype of the abnormal movements which could appear with causalgia. Bhatia et al. (1993) underscored the level of severity of abnormal postures in such patients, described as "fixed dystonia," the absence of peripheral nerve damage, the clinical differences of patients with fixed dystonic postures from those with primary torsion dystonia, and the unusual distribution and spread of symptoms over time.

During this period functional/psychogenic movement disorders were being reintroduced in the differential diagnosis of movement disorders, but for focal dystonias, the diagnosis remained difficult (Table 41.1: Marsden, 1976) and clinicians were becoming aware of the great harm done in affected individuals and families by diagnostic mislabeling to one or the other category. In fact, in the first etiologic classification of dystonias by Fahn and Eldridge in 1976, the diagnostic anxiety of mislabeling patients who had primary (or organic) focal dystonias as functional (or psychogenic at that time) had led to the inclusion of "psychogenic dystonia" only at the end of their list, just "for the sake of completeness," as it was unclear whether this diagnosis would have existed at all.

Several factors contributed to this development. First, familial and epidemiologic studies allowed the delineation of the main features of typical (or organic) syndromes and differentiated them from less common, atypical forms. Second, neurophysiology aided assessing basic characteristics of most abnormal movements and establishing differences between organic and functional forms. Third, it became clear that treatments that focused solely on psychologic factors were not successful. As a result, the first reports on patients with functional/psychogenic dystonia emerged (Lesser and Fahn, 1978; Fahn et al., 1983) and diagnostic criteria emphasizing neurologic, rather than psychiatric, parameters were proposed (Fahn and Williams, 1988). In fact, elaborating on these criteria, Bhatia and colleagues (1993) suggested that some patients with the clinical syndrome of (fixed) dystonia and causalgia might have underlying functional (psychogenic), rather than purely organic causes, a notion that had already been supported by Lang and Fahn (1990) in their reply to Schwarzmann and Kerrigan's (1990) case series (see above).

Table 41.1

Characteristics of focal dystonias that have contributed in their mislabeling as psychogenic

1	The bizarre nature of the dyskinesias
2	Their appearance frequently only on certain actions; other motor acts employing the same muscles are carried out normally
3	Their relief by certain inexplicable trick actions
4	Their exquisite sensitivity to social and mental stress
5	The failure so far to find any anatomic, physiologic, or biochemical abnormality in any of these conditions
6	The belief that such patients show overt psychiatric disturbance
7	A psychopathologic interpretation of the significance of, for example, eye closure or neck turning

Reproduced from Marsden (1976).

DISTINCT PHENOTYPES OF MOVEMENT DISORDERS FOLLOWING PERIPHERAL TRAUMA AND THEIR OVERLAP WITH FUNCTIONAL MOVEMENT DISORDERS

The definition of PTMD is difficult, as no validated criteria exist. Moreover, the process of definition is hampered by the absence of any pathophysiologic consensus (see below). Hence, the only approach to classify patients as to whether their movement disorder is induced by peripheral trauma or not is an empiric one. According to Cardoso and Jankovic, three criteria of PTMD must be met: (1) trauma severity, which causes local symptoms for more than 2 weeks or requires medical evaluation within the first 2 weeks; (2) trauma location and movement disorder are co-localized; and (3) the movement disorder appears within 1 year after the traumatic event (Cardoso and Jankovic, 1995; Jankovic, 2009). However, these criteria are rather arbitrary (e.g., the poor definition of peripheral trauma in itself, as well as trauma severity, the wide timeframe of 1 year between trauma and onset of movement disorder), therefore susceptible to criticism (Weiner, 2001; Hawley and Weiner, 2011), and have not found general acceptance. Irrespective of the exact criteria applied, distinct phenotypic forms of PTMD, notably dystonia, have been recognized. These include peripheral trauma-induced fixed limb dystonia, posttraumatic painful torticollis, and further, less common presentations, such as trauma-induced axial jerks or painful-legs/moving-toes syndrome.

As will be clear from the descriptions below, PTMD commonly co-occurs with chronic pain, typically in the affected part of the body, but sometimes more generalized. Thus, there is a clear overlap between complex regional pain syndrome (CRPS) – a syndrome dominated by chronic pain following (typically minor) injury – and PTMD.

CRPS is a syndrome that, like PTMD, creates controversy regarding etiology and classification. The term CRPS was coined in 1995 by the International Association for the Study of Pain to unify previous descriptive labels as reflex sympathetic dystrophy, Sudeck's atrophy, or causalgia (Merskey and Bogduk, 1994). Although initial criteria distinguished two types of CRPS according to the presence or absence of nerve injury (CRPS types II and I, respectively), current criteria rather focus on the presence of continuous regional pain (not confined in a specific nerve territory or dermatome) that is disproportionate to any type of inciting injury with sensory, sudomotor/edema, vasomotor, and motor/trophic changes (Harden et al., 2007). It is of interest that motor symptoms are commonly reported in case series of patients with CRPS, and such motor symptoms are reported by some to have characteristics that are typical of patients with functional movement disorders (Veldman et al., 1993). In addition, malingering has been reported as being the diagnosis in 2 patients diagnosed with CRPS (Verdugo and Ochoa, 2000).

Peripheral trauma-induced fixed limb dystonia

Following the first few reports on peripheral trauma-induced dystonic posturing of the limbs, one of the most controversial phenotypes in movement disorders was gaining increasing recognition. There were two main shared features in all original reports: a peripheral traumatic event, usually associated with some period of limb immobilization, was in close temporal association with the manifestation of (1) tonic (or fixed) dystonic posturing with superimposed spasms and difficulties in performing voluntary actions, and (2) disabling pain. Both features were unusual for primary dystonia (including idiopathic and/or inherited forms of dystonia, according to the new dystonia classification: Albanese et al., 2013), which is largely mobile (i.e., joint mobility is not reduced from dystonic posturing) and pain, although it may be present, is usually not as disabling. Other differences in the syndrome of fixed dystonia include the absence of sensory tricks, an abrupt to subacute symptom onset following injury and/or immobilization, and a poor long-term response to treatment, including botulinum toxin injections (Bhatia et al., 1993; Schrag et al., 2004; Hawley and Weiner, 2011).

Schrag et al. (2004) provided a detailed account of the clinical characteristics of 103 patients with the syndrome of fixed dystonia (41 patients were studied prospectively), most of whom had a physical traumatic event preceding symptom onset. Syndromic descriptions overlapped with previous reports. For the most commonly affected lower limb, initial resting dystonia soon developed to fixed dystonic posturing with foot inversion, plantar flexion, and toe curling (Fig. 41.1 A and B). In more than half of patients dystonia spread to involve other (ipsi- and contralateral) parts of the body. For the upper limb, wrist and finger flexion at the metacarpo- and/or interphalangeal joints with sparing of the thumb and forefinger was typically observed. Continuous pain was present in all prospectively studied patients except 3. However, only a fifth of those patients met the criteria for CRPS.

Schrag et al. (2004) highlighted that "psychogenic signs" had been documented in a large number of patients (46% for the prospectively examined group) and further emphasized that in only 10% of patients of the prospective group were Fahn and Williams' criteria for functional (at the time labeled as psychogenic) dystonia (Fahn and Williams, 1988) not fulfilled. Moreover, the prevalence of affective, somatization, and dissociative disorders (*Diagnostic and Statistical Manual of Mental Disorders*, fourth edition (DSM-IV) criteria: American Psychiatric Association, 1994) was compared between patients with either fixed or primary dystonia, and was found to be significantly higher for fixed dystonia.

Clinical follow-up 7.6 (±3.6) years later in a proportion of these patients ($n = 35$) showed that in approximately one-fifth of cases ($n = 8$) symptoms largely remitted (Ibrahim et al., 2009). None of these patients had CRPS at baseline. On the other hand, about one-third of patients ($n = 11$; 8 with features of CRPS at onset) experienced clinical worsening. Two of these patients underwent above-knee amputation, which was complicated by phantom-limb pain. One further patient was rediagnosed with corticobasal syndrome. Among the 16 patients who remained unchanged, 6 had signs of

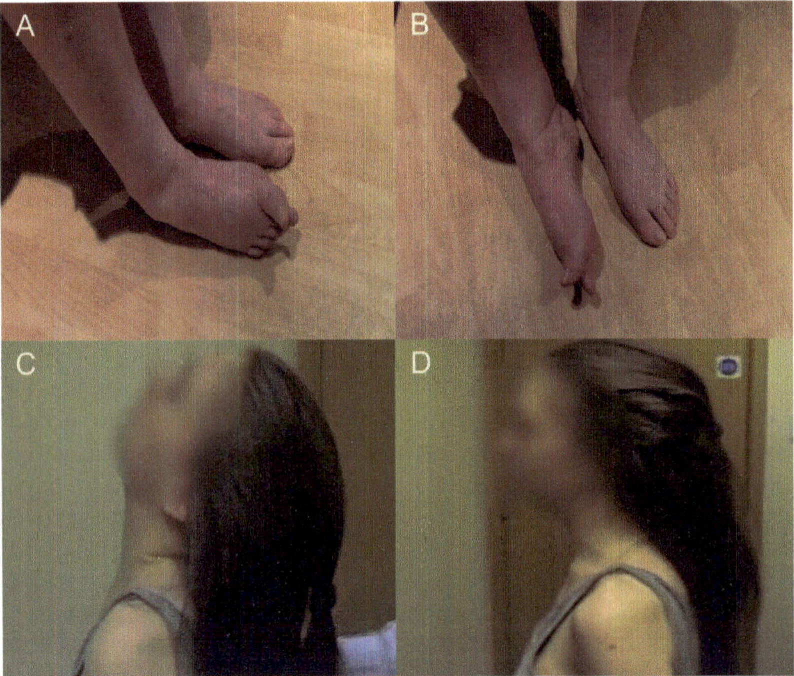

Fig. 41.1. **(A, B)** Posttraumatic fixed dystonia of the right foot. Two months after a minor surgical procedure at the right popliteal fossa, there was an initial tonic extension of the right big toe. This was shortly followed by inward rotation and plantar flexion of the foot with severe pain and subsequent immobilization, leading to the fixed posture shown here. The patient also more recently complained of intermittent "shakes" and sensory disturbance affecting both arms. **(C, D)** A day after a very painful chiropractic neck treatment, this then-22-year-old female developed painful involuntary posturing of the neck with severe retrocollis, which has been present for 4 years **(C)**. Immediate (<5 minutes; placebo) response to botulinum toxin injected to both semispinalis capitis muscles **(D)**.

CRPS at baseline. Patients without clinical improvement scored higher on ratings of depression and dissociative/somatoform disorders. The presence of CRPS was found to be the only significant predictor of poor outcome in this study. Notably, 31 of 35 cases fulfilled Fahn and Williams' criteria for psychogenic dystonia (Fahn and Williams, 1988).

Of note, some patients with fixed dystonia have been reported to have an excellent immediate, and therefore placebo, response to botulinum toxin (Edwards et al., 2011b). Also, in patients with either the diagnosis of functional dystonia or posttraumatic fixed dystonia, functional neurologic signs, such as give-way weakness, functional tremor, and jerks, may be seen in affected and nonaffected body parts (Ganos et al., 2014a).

Posttraumatic painful torticollis

Truong et al. (1991) described 6 patients who, within 4 days following a minor cranial/neck injury, developed abnormal persistent neck posturing. All patients had continuous (or fixed) abnormal neck/shoulder posturing with marked limitation of range of motion. There was no *geste antagoniste* and no overflow dystonia. All patients had disabling pain and in 1 patient features resembling those of CRPS were noted. Truong et al. highlighted the unusual character of the syndrome, drew a parallel with functional dystonic cervical posturing, and concluded that reported cases might represent a distinct entity, different from primary cervical dystonia. Subsequently, and by applying a temporal cutoff of 3 months between traumatic event and onset of symptoms, further larger case series reiterated syndromic findings (Goldman and Ahlskog, 1993; Tarsy, 1998; Sa et al., 2003; Frei et al., 2004). In light of this distinctive clinical features, the term "posttraumatic painful torticollis" was proposed, to separate this syndrome from that of primary cervical dystonia (Sa et al., 2003) (Fig. 41.1C and D). Of note, some patients also exhibited further functional neurologic signs on examination, such as give-way weakness, nonanatomic sensory changes, and also had an excellent response to amytal infusion (Sa et al., 2003). Moreover, psychologic evaluation of 11 patients with the syndrome of posttraumatic painful torticollis revealed profiles consistent with conversion disorder (Sa et al., 2003).

In summary, despite the difference in anatomic location, the syndrome of posttraumatic painful torticollis bears striking similarities with that of fixed dystonia in terms of clinical phenomenology (fixed posturing with prominent pain), but also presence of additional functional neurologic signs and (poor) response to established treatments. Although there is some heterogeneity among patients classified with posttraumatic painful torticollis (Frei et al., 2004), it appears that, at least for many patients, the aforementioned clinical characteristics should prompt the consideration of a functional movement disorder. Indeed, it is difficult to see a clear alternative diagnosis in the majority of reported patients.

Other movement disorders induced by peripheral trauma

Although there are sparse reports for characteristic and well-delineated posttraumatic presentations of movement disorders other than the aforementioned dystonic phenotypes, onset of tremulous and jerky movements, as well as the syndrome of painful legs/moving toes, has been found to present in patients following a posttraumatic event (van Rooijen et al., 2011). Indeed, a systematic review found tremor to be the second most common presentation of PTMD (Cardoso and Jankovic, 1995; Jankovic, 2009; van Rooijen et al., 2011). Notably, however, a large proportion of these patients was found to also have different PTMD, commonly dystonia (Jankovic, 2009). In some reports, which examined the clinical features of both phenomena, characteristics such as tremor distractibility were found (Schwartzman and Kerrigan, 1990; Sa et al., 2003; Schrag et al., 2004), whereas in others this was not tested/reported. Also, some patients diagnosed with peripheral trauma-induced tremor were additionally diagnosed with a functional movement disorder due to the presence of other abnormal movements (van Rooijen et al., 2011).

Jerky movements are another common phenotypic presentation of posttraumatic movement disorders. These are commonly jerks of the axial muscles, also labeled as axial or propriospinal myoclonus. A recent systematic meta-analysis of patients with propriospinal myoclonus, however, highlighted that the majority of cases with this diagnosis have a functional movement disorder (van der Salm et al., 2014). Furthermore, a large retrospective series of 76 patients with functional axial jerks showed that 36.8% had minor physical precipitants associated with the onset of the abnormal jerky movements (Erro et al., 2014). Similarly, in other more rare presentations of PTMD, such as painful legs/moving toes (Schott, 1981), adult-onset tic disorders (Singer et al., 1989; Factor and Molho, 1997; Erer and Jankovic, 2008), or posttraumatic shoulder movement disorders (Pandey et al., 2014), there are clinical features of a functional movement disorder (Ganos et al., 2014b; Stone and Erro, 2014; Demartini et al., 2015). However, we also acknowledge that it is often difficult in some of these cases, in the absence of objective biomarkers and due to the similarities of movement physiology to voluntary actions (for example, in patients with tics), to make a definitive general argument with regard to etiology in all cases. Furthermore, the lack of specificity of the nonvalidated criteria to diagnose PTMD allows for type I errors, i.e., diagnostic mislabeling of movement disorders incidentally occurring within the timeframe of 1 year following or even being the cause of a traumatic event (e.g., patient with a parkinsonian condition leading to fall with fracture of the right arm, and incidental manifestation of a right-arm tremor within 12 months after the injury). This notwithstanding, it appears that the majority of posttraumatic and functional movement disorders are closely linked on clinical grounds.

PATHOPHYSIOLOGIC CONSIDERATIONS

When considering PTMD, one of the very first questions to pose is that of definition, in other words to understand which trauma severity and timeframe are necessary for the development of abnormal movements following minor peripheral injury. Although an attempt to answer this question, in order to set a diagnostic framework for such disorders, has been made (Cardoso and Jankovic, 1995; Jankovic, 2009), the arbitrary character of chosen criteria in the absence of any pathophysiologic basis has not led to wide acceptance. Therefore, parallel to setting criteria of definition, one different question to pose would be related to understanding how peripheral trauma leads to abnormal movements.

Here, we will explore two main possibilities. One of these possibilities relates to the notion of environmental triggers, such as minor traumatic events, unmasking a pre-existing vulnerability of the central nervous system to develop abnormal movements (Fletcher et al., 1991). This hypothesis largely adheres to knowledge from primary adult-onset dystonias. Two large case-control studies have shown an association between the incidence of head trauma (with loss of consciousness) and the development of typical mobile cervical dystonia and writer's cramp (Defazio et al., 1998; Roze et al., 2009). Interestingly, neck and trunk trauma was increased in cervical dystonia patients in one of these studies (Defazio et al., 1998). An additional study showed a similar association between the incidence of traumatic events (e.g., following car accidents with hospital attendance) and the risk of development of cervical dystonia (Molloy et al., 2015). For laryngeal dystonia, longstanding history of occupational voice use, as well as recurrent viral exposures of the upper respiratory tract, was associated with increased risk of symptom manifestation compared to patients with other voice disorders (Tanner et al., 2012). Also, the incidence of eye disease at the anterior eye segment was associated with the incidence of blepharospasm in two further studies (Defazio et al., 1998; Martino et al., 2005). Moreover, according to a rat model of blepharospasm, the onset of the movement disorder occurred only after a superimposed environmental stressor on a pre-existing vulnerable (i.e., dopamine-depleted) brain (double-hit hypothesis) (Schicatano et al., 1997). Finally, although different than aforementioned dystonic phenotypes, in genetically proven cases of rapid-onset dystonia-parkinsonism, but also in mitochondrial disorders, minor physical precipitants may trigger or aggravate neurologic symptoms (Berkovic et al., 1989; Brashear et al., 2007).

On the other hand, not all results from case-control studies in adult-onset primary dystonia have been replicated, casting doubt on the presumed pathophysiologic significance of peripheral trauma in the precipitation of at least some focal forms of adult-onset primary dystonias (Martino et al., 2007; Roze et al., 2009). Martino et al. (2007) did not find an association between any type of head trauma and cranial dystonia, and Roze et al. (2009) showed that the incidence of injuries of the affected limb was not associated with increased risk of developing writer's cramp.

Moreover, the temporal association between symptom onset in the aforementioned positive case-control studies and traumatic event is different and clearly much longer from that conceptualized in PTMD, described in this chapter. For example, Defazio et al. (1998) showed that head trauma with loss of consciousness preceded the onset of cervical dystonia by an average of 4.7 years, whereas neck injury was on average 4.3 years earlier, as opposed to the temporal criterion of 1 year proposed by Cardoso and Jankovic (Cardoso and Jankovic, 1995; Jankovic, 2009). Finally, it is unclear whether knowledge gained from the study of adult-onset primary dystonia should apply at all to the spectrum of movement disorders presented here, as it presumes pathophysiologic similarities on the basis of a phenomenologic analogy of similar, but not identical, movement disorders (Schrag, 2006).

A different possibility relates to the clear phenotypic overlap of many cases of movement disorders following peripheral trauma with functional movement disorders. A pathophysiologic framework in this regard would incorporate the circumstances and mechanisms that allow a physical precipitant to lead to the expression of abnormal functional somatic events. In fact, this consideration dates back to Charcot's clinical lectures on hysteria, where he argued the improbability of peripheral traumatic events leading to organic movement disorders (Charcot, 1877). Indeed, following a large gap throughout the 20th century, during which the psychoanalytic theories of dissociation and symptom conversion emphasized the importance of psychologic rather than physical trauma (Trimble, 2004), more recent work attempted to create a neurobiologic framework of understanding of functional neurologic symptoms (Edwards et al., 2012, 2013), including those associated with physical precipitators (Pareés et al., 2014) in the absence of identifiable psychologic stressors (Kranick et al., 2011). Indeed, a study that compared psychologic profiles and self-reported life events of physical/sexual abuse failed to identify major differences between patients with functional movement disorders, healthy controls, and patients with organic movement disorders (Kranick et al., 2011). It is important to note that other studies have found traumatic life events and psychopathology to be present at higher rates in patients with functional neurologic symptoms in general than in the healthy population or disease controls (Anderson et al., 2007; Feinstein et al., 2001).

On the other hand, a study that assessed the circumstances preceding the onset of functional movement disorders found that physical precipitants were present in 44 of 50 patients (Pareés et al., 2014). Moreover, most patients ($n=40$) reported a physical precipitating event in close temporal proximity to the onset of the abnormal movements (ranging from minutes to less than 3 months). Peripheral injuries, ranging from minor soft-tissue damage to bone fractures with subsequent immobilization, and viral infections, such as flu-like illness, were the most frequent physical precipitants. Of note, a majority of patients also reported symptoms of panic related to the onset of the abnormal movements, with a substantial proportion (38%) fulfilling criteria for a panic attack. Importantly, physical precipitants are not only confined in the spectrum of functional movement disorders, but are encountered for the entire range of functional neurologic symptoms. Indeed, a study on symptoms associated with onset of functional paralysis identified the presence of preceding physical injury to the relevant limb in 20% of cases (Stone et al., 2012). Moreover, a systematic meta-analysis of physical events preceding the onset of functional motor and sensory symptoms found their presence in 37% of patients (324/869 cases) (Stone et al., 2009).

With a shift away from "pure" psychodynamic interpretations of "psychogenic" neurologic symptoms, it becomes apparent that opposing viewpoints of pathophysiology of PTMD may be closer together than once thought. It is clear to us that many patients with PTMD have physical signs and in some cases response to treatment (e.g., dramatic placebo response) that provide positive evidence that they have a functional movement disorder. It does not concern us particularly that these patients may not have emotionally traumatic life events in childhood or the more recent past or other supposedly triggering psychopathology, as we recognize that many patients with functional movement disorders in general do not have such features. While we cannot state with complete confidence that all PTMDs are best considered as functional movement disorders, the evidence to us points clearly to this in the majority of reported cases and those from our own clinical practice. This has important implications for diagnostic explanation and treatment, which we discuss below.

MANAGEMENT OF MOVEMENT DISORDERS INDUCED BY PERIPHERAL TRAUMA <LIZ>

There are no systematic studies on appropriate management of PTMD. However, we have argued that most can be classified within the diagnostic category of functional movement disorders, and therefore, knowledge from this disorder spectrum might prove helpful. Although part IV of this volume provides extensive accounts of treatment methods for functional movement disorders, here we will briefly discuss basic, but important, aspects of management that in our experience are helpful and can improve prognosis.

The first step of management is providing the patient with a reasoned and reasonable explanation of how the symptoms have developed. Patients frequently have a long route to receiving a diagnosis, and along the way may become very sensitized to the implication that their symptoms are "different" from typical structural or degenerative disease; for many patients this implies that the doctor is suggesting their symptoms are "made up" or "imagined." Patients, particularly those with significant pain, are often burdened with multiple medications, many of which have significant side-effects. Clinicians ought though not to be discouraged, but should attempt to establish a clear and effective communication with their patients, as this is paramount for any further interventions. In this way, patients can be informed about their condition in detail and understand its potential reversibility. In turn, clinicians may gain additional information, such as important contextual factors that may not be consciously perceived by patients and may further facilitate the selection of appropriate treatments. Of note, some patients may have pending litigation, which could by itself further complicate treatment outcome.

For patients with fixed dystonic presentations, the following aspects need to be considered. Re-establishment of movement as soon as possible following traumatic injury is of paramount importance, as any delay between symptom and treatment onset, which may also result in prolonged periods of immobilization, is associated with poor outcome and the development of contractures (Schrag et al., 2004; Thomas et al., 2006). As pain is often a prominent element of posttraumatic functional fixed dystonia, which may also limit physiotherapeutic attempts to reinstate movement, holistic pain management is necessary. This involves the implementation of cognitive-behavioral and physical aspects of pain management paralleled by a gradual reduction of any opiate-based pain medication. Comorbidities, such as anxiety or depression, should also be adequately addressed, and pharmacologic treatments may often be necessary (Voon and Lang, 2005).

In more challenging, severe cases, an inpatient rehabilitation plan, which would include input from physiotherapy, cognitive-behavioral and occupational therapy, as well as neuropsychiatry and neurology, may be particularly helpful (Saifee et al., 2012; Demartini et al., 2014). Conversely, oral pharmacologic agents, established in the treatment of organic movement disorders, are usually unhelpful in these patients. Although small injections of botulinum toxin might temporarily improve symptoms in some patients, ethical issues complicate their usage, and evidence on their long-term efficacy is lacking. Invasive procedures, including limb amputation, should be avoided, as outcome is poor and may be complicated by local infections, the presence of phantom-limb pain, as well as the migration of symptoms to other body parts (Schrag et al., 2004; Bramstedt and Ford, 2006; Ibrahim et al., 2009; Bodde et al., 2011; Edwards et al., 2011a).

CONCLUSION

Peripheral trauma has been associated with the onset of a wide range of movement disorders, notably hyperkinesias and in particular (fixed) dystonic posturing. The difficulties in the syndromic definition of PTMD paralleled with the lack of consensus on pathophysiologic models of their emergence have perpetuated a divide in neurology as to the exact nature of abnormal movements. However, for at least many of the established PTMD phenotypes, a functional cause should be considered. In these cases, prompt multidisciplinary treatment, including physical and psychologic support, is necessary in order to ensure best possible outcome, while invasive procedures should be avoided.

References

Albanese A, Bhatia K, Bressman SB et al. (2013). Phenomenology and classification of dystonia: a consensus update. Mov Disord 28: 863–873.

American Psychiatric Association (1994). Diagnostic and statistical manual of mental disorders : DSM-IV. American Psychiatric Association, Washington, DC.

Anderson KE, Gruber-Baldini AL, Vaughan CG et al. (2007). Impact of psychogenic movement disorders versus Parkinson's on disability, quality of life, and psychopathology. Mov Disord 22: 2204–2209.

Berkovic SF, Carpenter S, Evans A et al. (1989). Myoclonus epilepsy and ragged-red fibres (MERRF). 1. A clinical, pathological, biochemical, magnetic resonance spectrographic and positron emission tomographic study. Brain 112 (Pt 5): 1231–1260.

Bhatia KP, Bhatt MH, Marsden CD (1993). The causalgia-dystonia syndrome. Brain 116 (Pt 4): 843–851.

Bodde MI, Dijkstra PU, Den Dunnen WF et al. (2011). Therapy-resistant complex regional pain syndrome type I: to amputate or not? Journal of bone and joint surgery. American volume 93: 1799–1805.

Bramstedt KA, Ford PJ (2006). Protecting human subjects in neurosurgical trials: the challenge of psychogenic dystonia. Contemp Clin Trials 27: 161–164.

Brashear A, Dobyns WB, de Carvalho Aguiar P (2007). The phenotypic spectrum of rapid-onset dystonia-parkinsonism (RDP) and mutations in the ATP1A3 gene. Brain 130: 828–835.

Cardoso F, Jankovic J (1995). Peripherally induced tremor and parkinsonism. Arch Neurol 52: 263–270.

Charcot J-M (1877). Lectures on the Diseases of the Nervous System delivered at La Salpetriere (1877), New Sydenham Society, London.

Defazio G, Berardelli A, Abbruzzese G et al. (1998). Possible risk factors for primary adult onset dystonia: a case-control investigation by the Italian Movement Disorders Study Group. J Neurol Neurosurg Psychiatry 64: 25–32.

Demartini B, Batla A, Petrochilos P et al. (2014). Multidisciplinary treatment for functional neurological symptoms: a prospective study. J Neurol 261: 2370–2377.

Demartini B, Ricciardi L, Parees I et al. (2015). A positive diagnosis of functional (psychogenic) tics. Eur J Neurol 22: 527–536.

Edwards MJ, Alonso-Canovas A, Schrag A et al. (2011a). Limb amputations in fixed dystonia: a form of body integrity identity disorder? Mov Disord 26: 1410–1414.

Edwards MJ, Bhatia KP, Cordivari C (2011b). Immediate response to botulinum toxin injections in patients with fixed dystonia. Mov Disord 26: 917–918.

Edwards MJ, Adams RA, Brown H et al. (2012). A Bayesian account of 'hysteria'. Brain 135: 3495–3512.

Edwards MJ, Fotopoulou A, Parees I (2013). Neurobiology of functional (psychogenic) movement disorders. Curr Opin Neurol 26: 442–447.

Erer S, Jankovic J (2008). Adult onset tics after peripheral injury. Parkinsonism Relat Disord 14: 75–76.

Erro R, Edwards MJ, Bhatia KP et al. (2014). Psychogenic axial myoclonus: clinical features and long-term outcome. Parkinsonism Relat Disord 20: 596–599.

Factor SA, Molho ES (1997). Adult-onset tics associated with peripheral injury. Mov Disord 12: 1052–1055.

Fahn S, Eldridge R (1976). Definition of dystonia and classification of the dystonic states. Adv Neurol 14: 1–5.

Fahn S, Williams DT (1988). Psychogenic dystonia. Adv Neurol 50: 431–455.

Fahn S, Williams D, Reches A et al. (1983). Hysterical dystonia, a rare disorder: Report of five documented cases. Neurology 33 (suppl. 2): 161.

Feinstein A, Stergiopoulos V, Fine J et al. (2001). Psychiatric outcome in patients with a psychogenic movement disorder: a prospective study. Neuropsychiatry Neuropsychol Behav Neurol 14: 169–176.

Fletcher NA, Harding AE, Marsden CD (1991). The relationship between trauma and idiopathic torsion dystonia. J Neurol Neurosurg Psychiatry 54: 713–717.

Frei KP, Pathak M, Jenkins S et al. (2004). Natural history of posttraumatic cervical dystonia. Mov Disord 19: 1492–1498.

Ganos C, Edwards MJ, Bhatia KP (2014a). The phenomenology of functional (psychogenic) dystonia. Mov Disord Clin Pract: 36–44.

Ganos C, Aguirregomozcorta M, Batla A et al. (2014b). Psychogenic paroxysmal movement disorders – clinical features and diagnostic clues. Parkinsonism Relat Disord 20: 41–46.

Goldman S, Ahlskog JE (1993). Posttraumatic cervical dystonia. Mayo Clin Proc 68: 443–448.

Gowers W (1888). A manual of diseases of the nervous system. Churchill, London.

Harden RN, Bruehl S, Stanton-Hicks M et al. (2007). Proposed new diagnostic criteria for complex regional pain syndrome. Pain Med 8: 326–331.

Hawley JS, Weiner WJ (2011). Psychogenic dystonia and peripheral trauma. Neurology 77: 496–502.

Headley B (1987). Historical perspective of causalgia. Management of sympathetically maintained pain. Phys Ther 67: 1370–1374.

Ibrahim NM, Martino D, Van de Warrenburg BP et al. (2009). The prognosis of fixed dystonia: a follow-up study. Parkinsonism Relat Disord 15: 592–597.

Jankovic J (2009). Peripherally induced movement disorders. Neurol Clin 27: 821–832. vii.

Jankovic J, Van der Linden C (1988). Dystonia and tremor induced by peripheral trauma: predisposing factors. J Neurol Neurosurg Psychiatry 51: 1512–1519.

Kranick S, Ekanayake V, Martinez V et al. (2011). Psychopathology and psychogenic movement disorders. Mov Disord 26: 1844–1850.

Lang AE, Fahn S (1990). Movement disorder of RSD. Neurology 40: 1476–1477.

Lesser RP, Fahn S (1978). Dystonia: a disorder often misdiagnosed as a conversion reaction. Am J Psychiatr 135: 349–352.

Marsden CD (1976). The problem of adult-onset idiopathic torsion dystonia and other isolated dyskinesias in adult life (including blepharospasm, oromandibular dystonia, dystonic writer's cramp, and torticollis, or axial dystonia). Adv Neurol 14: 259–276.

Marsden CD, Obeso JA, Traub MM et al. (1984). Muscle spasms associated with Sudeck's atrophy after injury. Br Med J (Clin Res Ed) 288: 173–176.

Martino D, Defazio G, Alessio G et al. (2005). Relationship between eye symptoms and blepharospasm: a multicenter case-control study. Mov Disord 20: 1564–1570.

Martino D, Defazio G, Abbruzzese G et al. (2007). Head trauma in primary cranial dystonias: a multicentre case-control study. J Neurol Neurosurg Psychiatry 78: 260–263.

Merskey H, Bogduk N (1994). Classification of chronic pain: pain syndromes and definition of pain terms, 2nd edn. IASP Press, Seattle.

Molloy A, Kimmich O, Williams L et al. (2015). An evaluation of the role of environmental factors in the disease penetrance of cervical dystonia. J Neurol Neurosurg Psychiatry 86: 331–335.

Pandey S, Nahab F, Aldred J et al. (2014). Post-traumatic shoulder movement disorders: a challenging differential diagnosis between organic and functional. Movmnt Disord Clin Pract 1: 102–105.

Pareés I, Kojovic M, Pires C et al. (2014). Physical precipitating factors in functional movement disorders. J Neurol Sci 338: 174–177.

Roze E, Soumare A, Pironneau I et al. (2009). Case-control study of writer's cramp. Brain 132: 756–764.

Sa DS, Mailis-Gagnon A, NICHOLSON K (2003). Posttraumatic painful torticollis. Mov Disord 18: 1482–1491.

Saifee TA, Kassavetis P, Parees I et al. (2012). Inpatient treatment of functional motor symptoms: a long-term follow-up study. J Neurol 259: 1958–1963.

Scherokman B, Husain F, Cuetter A et al. (1986). Peripheral dystonia. Arch Neurol 43: 830–832.

Schicatano EJ, Basso MA, Evinger C (1997). Animal model explains the origins of the cranial dystonia benign essential blepharospasm. J Neurophysiol 77: 2842–2846.

Schott GD (1981). "Painful legs and moving toes": the role of trauma. J Neurol Neurosurg Psychiatry 44: 344–346.

Schott GD (1986). Induction of involuntary movements by peripheral trauma: an analogy with causalgia. Lancet 2: 712–716.

Schrag A (2006). Psychogenic dystonia and reflex sympathetic dystrophy. In: M Hallett, S Fahn, J Jankovic et al. (Eds.), Psychogenic movement disorders: neurology and neuropsychiatry, Lippincott Williams & Wilkins, Philadelphia, PA.

Schrag A, Trimble M, Quinn N et al. (2004). The syndrome of fixed dystonia: an evaluation of 103 patients. Brain 127: 2360–2372.

Schwartzman RJ, Kerrigan J (1990). The movement disorder of reflex sympathetic dystrophy. Neurology 40: 57–61.

Sheehy MP, Marsden CD (1980). Trauma and pain in spasmodic torticollis. Lancet 1: 777–778.

Singer C, Sanchez-Ramos J, Weiner WJ (1989). A case of post-traumatic tic disorder. Mov Disord 4: 342–344.

Stone J, Erro R (2014). Functional (psychogenic) painful legs moving toes syndrome. Mov Disord 29: 1701–1702.

Stone J, Carson A, Aditya H et al. (2009). The role of physical injury in motor and sensory conversion symptoms: a systematic and narrative review. J Psychosom Res 66: 383–390.

Stone J, Warlow C, Sharpe M (2012). Functional weakness: clues to mechanism from the nature of onset. J Neurol Neurosurg Psychiatry 83: 67–69.

Tanner K, Roy N, Merrill RM et al. (2012). Case-control study of risk factors for spasmodic dysphonia: a comparison with other voice disorders. Laryngoscope 122: 1082–1092.

Tarsy D (1998). Comparison of acute- and delayed-onset posttraumatic cervical dystonia. Mov Disord 13: 481–485.

Thomas M, Vuong KD, Jankovic J (2006). Long-term prognosis of patients with psychogenic movement disorders. Parkinsonism Relat Disord 12: 382–387.

Trimble MR (1981). Traumatic neurosis: from railway spine to the whiplash, John Wiley, Chichester, UK.

Trimble MR (2004). Somatoform disorders – a medico legal guide, Cambridge University Press, Cambridge.

Truong DD, Dubinsky R, Hermanowicz N et al. (1991). Posttraumatic torticollis. Arch Neurol 48: 221–223.

Van der Salm SM, Erro R, Cordivari C et al. (2014). Propriospinal myoclonus: clinical reappraisal and review of literature. Neurology 83: 1862–1870.

Van Rooijen DE, Geraedts EJ, Marinus J et al. (2011). Peripheral trauma and movement disorders: a systematic review of reported cases. J Neurol Neurosurg Psychiatry 82: 892–898.

Veldman PH, Reynen HM, Arntz IE et al. (1993). Signs and symptoms of reflex sympathetic dystrophy: prospective study of 829 patients. Lancet 342: 1012–1016.

Verdugo RJ, Ochoa JL (2000). Abnormal movements in complex regional pain syndrome: assessment of their nature. Muscle Nerve 23: 198–205.

Voon V, Lang AE (2005). Antidepressant treatment outcomes of psychogenic movement disorder. J Clin Psychiatr 66: 1529–1534.

Weiner WJ (2001). Can peripheral trauma induce dystonia? No! Mov Disord 16: 13–22.

Handbook of Clinical Neurology, Vol. 139 (3rd series)
Functional Neurologic Disorders
M. Hallett, J. Stone, and A. Carson, Editors
http://dx.doi.org/10.1016/B978-0-12-801772-2.00042-4

Chapter 42

Factitious disorders and malingering in relation to functional neurologic disorders

C. BASS[1]* AND P. HALLIGAN[2]
[1]*Department of Psychological Medicine, John Radcliffe Hospital, Oxford, UK*
[2]*School of Psychology, Cardiff University, Cardiff, UK*

Abstract

Interest in malingering has grown in recent years, and is reflected in the exponential increase in academic publications since 1990. Although malingering is more commonly detected in medicolegal practice, it is not an all-or-nothing presentation and moreover can vary in the extent of presentation. As a nonmedical disorder, the challenge for clinical practice remains that malingering by definition is intentional and deliberate. As such, clinical skills alone are often insufficient to detect it and we describe psychometric tests such as symptom validity tests and relevant nonmedical investigations. Finally, we describe those areas of neurologic practice where symptom exaggeration and deception are more likely to occur, e.g., postconcussional syndrome, psychogenic nonepileptic seizures, motor weakness and movement disorders, and chronic pain.

Factitious disorders are rare in clinical practice and their detection depends largely on the level of clinical suspicion supported by the systematic collection of relevant information from a variety of sources. In this chapter we challenge the accepted DSM-5 definition of factitious disorder and suggest that the traditional glossaries have neglected the extent to which a person's reported symptoms can be considered a product of intentional choice or selective psychopathology largely beyond the subject's voluntary control, or more likely, both. We present evidence to suggest that neurologists preferentially diagnose factitious presentations in healthcare workers as "hysterical," possibly to avoid the stigma of simulated illness.

A lie is as good as the truth if you can get somebody to believe it.

INTRODUCTION

Controversial and ubiquitous, deception describes a common pervasive form of episodic human behavior that understandably raises concerns and prejudices when found and/or thought to occur in medical settings (Conroy and Kwartner, 2006). Considered by some to be evolutionarily adaptive (Spence, 2004), it is important from the outset to locate illness deception within a wider context of human deception. In a study of absenteeism in Canada of hospital workers who had just returned from a scheduled day off or an unscheduled day off classified by the employer as due to sickness absence, 72% admitted not being sick on their (sick) day off (Haccoun and DuPont, 1987).

The key issue (and source of much controversy) in medicine remains the extent to which a person's reported symptoms can be considered a product of conscious choice, a form of psychopathology (beyond the person's volitional making), and/or perhaps both. Notwithstanding recent experimental findings using functional brain imaging, the diagnosis established is frequently

*Correspondence to: Dr. Christopher Bass, MA MD FRCPsych, Consultant Liaison Psychiatrist, Department of Psychological Medicine, John Radcliffe Hospital, Oxford OX3 9DU, UK. E-mail: c.bass1@btinternet.com

"influenced by circumstantial factors and the physician's opinion of the patient's personality or background" (Spence, 2004).

According to Rogers (1997):

> *If we never investigate dissimulation [e.g., deceit subterfuge, falsification], then we may never find it. I believe that our working assumption in clinical practice should be that an appreciable minority of evaluatees engage, at some time, in a dissimulate response style. If we accept this working assumption, then we also accept the responsibility to screen all referrals and activity to consider the possibility of malingering and other forms of deception.*

We have argued elsewhere (Halligan et al., 2003b; Bass and Halligan, 2014) that illness deception (e.g., factitious disorder and malingering as defined in DSM-5) is probably underestimated and is better understood within a wider biopsychosocial model. At the heart of the DSM-5 definition is falsification of symptoms and/or signs associated with deception, in the absence of external rewards. The behavior is not accounted for by another mental disorder such as delusional disorder.

We suggest that the medicalization of illness deception (such as factitious disorders and compensation neurosis) arose largely as an attempt to create a way of bridging or linking diagnoses between unconsciously mediated psychiatric disorder and consciously mediated malingering (Bass and Halligan, 2014). Moreover, we believe that the current DSM diagnosis of factitious disorder has little clinical validity (Bass and Halligan, 2007).

This is not to argue that medical factors involving deception are not relevant, but that medical education needs to provide doctors with a broad conceptual, developmental, and management framework from which to better understand and manage deception in patient–doctor interactions. It is equally important however, to ensure that medical disorders are not ignored where symptoms-based illness behavior provides for an alternative working hypothesis. A study in the Israeli military showed that two dozen conscripts repeatedly considered to be malingering were in fact suffering from serious psychiatric disorders (Witztum et al., 1996).

A growing challenge for dealing with illness deception is the increasing acceptance that many medical illnesses cannot be exclusively diagnosed or validated on the basis of the biomedical model. Medically unexplained symptoms (MUS) continue to form one of the most expensive diagnostic categories in Europe and are the fifth most common reason for visiting doctors in the USA (Creed et al., 2011). Interest in functional neurologic disorders has also grown steadily over the last decade, and recent conferences on conversion disorders and psychogenic movement disorders (PMD) have led to the publication of a number of books (Halligan et al., 2001; Hallett et al., 2011) and in the UK the formation of an interdisciplinary Functional Neurology Group (Carson et al., 2011a). In tandem, there has been a growing neuropsychologic interest in illness deception and malingering (e.g., Halligan et al., 2003a; Rogers, 2008; Bass and Halligan, 2014; Young, 2014), with neuropsychologists and clinicians introducing and refining novel methods of assessment in patients suspected of simulating illness.

In addition to a brief historic review, this chapter considers some current themes and outlines the main areas of clinical practice where deception can complicate the clinical presentation and its subsequent management, with particular reference to neurologic practice.

HISTORIC CONTEXT

The practice of illness deception by feigning illness has a long history, with illustrative cases from Greek, biblical and classic literature. Before the 1880s there are several isolated reports on malingering (e.g., Gavin, 1838), listing motives such as the need to "to obtain the ease and comfort of a hospital" and the "avoidance of duties." Similar motives were ascribed to the behavior of soldiers in the American Civil War, including "choosing a career diversion as a patient rather than a soldier" (Bartholow, 1863). But, as Wessely (2003) argues, a key catalyst behind the growth in illness deception was the introduction of the social welfare state and in particular the rise in workmen's compensation schemes in the postindustrial revolution societies of North America and Western Europe. Fallik (1972) goes so far as to suggest that:

> *laws of social welfare and work insurance were made mostly for law-abiding people who really are in need. Therefore it is not the individual who causes the problem of simulation and malingering but the society which created the legal framework for exploitation.*

The introduction of social insurance schemes and of steam-driven train accidents led to an increase in illness deception and moved from the social, moral, and political to the medical sphere (Mendelson and Mendelson, 1993).

In the UK in 1913, Sir John Collie published a book on malingering and feigned sickness (including hysteria), where the doctor was cast in the role of detective, utilizing a number of tricks, signs, and traps to detect the malingering patient.

Malingering and the military have always been closely linked (Palmer, 2003). The advent of the First World War, with its focus on "psychotraumatology," including "shellshock," provided a fertile ground for revisiting non-medical etiologies and diagnostic challenges for psychiatrists (Crocq and Crocq, 2000). Given that the military and the governments at the time were ill prepared to accept the large number of psychiatric casualties, "psychiatrists were often viewed as a useless burden" (Crocq and Crocq, 2000). This was well illustrated in a memorandum addressed by Winston Churchill to the Lord President of the Council in December 1942, where he wrote:

> *I am sure it would be sensible to restrict as much as possible the work of these gentlemen [psychologists and psychiatrists]... it is very wrong to disturb large numbers of healthy, normal men and women by asking the kind of odd questions in which the psychiatrists specialize (Ahrenfeldt, 1958).*

In the UK, detecting malingering became part of the war effort, and when Collie's textbook was reissued in 1917, the second edition was nearly twice as long. After the First World War, the focus of illness deception moved from military to civilian settings, with medical practitioners as the main gatekeepers.

Gavin introduced the term "factitious disorder" in 1838 in a book on military malingering, to delineate a subtype of malingering where the clinical evidence was tampered with or faked. The term was used sporadically over the next 100 years, but it was not until Richard Asher's paper in 1951 involving 5 cases described as "Munchausen's syndrome" that greater awareness of illness deception was raised. However, factitious disorder first entered the psychiatric glossaries in 1980 (American Psychiatric Association, 1980) and was used to describe (diagnose) those patients considered to differ from hysteria, in whom the symptoms were produced consciously rather than unconsciously (Hyler and Spitzer, 1978). In their essay on the origins of factitious disorder, Kanaan and Wessely (2010a) suggest that the term developed as a "mediating diagnosis" between hysteria and malingering, whilst recognizing that some of the diagnoses classified as such would have been previously subsumed within the category of hysteria. One of the main consequence of the new nosology was appropriating a form of illness deception as a legitimate, medical diagnosis (Bass and Halligan, 2014).

DIAGNOSIS OF SIMULATED ILLNESS

Despite general acceptance that malingering is not a medical diagnosis "it is clear from medical literature and the examination of law reports that many doctors consider detection of malingering as an integral part of the medical enterprise" (Mendelson, 1995). From a clinical and diagnostic perspective, however, there is also evidence that most people, including clinicians, are unable to reliably and consistently detect the contributory role of deception (Ekman, 1985; Rosen et al., 2004). Unlike more established medical conditions there is evidence that factitious disorders and malingering behaviors are episodic, situation-specific, and dependent on selective interactions with medical, social, or legal professionals governed by a cost–benefit analysis (Rogers, 1990).

Moreover, feigning illness is not as difficult as some doctors appear to imagine, "The possibility that an individual would ever feign illness runs contrary to the empathetic, trusting nature of the physician, so the issue often never reaches the threshold of consideration" (Lande, 1989). According to Barrow (1971), who developed the use of "standardized" patient programs in North America,

> *A wide range of psychiatric problems can be simulated, such as depression, agitation, psychosis, neurotic reactions and thought aberrations, with little problem. In neurology, the simulated patients can show a variety: paralysis, sensory losses, reflex changes, extensor plantar responses, gait abnormalities, cranial nerve palsy, altered levels of consciousness, coma, seizures, hyperkinesias, and so forth.*

Even after being warned that these "simulated patients" were among the examinees, experienced clinicians found it difficult to detect them (Halligan et al., 2003a).

According to Eagles et al. (2007), "simulated patients are now deployed for teaching purposes in almost all areas of medicine where students and healthcare professionals interact with conscious patients." At Aberdeen, Eagles and colleagues (2007) employed professional actors and used live performances informed by detailed life histories and scripts. Psychiatric conditions presented by these actors included depression, anxiety, alcohol misuse/dependence, hypomania, schizophrenia, psychosis with aggression, obsessive-compulsive disorder, overdose in adolescence, and early dementia. In their final year, students have "a week of joint teaching from psychiatrists and general practitioners, during which actors portray somatisation, life crisis/depression, the spouse of a dementia sufferer, adolescent crisis and alcohol misuse." With actors portraying a wide range of presentations with "flair and professionalism," students generally found that they could not distinguish them from "real" patients (Eagles et al., 2007).

GROWING INTEREST IN ILLNESS DECEPTION

After World War II medical efforts to detect deception moved from clinical "intuition" to the more active search for new techniques to detect it. Understanding deception in the medical context was further facilitated by the introduction of concepts such as abnormal illness behavior (Pilowsky, 1969; Mechanic, 1978). The introduction of quantitative testing by clinical psychologists however arrived relatively late, with the first modern textbook on malingering published as late as 1988 (Rogers, 1988), but now in its third edition (Rogers, 2008).

Identifying the number of published papers using key illness deception terms provides a simple way to capture the growing interest in the field. A bibliometric scan (Fig. 42.1) of the published journal papers listing the terms "malingering" using Scopus (the largest abstract and citation database of English-language peer-reviewed literature) over the past 123 years (accessed December 2014) lists nearly 4000 documents and shows a slow and relatively modest interest until the 1990s. By 2000 the number of documents pertaining to malingering was approaching 150 per year (Berry and Nelson, 2010).

A similar bibliometric scan of the published journal papers listing the terms "factitious disorder" again using Scopus (accessed December 2014) showed an understandably slower uptake. Since 1891, Scopus listed a total of nearly 2000 documents but shows a slow but growing interest, with approximately 50 papers per year since 1980.

Finally, a bibliometric scan of the published journal papers listing the specific illness deception term "Munchausen's syndrome," coined by Asher in 1951 (accessed December 2014) lists over 500 documents demonstrating variable interest, with an average of 15 papers per year since 1997.

PSYCHOSOCIAL CONTEXT

The clinical dilemmas presented by patients with illnesses without definable biomedical causes are well established (Hatcher and Arroll, 2008; Sharpe, 2013). In general practice, one-fifth of consultations constitute medical unexplained symptoms (MUS) (Burton, 2003) and estimates of those without confirmed disease seen in hospital outpatient clinics range from 35% to 53% (Stone et al., 2010; Creed et al., 2011). These figures are likely to be an underestimate, as many doctors understandably remain cautious about excluding physical disease and presenting a patient with a "psychogenic," less than definitive diagnosis (Espay et al., 2009).

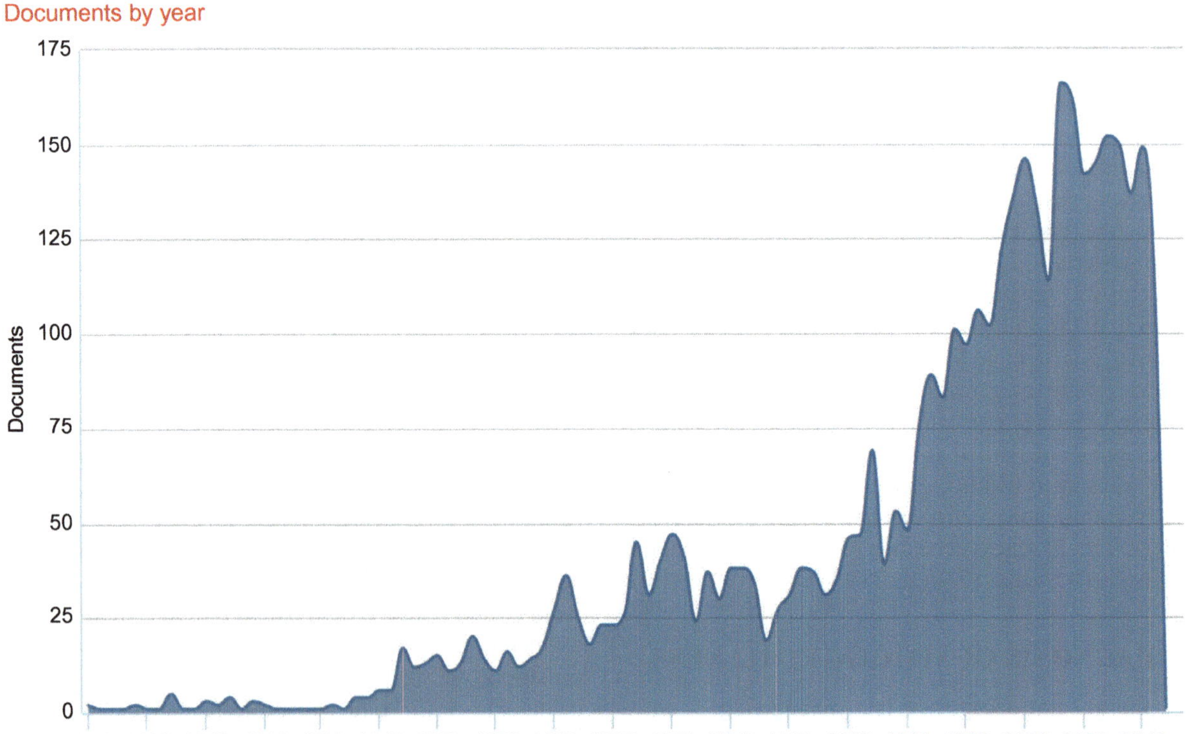

Fig. 42.1. Number of published papers on malingering (Scopus December 2014).

Whereas disease is typically dependent on objective abnormalities of physical structure or function, illness relates to the patient's experience, including what the individual reports to be involuntary behaviors. This, in turn, has led to the growing inclusion of a number of illness-based conditions such as "functional somatic symptoms/syndromes," particularly within psychiatry, where many of the mental disorders already described by DSM-5 currently remain biomedically unexplained.

In response to the perceived and growing need to consider more complex, interactional, and contextual paradigms, "biopsychosocial models" applied to health sciences emerged in the 1970s (Engel, 1977; White, 2005). These biopsychologic models, however, were not specifically etiologic but rather argued for a more holistic process model of illness (Halligan and Aylward, 2006), where the person, and not the disease, is the central focus when defining ill health. Acute and chronic symptoms originating from benign or mild forms of physical or mental impairment were considered to be re-experienced as amplified perceptions with accompanying distress which, when filtered through the presenting patient's attitudes, beliefs, coping skills, and occupational or cultural social context, were seen to affect patients' perceptions of their impairment and associated disability (Petrie and Weinman, 2006).

FACTITIOUS DISORDERS

Definition

It was recently suggested that factitious disorders should be considered a variant of somatoform disorders (Krahn et al., 2008), as both conditions provide patients with the opportunity to "organize their lives around seeking medical services in spite of having primarily a psychiatric condition." This latter model has been adopted by DSM-5, with factitious disorders recategorized as somatic symptom disorders with two types: factitious disorder imposed on self and factitious disorder imposed on the other. Although the motivation for the behavior has attracted less emphasis in this definition, which tends to focus more on observed behavior, there remains little recognition that patients as people can and do exercise choices which can, and often includes being influenced by personal gain or benefit (Bass and Halligan, 2014).

Epidemiology

Factitious disorders are relatively uncommon but, like many conditions remain largely based on patient feedback, and probably remains underdiagnosed. A survey of referrals to a psychiatric liaison service in a North American general hospital found that 0.8% had factitious disorder (Sutherland and Rodin, 1990). Surveys of physicians demonstrate a wide range of prevalence estimates, with a mean estimated prevalence of 1.3%, with dermatologists and neurologists giving the highest estimations (Fliege et al., 2007).

Recognizing simulation remains largely a function of experience and the predisposing attitudes of the observer, especially neurologists (Miller and Cartilidge, 1972). In a review of factitious disorders in neurology, Kanaan and Wessely (2010b) found that neurology patients were strikingly different from those in other specialties in terms of their demographics. Considering 90 patients from a total of 45 published reports, they found a wide range of neurologic presentations, the most common of which was functional motor symptoms/simulated strokes, and seizures/blackouts. They found that proportionately more of the patients were male (56%) and only 17% were healthcare workers, which was surprising, given that the majority of patients with factitious disorders are women and many are involved in the healthcare professions. The authors speculated that "factitious nurses" (or, more properly, nurses presenting with factitious disorders) are typically diagnosed with conversion disorder. They also speculated that there was evidence that neurologists preferentially diagnosed factitious presentations in nurses as "hysterical," presumably to avoid the stigma of simulated illness.

Factitious disorders: clinical features

Clinical features remain diverse, but the majority of patients with factitious disorders are nonperipatetic, socially conforming young women with relatively stable social networks (Krahn et al., 2003). Evidence of fabrication can be derived from multiple sources, e.g., inexplicable laboratory results, an inconsistent or implausible history, admission of an induced illness (rare), scrutiny of outside records, observed tampering with syringes, and finding hidden medications. Deputing a clinician to construct a medical chronology is invaluable.

Most patients enact their deceptions in general hospitals, especially Accident and Emergency departments. In a large case series 72% were women, of whom two-thirds had an affiliation with health-related professions (Krahn et al., 2003). In this study the initial presentation of factitious disorders typically began before the age of 30 years, but there is often evidence of simulation in childhood and adolescence. Close enquiry and examination of medical records often reveal an unexpectedly large number of childhood illnesses and operations, and high rates of substance abuse, mood disorder, and personality disorder (Bass and Halligan, 2014). There is also increasing evidence to suggest that a high proportion of patients with factitious disorders have so-called cluster B personality disorders, in particular borderline personality disorder (Goldstein, 1998; Gordon and Sansone, 2013). Recent case reports of suicide suggest that deceptive behavior does not preclude the presence of serious psychopathology (Binder and Grieffenstein, 2012).

There is a suggestion that factitious behavior can be "communicated" from one generation to another (Libow, 1995). For example, of children with illnesses induced by their carers (often the mothers), a proportion present with pseudoneurologic symptoms such as anoxic episodes and epilepsy. Examination of their mother's medical records reveals that pseudoseizures are often a key component of their somatoform presentation (Bass and Jones, 2011). This is an important observation, and neurologists should be alert to it, especially as seizures have been reported to be the most common presentations of fabricated and induced illness in children (Barber and Davis, 2002).

Table 42.1

Supportive confrontation: preparation and process (for nonpsychiatrists)

- Collect firm evidence of fabrication, e.g., catheter, syringe, ligature
- Discuss with psychiatrist (or member of hospital legal team if no psychiatrist is available)
- Arrange meeting to marshal the facts, discuss strategy, discuss with primary care doctor
- Confrontation with the patient should be nonjudgmental and nonpunitive, and include a proposal of ongoing support and follow-up
- Discuss the outcome of the confrontation with the primary care doctor
- If the patient is a healthcare worker, the doctor should discuss with a member of his/her defense organization
- Document a full record of the meeting and its outcome in the patient record

Management

Management of simulated disorders can be divided into two phases: the acute management in the hospital, which could be an emergency room or an inpatient infectious diseases unit, or the chronic process of engaging the patient in outpatient management with some form of psychotherapy (McCullumsmith and Ford, 2011). Management in both phases must focus on negotiating the diagnosis with the patient and then engaging the patient into treatment.

The initial diagnosis of factitious disorder (in hospital) is nearly always made by a nonpsychiatrist, who may wish to involve a psychiatric college in a supportive confrontation of the patient. This process requires careful preparation (Table 42.1).

There is no robust research evidence to support the effectiveness of any management strategy for factitious illness (Eastwood and Bisson, 2008). Despite this, the authors of this chapter recommend supportive confrontation, which should always involve at least two members of staff, with an emphasis on the patient being a sick person in need of help. For some patients a more nuanced approach may be preferred, with nonconfrontational approaches. Face saving is a key element, and it is important for patients to subsequently explain their disclosures to other people as "recoveries," without admitting that their original problems were fabricated.

Course and prognosis

Recovery from factitious disorder is extremely rare as few patients agree to comply with treatment. In the 93 patients described by Krahn et al. (2003), three-quarters were confronted with their diagnosis; however, only 17% acknowledged that their illness was self-induced or simulated, and a small number agreed to have psychiatric treatment, but the outcomes were not published. Despite this, recent accounts of patients wishing to engage in treatment have demonstrated that, with appropriate management, these individuals can be helped (Avignal and Hall, 2012; Bass and Taylor, 2013). In a fascinating study using a novel method of accessing first-hand experiences of an online community of factitious disorder sufferers, Lawlor and Kirakowski (2014) found that members were aware of their motivations, were upset by their behavior, and claimed to want to recover, but were deterred by fear. The enormous cost to the healthcare system has been extensively documented (Hoertel et al., 2012).

MALINGERING

Conceptual and definitional problems

Rogers (1990) considers malingering to be a behavior governed by a cost–benefit analysis. Psychiatric glossaries have struggled to define malingering, and the shortcomings of the DSM-5 definition have been described elsewhere (Bass and Halligan, 2014). In essence, the diagnostic glossary presents malingering as a categoric condition ("the intentional production of false or grossly exaggerated physical or psychological symptoms, motivated by external incentives" and where this external gain may take the form of financial rewards, or evading criminal responsibility), while much of the evidence supports the view that it is a dimensional construct. As Lipman (1962) pointed out, the behavior is not a binary

Table 42.2

Malingering – best viewed as a continuum disorder

1. Exaggeration: symptoms and/or disabilities magnified or embellished
2. Dissimulation (concealment): patient denies the existence of problems that would account for the symptoms (e.g., presenting to doctors repeatedly with gastric bleeding whilst deliberately withholding the fact that he/she is prescribed nonsteroidal anti-inflammatory drugs)
3. Symptom feignings only (subjective states, e.g., abdominal pain)
4. Misattribution/false imputation of cause: attributing real symptoms to a false cause (e.g., patient reports symptoms that were formerly present and ceased, but are alleged to continue; alternatively, genuine symptoms are fraudulently attributed to a particular injury)
5. Invention: creating symptoms and signs when none exist (e.g., smash fist on wall and present to Accident and Emergency, stating that hand was damaged in a road traffic accident)

characteristic of being "present" or "absent": an individual might, for example, be exaggerating genuine difficulties (Table 42.2).

Epidemiology

A frequently cited study (Mittenberg et al., 2002) found that experienced neuropsychologists estimate the prevalence of malingering in patient referrals from civil (i.e., personal injury cases) and criminal legal settings to be in the 10–30% range. Further evidence to support the nontrivial prevalence of malingering comes from studies that have administered symptom validity tests (SVTs) to patients involved in litigation or disability-related evaluation (discussed further below). Many of these studies concluded that the prevalence of suspicious performance on SVTs exceeds the 10–30% range in those seeking compensation who report a diverse range of clinical disorders, e.g., mild traumatic brain injury, whiplash neck injury, and psychogenic nonepileptic seizures (PNES). The feigning of disabling illness for the purpose of disability compensation has been reported to occur in 45–59% of adult cases, with an estimated cost of $20 billion for adult mental disorder claimants (Chafetz and Underhill, 2013).

Assessment

The clinical cornerstone of detection as opposed to diagnosis of malingering is the well-prepared clinical interview, having reviewed available documents and incorporating available forensic materials. Further evidence includes lying from differing accounts to people, evidence of tampering with wounds, and avoiding investigations that might confirm their stated diagnosis. Typically, diagnosis requires collating evidence from multiple sources over time, including both structured and unstructured clinical interviews, psychometric testing, and information collected from third parties (Iverson, 2007).

A longitudinal health record is invaluable, as medical records provide objective evidence of reported complaints and clinic attendances that help illuminate the relationship between an accident/injury/life event and any subsequent symptoms attributed by the patient to the putative causal event. A chronologic summary or "chronology" often pays dividends in the assessment of health documents.

Special investigations

Probably the most widely encountered is video surveillance and evidence from social media sites, typically provided by the insurance companies/lawyers. Usually this provides information about both the reported and observed physical abilities of the claimant. Marked or unexpected differences between the claimant's reported/observed behaviors and what he/she claims not to be able to do can understandably raise serious doubts as to the credibility of a claimant's report.

Psychologic approaches

Clinical psychologists and neuropsychologists have developed tests that claim to provide for a more precise assessment of the credibility of verbally claimed symptoms. In this context symptom validity refers to the accuracy or veracity of a person's behavioral presentation, self-reported symptoms, or performance on neuropsychologic tests (Larrabee, 2012; Tracy, 2014). SVTs typically comprise a simple memory or recognition task in which a wide range of people with neurologic or psychiatric problems can achieve near-perfect performance (Guidotti Breting and Sweet, 2013). The basic premise behind this approach is establishing a finding of "below-chance" (i.e., less than 50%) performance on a forced-choice test. Here voluntary endorsement of incorrect answers (Bush et al., 2005) is taken by some as "tantamount to confession of malingering" (Larrabee, 2004), but by others to help the expert to differentiate between credible and noncredible symptom presentations (Merten and Merckelbach, 2013). Professional bodies and guidelines have stressed the importance of SVTs (Heilbronner et al., 2009).

When patients present with dissociative and somatoform disorders or MUS, clinicians may administer SVTs to determine whether or not the patient exhibits negative response bias. Although some authors have argued that psychologic problems (e.g., unconscious conflicts and depression) and life circumstances (e.g., a cry for help) may explain such bias, Merten and Merckelbach (2013) have argued that there is no empiric evidence to support the view that psychiatric disorders such as somatoform and dissociative disorders lead to SVT failure. These authors have argued that it is not unreasonable to conclude that the patient's self-reported symptoms and life history can no longer be accepted at face value.

CLINICAL PRESENTATIONS RELATING TO NEUROPSYCHIATRIC PRACTICE

Malingered cognitive deficit (e.g., postconcussional syndrome)

A significant proportion (15–30%) of patients with mild traumatic brain injury seem at risk of developing postconcussional syndrome, with symptoms such as headache, distress, cognitive problems, and dizziness (Hou et al., 2012). It has also been shown that there is an association between patient concern (i.e., expectations) that symptoms will have adverse consequences, and the reporting of major and enduring complaints (Whittaker et al., 2007; Ferrari, 2011).

In their influential paper, Miller and Cartilidge (1972) suggested that many patients malingered their memory and other cognitive symptoms and those symptoms were in inverse proportion to injury severity and were only resolved with receipt of compensation. Recent findings tend to support the authors' original observations that embellishment rises as injury severity decreases in a compensable context (Greiffenstein and Baker, 2005). The American Academy of Neuropsychologists recently published a consensus statement which concluded that "Symptom exaggeration or fabrication occurs in a sizeable minority of neuropsychological examinees, with greater prevalence in forensic contexts," and that the use of effort testing is mandatory in neuropsychologic assessments (Heilbronner et al., 2009). By contrast, in individuals with moderate to severe brain injury, Gouse et al. (2013) found no evidence that subjects malingered or delivered suboptimal effort during neuropsychologic testing in the context of litigation.

Silver (2012) has recently argued against excessive reliance on the results of effort testing as evidence of malingering. He pointed out that poor effort and exaggeration are not categoric values, but are complex and multidetermined and have a differential diagnosis of their own. Some factors, he suggests, are intrinsic to the circumstances of the injury or the assessment process, such as expectations and beliefs about illness duration and consequences, the pressure to perform well under "threat conditions," and anger and revenge.

Similar views have been expressed by Bender and Matusewicz (2013), who cited work suggesting that deception in the medicolegal arena may not be a one-dimensional construct but instead involves at least two dimensions: self and other. Each separate dimension may involve varying degrees, such that high self-deception and low other-deception would reflect pure MUS, and vice versa for pure malingering (Merckelbach and Merten, 2012). Further research is needed to describe this paradigm and how it applies to the boundaries between somatoform disorders, factitious disorders, and malingering.

Somatoform and dissociative disorders

It is well established that approximately one-third of all referrals to outpatient services in neurology have symptoms unexplained by disease (e.g., conversion symptoms such as paralysis or blackouts; Carson et al, 2011b). Furthermore, follow-up studies of these patients have shown that two-thirds had a poor outcome after 1 year (Sharpe et al., 2010). Significantly, illness beliefs and receipt of financial benefits were more useful in predicting poor outcome than the number of symptoms, disability, and distress.

It has recently been demonstrated that, in nonlitigant patients presenting to neurology outpatients, 11% failed effort tests (Kemp et al., 2008). It is possible that some patients with somatoform disorders are likely to fail effort testing due to consciously feigning or symptom exaggeration (i.e., factitious disorder or malingering) and that, if this is the case, then the patient's self-report can no longer be taken at face value (Merten and Merckelbach, 2013). An alternative explanation is that, for various nonspecific reasons, such as fatigue, pain, general malaise, or the presence of medical symptoms (regardless of etiology), patients could have underperformed on effort tests in the absence of intention to feign or exaggerate. The authors of this paper urged clinicians to acquire the tools to identify patients who do exaggerate and base rate data that assist them in making judgments that do not prejudice patients in genuine clinical need. In an accompanying commentary to this paper, Stone (2008) pointed out that cognitive effort testing is only a proxy measure of the degree of motoric "effort failure" that may underlie other physical symptoms, such as weakness and fatigue, and furthermore that the study did not reveal whether patients with weakness, for example, had "effort failure" when attempting to move their weak limb.

It is possible that the emergence of effort testing may cast new light on the area of unexplained physical symptoms. For example, the concept of somatoform disorders assumes that the symptoms are not consciously produced

(Creed et al., 2011). However, to date studies of patients with functional neurologic disorders have yielded equivocal results. Heintz et al. (2013) compared patients with PMD and those with Gilles de la Tourette syndrome using an SVT to measure noncredible test performance. No evidence of neuropsychologic impairments was found in the PMD sample: the only differences to emerge were noncredible cognitive symptoms in the PMD patients. The authors concluded that noncredible response might help to differentiate PMD from other movement disorders.

Psychogenic nonepileptic seizures

Drane et al. (2006) first raised the possibility that patients with PNES performed poorly on effort tests, especially when compared to patients with epilepsy. These findings were not replicated by Dodrill (2008), whose patients were recruited over a consecutive period, none of whom had received epilepsy surgery. In keeping with the findings of Cragar et al. (2006), these authors founds a high failure rate on effort test scores for the epilepsy patients, and point out that the failure rate in unselected epilepsy patient samples may be much higher than is commonly believed.

In a recent study of 91 participants with PNES, Williamson et al. (2012) found a relationship between failure rates on SVTs and reported histories of abuse, but, contrary to expectation, was not associated with the presence of financial incentives or severity of reported psychopathology. This finding was unexpected, and the extent to which SVT failure is related to reports of abuse in other groups of patients with MUS is unclear. It has been argued that large-scale studies that dissect incentive, motivation, and effort (as opposed to effort tests) are needed to answer these questions (Bender and Matusewicz, 2013).

Complex regional pain syndrome

The phenomenon of complex regional pain syndrome type I (CRPS I) can arise after an injury to a limb (Goebel, 2011). It is often diagnosed on the basis of nonspecific, often subjective observations, and in 85% of patients the symptoms resolve within 18 months (de Mos et al., 2009). It has been shown that certain "diagnostic" features, such as skin temperature and color differences between limbs, can be produced and maintained by short-term immobilization and dependency of the limb (Singh and Davis, 2006). Iatrogenic complications are common and can lead to amputation in some cases (de Asla, 2011). Self-induced symptoms have been reported (Mailis-Gagnon et al., 2008) and, in a recent survey of 73 patients with CRPS, potentially incentivized by disability-seeking contexts, at least 75% of the sample failed one performance validity indicator and over half showed at least one positive symptom validity score (Grieffenstein et al., 2013). These findings suggest that doctors need to be vigilant when confronted with this diagnosis, especially in medicolegal settings (Ochoa and Verdugo, 2010; Crick and Crick, 2011; Bass, 2014).

Prognosis and outcome

The levels of physical disability and psychologic comorbidity in follow-up studies of patients with functional motor symptoms (weakness and movement disorder) are generally high (Gelauff et al., 2014). The prognosis for malingered neurologic disorders, however, is unknown, but clinical experience suggests that patients with longstanding disability, even if partly or wholly nonorganic, do not always recover after settlement (Mendelson, 1995). Outcomes following the completion of litigation require more systematic evaluation.

CONCLUSIONS

Sensitivities surrounding the nature of illness deception will no doubt continue to be a challenging issue for modern medicine given the growing recognition that many medical illnesses are not exclusively diagnosed or validated on the basis of the biomedical model. Given the personal, financial, and social benefits provided by sick role and the low risk of detection (Halligan et al., 2003b), it seems reasonable that illness deception is more prevalent than previously presumed or detected. Much of the controversy surrounding illness deception reflects the conflict of strongly held beliefs regarding human nature and the motivation of people seeking medical attention. Unlike the traditional biomedical model, the expanded World Health Organization International Classification of Functioning model, which highlights the role of the person when defining illness (Wade and Halligan, 2003), provides a more comprehensive and pragmatic model that includes the capacity for people as patients to knowingly engage in deception for the purpose of personal gain or avoidance of responsibility.

References

Ahrenfeldt R (1958). Psychiatry in the British army in the Second World War. Columbia University Press, New York, NY26.

American Psychiatric Association (1980). Diagnostic and Statistical manual of mental Disorders, 3rd edn. American Psychiatric Association, Washington, DC.

Asher R (1951). Munchausen's syndrome. Lancet 1: 339–341.

Avignal A, Hall T (2012). Secrets unraveled. Overcoming Munchausen syndrome (ebook).

Barber M, Davis P (2002). Fits, faints, or fatal fantasy? Fabricated seizures and child abuse. Arch Dis Child 86: 230–233.

Barrow H (1971). Simulated patients, Charles C Thomas, Springfield, IL.

Bartholow R (1863). A Manual of Instructions for Enlisting and Discharging Soldiers, J. B. Lippincott, Philadelphia, PA.

Bass C (2014). Complex regional pain syndrome medicalises limb pain. Br Med J 348: g2361.

Bass C, Halligan P (2007). Illness related deception: social or psychiatric problem? J R Soc Med 100: 81–84.

Bass C, Halligan P (2014). Factitious disorders and malingering: challenges for clinical assessment and management. Lancet 383: 1422–1432.

Bass C, Jones D (2011). Psychopathology of perpetrators of fabricated or induced illness: a case series. Br J Psychiatr 199: 113–118.

Bass C, Taylor M (2013). Recovery from chronic factitious disorder (Munchausen's syndrome): a personal account. Pers Ment Health 7: 80–83.

Bender S, Matusewicz M (2013). PCS, iatrogenic symptoms, and malingering following concussion. Psychol Inj Law 6: 113–121.

Berry D, Nelson N (2010). DSM-5 and malingering: a modest proposal. Psychol Inj Law 3: 295–303.

Binder L, Grieffenstein M (2012). Deceptive examinees who committed suicide: report of two cases. Clin Neuropsychol 26: 116–128.

Burton C (2003). Beyond somatization: a review of the understanding and treatment of patients with medically unexplained physical symptoms (MUPS). Br J Gen Pract 53: 231–239.

Bush S, Ruff RM, Troster AI et al. (2005). Symptom validity assessment: practical issues and medical necessity: NANN policy and planning committee. Arch Clin Neuropsychol 20: 419–426.

Carson A, Brown R, David A et al. (2011a). Functional (conversion) neurological symptoms: research since the millennium. J Neurol Neurosurg Psychiatry 83: 842–850.

Carson A, Stone J, Hibberd C et al. (2011b). Disability, distress and unemployment in neurology outpatients with symptoms "unexplained by organic disease". J Neurol Neurosurg Psychiatry 82: 810–813.

Chafetz M, Underhill J (2013). Estimated costs of malingered disability. Arch Clin Neuropsychol 28: 633–639.

Collie J (1913). Malingering and Feigned Sickness, Edward Arnold, London.

Conroy MA, Kwartner P (2006). Malingering. Appl Psychol Crim Justice 2 (3): 29–51.

Cragar D, Berry D, Fakhoury T et al. (2006). Performance of patients with epilepsy or psychogenic non-epileptic seizures on four measures of effort. Clin Neuropsychol 20: 552–556.

Creed F, Barsky A, Leiknes K (2011). Epidemiology: prevalence, causes and consequences. In: F Creed, P Henninngsen, P Fink (Eds.), Medically Unexplained Symptoms, Somatisation and Bodily Distress, Cambridge University Press, Cambridge, pp. 1–42.

Crick B, Crick J (2011). Lawsuit verdicts and settlements involving reflex sympathetic dystrophy and complex regional pain syndrome. J Surg Orthop Adv 20: 153–157.

Crocq M, Crocq L (2000). From shell shock and war neurosis to posttraumatic stress disorder: a history of psychotraumatology. Dialogues Clin Neurosci 2: 47–55.

de Asla R (2011). Complex regional pain syndrome type 1: disease or illness construction? J Bone Surg Am 93 (19): e116 (1).

de Mos M, Huygen F, van der Hoeven-Borgman M et al. (2009). Outcome of the complex regional pain syndrome. Clin J Pain 25: 590–597.

Dodrill C (2008). Do patients with psychogenic nonepileptic seizures produce trustworthy findings on neuropsychological tests? Epilepsia 49: 691–696.

Drane D, Williamson D, Stroup E et al. (2006). Cognitive impairment is not equal in patients with epileptic and psychogenic nonepileptic seizures. Epilepsia 47: 1879–1886.

Eagles J, Calder S, Wilson S et al. (2007). Simulated patients in undergraduate education in psychiatry. Psychiatr Bull 31: 1878–1890.

Eastwood S, Bisson J (2008). Management of factitious disorders: a systematic review. Psychother Psychosom 77: 209–218.

Ekman P (1985). Telling Lies: Clues to Deceit in the Marketplace, Politics, and Marriage. W.W. Norton, New York.

Engel G (1977). The need for a new medical model: a challenge for biomedicine. Science 196: 129–136.

Espay A, Goldenhar L, Voon V et al. (2009). Opinions and clinical practices related to diagnosing and managing patients with psychogenic movement disorders: an international survey of movement disorder society members. Mov Disorders 24: 1366–1374.

Fallik A (1972). Simulation and malingering after injuries to the brain and spinal cord. Lancet 7760: 1126.

Ferrari R (2011). Minor head injury: do you get what you expect? J Neurol Neurosurg Psychiatry 82: 826.

Fliege H, Grimm A, Eckhardt-Henn A et al. (2007). Frequency of ICD-10 factitious disorder: survey of senior hospital consultants and physicians in private practice. Psychosomatics 48: 60–64.

Gavin H (1838). On feigned and factitious diseases, Edinburgh University Press, Edinburgh.

Gelauff J, Stone J, Edwards M et al. (2014). The prognosis of functional (psychogenic) motor symptoms: a systematic review. J Neurol Neurosurg Psychiatry 85: 220–226.

Goebel A (2011). Complex regional pain syndrome in adults. Rheumatology 50: 1739–1750.

Goldstein AB (1998). Identification and classification of factitious disorders: an analysis of cases reported during a 10-year period. Int J Psychiatry Med 28: 221–241.

Gordon D, Sansone R (2013). A relationship between factitious disorder and borderline personality disorder. Innov Clin Neurosci 10: 10–14.

Gouse H, Thomas K, Solms M (2013). Neuropsychological, functional, and behavioural outcome in South African traumatic brain injury litigants. Arch Clin Neuropsychol 28: 38–51.

Greiffenstein M, Baker J (2005). Miller was (mostly) right: head injury severity inversely related to simulation. Legal Crim Psychol 10: 1–16.

Grieffenstein M, Gervais R, Baker W et al. (2013). Symptom validity testing in medically unexplained pain: a chronic regional pain syndrome type 1 case series. Clin Neuropsychol 27: 138–147.

Guidotti Breting L, Sweet J (2013). Freestanding cognitive symptom validity tests: use and selection in mild traumatic brain injury. In: D Carone, S Bush (Eds.), Mild traumatic brain injury, symptom validity assessment and malingering, Springer, New York, pp. 145–158.

Haccoun R, DuPont S (1987). Absence research: a critique of previous approaches and an example for a new direction. Can J Admin Sci 15: 143–156.

Hallett M, Lang A, Jankovic J et al. (Eds.), (2011). Psychogenic Movement Disorders and other conversion disorders, Cambridge University Press, Cambridge.

Halligan P, Aylward M (Eds.), (2006). The Power of belief. Psychosocial influences on illness, disability, and medicine. Oxford University Press, Oxford.

Halligan P, Bass C, Marshall J (2001). Contemporary approaches to the study of hysteria, Oxford University Press, Oxford.

Halligan P, Bass C, Oakley D (2003a). Malingering and Illness Deception, Oxford University Press, Oxford.

Halligan P, Bass C, Oakley D (2003b). Willful deception as illness behaviour. In: P Halligan, C Bass, D Oakley (Eds.), Malingering and Illness Deception. Oxford University Press, Oxford, pp. 3–30.

Hatcher S, Arroll B (2008). Assessment and management of medically unexplained symptoms. Br Med J 336: 1124–1128.

Heilbronner R, Sweet J, Morgan J et al. (2009). American Academy of Clinical Neuropsychology Consensus Conference Statement on the neuropsychological assessment of effort, response bias, and malingering. Clin Neuropsychol 23: 1093–1129.

Heintz C, van Tricht M, van der Salm SA et al. (2013). Neuropsychological profile of psychogenic jerky movement disorders: importance of evaluating non-credible cognitive performance and psychopathology. J Neurol Neurosurg Psychiatry 84: 862–867.

Hoertel N, Levand P, Le Strat Y et al. (2012). Estimated cost of a factitious disorder patient with 6-year follow up. Psychiatry Res 200: 1077–1078.

Hou R, Moss-Morriss R, Peveler R et al. (2012). When a minor head injury results in enduring symptoms: a prospective investigation of risk factors for postconcussional syndrome after mild traumatic brain injury. J Neurol Neurosurg Psychiatry 83: 217–223.

Hyler S, Spitzer R (1978). Hysteria split asunder. Am J Psychiatr 135: 1500–1504.

Iverson G (2007). Identifying exaggeration and malingering. Pain Pract 7: 94–102.

Kanaan R, Wessely S (2010a). The origins of factitious disorder. Hist Hum Sci 23: 68–85.

Kanaan R, Wessely S (2010b). Factious disorders in neurology: an analysis of reported cases. Psychosomatics 51: 47–54.

Kemp S, Coughlan A, Rowbotham C et al. (2008). The base rate of effort test failure in patients with medically unexplained symptoms. J Psychosom Res 65: 319–325.

Krahn L, Honghzhe L, O'Connor K (2003). Patients who strive to be ill: factitious disorder with physical symptoms. Am J Psychiatr 160: 1163–1168.

Krahn L, Bostwick J, Stonnington C (2008). Looking towards DSM-5: should factitious disorder become a subtype of somatoform disorder? Psychosomatics 49: 277–282.

Lande R (1989). Malingering. J Am Osteopath Assoc 89: 483–488.

Larrabee G (2004). Differential diagnosis of mild head injury. In: J Ricker (Ed.), Differential diagnosis in adult neuropsychological assessment, Springer, New York, pp. 243–275.

Larrabee G (2012). Performance validity and symptom validity in neuropsychological assessment. J Int Neuropsychol Soc 18: 625–630.

Lawlor A, Kirakowski J (2014). When the lie is the truth: grounded theory analysis of an online support group for factitious disorder. Psychiatry Res 218: 209–218.

Libow J (1995). Munchausen by proxy victims in adulthood: a first look. Paediatrics 19: 1131–1142.

Lipman F (1962). Malingering in personal injury cases. Temple Law Q 35: 141–162.

Mailis-Gagnon A, Nicholson K, Blumberger D et al. (2008). Characteristics and period prevalence of self-induced disorder in patients referred to a pain clinic with the diagnosis of complex regional pain syndrome. Clin J Pain 24: 176–185.

McCullumsmith C, Ford C (2011). Simulated illness: the factious disorders and malingering. Psychiatr Clin North Am 34: 621–641.

Mechanic D (1978). Medical Sociology, 2nd edn. Free Press, New York.

Mendelson G (1995). Compensation neurosis revisited: outcome studies of the effects of litigation. J Psychosom Res 39: 695–706.

Mendelson G, Mendelson D (1993). Legal and psychiatric aspects of malingering. J Law Med 1: 28–34.

Merckelbach H, Merten T (2012). A note on cognitive dissonance and malingering. Clin Neuropsychol 26: 1217–1229.

Merten T, Merckelbach H (2013). Symptom validity testing in somatoform and dissociative disorders: a critical review. Psychol Inj Law 6: 122–137.

Miller H, Cartilidge N (1972). Simulation and malingering after injuries to the brain and spinal cord. Lancet 1: 580–585.

Mittenberg W, Patton C, Vanyock E et al. (2002). Base rates of malingering and symptom exaggeration. J Clin Exp Neuropsychol 24: 1094–1102.

Ochoa J, Verdugo R (2010). Neuropathic pain syndrome displayed by malingerers. J Neuropsychiatry Clin Neurosci 22: 278–286.

Palmer I (2003). Malingering, shirking, and self-inflicted injuries in the military. In: P Halligan, C Bass, D Oakley (Eds.), Malingering and Illness Deception. Oxford University Press, Oxford, pp. 42–53.

Petrie K, Weinman J (2006). Why illness perceptions matter. Clin Med 6: 536–539.

Pilowsky I (1969). Abnormal Illness behaviour. Br J Med Psychol 42: 347–351.

Rogers R (Ed.), (1988). Clinical assessment of Malingering and Deception, Guilford Press, New York.

Rogers R (1990). Development of a new classificatory model of malingering. Bull Am Acad Psychiatry law 18: 323–333.

Rogers R (1997). Introduction. In: R Rogers (Ed.), Clinical Assessment of Malingering and Deception, 2nd edn. Guilford Press, New York, pp. 1–19.

Rogers R (Ed.), (2008). Clinical assessment of Malingering and Deception, 3rd edn. Guilford Press, New York.

Rosen J, Mulsant B, Bruce M et al. (2004). Actors' portrayals of depression to test interrater reliability in clinical trials. Am J Psychiatr 161: 1909–1911.

Sharpe M (2013). Somatic symptoms: beyond "medically unexplained". Br J Psychiatr 203: 320–321.

Sharpe M, Stone J, Hibberd C et al. (2010). Neurology outpatients with symptoms unexplained by disease: illness beliefs and financial benefits predict 1-year outcome. Psychol Med 40: 689–698.

Silver JM (2012). Effort, exaggeration and malingering after concussion. J Neurol Neurosurg Psychiatr 83: 836–841.

Singh H, Davis T (2006). The effect of short term dependency and immobility on skin temperature and colour in the hand. J Hand Surg [Br] 31: 611–615.

Spence S (2004). The deceptive brain. J R Soc Med 97: 6–9.

Stone J (2008). Effort testing in patients with neurological symptoms unexplained by disease. J Psychosom Res 65: 327–328.

Stone J, Carson A, Duncan R et al. (2010). Who is referred to neurology clinics? The diagnoses made in 3781 new patients. Clin Neurol Neurosurg 112: 747–757.

Sutherland AJ, Rodin GM (1990). Factitious disorders in a general hospital setting: clinical features and review of the literature. Psychosomatics 31: 392–399.

Tracy T (2014). Evaluating malingering in cognitive and memory examinations: a guide for clinicians. Adv Psychiatr Treat 20: 405–412.

Wade D, Halligan P (2003). New wine in old bottles: the WHO ICF as an explanatory model of human behaviour. Clin Rehabil 17: 349–354.

Wessely S (2003). Malingering: historical perspectives. In: P Halligan, C Bass, D Oakley (Eds.), Malingering and Illness Deception. Oxford University Press, Oxford, pp. 31–41.

White P (2005). Biopsychosocial Medicine. Oxford University Press, Oxford.

Whittaker R, Kemp S, House A (2007). Illness perceptions and outcome in mild head injury: a longitudinal study. J Neurol Neurosurg Psychiatry 8: 644–646.

Williamson D, Holsman M, Chaytor N et al. (2012). Abuse, not financial incentive, predicts non-credible cognitive performance in patients with psychogenic non-epileptic seizures. Clin Neuropsychol 26: 588–598.

Witztum E, Grinshpoon A, Margolin J et al. (1996). The erroneous diagnosis of malingering in a military setting. Mil Med 47: 998–1000.

Young G (2014). Malingering, feigning, and response bias in psychiatric/psychological injury. Implications for practice and court, Springer, Dordrecht.

Section 4

Treatment

Handbook of Clinical Neurology, Vol. 139 (3rd series)
Functional Neurologic Disorders
M. Hallett, J. Stone, and A. Carson, Editors
http://dx.doi.org/10.1016/B978-0-12-801772-2.00043-6

Chapter 43

Prognosis of functional neurologic disorders

J. GELAUFF[1] AND J. STONE[2]*

[1]*Department of Neurology, University Medical Center Groningen, University of Groningen, Groningen, The Netherlands*

[2]*Department of Clinical Neurosciences, Centre for Clinical Brain Sciences, University of Edinburgh, Edinburgh, UK*

Abstract

The prognosis of functional (psychogenic) neurologic disorders is important in being able to help answer patients' and carers' questions, determine whether treatment is worthwhile, and to find out which factors predict outcome. We reviewed data on prognosis of functional neurologic disorders from two systematic reviews on functional motor disorders and dissociative (nonepileptic) seizures as well as additional studies on functional visual and sensory symptoms.

Methodologic problems include heterogeneity in studied samples and outcome measures, diagnostic suspicion and referral bias, small size and retrospective design of available studies, possible treatments during follow-up, and literature review bias.

With these caveats, the prognosis of functional neurologic disorders does appear to be generally unfavorable. In most studies, functional motor symptoms and psychogenic nonepileptic attacks remain the same or are worse in the majority of patients at follow-up. Measures of quality of life and working status were often poor at follow-up. Frequency of misdiagnosis at follow-up was as low as other neurologic and psychiatric disorders.

Long duration of symptoms was the most distinct negative predictor. Early diagnosis and young age seem to predict good outcome. Emotional disorders and personality disorders were inconsistent predictors. Litigation and state benefits were found to be negative predictors in some studies, but others found they did not influence outcome.

INTRODUCTION

The prognosis of any disorder is important in being able to help answer patients' and carers' common questions about the future, determine whether treatment is worthwhile, and to find out which factors determine poor and good outcome.

Views about prognosis of functional neurologic symptoms expressed in the literature are markedly variable. Historically the neurologist's view has often wavered around optimism, mostly based on the conviction that symptoms that occur without any assignable pathology should disappear as quickly as they arise. This view has sometimes been confused with an overall treatment approach of some neurologists involving a feeling that they must reassure patients that they will get better, with the view that doing so will help that outcome to occur.

However, in clinical practice and especially in tertiary centers, neurologists encounter many patients who suffer from chronic, disabling symptoms, resistant to many forms of treatment. Overly optimistic views of physicians who treat these patients can discourage both patient and physician in the long run, when symptoms do not resolve. On the other hand, too little optimism in a disorder that may be dependent in part on abnormal focused attention and "habit" may lead to an outcome that is worse than it otherwise might be.

In this chapter, we discuss the prognosis of functional neurologic symptoms in adults and children, starting

*Correspondence to: Jon Stone, Consultant Neurologist and Honorary Senior Lecturer, Department of Clinical Neurosciences, Centre for Clinical Brain Sciences, University of Edinburgh, Edinburgh EH4 2XU, UK. Tel: +44-131-537-1167, Fax: +44-131-537-1132, E-mail: Jon.Stone@ed.ac.uk

with methodologic issues, then discussing the data by symptom type, as well as prognostic factors, misdiagnosis and symptom cross-over. We have drawn on data from two systematic reviews, one on motor disorders co-written by the authors of this chapter (Gelauff et al., 2014), and another on nonepileptic seizures (Durrant et al., 2011). We supplemented this with a further literature search to update these reviews and describe studies of other functional neurologic symptoms, especially those older studies where symptoms were grouped together.

We present data of studies with at least 8 patients in follow-up, that report on follow-up duration of 3 months or more, and in which a majority of patients had functional neurologic symptoms.

METHODOLOGIC ISSUES

There are a number of difficulties in determining overall outcome of functional neurologic symptoms, some of which are listed below.

Heterogeneity

Arguably the only thing that patients with functional neurologic disorders really have in common with each other is their symptoms. Some patients have symptoms for a few hours, others for their whole life. Some have complex psychologic and physical comorbidity, some present with a single transient symptom. Patients often want to know: "How long will I have this for?" The studies we have can only hint at the answer to that question. Clinical experience also teaches us that some patients who on paper may have several poor prognostic factors can do surprisingly well, sometimes in relation to nonmedical life events such as divorce or a change of job. Patients who theoretically are in the best prognostic group may do surprisingly badly.

Diagnostic suspicion bias

Patients with comorbidities, especially psychologic ones, that may predict poor outcome are perhaps more likely to be given a diagnosis of a functional disorder in the first place, thus altering long-term outcome.

Secondary and tertiary care referral bias

It would be hard to carry out a truly population-based study of functional neurologic disorders since they usually require diagnosis in secondary care. Patients may be sampled in neurology services, specialist neurology clinics, videotelemetry lists, psychiatry services, or tertiary centers draining the most complex patients from a wide area. Many studies described in this chapter were performed in tertiary centers, while patients who present at an emergency department or in general practice with functional symptoms of short duration probably have a better outlook.

Study size and design

Many studies are relatively small and potentially prone to the play of chance. Retrospective studies dominate the literature. These are problematic as they are more likely to be nonconsecutive and so less representative. Individual studies measure different prognostic factors. Statistical analysis for prognostic factors can sometimes seem more like "data mining" and may depend on the biases of the authors of the study.

Follow-up rates

Follow-up rates in studies range between 50% and 100%, with most studies sitting at around 70%. There is an obvious bias here, although whether this favors patients with a better outcome or those with a worse outcome is uncertain.

Assessing natural history vs. treatment studies

Most of the studies in this chapter describe "natural history." However, many of these patients have had treatment which may have confounded the outcome.

Measuring outcome

Prognostic and treatment studies and anecdotal experience suggest that patients' wellbeing is not always correlated with improvement of symptoms. Either patients' symptoms have resolved but quality of life hasn't improved, or vice versa. A study of 147 patients with nonepileptic seizures casts doubt on whether measuring seizure frequency, for example, is the most meaningful outcome measure by showing that equal proportions of patients were receiving state-related benefit in the 29% who had seizure remission at 4 years compared to those who still had seizures (Reuber et al., 2005). Outcome may objectively appear better, but from the patients' perspective, may be no different. In a study of multidisciplinary inpatient treatment, the objectively rated Health of the Nation outcome scale was the most sensitive to change over time, whereas subjectively rated measures performed less well (Demartini et al., 2014), perhaps because patients have an inherent difficulty in rating themselves accurately (Ricciardi et al., 2015).

Literature review bias

Most of the data in this chapter comes from a systematic review. Nonetheless, there are potentially issues with missing studies, especially from non-English sources, and from studies using different terminology. It should be noted that studies that were used in this chapter are heterogeneous in their study approach and numbers of included patients are small, so strong conclusions cannot be drawn.

SYMPTOM OUTCOME

With all of the caveats and potential confounders listed above, the prognosis of functional neurologic disorders does appear to be generally unfavorable. Tables 43.1–43.3 show data from prognostic studies grouped by symptom type. In a large number of studies symptoms remain the "same or worse" in the majority of patients. Producing a meaningful "bottom-line" figure is not really possible due to the above-mentioned heterogeneity between studies.

In recent years research has evolved to categorize studies according to symptom type (e.g., nonepileptic seizures, functional movement disorder), in contrast with earlier studies that looked at "conversion disorder" or "hysteria" as a whole. We therefore discuss prognosis by symptom type but also present data from older studies of all functional neurologic disorders.

Motor symptoms

We have previously systematically reviewed the prognosis of functional motor symptoms, consisting of movement disorders, paresis, and gait disorders (Gelauff et al., 2014). This review covered studies between 1940 and 2013. We found 24 studies in total ($n=2069$ patients, two of these studies with overlapping data excluded) where there was follow-up data of at least 6 months and there were more than 8 patients reported (Table 43.1). The functional motor symptoms studied were tremor ($n=5$ studies), dystonia ($n=3$ studies), weakness ($n=5$ studies), parkinsonism ($n=1$ study), and mixed motor ($n=11$ studies).

The overall prognosis of motor symptoms appeared unfavorable from the studies in this review. The mean duration of follow-up was 7.4 years. An analysis of all studies weighted according to the size of the study found an overall figure of 40% of patients with the same or worse outcome at follow-up with only 20% of patients in the whole cohort showing complete remission. In four studies with 135 patients, 66–100% of patients had the same or worse symptoms at follow-up. In 14 studies with 533 patients, 33–66% of patients had the same or worse symptoms at follow-up and in only five studies with 464 patients, 33% of patients or fewer had symptoms the same or worse at follow-up.

The review showed there is variability in outcome between different functional motor symptoms, but no clear relationship between outcome and symptom type was found. Studies in functional dystonia showed worst prognosis: 73% and 78% of patients had the same or worse symptoms (Schrag et al., 2004; Ibrahim et al., 2009). Functional tremor also has a relatively poor prognosis, with 44–90% of patients the same or worse at follow-up (Ljungberg, 1957; Deuschl et al., 1998; Kim et al., 1999; Jankovic et al., 2006; McKeon et al., 2009). The outcome of weakness/paralysis seemed to be more favorable. These differences might be explained by selection bias: many studies of movement disorders (like tremor and dystonia) were performed in tertiary specialized clinics, while limb weakness is more often seen in general neurology clinics. However, Ljungberg (1957), in a single-author study which methodologically is still one of the best, even if its 1950s diagnostic certainty is potentially problematic, compared different symptoms within one large ($n=381$) prospective study. He also found that tremor had the poorest outcome, compared to gait disorder and weakness at 5-year follow-up. On the other hand, two other studies ($n=69$ in follow-up) found no correlation between motor symptom type and outcome (Williams et al., 1995; Feinstein et al., 2001).

Two additional articles of functional axial myoclonus and paroxysmal movement disorder were published after the systematic review with 93 patients in follow-up (Ganos et al., 2013; Erro et al., 2014). Their results are in line with above-mentioned findings.

Dissociative (nonepileptic) seizures

The prognosis of dissociative (nonepileptic) seizures has also been subject to a systematic review (Durrant et al., 2011). This review, of 15 studies, suggested the overall prognosis was poor. In 11 studies, 40% patients or fewer achieve seizure remission in the follow-up period (Meierkord et al., 1991; Ettinger et al., 1999; Kanner et al., 1999; Selwa et al., 2000; Silva et al., 2001; Carton et al., 2003; Reuber et al., 2003; Arain et al., 2007; Bodde et al., 2007; O'Sullivan et al., 2007; McKenzie et al., 2010).

Our own search of the literature found an additional 10 studies both before and after the publication of the Durrant et al. review, giving a total of 25 studies (Table 43.2). Looking at these 25 studies (Table 43.2), 20 found $<50\%$ of the patients had completely recovered at follow-up. The total weighted remission rate in nonepileptic seizure studies was 33%. This number is not corrected for follow-up duration or follow-up rate. In the largest study of 260 patients, 19% of patients actually had an increase in the frequency of

Table 43.1

Study characteristics of follow-up studies in functional motor symptoms

Article characteristics								Symptom outcome				Disability/functioning	
Author and year	Symptom	*n* in follow-up	Follow-up duration	Follow-up rate (%)	Mean age (years)	Symptom duration (years)	Female (%)	Worse	Same	Improved	Complete remission	Disability	Work
McKeon et al., 2009	Tremor	33	3.2 years	53	50[o]	0.1–15[b]	70	64		36		40% severe, 24% moderate, 36% mild	–
Jankovic et al., 2006*	Tremor	127	3.4 years	60	44[b]	4.6[b]	73	43		57	0	–	–
Kim et al., 1999	Tremor	10	1.5 years	14	41[b]	4.1[b]	66	30	60	10	0	–	–
Deuschl et al., 1998	Tremor	16	0.5–8 years	64	42[b]	2.5[ttd]	80	25	38	0	37	If symptoms remained: 75% moderately and 25% severely impaired	44% retired
Carter, 1949	Tremor	8	4–6 years	80	–	–	–	0	50	0	50	–	–
Ibrahim et al., 2009[†]	Fixed dystonia	35	7.6 years	73	43[b]	11.8[b]	83	31	46	23	0		–
Schrag et al., 2004[†]	Fixed dystonia	69	3.3 years	67	30[b]	5[b]	83	73		19	8	All on allowance	–
Lang, 1995	Dystonia	8	?	4	35.5[o]	3.8[ttd]	72	0	37	38	25		–
Erro et al., 2014	Axial myoclonus	76	2.2 years	10	40[b]	5.9[b]	51	17	45	16	22	–	–
Lang et al., 1995	Parkinsonism	14	?	100	43[o]		50	0	79	7	14	7% moderate, 57% heavy, 36% fully disabled	79% unable to work, 14% early retired, 7% unemployed
Ganos et al., 2013	Mixed movement disorder	17	2.3 years	65	39[o]	–	73	18		82		–	–
Munhoz et al., 2011	Mixed movement disorder	58	0.5 years	70	39[o]	–	88	40		22	38	–	–
Ertan et al., 2009	Mixed movement disorder	26	15 days–2 years	53	7–70[o]	4.4[†]	70	–	–	46	–	–	–
Thomas et al., 2006*	Mixed movement disorder	122	3.4 years	24	43[b]	4.7[†]	73	22	21	57	0		33% employed, 30% on disability, 4% unemployed
Feinstein et al., 2001	Mixed movement disorder	42	3.2 years	48	45[b]	–	62	33	24	33	10	–	17% at work, 76% unemployed

Williams et al., 1995	Mixed movement disorder	21	1.8 years	88	36.5^{o}	4.9 ^{ttd}	79	14		57	29	27% disabled	27% at work
Factor et al., 1995	Mixed movement disorder	20	0–6 years	71	51^{-}	2.8 ^{ttd}	60	50		0	50	–	–
Stone et al., 2003	Weakness	42	12.5 years	70	36^{b}	–	81	69		31		38% limited in moderate activities	30% disability leave
Binzer and Kullgren, 1998	Weakness	30	3.5 years	86	39°	0,2†	60	10		27	63	–	57% at work
Knutsson and Martensson, 1985	Weakness	25	0.5–9 years	100	19–47^{-}	1 day–5 years	76	0	56	44		–	–
Brown and Pisetsky, 1954	Weakness	10	1–6 years	91	26^{b}	–	10	10	20	20	50		
Carter, 1949	Weakness	22	4–6 years	96	–	–	–	4	14	4	78		
Crimlisk et al., 1998	Mixed motor	64	5–7 years	88	37^{b}	1.5 ^{ttd}	48	38	14	20	28	–	33% at work, 47% health-related retirement
Mace and Trimble, 1996	Mixed motor	31	9.8 years	?	?	–	78	44		56			
Couprie et al., 1995	Mixed motor	56	4.5 years	93	36^{b}	–	64	43		16	41	34% from small restrictions in lifestyle to severely impaired independence, 7% total dependence	
Gatfield and Guze, 1962	Mixed motor	24	2.5–10 years	65	14–67^{b}		83	62		–	38		
Ljungberg, 1957	Mixed motor	381	11.9 years	?	28.5^{o}	–	65	0	20	80			65% at work, 14% health-related pension
Total number of patients in follow-up	1387		Weighted mean complete remission rate:								20%		

Partly adapted from Gelauff et al. (2014).

*and † indicate studies with overlapping data.

n = number of patients at follow-up.

Follow-up rate in percentages. Age: mean age, measured at onset of symptoms (o), baseline of the study (b) or unknown (–). Symptom duration in years, either measured at baseline of the study or reported as the time between onset and diagnosis "time to diagnosis" (ttd). Percentage of females in the study, mainly from the baseline population (not at follow-up). Symptom outcome in percentage of patients with improved, same, worse, or remitted symptoms at follow-up. Only studies that reported specifically on complete remission were used to calculate the mean weighted complete remission rate.

Table 43.2

Study characteristics of follow-up studies in nonepileptic attacks

Nonepileptic attacks												
Article characteristics							Symptom outcome				Disability/functioning	
Author and year	*n* in follow-up	Follow-up duration	Follow-up rate (%)	Mean age (years)	Symptom duration (years)	Female (%)	Worse (%)	Same (%)	Improved (%)	Complete remission (%)	Disability (%)	Work (%)
Sadan et al., 2016	51	4.6 years	70	27[o]	7.8[ttd]	71				39	–	–
Duncan et al., 2014	188	8.7 years	72	30.5[o]	6.7[ttd]	75.5	31.9% attendance with seizures			–	–	22.8% of 114 patients in employment
Chen et al., 2012	47	6–9 months	71	–	–	–	62		38		–	–
Duncan et al., 2011	47	6 months	87	30[o]	1.7[ttd]	82	36		13	51	–	–
Jones et al., 2010	57	4.1 years	26	39[D]	6.7[ttd]	61	16	35	42	7		
McKenzie et al., 2010	187	6–12 months	72	38[b]	7[ttd]	76	62		38		Good 11,5%, intermediate 47,5%, poor 36%	23,5% employed (10% at baseline)
An et al., 2010	52	15.7 months	81	21[o]	0.5[ttd]	50	–	46		54	–	–
Arain et al., 2007	48	3 months	29	30[o]	9[ttd]	63	65			35	–	50% employed at f-u
Bodde et al., 2007	22	4–7 years	96	30[D]	7.2[ttd]	86	–	36	32	32	–	–
O'Sullivan et al., 2007	38	21 months	76	34[o]	1.7–3.8[ttd]	61	84			16	–	–
Carton et al., 2003	78	0.5–7 years	93	23[o]	10[ttd]	77	11	13	48	28	–	–
Reuber et al., 2003	164	4.1 years	50	27[o]	7.7[ttd]	79	71			29	56.4% dependent	40.5% employment or school, 12.4% unemployed, 41.4% retired on health grounds, 4.8% retired on age grounds
Selwa et al., 2000	57	1.9–4 years	67	40[–]	?	74	4		56	40	–	–
Silva et al., 2001	17	0.5–3 years	100	25[o]	9[ttd]	70	77			23	–	–
Ettinger et al., 1999	43	6–9 months	78	34[o]	–	91	9	16	56	19	–	–
Jongsma et al., 1999	28	23–67 months	85	31[D]		75	21	43	11	25	Overall functioning self-rated: 75% improved	No improvement
Kanner et al., 1999	45	14 months	100	30[b]	1.7[b]	69	–	71		29	–	–
Riaz et al., 1998	15	14 months	60	16[o]	17.2[ttd]	80	13	7	53	27	–	–
Ramani et al., 1996	21	4.7 years	62	–	–		5	14	81			Improved in 24%

Lancman et al., 1993	63	60 months	86	32°	–	84	75			25	–	–
Buchanan and Snars, 1993 acute/chronic group	50	2.5–3.4 years	100	18 / 28	–	72	42			58	–	–
Walczak et al., 1995	51	16 months	71	36^{D}	–	84	0	0	65	35		Improved 20%
Kristensen and Alving, 1992	22	5.8 years	79	28^{D}	9 ^{ttd}	86	(2 patients died)			45	–	–
Meierkord et al., 1991	70	1–14 years	64	7–71°	1–20 ^{ttd}	78	60			40	–	–
Lempert and Schmidt, 1990	40	24 months	80	38^{b}	–	64	–	42.5	22.5	35	Good 3 patients, fair 15, poor 18, very poor 5	28% at work, 42% out of work
Total number of patients in follow-up	1058											
		Weighted mean complete remission rate:								33%		

n = number of patients at follow-up.

Age: mean age, measured at onset of symptoms (o), diagnosis (D), baseline of the study (b), or unknown (–). Symptom duration in years, either measured at baseline of the study (b) or reported as the time between onset and diagnosis "time to diagnosis" (ttd). Percentage of females in the study, mainly from the baseline population (not at follow-up). Symptom outcome in percentage of patients with improved, same, worse, or remitted symptoms at follow-up. Only studies that reported specifically on complete remission were used to calculate the mean weighted complete remission rate.

Table 43.3

Study characteristics of follow-up studies in sensory symptoms, visual symptoms, and studies with mixed neurologic symptoms

Article characteristics								Symptom outcome				Disability (%)
Author and year	Symptom	*n* in follow-up	Follow-up duration	Follow-up rate (%)	Mean age (years) (baseline/ follow-up)	Symptom duration (years)	Female (%)	Worse	Same	Improved	Complete remission	
Toth, 2003	Hemisensory	30	16 months	88	35 ⁻	2 days	74	20		–	80	–
Sletteberg et al., 1989	Visual symptoms	24	7 years	54	24 [b]	–	72	55			45	
Barris et al., 1992	Visual symptoms	45	–	63	26 ⁻	–	67	22		78		
Kathol et al., 1983	Visual symptoms	42	53 months	53	32 [b]	–	78	55			45	Living incapacities confounded by other symptoms. 19% visually disabled
Friesen and Mann, 1966	Visual symptoms	11	6–32 years	20	–	–	–	54		46		–
Behrman and Levy, 1970	Visual symptoms	10	1–4 years	71	–	16 months [b]	86	40		60		–
Sharpe et al., 2010	Mixed	716	12 months	63	46 [b]	–	68	19	48	33		–
Carson et al., 2003	Mixed	66	8 months	73		–	64	14	41	45		
Kent et al., 1995	Mixed	32	4.5 years	71	42 [follow-up]	-	75	72			28	–
Chandrasekaran et al., 1994	Mixed	38	5 years	51	–	–	100	37			63	–
Wig and Mangalwedhe, 1982	Mixed	54	5 years	67	–	–	83	7	19	19	54	–

n = number of patients at follow-up. Follow-up rate in percentages. Age: mean age, measured at onset of symptoms (o), diagnosis (D), baseline of the study (b), or unknown (–). Symptom duration in years, either measured at baseline of the study or reported as the time between onset and diagnosis, "time to diagnosis" (ttd). Percentage of females in the study, mainly from the baseline population (not at follow-up). Symptom outcome in percentage of patients with improved, same, worse, or remitted symptoms at follow-up. Only studies that reported specifically on complete remission were used to calculate the mean weighted complete remission rate. None of the studies reported on work at follow-up.

seizures at a follow-up duration of 6–12 months (McKenzie et al., 2010).

However, more promising outcomes have also been reported, and it is perhaps useful to look at these studies in more detail to understand why. One study found relatively good outcome in dissociative seizures (Buchanan and Snars, 1993). The researchers divided patients into two groups: acute ($n = 18$) and chronic ($n = 32$). In the acute group, a very high number (83%) of patients completely recovered after a mean of 2.3 years of follow-up. In the chronic group, 38% of 8 patients in total remained the same.

Some studies (Walczak et al., 1995; Ramani et al., 1996; An et al., 2010; Duncan et al., 2011) found that >50% of patients improved at follow-up. Although some of these can be explained by short duration (Duncan et al., 2011) or young age (An et al., 2010), in other studies this outcome is harder to understand.

Sensory symptoms

Functional sensory symptoms like numbness or paresthesia are mostly reported in combination with motor symptoms or nonepileptic attacks. Only two studies report specifically on the prognosis of sensory symptoms (Table 43.3).

Stone et al. (2003) carried out 12-year follow-up on 42 from 70 baseline patients with weakness, sensory disturbance, or both. At baseline 57% of patients experienced numbness; 48% of patients still reported this symptom 12.5 years later. A high proportion of patients crossed over from weakness to numbness and vice versa in this study. However, the 45% of patients with solely sensory symptoms at outset had a better outcome on pain, physical and social functioning than patients who complained of weakness.

Another study followed up 26 from 34 patients with unexplained hemisensory disturbance with numbness and tingling, but excluding patients with chronic pain (Toth, 2003). One-third of these patients had motor symptoms with heaviness or clumsiness, and other symptoms, including intermittent blurring of vision (28%) and ipsilateral disturbance of hearing (16%), were also recorded. At 16-month follow-up in 30 patients, 17% of patients had the same severity of symptoms and 83% of patients' symptoms were completely resolved. A cautious conclusion from this limited amount of data could be that isolated sensory symptoms seem to have a relatively good prognosis, while outcome of sensory symptoms within a broader spectrum of functional neurologic symptoms remains undetermined.

Visual symptoms

The prognosis of functional visual symptoms also appears somewhat better than for motor symptoms. Five studies, in 132 patients, have found a frequency of 46–78% of patients with improved or remitted symptoms at follow-up (Table 43.3) (Friesen and Mann, 1966; Behrman and Levy, 1970; Kathol et al., 1983; Sletteberg et al., 1989; Barris et al., 1992) (Table 43.1). Follow-up rate in these studies was low, ranging from 20% to 71%.

Hearing loss

Functional hearing loss is rare and literature on the topic is scarce. There are no studies that met our quality demands with respect to number of patients and follow-up duration. Oishi et al. (2009) and Ban and Jin (2006) found in 13 patients in total that patients who were diagnosed early and were treated with steroid injections and psychotherapy seemed to have a good prognosis, but follow-up duration was not stated.

Mixed studies

The largest prospective follow-up study in mixed functional neurologic symptoms is a cohort study of 716 patients followed up over a 1-year period from 1144 seen by 41 neurologists across Scotland (Scottish Neurological Symptoms Study: SNSS) (Sharpe et al., 2010). Patients were included if the neurologist rated their symptoms as "not at all explained" or "somewhat explained" by disease. The symptoms included "conversion disorder" symptoms (sensory and motor symptoms), but also fatigue and pain disorders, and patients who had a neurologic disease but the neurologist viewed the symptoms as unexplained by that disease. Poor outcome, defined as unchanged, worse, or much worse symptoms, was reported by 67% of the 716 patients at 1-year follow-up. This study confirmed findings of an earlier study in a comparable population (Carson et al., 2003), that found 54% of 66 patients were the same or worse at follow-up.

Some older studies are still relevant. Carter (1949) found relatively favorable results. Apart from the results in paresis and tremor (Table 43.1), it was reported that 20 out of 24 patients with amnesia recovered completely within 1 week after hypnosis or suggestion and stayed well in the following 4–6 years. Only 1 patient relapsed and developed tremor additionally; the others were untraced. From 29 patients with aphonia, 19 remained well at follow-up, while 7 kept losing their voice in stressful circumstances. Three patients with blindness completely recovered after hypnosis.

QUALITY OF LIFE AND FUNCTIONING AT FOLLOW-UP

Persistence of functional symptoms at follow-up is not the only relevant measure for prognosis. Arguably, quality of life (Jones et al., 2016) and functioning at follow-up provide a better indication of long-term outcome of patients suffering from functional neurologic symptoms. As Kathol et al. (1983) pointed out in their study with visual impairment, the difficulty in interpreting these data is knowing how much of the impairment relates to the specific neurologic symptom compared to other comorbidities commonly found in these patients, such as pain, fatigue, and emotional disorders.

Studies have reported on several different outcome measures, but again outcome is generally unfavorable, with high percentages of disabled and impaired patients. A study in weakness found 38% of patients were limited in moderate activities at follow-up (Stone et al., 2003); another study in tremor reported daily activities were moderately (75%) or markedly (25%) impaired in patients with the same or worse symptoms (Deuschl et al., 1998). Couprie et al. (1995) found 41% of the patients were disabled (grade 2–5 Modified Rankin) at follow-up and 26% still regularly visited a specialist. McKeon et al. (2009) found 40% of patients were severely impaired in at least one activity.

In nonepileptic seizures comparable numbers were reported. Lempert and Schmidt (1990) found the impact of psychogenic nonepileptic seizures at 8–39 months of follow-up on daily life was minor in 32% of patients, moderate in 37%, and serious in 29% within a sample of 41 patients. One study investigated the outcome on a epilepsy scale and found global measures to be lower than quality of life in a typical epilepsy cohort (Jones et al., 2010). It was found patients had poor physical function, physical symptoms (like energy/fatigue and pain), poor emotional wellbeing, and negative health perception. Another study found 36% of patients rated their general quality of life as being poor (McKenzie et al., 2010).

WORKING STATUS

The frequency of patients in work at follow-up also provides a marker of the overall outcome. Several studies report a high rate of patients not working, ranging from 43% to 89% (Binzer and Kullgren, 1998; Crimlisk et al., 1998), and 20–47% of patients taking medical retirement who had motor symptoms (Ljungberg, 1957; Crimlisk et al., 1998; Stone et al., 2003). One study in fixed dystonia even found all patients were on disability benefits at follow-up (Schrag et al., 2004). Similar numbers are seen in nonepileptic seizures (Reuber et al., 2003). Two studies in seizures found numbers of patients in work had increased after the follow-up period, but at baseline this number was already very low in both cases (10% increased to 24% at follow-up in McKenzie et al., 2011; rates increased from 15% at baseline to 23% at follow-up in Duncan et al., 2014). All of these studies suffer from a lack of a control group to gain an understanding both of rates of working in disease controls and also in the general population of similar age and gender.

CROSS-OVER

As patients with functional neurologic symptoms often have more than one symptom and having a functional symptom is a risk factor for developing other functional symptoms, it would be conceivable that symptoms might interchange during the follow-up period. Especially in a therapeutic setting, this can be a cause for concern: if patients recover from the initial symptoms only to develop new functional symptoms, their functional disorder as a whole has not improved. There is not much evidence that symptoms are replaced in such a manner. In motor symptoms, for example, many studies looked at comorbid functional symptoms, but none compared follow-up with baseline symptom count (Gelauff et al., 2014).

One study has specifically looked into symptom cross-over in a cohort of 187 patients with psychogenic nonepileptic attacks at an average follow-up duration of 6–12 months (McKenzie et al., 2011). A high number of "unexplained" (functional) symptoms was reported at baseline. At follow-up it was found that the total number of patients with other "unexplained" (functional) symptoms had increased by 6.4%, but this was not statistically significant. New symptoms were recorded in 23.5% of patients. No correlation was found between recovery from the nonepileptic attacks and an increase in other functional symptoms. Those who continued to have attacks were just as likely to have new "medically unexplained symptoms" as patients who were attack-free. Feinstein et al. (2001) found 38% of patients developed other physical symptoms at follow-up, in addition to their original abnormal movements. This was not correlated with good outcome of the initial movement disorder. Stone et al. (2003) found 58% of those who only had sensory symptoms initially went on to develop weakness. These findings generally oppose the idea that cross-over occurs when symptoms resolve; many studies do show a high rate of functional symptoms at follow-up and symptom replacement is undoubtedly a relatively common clinical experience.

PROGNOSTIC FACTORS

In clinical practice, prognostic factors can be useful to guide treatment in individuals. Studies report on several different factors that are correlated with good or bad outcome in prognostic studies. Table 43.4 summarizes studies looking at prognostic factors.

Gender

Gender does not influence outcome of functional neurologic disorders. In motor symptoms no correlation was found between gender and symptom outcome (Gelauff et al., 2014). In the SNSS cohort no effect of gender was found either (Sharpe et al., 2010). The only two studies in nonepileptic attacks that found a predictive effect of age were contradicting: one study found a positive predictive effect of male gender (McKenzie et al., 2010), while another found a positive predictive effect of female gender (Meierkord et al., 1991).

Age at onset

As will be discussed in more detail below, prognosis in children with functional symptoms seems to be better than prognosis in adults. Therefore, Durrant et al. (2011) concluded that age has a strong effect on outcome. However, studies that only include adults with nonepileptic attacks, general unexplained neurologic symptoms, and motor symptoms show heterogeneous results.

In the SNSS cohort of unexplained symptoms ($n=716$), older age predicted poor outcome (Sharpe et al., 2010). Two studies in nonepileptic attacks ($n=268$) found older age predicted poor outcome (Reuber et al., 2003; An et al., 2010), as did four studies in motor symptoms ($n=211$) (Mace and Trimble, 1996; Deuschl et al., 1998; Stone et al., 2003; Thomas et al., 2006). Two studies in sensory symptoms found a correlation between age and outcome, but they included both adults and children (Sletteberg et al., 1989; Barris et al., 1992). Eight studies in motor symptoms ($n=670$) (Ljungberg, 1957; Couprie et al., 1995; Williams et al., 1995; Binzer and Kullgren, 1998; Crimlisk et al., 1998; Feinstein et al., 2001; Ibrahim et al., 2009; Erro et al., 2014) and five studies in nonepileptic attacks ($n=410$) (Lempert and Schmidt, 1990; Lancman et al., 1993; Carton et al., 2003; Arain et al., 2007; Duncan et al., 2014) found no correlation between age and outcome. All in all, the effect of age on outcome is not evident from these studies.

Health-related benefits

Not many prognostic studies have looked at health-related benefits as a prognostic factor. Within the SNSS cohort it was found that receiving health-related benefits at initial consultation had a negative effect on outcome (Sharpe et al., 2010). McKenzie et al. (2010) (nonepileptic attacks) found that not receiving social payment predicted good outcome. In motor symptoms one study confirms this (Crimlisk et al., 1998), while three other (partly overlapping) studies found no correlation between litigation and outcome (Feinstein et al., 2001; Jankovic et al., 2006; Thomas et al., 2006).

The concept of secondary gain, such as the receipt of health-related benefits or other benefits of being ill, has a firm foothold in many people's thinking about functional neurologic disorders. There are several alternative possible explanations for a positive relationship between health benefits and poor outcome: (1) those with the worst severity are more likely to receive benefits; (2) given that few cohorts are inception cohorts, there is a bias towards patients with chronic disorders already on benefits; (3) some patients on health-related benefits become poorly motivated to improve, as they may not earn a great deal more if they did so; and (4) some patients on health-related benefits may be malingering. The data on litigation are surprising, since most larger studies in disorders such as posttraumatic symptoms after whiplash injury do seem to conclude that ongoing litigation or the effect of changes to the tort system influences outcome strongly (Obelieniene et al., 1999; Cassidy et al., 2000).

Employment and educational status

Other socioeconomic factors that have been studied are employment, which was found to be correlated with good outcome in two studies in nonepileptic attacks ($n=125$) (Carton et al., 2003; Duncan et al., 2011), or higher educational status/IQ, which has been found to have a positive predictive effect in nonepileptic attacks (Reuber et al., 2003; Arain et al., 2007; McKenzie et al., 2010). However, a higher number of studies with more patients in total in nonepileptic attacks, motor symptoms, and mixed symptoms found no correlation between employment or educational status and outcome (Table 43.3).

Comorbidity

Comorbidity, both psychiatric and neurologic, is high in functional neurologic disorders, but the influence of comorbidity on outcome of the presenting symptoms remains unclear.

In one study in functional tremor it was found that any kind of comorbidity, whether psychiatric, somatic, or functional, was associated with poor outcome (Jankovic et al., 2006). In combination with another five studies it was found in a total of 633 patients with motor

Table 43.4

Prognostic factors at baseline predicting outcome. Studies mostly calculated prognostic factors that predict symptom outcome

		Positive		Negative		No correlation found	
Factor		Studies	Number of patients	Studies	Number of patients	Studies	Number of patients
Young age	Motor	Mace and Trimble, 1996; Deuschl et al., 1998; Stone et al., 2003; Thomas et al., 2006	175	–	–	Ljungberg, 1957; Couprie et al., 1995; Williams et al., 1995; Binzer and Kullgren, 1998; Crimlisk et al., 1998; Feinstein et al., 2001; Ibrahim et al., 2009; Erro et al., 2014	670
	NES	Reuber et al., 2003; An et al., 2010	233	–	–	Lempert and Schmidt, 1990; Lancman et al., 1993; Carton et al., 2003; Arain et al., 2007; Duncan et al., 2014	410
	Mixed	Sharpe et al., 2010	716	–	–	Carson et al., 2003; Chandrasekaran et al., 1994	104
	Sensory	Sletteberg et al., 1989; Barris et al., 1992	74	–	–	–	–
	Total:	9 studies	1198	0 studies	–	15 studies	1184
Female	Motor	–		–	–	Ljungberg, 1957; Williams et al., 1995; Binzer and Kullgren, 1998; Crimlisk et al., 1998; Stone et al., 2003; Ibrahim et al., 2009; Erro et al., 2014	649
	NES	Meierkord et al., 1991	70	McKenzie et al., 2010	187	Lempert and Schmidt, 1990; Lancman et al., 1993; Silva et al., 2001; Arain et al., 2007; Duncan et al., 2014	356
	Mixed	–	–			Carson et al., 2003; Sharpe et al., 2010	782
	Total:	1 study	70	1 study	187	14 studies	1787
Early diagnosis	Motor	Couprie et al., 1995; Factor et al., 1995; Crimlisk et al., 1998; McKeon et al., 2009; Munhoz et al., 2011; Erro et al., 2014	307	–	–	–	–
	NES	Duncan et al., 2011	47	–	–	Meierkord et al., 1991; Lancman et al., 1993; Duncan et al., 2014	321
	Mixed	–					
	Total	7 studies	354	0 studies	–	3 studies	321
Positive reaction to diagnosis	Motor	Thomas et al., 2006 (believe in treatment outcome)	122				
	NES	Silva et al., 2001; Carton et al., 2003 (also: understanding diagnosis)	95	–	–	Ettinger et al., 1999	43
	Total	3 studies	217			1 study	43

Patient believe of nonrecovery	Mixed	–	–	Sharpe et al., 2010	716	–	–
	Total	0 studies	–		716		
Short duration of illness	Motor	Knutsson and Martensson, 1985; Williams et al., 1995; Mace and Trimble, 1996; Feinstein et al., 2001; Thomas et al., 2006	241	–	–	Ibrahim et al., 2009	35
	NES	Lempert and Schmidt, 1990; Walczak et al., 1995; Selwa et al., 2000	148	–	–	–	–
	Mixed	–	–	–	–	Chandrasekaran et al., 1994	38
	Total:	8 studies	389	0 studies	–	2 studies	73
Personality disorder	Motor	–	–	Ljungberg, 1957; Mace and Trimble, 1996; Binzer and Kullgren, 1998	442	–	–
	NES	–	–	Kanner et al., 1999; Reuber et al., 2003 (trait:inhibitedness)	45 164	–	–
	Mixed	–	–	Chandrasekaran et al., 1994	38		
	Total:	1 study	–	5 studies	689	0 studies	–
Psychiatric disorder (axis 1)	Motor	Crimlisk et al., 1998; Thomas et al., 2006	186	Mace and Trimble, 1996; Binzer and Kullgren, 1998; Feinstein et al., 2001; Ibrahim et al., 2009	138	Erro et al., 2014	76
	NES	Kanner et al., 1999 (Kanner: single episode of major depression); Bodde et al., 2007	76	Walczak et al., 1995; Kanner et al., 1999 (Kanner: recurrent depression); McKenzie et al., 2010	283	Meierkord et al., 1991; Lancman et al., 1993; Ettinger et al., 1999; Silva et al., 2001; Carton et al., 2003; Duncan et al., 2014	459
	Mixed	–	–	Sharpe et al., 2010	716	Carson et al., 2003	66
	Sensory	–	–	Barris et al., 1992	45	–	–
	Total	3 studies	140	9 studies	1182	8 studies	601
Somatoform disorder	Motor	–	–	–	–	Crimlisk et al., 1998; Ibrahim et al., 2009	99
Other MUS/ functional symptoms	NES	McKenzie et al., 2010	187	–	–	Lempert and Schmidt, 1990; Kanner et al., 1999; Duncan et al., 2014	273
	Total:	1 study	187	0 studies	–	5 studies	372
Somatic diagnosis	Motor	Thomas et al., 2006	122	Binzer and Kullgren, 1998	30	–	–
	NES	–	–	Meierkord et al., 1991; Reuber et al., 2003; Duncan et al., 2014	442	Lancman et al., 1993	63
	Mixed	–	–	Sharpe et al., 2010	716	–	–
	Total	1 study	122	5 studies	1188	1 study	63

Continued

Table 43.4

Continued

Factor		Positive		Negative		No correlation found	
		Studies	Number of patients	Studies	Number of patients	Studies	Number of patients
Disability	Motor	–	–	–	–	Binzer and Kullgren, 1998; Thomas et al., 2006	152
	NES	–	–	–	–	–	–
	Mixed	–	–	–	–	Carson et al., 2003	66
	Total	0 studies	–	0 studies	–	3 studies	218
Litigation/ benefits	Motor	–	–	Crimlisk et al., 1998	64	Feinstein et al., 2001; Thomas et al., 2006	164
	NES	–	–	Ettinger et al., 1999; McKenzie et al., 2010	230	Duncan et al., 2014	188
	Mixed	–	–	Sharpe et al., 2010	716	–	–
	Total	0 studies	–	4 studies	1010	3 studies	352
High-level education/ IQ	Motor	–	–	–	–	Ljungberg, 1957; Williams et al., 1995; Binzer and Kullgren, 1998; Feinstein et al., 2001	474
	NES	Reuber et al., 2003; Arain et al., 2007; McKenzie et al., 2010	399	–	–	Kanner et al., 1999	45
	Mixed	–	–	–	–	Chandrasekaran et al., 1994	38
	Total	3 studies	399	0 studies	–	6 studies	557
Employment	Motor	–	–	–	–	Feinstein et al., 2001	42
	NES	Carton et al., 2003; Duncan et al., 2011	125	–	–	Ettinger et al., 1999; Arain et al., 2007; Duncan et al., 2014	279
	Total:	2 studies	125	–	–	4 studies	321
Marital status	Motor	Crimlisk et al., 1998 (change in marital status)	64	–	–	Feinstein et al., 2001	42
	NES	–	–	–	–	Arain et al., 2007	48
	Total	1 study	64	0 studies	–	2 studies	90
Social background	Motor	–	–	–	–	Crimlisk et al., 1998	64
	NES	Ettinger et al., 1999 (having many friends)	43	–	–	Lancman et al., 1993; Silva et al., 2001; Reuber et al., 2003	244
	Total	1 study	43	0 studies	–	4 studies	308

NES, nonepileptic seizure; MUS, medically unexplained symptoms.

symptoms that psychiatric comorbidity (anxiety, depression, or personality disorders) predicted worse outcome (Ljungberg, 1957; Mace and Trimble, 1996; Binzer and Kullgren, 1998; Feinstein et al., 2001; Ibrahim et al., 2009).

Two studies in nonepileptic attacks (Kanner et al., 1999; McKenzie et al., 2010) and two studies in visual symptoms (Sletteberg et al., 1989; Barris et al., 1992) found the same relationship between depression and outcome. One study showed that inhibitedness as a personality trait predicted poor outcome (Reuber et al., 2003). Interestingly, two studies, one in motor symptoms (Thomas et al., 2006) and one study in nonepileptic attacks (Kanner et al., 1999) found depression or anxiety at baseline was correlated with better outcome. This is most probably due to synergistic effect of improvement of the functional disorder and the psychiatric disorder.

Only a few studies investigated the effect of comorbid functional symptoms or "unexplained symptoms" on outcome; one study found a low somatization score predicted good outcome (Reuber et al., 2003). Another study found unexplained symptoms other than nonepileptic seizures predicted poor outcome (McKenzie et al., 2010), but a study in motor symptoms and one in nonepileptic seizures found it had no influence on outcome (Crimlisk et al., 1998; Duncan et al., 2014).

The influence of organic comorbidity on outcome is also indistinct. For example, epilepsy alongside nonepileptic attacks was found to predict poor outcome in three studies (Meierkord et al., 1991; Reuber et al., 2003; Duncan et al., 2014), although Duncan et al. (2014) reported attendance with seizures as an outcome variable, which could refer to epileptic seizures too. In another study this effect was not found (Lancman et al., 1993). In motor studies conflicting results were reported (Binzer and Kullgren, 1998; Thomas et al., 2006).

Duration of symptoms

Longer duration of symptoms was found to be correlated with negative outcome in many studies. In nonepileptic attacks this association was found in three studies (Lempert and Schmidt, 1990; Selwa et al., 2000; Reuber et al., 2003) and in motor symptoms in five studies (Knutsson and Martensson, 1985; Mace and Trimble, 1996; Feinstein et al., 2001; Jankovic et al., 2006; Thomas et al., 2006). Two other studies in motor symptoms did not find an effect of duration of symptoms on outcome (Williams et al., 1995; Ibrahim et al., 2009). All in all, longer duration of symptoms seems to be one of the most consistent negative predictors of outcome in functional neurologic disorders. Many explanations for this effect have been proposed, but irrespective of the mechanism, it is important to prevent symptoms from becoming chronic.

Early diagnosis and confidence in the diagnosis

In motor symptoms the only predictor that is tested in more than two studies and also correlates consistently with poor outcome is a long duration between start of symptoms and patients receiving a diagnosis ($n = 307$) (Couprie et al., 1995; Factor et al., 1995; Crimlisk et al., 1998; McKeon et al., 2009; Munhoz et al., 2011; Erro et al., 2014).

In nonepileptic attacks only one study found an early diagnosis to be predictive of good outcome (Duncan et al., 2011), while two others did not find any correlation (Meierkord et al., 1991; Lancman et al., 1993).

Also, two partially overlapping studies in motor symptoms (Jankovic et al., 2006; Thomas et al., 2006) and two studies in nonepileptic attacks (Silva et al., 2001; Carton et al., 2003) found confidence in the diagnosis to positively influence prognosis. SNSS found that beliefs about illness were of key importance in predicting outcome (Sharpe et al., 2010). Expectation of nonrecovery and nonattribution of symptoms to psychologic factors predicted poor outcome.

Crimlisk et al. (2000) showed in 64 patients with unexplained neurologic symptoms that the referral pattern is often extensive. After consultation at the National Hospital for Neurology and Neurosurgery in London, 48% were seen by a neurologist, and 27% by another specialist. A total of 42 (66%) had been admitted to hospital (the number of admissions ranged from 0 to 11). Furthermore, 34% of patients had been referred to rheumatologists, general physicians, and specialists in infectious diseases, orthopedics, and immunology for their functional symptoms. This referral behavior can result in iatrogenic damage and undermines understanding and belief of the diagnosis of a functional neurologic disorder. Patients who were not referred had a better chance of improvement in this study.

These findings are clinically highly relevant, because they support the idea that an early, tangible, positive diagnosis is essential in the approach of patients with functional neurologic disorders. This has been argued in the literature (Carton et al., 2003; Stone and Carson, 2011).

MISDIAGNOSIS

Both patients and physicians can remain unconvinced of the diagnostic certainty of functional neurologic disorders. They think symptoms that are diagnosed as being a functional neurologic disorder often prove to be part of neurologic disease eventually. In medical literature this concern has been strongly influenced by one paper on prognosis, in which a misdiagnosis rate of more than 50% at 10-year follow-up was found in patients with hysteria (Slater and Glithero, 1965). Based on these findings, the author concluded that the concept of hysteria as a syndrome "was based entirely on tradition and lacked evidential support" (Slater, 1965).

However, Stone (2005) have shown, in their systematic review on misdiagnosis that included 27 studies and 1466 patients with motor and seizure conversion disorder, that since the 1970s the rate of misdiagnosis of functional symptoms has only been 4% (Adler et al., 2014). This is similar to the rate of misdiagnosis for other neurologic and psychiatric disorders (Fig. 43.1). There was no difference between motor symptoms (4%) and seizures (2.6%) overall. There was some suggestion that movement disorders and gait disorders specifically were more prone to error. The higher rate of misdiagnosis seen in earlier studies such as Slater's appears to relate more to poorly defined cohorts and outcomes than clearly worse diagnosis. The data are compatible with a view that functional neurologic disorders are a clinical bedside diagnosis that has been reliably made since before computed tomography scans and videotelemetry.

Within a prospective large sample of patients ($n=1030$ followed up from 1144) with unexplained neurologic symptoms from the SNSS, it was found that, after 1 year and 7 months of follow-up, only 4 patients acquired a diagnosis of new organic disease that was unexpected at initial assessment and provided a better explanation for the symptoms (Stone et al., 2009). In movement disorders a comparable low rate of 0–3% was found in 195 patients (Jankovic et al. 2006; Ibrahim et al., 2009; McKeon et al., 2009).

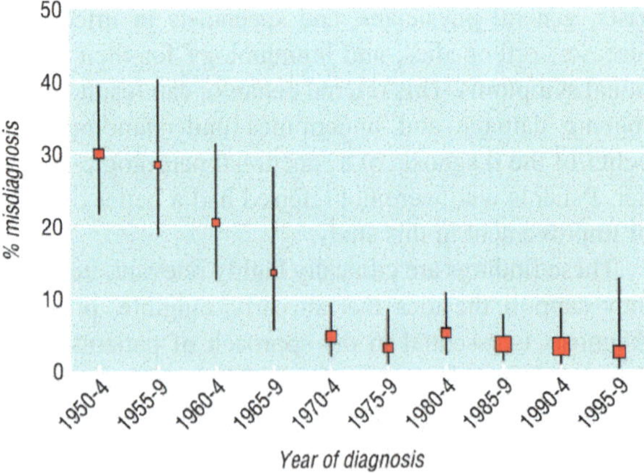

Fig. 43.1. Misdiagnosis of functional neurologic disorders (mean %, 95% confidence intervals, random effects) plotted at midpoint of 5-year intervals according to when patients were diagnosed. Size of each point is proportional to number of subjects at each time point (total $n=1466$, 27 studies). (Reproduced from Stone (2005), with permission from BMJ Publications.)

One of the reasons for the discrepancy between these recent findings and early findings is the interpretation of the definition of misdiagnosis. A change of diagnosis at follow-up does not necessarily explain the original symptoms better; it could simply mean narrowing of the differential diagnosis, a difference in opinion between the initial neurologist and the subsequent physician, or a comorbid neurologic diagnosis that does not account for earlier symptoms, but might explain symptoms at follow-up. Earlier studies did not take these subtleties into account (Stone et al., 2009).

Misdiagnosis is a pitfall in many neurologic disorders, but undoubtedly physicians have traditionally been more worried to miss an organic diagnosis than a functional disorder, although the consequences for the patient are considerable in both situations.

PEDIATRIC STUDIES

On average, children with a functional neurologic disorder seem to have a better prognosis than adults with the same symptoms.

Although numbers of patients are low, pediatric studies in nonepileptic attacks show relatively high percentages of completely remitted symptoms. Reilly et al. (2013) reviewed the available literature on nonepileptic seizures in children and found remission rates ranging from 43% to 81% in studies with 15–50 patients in follow-up. The proportion of patients with improved or remitted symptoms (71–100%) is impressive compared to the numbers in adults (Durrant et al., 2011; Reilly et al., 2013). It is hypothesized that perhaps the shorter duration of symptoms at presentation or possibly more effective local treatment interventions could explain this difference, but no evidence is available.

In a 1-year follow-up study with motor symptoms, sensory symptoms, and/or nonepileptic attacks, 75–100% of 147 children (median age 12.5 years) had improved symptoms (Ani et al., 2013). In this study motor symptoms and nonepileptic attacks had a more favorable outcome (90–100% improved) than sensory symptoms like visual loss, hearing loss, speech problems, and paresthesia. Many of these children received some kind of psychotherapy. Despite the favorable outcome for the neurologic symptom, a quarter of the children developed a new psychiatric disorder during follow-up, especially anxiety and depressive disorders. Another pediatric study of mixed functional neurologic symptoms reported outcome of 30 children who were seen at the emergency department with relatively short duration of symptoms. Symptoms had resolved at follow-up of 3–6 months in 83% of cases (De Gusmão et al., 2014). Despite this, patients on average missed 22.3 days of school, parents missed 8 days of work, and patients visited the emergency department twice during the follow-up period.

In a study of 15 children with functional movement disorder with a 3.1-year follow-up, 12 had substantially improved or remitted symptoms. The three children who did not recover remained highly disabled (Schwingenschuh et al., 2008). Another study summarized findings of outcome in visual symptoms in childhood. In their own series of 58 patients and in the existing literature, outcome was good, with almost all patients completely recovered (Toldo et al., 2010).

Prognostic factors in pediatric studies that correlated with bad outcome are longer duration of symptoms before diagnosis (Pehlivantürk and Unal, 2002; Schwingenschuh et al., 2008), and premorbid conduct problems (such as behavior that expressed disrespectfulness, difficulty getting along, arrogance, or aggression) (Pehlivantürk and Unal, 2002). Comorbid neurologic disease (such as epilepsy) was found to be correlated with poor outcome in some, but not all, studies (Durrant et al., 2011).

CONCLUSION

There are many methodologic problems in studying the prognosis of functional neurologic disorders but in general they appear to have a poor prognosis, with low remission rates at follow-up. Patients with pure sensory symptoms and pediatric populations appear to have a better outcome, although numbers are low. In nonepileptic attacks and motor symptoms differences between symptoms remain unclear.

High frequency of psychologic and physical comorbidity is typically reported at baseline and follow-up. From the small number of studies that looked into cross-over at follow-up there was no obvious indication that symptoms are replaced by other symptoms after they have resolved, but this is an unresolved epidemiologic question. Perhaps unsurprisingly, quality of life, general functioning, and working status at follow-up are often found to be poor in many cases.

The most consistent negative prognostic factor is long duration of symptoms. Psychiatric comorbidity was not looked at in many studies, but was found to be an inconsistent predictor of poor outcome. The effect of other comorbidities on outcome remains uncertain. The effect of age is highly dependent on the population. Pediatric studies have shown better outcome than adult studies, so age is clearly predictive of outcome. But within the adult population, varying results were found. Socioeconomic factors, including health-related benefits, were too variable to draw a conclusion but may be relevant. Gender does not influence outcome. Larger studies with multivariate regression suggest the relevance of illness beliefs in particular.

References

Adler CH, Beach TG, Hentz JG et al. (2014). Low clinical diagnostic accuracy of early vs advanced Parkinson disease: clinicopathologic study. Neurology 83: 406–412.

An D, Wu XT, Yan B et al. (2010). Clinical features of psychogenic nonepileptic seizures: a study of 64 cases in southwest China. Epilepsy Behav: E&B 17 (3): 408–411.

Ani C, Reading R, Lynn R et al. (2013). Incidence and 12-month outcome of non-transient childhood conversion disorder in the U.K. and Ireland. Br J Psychiatr 202: 413–418.

Arain AM, Hamadani AM, Islam S et al. (2007). Predictors of early seizure remission after diagnosis of psychogenic nonepileptic seizures. Epilepsy Behav 11: 409–412.

Ban JH, Jin SM (2006). A clinical analysis of psychogenic sudden deafness. Otolaryngol Head Neck Surg 134: 970–974.

Barris MC, Kaufman DI, Barberio D (1992). Visual impairment in hysteria. Doc Ophthalmol 82: 369–382.

Behrman J, Levy R (1970). Neurophysiological studies on patients with hysterical disturbances of vision. J Psychosom Res 14 (2): 187–194.

Binzer M, Kullgren G (1998). Motor conversion disorder. A prospective 2- to 5-year follow-up study. Psychosomatics 39 (6): 519–527.

Bodde NMG, Janssen AM, Theuns C et al. (2007). Factors involved in the long-term prognosis of psychogenic nonepileptic seizures. J Psychosom Res 62: 545–551.

Brown W, Pisetsky J (1954). Sociopsychologic factors in hysterical paraplegia. J Nerv Ment Dis 119: 283–298.

Buchanan N, Snars J (1993). Pseudoseizures (non epileptic attack disorder) – clinical management and outcome in 50 patients. Seizure 2 (2): 141–146.

Carson AJ, Best S, Postma K et al. (2003). The outcome of neurology outpatients with medically unexplained symptoms: a prospective cohort study. J Neurol Neurosurg Psychiatry 74 (7): 897–900.

Carter AB (1949). The prognosis of certain hysterical symptoms. BMJ i: 1076–1079.

Carton S, Thompson PJ, Duncan JS (2003). Non-epileptic seizures: patients' understanding and reaction to the diagnosis and impact on outcome. Seizure 12: 287–294.

Cassidy JD, Carroll LJ, Côté P et al. (2000). Effect of eliminating compensation for pain and suffering on the outcome of insurance claims for whiplash injury. New Engl J Med 342 (16): 1179–1186.

Chandrasekaran R, Goswami U, Sivikurnar V et al. (1994). Hysterical neurosis: a follow-up study. Acta Psychiatr Scand 89 (9): 78–80.

Chen DK, Izadyar S, Wisdom NM et al. (2012). Intact vs. impaired ictal sensorium: does it affect outcome of psychogenic nonepileptic events following disclosure of diagnosis? Epilepsy Behav 24 (1): 30–35.

Couprie W, Wijdicks EF, Rooijmans HG et al. (1995). Outcome in conversion disorder: a follow up study. J Neurol Neurosurg Psychiatry 58 (6): 750–752.

Crimlisk HL, Bhatia KP, Cope H et al. (1998). Slater revisited: 6 year follow up study of patients with medically unexplained motor symptoms. BMJ 316 (7131): 582–586.

Crimlisk HL, Bhatia KP, Cope H et al. (2000). Patterns of referral in patients with medically unexplained motor symptoms. J Psychosom Res 49: 217–219.

De Gusmão CM, Guerrierio RM, Bernson-Leung ME et al. (2014). Functional neurological symptom disorders in a pediatric emergency room: diagnostic accuracy, features, and outcome. Pediatr Neurol 51 (2): 233–238.

Demartini B, Bhatia A, Petrochilos P et al. (2014). Multidisciplinary treatment for functional neurological symptoms: a prospective study. J Neurol 261 (12): 2370–2377.

Deuschl G, Köster B, Lücking CH et al. (1998). Diagnostic and pathophysiological aspects of psychogenic tremors. Mov Disord 13: 294–302.

Duncan R, Razvi S, Mulhern S (2011). Newly presenting psychogenic nonepileptic seizures: incidence, population characteristics, and early outcome from a prospective audit of a first seizure clinic. Epilepsy Behav: E&B 20 (2): 308–311.

Duncan R, Graham CD, Oto M et al. (2014). Primary and secondary care attendance, anticonvulsant and antidepressant use and psychiatric contact 5–10 years after diagnosis in 188 patients with psychogenic non-epileptic seizures. J Neurol Neurosurg Psychiatry 85 (9): 954–958.

Durrant J, Rickards H, Cavanna AE (2011). Prognosis and outcome predictors in psychogenic nonepileptic seizures. Epilepsy Res Treat 2011: 1–7.

Erro R, Edwards MJ, Bhatia KP et al. (2014). Psychogenic axial myoclonus: clinical features and long-term outcome. Parkinsonism Relat Disord 20 (6): 596–599.

Ertan S, Uluduz D, Ozekmekçi S et al. (2009). Clinical characteristics of 49 patients with psychogenic movement disorders in a tertiary clinic in Turkey. Mov Disord 24 (5): 759–762.

Ettinger AB, Dhoon A, Weisbrot DM et al. (1999). Predictive factors for outcome of nonepileptic seizures after diagnosis. J Neuropsychiatry Clin Neurosci 11 (4): 458–463.

Factor SA, Podskalny GD, Molho ES (1995). Psychogenic movement disorders: frequency, clinical profile, and characteristics. J Neurol Neurosurg Psychiatry 59 (4): 406–412.

Feinstein A, Stergiopoulos V, Fine J et al. (2001). Psychiatric outcome in patients with a psychogenic movement disorder: a prospective study. Neuropsychiatry Neuropsychol Behav Neurol 14 (3): 169–176.

Friesen H, Mann WA (1966). Follow-up study of hysterical amblyopia. Am J Ophthalmol 62 (6): 1106–1115.

Ganos C, Aguirregomozcorta M, Batla A et al. (2013). Psychogenic paroxysmal movement disorders - Clinical features and diagnostic clues. Parkinsonism Relat Disord 20 (1): 41–46.

Gatfield PD, Guze SB (1962). Prognosis and differential diagnosis of conversion reactions. Dis Nerv Syst 23: 623–631.

Gelauff J, Stone J, Edwards M et al. (2014). The prognosis of functional (psychogenic) motor symptoms: a systematic review. J Neurol Neurosurg Psychiatry 85 (2): 220–226.

Ibrahim NM, Martino D, van de Warrenburg BP et al. (2009). The prognosis of fixed dystonia: a follow-up study. Parkinsonism Related Disorders 15 (8): 592–597.

Jankovic J, Vuong KD, Thomas M (2006). Psychogenic tremor: long-term outcome. CNS Spectr 11 (7): 501–508.

Jones SG, O'Brien TJ, Adams SJ et al. (2010). Clinical characteristics and outcome in patients with psychogenic nonepileptic seizures. Psychosom Med 72: 487–497.

Jones B, Reuber M, Norman P (2016). Correlates of health-related quality of life in adults with psychogenic nonepileptic seizures: a systematic review. Epilepsia 57: 171–181.

Jongsma MJ, Mommers JM, Renier WO et al. (1999). Follow-up of psychogenic, non-epileptic seizures: a pilot study – experience in a Dutch special centre for epilepsy. Seizure 8 (3): 146–148.

Kanner AM, Parra J, Frey M et al. (1999). Psychiatric and neurologic predictors of psychogenic pseudoseizure outcome. Neurology 53 (5): 933–938.

Kathol RG, Cox TA, Corbett JJ et al. (1983). Functional visual loss – follow up on 42 cases. Arch Ophthalmol 101: 729–735.

Kent DA, Tomasson K, Coryell W (1995). Course and outcome of conversion and somatization disorders. A four-year follow-up. Psychosomatics 36 (2): 138–144.

Kim YJ, Pakiam AS, Lang AE (1999). Historical and clinical features of psychogenic tremor: a review of 70 cases. Can J Neurol Sci 26 (3): 190–195.

Knutsson E, Martensson A (1985). Isokinetic measurements of muscle strength in hysterical paresis. Electroencephalogr Clin Neurophysiol 61 (5): 370–374.

Kristensen O, Alving J (1992). Pseudoseizures – risk factors and prognosis. Acta Neurol Scand 85: 177–180.

Lancman ME, Brotherton TA, Asconapé JJ et al. (1993). Psychogenic seizures in adults: a longitudinal analysis. Seizure 2 (4): 281–286.

Lang AE (1995). Psychogenic dystonia: a review of 18 cases. Can J Neurol Sci 22 (2): 136–143.

Lang AE, Koller WC, Fahn S (1995). Psychogenic parkinsonism. Arch Neurol 52 (8): 802–810.

Lempert T, Schmidt D (1990). Natural history and outcome of psychogenic seizures: a clinical study in 50 patients. J Neurol 237 (1): 35–38.

Ljungberg L (1957). Hysteria: a clinical, prognostic and genetic study. Acta Psychiat Neurol Scand, Suppl 112: 1–162.

Mace CJ, Trimble MR (1996). Ten-year prognosis of conversion disorder. Br J Psychiatr 169 (3): 282–288.

McKenzie P, Oto M, Russell A et al. (2010). Early outcomes and predictors in 260 patients with psychogenic nonepileptic attacks. Neurology 74 (1): 64–69.

McKenzie PS, Oto M, Graham CD et al. (2011). Do patients whose psychogenic non-epileptic seizures resolve, "replace" them with other medically unexplained symptoms? Medically unexplained symptoms arising after a diagnosis of psychogenic non-epileptic seizures. J Neurol Neurosurg Psychiatry 82 (9): 967–969.

McKeon A, Ahlskog JE, Bower JH et al. (2009). Psychogenic tremor: long-term prognosis in patients with electrophysiologically confirmed disease. Mov Disord 24 (1): 72–76.

Meierkord H, Will B, Fish D et al. (1991). The clinical features and prognosis of pseudoseizures diagnosed using video-EEG telemetry. Neurology 41 (10): 1643–1646.

Munhoz RP, Zavala JA, Becker N et al. (2011). Cross-cultural influences on psychogenic movement disorders – a comparative review with a Brazilian series of 83 cases. Clin Neurol Neurosurg 113 (2): 115–118.

O'Sullivan SS, Spillane JE, McMahon EM et al. (2007). Clinical characteristics and outcome of patients diagnosed with psychogenic nonepileptic seizures: a 5-year review. Epilepsy Behav: E&B 11: 77–84.

Obelieniene D, Schrader H, Bovim G et al. (1999). Pain after whiplash: a prospective controlled inception cohort study. J Neurol Neurosurg Psychiatry 66: 279–283.

Oishi N, Kanzaki S, Kataoka C et al. (2009). Acute-onset unilateral psychogenic hearing loss in adults: report of six cases and diagnostic pitfalls. ORL; journal for oto-rhino-laryngology and its related specialties 71 (5): 279–283.

Pehlivantürk B, Unal F (2002). Conversion disorder in children and adolescents: a 4-year follow-up study. J Psychosom Res 52 (4): 187–191.

Ramani V, Girgenti L, Hickling E (1996). Outcome after diagnosis of psychogenic nonepileptic seizures (PNES). Epilepsia 37 (4): 416–417.

Reilly C, Menlove L, Fenton V et al. (2013). Psychogenic nonepileptic seizures in children: a review. Epilepsia 54 (10): 1715–1724.

Reuber M, Pukrop R, Bauer J et al. (2003). Outcome in psychogenic nonepileptic seizures: 1 to 10-year follow-up in 164 patients. Ann Neurol 53: 305–311.

Reuber M, Mitchell AJ, Howlett S et al. (2005). Measuring outcome in psychogenic nonepileptic seizures: how relevant is seizure remission? Epilepsia 46 (11): 1788–1795.

Riaz H, Cornish S, Lawton L et al. (1998). Non-epileptic attack disorder and clinical outcome: a pilot study. Seizure 7 (5): 365–368.

Ricciardi L, Demartini B, Morgante F et al. (2016). Symptom severity in patients with functional motor symptoms: Patient's perception and doctor's clinical assessment. Parkinsonism Relat Disord 21 (5): 529–532.

Sadan O, Neufeld MY, Parmet Y et al. (2016). Psychogenic seizures: long-term outcome in patients with and without epilepsy. Acta Neurol Scand 133: 145–151.

Schrag A, Trimble M, Quinn N et al. (2004). The syndrome of fixed dystonia: an evaluation of 103 patients. Brain 127 (Pt 10): 2360–2372.

Schwingenschuh P, Pont-Sunyer C, Surtees R et al. (2008). Psychogenic movement disorders in children: a report of 15 cases and a review of the literature. Mov Disord 23 (13): 1882–1888.

Selwa LM, Geyer J, Nikakhtar N et al. (2000). Nonepileptic seizure outcome varies by type of spell and duration of illness. Epilepsia 41 (10): 1330–1334.

Sharpe M, Stone J, Hibberd C et al. (2010). Neurology outpatients with symptoms unexplained by disease: illness beliefs and financial benefits predict 1-year outcome. Psychol Med 40 (1): 689–698.

Silva W, Giagante B, Saizar R et al. (2001). Clinical features and prognosis of nonepileptic seizures in a developing country. Epilepsia 42 (3): 398–401.

Slater ET (1965). Diagnosis of 'hysteria'. BMJ : Br Med J i: 1395–1399.

Slater ET, Glithero E (1965). A follow up study of patients diagnosed with hysteria. J Psychosom Res 9: 9–13.

Sletteberg O, Bertelsen T, Høvding G (1989). The prognosis of patients with hysterical visual impairment. Acta Ophthalmol 67 (2): 159–163.

Stone J (2005). Systematic review of misdiagnosis of conversion symptoms and "hysteria". BMJ 331 (7523): 989–990.

Stone J, Carson A (2011). Functional neurologic symptoms: assessment and management. Neurol Clin 29 (1): 1–18.

Stone J, Sharpe M, Rothwell PM et al. (2003). The 12 year prognosis of unilateral functional weakness and sensory disturbance. J Neurol Neurosurg Psychiatry 74 (5): 591–596.

Stone J, Carson A, Duncan R et al. (2009). Symptoms "unexplained by organic disease" in 1144 new neurology out-patients: how often does the diagnosis change at follow-up? Brain 132 (Pt 10): 2878–2888.

Thomas M, Vuong KD, Jankovic J (2006). Long-term prognosis of patients with psychogenic movement disorders. Parkinsonism Relat Disord 12 (6): 382–387.

Toldo I, Pinello L, Suppiej A et al. (2010). Nonorganic (psychogenic) visual loss in children: a retrospective series. J Neuroophthalmol 30: 26–30.

Toth C (2003). Hemisensory syndrome is associated with a low diagnostic yield and a nearly uniform benign prognosis. J Neurol Neurosurg Psychiatry 74 (8): 1113–1116.

Walczak TS, Papacostas S, Williams DT et al. (1995). Outcome after diagnosis of psychogenic nonepileptic seizures. Epilepsia 36 (11): 1131–1137.

Wig N, Mangalwedhe K (1982). A follow up study of Hysteria. Indian J Psychiatr 24: 120–125.

Williams DT, Ford B, Fahn S (1995). Phenomenology and psychopathology related to psychogenic movement disorders. Adv Neurol 65: 231–257.

Handbook of Clinical Neurology, Vol. 139 (3rd series)
Functional Neurologic Disorders
M. Hallett, J. Stone, and A. Carson, Editors
http://dx.doi.org/10.1016/B978-0-12-801772-2.00044-8

Chapter 44

Explanation as treatment for functional neurologic disorders

J. STONE[1]*, A. CARSON[2], AND M. HALLETT[3]

[1]*Department of Clinical Neurosciences, Centre for Clinical Brain Sciences, University of Edinburgh, Edinburgh, UK*

[2]*Departments of Clinical Neurosciences and of Rehabilitation Medicine, NHS Lothian and Centre for Clinical Brain Sciences, University of Edinburgh, Edinburgh, UK*

[3]*Human Motor Control Section, National Institute of Neurological Disorders and Stroke, Bethesda, MD, USA*

Abstract

There is widespread agreement that the way health professionals communicate the diagnosis of functional neurologic disorders (FND) has a central role in treatment, as it does arguably for most conditions.

In this chapter we discuss barriers to effective diagnosis, different models of explanation and evidence regarding the importance of effective communication of the diagnosis in FND, especially movement disorders, and dissociative (nonepileptic) seizures. Debates and disagreements about how to go about this task often reflect different theoretic models held by health professionals rather than evidence. More evidence is required to know whether an initial emphasis on one model is more or less effective than another (e.g., a functional model vs. a psychologic model).

We conclude, however, that there are a number of generic components to effective explanation shared by most authors on the topic that form the basis of a consensus. These include taking the patient seriously, giving the problem a diagnostic label, explaining the rationale for the diagnosis, some discussion of how the symptoms arise, emphasis on the potential for reversibility (rather than damage), and effective triage and referral for other treatment where appropriate. Although explanation can sometimes be therapeutic on its own, its role is probably more important as a facilitator to other therapy, including self-help, physical treatments, and psychotherapy.

INTRODUCTION

If you gather a group of interested doctors or other health professionals together to discuss how they treat functional disorders, the conversation quickly turns to discussion of communication of the diagnosis. Views are often strongly held and tied to underlying thoughts about the etiology and nature of the disorder, which in turn may reflect ongoing controversies about these conditions. What is clear is that health professionals believe it to be important. In an international survey of 519 members of the Movement Disorders Society, "educating the patient" was felt to be the second most important intervention (after avoiding iatrogenic harm) (Espay et al., 2009). In a separate survey, 87% of 343 Dutch neurologists thought explanation was part of the treatment they should offer (de Schipper et al., 2014).

In this chapter we attempt an impartial look at the subject of communication, looking at potential barriers to explanation, types of explanation that have been used, and evidence for how communication techniques affect patients with functional neurologic disorders (FND) seen in neurologic practice, both good and bad.

We especially focus on areas of common ground between various authors and highlight areas that could usefully be subject to more rigorous research.

*Correspondence to: Jon Stone, Department of Clinical Neurosciences, Western General Hospital, Crew Rd, Edinburgh EH4 2 XU, UK. Tel: +44-131-5371167, E-mail: Jon.Stone@ed.ac.uk

EVIDENCE FOR THE IMPORTANCE OF GOOD COMMUNICATION / EXPLANATION

It should perhaps go without saying that if you want patients to benefit from treatment, it's important that they have a diagnosis that they can understand, have some confidence in, and for which they can access appropriate information. It is also worth noting that complaints and litigation more often arise from poor communication than poor medical practice.

Indirect evidence for this comes from studies that have looked at the outcome of FND. In overlapping longitudinal studies of functional tremor, early diagnosis and patient confidence in the diagnosis were associated with a better outcome (Jankovic et al., 2006; Thomas et al., 2006). Other studies have also found that early diagnosis is associated with better outcome, although do not inform the question of whether a good communication of that diagnosis is important (Couprie et al., 1995; Mace and Trimble, 1996; Crimlisk et al., 1998). Studies of dissociative nonepileptic seizures found that relief (Carton et al., 2003) or acceptance (Ettinger et al., 1999) of the diagnosis predicted positive outcome.

This is a process that we often take for granted in neurology. Patients and their families have heard of epilepsy, multiple sclerosis, and migraine, and there are websites and some support structures for them to find out more after the consultation. The situation is different for functional disorders. Although there are exceptions, and there are now online resources such as www.nonepilepticattacks.info and www.neurosymptoms.org and patient organizations such as www.fndhope.org, many patients with functional disorders are not given a specific diagnosis, and not directed to any information.

In an article called "Psychogenic disorders; the need to speak plainly," Friedman and LaFrance (2010) drew attention to how commonly neurologists seeing patients with functional disorders will simply fail to provide a diagnosis at all; e.g., "I can't explain this problem on physiologic grounds," or will use coded jargon that fails to provide a positive diagnosis. Another approach that avoids the diagnosis focuses on the negative: "Good news, you don't have multiple sclerosis." Patients might leave knowing what they don't have, but not what they have. Many doctors believe that having a functional disorder is somehow "good news," whereas for patients that is not the case (McWilliams et al., 2016).

Our own experience is that audiences and readers are often keen to hear about how to communicate a diagnosis of functional disorder, as it's something they find difficult. In a study of 299 neurology outpatient encounters we demonstrated that the more the symptom was not explained by a disease process, the more "difficult" the neurologist found the patient to help (Carson et al., 2004): 82% of patients with predominantly functional disorders were rated as at least somewhat difficult, compared to 25% in the group with clearcut neurologic diseases.

BARRIERS TO EXPLANATION

These can be broadly divided in to those arising primarily in the health professional and those from the patient. Clearly factors within society in general influence both groups.

Barriers to successful explanation from health professionals

Lack of interest/negative attitudes

Surveys of a variety of health professionals have demonstrated how commonly negative views are held about patients with functional disorders (Stone, 2014). These range from the topic to the character of the patients themselves. A study of the "likeability" of various neurologic disorders among 205 Texan neurologists placed "psychogenic (functional) neurologic disorders" rock bottom, by some distance, in a list of 20 disorders. Dizziness, low-back pain, insomnia, and whiplash injuries were the only other conditions neurologists actively disliked treating (Evans and Evans, 2010). Dislikeability was rated as a useful diagnostic feature of functional disorders by 13% of UK neurologists in a survey (Kanaan et al., 2011). A survey of 519 Movement Disorders Society members painted a more positive picture. They were not asked about their attitudes to patients, but 92% responded that they believed their role extended beyond diagnosis to coordinate long-term management or triage to other professionals.

Attitudes and interests may vary between professions. We were surprised at how positively 702 neurophysiotherapists in the UK felt towards patients with functional disorder (Edwards et al., 2012). They ranked them sixth out of a list of 10 conditions they liked to treat, even though they judged their own knowledge as low, and only 25% felt support from neurologists in treatment.

Lack of education

It seems likely that some of the lack of interest stems from a lack of training. In a survey of neurologic textbooks over the last century it is evident that functional disorders have gradually been cleared out of the neurologic curriculum. Whereas Gowers' famous textbook of 1892 had an excellent 50-page chapter on the topic, most well-known textbooks of the 1990s had no section at all (Stone et al., 2008), although happily that is a situation that is changing. The venerable series, Handbook of Clinical Neurology, started in 1968, in which this chapter appears, has never previously had a volume on functional disorders.

The issue of malingering

FNDs, by their very nature, usually have the quality of voluntary movement. As such, it is perhaps understandable that issues of how much conscious control patients have over their symptoms present a considerable barrier to effective communication. In a series of indepth interviews with 22 neurologists on this topic, Richard Kanaan and colleagues exposed considerable ambivalence among many neurologists (Kanaan et al., 2009b). They suggested that neurologists use the diagnosis of functional disorder in a deceptive way because they were often "agnostic" about whether the patient is or is not genuinely experiencing the symptoms. Even if health professionals do not aggressively disbelieve patients, everyday language such as use of the terms "real/not real" or "genuine seizures" betray underlying assumptions. They suggest that this agnosticism often leads to an avoidance of treatment and engagement by doctors. The authors concluded that "the patient behaves 'as though' feigning, but the painful business of deciding quite how that is explained is someone else's problem." The avoidance of discussion of psychologic explanations and neurologists' doubts about the genuineness of the symptoms was framed in a subsequent paper as "limits to truth telling," although of course this is only the truth as those neurologists saw it (Kanaan et al., 2009a). Our own survey among 68 neuroscience nurses found quite high rates of similarly negative views (Stone et al., 2003). Sixteen percent disagreed that functional disorders were "real," 46% thought the patients were manipulative, and 34% disagreed that a neuroscience unit was an appropriate place for the patients.

Uncertainty over which model / terminology is correct

A less negative, but still mixed, picture emerged from a survey of 343 neurologists and 64 psychiatrists in the Netherlands from 2013. Less than 1% of neurologists thought that feigning explained the etiology of functional disorders. Most (60%) preferred a model in which psychologic factors and disordered nervous system functioning were relevant and only 22% viewed the problem as purely psychogenic (de Schipper et al., 2014), although hardly any (3%) preferred a purely psychogenic explanation. Such heterogeneity is a problem for a young doctor learning about this patient group. There would be little controversy about how to explain the diagnosis of multiple sclerosis as inflammation of the brain, but with functional disorders, which is the correct model? Furthermore, hypothetically speaking, if our understanding of the mechanism of multiple sclerosis were to change and inflammation was no longer part of the etiology, the name itself would be unaffected, but one cannot say the same of "psychogenic movement disorder." The model is intrinsically bound into much of the terminology.

Alteration of the normal order of explanation

Evidence from qualitative studies points to a problem that seems relatively unique to functional disorders (Thompson et al., 2009). In explaining the diagnosis, health professionals tend to invert the normal order in which information is presented. Most explanations of Parkinson's disease, for example, would start with a statement: "You have Parkinson's disease," and be followed up with an explanation of how that information is known (e.g., the examination is in keeping with Parkinson's disease) and something of the mechanism (e.g., not enough dopamine). It is unlikely the doctor would stray into etiology at an early stage, partly because the etiology is uncertain and multifactorial. For functional disorders, the opening statement is often a negative one: "You don't have multiple sclerosis," which is then often quickly followed by some speculation on the etiology. It is hard to think of other neurologic diagnoses being presented in this odd way, and it seems likely that patients pick up early that something is amiss in the presentation of the problem.

Lack of diagnostic certainty

The patient cannot receive a diagnosis of a functional disorder if the neurologist fails to make one. This is also potentially a training issue, but is undoubtedly one that has a significant influence. One of our colleagues who worked in a capital city in Eastern Europe told us that no one in his department made a diagnosis of a functional disorder. This was a diagnosis left exclusively to the head of the department as it was considered too risky for others to make.

There is a perception that to misdiagnose a patient with an "organic" condition as functional is much more of a sin than the other way round. Studies from the 1960s of misdiagnosis, especially that of Eliot Slater (see Chapter 43), were particularly influential in persuading some doctors that the diagnosis of "hysteria" was a "delusion and a snare" (Stone et al., 2005). We discuss the issue of clinical uncertainty and investigations further at the end of this chapter.

Lack of diagnostic codes

A parallel issue in many countries is that neurologists who see patients with functional disorders may not get paid if they try to make a functional diagnosis, or at least try to code it. In the International Classification of Diseases, 10th edition (ICD-10: World Health Organization, 2010), functional disorders are only coded in the psychiatric section, which some neurologists are not able to bill for. They therefore resort to vague codes, such as "leg weakness," when they know fully that the patient has functional leg weakness (personal communication from a US doctor) or "encephalopathy," when they know that the patient has dissociative (nonepileptic) seizures (personal communication from a Russian doctor). This is one compelling reason for allowing FNDs to have codes within the neurologic classification in ICD-11, as well as the psychiatric one, or even better, to argue for abandoning the two separate systems altogether and have a section encompassing neurology and psychiatry (Stone et al., 2014).

Barriers to successful explanation from patients

Health professionals have often had a tendency to blame patients for how difficult it is to explain functional disorders – an interesting situation, since it's not the patient that is doing the explaining! There are, however, some important patient-related and societal-related barriers to explanation for these disorders in particular.

Lack of public awareness

This is arguably not the fault of the patient either, but it is much harder to explain a condition someone has never heard of than one that is known. In fact, patients with functional disorders often express a feeling that the whole process would have been much easier if they had a disease like multiple sclerosis (Wessely, 2000).

Lack of supporting radiologic or laboratory abnormalities

The presence of such abnormalities provides an "instant short cut" to validity and acceptance in situations where the diagnosis is new to the patient or family.

Strong views of alternative diagnoses

Patients with functional disorders may have already come to a view prior to the consultation that they have a particular disease diagnosis. Sometimes these views are held so strongly that they are insurmountable. Usually, however, the patient has arrived at these views by a process of fairly reasonable assumptions in the face of no alternative diagnosis, and a media and internet environment rich with cues for self-diagnosis.

Societal unacceptability of psychologic factors/psychosomatic concepts

Although there are competing models, which we discuss below, it remains the case that most health professionals believe that psychologic factors are of key importance in functional disorders. If a health professional starts to explain this to a patient, there is an immediate problem. The general public are also ambivalent about physical symptoms that are variable and in which psychologic factors may be relevant. A study of the word "psychosomatic" in US and UK newspapers found that it was used in a negative way, such as "made up" or "imaginary" 34% of the time it was used (Stone et al., 2004). Although there are stigma and negativity surrounding mental health, there seems to be particular antipathy towards physical symptoms associated with psychologic factors. Well-known celebrities may declare their history of depression and patronage of mental health charities, but they are unlikely to own up to having a functional paralysis. This appears to relate to the same ambivalence about malingering seen among neurologists. If it can be faked, then how can we know if it's real?

Several studies have investigated this issue among patients. Studies of neurology outpatients show that they frequently equate several words for limb weakness, including "hysterical," "psychosomatic," and, surprisingly, "medically unexplained" with offensive concepts such as "putting it on," "not a good reason to be off work," and "mad" (Stone et al., 2002). One of us (JS) derived an offense score from this data to show that the "number needed to offend" for these words (i.e., the number of patients you would have to use this word with before one of them was offended) ranged between 2 and 3. The terms functional and stroke fared better (number needed to offend was 9). A study of terms for dissociative nonepileptic seizures found similar results for the terms "pseudoseizures" and "psychogenic seizures" (Stone et al., 2003). Studies in the Netherlands replicated these findings for patients with chronic fatigue syndrome. Psychosomatic fatigue was offensive to 1 in 3; chronic fatigue syndrome and "functional fatigue" was offensive to 1 in 11 (Kingma et al., 2012). A qualitative study of neurologists delivering diagnoses of functional disorders used conversation analysis to dissect some of these issues (Monzoni et al., 2011a). The doctors in this study offered a psychosocial explanatory model which was, in turn, often met with resistance by patients. This resistance took the form of overt disagreement and challenge but also passive responses, such as lack of engagement, silences, and minimal responses. Doctors in turn, provided formulation effort, which the authors proposed reflected the difficulties doctors faced in these encounters (Monzoni et al., 2011b). Somewhat in contrast, patients in primary care with functional disorders have shown that they do offer psychologic cues during consultations, even if doctors often fail to pick up on them (Ring et al., 2005).

Individual sensitivity regarding psychologic factors

Although there are societal barriers to understanding functional disorders, there may also be factors particular to patients with functional disorders. Studies of patients with FNDs have shown that they tend to view psychologic factors as less relevant than patients with disease (Table 44.1).

The difficulty in interpreting such data is that it is unclear whether patients with functional disorders, a priori, are particularly hostile or averse to the idea of psychologic factors, or whether those views are shaped by negative interactions with health professionals. However, in the end, regardless of the reasons, many patients do not want to hear that they have a psychiatric condition. This is usually interpreted as "it's all in my head" or "the doctor thinks I'm crazy." They would often rather try to find a doctor who can validate their distress with a disease diagnosis.

Our own experience, mirrored in some qualitative research, is that patients with functional disorders may sometimes be aware of the variability of their symptoms to the point where they often wonder if they are "imagining" it themselves (Karterud et al., 2015). It also remains plausible that individuals who have had adverse experiences or psychologic difficulties would actively prefer not to consider the possibility that the new difficulties they experience may have a link to those vulnerabilities. The alternative, of a disease process, tends to be viewed as less "blaming."

Even allowing for an absence of blame, a further factor may relate to who is going to cure the symptom. If one has a neurologic disease, it could be considered as having an external locus of control and it being the doctor's problem to treat, whereas if the symptom is psychogenic, it implies an internal locus of control and puts the onus on the patient to change and sort the problem out.

It is often speculated that some family members reinforce "antipsychologic" views of patients with functional disorders. Data from both functional limb weakness and dissociative seizures suggest the opposite – that relatives tend to see psychologic factors as more relevant, in keeping with the notion that the patients themselves are especially sensitive to this idea (Whitehead et al., 2015). It appears likely that sensitivities to psychologic formulations are multifactorial, arising in the doctor, patient, and society.

Table 44.1

Studies examining illness beliefs in patients with conversion symptoms show that only a minority endorse psychologic causation, and often less so than disease controls

Study	Patients (no.)	Findings
Kapfhammer et al. (1998)	Motor/nonepileptic attacks (103)	76% believed there was a somatic cause, 15% thought there was a psychologic cause, and only 7% thought stress was the main cause
Ewald et al. (1994)	Neurology inpatient "somatizers" (40) vs. disease controls (60)	36% of neurology inpatients with conversion symptoms thought psychologic factors were of importance vs. 76% of neurology inpatients with disease
Binzer et al. (1998)	Paralysis (30) vs. disease controls (30)	Patients with conversion had greater disease conviction (Illness Behaviour Questionnaire) and a more external locus of control than controls with disease
Crimlisk et al. (2000)	Weakness/movement disorder (64)	5% thought that psychologic factors were important, 22% thought psychologic factors had played a part (e.g., stress), 73% thought psychologic factors irrelevant
Stone et al. (2003)	Nonepileptic attacks (20) vs. epilepsy (20)	Patients with nonepileptic attacks had greater disease conviction (Illness Behaviour Questionnaire) and a more external locus of control than controls with epilepsy
Stone et al. (2010)	Weakness (107) vs. disease controls (85)	24% thought that stress was a potential factor vs. 56% of neurologic controls

EVIDENCE ABOUT EXPLANATIONS IN CLINICAL PRACTICE

What evidence do we have regarding the actual experience of patients with functional disorders in neurologic practice, and what lessons can we draw from them?

Patient experiences of diagnosis and predictors of outcome

In a qualitative study, Peter Salmon and colleagues looked at the experience of 228 patients in primary care with somatization disorders. They divided patient responses into three: (1) rejection – in which patients felt that the doctor was simply dismissing the symptoms as imaginary or dismissing them as related to anxiety or depression; (2) collusion – in which the patient was given a diagnosis such as fibromyalgia or myalgic encephalomyelitis but without a clear understanding of how that problem could be treated; and, least commonly, (3) empowering – in which the explanation contained a tangible mechanism that could link to self-management (Salmon et al., 1999). Studies of US ambulatory care have also shown that patients who do not receive an explanation or have "unmet expectations" are less satisfied than those who do (Jackson et al., 2001).

Several qualitative studies have examined the experiences patients with FNDs have had receiving their diagnoses. A qualitative study of 18 patients highlighted the difficulty they had when not presented with a medical theory to engage with and how this often led to fears that their illness was regarded as "imagined" or "fake," because "society does not readily grant permission to be ill in the absence of disease" (Nettleton et al., 2004).

A series of studies from Markus Reuber's group have explored the experience of diagnosis in patients with dissociative seizures from both the doctors' and patients' perspective (Thompson et al., 2009; Hall-Patch et al., 2010; Monzoni et al., 2011a, b; Baxter et al., 2012). An early qualitative study highlighted themes from interviews with patients, including the importance of the confidence with which neurologists made the diagnosis, and the way in which positive behavior from a neurologist could overcome self-doubt and doubt by others. This and a subsequent study exploring treatment highlighted considerable heterogeneity in patients' responses (Baxter et al., 2012). A study of 50 patients undergoing standardized protocol for communication found that reasonably high levels of acceptability and effective communication could be achieved using a training protocol and crib sheet in 23 neurologists (Hall-Patch et al., 2010). This emphasized that the attacks were real, had a name, had multiple etiologic factors which included psychologic factors, and could be treated with psychologic therapy. Feelings of anger were rare and most patients felt listened to and relieved. Although a case series, there was significant improvement in seizure frequency as well, with 14% seizurefree and 63% with a greater than 50% seizure reduction at 3 months.

A study from Nashville found that, of 75 patients with dissociative seizures, 70 were satisfied with the diagnosis, but of these, 19 thought there was no hope of treatment, 25 thought the diagnosis meant "being crazy," and 9 disagreed that psychologic factors were relevant (Arain et al., 2016). Studies from Norway and South Africa collected a higher proportion of angry, stigmatized, and disappointed outcomes from patients with dissociative seizures, suggesting a potential difference in clinical practice (Karterud et al., 2010; Pretorius, 2016).

A review of literature taken more widely across other disorders such as fibromyalgia and irritable-bowel syndrome emphasized the importance of perceiving patients' expectations and beliefs correctly (Weiland et al., 2012).

Overall, the data confirm significant barriers to communication, but that these can potentially be overcome with attention paid to common issues faced by patients. Varying outcomes in studies do suggest that some practitioners or methods may be better than others. However, it is unlikely that one method will be good for all patients, and the physician has to take into account individual differences.

Can training health professionals improve patient satisfaction with communication?

In the late 1980s David Goldberg, a psychiatrist, and colleagues, including Linda Gask, promoted a model of reattribution for "medically unexplained symptoms" on the basis that patients could benefit from learning how their emotions linked to their physical symptoms and thus manage them better. Large studies showed that doctors could be trained in reattribution, but a randomized controlled trial of 141 patients showed no ultimate benefit to patients in terms of outcome; in fact, their overall health may have even been slightly worse (Morriss et al., 2007). Another similar trial in 478 patients in secondary care in the Netherlands showed no effect on patient outcome despite 14 hours of "medically unexplained physical symptom" training, again with an emphasis on psychosocial factors (Weiland et al., 2016). Linda Gask and colleagues have reflected on their efforts and concluded that a reattribution model was too simplistic (Gask et al., 2011). They suggested that the model should move to one in which patients with symptoms should be approached with "no certainties about the presence or absence of organic pathology." In the field of functional disorders in neurology, however, it is clear that a diagnosis can be reached positively and clearly. This direction of travel, as epitomized in the somatic symptom disorder diagnosis in the Diagnostic and Statistical Manual of Mental Disorders, 5th edition (DSM-5: American Psychiatric Association, 2013), in which symptoms can be explained or not explained by disease, therefore also seems unhelpful in this context.

Evidence about explaining and arranging investigations

Patients with functional disorders will typically require investigations because of diagnostic uncertainty or to look for comorbid neurologic disease. Contrary to expectation, a study in primary care found that it is more often doctors than patients who tend to push for physical interventions in these situations, and doctors often fail to pick up on relevant psychosocial cues (Ring et al., 2004, 2005). It is not clear whether the same holds in secondary care.

There is evidence that preparing patients that their investigations are likely to be negative can have a positive effect on outcome. One of the best studies in this area is of noncardiac chest pain, where preparing patients for this outcome not only improved satisfaction with their diagnosis, but also reduced symptomatic outcome (Petrie et al., 2007). For patients with health anxiety, investigations only have a short-lived effect, as demonstrated by a study of patients undergoing endoscopy for dyspepsia. Those with low health anxiety were reassured; those with high health anxiety were only reassured for a week (Lucock et al., 1997). In headache, computed tomography head scans do provide short-term reassurance, but the effect is lost (unlike their headache) at 1 year (Howard et al., 2005). Many doctors believe reassurance is a goal of treatment, but fail to realize that: (1) the best form of reassurance is to provide an explanatory model of what has happened (Coia and Morley, 1998); and (2) in patients with health anxiety, reassurance is a "drug" that provides short-term relief but fuels the problem.

A consensus of core features of explanation

The last time two of us (JS and AC) wrote a chapter on this topic, we presented arguments for and against various ways of approaching explanation of functional disorders (Stone et al., 2011). This had a particular emphasis on whether to adopt a primarily "functional" explanation or a "psychologic" one.

Our review of the barriers to successful explanation and research in this area has highlighted questions that do relate to this dilemma. However, it is also clear from the way that numerous authors have grappled with and researched this problem that there are many important features of a good explanation that they share. Arguably, it is easy to lose sight of these core features when arguing about etiologic models and terminology.

In the time since that chapter, we have reflected on the fact that most of the core ingredients of an explanation for functional disorder, and for that matter, any problem in clinical practice, do not hinge on choosing one or other of these models (Carson et al., 2016). There is, of course, no "one-size-fits-all" solution. A patient with transient and improving isolated symptom requires a different approach to someone with severe health anxiety or someone else in a wheelchair. The more we have thought about this issue, the more we notice that the simplest solution to explaining functional disorders is to try as much as possible to replicate what happens with any other problem in neurology:

1. Take the problem seriously. In practical terms this may translate to saying to the patient during the assessment, "this is familiar, I'll explain at the end" or "this is a genuine problem/I believe you" during the explanation. Such explicit statements of belief may be necessary during an explanation of a disorder which the patient won't have heard of and which cannot be seen on a test. Such simple measures may overcome barriers of health professional interest and questions of malingering in patients who may have had previous experience of being dismissed or held in contempt. Clearly, such an approach will probably not be successful if delivered by a doctor who holds an ambivalent attitude.
2. Make it clear that there is a diagnosis. As discussed above, there is a tendency for doctors to overemphasize the diagnoses that patients do not have, often by introducing these before the actual diagnosis. This inversion of the normal order is often jarring for patients. If you have a diagnosis, then the diagnoses that you do not have are of lesser importance. Sometimes this problem is embodied in the diagnosis; for example, "you don't have epilepsy, you have nonepileptic attacks" is arguably an oxymoron. Many neurologists still give no diagnosis or may attempt a formulation instead. We would argue that a diagnostic label, whether functional or psychogenic is an essential signpost to direct the patient to information, explain the condition to family, friends, and employer, and access correct treatment. In some situations, especially where symptoms are mild, patients may not be looking for a diagnosis and may want to have their symptoms normalized or formulated. Diagnostic labels in that scenario may be iatrogenic. Common sense is required.
3. Demonstrate the rationale for the diagnosis. Much of the literature from primary care on "explaining medically unexplained symptoms"

(another oxymoron) emphasizes sharing clinical uncertainty about the presence of disease. In neurologic practice, however, functional disorders should be diagnosed on the basis of positive features and the patient can be invited to understand this process. Our own experience is that sharing clinical signs such as the tremor entrainment test or Hoover's sign with patients is a powerful way of persuading the patient that the diagnosis is correct, that there is the potential for reversibility, and that the consultation is a transparent process (Stone and Edwards, 2012).

4. Convey the potential for reversibility. A diagnosis of functional disorder can be presented in an empathetic and transparent way, but has arguably failed if the patient is left feeling that there is no potential for improvement. Feelings of irreversibility can be engendered by all models of functional disorder. A functional diagnosis can be interpreted as "something in the brain I can't influence" and a psychogenic diagnosis can be interpreted as "it's all down to me and my personality and there's no changing that." Patients and doctors often fixate on whether the problem is psychologic or neurologic when arguably it is more useful to consider whether the problem is reversible or not reversible, software or hardware.
5. Provide written information. Most patients recall only a fraction of the medical consultation (Kessels, 2003). As a generic recommendation, therefore, and arguably especially when there is complex and new information, it is essential to provide written information (Walker et al., 2015). This may take the form of a copy of the clinic letter supplemented with printed or online information specific for FNDs, e.g., www.neurosymptoms.org or www.nonepilepticattacks.info. In the last few years, patient organizations such as www.fndhope.org have also appeared, providing a perspective that has been missing in comparison to other conditions seen in neurologic practice.
6. Triage for further treatment. There appears to have been a shift in practice, with many neurologists in surveys, at least, indicating that they feel they do have a role in the treatment as well as diagnosis of functional disorders. Once again, using a model from other conditions seen in neurology, it would be standard for neurologists to review a patient with a new and complex condition and to consider which directions of treatment would be useful, even if they are not delivering those treatments themselves. Neurologists should continue to play a role in the treatment of patients with FND and are arguably in the best position to continue that role.

Psychogenic or functional?

We have relegated the discussion of whether a psychogenic or functional model and terminology is most helpful after the discussion of the core features of explanation, in keeping with our view that this is a secondary issue.

Nonetheless, many of the barriers we have identified are relevant to this question. There is little research to guide us on which in practice is most helpful. There have been interventions using a functional model (Sharpe et al., 2011) and a psychogenic model (Goldstein et al., 2010; Hall-Patch et al., 2010), with good outcomes for patients in neurologic settings. This suggests it would take a substantial randomized trial to detect a difference between the two approaches.

In two articles in Movement Disorders and subsequent correspondence, these issues were recently rehearsed (Edwards et al., 2014a, b; Fahn and Olanow, 2014a, b; Jankovic, 2014; LaFaver and Hallett, 2014). It was striking how much consensus there was on the core features above, even if there was disagreement on the wording. Arguments for and against each term are summarized in Table 44.2.

There are other models, including, importantly, a dissociative model, which is especially pertinent for patients with seizures, has some of the advantages of the term functional, in that it describes a broad mechanism rather than etiology, and is already in use in ICD-10 (Brown et al., 2007). The term "medically unexplained" in our view fails at almost every level, both theoretically and practically, something that is now recognized from the discipline of liaison psychiatry that popularized it (Creed et al., 2010). The issues for models such as conversion and somatization are similar to those as psychogenic. The term nonorganic is popular among clinicians who are looking for a term which does not differentiate between genuinely experienced and feigned symptoms. Finally, there is the preferred solution of some clinicians, which is not to apply any diagnosis at all, whether because they consider that someone else's responsibility, because they think we don't really understand these disorders, or because they do not agree with "medicalizing" the problem.

Readers must make their own minds up on this issue, but we suggest that the debate should not obscure more important and settled features of an explanatory model, listed above.

Improving evidence for explanation

Literature on explanatory models is increasing, but how could it be improved? Although explanation is widely thought to be a key therapeutic step, there is still

Table 44.2

Arguments for and against functional vs. psychogenic models and terminology as an explanatory model for patients

Model	For	Against
Functional	• Emphasis on mechanism rather than etiology • In keeping with a genuinely biopsychosocial model in which biologic mechanisms and factors are accepted as important • Less likely to be equated with "faking" or "imagining" symptom • Consistent with referral to physiotherapy (to improve function)	• Ambiguous about absence of neurologic disease • Greater difficulty in linking to relevant psychologic factors and treatment • A vague and wide term which could be applied to other disorders of nervous system functioning, including migraine, epilepsy, and dystonia. • Issues of patient acceptability are irrelevant, since any term will acquire stigma and terms should be determined on the basis of science • The term should be "dysfunctional," not functional
Psychogenic	• Symptoms are powerfully determined by expectation/belief/ psychologic conditioning • Higher rates of psychologic comorbidity and difficulties in patients with these disorders • Consistent with referral to psychology/psychiatry • Label indicates lack of "organic" disease	• Presumes etiology within diagnostic label • Narrows etiologic discussion and excludes biopsychosocial model • Promotes dualistic thinking • Diagnosis can't be made on the basis of psychologic characteristics of the patient • Implies an external stressor must be present, when it may not be • Increased likelihood that patient will interpret diagnosis as "faking" or imagining symptoms • Harder for patient to communicate diagnosis with others • Greater potential for patient to self-blame

relatively little evidence to guide practitioners. If explanation is a "therapy," then it should be tested like other therapies, with randomized trials.

The difficulty in carrying out such trials is separating out elements that are repeatable and can be subject to training from those that rely on the personality or enthusiasm of the practitioner. Some elements of explanation, such as transparency and taking the problem seriously, should arguably not be subject to randomization. Explanation as a therapy is not usually something to consider in isolation without backup from educational materials, consistent messages within a multidisciplinary team, further follow-up, and a change in societal awareness of functional disorders.

Nonetheless, it should be possible to design trials and interventions which do test component elements of explanation, especially educational parts and those in which clinicians themselves have equipoise.

References

American Psychiatric Association (2013). Diagnostic and statistical manual of mental disorders, 5th edn. American Psychiatric Association, Washington, DC.

Arain A, Tammaa M, Chaudhary F et al. (2016). Communicating the diagnosis of psychogenic nonepileptic seizures: the patient perspective. J Clin Neurosci 28: 67–70.

Baxter S, Mayor R, Baird W et al. (2012). Understanding patient perceptions following a psycho-educational intervention for psychogenic non-epileptic seizures. Epilepsy and Behavior 23: 487–493.

Binzer M, Eisemann M, Kullgren G (1998). Illness behavior in the acute phase of motor disability in neurological disease and in conversion disorder: a comparative study 44: 657–666.

Brown RJ, Cardena E, Nijenhuis E et al. (2007). Should conversion disorder be reclassified as a dissociative disorder in DSM V? Psychosomatics 48: 369–378.

Carson AJ, Stone J, Warlow C et al. (2004). Patients whom neurologists find difficult to help. J Neurol Neurosurg Psychiatry 75: 1776–1778.

Carson A, Lehn A, Ludwig L et al. (2016). Explaining functional disorders in the neurology clinic: a photo story. Pract Neurol 16: 56–61.

Carton S, Thompson PJ, Duncan JS (2003). Non-epileptic seizures: patients' understanding and reaction to the diagnosis and impact on outcome. Seizure 12: 287–294.

Coia P, Morley S (1998). Medical reassurance and patient's responses. J Psychosom Res 45: 377–386.

Couprie W, Wijdicks EF, Rooijmans HG et al. (1995). Outcome in conversion disorder: a follow up study. J Neurol Neurosurg Psychiatry 58: 750–752.

Creed F, Guthrie E, Fink P et al. (2010). Is there a better term than "medically unexplained symptoms"? J Psychosom Res 68: 5–8.

Crimlisk HL, Bhatia K, Cope H et al. (1998). Slater revisited: 6 year follow up study of patients with medically unexplained motor symptoms. BMJ 316: 582–586.

Crimlisk HL, Bhatia KP, Cope H et al. (2000). Patterns of referral in patients with medically unexplained motor symptoms. J Psychosom Res 49: 217–219.

de Schipper LJ, Vermeulen M, Eeckhout AM et al. (2014). Diagnosis and management of functional neurological symptoms: The Dutch experience. Clin Neurol Neurosurg 122: 106–112.

Edwards MJ, Stone J, Nielsen G (2012). Physiotherapists and patients with functional (psychogenic) motor symptoms: a survey of attitudes and interest. J Neurol Neurosurg Psychiatry 83: 655–658.

Edwards MJ, Stone J, Lang AE (2014a). From psychogenic movement disorder to functional movement disorder: it's time to change the name. Mov Disord 29: 849–852.

Edwards MJ, Stone J, Lang AE (2014b). Functional/psychogenic movement disorders: do we know what they are? Mov Disord 29: 1696–1697.

Espay AJ, Goldenhar LM, Voon V et al. (2009). Opinions and clinical practices related to diagnosing and managing patients with psychogenic movement disorders: an international survey of Movement Disorder Society members. Mov Disord 24: 1366–1374.

Ettinger AB, Dhoon A, Weisbrot DM et al. (1999). Predictive factors for outcome of nonepileptic seizures after diagnosis. J Neuropsychiatry Clin Neurosci 11: 458–463.

Evans RW, Evans RE (2010). A survey of neurologists on the likeability of headaches and other neurological disorders. Headache 50: 1126–1129.

Ewald H, Rogne T, Ewald K et al. (1994). Somatization in patients newly admitted to a neurological department. Acta Psychiatr Scand 89: 174–179.

Fahn S, Olanow CW (2014a). "Psychogenic movement disorders": they are what they are. Mov Disord 29: 853–856.

Fahn S, Olanow CW (2014b). Reply to: Psychogenic movement disorders: What's in a name? Move Disord : Official Journal of the Movement Disorder Society 29: 1699–1701.

Friedman JH, LaFrance WC (2010). Psychogenic disorders: the need to speak plainly. Arch Neurol 67: 753–755.

Gask L, Dowrick C, Salmon P et al. (2011). Reattribution reconsidered: narrative review and reflections on an educational intervention for medically unexplained symptoms in primary care settings. J Psychosom Res 71: 325–334.

Goldstein LH, Chalder T, Chigwedere C et al. (2010). Cognitive-behavioral therapy for psychogenic nonepileptic seizures: a pilot RCT. Neurology 74: 1986–1994.

Gowers WR (1892). Hysteria. In: A Manual of diseases of the Nervous System, Churchill, London, pp. 903–960.

Hall-Patch L, Brown R, House A et al. (2010). Acceptability and effectiveness of a strategy for the communication of the diagnosis of psychogenic nonepileptic seizures. Epilepsia 51: 70–78.

Howard L, Wessely S, Leese M et al. (2005). Are investigations anxiolytic or anxiogenic? A randomised controlled trial of neuroimaging to provide reassurance in chronic daily headache. J Neurol Neurosurg Psychiatry 76: 1558–1564.

Jackson JL, Chamberlin J, Kroenke K (2001). Predictors of patient satisfaction. Soc Sci Med 52: 609–620.

Jankovic J (2014). "Psychogenic" versus "functional" movement disorders? That is the question. Mov Disord 29: 1697–1698.

Jankovic J, Vuong KD, Thomas M (2006). Psychogenic tremor: long-term outcome. CNS Spectr 11: 501–508.

Kanaan R, Armstrong D, Wessely S (2009a). Limits to truth-telling: neurologists' communication in conversion disorder. Patient Educ Couns 77: 296–301.

Kanaan R, Armstrong D, Barnes P et al. (2009b). In the psychiatrist's chair: how neurologists understand conversion disorder. Brain 132: 2889–2896.

Kanaan RA, Armstrong D, Wessely SC (2011). Neurologists' understanding and management of conversion disorder. J Neurol Neurosurg Psychiatry 82: 961–966.

Kapfhammer HP, Dobmeier P, Mayer C et al. (1998). Konversionssyndrome in der Neurologie—eine psychopathologische und psychodynamische Differenzierung in Konversionsstörung, Somatisierungsstörungen und artifizielle Störung. Psychosom Psychother Med Psychol 48: 463–474.

Karterud HN, Knizek BL, Nakken KO (2010). Changing the diagnosis from epilepsy to PNES: patients' experiences and understanding of their new diagnosis. Seizure 19: 40–46.

Karterud HN, Risør MB, Haavet OR (2015). The impact of conveying the diagnosis when using a biopsychosocial approach: a qualitative study among adolescents and young adults with NES (non-epileptic seizures). Seizure 24: 107–113.

Kessels RPC (2003). Patients' memory for medical information. JRSM 96: 219–222.

Kingma EM, Moddejonge RS, Rosmalen JGM (2012). How do patients interpret terms for medically unexplained symptoms? Nederlands Tijdschrift Voor Geneeskunde 156: A4541.

LaFaver K, Hallett M (2014). Functional or psychogenic: what's the better name? Mov Disord 29: 1698–1699.

Lucock MP, Morley S, White C et al. (1997). Responses of consecutive patients to reassurance after gastroscopy: results of self administered questionnaire survey. BMJ 315: 572–575.

Mace CJ, Trimble MR (1996). Ten-year prognosis of conversion disorder. Br J Psychiatry 169: 282–288.

McWilliams A, Reilly C, McFarlane FA et al. (2016). Nonepileptic seizures in the pediatric population: a qualitative study of patient and family experiences. Epilepsy and Behavior 59: 128–136.

Monzoni CM, Duncan R, Grünewald R et al. (2011a). Are there interactional reasons why doctors may find it hard to tell patients that their physical symptoms may have emotional causes? A conversation analytic study in neurology outpatients. Patient Educ Couns 85: e189–e200.

Monzoni CM, Duncan R, Grünewald R et al. (2011b). How do neurologists discuss functional symptoms with their patients: a conversation analytic study. J Psychosom Res 71: 377–383.

Morriss R, Dowrick C, Salmon P et al. (2007). Cluster randomised controlled trial of training practices in reattribution for medically unexplained symptoms. Br J Psychiatry 191: 536–542.

Nettleton S, Watt I, O'Malley L et al. (2004). Enigmatic illness: narratives of patients who live with medically unexplained symptoms. Soc Theory Health 2: 47–66.

Petrie KJ, Muller JT, Schirmbeck F et al. (2007). Effect of providing information about normal test results on patients' reassurance: randomised controlled trial. BMJ 334: 352.

Pretorius C (2016). Barriers and facilitators to reaching a diagnosis of PNES from the patients' perspective: preliminary findings. Seizure 38: 1–6.

Ring A, Dowrick C, Humphris G et al. (2004). Do patients with unexplained physical symptoms pressurise general practitioners for somatic treatment? A qualitative study. BMJ 328: 1057.

Ring A, Dowrick CF, Humphris GM et al. (2005). The somatising effect of clinical consultation: what patients and doctors say and do not say when patients present medically unexplained physical symptoms. Soc Sci Med 61: 1505–1515.

Salmon P, Peters S, Stanley I (1999). Patients' perceptions of medical explanations for somatisation disorders: qualitative analysis. BMJ 318: 372–376.

Sharpe M, Walker J, Williams C et al. (2011). Guided self-help for functional (psychogenic) symptoms: a randomized controlled efficacy trial. Neurology 77: 564–572.

Stone L (2014). Managing the consultation with patients with medically unexplained symptoms: a grounded theory study of supervisors and registrars in general practice. BMC Fam Pract 15: 192.

Stone J, Edwards M (2012). Trick or treat? Showing patients with functional (psychogenic) motor symptoms their physical signs. Neurology 282–284.

Stone J, Wojcik W, Durrance D et al. (2002). What should we say to patients with symptoms unexplained by disease? The "number needed to offend". BMJ 325: 1449–1450.

Stone J, Campbell K, Sharma N et al. (2003). What should we call pseudoseizures? The patient's perspective. Seizure 12: 568–572.

Stone J, Colyer M, Feltbower S et al. (2004). 'Psychosomatic': a systematic review of its meaning in newspaper articles. Psychosomatics 45: 287–290.

Stone J, Warlow C, Carson A et al. (2005). Eliot Slater's myth of the non-existence of hysteria. J R Soc Med 98: 547–548.

Stone J, Hewett R, Carson A et al. (2008). The "disappearance" of hysteria: historical mystery or illusion? J R Soc Med 101: 12–18.

Stone J, Warlow C, Sharpe M (2010). The symptom of functional weakness: a controlled study of 107 patients. Brain 133: 1537–1551.

Stone J, Carson AJ, Sharpe M (2011). Psychogenic movement disorders: explaining the diagnosis. In: M Hallett, AE Lang, J Jankovic et al. (Eds.), Psychogenic Movement Disorders and Other Conversion Disorders. Cambridge University Press, Cambridge, pp. 254–266.

Stone J, Hallett M, Carson A et al. (2014). Functional disorders in the Neurology section of ICD-11: a landmark opportunity. Neurology 83: 2299–2301.

Thomas M, Vuong KD, Jankovic J (2006). Long-term prognosis of patients with psychogenic movement disorders. Parkinsonism Relat Disord 12: 382–387.

Thompson R, Isaac CL, Rowse G et al. (2009). What is it like to receive a diagnosis of nonepileptic seizures? Epilepsy Behav 14: 508–515.

Walker J, Meltsner M, Delbanco T (2015). US experience with doctors and patients sharing clinical notes. BMJ 350: g7785.

Weiland A, Van de Kraats RE, Blankenstein AH et al. (2012). Encounters between medical specialists and patients with medically unexplained physical symptoms; influences of communication on patient outcomes and use of health care: a literature overview. Perspect Med Edu 1: 192–206.

Weiland A, Blankenstein AH, Van Saase JLCM et al. (2016). Training medical specialists in communication about medically unexplained physical symptoms: patient outcomes from a randomized controlled trial. Int J Pers Cent Med 6.

Wessely S (2000). To tell or not to tell? The problem of medically unexplained symptoms. In: A Zeman, L Emmanuel (Eds.), Ethical Dilemmas in Neurology, W.B. Saunders, London, pp. 41–53.

Whitehead K, Stone J, Norman P et al. (2015). Differences in relatives' and patients' illness perceptions in functional neurological symptom disorders compared with neurological diseases. Epilepsy and Behavior 42: 159–164.

World Health Organization (2010). The ICD-10 classification of mental and behavioural disorders: clinical descriptions and diagnostic guidelines, World Health Organization, Geneva.

Handbook of Clinical Neurology, Vol. 139 (3rd series)
Functional Neurologic Disorders
M. Hallett, J. Stone, and A. Carson, Editors
http://dx.doi.org/10.1016/B978-0-12-801772-2.00045-X

Chapter 45

Physical treatment of functional neurologic disorders

G. NIELSEN*

Sobell Department of Motor Neuroscience and Movement Disorders, UCL Institute of Neurology and Therapy Services, National Hospital for Neurology and Neurosurgery, Queen Square, London, UK

Abstract

Physical interventions are widely considered an important part of treatment of functional neurologic disorders (FNDs). The evidence base for physical interventions has been limited to a collection of case series, but the recent publication of several large cohort studies and a randomized controlled trial have provided stronger evidence to support its use. While the evidence for efficacy appears to be promising, details on how this should be delivered remain limited, perhaps due to the dominance of psychologically focused etiologic models. A move towards understanding how the symptoms of FND are generated on a neurobiologic level has resulted in an expansion of pathophysiologic models providing a clearer rationale for physical treatment. In this context, the motor symptoms of FND can be considered as learnt patterns of movement, driven by attention and belief. Physical treatment aims to retrain movement by redirecting attention and addressing unhelpful illness beliefs and behaviors. The patient's problems should be considered in a broad biopsychosocial framework where symptom-predisposing, precipitating, and perpetuating factors can be addressed within a multidisciplinary environment as a gold standard. Further research is required to refine interventions and create evidence-based treatment guidelines.

INTRODUCTION

Functional neurologic disorders (FNDs) have been predominantly understood from a psychologic standpoint and etiologic models to explain symptoms have emphasized psychologic disturbance and emotionally traumatic events as key factors. This has placed physical treatment in uncertain territory and its rationale is unclear or indeed considered more as an opportunity for face saving (Nielsen et al., 2015a). However, in recent years a number of successful treatments with a more physical approach have been described, including the first randomized controlled study (Jordbru et al., 2014). The evidence base is limited, but there is a suggestion that specific physical treatment approaches are effective for some patients.

This chapter will explore the topic of physical-based treatments for FNDs. Rather than a discipline-specific instruction guide, the intention is to describe the rationale for physical treatment, then describe treatment principles and strategies based on the evidence and published expert opinion.

PATHOPHYSIOLOGIC MODEL AND RATIONALE FOR PHYSICAL TREATMENT

The starting point for treatment should be to consider FND within a biopsychosocial framework. For each patient there will be a heterogeneous mixture of predisposing, precipitating, and perpetuating factors that may need to be addressed as part of treatment. Relevant factors will differ between individuals. For some patients psychologic and social factors may be significant and require specific treatment; for others, a physical approach may be equally or more relevant. The rationale for physical treatment is that it can be used to retrain abnormal movement patterns. Central to this rationale is that symptoms are conceived as learnt patterns of movement that are outside the patient's control.

*Correspondence to: Glenn Nielsen, Box 146, Sobell Department of Motor Neuroscience and Movement Disorders, UCL Institute of Neurology, Queen Square, London WC1N 3GB, UK. Tel: +44-20-3448-3718, E-mail: g.nielsen@ucl.ac.uk

Emphasizing the biologic sphere of the biopsychosocial framework, and therefore physical treatment, is that symptoms are commonly precipitated by physical triggering events – most typically, injury, illness, and the somatosensory consequences of states of heightened arousal (Edwards et al., 2012; Stone et al., 2012; Pareés et al., 2014). Further validating physical treatment are etiologic models that seek to describe the neurobiologic mechanisms that account for functional neurologic symptoms. Clinical and laboratory studies have demonstrated that illness belief and attention directed towards the body are key mechanistic factors that drive symptoms (Edwards et al., 2013). The importance of illness belief is illustrated in the reports of dramatic curative responses to placebo treatment (Edwards et al., 2011). To this end, a change in illness belief or redirection of a patient's attention (distraction) can temporarily resolve symptoms or normalize movement.

A clear rationale for physical treatment can therefore be argued, particularly where symptoms are triggered by physical events. These events or their somatosensory consequences result in abnormally high levels of self-directed attention and a particular illness belief. This in turn leads to altered patterns of movement or maladaptive compensatory movements that become habitual. Theoretically, this may be associated with neuroplastic changes in the central nervous system. Physical treatment therefore seeks to retrain movement, with redirected attention, and to positively influence illness belief.

EVIDENCE FOR PHYSICAL REHABILITATION

A systematic review from 2013 highlighted the paucity of evidence for physical treatment for FND (Nielsen et al., 2013). To date there have been 33 published studies inclusive of physical treatment and only 12 studies with numbers greater than 10 (Table 45.1). Seven of the 12 studies are multidisciplinary interventions, including physical and psychologic therapies with medical oversight. The remaining five studies are treatments with a physical focus: these are inpatient rehabilitation (Czarnecki et al., 2012; Jordbru et al., 2014); a physiotherapy-delivered education and movement retraining program (Nielsen et al., 2015b); a walking-for-exercise program (Dallocchio et al., 2010); and a transcutaneous electric nerve stimulation (TENS) treatment (Ferrara et al., 2011). Interventions tend to be multifaceted, with cognitive, behavioral, and physical components. Physical treatment descriptions usually involve an overarching conceptual approach or principles that support rehabilitation (Table 45.2).

The only controlled study of physical treatment for FND is a delayed-start design, where 60 patients with a functional gait disorder were randomized to receive treatment (3-week inpatient rehabilitation) immediately or after a 4-week delay (Jordbru et al., 2014). The multidisciplinary team consisted of a physician, physiotherapist, occupational therapist, nurse, and an educator in adapted physical activity. The diagnosis was explained to patients as a disconnection between the nervous system and muscles, and it was not clear exactly why this had happened but that it commonly occurred after stressful life events. Positively reinforcing normal function with praise and attention was an important principle. The physical treatment included sporting activity, such as riding a bicycle, canoeing, and indoor climbing, with the aim of shifting attention to mastering the activity. At the end of treatment, the intervention group had significant improvements in the Functional Independence Measure, Functional Mobility Scale, and Short Form-12. Improvement was carried over 12 months, except for the mental health scale of the Short Form-12. The delayed-start design in this study limits the control period to 4 weeks and thus it cannot be ruled out that the long-term effects are due to spontaneous recovery over the 12-month follow-up period. Another limitation with this pragmatic and ethically pleasing experimental design is that the absence of intervention in a waiting-list condition does not control for placebo effects of the intervention and it has been suggested that waiting-list controls may have nocebo effects that inflate the effect size (Furukawa et al., 2014).

Nielsen et al. (2015b) report the outcomes of a prospective cohort of 47 consecutive patients with FND who completed an intensive 5-day physiotherapy treatment. The treatment was based on a symptom model for FND, highlighting self-focused attention and expectations about movements as key mechanisms. Education on the symptom model formed the basis of the treatment and physical retraining aimed to normalize movement by progressive task retraining with redirected attention. Sixty-five percent of patients were judged to have had a good outcome with treatment (a self-rating of much improved or very much improved). This was reduced to 55% at 3-month follow-up. There was also a corresponding change in physical and self-reported outcome measures. These improvements occurred in a cohort with characteristics that are typically regarded as indicators of poor prognosis, such as long symptom durations (median 44 months) and high rates of unemployment due to ill health (64%).

Czarnecki et al. (2012) presented the results of an innovative 5-day physical-based rehabilitation program for functional motor symptoms. The treatment was overseen by a physiatrist and patients were assessed by a psychiatrist; the treatment however was carried out by physiotherapists, occupational therapists, and, if

Table 45.1

Studies of rehabilitation of functional neurologic symptoms inclusive of physical treatment: $n > 10$

Reference	Subjects	Study design	Treatment	Outcome
Nielsen et al. (2015b)	$n = 48$ Functional motor symptoms Mean symptom duration 5.5 years	Prospective cohort study	5-day specialist physiotherapy-based program consisting of education and movement retraining with a self-management focus	65% rated their symptoms as "very much improved" or "much improved" on a 7-point CGI at the end of treatment. This reduced to 55% at 3-month follow-up. This corresponded with significant improvement in physical scales and self-reported outcome measures
Demartini et al. (2014)	$n = 66$ Functional motor symptoms Mean symptom duration 4.8 years	Prospective case series	4-week inpatient multidisciplinary rehabilitation involving physiotherapists, occupational therapists, cognitive-behavioral therapists and nursing, overseen by psychiatry with input from neurology	Two-thirds of patients rated their general health as better or much better on a 5-point CGI at discharge, which was maintained at 12-month follow-up. 45% of patients were lost to follow-up
McCormack et al. (2013)	$n = 33$ Motor conversion disorder Median symptom duration 48 months	Retrospective case series of consecutive patients	Multidisciplinary rehabilitation on a specialist neuropsychiatric unit, median length of stay was 101 days. The core treatment was from neuropsychiatrists, psychologists, physiotherapists, occupational therapists, and speech therapists if needed	Significant improvement in Modified Rankin Scale. There was also an increase in the proportion of patients mobilizing unaided or with a stick/crutches, and an increase in proportion of patients independent in personal activities of living. There was no follow-up
Jordbru et al. (2014)	$n = 60$ Functional gait disorder Mean symptom duration 10 months	Randomized cross-over design (4-week waiting-list control)	3-week inpatient rehabilitation described as adapted physical activity within a cognitive behavioral framework. The intervention was carried out by physicians, physiotherapists, occupational therapists, nurses, and an educator in adapted physical activity	Treatment resulted in significant improvement in physical function (FMS and FIM) and quality of life (SF12). Improvements were sustained at 1-month and 1-year follow-up (except for the mental health domains of the SF12)
Czarnecki et al. (2012)	$n = 60$ Functional motor symptoms Median symptom duration 17 months	Retrospective case series of consecutive patients (with historic control group)	5-day intensive physical rehabilitation based on the concept of motor reprogramming. The intervention was carried out by a physiatrist, physiotherapist, occupational therapist, and speech therapist where needed	68.8% of patients rated themselves as markedly improved or almost completely normal immediately after treatment. This reduced to 60.4% at 2-year follow-up
Saifee et al. (2012)	$n = 26$ Functional motor symptoms Symptom duration not stated	Retrospective case series with postal follow up	This paper is from the same rehabilitation programme as Demartini et al. (2014), above, but with a different cohort	At long-term follow-up of 7 years, 58% reported the program had been helpful or very helpful

Continued

Table 45.1

Continued

Reference	Subjects	Study design	Treatment	Outcome
Ferrara et al. (2011)	$n = 19$ Functional motor symptoms Mean symptom duration 46 months	Prospective case series	Use of TENS for 30 minutes a day, administered in an outpatient setting	Only 15 patients elected to continue with TENS and 11 were followed up at a mean of 6.9 months. Improvements were reported in the PMDRS and all self-rated outcome measures. 5 patients had no visible abnormal movements at follow-up
Dallocchio et al. (2010)	$n = 16$ Functional motor symptoms Mean symptom duration 15.5 months	Prospective case series	Walking exercise program for sedentary patients with mild to moderate symptoms	14 subjects completed the full 12-week trial. Marked improvement in 62% of patients (defined as complete resolution to 48% reduction in the PMDRS)
Shapiro and Teasell (2004)	$n = 39$ Weakness and gait disorder Symptom duration: 9 acute (less than 2 months) 28 chronic (more than 6 months)	Prospective case series of consecutive patients	Treatment in the first instance was progressive gait and posture retraining. If unsuccessful, a strategic-behavioral intervention was commenced, where patients were presented with two scenarios. Either there needed to be some adjustment to their program that would result in complete recovery or the problem was due to a psychiatric disorder requiring long-term psychiatric treatment	Physical-based treatment was effective for acute presentations only with recovery in 8/9 acute patients and 1/28 patients with chronic symptoms. The strategic protocol resulted in recovery in 14/22 patients (20 of whom did not improve without the strategic protocol)
Moene et al. (2002)	$n = 45$ Motor conversion disorder Mean symptom duration 3.9 years	RCT of the addition to hypnosis to multidisciplinary rehabilitation	12-week comprehensive multidisciplinary rehabilitation including physical therapists and psychologists. Patients were randomized to receive additional hypnosis	65% of patients from both groups were substantially to very much improved postretreatment and 83.7% at follow-up of 6 months. The addition of hypnosis did not affect outcome
Heruti et al. (2002)	$n = 34$ Weakness	Retrospective case series of consecutive patients	Multidisciplinary rehabilitation in a spinal rehabilitation unit, involving physiatrists, nurses, physiotherapists, occupational therapists, social workers, and psychologists, with consultation from a psychiatrist	At the end of treatment, 26% had complete recovery, 29% had partial recovery, and 44% were unchanged
Speed (1996)	$n = 10$ Weakness Symptom duration from days to 112 weeks	Retrospective case series of consecutive patients	Multidisciplinary rehabilitation lasting 4–22 days (mean 12 days). Treatment included physical therapy, occupational therapy, recreation therapy, and psychology	All patients improved on the FIM gait score. At follow-up of 7–36 months, 7/9 patients had maintained improvements

CGI, Clinical Global Impression; FMS, Functional Mobility Scale; FIM, Functional Independence Measure; SF12, Short Form 12; TENS, transcutaneous electric nerve stimulation; PMDRS, Psychogenic Movement Disorders Rating Scale; RCT, randomized controlled trial.

Table 45.2

Treatment principles commonly described in the literature

Build trust and rapport before challenging the patient
Create an expectation of recovery
Open and consistent communication
Involve family members
Avoid passive treatments
Encourage early weight bearing
Foster independence and self-management
Goal-directed rehabilitation
Avoid adaptive equipment
Use principles of behavioral management
Recognize and challenge unhelpful thoughts and behaviors
Develop a relapse prevention and management plan

Reproduced from Nielsen et al. (2015a), with permission from BMJ Publishing Group.

relevant, speech therapists. The intervention was described as relearning normal movement, starting with establishing elementary movements and building on them. Distraction strategies were utilized to extinguish abnormal movements. Repetition and positive reinforcement of gains were described as important principles. At the end of the 5 days, 70% of 60 patients rated themselves as markedly improved or almost completely normal. This reduced to 60% at 2 years.

The interventions described in the above studies are complex interventions with a number of components or multidisciplinary treatments. In contrast, Dallocchio et al. (2010) describe an intervention that on the surface appears very simple: a progressive walking exercise program for patients with mild to moderate symptoms. This 10-week program of supervised walking resulted in improvement in symptom severity according to blinded video rating. As with the other examples of physical treatment, the apparent simplicity here may belie multiple therapeutic ingredients that are in addition to improved general health and physical fitness, such as the effect of exercise on mood, peer support, and re-engagement with activity and community.

Physical treatment has been described as an integral part of established multidisciplinary inpatient rehabilitation programs (McCormack et al., 2013; Demartini et al., 2014). This is described further in Chapter 51. These programs usually accept the patients with more complex presentations and comorbidities (such as psychiatric treatment needs) that are excluded in the studies described above. While relapse of symptoms may be common and symptom resolution rare, ongoing benefit from treatment was reported in the majority of one cohort at 7-year follow-up (Saifee et al., 2012).

The limitations of the literature are clear. There are few large studies and only one with a randomized controlled design, albeit with a 4-week control period. Outcome measures are used inconsistently and it is not clear which are the most useful, valid, and reliable. The lack of controlled designs and multifaceted nature of interventions make it impossible to determine which are the more important ingredients of physical treatment. Finally, the treatment effect size is unclear, due to the heterogeneous characteristics of subjects and limitations of the outcome measures used. Despite these limitations, outcomes from physical treatment are promising. The majority of patients selected for specialized treatment demonstrate improvement on subjective and objective measures (Czarnecki et al., 2012; Nielsen et al., 2013, 2015b; Jordbru et al., 2014). The number who report symptom resolution is low, but the majority of patients report sustaining at least some benefit from treatment at follow-up of 1–2 years and beyond (Czarnecki et al., 2012; Saifee et al., 2012; Jordbru et al., 2014).

REFERRAL TO PHYSICAL TREATMENT

Given the link between chronicity of symptoms and poor outcome (Gelauff et al., 2014), referral to physical treatment should not be delayed. The referral should be made in a way that facilitates physical treatment specific to FND. This includes an honest and open explanation of the diagnosis to the patient, an explanation of the rationale for physical treatment, and good communication between treating clinicians. It is usually advised that investigations are completed prior to commencement of rehabilitation in order to reduce doubt in the diagnosis. However, it may be appropriate to proceed when investigations are delayed. In addition, an assessment from a physiotherapist or similar clinician may provide further evidence of a functional diagnosis.

ASSESSMENT

A comprehensive subjective history and physical assessment are important to understand the patient's problems, to recognize predisposing, precipitating, and perpetuating factors, and identify the problems that may be amenable to a physical treatment approach.

Helpful components of assessment include the following:

1. Create a comprehensive list of current symptoms. For each problem, enquire about frequency, severity (at worst and at best), exacerbating and easing factors.
2. Enquire about the onset of symptoms. This may highlight precipitating factors that can help to formulate an understanding of the diagnosis.
3. Establish the patient's general health condition prior to the onset of symptoms and the patient's past medical history.

4. If not already discussed, ask about pain and fatigue. Irritable pain and fatigue may influence decisions on the most appropriate treatment approach, setting, and intensity.
5. Ask about falls. Clarify differences between "near misses" and uncontrolled falls to the ground.
6. Create an impression of the impact of symptoms on daily life. This can be achieved by charting a 24-hour routine, enquiring about the need for personal assistance, use of adaptive aids and social support. A 24-hour routine may reveal symptom-perpetuating behaviors that can be addressed as part of treatment.
7. Find out about social history, work, and leisure.
8. Find out about experience of previous treatments.
9. Explore the patient's beliefs and understanding of the diagnosis, the patient's goals and expectations of treatment.
10. Complete a physical assessment, observing symptoms, their effect on activity and function, such as posture, transfers, gait, and upper-limb tasks. Variations in symptom severity with distraction and any maneuvers where symptoms dampen should be noted as potential starting points for education and movement retraining. Assessment at the level of impairment (e.g., power, coordination) rarely correlates with ability.

TREATMENT AGREEMENT

A treatment agreement or contract negotiated at an early stage can facilitate a smooth discharge and may pre-empt problems that can arise during treatment. The agreement can outline the number, duration, and frequency of sessions as well as expectations of the patient.

COMPONENTS OF TREATMENT

Based on the pathophysiologic model described above, physical treatment can be seen to have three main components: (1) education; (2) movement retraining; and (3) supporting self-management.

Education

Developing an understanding of the diagnosis and an insight into symptoms is an important first step to prepare the patient for physical treatment. This is arguably important for any condition, but it takes on a special significance in FND, due to the etiologic role of belief. The patient and clinician should come to a shared understanding of the problem, in order to collaborate on a treatment and management approach. Education-based interventions (guided self-help cognitive-behavioral therapy) for FND have been shown to improve self-reported health, symptom burden, and anxiety (Sharpe et al., 2011). Studies of physiotherapy-delivered education in patients with chronic pain, fatigue, and fibromyalgia have demonstrated improvements in symptom severity and functional outcome (Moseley, 2004; Meeus et al., 2010; Van Oosterwijck et al., 2013).

Explaining the diagnosis to the patient is not an easy or quick task. Firstly, understanding a diagnosis known by many names, with many different interpretations about the causes, sometimes tainted with unfavorable views, is understandably difficult. Secondly, understanding the value of a self-management treatment approach often requires a shift in the patient's concept of illness from a traditional biomedical model, where the patient is the passive recipient of treatment, to a biopsychosocial model, where the patient is expected to understand the problem and "administer the solution."

An important outcome of education is the understanding that symptoms are not caused by structural damage or a degenerative disease process. Symptoms can be described as "unconsciously" learnt patterns of movement, related to an abnormally high level of self-directed attention, often triggered by a specific event. This explanation can help to lower the threat value of symptoms and provides a rationale for physical treatment to retrain movement. It may be helpful for some patients to express some degree of optimism of the chances of improvement, but this should be balanced by a realistic impression of the prognosis. For example, it could be explained that most patients make at least some improvement with specific treatment, but that rehabilitation is often a long process requiring ongoing effort. Education starts with the diagnosing clinician. Information should then be reinforced and built on during physical treatment. Explanations should be backed up with written or online information (e.g., www.neurosymptoms.org). Table 45.3 gives examples of ways to discuss and explain the diagnosis with the patient.

Movement retraining

It has been suggested that the physical components of treatment can be similar to those used in "analogous neurological conditions" (Speed, 1996). Here a case is put forward that movement retraining is more effective when it is specific to FND and directed towards mechanisms responsible for driving symptoms, specifically:

1. belief (including expectations of abnormal movement)
2. abnormal self-directed attention
3. compensatory maladaptive habitual postures, movement patterns and behaviors.

Table 45.3

Examples of how to discuss and explain the diagnosis with patients

Potential components of patient education	Examples
Acknowledge the diagnosis	You have been referred to me for management/advice/treatment of functional neurologic disorder
Find out what their understanding of the diagnosis is	What do you understand about this diagnosis? What did the doctor tell you about this problem?
Explain what they have	You have functional weakness/tremor/dystonia/gait disorder
Explain what this means and that it is real	This is a type of functional neurologic disorder In functional neurologic disorder there is a problem with the ability to access normal movement This is quite a common neurologic diagnosis It is very real; I know that you are not making it up and that it is not "all in your head"
Explain what this does not mean	Unlike some other neurologic conditions, functional neurologic disorder is not caused by structural damage to the nervous system or neurologic disease The symptoms you are experiencing are not caused by damage to the structure of your brain, spinal cord, nerves, or muscles. However some people may have other problems in addition to functional neurologic disorder that can contribute to their symptoms, such as arthritis, migraine, or spinal stenosis
Explain how the diagnosis is made or how the symptoms differ from those caused by neurologic disease	Functional neurological symptoms are different from other neurologic symptoms in that they change with attention and distraction You have a Hoover's sign – this means that when you try to push down on your leg, you are unable to do it. However, when you push your other leg up against my hand, the muscle turns on via a reflex. This means that the "wiring" is intact and the problem lies with your ability to access movement when you try Your tremor changes when you do a competing movement. When you tap your fingers of your other hand, the tremor subsides or goes away. Or when you do a sudden ballistic movement, the tremor pauses There are fluctuations in the severity of your symptoms; sometimes they are much more severe than at other times This variability is typical for functional neurologic disorder and it is used to help make the diagnosis This type of variability in symptoms is usually not possible in symptoms caused by structural neurologic disease
Explain what variability and distractibility mean	The variability/Hoover's sign/distractibility is related to where the brains attention or "spotlight" is directed When attention is directed towards the body part or symptom, usually the symptom gets worse. Some people find that the harder they try to move normally or suppress the symptom, the worse it becomes. Most people find this very frustrating Usually more automatic movements are performed better and the harder someone tries to move, the more difficult the movement becomes The worsening of a movement with attention is similar to when a sports person "chokes under pressure"; for example, when a tennis player thinks too much about her serve or a golfer thinks about his swing, rather than using "muscle memory"
Discuss reinforcement of the movement problem	This seems to cause a new "motor program" which gets stuck Repetition of the movement/symptom/problem over time causes reinforcement of the motor program The problem becomes a "subconsciously learnt" pattern of movement The brain can start to expect movement to go wrong, which can result in abnormal movement; for example, when lifting an object that you expect to be heavy but which turns out to be very light. The movement output is "wrong," created by a false expectation
Discuss secondary problems	The movement problems themselves often cause other secondary problems, such as musculoskeletal pain and hypersensitivity, muscle and joint stiffness or contracture, tiredness and fatigue, sleep disturbance, loss of physical fitness, problems with concentration These secondary problems become another source of disability that can worsen or perpetuate the problems
Discuss what we know about why people get FNS	We are still not certain exactly what causes someone to develop functional neurologic disorder, in the same way that we are not certain why some people develop multiple sclerosis or Parkinson's disease The causes are likely to be different in every case

Continued

Table 45.3

Continued

Potential components of patient education	Examples
	The cause is most likely multifactorial, meaning that a number of different things have happened and interacted to result in functional neurologic disorder
Discuss triggering factors, if relevant	It is common for people to identify an event that triggered their symptoms; common triggers include illness, injuries, surgery, shock, or panic
	For some people psychologic factors are important and, where this is the case, it is usually helpful to speak to someone in this field for advice. This does not mean that the symptoms are any less real; it is just another part of rehabilitation
Introduce the role of physical rehabilitation	Physical rehabilitation can help you retrain your movement, helping you get access to and control of your movement
	Physical rehabilitation is not easy and it involves a lot of work
	Understanding is an important part of physical rehabilitation
	It is important for you to understand what things you can do to help get yourself better and to know what things might be slowing down your progress
	Physical rehabilitation can help by changing what you do and how you do it; the 23 hours you spend outside of therapy are more important than the hour you spend in therapy
Express confidence in ability to improve, but acknowledge that it is not easy	Physical rehabilitation is not a quick fix, but most people get at least some benefit from it

Addressing belief and expectation by demonstrating normal movement

Demonstrating to patients that their movement can be normal is a powerful way of convincing them of the diagnosis and helping them understand their symptoms (Stone and Edwards, 2012). Normal movement can be elicited with clinical tests, such as Hoover's sign or entrainment of a tremor. Normal movement can also be produced in the context of more meaningful activity. For example, a functional gait disturbance may appear normal when the patient walks backwards or advances forward by sliding the feet along the ground. Tasks that normalize movement are likely to be novel or unfamiliar and redirection of attention is required to achieve the task. Asking patients to observe their movement in a mirror or on video can reinforce this with visual evidence. Strategies and maneuvers that reduce symptoms can be used to help retrain movement.

Strategies to retrain movement (with redirected attention)

Sequential learning is the most common approach to movement retraining described in the physical treatment literature. This starts by establishing elementary (symptom-free) components of a movement, which are then built on in successive stages to reshape normal movement patterns (Trieschmann et al., 1970; Czarnecki et al., 2012). An example of putting this into action for a functional gait disturbance might start by retraining the sit-to-stand movement, in order to achieve an appropriate standing posture. The patient can then be progressed to standing with gentle lateral weight shift, which can be progressed to "de-weighting" the feet reciprocally. The patient is instructed to keep the attention on maintaining smooth rhythmic weight shift. The de-weighted foot is then allowed to advance forward, not by encouraging an active (consciously considered) step, but by introducing some forward momentum to the lateral weight shift (the center of mass is directed towards the front of the weight-bearing foot) so that the de-weighted foot "relaxes forward." Slow progressions in this way can introduce stepping without specifically instructing patients to step or drawing excessive attention to their lower limbs. Progressions may occur within a single treatment session or across multiple sessions as required. A sequential approach has appeal, as movement retraining can occur while minimizing reinforcement of symptomatic movement patterns.

Exploring symptoms and movement with the patient may reveal other useful strategies to help retrain movement. Often patients have identified their own "tricks" to control movement. For example, some people find cognitive distraction helpful, such as having a conversation, listening to music, or singing. Changing the speed of movement (increasing or decreasing), tapping an unaffected hand or foot, or bouncing a ball might be helpful. Table 45.4 lists examples of ways to normalize and retrain movement.

Applying principles of motor learning

Principles of motor learning have been described that aim to accelerate skill acquisition and associated adaptive plastic changes in the central nervous system. Important components of effective motor learning are repetition, task-oriented exercises, task shaping (gradually increasing the difficulty of the task), and feedback (Homberg, 2013). Task-oriented exercise allows for more direct translation into improved ability and for attention to be directed away from the mechanics of movement (e.g., generating sufficient power to extend the knees) and towards the goal of movement (e.g., standing up). Feedback is important to facilitate motor learning. Feedback from a mirror, video, or electromyography (EMG) may help patients identify maladaptive movement patterns that they had been unaware of. Feedback may also help to redirect the patient's attention to normalize movement. However, feedback also has the potential to exacerbate symptomatic movement by increasing self-focused attention.

Consolidation and generalization of motor learning are important to consider as part of treatment. These are the degree to which a "motor memory" is resistant to interference by another task and how the training translates to different contexts (Kitago and Krakauer, 2013). This is facilitated by increasing the difficulty of tasks and introducing variability. This can include a change in context (e.g., upper-limb activities in personal care, eating, and writing), a change in environment (walking indoors, outdoors, on uneven surfaces, and busy environments), varying speeds, and multitasking.

Supporting self-management

The self-management approach recognizes that FNDs are often chronic conditions with multiple contributing factors that can require ongoing attention in order to sustain or continue to make progress. Relapses or periods of symptom exacerbation are common following discharge and it is important for the patient to be prepared to manage this situation. A useful treatment device to foster self-management is to support the patient to complete a rehabilitation workbook that includes a personal management plan. The contents of a workbook may include:

1. an explanation of the diagnosis, with reference to the patient's personal experience
2. relevant symptom-precipitating and perpetuating factors with management strategies
3. reflections from treatment sessions
4. strategies employed during treatment that help to normalize movement
5. markers of progress, including achieved goals and scores from outcome measures
6. future goals and plans to achieve them
7. plans for managing difficult days and setbacks.

Precipitating and perpetuating factors relevant to physical treatment

A self-management plan should help the patient identify, understand, and change maladaptive habitual behaviors that act as symptom-precipitating or perpetuating factors. Maladaptive behaviors may include:

1. habitual postures, such as sitting with a lower limb resting in an end-of-range "dystonic" position (this is particularly common in fixed functional dystonia)
2. habitual movement patterns
3. learnt nonuse of an upper limb

Table 45.4

Examples of strategies to normalize and retrain movement

Symptom	Movement strategy
Leg weakness	Early weight bearing with progressively less upper-limb support, e.g., "fingertip" support Standing in a safe environment with side-to-side weight shift Crawling in four-point then two-point kneeling Increase walking speed Treadmill walking (with or without a body weight support harness and feedback from a mirror)
Ankle weakness	Elicit ankle dorsiflexion activity by asking patient to walk backwards, with anterior/posterior weight shift while standing or by walking by sliding feet along the floor Use of electric muscle stimulation to initiate movement during treatment
Upper-limb weakness	Weight bear through the upper limbs, weight bearing with weight shift or crawling Minimize habitual nonuse by using the affected upper limb in tasks (e.g., while showering or to stabilize a plate when eating)

Continued

Table 45.4

Continued

Symptom	Movement strategy
	Practice tasks that are very familiar or important to the individual, that may not be associated with symptoms (e.g., use of mobile phone, computer, tablet)
	Stimulate automatic upper-limb postural response by sitting on an unstable surface such as a therapy ball, resting upper limbs on a supporting surface
Gait disturbance	Speed up walking (in some cases this may worsen walking pattern)
	Slow down walking speed
	Walk by sliding feet forward, keeping plantar surface of foot in contact with the ground. (i.e., like wearing skis). Progress towards normal walking in graded steps
	Build up a normal gait pattern from simple achievable components that progressively approximate normal walking
	Walk carrying small weights/dumbbells in each hand
	Walk backwards or sideways, progressing towards forwards walking
	Walk to a set rhythm (e.g., in time to music, counting: 1, 2, 1, 2 …)
	Exaggerated movement (e.g., walking with high steps)
	Walking up or down stairs (this is often easier than walking on flat ground)
Upper-limb tremor	Make the movement "voluntary" by actively imposing a movement that interferes with the tremor, change the movement to a larger amplitude and slower frequency, then slow the movement to stillness
	Teach the patient how to relax the muscles by actively contracting muscles for a few seconds, then relaxing
	Change habitual postures and movement relevant to symptom production (e.g., discourage using excessive muscle tension to supress a tremor)
	Perform a competing movement. For example, clap to a rhythm or large flowing movements of the symptomatic arm as if conducting an orchestra
	Focus on another body part, for example, tapping the other hand or a foot
	Muscle relaxation exercises. For example, progressive muscle relaxation techniques, electromyogram biofeedback, or using mirror feedback
Lower-limb tremor	Side-to-side or anterior–posterior weight shift to entrain or interfere with the tremor. When the tremor has reduced, slow weight shift to stillness
	Competing movements such as toe tapping
	Ensure even weight distribution when standing. This can be helped by using weighing scales and/or a mirror for feedback
	Change habitual postures relevant to symptom production. For example, reduce forefoot weight bearing
Fixed dystonia	Change habitual sitting and standing postures to prevent prolonged periods in end-of-range joint positions and promote postures with good alignment
	Normalize movement patterns (e.g., sit to stand, transfers, walking) with an external or altered focus of attention (i.e., not the dystonic limb)
	Discourage unhelpful protective avoidance behaviors and encourage normal sensory experiences (e.g., wearing shoes and socks, weight bearing as tolerated, not having the arm in a "protected" posture)
	Prevent or address hypersensitivity and hypervigilance
	Teach strategies to turn overactive muscles off in sitting and lying (e.g., by allowing the supporting surface to take the weight of a limb. Cushions or folded towels may be needed to bring the supporting surface up to the limb where contractures are present)
	The patient may need to be taught to be aware of maladaptive postures and overactive muscles in order to use strategies
	Consider examination under sedation, especially if completely fixed or concerned about contractures
	Consider a trial of electric muscle stimulation or functional electric stimulation to normalize limb posture and movement (e.g., stimulation of tibialis anterior muscle to align the foot and ankle to allow weight bearing or stimulation of wrist and finger extensors for a clenched fist)
Functional jerks/ myoclonus	Movement retraining may be less useful for intermittent sudden jerky movements. Instead, look for self-focused attention or premonitory symptoms prior to a jerk that can be addressed with education and distraction or redirected attention
	When present, address pain, muscle overactivity, or altered patterns of movement that may precede a jerk

Adapted from Nielsen et al. (2015a), with permission from BMJ Publishing Group.

4. boom-and-bust activity patterns (all-or-nothing behavior)
5. sedentariness
6. passive coping strategies, such as excessive rest
7. lack of structure and routine
8. poor sleep hygiene
9. pain avoidance behavior
10. relying on excessive support from others.

COMPONENTS OF PHYSICAL TREATMENT AND THERAPEUTIC ADJUNCTS

Mirror and video feedback

Visual feedback may facilitate movement retraining. Paradoxically, visual feedback from a mirror during movement may reduce self-focused attention in some patients. Video can be used to demonstrate to patients how their movement normalizes with distraction or a treatment strategy. Conversely, video can demonstrate how symptoms are exacerbated with increased attention to the body. In this way, videos are a useful tool to help patients understand their symptoms, how they may learn to control their movement, and provide convincing evidence if they are doubtful of the diagnosis. Treatment using mirrors may also help to address distortions in cortical somatotopic maps, though more research is needed to support this idea in FND.

Nonspecific exercise

There is some evidence that general exercise in groups can be beneficial for FND in people with mild to moderate symptoms (Dallocchio et al., 2010). Also highly relevant is the evidence that graded-exercise therapy can moderately improve outcomes in chronic fatigue syndrome and is superior in a trial setting to usual care or adaptive pacing (White et al., 2011). The ability to engage in exercise is restricted in patients with more severe symptoms, particularly pain and fatigue. In this situation the concept of exercise is expanded to include re-engagement with the community and incidental activity, such as personal care and housework. Enjoyable leisure activities are scheduled with equal priority as rest. Activity level is stabilized with planning and increased in small gradations by setting goals.

Electrotherapies

Electric therapies have a long history in the treatment of FND. Early applications were used as aversive stimulus and were often brutal (Broussolle et al., 2014). Modern descriptions of electrotherapies include the use of TENS for sensory stimulation (Ferrara et al., 2011), and EMG biofeedback (Withrington and Wynn Parry, 1985; Klonoff and Moore, 1986; Fishbain et al., 1988; Hughes and Alltree, 1990). Functional electric muscle stimulation, for example, stimulating ankle dorsiflexion via surface electrodes during gait, holds promise as a treatment strategy in some types of symptoms, such as weakness and fixed functional dystonia (Nielsen et al., 2015b).

Other treatment adjuncts

Other novel treatments have been suggested for FND, such as visualization and mirror-box (Nielsen et al., 2015a). Treadmill training and use of an overhead body weight support harness have been used as part of gait rehabilitation (Nielsen et al., 2015b). One study described using a therapy ball as an unstable surface to help stimulate automatic postural responses in functional weakness (Delargy et al., 1986).

Addressing pain and fatigue

Pain and fatigue are a common part of many, if not most, patients' symptom presentation (Stone et al., 2010; Saifee et al., 2012; Nielsen et al., 2015b). Both can act as predisposing, precipitating, or perpetuating factors and should be addressed as part of treatment with education and graded exercise. Treatments have been well described in the literature (Butler and Moseley, 2003; Hansen et al., 2010; Nijs et al., 2011; White et al., 2011; Moss-Morris et al., 2013; Kamper et al., 2014).

Falls prevention in symptoms affecting mobility

There is a common but unsubstantiated perception that patients with FND are at low risk of falling and sustaining an injury, and that near misses and controlled descents are more common. In this case it may be appropriate to encourage graded independent ambulation in order to progress rehabilitation and avoid unnecessary mobility restrictions delaying recovery. Conversely, injuries have been reported (Nielsen et al., 2015b), and rushing the patient can be counterproductive, therefore a balance should be negotiated with the patient. The situation is more complex when the patient has a history of self-harm, where injury may be an expression of distress or initiated to relieve unbearable tension. When there is a history of serious falls, the role of "voluntary" or "involuntary" self-harm should be considered and additional support from a multidisciplinary team should be sought.

ADAPTIVE AIDS, EQUIPMENT, AND ENVIRONMENTAL MODIFICATIONS

Where possible, walking aids, adaptive equipment, splints, and braces should be avoided. Equipment leads to adaptive movement patterns, which may prevent the return of normal "automatic" movement and result in secondary problems such as pain and deconditioning. For example, excessive upper-limb weight bearing through crutches can perpetuate functional lower-limb weakness and result in shoulder joint pain. Immobilization of joints in splints and casts (such as serial casting) has been reported as being harmful, linked to the development or deterioration of fixed dystonia (Schrag et al., 2004), and should be avoided.

In some cases aids and environmental adaptations may be necessary or unavoidable. Where this is the case, it is recommended that the patient is involved in the decision-making process, having been made aware of the potential negative consequences. A plan should be in place to minimize the potential harmful impact of the equipment and, if relevant, to wean the patient off its use. In the situation where the patient has had appropriate attempts at rehabilitation without benefit, adaptations should be considered to increase independence, safety, and quality of life.

SETTING INTENSITY AND DURATION

Optimal treatment setting, intensity, and duration are not known and likely to be dependent upon individual characteristics. The majority of the physical treatment research has been on inpatient settings, which have the advantage of control over social and environmental factors that may be working to perpetuate the patient's symptoms. It also allows for greater intensity of treatment. Conversely, outpatient and domiciliary treatment may address relevant environmental factors more directly, while allowing for slower stream and longer duration treatment. This may be important with irritable pain and fatigue. There is some suggestion that higher intensity of treatment over a short duration may be effective (Czarnecki et al., 2012; Nielsen et al., 2015b). Providing a time-defined treatment duration is a common feature of some established programs (Czarnecki et al., 2012; Demartini et al., 2014; Nielsen et al., 2015b). This may help focus treatment, and provide an impetus for change, while rationing a limited resource.

MEASURING OUTCOME

Accurate measurement of outcome with physical treatment remains challenging. A battery of measures is required to capture the biopsychosocial domains of FND. Objective physical scales are arguably important for physical symptoms to quantify disability, but they are vulnerable to inaccuracy and reliability issues due to the variable nature of functional symptom severity. Patient-reported outcome measures with a set recall period might counteract this issue, at the cost of objectivity and sensitivity.

DISCHARGE

Concluding a treatment episode can be difficult when the patient remains symptomatic. To minimize problems, discharge planning can commence at the onset of treatment, starting with an explicit treatment contract (as described above) and concluding with creating a self-management plan. Tapering the frequency of therapy sessions towards the end of a block of treatment can help prepare the patient for self-management and a follow-up session several weeks after discharge may provide an opportunity to iron out any problems encountered. Sending the patient a comprehensive discharge report can be an opportunity to reinforce information and educate others.

SYMPTOM-SPECIFIC TREATMENT APPROACHES

Lower-limb weakness

Early standing and weight bearing with support are important. The patient can be encouraged to use the environment for light touch support. Hands-on treatment is probably best kept to a minimum, but during treatment sessions, the patient can be supported and guided with facilitative handling (fingertip support) for confidence. The therapist should prevent the patient from taking excessive support, as this is likely to generate symptomatic movement. Fear of falling can be addressed by grading exposure to more challenging tasks and environments. Potentially useful treatment adjuncts include a treadmill, body weight support harness, and functional electric muscle stimulation. The patient should be progressed from rehabilitation equipment early and prior to discharge (Fig. 45.1).

Tremor

Entrainment with biofeedback as a treatment for functional tremor has been tested in a small proof-of-concept study (Espay et al., 2014). The aim was to help the patient to develop volitional control over the movement and bring it to a stop. This small study of 10 patients demonstrated improvements in tremor after three 2-hour retraining sessions. Six patients reported lasting improvement at 6 months. Others have described physical strategies to retrain a tremor, where an active movement is imposed

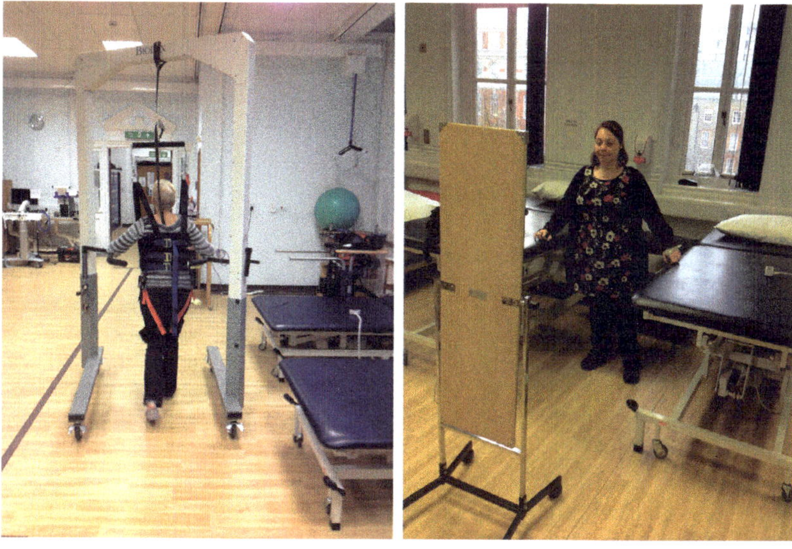

Fig. 45.1. (**A**, **B**). Gait retraining with a body weight support harness and treatment of lower-limb weakness.

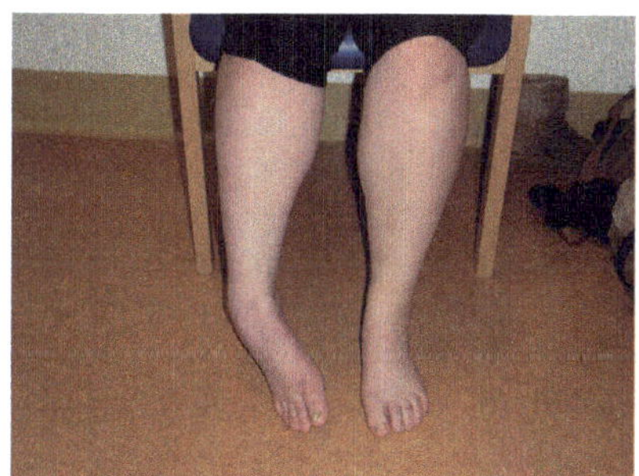

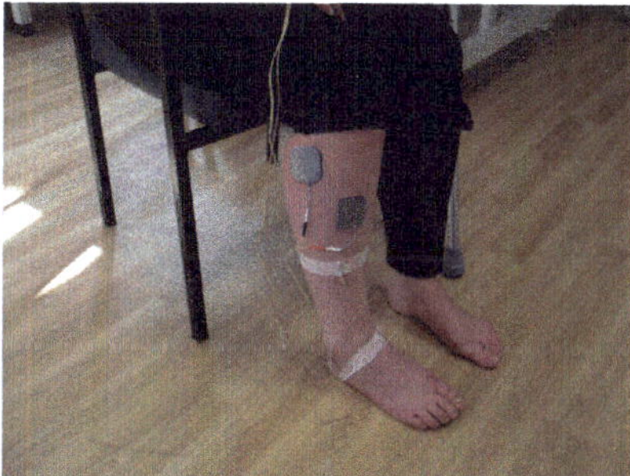

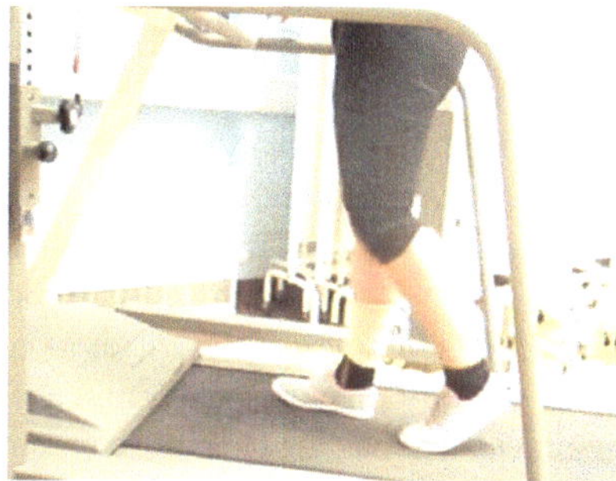

Fig. 45.2. (**A**–**C**). Use of functional electric stimulation and a treadmill for fixed functional dystonia.

on top of the tremor, with the aim of gaining control of the movement (Nielsen et al., 2015a).

In the absence of biofeedback equipment, the use of a mirror may be a useful and more accessible source of feedback. Maladaptive behaviors or compensatory strategies seem to be important in generating or perpetuating functional tremor and should be addressed in treatment. Some examples include a "heel-bouncing" tremor generated by forefoot contact with the ground, attempting to suppress a tremor by increasing muscle rigidity, and nonuse of an affected upper limb.

The special case of fixed functional dystonia and joint contractures

Functional dystonia typically presents as a fixed abnormal joint posture (commonly ankle plantar flexion and inversion), accompanied by significant pain. It often overlaps with the diagnosis of complex regional pain syndrome (Schrag et al., 2004). Evaluation under sedation helps diagnosis and treatment planning. It may reveal a contracture, but sometimes joint range of motion is unexpectedly preserved. Management involves early but graded restoration of movement, weight bearing, and function, following the principles of pain management, including desensitizing hypersensitive areas (Harden et al., 2013). Habitual postures and movement patterns that reinforce the "dystonic" position should be identified and addressed through education, postural advice, and movement retraining. Exacerbation of pain is usually associated with more extreme posturing; therefore painful interventions such as passive stretches are usually counterproductive. A contracture can be addressed by changing maladaptive habitual movements and postures. Consider gentle therapeutic positions over the 24-hour routine and therapeutic purposeful movement through available range during normal activity (e.g., optimizing sit-to-stand pattern). Functional electric muscle stimulation may be a useful adjunct to treatment to encourage movement, distract from pain, align a foot and ankle to be able to weight bear, or facilitate gait (e.g., dorsiflexion stimulation with a foot switch: Fig. 45.2).

CONCLUSIONS

Physical treatment is recognized as an integral component of the rehabilitation of FND. There is growing evidence that supports its use, including a randomized controlled study. However the literature is limited when it comes to describing how physical treatment should be delivered. Here it is argued that physical treatment of FND is a complex intervention that involves education, movement retraining, and self-management. The movement retraining can be based on the principles of motor learning theory and should be delivered in a way that redirects attention away from the body. As part of treatment, the clinician can challenge illness beliefs by demonstrating to the patient that normal movement is possible.

The unfavorable prognosis that accompanies FND may yet be revised as our understanding of the pathology improves. Research directed towards understanding the mechanisms by which physical treatment works, including identifying mediators of change, will help to refine interventions and allow for the development of evidence-based treatment guidelines. Further research should be directed towards developing valid and reliable outcome measures and identifying subpopulations that may be suited to a particular treatment approach. Outcomes may also be improved with better utilization of existing services structures, such as a system that provides an early diagnosis and rapid access to specialized treatment that has the flexibility to suit the needs of the individual with interdisciplinary cooperation.

FINANCIAL DISCLOSURES

GN is supported by a National Institute for Health Research/Health Education England clinical doctoral research fellowship.

ACKNOWLEDGMENT

Thank you to specialist occupational therapist Clare Nicholson for her advice in the preparation of this manuscript.

References

Broussolle E, Gobert F, Danaila T et al. (2014). History of physical and 'moral' treatment of hysteria. Front Neurol Neurosci 35: 181–197.

Butler DS, Moseley GL (2003). Explain Pain, Noigroup Publications, Adelaide.

Czarnecki K, Thompson JM, Seime R et al. (2012). Functional movement disorders: successful treatment with a physical therapy rehabilitation protocol. Parkinsonism Relat Disord 18: 247–251.

Dallocchio C, Arbasino C, Klersy C et al. (2010). The effects of physical activity on psychogenic movement disorders. Mov Disord 25: 421–425.

Delargy MA, Peatfield RC, Burt AA (1986). Successful rehabilitation in conversion paralysis. Br Med J (Clin Res Ed) 292: 1730–1731.

Demartini B, Batla A, Petrochilos P et al. (2014). Multidisciplinary treatment for functional neurological symptoms: a prospective study. J Neurol 261: 2370–2377.

Edwards MJ, Bhatia KP, Cordivari C (2011). Immediate response to botulinum toxin injections in patients with fixed dystonia. Mov Disord 26: 917–918.

Edwards MJ, Adams RA, Brown H et al. (2012). A Bayesian account of 'hysteria'. Brain 135: 3495–3512.

Edwards MJ, Fotopoulou A, Parees I (2013). Neurobiology of functional (psychogenic) movement disorders. Curr Opin Neurol 26: 442–447.

Espay AJ, Edwards MJ, Oggioni GD et al. (2014). Tremor retrainment as therapeutic strategy in psychogenic (functional) tremor. Parkinsonism Relat Disord 20: 647–650.

Ferrara J, Stamey W, Strutt AM et al. (2011). Transcutaneous electrical stimulation (TENS) for psychogenic movement disorders. J Neuropsychiatry Clin Neurosci 23: 141–148.

Fishbain D, Goldberg M, Khalil T et al. (1988). The utility of electromyographic biofeedback in the treatment of conversion paralysis. Am J Psychiatry 145: 1572.

Furukawa TA, Noma H, Caldwell DM et al. (2014). Waiting list may be a nocebo condition in psychotherapy trials: a contribution from network meta-analysis. Acta Psychiatr Scand 130: 181–192.

Gelauff J, Stone J, Edwards M et al. (2014). The prognosis of functional (psychogenic) motor symptoms: a systematic review. J Neurol Neurosurg Psychiatry 85: 220–226.

Hansen Z, Daykin A, Lamb SE (2010). A cognitive-behavioural programme for the management of low back pain in primary care: a description and justification of the intervention used in the Back Skills Training Trial (BeST; ISRCTN 54717854). Physiotherapy 96: 87–94.

Harden RN, Oaklander AL, Burton AW et al. (2013). Complex regional pain syndrome: practical diagnostic and treatment guidelines, 4th edition. Pain Med 14: 180–229.

Heruti RJ, Reznik J, Adunski A et al. (2002). Conversion motor paralysis disorder: analysis of 34 consecutive referrals. Spinal Cord 40: 335–340.

Homberg V (2013). Neurorehabilitation approaches to facilitate motor recovery. Handb Clin Neurol 110: 161–173.

Hughes S, Alltree J (1990). A behavioural approach to the management of functional disorders. Physiotherapy 76: 255–258.

Jordbru AA, Smedstad LM, Klungsøyr O et al. (2014). Psychogenic gait disorder: a randomized controlled trial of physical rehabilitation with one-year follow-up. J Rehabil Med 46: 181–187.

Kamper SJ, Apeldoorn AT, Chiarotto A et al. (2014). Multidisciplinary biopsychosocial rehabilitation for chronic low back pain. Cochrane Database Syst Rev 9. Cd000963.

Kitago T, Krakauer JW (2013). Motor learning principles for neurorehabilitation. Handb Clin Neurol 110: 93–103.

Klonoff EA, Moore DJ (1986). "Conversion reactions" in adolescents: a biofeedback-based operant approach. J Behav Ther Exp Psychiatry 17: 179–184.

McCormack R, Moriarty J, Mellers JD et al. (2013). Specialist inpatient treatment for severe motor conversion disorder: a retrospective comparative study. J Neurol Neurosurg Psychiatry 85: 895–900.

Meeus M, Nijs J, Van Oosterwijck J et al. (2010). Pain physiology education improves pain beliefs in patients with chronic fatigue syndrome compared with pacing and self-management education: a double-blind randomized controlled trial. Arch Phys Med Rehabil 91: 1153–1159.

Moene FC, Spinhoven P, Hoogduin KA et al. (2002). A randomised controlled clinical trial on the additional effect of hypnosis in a comprehensive treatment programme for in-patients with conversion disorder of the motor type. Psychother Psychosom 71: 66–76.

Moseley GL (2004). Evidence for a direct relationship between cognitive and physical change during an education intervention in people with chronic low back pain. Eur J Pain 8: 39–45.

Moss-Morris R, Deary V, Castell B (2013). Chronic fatigue syndrome. Handb Clin Neurol 110: 303–314.

Nielsen G, Stone J, Edwards MJ (2013). Physiotherapy for functional (psychogenic) motor symptoms: a systematic review. J Psychosom Res 75: 93–102.

Nielsen G, Stone J, Matthews A et al. (2015a). Physiotherapy for functional motor disorders: a consensus recommendation. J Neurol Neurosurg Psychiatry 86: 1113–1119.

Nielsen G, Ricciardi L, Demartini B et al. (2015b). Outcomes of a 5-day physiotherapy programme for functional (psychogenic) motor disorders. J Neurol 262: 674–681.

Nijs J, Paul van Wilgen C, Van Oosterwijck J et al. (2011). How to explain central sensitization to patients with 'unexplained' chronic musculoskeletal pain: practice guidelines. Man Ther 16: 413–418.

Pareés I, Kojovic M, Pires C et al. (2014). Physical precipitating factors in functional movement disorders. J Neurol Sci 338: 174–177.

Saifee TA, Kassavetis P, Parees I et al. (2012). Inpatient treatment of functional motor symptoms: a long-term follow-up study. J Neurol 259: 1958–1963.

Schrag A, Trimble M, Quinn N et al. (2004). The syndrome of fixed dystonia: an evaluation of 103 patients. Brain 127: 2360–2372.

Shapiro AP, Teasell RW (2004). Behavioural interventions in the rehabilitation of acute v. chronic non-organic (conversion/factitious) motor disorders. Br J Psychiatry 185: 140–146.

Sharpe M, Walker J, Williams C et al. (2011). Guided self-help for functional (psychogenic) symptoms: a randomized controlled efficacy trial. Neurology 77: 564–572.

Speed J (1996). Behavioral management of conversion disorder: retrospective study. Arch Phys Med Rehabil 77: 147–154.

Stone J, Edwards M (2012). Trick or treat? Showing patients with functional (psychogenic) motor symptoms their physical signs. Neurology 79: 282–284.

Stone J, Warlow C, Sharpe M (2010). The symptom of functional weakness: a controlled study of 107 patients. Brain 133: 1537–1551.

Stone J, Warlow C, Sharpe M (2012). Functional weakness: clues to mechanism from the nature of onset. J Neurol Neurosurg Psychiatry 83: 67–69.

Trieschmann RB, Stolov WC, Montgomery ED (1970). An approach to the treatment of abnormal ambulation resulting from conversion reaction. Arch Phys Med Rehabil 51: 198–206.

Van Oosterwijck J, Meeus M, Paul L et al. (2013). Pain physiology education improves health status and endogenous pain inhibition in fibromyalgia: a double-blind randomized controlled trial. Clin J Pain 29: 873–882.

White P, Goldsmith K, Johnson A et al. (2011). Comparison of adaptive pacing therapy, cognitive behaviour therapy, graded exercise therapy, and specialist medical care for chronic fatigue syndrome (PACE): a randomised trial. Lancet 377: 823–836.

Withrington RH, Wynn Parry CB (1985). Rehabilitation of conversion paralysis. J Bone Joint Surg Br 67: 635–637.

Handbook of Clinical Neurology, Vol. 139 (3rd series)
Functional Neurologic Disorders
M. Hallett, J. Stone, and A. Carson, Editors
http://dx.doi.org/10.1016/B978-0-12-801772-2.00046-1

Chapter 46

Psychologic treatment of functional neurologic disorders

L.H. GOLDSTEIN[1] AND J.D.C. MELLERS[2]*

[1]*Department of Psychology, Institute of Psychiatry, Psychology and Neuroscience, King's College London, De Crespigny Park, London, UK*

[2]*Department of Neuropsychiatry, Maudsley Hospital, South London and Maudsley NHS Foundation Trust, Denmark Hill, London, UK*

Abstract

The management of patients with functional neurologic disorders poses many challenges. Psychologic treatments may well start at the point of delivery of the diagnosis, when careful explanations about the nature of the disorder have to be given to the patient and possibly also relatives/carers. Different conceptual models may assist in explaining the factors underlying the presentation, two of which (functional and dissociative) are briefly outlined here. The challenges for neurologists and psychiatrists of delivering a psychologic formulation as part of the diagnosis delivery are considered, along with the importance of clear communication between professionals involved in the patient's care. Existing literature on treatments incorporating psychologic components suggests that, despite limitations in the study designs and the potential bias in some outcome evaluations, there is evidence to support the use of psychologic interventions for at least some functional neurologic disorders, although larger and better-designed studies are required in this area.

INTRODUCTION

Treatment begins with an explanation of diagnosis. While different approaches to delivering a diagnosis of psychogenic nonepileptic seizures have been summarized (e.g., LaFrance et al., 2013), how do we explain "medically unexplained" symptoms more generally (Table 46.1; Chapter 44)?

The "easy" part is telling patients what they do not have. Slightly more challenging, perhaps, is an explanation of why this conclusion has been reached. It is probably helpful to describe the clinical reasons for diagnosis as well as investigation results so that patients are not left with the impression they just need more tests and so that the diagnosis is not presented purely as one made by excluding disease. If symptoms or signs are inconsistent with neurologic disease, this can be explained. Positive findings on examination can be demonstrated to patients and used to illustrate the role of attention in symptom generation (Stone and Edwards, 2012). The "difficult" aspect of conveying diagnosis undoubtedly begins when we try to explain what the patient does have. A good start is to emphasize that patients are not being accused of putting on their symptoms; that most patients experience these symptoms as something that "happens to them," not as something they "do." Many patients will have encountered negative, even hostile, reactions from healthcare staff and will be very sensitive about whether the clinician seems to believe them or is "just like all the rest." The name we give the disorder is important. Some terms, such as hysteria and pseudoseizures, are viewed by patients as pejorative (Stone et al., 2002). Others, notably dissociative and functional, while not new are, as yet, untainted with stigma. They also provide a useful springboard for discussing mechanism and treatment. In each case, this can be done without any explicit mention

*Correspondence to: John D.C. Mellers, Department of Neuropsychiatry, Maudsley Hospital, South London and Maudsley NHS Foundation Trust, Denmark Hill, London SE5 8AZ, UK. Tel: +44-020-3228-2330, E-mail: john.mellers@slam.nhs.uk

Table 46.1

Conveying a diagnosis of functional neurologic disorder

Explanation
Describe what the patient doesn't have (e.g., epilepsy, stroke) and the reasons for drawing this conclusion
Describe what the patient does have – give the condition a name and a description
Reassurance
Tell the patient that this condition is common
Tell the patient that s/he is not being accused of "putting on" the symptoms
Mechanism
Describe dissociation
Describe the role of attention
Cause
Often not clear, complex
Summarize predisposing/triggering/maintaining factors that have emerged in history taking and provide a description of how these might be relevant and related to symptoms
Treatment
The patient's symptoms are potentially fully reversible
Direct the patient to self-help websites
Initiate medication withdrawal where appropriate (e.g., antiepileptic drugs)
Describe distraction techniques
Describe treatment

of psychologic factors. Both models can be described in the clinic without any mention of what might have caused the symptoms, psychologic or otherwise.

Functional model

This model begins with the idea that symptoms and signs have their origins in a disorder of function without any underlying disease process or structural abnormality of the nervous system. Symptoms are seen as arising from alterations in attention, with the form symptoms take and the course the disorder follows being shaped by beliefs about illness. This model has a growing evidence base (Edwards et al., 2013) and provides an especially useful template for explaining motor disorders, including paresis and movement disorder. Functional motor disorders can be described as the product of misdirected attention in processes that normally happen without having to think about them. The notion that the "automatic" processes that usually control movement break down when they become the focus of conscious effort has intuitive face validity. Symptoms are maintained by a set of beliefs regarding the symptoms and by associated maladaptive behavior. Treatment is construed as learning to reinstate automatic neurologic control, with distraction techniques to redirect unhelpful movement-focused attention. Cognitive-behavioral techniques target beliefs and avoidant behavior. In this way, a clear rationale for treatment, which may combine physical and psychologic therapies, can be outlined without addressing psychologic causes at all.

Dissociative model

Dissociation is both a mental state, characterized by a subjective sense of detachment, and a putative mechanism whereby an altered state of awareness, responsiveness, and/or control over neurologic function arises as a result of psychologic processes (Holmes et al., 2005; Stone, 2006; Nijenhuis, 2009). This model is especially helpful in describing psychogenic nonepileptic seizures. Examples of normal "dissociation" can be used to illustrate how, through focused attention, for example, we may have a reduced awareness of our surroundings or, indeed, carry out quite complex automatic, purposeful motor sequences without having to think about them. Peritraumatic dissociative states – in lay terms, a state of "shock" – are particularly useful to illustrate how profound, involuntary, and reversible alterations in awareness, memory, and motor control can be triggered in the form of a trance-like state by a sudden frightening experience. This latter example does bring a psychologic element into the explanation, but this can be left implicit. Evidence of physiologic arousal, with or without a heightened emotional state, occurring before or during paroxysmal symptoms, exemplified by dissociative seizures, suggests that these symptoms can be seen as a dissociative response to arousal. Patients are often aware of this at some level and, with careful questioning, many are aware of the symptoms effect of reducing tension such that they may sometimes fully submit to the episode as it brings a sense of relief (Stone and Carson, 2013; Pick et al., 2016). If patients have any of these experiences as part of their seizures, these symptoms can form the basis of a description of mechanisms underlying seizures. As in the functional model, etiologic factors do not have to be mentioned explicitly.

"Psych": what to leave in?

What, if anything, should we mention about "psychology"? This question seems particularly important if we are planning to recommend psychologic treatment to a patient. At the very least, an explanation of functional disorders should include a clear rationale for treatment (Mellers, 2005; LaFrance et al., 2013). There are plenty of reasons why neurologists, the professional group most commonly charged with discussing diagnosis, find the "management interview" difficult (Kanaan et al., 2009). Many have learned that even a cautious attempt to introduce psychologic concepts may lead to an acrimonious end of the therapeutic relationship.

When no psychologic factors have emerged in routine (neurologic) history taking, as is often the case, a simple explanation of symptoms in terms of "stress" has no credibility. When "stress" is present and acknowledged by patients, they may quite reasonably argue that this has occurred because of their symptoms, not the other way round. Even when there is a clear psychosocial background, how events in the past might be related to a more recent physical symptom requires some explanation. And, casting an ever-present shadow over the management interview, stigma associated with psychiatric disorder may be an unsurmountable barrier to accepting the diagnosis and treatment for some patients. Psychologic explanations are often interpreted as meaning symptoms are "all in the mind" – shorthand for "not real" or "put on." One possibility is to leave it to the psychiatrist or therapist, but neurologists complain that patients are often sent back to them having received a clean bill of health from the "psych" professional (Espay et al., 2009).

An obvious problem is that many of the psychologic concepts historically linked to conversion disorder have no evidence base and have little face validity in the majority of cases. They can also be rather difficult to discuss with nonpsychologically minded patients. The concept of conversion itself, and the notion of conflict, can sound rather theoretic and far-fetched. It would also be a highly skilled (and brave) clinician who attempted to explain secondary gain while managing to distinguish it from malingering/factitious disorder.

The presence of a psychosocial explanation of symptom generation has quite rightly been dropped from current diagnostic criteria (American Psychiatric Association, 2013). However, it is worth reminding ourselves that this does not mean that psychologic factors are not relevant, nor does it mean that discussing them with patients should be filed under "too difficult" and consigned to history. The fact remains that antecedent and maintaining psychologic factors are clearly associated with these disorders and psychiatric comorbidity is common (Binzer et al., 2004; Tull et al., 2004; Reuber et al., 2007b). Where these factors are present (in psychiatric assessment), they can be discussed in a straightforward, meaningful way that relates to a growing body of evidence. Where a history of adverse or traumatic experiences is present, for example, an explanation of how this may be associated with changes in the way people are aware of their own emotional state, deal with emotional situations, and cope with stress is fairly straightforward and relates to evidence concerning alexithymia, emotional processing, avoidant coping styles, and dissociative traits/suggestibility (Goldstein et al., 2000; Salmon et al., 2003; Bakvis et al., 2009; Espirito-Santo and Pio-Abreu, 2009; Kaplan et al., 2013). The possibility that triggers for the onset of the disorder may involve the coincidence of a number of stresses in different aspects of the patient's life may make more sense for many patients than misguided efforts to identify a single "causative" stressor. A description of maintaining factors is especially important when antecedent factors are not obvious and can be used to explain how paroxysmal symptoms may occur at times when the patient feels free of stress.

As yet there is no evidence that discussing a psychologic formulation to account for how, why, and when symptoms developed is necessary as part of treatment or encourages engagement in psychiatric/psychologic treatment, although suggestions of how such formulations may be delivered have been outlined (Carson et al., 2016). Research into who is best placed to communicate a detailed formulation might help inform how to facilitate the treatment process. However, it is possible to discuss these issues with patients using everyday language in a way that draws on established associations between psychosocial factors and functional disorders. Certainly it is important that therapists, wherever possible, are made aware in advance of the nature of the explanations that patients have been previously given by clinicians for their disorders. Similarly, it is important that patients arrive for psychotherapeutic interventions having been told clearly by their neurologist/psychiatrist what conditions they do and do not have so that, while patients may not always retain/accept what they have been told, there is potentially less scope for perpetuation of misunderstanding and contradiction between professionals, and less scope for antagonism between the patient and the therapist. It is also very important, therefore, that therapists familiarize themselves with and understand the reasons why the patients' presentations are considered not to be characteristic of an organic disorder, so that they can avoid being side-tracked during therapy.

WHAT IS THE TREATMENT EVIDENCE BASE?

The models and approaches to conceptualizing functional neurologic disorders described above influence much of the current thinking and design of psychotherapeutic and other interventions for this range of disorders. Much of the existing evidence base, however, predates these specific conceptualizations and explanatory models. It is likely that novel treatment approaches will take into account attentional models, for example, in greater depth. However, the existing literature does add support to advocating psychotherapeutic interventions for functional neurologic disorders and some of this literature will be reviewed below.

Psychologic interventions

One of the difficulties in identifying effective treatments for functional neurologic symptoms is that the majority of systematic reviews investigating psychologic interventions have focused more generally on somatoform disorders rather than specifically on conversion disorders, most likely reflecting the paucity of the available literature on interventions for conversion disorder. However, given the high comorbidity with other somatoform disorders (e.g., irritable-bowel syndrome, chronic fatigue syndrome) as well as other chronic complaints such as pain accompanying conversion disorders, this literature may nonetheless be informative. More recent developments, such as attempts to evaluate the effectiveness of physiotherapy or multidisciplinary treatments, will also be considered here. Of note, however, is the inherent bias in psychologic intervention studies. As noted by van Dessel et al. (2014) and others, intervention studies inevitably only include individuals who accept the offer of psychologic treatment. Thus the reviews will never include those people who explicitly reject a psychologic formulation of their difficulties. Therefore, it is unclear how representative those individuals entering such psychologic studies are of the population of people with somatoform/conversion disorders as a whole, and as a result what the potential broader benefit of such interventions might be.

Early reviews of interventions

One of the earlier systematic reviews (Kroenke, 2007) summarized 34 randomized controlled trials (RCTs) that were reported in English between 1966 and 2006 and which involved psychotherapy or pharmacotherapy for somatoform disorders, somatization disorder, undifferentiated somatoform disorder, hypochrondriasis, conversion disorder, pain disorder, and body dysmorphic disorder. Cognitive-behavioral therapy (CBT) was effective in 11/13 studies; antidepressants were found to be effective in four of five studies. The effect size for antidepressants (0.92; involving either selective serotonin reuptake inhibitors or clomipramine) was, however, lower than for behavioral therapy (1.43) or CBT (1.78). Where other treatments were concerned, Kroenke (2007) summarized findings from RCTs as having demonstrated benefit in eight of 16 studies; of note here, the most consistent evidence existed for the provision of a clinic letter about the consultation to the physician providing the patient's primary care. Kroenke (2007) concluded that it had been possible to identify evidence for effective treatments for all somatoform disorders with the exception of conversion disorder (where only one of three studies included in his review indicated beneficial outcomes). The three studies of conversion disorder (Moene et al., 2002, 2003; Ataoglu et al., 2003) included in his review feature in several systematic reviews (e.g., Ruddy and House, 2005) and later in Martlew et al.'s (2014) review. Ataoglu et al. (2003) had compared inpatient paradoxic intention therapy with outpatient follow-up and diazepam for dissociative seizures; Moene et al. (2002) compared an inpatient treatment program for motor conversion disorder with the same treatment program plus hypnosis and Moene et al. (2003) compared outpatient hypnosis with a waiting-list control for motor conversion disorder patients (hypnosis as a treatment modality is considered in depth in Chapter 47). Kroenke's (2007) review also found that, where measured, 10/11 studies indicated a beneficial outcome in terms of a reduction in healthcare use or costs (five trials each). Kroenke (2007) reported, however, a lack of treatment studies demonstrating effectiveness for pain disorder.

More recent reviews of interventions for somatoform disorders

A more recent Cochrane review for interventions for what were termed medically unexplained physical symptoms (van Dessel et al., 2014) similarly evaluated studies focusing on the treatment of somatoform disorder, undifferentiated somatoform disorder, somatoform disorders unspecified, somatoform autonomic dysfunction, pain disorder and alternative somatoform disorders. They considered studies where interventions were compared with treatment as usual, waiting-list controls, either attention or psychologic placebos, and studies incorporating enhanced or structured care and or other physical/psychologic therapies. In general it was considered that the treatments were being trialed for patients with chronic symptoms. Their final review focused on 21 studies; two-thirds of the studies had tested variations of CBT while others had evaluated variants of behavior therapy, mindfulness, psychodynamic interventions, and what was referred to as integrative therapy. Fifteen studies compared the studied psychologic therapy with usual care or a waiting list. Five studies compared the intervention to enhanced or structured care. Only one study compared CBT with behavior therapy.

Across the 21 studies, there was considerable variation in the number of sessions involved and the time across which the treatment took place, with a range of follow-up assessments taking place between 2 weeks and 2 years. A representative example of studies they included was that by Allen et al. (2006), where 84 patients with somatization disorder were randomized to receive either standard medical care plus a psychiatric consultation intervention, or 10 sessions of a manualized CBT package plus the psychiatric consultation intervention. Allen et al. found that, 15 months after the baseline assessment, the CBT group demonstrated significantly less severe symptoms of somatization and were more likely to be rated as much improved or very much improved than were patients treated with the enhanced standard medical care. The CBT group also reported greater improvements in everyday functioning and a greater decrease in healthcare costs, indicating that the effects of the CBT intervention were not limited to subjective self-report but extended to objective measures of improvement.

Despite a range of methodologic weaknesses in the studies, and little information on adverse events, van Dessel et al.'s (2014) meta-analysis indicated that the tested psychologic therapy was generally found to result in less severe symptoms following treatment, with small to medium effect sizes. van Dessel et al. (2014) indicated that the findings for those studies comparing CBT with standard care mirrored those for the entire group of studies. Interestingly, in comparison with standard medical care, psychologic therapies were found to be associated with a 7% higher proportion of drop-outs during treatment.

Of note, the review demonstrated early benefits of what was described as enhanced standard care when compared to a psychologic intervention. Enhanced care incorporated, in addition to care as usual (most likely provided by the patient's general practitioner), additional features such as education, a psychiatric assessment, brief use of counseling components, or reattribution training (Rosendal et al., 2013). Thus, when comparing a psychologic therapy against enhanced care, the five studies evaluating symptom severity as their outcome found no clear difference between these interventions at the end of treatment. However, at longer-term follow-up there was a small but significant benefit of psychologic interventions over enhanced care, suggesting that the psychologic interventions may have provided longer-term strategies to assist individuals in overcoming their difficulties. In terms of functional disability and quality of life, the review similarly revealed no clear evidence of a difference at the end of treatment when CBT was compared to enhanced care, but there was a small significant benefit from CBT within 1 year of follow-up. There were no apparent differences in healthcare use as a result of psychologic therapies compared with enhanced care.

van Dessel et al. (2014) concluded that, when all psychologic therapies evaluated in their review were considered together, there was evidence for better outcomes compared to standard care or waiting-list controls in terms of reductions in symptom severity; they noted, however, that overall effect sizes for treatment outcomes were small. The majority of evidence came from studies of CBT which, when evaluated against standard care or waiting-list controls was seen to decrease somatic symptoms, although there were considerable variations in study findings. However, the review demonstrated potential durability of findings up to 1 year of follow-up. Nonetheless, the early impact of enhanced or structured care was a notable finding and has some practice implications.

Interestingly, in view of likely psychologic/psychiatric comorbidities, the review failed to elicit evidence for a clear difference between the groups in terms of improvement in anxiety and/or depressive symptoms either at the end of treatment and/or up to 1 year after treatment; this was also the case even when psychologic therapies were compared with enhanced care. In relation to this, van Dessel et al. (2014) also found no clear evidence of a difference between the groups in terms of dysfunctional cognitions, emotions, and behaviors at end of treatment; however, at follow-up within 1 year of treatment there was a small effect in favor of psychologic therapy over enhanced care. As with Kroenke's (2007) review, van Dessel et al. (2014) found insufficient reporting by studies of adverse events, which minimizes the extent to which any negative outcomes might be evaluated.

van Dessel et al. were not alone in publishing a systematic review and meta-analysis showing benefits of psychotherapeutic interventions for somatoform disorders in 2014. Koelen et al. (2014) concluded that there were positive benefits from psychotherapeutic interventions in terms of physical symptoms and functional impairment, but not for psychologic symptoms, although better psychologic outcome was found for men, younger patients, people with somatization disorder, and in studies judged to have been less methodologically rigorous. However, their review suffered from potential selectivity as a result of having limited their search period to 4 years prior to publication as well as from omitting discussion of therapeutic outcomes for individual functional somatic disorders (Stone, 2014).

Specific nonmotor conversion disorders

Chronic pain

Although not featuring prominently in the above reviews, studies of behavioral therapy and CBT interventions for chronic pain, again, highly relevant to many patients with functional neurologic symptoms, have been reviewed systematically (Williams et al., 2012). The reviewers concluded that, on the basis of poor-quality interventions, there is little evidence for the beneficial effects of behavior therapy, except for a small improvement in mood immediately following treatment, when compared with an active control. They found that the reported benefits of CBT derived almost entirely from studies where it was compared with treatment as usual/waiting-list controls, but not with an active control intervention. CBT was shown to have small to moderate beneficial effects on pain, disability, mood, and negative cognitions (namely catastrophizing) at the end of treatment, in comparison to benefits from standard care/waiting-list controls, but Williams et al. found that only a small beneficial effect on mood remained at follow-up. CBT appeared to give rise to small benefits (in terms of reducing disability and catastrophizing), but, perhaps surprisingly, not on pain or mood, in comparison to other active control conditions.

Dizziness

The importance of developing effective interventions for dizziness, which is not medically fully explained or associated with a psychiatric disorder, has been highlighted by the results of a systematic review (Schmid et al., 2011). This review elicited three controlled trials, of which two were prospective and incorporated randomized allocation of patients; these two studies included a waiting-list control condition compared to a package consisting of CBT and individualized vestibular rehabilitation (as well as relaxation in one study). Schmid et al. (2011) indicate that the rationale of including vestibular rehabilitation alongside CBT was to help encourage participants experience movement and to provide them with strategies to deal with their cognitions about dizziness. The third study incorporated CBT (including relaxation) compared to self-exposure to provoke dizziness but participants were not allocated to treatment groups at random. Schmid et al. (2011) concluded that all three studies demonstrated that CBT offered in combination with vestibular rehabilitation and/or relaxation led to some improvement, measured in terms of functional ability and/or psychologic state. However, the studies involved small and unrepresentative samples, and in the only study that included a follow-up there was no lasting benefit of the psychotherapeutic intervention at 1 year. Thus, while the preliminary evidence is encouraging, more robust evaluations in this area are required.

Psychotherapeutic and psychoeducational interventions for dissociative (nonepileptic) seizures

Interventions for nonmotor conversion symptoms, specifically dissociative seizures, were reviewed systematically by Martlew et al. (2014), who considered four RCTs and eight open-label noncontrolled studies. Of the RCTs identified by the authors only one examined patients exclusively with dissociative (nonepileptic) seizures (Goldstein et al., 2010), while three (Moene et al., 2002, 2003; Ataoglu et al., 2003) had enrolled patients with mixed diagnoses (i.e., dissociative seizures, conversion disorder, and somatization disorder) and the studies by Moene and colleagues investigated hypnosis rather than more mainstream psychologic therapies. Most of the nonrandomized studies included in the review studied patients with only dissociative seizures. While a meta-analysis was not feasible due to the diversity of study designs and interventions, the majority of studies did report improved outcomes for the treatment being delivered. Martlew et al. (2014) concluded that, despite certain weaknesses, one RCT (Goldstein et al., 2010) provided the strongest evidence to date for an effective intervention for people with dissociative seizures.

Goldstein et al. (2010) reported beneficial outcomes in terms of reduced dissociative seizures frequency in a pilot RCT that compared CBT plus standard medical care (provided in an outpatient neuropsychiatry service) compared to standard medical care alone. Sixty-six patients without comorbid epilepsy, without an IQ below 70, and not taking more than the benzodiazepine equivalent of 10 mg diazepam daily but experiencing at least two dissociative seizures per month, were randomized across the two treatment arms (33 to each). At the end of treatment, an intention-to-treat analysis indicated that seizure frequency reduction was greater in the CBT plus standard medical care group than in the group receiving standard medical care alone. At a 6-month follow-up there was a trend for this beneficial effect of CBT (in terms of seizure reduction) to have been maintained and the CBT group were around three times more likely than the standard medical care group to have been seizure-free for the previous 3 months, although loss to follow-up reduced statistical power ($p = 0.086$). There was some improvement in both groups in terms of health service use and on the Work and Social Adjustment Scale, although there was no differential effect of treatment on employment status or mood. To date this study remains the largest completed RCT of a psychotherapeutic intervention specifically for dissociative seizures.

Omitted from the review by Martlew et al. (2014) was a small study of a behavior therapy intervention evaluated in a mainly rural Pakistani sample (Aamir et al., 2011). The authors assessed the impact of 15 - sessions of behavior therapy on seizure occurrence and mood in dissociative seizure patients over a 2½-month period and compared its efficacy with treatment as usual (described as pharmacotherapy and outpatient review). The active intervention comprised positive reinforcement on a variable ratio and variable interval schedule with the intention of increasing seizure-free behavior; the intervention also included the withdrawal of privileges (construed within an operant approach as punishment) to reduce maladaptive (presumably seizure-related) behavior and to minimize opportunities for negative reinforcement to occur. The protocol involved initial inpatient treatment over a 1-week period; following discharge patients received follow-up for 15 weeks. Caregivers of the behavior therapy group also received intensive training so that they could act as behavior therapists to their family member outside of the hospital environment. At the end of the study, the group treated with behavior therapy reported significantly fewer seizures and lower anxiety and depression scores. Despite the small sample size, the extension of studies of this nature to non-Western settings makes the findings all the more interesting and worthy of further consideration and replication.

A further, but still small, RCT comparing CBT-informed psychotherapy (CBT-ip), CBT-ip plus sertraline, sertraline, and standard medical care (LaFrance et al., 2014) has also attested to the potential benefit of CBT-informed psychotherapy for the treatment of dissociative seizures. This study extended previous open-label evaluations of a psychotherapeutic intervention (LaFrance et al., 2009) and a pilot double-blind RCT of flexible-dose sertraline versus placebo (LaFrance et al., 2010). LaFrance et al.'s (2014) intervention is manualized and designed to be delivered over 12 sessions, each 1 hour in length, and is strongly informed by CBT principles but adopts an eclectic approach incorporating, for example, mindfulness and some psychodynamic therapeutic techniques. In this relatively small study, 34 out of 38 patients randomized across the four treatment arms provided outcome data. The study was not powered for between-group analyses so primary outcomes were evaluated using within-group comparisons. At the end of treatment, the CBT-ip group demonstrated a significant (51.4%) reduction in seizure frequency, and improved affective state, quality of life, and global functioning scores. A statistically significant improvement in seizure occurrence of a broadly similar extent (59.3%) was seen in the CBT-ip + sertraline group, together with improvement in some secondary outcomes, including global functioning. The sertraline-only group demonstrated a nonsignificant trend towards reduced seizure frequency (26.5%) but there was no significant improvement in secondary outcomes. The standard medical care group showed no improvements in seizure frequency or secondary outcomes. The CBT-ip group also demonstrated reduced numbers of visits to emergency departments at the end of treatment compared to baseline.

Clearly the evidence for psychotherapeutic interventions remains limited in light of there being no adequately powered multicentered RCTs. To redress this balance, a considerably larger and adequately powered multicenter study comparing a manualized approach to CBT plus what might be considered to be enhanced medical care vs. enhanced medical care alone is now underway in the UK (Goldstein et al., 2015). This study extends the previous work by Goldstein et al. (2010), but incorporates an initial phase of diagnosis delivery in neurology/specialist epilepsy clinics and a requirement of continuing seizure occurrence for the 8-week period prior to psychiatric assessment and randomization.

Of course, the therapeutic interventions described above are costly and time-intensive. It is useful, therefore, that some preliminary data, not included in earlier reviews, are available on the impact of brief psychoeducational approaches. Some limited evidence from a small RCT (randomizing a total of 64 patients who had received their diagnosis of dissociative seizures in an epilepsy monitoring unit) has been reported by Chen et al. (2014). Diagnosis delivery adopted a standardized approach to all participants. Following this they found that a brief psychoeducation intervention conducted in three 1.5-hour-long group sessions conducted 1 month apart led to a significant improvement in psychosocial functioning as measured on the Work and Social Adjustment Scale at a 3- and 6-month follow-up, in comparison to outcome following the control condition, namely routine seizure follow-up clinic visits. Although there was no between-group difference in terms of seizure frequency, the intervention group showed a trend towards lower hospital service use (namely emergency room visits or hospitalizations). The study is encouraging, however, in that it demonstrated the possibility of providing a brief intervention within the same clinical service responsible for diagnosis delivery.

In the UK a broadly similar approach has been piloted within a feasibility (but not RCT) study (Mayor et al., 2013), wherein a four-session manualized psychoeducational package was delivered, this time by individuals with relatively little experience of working with dissociative seizure patients. Of promise was the observation that, at the 3-month follow-up, 4/13 patients reported complete seizure cessation and a further 3/13 reported at least a 50% reduction in seizure frequency.

Self-management approaches for functional neurologic symptoms (not specifically dissociative seizures)

Despite the absence of significant numbers of treatment studies for functional neurologic symptoms, interest has grown in self-management approaches that might supplement standard medical care for such patients, especially as CBT may not always be widely available for patients attending neurology clinics. Sharpe et al. (2011) devised a CBT-based guided self-help (GSH) approach and added this to the standard care received by patients, within an RCT based in two neurology services in the UK. They enrolled outpatients who presented with functional symptoms (including dissociative seizures) and randomized them to receive standard care or standard care plus GSH. Those receiving GSH were given a self-help manual and four 30-minute-long guidance sessions. The GSH group reported greater improvement in self-rated health at 3 months. However, at 6 months the primary treatment effect was no longer statistically significant but patients still had greater improvement in terms of their symptom profile and had less belief in the permanence of their symptoms; they also reported greater satisfaction with the care they had received. Sharpe et al. (2011) suggested that future investigation of such an approach might lead to better outcome with the addition of a maintenance phase to the GSH approach.

Multidisciplinary approaches

While the reviews and individual studies cited above have focused on psychologic interventions, interest has been growing in evaluating systematically the role of physiotherapy in improving physical status in patients with functional motor symptoms (i.e., motor conversion disorder). The application of such approaches, however, will likely incorporate a formulation that will undoubtedly and increasingly include psychologic factors (such as unhelpful movement-focused attention: Edwards et al., 2013) in the explanation of presenting symptoms. Indeed, Nielsen et al. (2015b) have highlighted the involvement of psychologic processes within a biopsychosocial etiologic model, when advocating the use of physiotherapy for functional motor disorders. For children and adolescents, only limited evidence exits as to the effectiveness of physiotherapy as a result of poor-quality studies that lack functional outcome measures (FitzGerald et al., 2015). In terms of studies focusing on adults, undertaking a systematic review of literature published between 1950 and September 2012, Nielsen et al. (2013) found only one controlled intervention study (but no RCTs); they also found 28 case series or reports where interventions were described. They noted that physiotherapy was most likely to form part of multidisciplinary inpatient treatment (making it hard to identify what might be the effective treatment component) and was applied for varying durations and with different intensities; however, approaches generally involved motor relearning combined with a behavioral approach. Other studies investigated the use of distraction techniques and transcutaneous electric nerve stimulation (TENS) machines. Nielsen et al. (2013) also noted the use in some studies of deceptive behavioral techniques. They documented some support for an approach whereby addressing erroneous illness beliefs was included as part of patients' rehabilitation; this was done by communicating the diagnosis and rationale for treatment.

Overall, despite the heterogeneous methods applied and the general lack of reliable and valid outcomes, Nielsen et al. (2013) concluded that the majority of studies found physical interventions to be beneficial, with improvement in 60–70% of patients, and they concluded that it would be helpful to develop a manualized approach that could then lead to an RCT of a physiotherapy treatment intervention in patients with motor conversion disorder. Further support for this comes from Nielsen et al.'s (2015a) open-label study report of improved physical outcomes following a specialist 5-day physiotherapy program that incorporated education and movement retraining that emphasized a long-term self-management approach (see Chapter 45).

However, as with identifying the effective component of CBT within a complex intervention for functional motor symptoms, the difficulty of identifying the specific role of physiotherapy in improving patient outcomes is of concern. This difficulty has been further demonstrated by two recent studies (Jordbru et al., 2014; McCormack et al., 2014). The former described a multidisciplinary treatment program for inpatients with chronic and severe motor conversion disorder receiving treatment on a neuropsychiatric inpatient unit (McCormack et al., 2014) (see Chapter 51). Here patients with median duration of illness of 4 years received individualized physiotherapy, predominantly CBT-informed psychotherapy and occupational therapy, in addition to neuropsychiatric input and nursing care. In this retrospective study, 33 patients, compared to patients with an organic brain injury, were evaluated in terms of their mobility, activities of daily living (ADLs) and their Modified Rankin Scale (MRS) score at admission and discharge. Twenty-eight of the 33 patients received psychotherapy. The conversion disorder patients showed significant improvements in their MRS scores, mobility, and ADLs following the inpatient treatment. While the data testify to the approach as a whole, it is not clear which specific aspects of the intervention might be enhanced to further improve outcomes.

A more powerfully designed study was described by Jordbru et al. (2014). In this RCT, 60 patients with psychogenic gait disorder were randomized consecutively in blocks of four, stratified by gender, to receive either an immediate, 3-week-long, inpatient rehabilitation program comprising adapted physical activity embedded within a CBT approach or to receive the program after spending 4 weeks on a waiting list. The intervention package was delivered by a multidisciplinary team comprising an occupational therapist, a physiotherapist, a nurse, an educator in adapted physical activity, and a doctor. The three main aspects of the intervention involved an explanation of symptoms (combined with an optimistic message about recovery), the positive reinforcement of normal function (gait or posture) both during therapy and other normal activities and not providing positive reinforcement for dysfunctional gait/posture; patients were also informed that the length of their admission would be reduced if no improvement was seen in the first week of their admission. Outcome measures were completed at baseline, admission, discharge, and at 1-month and 1-year follow-up intervals. The inpatient program led to improvements in the participants' mobility and functional independence, as well as most aspects of health-related quality of life, with improvements being maintained at the 1- and 12-month follow-up. The authors acknowledged the limitation of not having blinded outcome assessors, and the relatively short waiting-list time for the control group. They were also aware that they could not rule out the possibility of spontaneous remission in either group.

A brief outpatient-based interdisciplinary psychotherapeutic intervention (IPI) for 11 patients with conversion disorder and/or dissociative seizures and evaluated in a small RCT has also been described (Hubschmid et al., 2015). This comprised four to six sessions (based on a psychodynamic interpersonal therapy) over a period of about 2 months, led by a consultant liaison psychiatrist (with the first and final sessions including a neurologic consultation, a psychiatric consultation, and then a joint consultation). The control group ($n = 12$) received standard care, namely a single joint neurologic and psychiatric diagnosis communication lasting around 15 minutes. Following the intervention, outcomes were assessed at 2, 6, and 12 months; after 12 months the IPI group showed a reduction in physical symptoms (as measured by the Somatoform Dissociation Questionnaire-20) and improvement in terms of their Clinical Global Impression scale rating. There was also an improvement on the SF-36 (mental health domain) and a reduction in depression scores. Finally, there was evidence of improved health service use after the intervention. The standard care group, however, showed worsened mental health and lower levels of symptom improvement, as well as also reporting greater health service use at 12 months. The authors considered the joint neurologic and psychiatric input for patients to be a particularly important part of their approach, which they felt could be tailored to all patients with conversion disorder.

An open-label CBT-informed group intervention, which included weekly CBT-based group therapy sessions for patients with motor conversion symptoms or dissociative seizures, has also shown some potential efficacy, although the study was rather underpowered and lacked longer-term follow-up (Conwill et al., 2014).

Abreaction/sedative interviews (see Chapter 50)

Although individual or group psychotherapy may seem to be an appropriate treatment option for patients with functional neurologic symptoms, these options may not always be available or acceptable to patients. At an earlier stage in the management of the individual there is the potential to address either relevant psychologic content or attempt to manipulate the presenting symptoms through the use of abreaction or sedative interviews.

Recognizing that little was understood about the benefit of drug interviews in the treatment of conversion disorder, Poole et al. (2010) systematically reviewed studies published between 1920 and 2009 reporting (either quantitatively or qualitatively) on the use of drug interviews for treating conversion/dissociative disorder. They found 55 papers meeting their inclusion criteria, although no studies included a suitable control group and the data were generally of poor quality. They indicated, however, that two studies elicited high response rates in patients with previously treatment-resistant conversion disorder. In their meta-analysis, they found that, where studies used suggestion about potential recovery and reported what was described as emotional catharsis during the interview, there was a positive association with recovery. Poole et al. concluded that it was not possible to state which drug yielded best results and that psychiatric comorbidity should be treated independently rather than by use of abreaction. However, while further efficacy studies were felt to be needed (and indeed, the approach was felt to be amenable to a double-blind RCT), they felt sufficiently confident to conclude that drug interviews might be a useful intervention for individuals with both acute and treatment-resistant conversion disorder; they were not, however, able to comment on longer-term outcome. Nonetheless they considered that a temporary resolution of conversion symptoms might provide a window to permit treatment to be commenced that might address symptom-maintaining factors.

In contrast to the use of abreaction, Stone et al. (2014) describe the use of suggestion under the effects of propofol sedation to illustrate to patients that recovery from their symptoms might be possible. They undertook a retrospective analysis of their patients who underwent therapeutic sedation for functional neurologic symptoms between 2002 and 2012. Their cases were selected on the basis of patients having symptoms that could not be reversed on a temporary basis during a standard clinical examination. In addition, they had initiated a sedation-based interview when patients failed to demonstrate improvement despite psychotherapeutic input, physiotherapy, and/or hypnosis. They had also targeted this intervention at patients who accepted a functional diagnosis, had a positive relationship with the clinician, and who appeared motivated to improve. Stone et al. informed patients that sedation was not to help them arrive at a diagnosis and that the person would not be required to discuss new information while sedated; rather, sedation offered a means of helping the person start moving again or normalize the position of the affected limb. Of 11 patients studied (whose symptoms had a median duration of 14 months), 5 had symptoms that were cured or showed major improvement. In terms of maintenance, at a median follow-up of 30 months, 4 patients were symptom-free and 2 showed a significant improvement while a further individual demonstrated minor improvements. The limitations of this study (the lack of control participants, small sample size, and a lack of data documenting patients' own perspectives on the procedure) were acknowledged.

IMPLICATIONS OF TREATMENT STUDIES

In general the reviews and individual studies discussed suggest that, despite limitations in the quality of studies and the potential bias in some evaluations, there is evidence to support the effectiveness of psychologic interventions for at least some functional neurologic symptoms, although the evidence is stronger for somatoform disorders more widely than specifically for conversion disorders. McCormack et al. (2014) have highlighted the difficulties in undertaking treatment follow-up studies in patients with conversion disorders, which include evolving diagnostic criteria leading to differing patient samples across studies and diverse patient characteristics and places/modes of treatment delivery. They also question how best to measure outcome, i.e., whether this should be symptom-focused or focus on wider psychosocial or economic factors, an issue that has been raised also for dissociative seizures (Reuber et al., 2005), and they also highlight the difficulty in establishing an adequate control group. Additionally, adequately powered studies are still needed, although helpfully, in this respect, a large multicenter randomized controlled study is currently randomizing patients with multiple ($\geq$3) medically unexplained symptoms to receive either CBT or CBT plus emotion regulation training, with a view to evaluating whether the latter will enhance treatment effects (Kleinstauber et al., 2016).

A further limitation of the literature in general (and which has been highlighted when considering treatment effectiveness for pain: Williams et al., 2012) is the lack of clarity in data that permits an identification of who benefits from psychologic interventions. Furthermore, mediation analysis can assist in understanding how a treatment works, not just that it does. Thus, for example, Kroenke (2007) considered that the effect of CBT and antidepressants on somatic symptoms does not appear to be completely mediated through a reduction in depression and psychologic distress. A lack of analysis of potential mediators and moderators makes targeted service delivery very difficult and therefore differently designed studies, with more detailed analyses, may help researchers understand which components of a complex intervention are effective and for whom. Recent developments in mediational analyses offer hope in this regard (Chalder et al., 2015).

In the systematic reviews covered in this chapter, the majority of interventions undergoing evaluation have been variants of CBT. Kroenke (2007) and van Dessel et al. (2014) have highlighted the need to study the effectiveness of other, non-CBT psychotherapeutic interventions for somatoform (and by association therefore, for conversion) disorders. Indeed, some promising open-label work of this type has been undertaken for dissociative seizures (Mayor et al., 2010) and for functional motor disorders (Hinson et al., 2006; Reuber et al., 2007a). In Hinson et al.'s study only 10 patients received 12 sessions of psychodynamic psychotherapy plus, where appropriate, psychotropic medication. Reuber et al.'s (2007a) study incorporated a large sample size ($n=91$), although only 63 completed outcome measures at the end of treatment and 34 patients completed measures at 6-month follow-up. Nonetheless, improvements were seen on measures of psychologic functioning and health-related quality of life, and data suggested the potential cost-effectiveness of this approach. Kroenke (2007) also suggested the need to evaluate further possible pharmacologic approaches, and again, in the dissociative seizure field there has been interest in this approach (LaFrance et al., 2010).

Finally, most trials have effectively studied single treatments, whereas Kroenke (2007) suggested that combining treatments may be necessary in patients with chronic somatic conditions. However, even CBT is not really a "single" treatment, given the complexity of its components and the models on which a specific intervention might be based; in addition, the more recent multidisciplinary approaches (e.g., McCormack et al., 2014; Hubschmid et al., 2015) make identifying the critical components of therapy more difficult. Nonetheless, given the recent interest in the further evaluation of physiotherapy in treating functional neurologic symptoms a similar approach, i.e., identifying the critical therapeutic components and for whom they might work best, is likely to assume considerable importance in taking this field forward. As Nielsen et al. (2013) indicate, it will then be necessary to evaluate the relative effectiveness of physiotherapy compared to psychologic and other interventions or determine whether maximal benefit is derived from a multipronged approach. Such a comparative approach might similarly be necessary for nonmotor functional neurologic symptoms, such as functional visual loss (Pula, 2012; Egan and LaFrance, 2015) or functional dysphonia in adults (Ruotsalainen et al., 2007), where other interventions might be offered in addition to or instead of psychotherapy.

Finally, only recently has attention been paid to whether a stepped-care approach to treatment might be cost-effective (Healthcare Improvement Scotland, 2012). Work such as the evaluation of a brief psychoeducation package for dissociative seizures (Mayor et al., 2013) and GSH for functional neurologic symptoms more generally (Sharpe et al., 2011) could form the second care step if, following the delivery of the diagnosis there is no improvement, with a progression to a third treatment phase (complex care, provided by specialist psychology/psychiatry services, specialist physio/occupational/speech therapy services; specialist neurology; rehabilitation medicine; and chronic pain services) for patients with marked disability and complex comorbid psychiatric presentations.

While the development and evaluations of psychologic and related treatments continue to be important, clinicians are left with the day-to-day management challenges posed by this heterogeneous and challenging patient group. There is a marked need to convey clearly the diagnosis not only to patients but also to families and other primary- and secondary-level care providers to foster a consistent approach to management. In terms of professionals there may also be important benefit in the involvement in patients' management of both neurologists and psychiatrists (Hubschmid et al., 2015). Other interventions may well include the reduction of medication (analgesics or, for psychogenic nonepileptic seizure patients, the withdrawal of antiepileptic medication: Oto et al., 2010), though psychotropic medication may also have a role to play. What appears to be of paramount importance is that all professionals working with this patient group have training in the field, so that miscommunications are avoided and evidence-based treatments are delivered.

References

Aamir S, Hamayon S, Sultan S (2011). Behavior therapy in dissociative convulsion disorder. J Dep Anxiety 1.

Allen LA, Woolfolk RL, Escobar JI et al. (2006). Cognitive-behavioral therapy for somatization disorder: a randomized controlled trial. Arch Intern Med 166: 1512–1518.

American Psychiatric Association (2013). Diagnostic and statistical manual of mental disorders, 5th edn. American Psychiatric Publishing, Arlington, VA.

Ataoglu A, Ozcetin A, Icmeli C et al. (2003). Paradoxical therapy in conversion reaction. J Kor Med Sci 18: 581–584.

Bakvis P, Roelofs K, Kuyk J et al. (2009). Trauma, stress, and preconscious threat processing in patients with psychogenic nonepileptic seizures. Epilepsia 50: 1001–1011.

Binzer M, Stone J, Sharpe M (2004). Recent onset pseudoseizures – clues to aetiology. Seizure 13: 146–155.

Carson A, Lehn A, Ludwig L et al. (2016). Explaining functional disorders in the neurology clinic: a photo story. Practical Neurol 16: 56–61.

Chalder T, Goldsmith KA, White PD et al. (2015). Rehabilitative therapies for chronic fatigue syndrome: a secondary mediation analysis of the PACE trial. Lancet Psychiatry 2: 141–152.

Chen DK, Maheshwari A, Franks R et al. (2014). Brief group psychoeducation for psychogenic nonepileptic seizures: a neurologist-initiated program in an epilepsy center. Epilepsia 55: 156–166.

Conwill M, Oakley L, Evans K et al. (2014). CBT-based group therapy intervention for nonepileptic attacks and other functional neurological symptoms: a pilot study. Epilepsy Behav 34: 68–72.

Edwards MJ, Fotopoulou A, Parees I (2013). Neurobiology of functional (psychogenic) movement disorders. Curr Opin Neurol 26: 442–447.

Egan RA, LaFrance WC (2015). Functional vision disorder. Semin Neurol 35: 557–563.

Espay AJ, Goldenhar LM, Voon V et al. (2009). Opinions and clinical practices related to diagnosing and managing patients with psychogenic movement disorders: an international survey of movement disorder society members. Mov Disord 24: 1366–1374.

Espirito-Santo H, Pio-Abreu JL (2009). Psychiatric symptoms and dissociation in conversion, somatization and dissociative disorders. Aust New Zeal J Psychiatr 43: 270–276.

FitzGerald TL, Southby AK, Haines TP et al. (2015). Is physiotherapy effective in the management of child and adolescent conversion disorder? A systematic review. J Paed Child Health 51: 159–167.

Goldstein LH, Drew C, Mellers J et al. (2000). Dissociation, hypnotizability, coping styles and health locus of control: characteristics of pseudoseizure patients. Seizure 9: 314–322.

Goldstein LH, Chalder T, Chigwedere C et al. (2010). Cognitive-behavioral therapy for psychogenic nonepileptic seizures: a pilot RCT. Neurology 74: 1986–1994.

Goldstein LH, Mellers JDC, Landau S et al. (2015). Cognitive behavioural therapy vs standardised medical care for adults with dissociative non-epileptic seizures (CODES): a multicentre randomised controlled trial protocol. BMC Neurol 15.

Healthcare Improvement Scotland (2012). Stepped care for functional neurological symptoms – a new approach to improving outcomes for a common neurological problem in Scotland, NHS Scotland, Edinburgh.

Hinson VK, Weinstein S, Bernard B et al. (2006). Single-blind clinical trial of psychotherapy for treatment of psychogenic movement disorders. Parkinsonism Relat Disord 12: 177–180.

Holmes EA, Brown RJ, Mansell W et al. (2005). Are there two qualitatively distinct forms of dissociation? A review and some clinical implications. Clin Psychol Rev 25: 1–23.

Hubschmid M, Aybek S, Maccaferri GE et al. (2015). Efficacy of brief interdisciplinary psychotherapeutic intervention for motor conversion disorder and nonepileptic attacks. Gen Hosp Psychiatry 37: 448–455.

Jordbru AA, Smedstad LM, Klungsoyr O et al. (2014). Psychogenic gait disorder: a randomized controlled trial of physical rehabilitation with one-year follow-up. J Rehab Med 46: 181–187.

Kanaan R, Armstrong D, Wessely S (2009). Limits to truth-telling: neurologists' communication in conversion disorder. Patient Educ Counsel 77: 296–301.

Kaplan MJ, Dwivedi AK, Privitera MD et al. (2013). Comparisons of childhood trauma, alexithymia, and defensive styles in patients with psychogenic non-epileptic seizures vs. epilepsy: implications for the etiology of conversion disorder. J Psychosom Res 75: 142–146.

Kleinstauber M, Gottschalk J, Berking M et al. (2016). Enriching cognitive behavior therapy with emotion regulation training for patients with multiple medically unexplained symptoms (ENCERT): design and implementation of a multicenter, randomized, active controlled trial. Contemp Clin Trials 47: 54–63.

Koelen JA, Houtveen JH, Abbass A et al. (2014). Effectiveness of psychotherapy for severe somatoform disorder: meta-analysis. Br J Psychiatry 204: 12–19.

Kroenke K (2007). Efficacy of treatment for somatoform disorders: a review of randomized controlled trials. Psychosom Med 69: 881–888.

LaFrance Jr WC, Miller IW, Ryan CE et al. (2009). Cognitive behavioral therapy for psychogenic nonepileptic seizures. Epilepsy Behav 14: 591–596.

LaFrance Jr WC, Keitner GI, Papandonatos GD et al. (2010). Pilot pharmacologic randomized controlled trial for psychogenic nonepileptic seizures. Neurology 75: 1166–1173.

LaFrance Jr WC, Reuber M, Goldstein LH (2013). Management of psychogenic nonepileptic seizures. Epilepsia 54: 53–67.

LaFrance WC, Baird GL, Barry JJ et al. (2014). Multicenter pilot treatment trial for psychogenic nonepileptic seizures: a randomized clinical trial. JAMA Psychiatry 71: 997–1005.

Martlew J, Pulman J, Marson AG (2014). Psychological and behavioural treatments for adults with non-epileptic attack disorder. Cochrane Database Syst Rev 2: CD006370.

Mayor R, Howlett S, Grunewald R et al. (2010). Long-term outcome of brief augmented psychodynamic interpersonal therapy for psychogenic nonepileptic seizures: seizure control and health care utilization. Epilepsia 51: 1169–1176.

Mayor R, Brown RJ, Cock H et al. (2013). A feasibility study of a brief psycho-educational intervention for psychogenic nonepileptic seizures. Seizure 22: 760–765.

McCormack R, Moriarty J, Mellers JD et al. (2014). Specialist inpatient treatment for severe motor conversion disorder: a retrospective comparative study. J Neurol Neurosurg Psychiatry 85: 895–900.

Mellers JDC (2005). The approach to patients with 'non-epileptic seizures'. Postgrad Med J 81: 498–504.

Moene FC, Spinhoven P, Hoogduin KAL et al. (2002). A randomised controlled clinical trial on the additional effect of hypnosis in a comprehensive treatment programme for in-patients with conversion disorder of the motor type. Psychother Psychosom 71: 66–76.

Moene FC, Spinhoven P, Hoogduin KAL et al. (2003). A randomized controlled clinical trial of a hypnosis-based treatment for patients with conversion disorder, motor type. Int J Clin Exp Hypnosis 51: 29–50.

Nielsen G, Stone J, Edwards MJ (2013). Physiotherapy for functional (psychogenic) motor symptoms: a systematic review. J Psychosom Res 75: 93–102.

Nielsen G, Ricciardi L, Demartini B et al. (2015a). Outcomes of a 5-day physiotherapy programme for functional (psychogenic) motor disorders. J Neurology 262: 674–681.

Nielsen G, Stone J, Matthews A et al. (2015b). Physiotherapy for functional motor disorders: a consensus recommendation. J Neurol Neurosurg Psychiatry 86: 1113–1119.

Nijenhuis ER (2009). Somatoform dissociation and somatoform dissociative disorders. In: P Dell, J O'Neil (Eds.), Dissociation and the dissociative disorders: DSM-V and beyond, Routledge, New York.

Oto M, Espie CA, Duncan R (2010). An exploratory randomized controlled trial of immediate versus delayed withdrawal of antiepileptic drugs in patients with psychogenic nonepileptic attacks (PNEAs). Epilepsia 51: 1994–1999.

Pick S, Mellers JDC, Goldstein LH (2016). Emotion and dissociative seizures: a phenomenological analysis of patients' perspectives. Epilepsy Behav 56: 5–14.

Poole NA, Wuerz A, Agrawal N (2010). Abreaction for conversion disorder: systematic review with meta-analysis. Br J Psychiatry 197: 91–95.

Pula J (2012). Functional vision loss. Curr Opinion Ophthalmol 23: 460–465.

Reuber M, Mitchell AJ, Howlett S et al. (2005). Measuring outcome in psychogenic nonepileptic seizures: how relevant is seizure remission? Epilepsia 46: 1788–1795.

Reuber M, Burness C, Howlett S et al. (2007a). Tailored psychotherapy for patients with functional neurological symptoms: a pilot study. J Psychosom Res 63: 625–632.

Reuber M, Howlett S, Khan A et al. (2007b). Non-epileptic seizures and other functional neurological symptoms: predisposing, precipitating, and perpetuating factors. Psychosomatics 48: 230–238.

Rosendal M, Blankenstein AH, Morriss R et al. (2013). Enhanced care by generalists for functional somatic symptoms and disorders in primary care. Cochrane Database Syst Rev 10: CD008142.

Ruddy R, House A (2005). Psychosocial interventions for conversion disorder. Cochrane Database Syst Rev. (Online): CD005331.

Ruotsalainen JH, Sellman J, Lehto L et al. (2007). Interventions for treating functional dysphonia in adults. Cochrane Database Syst Rev: CD006373.

Salmon P, Al-Marzooqi SM, Baker G et al. (2003). Childhood family dysfunction and associated abuse in patients with nonepileptic seizures: towards a causal model. Psychosom Med 65: 695–700.

Schmid G, Henningsen P, Dieterich M et al. (2011). Psychotherapy in dizziness: a systematic review. J Neurol Neurosurg Psychiatry 82: 601–606.

Sharpe M, Walker J, Williams C et al. (2011). Guided self-help for functional (psychogenic) symptoms: a randomized controlled efficacy trial. Neurology 77: 564–572.

Stone J (2006). Dissociation: what is it and why is it important? Practical Neurol 6: 308–313.

Stone J (2014). Psychotherapy for severe somatoform disorder: problems with missing studies. Br J Psychiatry 204: 243–244.

Stone J, Carson AJ (2013). The unbearable lightheadedness of seizing: wilful submission to dissociative (non-epileptic) seizures. J Neurol Neurosurg Psychiatry 84: 822–824.

Stone J, Edwards M (2012). Trick or treat? Showing patients with functional (psychogenic) motor symptoms their physical signs. Neurology 79: 282–284.

Stone J, Wojcik W, Durrance D et al. (2002). What should we say to patients with symptoms unexplained by disease? The "number needed to offend". BMJ 325: 1449–1450.

Stone J, Hoeritzauer I, Brown K et al. (2014). Therapeutic sedation for functional (psychogenic) neurological symptoms. J Psychosom Res 76: 165–168.

Tull MT, Gratz KL, Salters K et al. (2004). The role of experiential avoidance in posttraumatic stress symptoms and symptoms of depression, anxiety, and somatization. J Nerv Ment Dis 192: 754–761.

van Dessel N, den Boeft M, van der Wouden JC et al. (2014). Non-pharmacological interventions for somatoform disorders and medically unexplained physical symptoms (MUPS) in adults. Cochrane Database Syst Rev 11: CD011142.

Williams ACDC, Eccleston C, Morley S (2012). Psychological therapies for the management of chronic pain (excluding headache) in adults. Cochrane Database Syst Rev. CD007407.

Handbook of Clinical Neurology, Vol. 139 (3rd series)
Functional Neurologic Disorders
M. Hallett, J. Stone, and A. Carson, Editors
http://dx.doi.org/10.1016/B978-0-12-801772-2.00047-3

Chapter 47

Hypnosis as therapy for functional neurologic disorders

Q. DEELEY*
Department of Forensic and Neurodevelopmental Sciences, Institute of Psychiatry, Kings College, London, UK

Abstract

Suggestion in hypnosis has been applied to the treatment of functional neurologic symptoms since the earliest descriptions of hypnosis in the 19th century. Suggestion in this sense refers to an intentional communication of beliefs or ideas, whether verbally or nonverbally, to produce subjectively convincing changes in experience and behavior. The recognition of suggestion as a psychologic process with therapeutic applications was closely linked to the derivation of hypnosis from earlier healing practices. Animal magnetism, the immediate precursor of hypnosis, arrived at a psychologic concept of suggestion along with other ideas and practices which were then incorporated into hypnosis. Before then, other forms of magnetism and ritual healing practices such as exorcism involved unintentionally suggestive verbal and nonverbal stimuli. We consider the derivation of hypnosis from these practices not only to illustrate the range of suggestive processes, but also the consistency with which suggestion has been applied to the production and removal of dissociative and functional neurologic symptoms over many centuries. Nineteenth-century practitioners treated functional symptoms with induction of hypnosis *per se*; imperative suggestions, or commands for specific effects; "medical clairvoyance" in hypnotic trance, in which patients diagnosed their own condition and predicted the time and manner of their recovery; and suggestion without prior hypnosis, known as "fascination" or "psychotherapeutics." Modern treatments largely involve different types of imperative suggestion with or without hypnosis. However, the therapeutic application of suggestion in hypnosis to functional and other symptoms waned in the first half of the 20th century under the separate pressures of behaviorism and psychoanalysis. In recent decades suggestion in hypnosis has been more widely applied to treating functional neurologic symptoms. Suggestion is typically applied within the context of other treatment approaches, such as cognitive-behavioral, rehabilitative, or psychodynamic therapy. Suggestions are generally symptom-focused (designed to resolve a symptom) or exploratory (using methods such as revivification or age regression to explore experiences associated with symptom onset). The evidence base is dominated by case studies and series, with a paucity of randomized controlled trials. Future evaluation studies should allow for the fact that suggestion with or without hypnosis is a component of broader treatment interventions adapted to a wide range of symptoms and presentations. An important role of the concept of suggestion in the management of functional neurologic symptoms is to raise awareness of how interactions with clinicians and wider clinical contexts can alter expectancies and beliefs of patients in ways that influence the onset, course, and remission of symptoms.

INTRODUCTION

In this chapter we will consider the application of suggestion in hypnosis to the treatment of functional symptoms. We begin by describing characteristics of hypnosis and suggestion, and then consider how hypnosis was derived from earlier healing practices to provide a broader insight into the links between suggestion and the treatment of functional symptoms. We go on to discuss the use of

*Correspondence to: Dr. Quinton Deeley, Department of Forensic and Neurodevelopmental Sciences, Institute of Psychiatry, De Crespigny Park, London SE5 8AZ, UK. E-mail: peter.q.deeley@kcl.ac.uk

suggestion and hypnosis in the treatment of hysteric symptoms by 19th-century pioneers of neurology and psychiatry, before considering their contemporary as well as prospective uses.

SUGGESTION, HYPNOSIS, AND FUNCTIONAL SYMPTOMS: A BRIEF HISTORY

Hypnosis involves controlled modulation of components of cognition – such as awareness, volition, perception, and belief – by an external agent (the hypnotist) or oneself (self-hypnosis) employing suggestion (Heap et al., 2001). Suggestions in hypnosis usually take the form of verbally expressed commands containing ideas and imagery relating to the intended effect. A typical hypnosis session begins with an induction procedure involving suggestions for attentional focusing and relaxation, followed by targeted suggestions aimed at producing specific alterations in some aspect of experience or behavior. Suggested effects include the production and removal of what would be regarded as hysteric or functional symptoms if they were encountered in a clinical context – symptoms such as aphonia, paralysis, involuntary movement, sensory loss or pain, amnesia or altered identity, and reductions of awareness (Kirsch, 1990; Oakley, 1999). The classic suggestion effect entails that the alterations in experience produced by suggestions should be experienced as involuntary and effortless (Weitzenhoffer, 1980). Hypnotic suggestibility refers to the number of suggestions that an individual responds to after the administration of a standard set of test suggestions, such as the Harvard Group Scale of Hypnotic Susceptibility (Shor and Orne, 1962) and the Stanford Scale of Hypnotic Susceptibility (Weitzenhoffer and Hilgard, 1962). Individual differences in hypnotic suggestibility may relate to variations in genes influencing executive function. For example, high hypnotic responsiveness is associated with variants of the catechol-*O*-metyltransferase polymorphism (Lichtenberg et al., 2000; Szekely et al., 2010).

While hypnosis is composed of particular uses of suggestion, suggestion itself is a much broader phenomenon. It has been defined as "a form or type of communicable belief capable of producing and modifying experiences, thoughts and actions. Suggestions can be (a) intentional/non-intentional, (b) verbal/non-verbal, or (c) hypnotic/non-hypnotic" (Halligan and Oakley, 2014). Interrogative suggestibility (compliance with leading questions under cross-examination) and placebo suggestibility (the tendency to experience a positive outcome after the administration of an inert substance or ineffective treatment) are also described, but do not correlate with hypnotic suggestibility (Kihlstrom, 2008; Oakley and Halligan, 2013). Suggestions in hypnosis are mainly verbal and intentional, although nonverbal, implicit features of hypnotic procedures also contribute to suggested effects. These nonverbal features of hypnosis range from the use of sensory cues to trigger suggested effects in posthypnotic suggestions, to the increase in response to suggestions when participants interpret an overall context as "hypnotic" (Gandhi and Oakley, 2005). Intentionally administered verbal suggestions can also produce suggested effects outside a hypnotic context – in other words, where no induction procedure has been administered and the context is not defined as "hypnotic" – a process termed "imaginative suggestibility" (Braffman and Kirsch, 1999). Yet historically and cross-culturally there is a far wider class of verbal and nonverbal religious and traditional healing practices that modify experience and behavior, including functional symptoms. These practices are not understood by local actors to work through the mere communication of ideas and beliefs as "suggestion," but by other powers and processes. From a psychologic perspective these practices involve unintentional suggestion, in the sense that suggestion is employed without being recognized as such. They form an essential part of the history of the hypnotic treatment of functional symptoms, because the techniques used in hypnosis were derived and adapted from these older practices. They illustrate the range of suggestive processes, and the consistency with which suggestion has been applied to the production and removal of dissociative and functional neurologic symptoms over many centuries.

The use and effects of unintentional suggestion in this sense are illustrated by the religious category of demonic possession and its cure through exorcism, which were central to the history of both hysteria and hypnosis (MacDonald, 1991; Ellenberger, 1994). Possession involves the apparent substitution of the ordinary self by a demon, which in psychologic terms would be described as dissociative identity change (Deeley, 2003). The identity change is typically accompanied by a range of other behavioral features which in a clinical setting would be considered functional symptoms, such as collapse, convulsions, aphonia or altered speech, and anesthesia. Signs of autonomic hyperarousal such as horripilation (hair standing on end) and trembling are also commonly described (Rouget, 1985). Possession was interpreted as hysteria by the English physician Edward Jorden as early as 1603 (MacDonald, 1991), while both Charcot and Janet explained it as a form of hysteria due to suggestion (Charcot and Richer, 1887; Janet, 1907).

While contemporary medical anthropologic and cultural neuroscience accounts also view possession as involving dissociative and functional changes in response to local beliefs and expectancies, greater emphasis is now placed on the social meanings and values attached to these phenomena than by authors of the 19th and early 20th centuries (Littlewood, 2002; Deeley, 2003; Seligman and Kirmayer, 2008). Nevertheless, religious practices of exorcism can still be understood as one of the major historic and cross-cultural methods of managing a widespread category of culturally influenced dissociative phenomena accompanied by loss or alteration in functioning.

Suggestive components of exorcism are evident in a report from 1775 about the Austrian exorcist Father Johann Joseph Gassner (1727–1779). Gassner described how he asked a nun suspected of possession whether she agreed that anything he should order would happen. She agreed, and then he ordered any possessing spirit to manifest itself – which it did. Gassner believed these effects were supernaturally caused, but his method resembles nonreligious applications of hypnosis in which a subject hands over executive control to a special agent (the "hypnotist") and conforms her behavior to expectations established within the hypnotic context.

The immediate precursor of hypnosis, animal magnetism, was itself derived from exorcism and related healing practices reinterpreted in terms of a theory originating in medieval science (Binet and Féré, 1887). Animal magnetism is central to understanding the treatment of functional symptoms with suggestion in hypnosis, given that – as Janet himself emphasized – the methods employed in hypnosis were largely developed by magnetizers in the late 18th century and first half of the 19th century (Janet, 1907; Ellenberger, 1994).

Animal magnetism began with a contemporary of Gassner, Anton Mesmer (1734–1815), who developed many techniques for the purpose of healing which recalled possession and exorcism. Mesmer's techniques included passes of the hand over the patient's body to produce "crises" (swooning, convulsions, shaking, crying, hysteric laughter, amongst other signs), followed by a stupor. Mesmer interpreted these effects in terms of his physical theory of "animal magnetism," based on ideas partially dating back to Paracelsus (1493–1541) and other medieval thinkers such as Cardan, who in 1584 described anesthesia produced by a magnet (Binet and Féré, 1887). Mesmer believed he had discovered a subtle force or fluid permeating the universe, forming a connecting medium between the heavenly bodies and humans, and between humans themselves. Akin to gravity, it could remotely cause or cure nervous illness depending on its balance in the body compared to the outside world. Mesmer believed he could accumulate and channel the "magnetic virtue" to "provoke and direct salutary crises, so as to completely control them" (Binet and Féré, 1887). The crisis was the manifestation of latent disease. As the patient was repeatedly provoked, the crises became less severe and eventually disappeared, at which point the patient was cured (Ellenberger, 1994, p. 62). Mesmer channeled magnetism not only through passes of his hands but with touching and eye contact, or through iron bars, water, or other objects he had previously "magnetized" by direct contact. Proximity to the magnetic source was essential, so Mesmer would place himself *en rapport* with the patient, directly touching or close to the patient – so introducing a term to describe the influence between therapist and patient that was eventually interpreted in more psychologic terms (Ellenberger, 1994, p. 152). Mesmer even believed that Gassner had unwittingly used animal magnetism to produce his cures, confiding to an associate that "Gassner possessed magnetism to an extraordinary degree and his own powers were not so great" (Ellenberger, 1994). While Mesmer applied his methods to the cure of any disease, descriptions of his practice provide many examples of his production as well as treatment of symptoms such as convulsions and aphonia that are often functional (Ellenberger, 1994, p. 64). Nevertheless, as with exorcism and faith healing, Mesmer's practices involved unintentional suggestion in the sense that he attributed their effects to processes other than beliefs and expectancies.

Successors such as the Marquis de Puysegur (1751–1825) developed Mesmer's techniques while introducing more psychologic accounts of magnetism which are the precursors of contemporary theories of hypnosis and suggestion (Binet and Féré, 1887; Ellenberger, 1994). Puysegur moved away from the dramatic crises of Mesmer, producing a more quiescent "perfect crisis" or "artificial somnambulism," comprising apparent wakefulness, obedience to the commands of the magnetizer, and then amnesia after being "disenchanted" by kissing a tree (Ellenberger, 1994). The wakefulness and obedience (suggestibility) of "artificial somnambulism" were the prototype of the hypnotic trance, although the techniques of induction and reversal, presence of subsequent amnesia, and interpretations of the condition have changed with time.

Puysegur's production of a state in which the patient became "obedient" to the commands of the magnetizer drew attention to the possibility of creating instructions for specific effects – marking the advent of intentional as opposed to unintentional suggestion. Puyseger came to view the real agent in cure as the magnetizer's will rather than the subtle fluid proposed by Mesmer (Ellenberger, 1994, p. 72). As Puysegur said in a lecture of August 1785, "I *believe* that I have the power to set into action the vital principle of my fellow men; I *want* to make use of it; this is all my science and all my means" (quoted in Ellenberger, 1994, p. 72). Puysegur's methods and teachings were applied to the treatment of a range of symptoms, including convulsions and paralysis, as well as the induction of surgical anesthesia (Binet and Féré, 1887).

Puysegur was later credited with arriving at the modern concept of suggestion (Binet and Féré, 1887).

While Pusyegur emphasized the role of the magnetizer's will in creating magnetic effects, another pioneer, the Abbé de Faria (1756–1819), taught that certain types of patient were susceptible to magnetization (Ellenberger, 1994, p. 75). Faria produced a similar condition to artificial somnambulism, "lucid sleep," with the command "sleep!" rather than mesmeric passes.

In effect, the early magnetizers established all of the major components of what would later be known as hypnosis. They produced artificial somnambulism as the prototype of hypnotic trance and discovered different methods of establishing it. They arrived at the concepts of suggestion and variation in suggestibility, recognized the reciprocal influence between magnetizer and patient in the concept of rapport, and applied their techniques to the treatment of a wide range of symptoms, including what would now be termed functional symptoms. Nevertheless, the interest of many magnetizers in otherworldly phenomena such as telepathy and clairvoyance led to caution and skepticism about animal magnetism in medical circles, preventing its widespread adoption (Ellenberger, 1994).

The medical concept of hypnotism was introduced by a Scottish doctor working in Manchester, James Braid (1795–1860), who had become interested in magnetism after seeing a demonstration by the French magnetizer Lafontaine (Braid, 1843). Braid described a way of establishing a hypnotic state by the subject staring at an object, producing "visual fatigue" and "nervous sleep" (Oakley, 2004, p. 416). Braid viewed hypnotism as a distinct physiologic state characterized by fixed stare, relaxation, suppressed breathing, and fixed attention to the words of the hypnotist (Ellenberger, 1994). He later came to view concentration by the patient on a single thought or idea, "monoideism," as the key factor in producing trance, so returning to a concept of suggestion. Braid was primarily a clinician who applied hypnotism to the treatment of a wide range of conditions, including tics, nervous headaches, neuralgia of the heart, epilepsy, paralysis, convulsions, and tonic spasms, amongst many other conditions (Binet and Féré, 1887).

Braid's ideas were not widely adopted in England. However, a French professor of surgery, Eugène Azam (1822–1899), applied Braid's methods to the investigation and treatment of cases of *dédoublement de la personalité* (what would now be termed dissociative identity disorder), as well as to surgical anesthesia with Paul Broca (Binet and Féré, 1887; Ellenberger, 1994). Azam's work became known at the Salpêtrière Hospital in Paris, where Charcot had developed an interest in hysteroepilepsy (nonepileptic seizures) and other hysteric conditions (Charcot, 1889; Charcot and Marie, 1892). Charcot viewed hypnosis as a model and treatment for hysteria (Charcot and Marie, 1892), in which both were pathologic states produced by suggestion or autosuggestion acting by as-yet unknown effects on brain function. This view was based on Charcot's observation of similarities between hysteric symptoms and suggested effects in hypnosis; that hysteric patients were susceptible to suggestion; and that hysteric symptoms could be produced and removed by suggestion in hypnosis (Charcot and Marie, 1892; Charcot and de la Tourette, 1892).

Despite Charcot's emphasis on the role of autosuggestion as the mechanism of hysteria, he retained the idea that there was some unexplained organic basis to hysteroepilepsy and other hysteric and hypnotic phenomena (Charcot and Marie, 1892; Charcot and de la Tourette, 1892). His theories and treatments were criticized for his fixed typologies and phases of hysteric and hypnotic symptoms by analogy with organic neurologic disorders, rather than recognizing the plasticity of symptoms in response to beliefs and expectancies (Janet, 1907). Charcot was also criticized for his retention of older "uterine," ideas, such as ovarian compression to treat hysteroepilepsy, and his belief in the existence of hypnogenetic points (Janet, 1907; Ellenberger, 1994). For his part, Charcot wrote of the treatment of hysteria that:

> *hypnotism may be of some service, but no so much as one might* a priori *expect; it may be applied against some local symptoms ... Suggestion may be applied without hypnotism, and may be quite as effective as hypnotic sleep (Charcot and Marie, 1892).*

Charcot's main critic within his lifetime was Hippolyte Bernheim (1837–1919), Professor of Medicine in Nancy, who argued that hypnosis is fully explained as the product of normal psychologic processes of suggestion and suggestibility (Oakley, 2004, p. 416). He defined suggestibility as "the aptitude to transform an idea into an act" (Ellenberger, 1994, p. 87). Bernheim and his associates at Nancy applied hypnosis to the treatment of functional and other symptoms on a large scale over many years, using the induction technique developed by the magnetizer Faria. However, as time passed, Bernheim made increasing use of suggestion in the waking state, which he termed "psychotherapeutics" (Ellenberger, 1994, p. 87).

Similarly, Josef Babinski, a former pupil of Charcot, renamed hysteria as "pithiatism," curable by suggestion (Broussolle et al., 2014). Janet noted how all of the major medical theorists of hypnosis in France in the latter part of the 19th century considered suggestion as central to hypnosis and hysteria, despite other theoretic differences (Janet, 1907, p. 324f). Also, all had applied suggestion within hypnosis or "the waking state" to its treatment (Broussolle et al., 2014).

Janet's own theories continue to influence current concepts of dissociation, hypnosis, and suggestion, including how suggestion can be used to treat functional symptoms (Janet, 1907; Moene and Roelofs, 2008). Janet originated the modern notion of dissociation as a "contraction of the field of consciousness," resulting in an abnormal compartmentalization of mental functions that are normally closely associated (Janet, 1907). Janet viewed dissociative symptoms as influenced by the suggestive effect of "fixed ideas," typically based on unresolved traumatic memories. The "ideas" that influence symptoms were not generally accessible to consciousness, but were "emancipated" in hysteric individuals who had an abnormal weakness of will and consciousness. The ideas were "systems of images" relating to movement, viscera, or other aspects of functioning. Hysteric individuals were suggestible, contributing to symptom formation but also rendering them amenable to therapeutic suggestion (Janet, 1907).

The period between 1775 and the early 1900s can therefore be considered a time in which theories and methods of magnetism and hypnosis, and their therapeutic applications, were developed and explored. It marks the shift from the unintentional application of suggestion in a variety of healing activities to awareness of suggestion itself as a therapeutic and experimental resource which can be intentionally used to produce specific effects. When reviewing this period Ellenberger (1994) identified four major therapeutic applications of hypnosis and suggestion.

Magnetizers and hypnotists used "magnetic" or "hypnotic sleep" (a state of deep relaxation and absorption produced by an induction procedure) as a therapy in its own right. A patient of the latter 19th century described hypnotic sleep as a:

> *most wonderful sensation, a feeling of concentration of one's self with one's body as if one were isolated within one's self. Everything disappears, only the I-consciousness is left. The concentration is like the most wonderful absolute rest one can imagine (quoted in Ellenberger, 1994).*

Yet the use of magnetic or hypnotic sleep sometimes rested on an assumption that it was a unitary state, rather than a product of suggestions and expectancies that introduced variable responses in the absence of more directive suggestion. For example, Braid himself observed that contradictory effects (such as anesthesia and hyperesthesia) could result from his induction procedure (Binet and Féré, 1887). Modern induction procedures use standardized verbal suggestions to establish more uniform effects (e.g., Oakley et al., 2007). Hypnotic induction *per se*, without the use of additional targeted suggestions, is not typical of modern therapeutic uses of hypnosis.

Magnetizers and early hypnotists made use of imperative suggestions involving commands, which are the forerunners of contemporary verbal suggestions in hypnosis. The magnetist Faria was an early proponent, and the technique was also used by both Charcot and colleagues at the Salpêtrière and the Nancy School. Imperative suggestions were considered to be most effective in people who occupied subordinate positions, such as soldiers and laborers. However, in an unwilling subject it was recognized that the symptoms would not resolve, or only temporarily recede before re-emerging or being replaced by another symptom. This phenomenon is still described in contemporary applications of suggestions to treat functional symptoms.

Another type of hypnotic cure involved a "kind of bargaining between the patient and the hypnotist" (Ellenberger, 1994, p. 151) when the patient was hypnotized. This recalled the long discussions between exorcist and demons in the case of possession, and the agreement of the demon or spirit to leave at a certain time and with certain conditions (for a modern example in India, see Deeley, 1999). Ellenberger comments that this kind of treatment was widespread in the first half of the 19th century, but was later replaced by the imperative suggestions used by both Charcot and colleagues at the Salpêtrière, and the Nancy School. However, even in this later period case histories record instances of "medical clairvoyance," in which the therapist suggested that a functional symptom would resolve at a time known to the patient, and the patient predicted the date on which he would subsequently recover (Ellenberger, 1994, p. 151).

Another type of therapy involved administration of suggestions without the use of a hypnotic induction procedure. This was called "fascination" in the early 19th century, "suggestion in the waking state" by the Nancy school, where it was employed by the 1880s, and, more recently, "imaginative suggestibility" (Braffman and Kirsch, 1999).

HYPNOSIS AND TREATMENT OF FUNCTIONAL SYMPTOMS IN THE 20TH CENTURY TO THE PRESENT

Scientific interest in hypnosis waned in the first half of the 20th century under the influence of behaviorism (Oakley, 2004). Therapeutic application of hypnosis also declined with the rise of Freudian psychoanalysis as the dominant form of psychotherapy. The main development of this period was the experimental work of the American psychologist Clark Hull (1933), who established valid and reproducible measures of suggested phenomena such as anesthesia and amnesia. Milton Erikson

(1901–1980), a student of Hull's, also developed a system of psychotherapy that included suggestive techniques (Oakley, 2004).

In 1955 the British Medical Association reported that hypnosis could be safely and effectively employed in medical and therapeutic settings (Oakley, 2004). In recent decades suggestion within and outside hypnosis has been applied to the treatment of functional symptoms along with other symptoms and illnesses (Nash, 2008). Suggestion in hypnosis is typically applied within the context of other treatment approaches, such as physiotherapy and occupational therapy, or cognitive-behavioral and psychodynamic therapy. For example, a report of the American Psychological Association in 1993 stated that "hypnosis is not a type of therapy, like psychoanalysis or behavior therapy. Instead it is a procedure that can be used to facilitate therapy." Adjunctive use of hypnosis and suggestion is supported by influential theoretic models of functional symptom formation and their links to suggestion and expectancy – for example, the cognitive neuropsychologic theory of Oakley (1999) and Brown and Oakley's (2004) model of medically unexplained symptoms based on cognitive psychology (see Chapter 9). These and other authors argue that treatment must involve detailed assessment of the patient's symptoms, including precipitating and maintaining factors, as part of a multidisciplinary approach (Moene and Roelofs, 2008).

The use of suggestion in hypnosis to treat functional symptoms has been mainly described in case studies or series. Oakley (2001) summarized 13 studies which used hypnotic techniques in the treatment of functional symptoms (Table 47.1). Most were single case studies, but one of them involved 8 patients (Moene et al., 1998). The studies illustrate how hypnotic techniques are variously integrated with cognitive-behavioral, rehabilitative, and psychodynamic approaches. Suggestions are generally symptom-focused (designed to resolve a symptom) or exploratory (using methods such as revivification or age regression to explore experiences associated with symptom onset). The choice of technique partly depends on the broader theoretic approach. For example, symptom-focused suggestions are commonly used with cognitive-behavioral therapy, while revivification (or age regression) has been particularly used with psychodynamic approaches to explore precipitating events and "unconscious" psychologic conflicts and motivations that may be relevant to symptom formation.

To date two randomized controlled trials on the treatment of functional symptoms (conversion disorder and somatoform disorder) have been conducted. Both involved an eclectic assessment and treatment model that included the use of hypnotic treatments for inpatients (Moene et al., 2002) and outpatients (Moene et al., 2003; see also Moene and Roelofs, 2008, for discussion of both studies together). The study of inpatients included 45 patients with motor conversion symptoms, and also patients with somatoform disorder, including motor conversion symptoms. A 2-month treatment program involved group therapy using cognitive-behavioral methods to increase problem solving. Treatment also included physiotherapy, individual exercise, and bed rest. Twenty-four patients also received hypnotic treatment with eight weekly 1-hour sessions using symptom-oriented and exploratory techniques. A control group of 21 patients received additional treatments which were not focused on conversion symptoms specifically. For the sample as a whole, statistically significant improvements were found in all outcome measures relating to symptoms and common physical activities, activities of daily living, and social functioning. The improvement in these measures was not only maintained at 6 months but improved overall. However, the hypnotic intervention did not appear to yield any additional benefit (Moene et al., 2002; Moene and Roelofs, 2008).

The second randomized controlled trial included 44 outpatients. This study reported that patients with functional (conversion motor) symptoms who had received a 10-week hypnosis treatment package significantly improved compared to baseline. The hypnotic treatments included symptom-oriented and exploratory techniques. The hypnotic treatment arm showed greater improvement than a waiting-list condition, and improvement was maintained at 6-month follow-up. This included 12 patients who were referred for further hypnotic treatment after the 10-week posttreatment assessment, receiving a mean number of 6.3 extra sessions. Consequently, of the two randomized controlled trials that have been conducted of hypnotic treatments in patients with functional (motor conversion) symptoms, only one has shown specific additional benefit from hypnotic treatment (Moene et al., 2002, 2003).

ASSESSMENT AND TREATMENT APPROACHES EMPLOYING HYPNOTIC TECHNIQUES

Moene and Roelofs (2008) provide a detailed description of hypnotic techniques and suggestions used in the treatment of functional and somatoform symptoms. Key features are summarized here (see Moene and Roelofs (2008) for fuller descriptions and case histories). Both symptom-oriented and exploratory hypnotic approaches employ direct suggestion as well as posthypnotic suggestion for symptom reduction. Some methods involve learning self-hypnosis to implement specific suggestions to reduce or resolve symptoms. Relaxation established through self-hypnosis has also been used to contribute to symptom reduction (Spinhoven, 1989, quoted in Moene and Roelofs, 2008).

Table 47.1

A summary of 13 studies in which hypnotic procedures were used in the treatment of conversion disorders

Study	Problem	Techniques used	Outcome
Braybrooke (1994) (single case, male)	Dislocation of shoulders	Direct and indirect hypnotic suggestion, hypnotic uncovering,* dream analysis, metaphors, face-saving strategies	Loss of symptoms after 33 sessions
Collinson (1972) (single case, female)	Paralysis, anesthesia	Spontaneous hypnotic state, indirect suggestion (story), face-saving strategy (confession)	Complete symptom removal
Davies and Wagstaff (1991) (single case, female)	Ataxia	"Physical" explanation of symptoms, cognitive-behavioral techniques, face-saving strategies, creative imagery, positive suggestion	Significant symptom loss after two sessions
Dunnet and Williams (1998) (single case, female)	Aphonia	Direct hypnotic suggestion, cognitive-behavioral techniques, speech therapy	Normal voice after 6 months of treatment
Giacalone (1981) (single case, 10-year-old female)	Dysphonia	Direct and indirect hypnotic suggestion, face-saving strategies, imagery	Normal voice after five weekly sessions
Horsley (1982) (single case, female)	Dysphonia	Hypnotic relaxation training, self-hypnosis, personal responsibility for recovery	Normal voice after two sessions and at 16-month follow-up
Little (1990) (single case, female)	Dysphonia	Hypnotic relaxation training, direct hypnotic suggestion	Normal voice after 2 sessions and at 5-month follow-up
Mander (1998) (single case, male)	Dysphonia	Hypnotic relaxation training, direct hypnotic suggestion, self-hypnosis, imagery	95% normal after five sessions. Normal at 2-month follow-up
McCue (1979) (single case, female)	Aphonia	Direct hypnotic suggestion, hypnotic uncovering,* symptom loss in hypnosis	Normal voice after one session and at 4-month follow-up
McCue and McCue (1988) (single case, female)	Aphonia	Direct hypnotic suggestion, symptom loss in hypnosis, face-saving strategies	Improved voice after five sessions. Normal after 11 sessions and at 2.5-year follow-up
Moene et al. (1998) (8 cases, all female)	Paralysis, gait disorder, contractures, tremor, nonepileptic seizures	A package including "physical" explanation of symptoms, face-saving strategies, direct and indirect hypnotic suggestion, hypnotic uncovering,* physiotherapy, supportive psychologic therapy	One patient dropped out. Seven completed with symptom removal, 3 relapsed
Neeleman and Mann (1993) (single case, female)	Aphonia	Direct hypnotic suggestion, challenge, symptom loss in hypnosis, face-saving strategies	Voice returned after 15 sessions. Relapse after 1 week and at 2-year follow-up
Pelletier (1997) (single case, female)	Aphonia	Direct and indirect hypnotic suggestion, hypnotic uncovering,* symptom loss in hypnosis, face-saving strategies	Normal voice after eight sessions. Relapse after 14 months

Reproduced from Oakley (2001), with permission from Oxford University Press.

*Where hypnotic uncovering is included in the techniques used, this refers to exploratory procedures employing hypnotic age regression or revivification to uncover psychologic factors underlying the presenting symptoms and reflects a more psychodynamic therapeutic approach. See text for further explanation.

SYMPTOM-ORIENTED TECHNIQUES

Moene and Roelofs (2008) summarized the types of suggestion used in the treatment of different functional symptoms (motor, sensory, and nonepileptic seizures).

Motor symptoms such as paralysis, contractures, and uncontrollable movements

Making use of the present rest capacity with flaccid paralysis

The patient's attention is directed to any sensations or movements within the affected limb. Sensations are strengthened by suggestions such as "the longer you concentrate on the tiny muscle spasms, the stronger they will become." Positive reinforcement (praise and encouragement) is used in response to evidence of increased movement, with progression to larger movements over treatment sessions.

The nonaffected limb helps the affected one

The patient is asked to concentrate on, name, and visualize sensations and movements in the unaffected limb. A suggestion is then made that the affected limb has forgotten to feel sensations or movements; the unaffected limb is going to retrain the affected one; and movement and sensation can flow from the unaffected to the affected limb (Hoogduin et al., 1993).

Relaxation and imagination

This technique has been employed for hand contracture. Suggestions for relaxation of the arm and hand muscles are made. An additional suggestion is made that a balloon inside the contracted hand is blown up and relaxed and that the hand moves with this (Hoogduin et al., 1993).

Imagination of normal functioning in the past

Under hypnosis suggestions are made that patients have returned to a time when they had voluntary movement in the affected limb. This technique has been used diagnostically as well as therapeutically for speech aphonia. Patients are taken back to a time when they could speak and are encouraged to do so in therapy. They are encouraged to "relearn" how to speak within a pleasant setting.

During sleep the symptoms are absent

This technique is applied to tremors or functional ataxia. This approach is based on a recognition that many functional symptoms remit during sleep. Suggestions are made that the patient has attained a state similar to sleep whereby the symptoms are removed. The patient is habituated to symptom removal through a succession of steps, from adopting a sleep-like position, to sitting, standing, and then normal movement. This approach is combined with self-hypnosis and practice of these techniques at home.

Letting go

This technique is applied to functional shaking and tremor. This technique rests on the observation that tensing muscles to increase control of involuntary movements can worsen them. "Letting go" involves progressive relaxation with or without hypnosis to enable patients to let go of their resistance to movement and so reduce the unwanted movement. Where hypnosis is employed, suggestions are given "not to resist the movements, to shake them off, and to make the body heavy and languid, whereby the movements will become increasingly slow and eventually shall stop."

Somatosensory symptoms

Making use of visual and auditory imagination in functional blindness or deafness

The patient is instructed to imagine pleasant sensory images (visual, auditory or tactile) during periods of relaxation at intervals during the day. The suggestion is then given that:

> *it is precisely from this positive and relaxed state of mind, that consciously* learning to see and hear will be facilitated*, and that one day it will manifest itself, initially just a bit, but after that, there will be more and more conscious awareness of images or sounds during longer periods of time (Moene and Roelofs, 2008).*

Seizures or convulsions

Hypnotic self-control procedures

Suggestion in hypnosis has been used to facilitate recovery of memory of events during nonepileptic seizures, which may also contribute to differential diagnosis of nonepileptic seizures and epilepsy given that suggested recall occurs in the former, but not the latter. The method may also help identify internal or external cues that precede or trigger seizure onset, potentially allowing patients to learn how to avoid seizure onset through cue conditioning. For example, if patients notices a precipitating sensation such as tingling, then they may be taught a rapid relaxation technique when tingling occurs. Moene and Roelofs (2008) provide the example of a patient who, when noting a tingling sensation:

> *stops doing whatever she is doing, she goes into a quick trance by thinking of her relax chair which is a synonym for deep relaxation and rest; she then takes a deep breath, holds it for a few seconds, breathes out and lets all tension leave her body.*

Prescribing the symptom as a self-controlled procedure

This technique is employed in situations where an attack is preceded and precipitated by anticipatory anxiety. A hypnotic recall technique is used to elicit a description of triggers for a recent attack. During hypnosis an attack is then precipitated. As the symptoms resolve, "the therapist emphasises that if the patient can 'turn on the attacks' by becoming anxious, he/she can learn to control them by becoming relaxed in the face of these situational triggers" (Moene and Roelofs, 2008).

EXPRESSIVE TECHNIQUES

Expressive techniques focus on the experience of emotional trauma. They are used with caution because of the potential for iatrogenic suggestion of false memories. These techniques can be applied in situations where the patient is otherwise too ashamed or anxious to acknowledge psychologically relevant events or conflicts. For example, Brady and Lind (1961) describe a case of hysteric (functional) blindness in which, during hypnosis, the patient, a young man, revealed his shame about leaving a house fire where his sister was injured before she was eventually rescued. A suggestion is given that he should discuss his inner conflict in psychotherapy and his vision can recover (Brady and Lind, 1961, quoted in Moene and Roelofs, 2008).

Hypnosis and suggestive techniques are generally considered safe, with a low incidence of significant side-effects, when applied in a principled way. False-memory induction through suggestive processes such as age regression is recognized. Patients can also misinterpret suggestions and respond in idiosyncratic ways – for example, raising both arms when a suggestion for unilateral arm levitation is administered (Moene and Roelofs, 2008).

FUTURE DIRECTIONS

Future evaluation studies should allow for the fact that suggestion with or without hypnosis is adapted to a wide range of symptoms and presentations as a component of broader treatment strategies. Hypnotic and suggestive treatments may prove to be more effective with some symptoms or treatment approaches than others. Equally, the effects of individual patient factors on response to hypnotic and suggestive treatments – such as motivation to change or hypnotizability – are important to clarify in order to target treatment. The concept of "suggestion" also points to how interactions with clinicians and wider clinical contexts can alter expectancies and beliefs of patients in ways that influence the onset, course, and remission of symptoms. This raises the possibility that communication guidelines should be employed with patients across interactions with different health professionals to enlist the therapeutic effects of beliefs and expectancies.

CONCLUSIONS

Suggestion in hypnosis has been applied to the treatment of functional neurologic symptoms since the earliest descriptions of hypnosis in the 19th century. Suggestion in this sense refers to an intentional communication of beliefs or ideas, whether verbally or nonverbally, to produce subjectively convincing changes in experience and behavior. The recognition of "suggestion" as a psychologic process with therapeutic applications was closely linked to the derivation of hypnosis from earlier healing practices. Animal magnetism, the immediate precursor of hypnosis, arrived at a psychologic concept of suggestion along with other ideas and practices which were then incorporated into hypnosis. Before then, other forms of magnetism and ritual healing practices such as exorcism involved unintentionally suggestive verbal and nonverbal stimuli. The derivation of hypnosis from these practices not only illustrates the range of suggestive processes, but also the consistency with which suggestion has been applied to the production and removal of dissociative and functional neurologic symptoms over many centuries. Janet observed that, by the latter half of the 19th century, all of the major theorists of hysteria saw suggestion as contributing to hysteric symptoms, whatever their theoretic differences. Also, suggestion with or without hypnosis was widely applied to its treatment. Nineteenth-century practitioners treated functional symptoms with induction of hypnosis *per se*; imperative suggestions, or commands for specific effects; the use of "medical clairvoyance" in hypnotic trance, in which patients diagnosed their own condition and predicted the time and manner of their recovery; and suggestion without prior hypnosis, known as "fascination" or "psychotherapeutics."

Modern treatments largely involve different types of imperative suggestion with or without hypnosis. However, the therapeutic application of suggestion in hypnosis to functional and other symptoms waned in the first half of the 20th century under the separate pressures of behaviorism and psychoanalysis. In recent decades suggestion in hypnosis has been more widely applied to treating functional neurologic symptoms. Suggestion is typically applied within the context of other treatment approaches, such as cognitive-behavioral, rehabilitative, or psychodynamic therapy. Suggestions are generally symptom-focused (designed to resolve a symptom) or exploratory (using methods such as revivification or age regression to explore experiences associated with symptom onset). The evidence base is dominated by case studies and series, with a paucity of randomized controlled trials. Future evaluation studies will have to allow for the fact that suggestion with or without hypnosis is a component of broader treatment interventions, adapted to a wide range of symptoms and presentations. An important role of the concept of "suggestion" to the management of functional neurologic symptoms is to raise awareness of how interactions with clinicians and wider clinical contexts can alter expectancies and beliefs of patients in ways that influence the onset, course, and remission of symptoms.

References

American Psychological Association (1993). Psychological Hypnosis: A Bulletin of Division 30,2, Division of Psychological Hypnosis, Executive Committee, American Psychological Association, Washington, DC.

Binet A, Féré C (1887). Animal magnetism, Kegan Paul, Trench, Trübner, London.

Brady JP, Lind DL (1961). Experimental analysis of hysterical blindness: Operant conditioning techniques. Arch Gen Psychiatry 4 (4): 331.

Braffman W, Kirsch I (1999). Imaginative suggestibility and hypnotizability: an empirical analysis. J Pers Soc Psychol 77 (3): 578.

Braid J (1843). Neurypnology; or, the rationale of nervous sleep, considered in relation with animal magnetism. Illustrated by cases of its application in the relief and cure of disease, John Churchill, London.

Braybrooke Z (1994). Hypnosis in the treatment of conversion hysteria. Aust J Clin Exp Hypn 22: 125–136.

Broussolle E, Gobert F, Danaiila T et al. (2014). History of physical and 'moral' treatment of hysteria. Front Neurol Neurosci 35: 181–197.

Brown RJ, Oakley DA (2004). An integrative cognitive theory of hypnosis and high hypnotizability. In: M Heap, RJ Brown, DA Oakley (Eds.), The highly hypnotizable person: Theoretical, experimental and clinical issues, Routledge, London, pp. 152–186.

Charcot JM (1889). Lectures on the Diseases of the Nervous System, Vol. 3. New Sydenham Society, London.

Charcot JM, de la Tourette G (1892). In: DH Tuke (Ed.), Dictionary of psychological medicine, Churchill, London.

Charcot JM, Marie P (1892). Hysteria. In: DH Tuke (Ed.), Dictionary of psychological medicine, Churchill, London.

Charcot JM, Richer PMLP (1887). Les démoniaques dans l'art. Delahaye et Lecrosnier, Paris.

Collinson DR (1972). Conversion paralysis: ancient and modern. Br J Clin Hypn 3: 43–45.

Davies AD, Wagstaff GF (1991). The use of creative imagery in the behavioural treatment of an elderly woman diagnosed as an hysterical ataxic. Contemp Hypn 8: 147–152.

Deeley Q (1999). Ecological understandings of mental and physical illness. Philos Psychiatr Psychol 6 (2): 109–124.

Deeley Q (2003). Social, cognitive, and neural constraints on subjectivity and agency: implications for dissociative identity disorder. Philos Psychiatr Psychol 10 (2): 161–167.

Dunnet CP, Williams JE (1998). Hypnosis in speech therapy. In: M Heap (Ed.), Hypnosis: Current Clinical, Experimental, and Forensic Practices. Croom Helm, London, pp. 246–256.

Ellenberger HF (1994). The discovery of the unconscious: the history and evolution of dynamic psychiatry, Fontana Press, New York.

Gandhi B, Oakley DA (2005). Does 'hypnosis' by any other name smell as sweet? The efficacy of 'hypnotic'inductions depends on the label 'hypnosis'. Conscious Cogn 14 (2): 304–315.

Giacalone AV (1981). Hysterical dysphonia: hypnotic treatment of a ten-year-old female. Am J Clin Hypn 23 (4): 289–293.

Halligan PW, Oakley DA (2014). Hypnosis and beyond: Exploring the broader domain of suggestion. Psychology of Consciousness: Theory, Research, and Practice 1 (2): 105.

Heap M, Alden P, Brown RJ et al. (2001). The nature of hypnosis: Report prepared by a working party at the request of the Professional Affairs Board of the British Psychological Society, British Psychological Society, Leicester.

Hoogduin K, Akkermans M, Oudshoorn D et al. (1993). Hypnotherapy and contractures of the hand. Am J Clin Hypn 36 (2): 106–112.

Horsley IA (1982). Hypnosis and self-hypnosis in the treatment of psychogenic dysphonia: a case report. Am J Clin Hypn 24 (4): 277–283.

Hull CL (1933). Hypnosis and suggestibility: An experimental approach. Appleton- Century Crofts, New York.

Janet P (1907). The major symptoms of hysteria. Classics of Psychiatry & Behavioral Sciences Library, Division of Gryphon Editions, New York.

Kihlstrom JF (2008). The domain of hypnosis, revisited. In: M Nash, AJ Barnier (Eds.), The Oxford handbook of hypnosis: Theory, research, and practice, Oxford University Press, Oxford.

Kirsch I (1990). Changing expectations: a key to effective psychotherapy. Pacific Grove, CA. Brooks.

Lichtenberg P, Bachner-Melman R, Gritsenko I et al. (2000). Exploratory association study between catechol-*O*-methyltransferase (COMT) high/low enzyme activity polymorphism and hypnotizability. Am J Med Genet 96 (6): 771–774.

Little ME (1990). Hypnosis in the treatment of a case of spastic dysphonia. Br J Exp Clin Hypn 7: 181–183.

Littlewood R (2002). Pathologies of the West: An anthropology of mental illness in Europe and America, Bloomsbury Publishing, London.

MacDonald M (1991). Witchcraft and Hysteria in Elizabethan London: Edward Jorden and the Mary Glover Case, Psychology Press, London.

Mander A (1998). Hypnosis in the treatment of dysphonia. Aust J Clin Exp Hypn 26: 43–48.

McCue PA (1979). A case of hysterical aphonia: Successful treatment with brief hypnotherapy. Bull Br Soc Exp Clin Hypn 1: 18–19.

McCue EC, McCue PA (1988). Hypnosis in the elucidation of hysterical aphonia: A case report. Am J Clin Hypn 30 (3): 178–182.

Moene FC, Roelofs K (2008). Hypnosis in the treatment of conversion and somatization disorders. In: M Nash, AJ Barnier (Eds.), The Oxford handbook of hypnosis: Theory, research, and practice, Oxford University Press, Oxford.

Moene FC, Hoogduin KA, Dyck RV (1998). The inpatient treatment of patients suffering from (motor) conversion symptoms: a description of eight cases. Int J Clin Exp Hypn 46 (2): 171–190.

Moene FC, Spinhoven P, Hoogduin KA et al. (2002). A randomised controlled clinical trial on the additional effect of hypnosis in a comprehensive treatment programme for in-patients with conversion disorder of the motor type. Psychother Psychosom 71 (2): 66–76.

Moene FC, Spinhoven P, Hoogduin KA et al. (2003). A randomized controlled clinical trial of a hypnosis-based treatment for patients with conversion disorder, motor type. Int J Clin Exp Hypn 51 (1): 29–50.

Nash M (2008). Foundations of clinical hypnosis. In: M Nash, AJ Barnier (Eds.), The Oxford handbook of hypnosis: Theory, research, and practice, Oxford University Press, Oxford.

Neeleman J, Mann AH (1993). Treatment of hysterical aphonia with hypnosis and prokaletic therapy. Br J Psychiatry 163 (6): 816–819.

Oakley DA (1999). Hypnosis and conversion hysteria: a unifying model. Cognit Neuropsychiatry 4 (3): 243–265.

Oakley DA (2001). Hypnosis and suggestion in the treatment of hysteria. In: P Halligan, C Bass, J Marshall (Eds.), Contemporary Approaches to the Study of Hysteria, Oxford University Press, Oxford, pp. 312–329.

Oakley DA (2004). Hypnosis. In: RL Gregory (Ed.), The Oxford Companion to the Mind, Oxford University Press, Oxford, pp. 415–419.

Oakley DA, Halligan PW (2013). Hypnotic suggestion: opportunities for cognitive neuroscience. Nat Rev Neurosci 14 (8): 565–576.

Oakley DA, Deeley Q, Halligan PW (2007). Hypnotic depth and response to suggestion under standardized conditions and during fMRI scanning. Int J Clin Exp Hypn 55 (1): 32–58.

Pelletier AM (1977). Hysterical aphonia: A case report. Am J Clin Hypn 20 (2): 149–153.

Rouget G (1985). Music and trance: A theory of the relations between music and possession, University of Chicago Press, Chicago.

Seligman R, Kirmayer LJ (2008). Dissociative experience and cultural neuroscience: narrative, metaphor and mechanism. Cult Med Psychiatry 32 (1): 31–64.

Shor RE, Orne EC (1962). Harvard Group Scale of Hypnotic Susceptibility, Form A, Consulting Psychologists Press, Palo Alto, CA.

Spinhoven Ph (1989). Hypnosis and Pain Control. Academic thesis, University of Leiden, Repro, Meppel, Leiden, pp. 17–18.

Szekely A, Kovacs-Nagy R, Bányai ÉI et al. (2010). Association between hypnotizability and the catechol-*O*-methyltransferase (COMT) polymorphism. Int J Clin Exp Hypn 58 (3): 301–315.

Weitzenhoffer AM (1980). Hypnotic susceptibility revisited. Am J Clin Hypn 22: 130–146.

Weitzenhoffer AM, Hilgard ER (1962). Stanford hypnotic susceptibility scale, form C, Vol. 27. Consulting Psychologists Press, Palo Alto, CA.

Handbook of Clinical Neurology, Vol. 139 (3rd series)
Functional Neurologic Disorders
M. Hallett, J. Stone, and A. Carson, Editors
http://dx.doi.org/10.1016/B978-0-12-801772-2.00048-5

Chapter 48

Nature of the placebo and nocebo effect in relation to functional neurologic disorders

E. CARLINO[1], A. PIEDIMONTE[1], AND F. BENEDETTI[1,2]*
[1]*Department of Neuroscience, University of Turin Medical School, Turin, Italy*
[2]*Plateau Rosa Labs, Breuil-Cervinia, Italy and Zermatt, Switzerland*

Abstract

Placebos have long been considered a nuisance in clinical research, for they have always been used as comparators for the validation of new treatments. By contrast, today they represent an active field of research, and, due to the involvement of many mechanisms, the study of the placebo effect can actually be viewed as a melting pot of concepts and ideas for neuroscience. There is not a single placebo effect, but many, with different mechanisms across different medical conditions and therapeutic interventions. Expectation, anxiety, and reward are all involved, as well as a variety of learning phenomena and genetic variants. The most productive models to better understand the neurobiology of the placebo effect are pain and Parkinson's disease. In these medical conditions, several neurotransmitters have been identified, such as endogenous opioids, cholecystokinin, dopamine, as well as lipidic mediators, for example, endocannabinoids and prostaglandins. Since the placebo effect is basically a psychosocial context effect, these data indicate that different social stimuli, such as words and therapeutic rituals, may change the chemistry of the patient's brain, and these effects are similar to those induced by drugs.

DEFINITION

Placebos are usually defined as inert substances. However, this definition is not completely correct, because placebos are made of words and rituals, symbols and meanings, and all these elements are active in shaping the patient's brain. Therefore, a better definition of placebo should embrace both the inert substance and the psychosocial context around the patient and the therapy. Inert substances, such as saline solution, have long been used in clinical trials and double-blind randomized protocols in order to assess the efficacy of new therapies, e.g., new pharmacologic agents. Although inert substances are of great validity in the clinical trial setting, the clinical trialist has always drawn attention to the inertness of the substance itself, thus diverting it from the real meaning of placebo (Moerman, 2002). If drawing attention to the inert substance is correct in pragmatic clinical trials, whereby the only purpose is to see whether drugs are better than placebos, this surely does not help us understand what a placebo is (Benedetti, 2014a).

Thus, a real placebo effect is a psychobiologic phenomenon occurring in the patient's brain following the administration of an inert substance, or of a sham physical treatment such as sham surgery, along with verbal suggestions (or any other cue) of clinical benefit (Price et al., 2008). It is important to stress that saline solutions or sugar pills do not, of course, intrinsically have therapeutic properties. Instead, the effect is due to the psychosocial context that surrounds the inert substance and the patient. In this sense, to the clinical trialist and to the neurobiologist, the term "placebo effect" has different meanings. Whereas the former is interested in any improvement that may occur in the group of patients

*Correspondence to: Fabrizio Benedetti, Department of Neuroscience, University of Turin Medical School, Corso Raffaello 30, 10125 Turin, Italy. Tel: +39-011-6708492, Fax: +39-011-6708174, E-mail: fabrizio.benedetti@unito.it

who take the inert substance, regardless of its origin, the latter is only interested in the improvement that derives from active processes occurring in the patient's brain. In fact, the improvement in patients who are given a placebo can be ascribed to a vast array of factors, such as spontaneous remission of the disease (the so-called natural history), regression to the mean (a statistic phenomenon due to selection biases), patient's and doctor's biases, and unidentified effects of co-interventions. In pragmatic clinical trials, the trialist is interested in the improvement irrespective of its cause, because s/he only needs to establish whether the patients who take the true treatment, be it pharmacologic or not, are better off than those who take the placebo. This pragmatic approach yields fruitful results in clinical trials. However, if we are interested in understanding what a real placebo effect is and how it works, we need to separate it from spontaneous remissions, regression to the mean, biases, and the like (Benedetti, 2014a).

Taking all these considerations into account, the true placebo effect is only the psychobiologic phenomenon taking place in the patient's brain. All the other phenomena can be ruled out by using the appropriate methodologic approach. For example, in order to rule out spontaneous remission, the placebo group must be compared with a no-treatment group which gives us information on the natural history of the disease. Likewise, in order to rule out biases, such as those which may occur in subjective symptoms like pain, objective outcome measures must be assessed. From this methodologic perspective, placebo research is not easy to perform, for it requires rigorous experimental protocols and plenty of control groups.

The real placebo response, i.e., the real psychobiologic phenomenon, is not irrelevant. Its contribution to the clinical improvement is substantial. For example, in antidepressant clinical trials, it has been shown that the natural history of the disease (i.e., spontaneous remission) accounts for 23.87% of the overall effect, the real placebo effect (i.e., expectations of benefit) for 50.97%, and the drug effect for 25.16% only (Kirsch and Sapirstein, 1998). Thus, placebo responses in depression are usually large and they have been found to increase over time, with larger placebo responses in more recent studies (Walsh et al., 2002). A similar increase over time has been found in neuropathic pain (Katz et al., 2008).

Today this experimental approach to the placebo effect is paying dividends and bodes well for the future (Finniss et al., 2010). We now know that there is not a single placebo effect, but many, with different mechanisms and in different diseases, systems, and therapeutic interventions (Enck et al., 2008; Benedetti, 2013, 2014a, b).

CHARACTERIZATION OF THE NEUROBIOLOGIC UNDERPINNINGS

Isolating the psychobiologic component from spontaneous remissions and methodologic biases allows for an excellent model to investigate several brain functions within the medical context. Two main mechanisms have been the focus of attention: expectation and learning. Expectation is a conscious event whereby the subject expects a therapeutic benefit (Kirsch, 1999). The link between expectation and clinical improvement is twofold. First, positive expectations may reduce anxiety, and anxiety is known to affect different symptoms, such as pain, in opposite directions, i.e., either decrease or increase, depending on the circumstances (Colloca and Benedetti, 2007). Second, expectation of a positive event, i.e., the therapeutic benefit, may activate reward mechanisms. Learning mechanisms, ranging from behavioral conditioning to social learning, are crucial, because the previous experience of effective treatments leads to powerful placebo responses. Expectation and learning are not necessarily mutually exclusive, since learning can lead to the reinforcement of expectations or can even create *de novo* expectations. Although today it is not always clear when and how expectations and learning are involved in different types of placebo responses, they may overlap in a number of conditions. The following is a brief description of the main mechanisms that have been characterized by using a neurobiologic approach (for a detailed description, see Benedetti, 2014a).

The opioid system activated by placebos is the most studied and understood (Fig. 48.1A). The μ-opioid antagonist, naloxone, prevents some types of placebo analgesia, thus indicating that the opioid system plays an important role (Levine et al., 1978; Amanzio and Benedetti, 1999; Eippert et al., 2009a). The cholecystokinin (CCK) antagonist, proglumide, enhances placebo analgesia on the basis of the antiopioid action of CCK (Benedetti et al., 1995; Benedetti, 1996), whereas the activation of the CCK type 2 receptors with the agonist pentagastrin disrupts placebo analgesia (Benedetti et al., 2011a). Therefore, the activation of the CCK type 2 receptors has the same effect as μ-opioid receptor blockade, indicating that the balance between CCK and opioids is crucial in placebo responsiveness in pain (Fig. 48.1A). Some brain regions in the cerebral cortex and the brainstem are affected by both a placebo and the opioid agonist remifentanil, which suggests a related mechanism in placebo-induced and opioid-induced analgesia (Petrovic et al., 2002). *In vivo* receptor-binding techniques show that placebos activate μ-opioid neurotransmission in the dorsolateral prefrontal cortex, the anterior cingulate cortex, the insula, and the nucleus

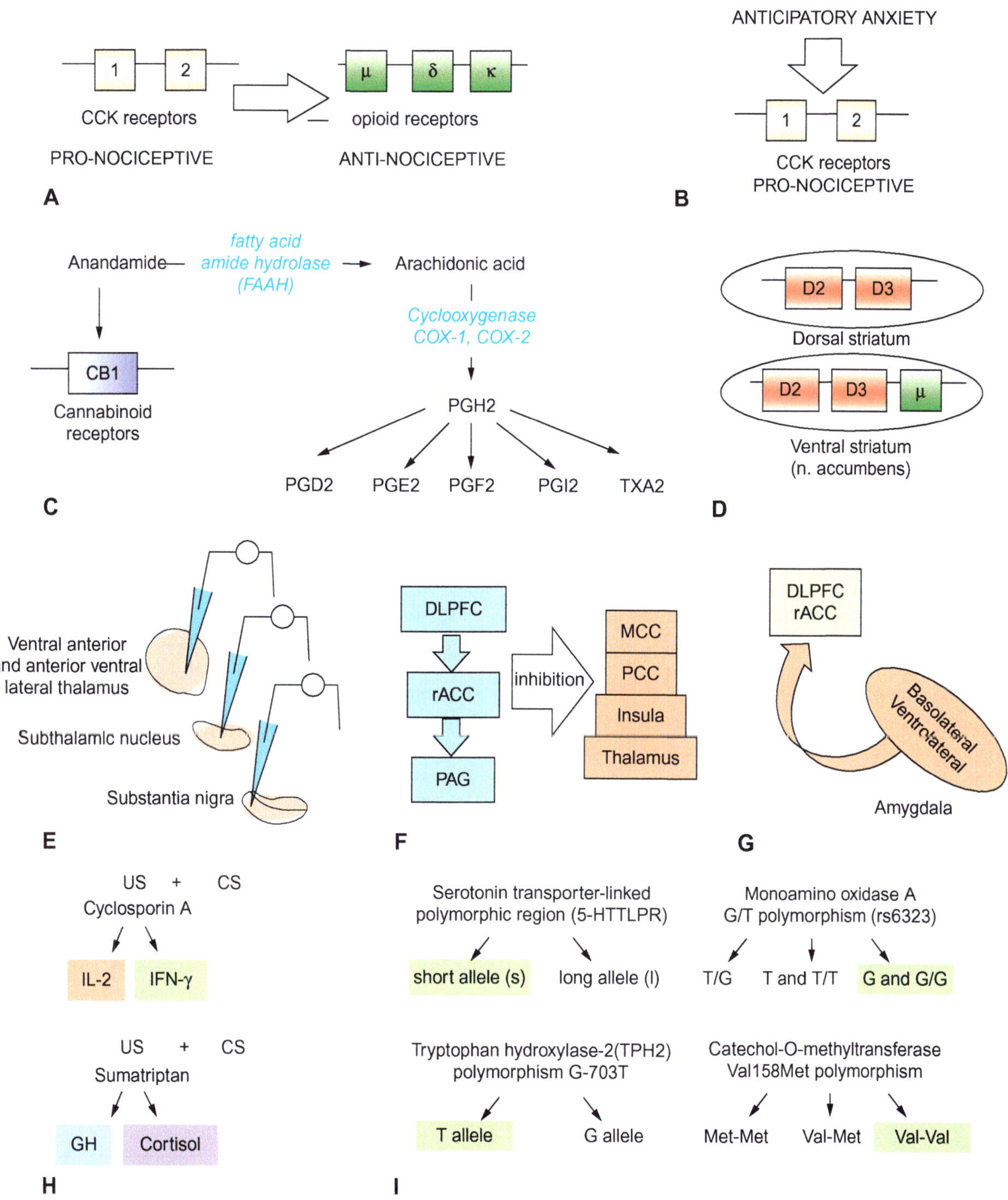

Fig. 48.1. Principal neurobiologic mechanisms of the placebo response that have been identified across a variety of conditions. (**A**) The antinociceptive opioid system is activated in placebo analgesia in some circumstances, and the μ – opiod receptors play a crucial role. The pronociceptive cholecystokinin (CCK) system antagonizes the opioid system, thus blocking placebo analgesia. (**B**) The pronociceptive CCK system is activated by anticipatory anxiety in nocebo hyperalgesia, with some evidence that the CCK-2 receptors are more important. (**C**) Different lipidic mediators have been identified in placebo analgesia and nocebo hyperalgesia. Whereas placebos activate the CB1 cannabinoid receptors and inhibit prostaglandins (PG) synthesis in some circumstances, nocebos increase PG synthesis. In addition, different genetic variants of fatty-acid amide hydrolase affect the magnitude of placebo analgesia. (**D**) The activation of D2–D3 dopamine receptors in the striatum is related to the placebo response in Parkinson's disease. Likewise, in placebo analgesia there is an activation of D2–D3 receptors and μ – opioid receptors in the nucleus accumbens, whereas in nocebo hyperalgesia there is a deactivation of D2–D3 and μ receptors. (**E**) Placebo administration

(*Continued*)

accumbens (Zubieta et al., 2005; Wager et al., 2007). Recent studies in rodents confirm these pharmacologic findings in humans (Guo et al., 2010; Nolan et al., 2012; Zhang et al., 2013). For example, by using different antagonists of different subtypes of opioid receptors (μ, δ, k), Zhang et al. (2013) found that placebo analgesia is mediated specifically by the μ-opioid receptors.

The CCK pronociceptive system has also been found to mediate nocebo hyperalgesia (Fig. 48.1B). The nocebo response is a phenomenon that is opposite to the placebo response, whereby negative expectations may lead to clinical worsening. For example, expectations of pain increase lead to nocebo hyperalgesia, and this increase can be blocked by the CCK antagonist proglumide (Benedetti et al., 1997, 2006a). Anticipatory anxiety plays a key role here, for nocebos are anxiogenic and induce negative expectations. Again, a social defeat model of anxiety in rats supports this view. In fact, CI-988, a selective CCK type 2 receptor antagonist, prevents anxiety-induced hyperalgesia (Andre et al., 2005).

When nonopioid drugs, like ketorolac, are administered for 2 days in a row and then replaced with a placebo on the third day, the placebo analgesic response is not reversed by naloxone, whereas the CB1 cannabinoid receptor antagonist, rimonabant, blocks this placebo analgesia completely (Benedetti et al., 2011b). Therefore, in some circumstances, for example, following previous exposure to nonopioid drugs, placebo analgesia is mediated by the CB1 cannabinoid receptors. Interestingly, there is compelling experimental evidence that the whole lipidic pathway, involving arachidonic acid, endogenous cannabinoid ligands (e.g., anandamide), and the synthesis of prostaglandins and thromboxane, is important in the modulation of the placebo response in pain (Fig. 48.1C). For example, the functional missense variant Pro129Thr of the gene coding fatty-acid amide hydrolase (FAAH), the major degrading enzyme of endocannabinoids, affects the analgesic responses to placebo as well as placebo-induced μ-opioid neurotransmission (Peciña et al., 2014). Moreover, cyclooxygenase, which is involved in prostaglandins and thromboxane synthesis (Fig. 48.1C), has been found to be modulated by both placebo and nocebo in hypobaric hypoxia, or high-altitude, headache with a mechanism similar to that of aspirin (Benedetti et al., 2014).

Dopamine is involved in placebo responsiveness in at least two conditions: pain and Parkinson's disease. In placebo analgesia, an increase in dopamine binding to D2/D3 receptors and in opioid binding to μ receptors occurs in the nucleus accumbens, whereas a decreased binding to the same receptors is present in nocebo hyperalgesia (Scott et al., 2007, 2008) (Fig. 48.1D). Likewise, dopamine receptors are activated in both ventral (nucleus accumbens) and dorsal striatum when a placebo is administered to patients with Parkinson's disease (de la Fuente-Fernandez et al., 2001, 2002; Lidstone et al., 2010) (Fig. 48.1D). The release of dopamine corresponds to a change of 200% or more in extracellular dopamine concentration, and is comparable to the response to amphetamine in subjects with an intact dopamine system. Dopaminergic activation in the nucleus accumbens in both pain and Parkinson's disease suggests that reward mechanisms could play an important role in many conditions.

Intraoperative single-neuron recording in placebo-treated parkinsonian patients during the implantation of electrodes for deep-brain stimulation (Fig. 48.1E) shows that the firing rate of the neurons in the subthalamic nucleus and substantia nigra pars reticulata decreases, whereas the firing rate of thalamic neurons in the ventral anterior and anterior ventral lateral thalamus increases, along with the disappearance of bursting activity in the subthalamic nucleus, when placebo is administered (Benedetti et al., 2004, 2009; Frisaldi et al., 2014). Although the dopamine findings and the electrophysiologic data were obtained in different studies (de la Fuente-Fernandez et al., 2001, 2002; Benedetti et al., 2004, 2009, respectively), the changes in firing pattern of the subthalamic and thalamic neurons are likely to be triggered by dopamine release.

Modern brain-imaging techniques have been fundamental in the understanding of the placebo response,

Fig. 48.1—Cont'd in Parkinson patients produces a decrease of firing rate and bursting activity of the subthalamic nucleus neurons. It also produces a decrease of firing rate in the substantia nigra pars reticulata and an increase in the ventral anterior and anterior ventral lateral thalamus. **(F)** The neuroanatomy of placebo analgesia has been described through brain imaging. Different regions are modulated by both placebos and nocebos, but the most studied and understood regions are the dorsolateral prefrontal cortex (DLPFC), the rostral anterior cingulate cortex (rACC), and the periaqueductal gray (PAG), which represent a descending pain-modulating network. This, in turn, inhibits those regions that are involved in pain processing, such as the mid and posterior cingulate cortex (MCC, PCC), insula, and thalamus. **(G)** In social anxiety disorder, placebos affect the basolateral and ventrolateral amygdala as well as its projections to DLPFC and rACC. **(H)** In the immune and endocrine system, the mechanism of the placebo response is classical conditioning, whereby an unconditioned stimulus (US) is paired with a conditioned stimulus (CS). For example, after pairing a CS with either cyclosporine A or sumatriptan, the CS alone can mimic the responses to cyclosporine and sumatriptan. IL-2, interleukin-2; IFN-γ, interferon-γ; GH, growth hormone. **(I)** Different polymorphisms have been found to be associated to low (squares) or high placebo responsiveness. (Reproduced from Benedetti, 2014b.)

particularly placebo analgesia, and many brain-imaging studies have been carried out to describe the functional neuroanatomy of the placebo analgesic effect (e.g., Petrovic et al., 2002; Wager et al., 2004; Zubieta et al., 2005; Bingel et al., 2006; Kong et al., 2006, 2007; Price et al., 2007; Scott et al., 2007, 2008; Eippert et al., 2009a, b; Lui et al., 2010; Tracey, 2010; Hashmi et al., 2012). A meta-analysis of brain-imaging data using the activation likelihood estimation method identified two phases: the expectation phase of analgesia and the pain inhibition phase (Amanzio et al., 2013). During expectation, areas of activation are found in the anterior cingulate, precentral and lateral prefrontal cortex, and in the periaqueductal gray. During pain inhibition, deactivations are found in the mid and posterior cingulate cortex, superior temporal and precentral gyri, in the anterior and posterior insula, in the claustrum and putamen, and in the thalamus and caudate body. Overall, many of the regions that are activated during expectation are likely to belong to a descending pain-inhibitory system that inhibits different areas involved in pain processing (Fig. 48.1 F).

In social anxiety disorder, positron emission tomography has been used to assess regional cerebral blood flow during an anxiogenic public speaking task, before and after 6–8 weeks of treatment with selective serotonin reuptake inhibitors (SSRIs) under double-blind conditions (Faria et al., 2012, 2014). Conjunction analysis reveals a common attenuation of regional cerebral blood flow from pre- to posttreatment in responders to SSRI and placebo in the left basomedial/basolateral and right ventrolateral amygdala, including amygdala-frontal projections to dorsolateral prefrontal cortex and rostral anterior cingulate cortices (Fig. 48.1G). This pattern correlates with behavioral measures of reduced anxiety and differentiates responders from nonresponders, with no differences between SSRI responders and placebo responders. Therefore, this pattern is capable of differentiating responders from nonresponders to both SSRI and placebos, suggesting that drugs and placebos act on common amygdalar targets and amygdala–frontal connections (Faria et al., 2012, 2014).

High temporal resolution techniques, such as electroencephalography, have also been used to better understand the effects of expectation and learning. In different studies on laser-evoked potentials (LEPs), placebos have been reported to affect both pain perception and the N2–P2 complex, which represents the largest LEP response, with peaks at approximately 200–350 ms after painful stimulation. These data show that placebo effects can be investigated at the electrophysiologic level, thus providing in the future an interesting approach to a more detailed temporal analysis (Wager et al., 2006; Colloca et al., 2008; Carlino et al., 2015).

Immune and endocrine responses can be behaviorally conditioned (Pacheco-López et al., 2005). When an unconditioned stimulus, e.g., the effect of a drug, is paired with a conditioned stimulus (CS), e.g., a gustatory stimulus, after repeated pairings the CS alone can mimic the effect of the drug (conditioned response). Since the CS is a neutral stimulus, it can be conceptualized as a placebo in all respects. Indeed, both immune mediators, like interleukin-2 (IL-2) and interferon-γ (IFN-γ), and hormones, like growth hormone (GH) and cortisol, can be conditioned in humans (Fig. 48.1H). After repeated associations of a CS with cyclosporine A or sumatriptan, which produces IL-2/IFN- γ decrease and GH increase/cortisol decrease, respectively, the CS alone can induce the same immune and hormonal responses (Goebel et al., 2002; Benedetti et al., 2003a).

An association of placebo responsiveness with some genetic variants has been described in some conditions (Fig. 48.1I). Patients with social anxiety disorder have been genotyped with respect to the serotonin transporter-linked polymorphic region (5-HTTLPR) and the G-703 T polymorphism in the tryptophan hydroxylase-2 (TPH2) gene promoter. Only patients homozygous for the long allele of the 5-HTTLPR or the G variant of the TPH2 G-703 T polymorphism show robust placebo responses and reduced activity in the amygdala, whereas carriers of short or T alleles do not show these effects (Furmark et al., 2008). In addition, in patients with major depressive disorder, polymorphisms in genes encoding the catabolic enzyme monoamine oxidase A are associated to the magnitude of the placebo response. Patients with monoamine oxidase A G/T polymorphisms (rs6323) coding for the highest activity form of the enzyme (G or G/G) show small placebo responses (Leuchter et al., 2009). Functional Val158Met polymorphism of the catabolic enzyme catechol-*O*-methyltransferase has been found to be associated with the placebo response in irritable-bowel syndrome. The lowest placebo responses occur in Val/Val homozygotes (Hall et al., 2012). As already described above, also the functional missense variant Pro129Thr of the gene coding FAAH has been found to affect the analgesic responses to placebo (Peciña et al., 2014).

DISRUPTION OF PLACEBO EFFECTS

Hidden administration of therapies has provided compelling evidence that expectation is a key element in therapeutic outcome (Colloca et al., 2004; Benedetti et al., 2011c). If the patient is unaware that a treatment is being performed and has no expectations about any clinical improvement, the therapy is not as efficacious. For example, the effectiveness of the benzodiazepine diazepam is reduced or completely abolished when it is administered unbeknownst to the patient (Benedetti et al., 2003b, 2011c; Colloca et al., 2004).

The same effects are present in other conditions, such as pain and Parkinson's disease (Benedetti et al., 2003b, 2011c; Colloca et al., 2004). In postoperative pain following the extraction of the third molar (Levine et al., 1981; Levine and Gordon, 1984), a hidden intravenous injection of 6–8 mg morphine corresponds to an open intravenous injection of saline solution in full view of the patient (placebo). In other words, telling the patient that a painkiller is being injected (with what is actually a saline solution) is as potent as 6–8 mg of morphine. This holds true for a variety of painkillers, such as morphine, buprenorphine, tramadol, ketorolac, metamizole, and remifentanil (Amanzio et al., 2001; Benedetti et al., 2003a; Colloca et al., 2004; Bingel et al., 2011).

A natural situation in which hidden therapies are delivered is represented by impaired cognition. Cognitively impaired patients do not have expectations about therapeutic benefits, so that the psychologic (placebo) component of a treatment is likely to be absent. On the basis of these considerations, Benedetti et al. (2006b) studied Alzheimer patients at the initial stage of the disease and after 1 year, in order to see whether the placebo component of the therapy is affected by the disease. The placebo component of an analgesic therapy was found to be correlated with both cognitive status and functional connectivity among different brain regions, according to the rule, "the more impaired the prefrontal connectivity, the smaller the placebo response" (Benedetti et al., 2006b).

To support this view, there are a number of studies which indicate that placebo responses are reduced when prefrontal functioning is impaired. First, the individual placebo analgesic effect is correlated with white-matter integrity indexed by fractional anisotropy, as assessed through diffusion tensor magnetic resonance imaging; stronger placebo analgesic responses are associated with increased mean fractional anisotropy values within white-matter tracts connecting the periaqueductal gray with the rostral anterior cingulate cortex and the dorsolateral prefrontal cortex (Stein et al., 2012). Second, inactivation of the frontal cortex with repetitive transcranial magnetic stimulation completely blocks the analgesic placebo response (Krummenacher et al., 2010). Third, the opioid antagonist naloxone blocks placebo analgesia, along with a reduction in the activation of the dorsolateral prefrontal cortex, suggesting that a prefrontal opioidergic mechanism is crucial in the placebo analgesic response (Eippert et al., 2009a). Therefore, both magnetic and pharmacologic inactivation of the prefrontal lobes have the same effects as those observed in prefrontal degeneration in Alzheimer's disease and reduced integrity of prefrontal white matter.

BEYOND THE HEALING CONTEXT

As for drug development, also in the assessment of efficacy of the many substances revolving around the sport world, there is a gray zone where placebos (and nocebos) can exert their influence. Here too, chemicals such as vitamins, ergogenic aids, or diet supplements are handed out, or physical treatments and manipulations of different kinds are delivered, and expectations about their effects are set in motion in the athlete's brain. In general, all available data indicate athletes' expectations as important elements of physical performance, in spite of the fact that very different experimental conditions have been investigated (Beedie and Foad, 2009; Pollo et al., 2011; Carlino et al., 2014a). These range from short anaerobic sprints to long aerobic endurance cycling, and many different outcome measures have been used, such as time, speed, and weight lifted. Indeed, many clinical trials of ergogenic and performance-boosting agents have been performed in a variety of sports.

In a simulation of sport competition in which subjects had to compete with each other in a competition of pain endurance, placebo administration on the day of competition was found to induce longer pain tolerance compared to an untreated group. However, if pharmacologic preconditioning is performed with morphine in the precompetition phase, the replacement of morphine with a placebo on the day of the competition induces an increase in pain endurance and physical performance that is significantly larger than placebo without prior morphine preconditioning. The placebo effect after morphine preconditioning can be prevented by administration of the opioid antagonist, naloxone, which suggests that this placebo response is opioid-mediated (Benedetti et al., 2007).

Similar findings can be obtained with a nonpharmacologic conditioning procedure (Pollo et al., 2008; Carlino et al., 2014b), in which the effects of an ergogenic placebo on the quadriceps muscle, which is responsible for extension of the leg relative to the thigh, can be assessed. A placebo, which the subjects believe to be caffeine at high doses, is administered twice in two different sessions. Each time the weight to be lifted with the quadriceps is reduced surreptitiously so as to make the subjects believe that the "ergogenic agent" is effective. After this conditioning procedure, the load is restored to the original weight, and both muscle work and fatigue are assessed after placebo administration. A robust placebo effect occurs with this procedure, with a significant increase in muscle work and a decrease in muscle fatigue.

Within the context of recent theories of muscle fatigue, these placebo responses acquire a very important meaning. In fact, central mechanisms would play a role in muscle performance and fatigue, as postulated early in the 1910s by Krogh and Lindhard (1913) through the concept of central command. The notion of central command, or central governor, implies that several physiologic parameters like heart rate, arterial blood pressure, pulmonary ventilation, and muscle performance could be altered by manipulating the subject's perception of exercise. Muscle fatigue has also been found to be affected by a central governor (St Clair Gibson et al., 2003, 2006; Lambert et al., 2005). In many studies, athletes are usually asked to perform at their limit, in an all-out effort. Placebos apparently act by pushing this limit forward. Therefore, it can be speculated that they could impact on a central governor of fatigue. The output of this center would continuously regulate exercise performance to avoid reaching maximal physiologic capacity. This would provide protection against damage on one hand, and constant availability of a reserve capacity on the other (Hampson et al., 2001; Lambert et al., 2005). By altering expectations, placebos could then represent a psychologic means to signal the central governor to release the brake, allowing an increase in performance in a manner not dissimilar from that achieved by pharmacologic means (for example, by amphetamines decreasing perceived fatigue).

It is interesting to note that the concept of a central governor has been applied to health as well, thus extending from fatigue and physical performance to the healing environment (Humphrey and Skoyles, 2012). To support this view, a recent study found that placebos modulate the anticipatory phase of movement, as assessed through the readiness potential, along with perceived fatigue, which suggests a central origin of fatigue and a central action of placebos (Piedimonte et al., 2015).

Nocebo effects are also important in physical performance. For example, in a 30-meter repeat-sprint protocol, placebo capsules coupled with different positive or negative instructions led to increased and decreased speed, respectively (Beedie et al., 2007). Likewise, it is possible to negatively modulate the performance of subjects carrying out a muscle exercise to volitional maximum effort by employing discouraging suggestions and negative conditioning (Pollo et al., 2012). These findings may have profound implications for training strategies, because negative expectations may counteract the positive effects of training programs.

A number of studies suggest that placebos and expectations also enhance, at least in part and in some circumstances, cognitive performance (Green et al., 2001; Oken et al., 2008; Parker et al., 2011; Weger and Loughnan, 2013) and other cognition-related tasks, such as reaction times (Anderson and Horne, 2008; Colagiuri et al., 2011), although nothing is known about the underlying mechanisms. However, it is interesting to note that a placebo, which subjects believed to be a memory-boosting drug, was found to increase short-term memory through the endogenous opioid system (Stern et al., 2011).

WHAT IS THE DIFFERENCE BETWEEN PLACEBOS AND DRUGS?

One of the most interesting concepts emerging today is that placebos and drugs may share common biochemical pathways, such as the endogenous opioid system, the endocannabinoid system, the cyclooxygenase pathway, and the dopaminergic system. For example, the analgesic morphine and the antiparkinsonian apomorphine act on opioid and dopamine receptors, respectively, but expectation of receiving morphine or apomorphine activates the same opioid and dopamine receptors, respectively. In spite of this similarity in the mechanism of action, placebos and drugs show many differences (Benedetti, 2014c).

Duration of action

In general, the duration of the effect of a drug is longer than that of a placebo. As far as we know today, this holds true for painkillers and antiparkinsonian agents, whereas much less is known about other therapeutic interventions. For example, the effect of the powerful antiparkinsonian drug apomorphine lasts on average much more than a placebo (Benedetti, 2014c).

Variability of effect

The larger variability in the response to placebos is present in many conditions, such as pain and Parkinson's disease. Thus, the response to a pharmacologic agent is usually more constant and less variable (Benedetti, 2014a, c).

Magnitude of effect

The effect following placebo administration can be as large as the effect following drug administration. For example, some good placebo responders may show a reduction of the Unified Parkinson's Disease Rating Scale of up to 50%, as occurs for drugs (Benedetti et al., 2004, 2009; Benedetti, 2014b; Frisaldi et al., 2014).

Similar differences are present in nocebo effects, whereby duration, variability, and magnitude of effects are comparable to those observed following the administration of placebos. Interestingly, in analgesic clinical trials for migraine, patients who receive the placebo often report a high frequency of adverse events, and these negative effects correspond to those of the antimigraine medication against which the placebo is compared (Amanzio et al., 2009). This is attributable to the important role of expectation in the placebo/nocebo phenomenon, such that sometimes patients get what they expect, for example, by reading the possible side-effects described in the informed consent.

CONCLUSIONS

Until a couple of decades ago, very little was known about the mechanisms and the very nature of both placebos and nocebos. What we have learned today, thanks to a more rigorous scientific approach and to modern neurobiologic tools, is that placebos modulate the very same biochemical pathways that are modulated by those drugs which are administered in routine clinical practice. The challenge for future research will be to characterize these placebo mechanisms across a variety of medical conditions and therapeutic interventions. For example, very little is known about the neurobiologic underpinnings of the placebo and nocebo effect in functional neurologic disorders, with the notable exception of some mechanisms in motor disorders and pain, as described throughout this chapter. However, it should be noted that functional disorders might represent a very nice model to better understand placebo and nocebo effects, because different psychologic factors may play a crucial role here. This warrants a more indepth analysis of all these functional conditions, which will certainly provide important information in the near future for a better understanding of human biology and medicine, as well as the design of clinical trials.

ACKNOWLEDGMENTS

This work was supported by grants from Compagnia di San Paolo Foundation, Giancarlo Quarta Foundation, Carlo Molo Foundation, and from the ICTH Initiative.

References

Amanzio M, Benedetti F (1999). Neuropharmacological dissection of placebo analgesia: expectation-activated opioid systems versus conditioning-activated specific subsystems. J Neurosci 19 (1): 484–494.

Amanzio M, Pollo A, Maggi G et al. (2001). Response variability to analgesics: a role for non-specific activation of endogenous opioids. Pain 90 (3): 205–215.

Amanzio M, Corazzini LL, Vase L et al. (2009). A systematic review of adverse events in placebo groups of anti-migraine clinical trials. Pain 146 (3): 261–269.

Amanzio M, Benedetti F, Porro CA et al. (2013). Activation likelihood estimation meta-analysis of brain correlates of placebo analgesia in human experimental pain. Hum Brain Mapp 34 (3): 738–752.

Anderson C, Horne JA (2008). Placebo response to caffeine improves reaction time performance in sleepy people. Hum Psychopharmacol 23 (4): 333–336.

Andre J, Zeau B, Pohl M et al. (2005). Involvement of cholecystokininergic systems in anxiety-induced hyperalgesia in male rats: behavioral and biochemical studies. J Neurosci 25 (35): 7896–7904.

Beedie CJ, Foad AJ (2009). The placebo effect in sports performance: a brief review. Sports Med 39 (4): 313–329.

Beedie CJ, Coleman DA, Foad AJ (2007). Positive and negative placebo effects resulting from the deceptive administration of an ergogenic aid. Int J Sport Nutr Exerc Metabol 17: 259–269.

Benedetti F (1996). The opposite effects of the opiate antagonist naloxone and the cholecystokinin antagonist proglumide on placebo analgesia. Pain 64 (3): 535–543.

Benedetti F (2013). Placebo and the new physiology of the doctor–patient relationship. Physiol Rev 93 (3): 1207–1246.

Benedetti F (2014a). Placebo effects, 2nd edn. Oxford University Press, New York.

Benedetti F (2014b). Placebo effects: from the neurobiological paradigm to translational implications. Neuron 84 (3): 623–637.

Benedetti F (2014c). Drugs and placebos: what's the difference? Understanding the molecular basis of the placebo effect could help clinicians to better use it in clinical practice. EMBO Rep 15 (4): 329–332.

Benedetti F, Amanzio M, Maggi G (1995). Potentiation of placebo analgesia by proglumide. Lancet 346 (8984): 1231.

Benedetti F, Amanzio M, Casadio C et al. (1997). Blockade of nocebo hyperalgesia by the cholecystokinin antagonist proglumide. Pain 71 (2): 135–140.

Benedetti F, Pollo A, Lopiano L (2003a). Conscious expectation and unconscious conditioning in analgesic, motor, and hormonal placebo/nocebo responses. J Neurosci 23 (10): b4315–b4323.

Benedetti F, Maggi G, Lopiano L et al. (2003b). Open versus hidden medical treatments: the patient's knowledge about a therapy affects the therapy outcome. Prev Treat 6 (1).

Benedetti F, Colloca L, Torre E et al. (2004). Placebo-responsive Parkinson patients show decreased activity in single neurons of subthalamic nucleus. Nat Neurosci 7 (6): 587–588.

Benedetti F, Amanzio M, Vighetti S et al. (2006a). The biochemical and neuroendocrine bases of the hyperalgesic nocebo effect. J Neurosci 26 (46): 12014–12022.

Benedetti F, Arduino C, Costa S et al. (2006b). Loss of expectation-related mechanisms in Alzheimer's disease makes analgesic therapies less effective. Pain 121 (1–2): 133–144.

Benedetti F, Pollo A, Colloca L (2007). Opioid-mediated placebo responses boost pain endurance and physical performance: is it doping in sport competitions? J Neurosci 27 (44): b11934–b11939.

Benedetti F, Lanotte M, Colloca L et al. (2009). Electrophysiological properties of thalamic, subthalamic and nigral neurons during the anti-parkinsonian placebo response. J Physiol (Lond) 587: 3869–3883.

Benedetti F, Amanzio M, Thoen W (2011a). Disruption of opioid-induced placebo responses by activation of cholecystokinin type-2 receptors. Psychopharmacology (Berl) 213 (4): 791–797.

Benedetti F, Amanzio M, Rosato R et al. (2011b). Nonopioid placebo analgesia is mediated by CB1 cannabinoid receptors. Nat Med 17: 1228–1230.

Benedetti F, Carlino E, Pollo A (2011c). Hidden administration of drugs. Clin Pharmacol Ther 90 (5): 651–661.

Benedetti F, Durando J, Vighetti S (2014). Nocebo and placebo modulation of hypobaric hypoxia headache involves the cyclooxygenase-prostaglandins pathway. Pain 155 (5): 921–928.

Bingel U, Lorenz J, Schoell E et al. (2006). Mechanisms of placebo analgesia: rACC recruitment of a subcortical antinociceptive network. Pain 120 (1–2): 8–15.

Bingel U, Wanigasekera V, Wiech K et al. (2011). The effect of treatment expectation on drug efficacy: imaging the analgesic benefit of the opioid remifentanil. Sci Transl Med 3 (70): 70ra14.

Carlino E, Piedimonte A, Frisaldi E (2014a). The effects of placebos and nocebos on physical performance. In: F Benedetti, P Enck, E Frisaldi et al. (Eds.), Placebo, Springer, Berlin, pp. 149–157.

Carlino E, Benedetti F, Pollo A (2014b). The effects of manipulating verbal suggestions on physical performance. Zeitschrift für Psychologie 222 (3): 154–164.

Carlino E, Torta DM, Piedimonte A et al. (2015). Role of explicit verbal information in conditioned analgesia. Eur J Pain 19: 546–553.

Colagiuri B, Livesey EJ, Harris JA (2011). Can expectancies produce placebo effects for implicit learning? Psychon Bull Rev 18 (2): 399–405.

Colloca L, Benedetti F (2007). Nocebo hyperalgesia: how anxiety is turned into pain. Curr Opin Anaesthesiol 20 (5): 435–439.

Colloca L, Lopiano L, Lanotte M et al. (2004). Overt versus covert treatment for pain, anxiety, and Parkinson's disease. Lancet Neurol 3 (11): 679–684.

Colloca L, Tinazzi M, Recchia S et al. (2008). Learning potentiates neurophysiological and behavioral placebo analgesic responses. Pain 139 (2): 306–314.

De la Fuente-Fernández R, Ruth TJ, Sossi V et al. (2001). Expectation and dopamine release: mechanism of the placebo effect in Parkinson's disease. Science 293 (5532): 1164–1166.

De la Fuente-Fernández R, Phillips AG, Zamburlini M et al. (2002). Dopamine release in human ventral striatum and expectation of reward. Behav Brain Res 136 (2): 359–363.

Eippert F, Bingel U, Schoell ED et al. (2009a). Activation of the opioidergic descending pain control system underlies placebo analgesia. Neuron 63 (4): 533–543.

Eippert F, Finsterbusch J, Bingel U et al. (2009b). Direct evidence for spinal cord involvement in placebo analgesia. Science 326 (5951): 404.

Enck P, Benedetti F, Schedlowski M (2008). New insights into the placebo and nocebo responses. Neuron 59 (2): 195–206.

Faria V, Appel L, Åhs F et al. (2012). Amygdala subregions tied to SSRI and placebo response in patients with social anxiety disorder. Neuropsychopharmacology 37 (10): 2222–2232.

Faria V, Ahs F, Appel L et al. (2014). Amygdala-frontal couplings characterizing SSRI and placebo response in social anxiety disorder. Int J Neuropsychopharmacol 17 (8): 1149–1157.

Finniss DG, Kaptchuk TJ, Miller F et al. (2010). Biological, clinical, and ethical advances of placebo effects. Lancet 375 (9715): 686–695.

Frisaldi E, Carlino E, Lanotte M et al. (2014). Characterization of the thalamic-subthalamic circuit involved in the placebo response through single-neuron recording in Parkinson patients. Cortex 60C (Nov): 3–9.

Furmark T, Appel L, Henningsson S et al. (2008). A link between serotonin-related gene polymorphisms, amygdala activity, and placebo-induced relief from social anxiety. J Neurosci 28 (49): 13066–13074.

Goebel MU, Trebst AE, Steiner J et al. (2002). Behavioral conditioning of immunosuppression is possible in humans. FASEB J 16 (14): 1869–1873.

Green MW, Taylor MA, Elliman NA et al. (2001). Placebo expectancy effects in the relationship between glucose and cognition. Br J Nutr 86 (2): 173–179.

Guo JY, Wang JY, Luo F (2010). Dissection of placebo analgesia in mice: the conditions for activation of opioid and non-opioid systems. J Psychopharmacol 24 (10): 1561–1567.

Hall KT, Lembo AJ, Kirsch I et al. (2012). Catechol-*O*-methyltransferase val158met polymorphism predicts placebo effect in irritable bowel syndrome. PLoS One 7 (10): e48135.

Hampson DB, St Clair Gibson A, Lambert MI et al. (2001). The influence of sensory cues on the perception of exertion during exercise and central regulation of exercise performance. Sports Med 31 (13): 935–952.

Hashmi JA, Baria AT, Baliki MN et al. (2012). Brain networks predicting placebo analgesia in a clinical trial for chronic back pain. Pain 153 (12): 2393–2402.

Humphrey N, Skoyles J (2012). The evolutionary psychology of healing: a human success story. Curr Biol 22 (17): R695–R698.

Katz J, Finnerup NB, Dworkin RH (2008). Clinical trial outcome in neuropathic pain: relationship to study characteristics. Neurology 70: 263–272.

Kirsch I (1999). How Expectancies Shape Experience, American Psychological Association, Washington, DC.

Kirsch I, Sapirstein G (1998). Listening to Prozac but hearing placebo: a meta-analysis of antidepressant medication. Prev Treat 1 (2).

Kong J, Gollub RL, Rosman IS et al. (2006). Brain activity associated with expectancy-enhanced placebo analgesia as measured by functional magnetic resonance imaging. J Neurosci 26 (2): 381–388.

Kong J, Kaptchuk TJ, Polich G et al. (2007). Placebo analgesia: findings from brain imaging studies and emerging hypotheses. Rev Neurosci 18 (3-4): 173–190.

Krogh A, Lindhard J (1913). The regulation of respiration and circulation during the initial stages of muscular work. J Physiol 47 (1–2): 112–136.

Krummenacher P, Candia V, Folkers G et al. (2010). Prefrontal cortex modulates placebo analgesia. Pain 148 (3): 368–374.

Lambert EV, St Clair Gibson A, Noakes TD (2005). Complex systems model of fatigue: integrative homoeostatic control of peripheral physiological systems during exercise in humans. Br J Sports Med 39 (1): 52–62.

Leuchter AF, McCracken JT, Hunter AM et al. (2009). Monoamine oxidase a and catechol-*o*-methyltransferase functional polymorphisms and the placebo response in major depressive disorder. J Clin Psychopharmacol 29 (4): 372–377.

Levine JD, Gordon NC (1984). Influence of the method of drug administration on analgesic response. Nature 312 (5996): 755–756.

Levine JD, Gordon NC, Fields HL (1978). The mechanism of placebo analgesia. Lancet 2 (8091): 654–657.

Levine JD, Gordon NC, Smith R et al. (1981). Analgesic responses to morphine and placebo in individuals with postoperative pain. Pain 10 (3): 379–389.

Lidstone SC, Schulzer M, Dinelle K et al. (2010). Effects of expectation on placebo-induced dopamine release in Parkinson disease. Arch Gen Psychiatry 67 (8): 857–865.

Lui F, Colloca L, Duzzi D et al. (2010). Neural bases of conditioned placebo analgesia. Pain 151 (3): 816–824.

Moerman DE (2002). Meaning, Medicine and the "Placebo Effect", Cambridge University Press, Cambridge.

Nolan TA, Price DD, Caudle RM et al. (2012). Placebo-induced analgesia in an operant pain model in rats. Pain 153 (10): 2009–2016.

Oken BS, Flegal K, Zajdel D et al. (2008). Expectancy effect: impact of pill administration on cognitive performance in healthy seniors. J Clin Exp Neuropsychol 30 (1): 7–17.

Pacheco-López G, Niemi M-B, Kou W et al. (2005). Neural substrates for behaviorally conditioned immunosuppression in the rat. J Neurosci 25 (9): 2330–2337.

Parker S, Garry M, Einstein GO et al. (2011). A sham drug improves a demanding prospective memory task. Memory 19 (6): 606–612.

Peciña M, Martínez-Jauand M, Hodgkinson C et al. (2014). FAAH selectively influences placebo effects. Mol Psychiatry 19 (3): 385–391.

Petrovic P, Kalso E, Petersson KM et al. (2002). Placebo and opioid analgesia – imaging a shared neuronal network. Science 295 (5560): 1737–1740.

Piedimonte A, Benedetti F, Carlino E (2015). Placebo-induced decrease in fatigue: evidence for a central action on the preparatory phase of movement. Eur J Neurosci 41: 492–497.

Pollo A, Carlino E, Benedetti F (2008). The top-down influence of ergogenic placebos on muscle work and fatigue. Eur J Neurosci 28 (2): 379–388.

Pollo A, Carlino E, Benedetti F (2011). Placebo mechanisms across different conditions: from the clinical setting to physical performance. Philos Trans R Soc Lond B Biol Sci 366 (1572): 1790–1798.

Pollo A, Carlino E, Vase L et al. (2012). Preventing motor training through nocebo suggestions. Eur J Appl Physiol 112 (11): 3893–3903.

Price DD, Craggs J, Verne GN et al. (2007). Placebo analgesia is accompanied by large reductions in pain-related brain activity in irritable bowel syndrome patients. Pain 127 (1–2): 63–72.

Price DD, Finniss DG, Benedetti F (2008). A comprehensive review of the placebo effect: recent advances and current thought. Annu Rev Psychol 59: 565–590.

Scott DJ, Stohler CS, Egnatuk CM et al. (2007). Individual differences in reward responding explain placebo-induced expectations and effects. Neuron 55 (2): 325–336.

Scott DJ, Stohler CS, Egnatuk CM et al. (2008). Placebo and nocebo effects are defined by opposite opioid and dopaminergic responses. Arch Gen Psychiatry 65 (2): 220–231.

St Clair Gibson A, Baden DA, Lambert MI et al. (2003). The conscious perception of the sensation of fatigue. Sports Med 33 (3): 167–176.

St Clair Gibson A, Lambert EV, Rauch LHG et al. (2006). The role of information processing between the brain and peripheral physiological systems in pacing and perception of effort. Sports Med 36 (8): 705–722.

Stein N, Sprenger C, Scholz J et al. (2012). White matter integrity of the descending pain modulatory system is associated with interindividual differences in placebo analgesia. Pain 153 (11): 2210–2217.

Stern J, Candia V, Porchet RI et al. (2011). Placebo-mediated, Naloxone-sensitive suggestibility of short-term memory performance. Neurobiol Learn Mem 95 (3): 326–334.

Tracey I (2010). Getting the pain you expect: mechanisms of placebo, nocebo and reappraisal effects in humans. Nat Med 16 (11): 1277–1283.

Wager TD, Rilling JK, Smith EE et al. (2004). Placebo-induced changes in FMRI in the anticipation and experience of pain. Science 303 (5661): 1162–1167.

Wager TD, Matre D, Casey KL (2006). Placebo effects in laser-evoked pain potentials. Brain Behav Immun 20 (3): 219–230.

Wager TD, Scott DJ, Zubieta JK (2007). Placebo effects on human mu-opioid activity during pain. Proc Natl Acad Sci U S A 104 (26): 11056–11061.

Walsh BT, Seidman SN, Sysko R et al. (2002). Placebo response in studies of major depression: variable, substantial, and growing. JAMA 287: 1840–1847.

Weger UW, Loughnan S (2013). Mobilizing unused resources: using the placebo concept to enhance cognitive performance. Q J Exp Psychol 66 (1): 23–28.

Zhang RR, Zhang WC, Wang JY et al. (2013). The opioid placebo analgesia is mediated exclusively through μ-opioid receptor in rat. Int J Neuropsychopharmacol 16 (4): 849–856.

Zubieta J-K, Bueller JA, Jackson LR et al. (2005). Placebo effects mediated by endogenous opioid activity on mu-opioid receptors. J Neurosci 25 (34): 7754–7762.

Handbook of Clinical Neurology, Vol. 139 (3rd series)
Functional Neurologic Disorders
M. Hallett, J. Stone, and A. Carson, Editors
http://dx.doi.org/10.1016/B978-0-12-801772-2.00049-7

Chapter 49

The role of placebo in the diagnosis and treatment of functional neurologic disorders

K.S. ROMMELFANGER*

Department of Neurology, Department of Psychiatry and Neuroethics Program, Center for Ethics, Emory University, Atlanta, GA, USA

Abstract

Placebo therapy can produce meaningful, clinical relief for a variety of conditions. While placebos are not without their ethically fraught history, they continue to be used, largely covertly, even today. Because the prognosis for psychogenic disorders is often poor and recovery may be highly dependent on the patient's belief in the diagnosis and treatment regimen, some physicians find placebo therapy for psychogenic disorders compelling, but also particularly contentious. Yet placebos also have a long tradition of being used for provocative diagnosis (wherein placebo is used to elicit and/or terminate the symptoms as a way of diagnosing symptoms as "psychogenic"). In this chapter we discuss cases describing placebo as therapy for psychogenic disorders and the challenges related to embedded Cartesian beliefs in Western medicine. The legitimate ethical reservations against placebo therapy, in general, have been related to assumptions about their "inertness" and a requirement for deception, both which are being refuted by emerging data. In this chapter, we also re-evaluate the concerns associated with placebo therapy for psychogenic disorders by asking, "Are we harming patients by withholding placebo treatment?"

EVOLVING CONTROVERSY OVER THERAPEUTIC PLACEBO

In the medical context, "placebo" is typically described as an innocuous treatment that is given to reinforce a patient's expectation to get well (Diederich and Goetz, 2008; Finniss et al., 2010). The gold standard of clinical trials includes a double-blind, placebo-controlled study wherein new treatment interventions must demonstrate greater benefit than placebo. However, placebos have effects that can rival new therapies. Discovering interventions devoid of or better than placebo effects can be challenging, a reminder that placebo controls are not used for their lack of effects; they are used because of their very strong effects. Just the act of taking medicine or providing a suggestion that medicine might work can impact patient outcomes. With such clinical effects one might wonder why the research and development of placebo therapies have not received more open conversation.

The therapeutic benefits of placebo have been long integrated into the popular imagination. This is perhaps part of its strength and popularity as well as its controversial evaluation and perhaps ethical demise. In 1621, Robert Burton wrote in The Anatomy of Melancholy that "a silly chirurgeon, doth more strange cures than a rational physician … because the patient puts his confidence in him" (Burton, 1621). In 1807 Thomas Jefferson had described therapeutic placebo as a "pious fraud" yet he still noted that "one of the most successful physicians … used more of bread pills, drops of colored water, and powders of hickory ashes, than all other medicines put together" (Ford, 1898). Arguments about the ethics of therapeutic placebos during the 19th and 20th centuries have remained fairly consistent. The problem can be summed as follows: placebos seem to "work," but not in the "right way." That is, patients report being better after placebo intervention (and this can be corroborated by an

*Correspondence to: Karen S. Rommelfanger, Department of Neurology, Emory University, 1531 Dickey Drive, Atlanta GA 30322, USA. E-mail: krommel@emory.edu

objective external observer). Yet placebos are by definition inert, their effects ostensibly achieved through deceptive manipulation of a vulnerable patient's mind or by implanting false beliefs about an inert remedy. Despite a pervasive view that it is categorically wrong to lie to patients (a violation of physicians' duty to be truthful both in their science and in their interaction with patients) – given the imbalance of power between the patient and physician and the vulnerable state of the patient – placebo use remains quite prevalent in medical practice.

Two independent studies report that 50% of US physicians have used placebo in clinical practice (Sherman and Hickner, 2008; Tilburt et al., 2008) for a variety of disorders, from gastrointestinal and immune disorders to cancer and neurologic disorders (Sherman and Hickner, 2008). Physicians include as placebo treatments items such as saline, sugar pills, vitamins, over-the-counter analgesics, antibiotics, and sedatives (Tilburt et al., 2008), and describe placebo therapy as "a substance that may help and will not hurt," "it is medication," "it is medicine with no specific effect," "a medicine not typically used for your condition but might benefit you," or say, "This may help you, but I am not sure how it works" (Sherman and Hickner, 2008; Tilburt et al., 2008). These statements reveal a method of communicating information that often falls on a spectrum somewhere between acceptable norms of simplifying explanations (where a physician states that a pill is simply an "antibiotic" or "antihistamine") to verbal misdirection to create a false impression of the treatment.

While the use of placebo has remained prevalent across the globe (Hrobjartsson and Norup, 2003; Tilburt et al., 2008; Fassler et al., 2010; Meissner et al., 2012; Howick et al., 2013), this practice does not reflect contemporary professional society values such as those of the American Medical Association (AMA: the AMA only in 2006 categorically prohibited deceptive placebo use) and the UK General Medical Council (Bostick et al., 2008; Blease, 2012). The popular use of therapeutic placebo also seems to prevail, even in the absence of a clear understanding of its precise mechanism: placebo helps somehow and, as for the mechanism, chalk it up to the mind (in this case, meaning imagination or expectation), as ethically unsatisfactory as that may be for some. So a consequentialist approach (because of the ultimate benefit to the patient, the end justifies the means) seems to explain placebo therapy's popularity amongst physicians, a deontologic view (the duty not to lie about a treatment that is inert) seems to drive ethical concerns, and ultimately the result is a relatively widespread use of placebo in a veiled manner (veiled to everyone, from physicians to their patients, except to the researchers who study the use of therapeutic placebo). Largely the arguments on whether to use placebo have come to a stalemate. While the ethical concerns are the same, the definition and what we know about placebos are evolving (Benedetti, 2014; Chapter 48), which necessitates that their utility and the contexts for their use be called into question once more.

One of the key concerns with placebo therapy is that the intervention involves a deceptive act because placebo is generally defined as being "inert" for the medical purpose for which it is prescribed (Ernst, 2007). However, a significant body of research has established neurophysiologic substrates of placebo activity (Enck et al., 2008), which challenges notions that placebos are truly inert. Placebo responses in disorders with established biochemical pathways have been quite prevalent: 16–55% of Parkinson's disease patients (Goetz et al., 2008), 30% of pain (migraine) patients (Bendtsen et al., 2003), and 50% of depressed patients (Dworkin et al., 2005). Studies have demonstrated enhanced endogenous release of neurotransmitters such as dopamine (de la Fuente-Fernandez et al., 2001; Mercado et al., 2006; Lidstone et al., 2010) as well as placebo-induced, therapeutically associated changes in neuronal activity (Benedetti et al., 2004). And placebo-induced opiate release (Zubieta et al., 2005; Wager et al., 2007) can be reversed with specific antagonists, such as naloxone (Amanzio and Benedetti, 1999), indicating that placebos can have specificity in their influence of endogenous neurochemistry. With the definition of placebo changing because of new insights into the mechanisms behind placebo, we start to see that even our use of the word placebo has become an anachronistic placeholder, or something akin to thingamajig, rather than an actually effectively representative word.

PLACEBO FOR PSYCHOGENIC DISORDERS

Placebo can produce meaningful, clinical relief for a variety of conditions. However, placebos also have a long tradition of being used for diagnosis, particularly in the case of psychogenic disorders.

For diagnosis

For psychogenic nonepileptic seizures (PNES), there is a rich literature of placebo use for diagnosing, so-called provocative testing, wherein placebo is used to elicit and/or terminate the symptoms. While not without its own ethical controversies and uncertainties (Stagno and Smith, 1997), diagnosing PNES with provocative testing can be done with a bit more confidence alongside data provided by subsequent video-electroencephalogram (EEG) monitoring (Devinsky et al., 2011). In these scenarios, patients can be kept in the hospital for observation and provoked with a suggestion or a placebo, hoping to induce a typical event (either seizure or PNES). The provocation involves a somewhat performative element with the healthcare team carefully narrating the procedure with positive suggestive statements for the seizure to occur, i.e., "when the episode occurs" versus "if the episode occurs" (Devinsky and Fisher, 1996). Other techniques are perhaps more simple, involving statements like, "hyperventilation might bring on attacks" (McGonigal et al., 2002). If the observed event is representative of their typical experiences, then physicians can determine whether those events were accompanied by abnormal EEG activity. If the saline, tuning fork, alcohol-soaked pad, etc., provokes an event and there is no abnormal EEG activity, physicians feel more confident in saying that these events were indeed psychogenic.

Patients with psychogenic movement disorders (PMDs) are often thought to be quite suggestible and the original diagnosis of PMD was based on a positive response to placebo as a therapy (Fahn and Williams, 1988; Factor et al., 1995). In the absence of a diagnostic tool, such as video-EEG for PNES, such placebo usage for PMD becomes enticing for physicians. While many neurologists currently report that placebo confirmation of PMD is useful, they do not endorse it (Espay et al., 2009), likely due to ethical reservations. Yet there are some who argue that placebo can be quite invaluable supportive evidence in assisting in a differential diagnosis. For example, one author notes the use of 25 mg carbidopa, which does not cross the blood–brain barrier, and so is not typically used for alleviation of motor symptoms. If patients respond favorably with a reduction in their motor symptoms, the patient is informed that carbidopa functioned as an inert placebo in this case and this opens up a discussion of the need to avoid iatrogenic harm from unnecessary pharmacotherapies (Jankovic, 2011).

Placebo diagnosis for PMD is also not without its caveats. A recent case study from Baik (2012) demonstrated that suggestion improved symptoms in a patient, leading the physicians to believe the patient had PMD. However, in this case, positron emission tomography imaging and the patient's responsiveness to levodopa indicated that the patient had Parkinson's disease, not PMD. In this case, the assessment for responsiveness to suggestion alone might have led to a misdiagnosis. Many movement disorders have no such diagnostic biomarkers. There is no consensus on how reliable placebo diagnosis is for PNES or PMD, only that it is frequently used (Espay et al., 2009).

The larger problem is that the diagnosis in the case of both PNES and PMD does not necessarily lead to a good strategy for care. In both cases, patients may not receive any follow-up and often lack access or financial resources to receive psychologic care. Others might suggest that the line between provocative placebo as a diagnostic or as a treatment is blurry, arguing that, with psychogenic disorders, the diagnosis also serves as the treatment in a way (Devinsky and Fisher, 1996; Burack et al., 1997; Stone and Edwards, 2012). Some might suggest this strategy (the diagnosis as the curative) provides a foundation for further treatment or can unravel subconscious beliefs that are somehow responsible for the manifestation of symptoms. However, the proposition that the information is the cure could easily be interpreted in a way that suggests psychogenic disorders are in some way under the patient's (conscious) control and patients informed of their diagnosis can stop being ill with conscious will. A recent report found that neurologists and psychiatrists view patients with PNES as having more control over their condition than patients with epilepsy (Whitehead and Reuber, 2012). This is particularly concerning, as the extent to which physicians view their patients' conscious control can impact their therapeutic strategy and the patients' blameworthiness for their symptoms (Kendell, 2001).

For treatment

Placebos used for treatment range from the more traditionally imagined placebo (i.e., saline, sugar pills) to so-called active or impure placebos, which might involve an intervention with some pharmacologic properties that are not relevant to the current condition, and is instead used for its psychologic rather than its pharmacologic effect. Some examples are described below.

Placebo treatment, such as placebo acupuncture and "digestive pills," has been explored and shown promise in individual case studies of PMD (Van Nuenen et al., 2007; Baik et al., 2009). In one case, a patient received placebo acupuncture (note that the authors refer to the acupuncture as placebo because the acupuncture was thought to be essentially inactive or inert as a treatment for movement disorders) (Van Nuenen et al., 2007). The patient with symptoms resembling myoclonus received repeated placebo treatment (the beneficial effects appeared to diminish across the time course of a month before the intervention again) for, at the time of the paper's publications, over a decade. In a second case, with digestive pills as placebo, a patient with paroxysmal kinesigenic dyskinesia had a positive dose–response to the placebo (Baik et al., 2009). The placebo dose was increased by suggestion. Once told that he had actually been given placebo pills, the patient was amenable to receiving psychotherapy and after psychotherapy was free of symptoms at follow-up 1 year later. In this case, the placebo was used for confirmation of the diagnosis and as a bridge to psychotherapeutic care.

The literature around PMD has repeatedly demonstrated that patients' beliefs that (1) they have PMD and (2) they will get better dictate the prognosis and success of treatment for PMD (Feinstein et al., 2001; Thomas and Jankovic, 2004; Hinson and Haren, 2006; Espay et al., 2009; Sharpe et al., 2010; Durrant et al., 2011; Gelauff et al., 2014). It is worth noting that the available literature is not without its own limitations, being largely retrospective and lacking baseline recording of prognostic factors and comorbidities that might provide better insight to the natural history of the disorder (Gelauff et al., 2014).

Given the poor prognosis and the lack of a standard of care, some neurologists advocate placebo therapy for PMD. They make a compelling case for this by conceptualizing PMD as a "belief" in having a sickness that is treatable with therapeutic placebo interventions whose efficacy is facilitated by the patient's belief in the therapy (Shamy, 2010). However, this notion still describes placebo and PMD in a kind of "black box" framework that warrants updating. Neuroimaging functional magnetic resonance imaging data have suggested that brain regions associated with psychogenic disorders, such as the dorsolateral prefrontal cortex and anterior cingulate (Ghaffar et al., 2006; Nowak and Fink, 2009), also mediate placebo effects for pain (Petrovic et al., 2002; Wager et al., 2004, 2007) and for depression (Mayberg et al., 2002; Benedetti et al., 2005); placebo administration may thus have a neurophysiologic basis for providing therapeutic benefit.

Our preliminary qualitative studies including interviews with neurologists and psychiatrists suggest that physicians who encounter patients with PNES and PMD utilize placebo in a variety of circumstances (Table 49.1): for diagnosis, as a tool for establishing a patient–physician relationship, and for acute and long-term treatment (Rommelfanger, 2013a). Their use of placebo involves, many times, "active" or "impure" placebos, wherein subthreshold doses or off-label use of "real" medications are prescribed to patients, a trend not unique to treatment of psychogenic disorders (Kolber, 2007; Harris and Raz, 2012; Rommelfanger, 2013a). In these scenarios, physicians slowly transition patients into accepting the diagnosis of psychogenic. Physicians feel they have circumvented the deception problem of placebos by not administering an "inert" substance like a sugar pill and instead administering an "active" substance (Rommelfanger, 2013a). When using placebo to build the patient–physician relationship, the physician continues to follow up with the patient, building a relationship by monitoring symptom evolution in response to placebo as part of a therapeutic strategy until the patient becomes more amenable or "ready" to accept the diagnosis and potentially receive care beyond the neurologist, which may or may not involve placebo. A part of this relationship building is to prescribe something that allows the patient to "get better gradually, and avoid the shame and embarrassment of having to recognize or having people recognize that it was "all in your head." This same physician also noted that "Humans' minds are complex, and you need to be able to access that complexity as long as it's for the good of the patient" (Rommelfanger, 2013a). These strategies may seem surprising and counterintuitive to those who believe placebos strictly deteriorate the patient–physician alliance. A bridging treatment, such as these, which initiates care early may be critical, as patients have poorer prognosis when treatment begins after a 6–12-month window of symptom onset (Gupta and Lang, 2009). A critical step prior to implementing these strategies is initiating an open community-wide discussion in order to optimize these effects and refine treatment strategies.

Table 49.1

Summary of themes in physician interviews on placebo for psychogenic disorders

Descriptions of placebo use or in support of placebo
1. Placebo helps save face and may ultimately be in the patient's best interest
2. We already deceive patients; if it works, who cares what the mechanism is?
3. Active placebos can act as a bridge for patient–physician engagement
4. I've used active placebo for long-term therapy
5. I've used active drugs for diagnosis vs. for therapeutic purposes, but active placebos are not really placebo
6. I learned to use placebo for acute benefit
Descriptions of ethical reservations against placebo usage
7. Suggestion is important, but placebo is unethical and I don't use it
8. Placebo is often used for diagnosis, but I don't think it's ethical

Reproduced from Rommelfanger (2013a).

One interesting feature of placebo use is how one comes to learn to use placebo therapeutically for psychogenic disorders, as there is surely no formal part of the neurologist's education to explicitly use placebo, not to mention a lack of formalized training on how to treat patients with psychogenic disorders. This training appears to follow an old model of apprenticeship: "see one, do one, teach one." One physician in my study recalled that a senior resident had explained that patients with PNES, given their suggestibility, could have their symptoms alleviated by a glass of water, leading the then junior resident to try their own techniques, such as saline eye drops for acute treatment and antidepressants as placebo for longer-term treatment (Rommelfanger, 2013a).

One unique feature of this scenario was setting – an already overburdened emergency room in a hospital of an underserved community. The physician in this case felt the placebo not only helped the patient in the short term, but also helped the emergency room patients whose care might be delayed by patients with psychogenic disorders that would otherwise take longer to assess without placebo. And because the physician knew that it was unlikely there would be any follow-up with the patient for the psychogenic disorder, the best that could be offered, following the eye drops administration, was a prescription for an antidepressant in the long term (notably not a recommendation or prescription for saline drops) that might elicit some nonspecific yet therapeutic effects in the longer term.

Conceptualizations of disease and medicine

The clearest ethical violation in the scenarios described in Table 49.1 is not the use of the placebo itself, but the hidden nature of this use. Hidden not just to the patient, but also from other physicians in the healthcare team. Of particular concern are the use of "impure" or active placebos and the introduction of iatrogenic harm. The secretive nature of these practices can largely be attributed to an entrenched belief in our medical care system that the mind is somehow separate from the body and that bodily disorders enjoy the privilege of being "legitimate" problems and as such avoid the stigma, blameworthiness, and illness invalidation that attend the stigma of a "psychological" disorder (Kendell, 2001; Miresco and Kirmayer, 2006).

Placebo therapy and psychogenic disorders both are subject to the mind–body dualist conceptual origin that is prevalent in Western medicine. Placebo effects and psychogenic symptoms are nonphysiologic or nonspecific and psychologic in origin, whereas "real" medicine works by physiologic mechanism for "real" disorders with a known physiologic origin (Lichtenberg et al., 2004). It is difficult to explain why an "unreal" treatment like placebo would give "real" relief. This becomes even more puzzling for diseases like PMD that have no clear neuropathologic features and thus fall into the category of psychologic or, to some, "not real" and "just in your head" (Espay et al., 2009). While some physicians call for the need to "elevate psychogenic disorder to the same level of neurological disorder," the current reality is that psychogenic disorders are typically not listed as an item on a list of differential diagnosis and in medical records are often described in nebulous terms, i.e., "not explained neurologically" (Friedman and LaFrance, 2010). There is a clear mind–body dualist entanglement with physicians who use placebo in diagnosis and treatment for psychogenic disorders, even by those who would say this Cartesian model is wrongheaded and outdated (Rommelfanger, 2013a). Conversations with patients with PNES and their physicians also reveal a gap in conceptual understanding: the physicians report a belief that their patients have a clearly psychologic, not physical, problem; patients tend to have less polarized views (Whitehead et al., 2013).

But frankly, with evolving neuroscience data, the bright line separating psychiatry and neurology is dissipating. Human psychologic states indeed are embodied and we see this exemplified in new detail by the neuroscience of placebo and psychogenic disorders. Central to the scientific enterprise is the revision of its tenets based on newer findings, often a consequence of new capabilities driven by technologic advances. And neuroscience data are now challenging perceived definitions of "real" medicine and "real" diseases. It is important to note that patient diagnosis and subsequent social realties are often at the mercy of the most recent advances in science. As prevalent as patients with psychogenic disorders are, they are marked by absence: lacking advocacy, support alliances, or even proper care.

ETHICAL AND LEGAL CONCERNS

A significant research effort and innovation in treatment and diagnosis, such as one that could be afforded with placebo therapy, could lead to important changes in attitudes towards PMD and psychogenic disorders in general. But first such a discussion must include the ethicolegal concerns attendant to the use of placebo therapy.

Deception and protecting patient autonomy

The dominating ethical concern with placebo therapy is not with the effects, but with the deception seemingly inherent to placebo therapy itself. As of 2006, the AMA Code of Medical Ethics prohibits the deceptive use of placebo. But what if deception was not required to gain benefit from placebo? A recent study has demonstrated that placebo effects are maintained even when patients are aware that they are being given an "inert" substance; this is contrary to the widespread assumption that placebo effects require deception (Kaptchuk et al., 2010). Researchers found that deception is not necessary for placebos to benefit patients with irritable-bowel syndrome who experienced relief from their symptoms despite being told they would be given "placebo (inert) pills, which were like sugar pills which had been shown to have self-healing properties." A study from 1965 demonstrated similar results in a nonblind placebo trial of a week's worth of sugar pills in patients with somatic symptoms (Park and Covi, 1965).

More recently, Sandler et al. (2010) used a "conditioned placebo dose reduction" in 99 children between the ages of 6 and 12 years with attention deficit hyperactivity disorder (ADHD). In this study, children began on their full optimal stimulant dose and were then given 50% of this dose for 1 month either with or without a placebo dose. Children and their parents were told that they would receive placebo as a "dose extender" and that the placebo contained no active pharmaceutical ingredient. Researchers found that the reduced dose plus placebo was not only more effective than the 50% dose alone, but also was just as effective as the full optimal dose. This study suggests that placebo can be used without deception to elicit positive therapeutic results and can also be used to modify existing treatments (in this case, reduce the dose of a potentially addictive drug to children).

In another model by Schafer et al. (2015), participants were first given deceptive placebo (a topical cream) for eliciting the placebo effect of analgesia. Participants continued to experience placebo-induced analgesia even after they were told explicitly and shown that the cream was simply petroleum jelly with blue food coloring. This study demonstrated that revealing that an intervention is a placebo, after patients experienced placebo effects during blinded administration, did not impact the placebo's future ability to elicit positive effects.

Note that the AMA's recommendation against placebo defines placebo as "a substance provided to a patient that the physician believes has no specific pharmacological effect upon the condition being treated." Importantly, the deceptive act in placebo therapy that is troubling is that physicians are knowingly using substances that they believe are "inert" to treat patients. Yet, placebos are not "inert." If physicians believe placebos are not inert, is it still a violation of AMA guidelines? Previous survey data reveal that, of physicians who utilize placebo, up to 96% believe that the placebo offers physiologic benefit to patients (Sherman and Hickner, 2008; Kermen et al., 2010). This is an important counterargument to placebo critics who voice concerns related to physicians' mal-intent: that they are trying to punish patients, relieve their own frustrations, or trick patients into revealing that their symptoms are not real (Purtilo, 1993). This is certainly a possibility that would need to be monitored were placebo to be adopted into routine use, but malintent may not be the driving force behind placebo therapy.

Another significant ethical concern around placebo practice concerns protecting patient autonomy. But, to avoid taking a paternalist tone, we must be sure of what our patients want; the answer to this question must be empirically driven. To date only a handful of studies report actual collected data on patient preferences about placebo treatment. One study from Sweden revealed that patients were stronger (25% of patients) advocates of deceptive placebo than physicians (7% of physicians) (Lynoe et al., 1993). Perhaps most surprising is that patients were substantially more placebo-friendly than their physicians.

In a more recent US study, respondents to a survey reported acceptability of placebos, with some respondents supporting use of deceptive placebo for themselves or others as patients, particularly if the patient is reporting benefit from the treatment (Hull et al., 2013). Bishop et al. (2014) reported that, while many patients reported supporting placebo usage (particularly if there were perceived beneficial outcomes), those who had negative views of placebo interpreted the term "placebo" as synonymous with "ineffective" and requiring deception, neither of which is necessarily true. Similar studies should be conducted before generalizing results, but this evidence should give us pause before categorically prohibiting placebo usage, deceptive or otherwise, on grounds of protecting patient autonomy.

Beneficence and nonmaleficence

A stated ethical stance in medical training and practice is that placebo usage can "cause patient harm, undermine trust in the medical profession, and destroy any possibility of a therapeutic alliance" (Hébert, 1995). But in light of the lack of successful standard treatments for PNES, and especially PMD, and the potential promise of placebo as a therapy for a disease that might otherwise have debilitating, costly effects over the course of a lifetime, we may need to ask a different ethical question (Rommelfanger, 2013b): "Does withholding placebo treatment harm patients and their families by depriving them of a treatment that might actually help alleviate suffering?"

The defensibility of placebo usage is more compelling for diseases such as PMD, which lack a successful standard of evidence-based treatment options (Singer, 2004). While studies are accumulating, there is a striking paucity of randomized placebo controlled studies exploring the efficacy of interventions for PMDs and PNES (Goldstein et al., 2010; Jordbru et al., 2014; LaFrance et al., 2014; Nielsen et al., 2015). Given the substantial costs accrued by patients and to the US healthcare system, placebo treatment could offer a relatively inexpensive alternative or complementary therapy to available treatment options for PMD and PNES and may also be revisited as a supplementary diagnostic tool for PMD. Moreover, given the reports of physicians using placebo in medical practice, neuroscience data will be critical for shaping guidelines for successful therapeutic placebo administration in medical contexts.

Deceptive placebos can be harmful, particularly in the case of active placebos. Engaging in open practices, which would include communication with the entire healthcare team, can minimize these harms. To protect against more long-term damages – which are a legitimate concern to the integrity of the physician–patient alliance – the practice of placebo therapy should be evaluated scientifically with transparent studies with a focus on dissemination of results to a public as well as an inclusive research process wherein the public and patient opinions are taken into account. In order to safely and effectively utilize placebo, empirical data will need to be collected on both clinical safety and efficacy, as well as contexts for placebo, and sociologic data to empirically assess patient preferences with regard to placebo. There is also a large body of evidence of beneficial placebo effects; patients may be equally susceptible to "nocebo effects," wherein a negative suggestion can negatively impact a patient's health (Enck et al., 2008). Researchers self-identified as the "Placebo Competence Team" suggest a professional imperative to decrease negative expectations of interventions (Bingel and Placebo Competence Team, 2014).

Legal considerations

Physicians report fear of litigious patients with psychogenic disorders, which hinders delivery of diagnosis (Espay et al., 2009). Understandably, physicians may have a similar concern with placebo therapy. To date there are very few cases filed by patients claiming damages from deceptive use of placebo (Kolber, 2007). This may be, in part, due to: (1) historic definitions indicating that placebos are inert and thus have a low side-effect profile; and (2) assumptions that any worsening of disease or illness progression in the presence of an "inert" intervention would simply be the natural course of the disease. Of course, because placebo can have powerful physiologic effects, the potential harms may need revisiting.

Of significant legal concern is giving appropriate informed consent. However, given that preliminary studies suggest that deception may not be required to obtain beneficial effects from placebo, patients may be openly informed of placebo treatments prior to administration. Another possibility is that patients could be provided waivers, wherein they request to not be made aware whether treatment is placebo or not. Again, informed-consent policies should largely be led by patient preference data as well as clinical data comparing the efficacy of deceptive versus nondeceptive placebo.

FUTURE DIRECTIONS

Clinical research and therapeutic discovery

Placebo therapy is a realm ripe for research. Examining physician attitudes, the contexts under which placebos are given, even the appearance, such as color of the placebo or mode of administration (Gracely et al., 1985; Di Blasi et al., 2001; Benedetti, 2008; Finniss et al., 2010), will be the first steps in exploring the viability of placebo for PMD and PNES (Gracely et al., 1985; de Craen et al., 1996; Kaptchuk and Eisenberg, 1998; Kaptchuk, 2002; Moerman and Jonas, 2002; Kaptchuk et al., 2006; Finniss et al., 2010). The context surrounding the clinical encounter can significantly impact the placebo effect, making each interaction between physicians and their patients an opportunity for a therapeutic moment (Di Blasi et al., 2001; Benedetti, 2008). Physicians may, unbeknownst to them, have demonstrable discomfort, especially revealed in their dialogue, that is detected by patients, when they are diagnosing patients who they believe may have a psychogenic disorder (Monzoni et al., 2011). Importantly, this research will need to be conducted and defined (i.e., What constitutes a placebo and a placebo effect?) by an interdisciplinary team of neuroscientists and clinicians and there must be a reciprocal flow of information between these parties to result in true therapeutic innovation.

Perhaps the greatest challenge will be handling the level of individual variability in response to the same placebo in similar contexts. Research will need to be conducted on which types of patients and which symptoms and disorders will be most amenable to placebo treatments. Some studies suggest that placebo effects are a conditioned response involving reward pathways, wherein the expectation to get well can be seen in the ventral striatum of patients susceptible to placebo effects (Lidstone et al., 2010). This would suggest that some patients may be more amenable than others to placebo therapy and could perhaps be pre-screened based on neuroimaging for biomarkers of reward expectancy tendencies or even suggestibility. Others suggest that it is important to recognize patients' "pre-cebo" states, referring to the set of life experiences (including previous experiences with a drug) and expectations (in part derived from the consent process) leading to amenability to a placebo response (Kim et al., 2012).

Recent studies revealed a possible genetic link to a variant of a gene coding for an enzyme involved in dopamine catabolism, to the catechol-*O*-methyltransferase gene and placebo response in patients with irritable-bowel syndrome (Hall et al., 2012), as well as with nocebo responses (Wendt et al., 2014). Such a link may aid in the development of a genetic screen.

Questions will also need to be asked about the extent and duration of treatment as well as what stage treatment should begin, initially as adjunct therapy or as part of a multidisciplinary effort. Studies should also address what are the neurophysiologic benefits from placebo from short- versus long-term placebo therapy and how placebos might impact physiology and disease course when administered during diagnosis or various stages of treatment.

More generally, because placebos can have specific effects, placebos may even serve as a research tool to help identify which biologic mechanisms might be responsible for generating psychogenic disorders. This raises novel opportunities for drug discovery. For disorders, like psychogenic disorders, which lack a clear mechanism for their symptoms, placebo might be helpful in testing specific hypotheses of candidate pharmacologic markers (i.e., if participants report subjective and objective benefits from placebos, and placebos can generate specific effects, candidate biomarkers can be examined before and after placebo administration). While finding an appropriate control for placebo studies is not without its challenges, one approach might be to perform a dose–response study. For example, in the Baik et al. (2009) study, researchers increased the dose of the medication by twice the amount through suggestion and found a corresponding reported benefit in the patient. Studies could also be conducted to look at additive paradigms (Enck et al., 2013), such as the model used in the ADHD study above (Sandler et al., 2010).

Important studies will also need to be conducted to assess patient preferences and efficacy with regard to deceptive placebo practices or nondeceptive placebo practices. To date, even recent studies have suggested perhaps a surprising acceptance of a paternalistic approach involving physician deception (Lynoe et al., 1993; Hull et al., 2013). Even fewer studies exist about general treatment preferences of patients with psychogenic disorders. For example, while physicians may consider psychotherapy a treatment of choice for patients with PNES (LaFrance et al., 2008) – despite the absence of robust (albeit developing) evidence of its efficacy (Baker et al., 2007; Gaynor et al., 2009; Goldstein et al., 2010; LaFrance et al., 2014) – patients state a strong preference against psychotherapy (Fairclough et al., 2014). It is also yet to be determined how efficacious psychotherapy may be for PMD or how desirable such treatment would be for patients (Hinson et al., 2006; Kompoliti et al., 2014).

Education of healthcare providers

Lack of suitable follow-up is a consistent problem for patients with PMD and in no small part is related to a lack of willing and able referral physicians. While there are numerous strong review articles, chapters in some neurology textbooks, and occasional workshops, by and large a formalized curriculum for medical students is in dire need of further development (although such programs are more advanced in the European Union, such as in the UK: Jon Stone, personal communication). Currently there is no standard or formalized education on how to treat psychogenic disorders for neurology or psychiatry students and physicians may more typically be learning on their own how to use placebo for PMD and PNES (Rommelfanger, 2013a). Education, like clinical care, should be empirically driven by data from the studies above and might even be best conducted by healthcare professionals who encounter these patients the most. Because neurologists and psychiatrists generally do not follow up with these patients – even if they may seem to be the most appropriate provider for care of patients with these disorders – patients land back in their primary care physicians' offices. Therefore, it might be equally important to train general internal medicine and primary care physicians in diagnosis and strategies for caring for patients with psychogenic disorders (with or without placebo) and apparently many of these primary care physicians are already administering placebo therapy for a variety of conditions (Sherman and Hickner, 2008; Tilburt et al., 2008).

Physicians' training must involve vigilance in challenging assumptions in identifying patients with psychogenic disorders. Especially in the Veterans Affairs, likely due to assumptions about the "type" of patient who might exhibit psychogenic symptoms (i.e., young, female, emotionally stressed), patients experience a three times greater delay for diagnosis and treatment (Salinsky et al., 2011). Learning to identify and treat patients with PMD and PNES early may facilitate any therapeutic strategy and placebo may especially help in early phases of treatment to bridge the gap before more long-term solutions can be found.

Finally, education should include the most current information on psychogenic disorders and on the neurophysiologic effects of placebo alongside an open discussion of placebo practices. These activities could not only reduce the discomfort of physicians encountering patients with psychogenic disorders but also perhaps lead to a deeper discussion of how to best treat psychogenic disorders and ultimately to better patient care.

CONCLUSIONS

Placebo and psychogenic disorders represent challenges for conceptualizing brain function and the mechanisms of "real" disease. Arguments about whether or not a disease is "only in your head" are outdated positions, as neuroscience continually illuminates new mechanisms for mental processes and mental illnesses. Indeed, abnormalities in the brain have begun to be identified in PMD patients as well as neurophysiologic mechanisms for placebo.

For a group of patients who largely have poor prognosis and limited resources for their care, placebo may play an important and untapped role in facilitating recovery. To be clear: placebo therapy need not trump all other interventions. Nor is this to say that a placebo intervention may provide some endpoint of physiologic impact superior to a psychologic intervention (which likely also ultimately has a downstream physiologic impact). Placebo therapy might also be best utilized as a bridging strategy or even as an adjunct therapy. These need not be theoretical arguments; questions of placebo therapy's utility (or how to maximize a placebo response) for psychogenic disorders are empirical ones. Psychogenic disorders require a truly interdisciplinary effort marked by active, transparent partnership between psychiatrists, neurologists, and primary care physicians. With this multidisciplinary partnership, diagnosis of patients as well as treatment plans and research strategies can be developed, and this is how we will truly develop a successful standard of care for patients with psychogenic disorders.

References

Amanzio M, Benedetti F (1999). Neuropharmacological dissection of placebo analgesia: expectation-activated opioid systems versus conditioning-activated specific subsystems. J Neurosci 19: 484–494.

American Medical Association (2006). Code of medical ethics. Available online at http://www.ama-assn.org/ama/pub/physician-resources/medical-ethics/code-medical-ethics.page.

Baik JS (2012). Attention in Parkinson's disease mimicking suggestion in psychogenic movement disorder. J Mov Disord 5: 53–54.

Baik JS, Han SW, Park JH et al. (2009). Psychogenic paroxysmal dyskinesia: the role of placebo in the diagnosis and management. Mov Disord 24: 1244–1245.

Baker GA, Brooks JL, Goodfellow L et al. (2007). Treatments for non-epileptic attack disorder. Cochrane Database Syst Rev: CD006370.

Bendtsen L, Mattsson P, Zwart JA et al. (2003). Placebo response in clinical randomized trials of analgesics in migraine. Cephalalgia 23: 487–490.

Benedetti F (2008). Mechanisms of placebo and placebo-related effects across diseases and treatments. Annu Rev Pharmacol Toxicol 48: 33–60.

Benedetti F (2014). Placebo effects: from the neurobiological paradigm to translational implications. Neuron 84: 623–637.

Benedetti F, Colloca L, Torre E et al. (2004). Placebo-responsive Parkinson patients show decreased activity in single neurons of subthalamic nucleus. Nat Neurosci 7: 587–588.

Benedetti F, Mayberg HS, Wager TD et al. (2005). Neurobiological mechanisms of the placebo effect. J Neurosci 25: 10390–10402.

Bingel U, Placebo Competence Team (2014). Avoiding nocebo effects to optimize treatment outcome. JAMA 312: 693–694.

Bishop FL, Aizlewood L, Adams AE (2014). When and why placebo-prescribing is acceptable and unacceptable: a focus group study of patients' views. PLoS One 9: e101822.

Blease C (2012). The principle of parity: the 'placebo effect' and physician communication. J Med Ethics 38: 199–203.

Bostick NA, Sade R, Levine MA et al. (2008). Placebo use in clinical practice: report of the American Medical Association Council on Ethical and Judicial Affairs. J Clin Ethics 19: 58–61.

Burack JH, Back AL, Pearlman RA (1997). Provoking nonepileptic seizures: the ethics of deceptive diagnostic testing. Hastings Cent Rep 27: 24–33.

Burton R (1621). The Anatomy of Melancholy, New York Review Books, New York.

de Craen AJ, Roos PJ, Leonard de Vries A et al. (1996). Effect of colour of drugs: systematic review of perceived effect of drugs and of their effectiveness. BMJ 313: 1624–1626.

de la Fuente-Fernandez R, Ruth TJ, Sossi V et al. (2001). Expectation and dopamine release: mechanism of the placebo effect in Parkinson's disease. Science 293: 1164–1166.

Devinsky O, Fisher R (1996). Ethical use of placebos and provocative testing in diagnosing nonepileptic seizures. Neurology 47: 866–870.

Devinsky O, Gazzola D, LaFrance Jr WC (2011). Differentiating between nonepileptic and epileptic seizures. Nat Rev Neurol 7: 210–220.

Di Blasi Z, Harkness E, Ernst E et al. (2001). Influence of context effects on health outcomes: a systematic review. Lancet 357: 757–762.

Diederich NJ, Goetz CG (2008). The placebo treatments in neurosciences: new insights from clinical and neuroimaging studies. Neurology 71: 677–684.

Durrant J, Rickards H, Cavanna AE (2011). Prognosis and outcome predictors in psychogenic nonepileptic seizures. Epilepsy Res Treat 2011: 274736.

Dworkin RH, Katz J, Gitlin MJ (2005). Placebo response in clinical trials of depression and its implications for research on chronic neuropathic pain. Neurology 65: S7–S19.

Enck P, Benedetti F, Schedlowski M (2008). New insights into the placebo and nocebo responses. Neuron 59: 195–206.

Enck P, Bingel U, Schedlowski M et al. (2013). The placebo response in medicine: minimize, maximize or personalize? Nat Rev Drug Discov 12: 191–204.

Ernst E (2007). Placebo: new insights into an old enigma. Drug Discov Today 12: 413–418.

Espay AJ, Goldenhar LM, Voon V et al. (2009). Opinions and clinical practices related to diagnosing and managing patients with psychogenic movement disorders: an international survey of movement disorder society members. Mov Disord 24: 1366–1374.

Factor SA, Podskalny GD, Molho ES (1995). Psychogenic movement disorders: frequency, clinical profile, and characteristics. J Neurol Neurosurg Psychiatry 59: 406–412.

Fahn S, Williams DT (1988). Psychogenic dystonia. Adv Neurol 50: 431–455.

Fairclough G, Fox J, Mercer G et al. (2014). Understanding the perceived treatment needs of patients with psychogenic nonepileptic seizures. Epilepsy Behav 31: 295–303.

Fassler M, Meissner K, Schneider A et al. (2010). Frequency and circumstances of placebo use in clinical practice – a systematic review of empirical studies. BMC Med 8: 15.

Feinstein A, Stergiopoulos V, Fine J et al. (2001). Psychiatric outcome in patients with a psychogenic movement disorder: a prospective study. Neuropsychiatry Neuropsychol Behav Neurol 14: 169–176.

Finniss DG, Kaptchuk TJ, Miller F et al. (2010). Biological, clinical, and ethical advances of placebo effects. Lancet 375: 686–695.

Ford PL (1898). The Writings of Thomas Jefferson, Putnam, New York.

Friedman JH, LaFrance Jr WC (2010). Psychogenic disorders: the need to speak plainly. Arch Neurol 67: 753–755.

Gaynor D, Cock H, Agrawal N (2009). Psychological treatments for functional non-epileptic attacks: a systematic review. Acta Neuropsychiatr 21: 158–168.

Gelauff J, Stone J, Edwards M et al. (2014). The prognosis of functional (psychogenic) motor symptoms: a systematic review. J Neurol Neurosurg Psychiatry 85: 220–226.

Ghaffar O, Staines WR, Feinstein A (2006). Unexplained neurologic symptoms: an fMRI study of sensory conversion disorder. Neurology 67: 2036–2038.

Goetz CG, Wuu J, McDermott MP et al. (2008). Placebo response in Parkinson's disease: comparisons among 11 trials covering medical and surgical interventions. Mov Disord 23: 690–699.

Goldstein LH, Chalder T, Chigwedere C et al. (2010). Cognitive-behavioral therapy for psychogenic nonepileptic seizures: a pilot RCT. Neurology 74: 1986–1994.

Gracely RH, Dubner R, Deeter WR et al. (1985). Clinicians' expectations influence placebo analgesia. Lancet 1: 43.

Gupta A, Lang AE (2009). Psychogenic movement disorders. Curr Opin Neurol 22: 430–436.

Hall KT, Lembo AJ, Kirsch I et al. (2012). Catechol-O-methyltransferase val158met polymorphism predicts placebo effect in irritable bowel syndrome. PLoS One 7: e48135.

Harris CS, Raz A (2012). Deliberate use of placebos in clinical practice: what we really know. J Med Ethics 38: 406–407.

Hébert PC (1995). Doing right: A practical guide to ethics for medical trainees and physicians, Oxford University Press, Toronto.

Hinson VK, Haren WB (2006). Psychogenic movement disorders. Lancet Neurol 5: 695–700.

Hinson VK, Weinstein S, Bernard B et al. (2006). Single-blind clinical trial of psychotherapy for treatment of psychogenic movement disorders. Parkinsonism Relat Disord 12: 177–180.

Howick J, Bishop FL, Heneghan C et al. (2013). Placebo use in the United Kingdom: results from a national survey of primary care practitioners. PLoS One 8: e58247.

Hrobjartsson A, Norup M (2003). The use of placebo interventions in medical practice – a national questionnaire survey of Danish clinicians. Eval Health Prof 26: 153–165.

Hull SC, Colloca L, Avins A et al. (2013). Patients' attitudes about the use of placebo treatments: telephone survey. BMJ 347: f3757.

Jankovic J (2011). Diagnosis and treatment of psychogenic parkinsonism. J Neurol Neurosurg Psychiatry 82: 1300–1303.

Jordbru AA, Smedstad LM, Klungsoyr O et al. (2014). Psychogenic gait disorder: a randomized controlled trial of physical rehabilitation with one-year follow-up. J Rehabil Med 46: 181–187.

Kaptchuk TJ (2002). The placebo effect in alternative medicine: can the performance of a healing ritual have clinical significance? Ann Intern Med 136: 817–825.

Kaptchuk TJ, Eisenberg DM (1998). The persuasive appeal of alternative medicine. Ann Intern Med 129: 1061–1065.

Kaptchuk TJ, Stason WB, Davis RB et al. (2006). Sham device v inert pill: randomised controlled trial of two placebo treatments. BMJ 332: 391–397.

Kaptchuk TJ, Friedlander E, Kelley JM et al. (2010). Placebos without deception: a randomized controlled trial in irritable bowel syndrome. PLoS One 5: e15591.

Kendell RE (2001). The distinction between mental and physical illness. Br J Psychiatry 178: 490–493.

Kermen R, Hickner J, Brody H et al. (2010). Family physicians believe the placebo effect is therapeutic but often use real drugs as placebos. Fam Med 42: 636–642.

Kim SE, Kubomoto S, Chua K et al. (2012). "Pre-cebo": an unrecognized issue in the interpretation of adequate relief during irritable bowel syndrome drug trials. J Clin Gastroenterol 46: 686–690.

Kolber A (2007). A limited defense of clinical placebo deception. Yale Law Policy Rev 26: 75–137.

Kompoliti K, Wilson B, Stebbins G et al. (2014). Immediate vs. delayed treatment of psychogenic movement disorders with short term psychodynamic psychotherapy: randomized clinical trial. Parkinsonism Relat Disord 20: 60–63.

LaFrance Jr WC, Rusch MD, Machan JT (2008). What is "treatment as usual" for nonepileptic seizures? Epilepsy Behav 12: 388–394.

LaFrance Jr WC, Baird GL, Barry JJ et al. (2014). Multicenter pilot treatment trial for psychogenic nonepileptic seizures: a randomized clinical trial. JAMA Psychiatry 71: 997–1005.

Lichtenberg P, Heresco-Levy U, Nitzan U (2004). The ethics of the placebo in clinical practice. J Med Ethics 30: 551–554.

Lidstone SC, Schulzer M, Dinelle K et al. (2010). Effects of expectation on placebo-induced dopamine release in Parkinson disease. Arch Gen Psychiatry 67: 857–865.

Lynoe N, Mattsson B, Sandlund M (1993). The attitudes of patients and physicians towards placebo treatment – a comparative study. Soc Sci Med 36: 767–774.

Mayberg HS, Silva JA, Brannan SK et al. (2002). The functional neuroanatomy of the placebo effect. Am J Psychiatry 159: 728–737.

McGonigal A, Oto M, Russell AJ et al. (2002). Outpatient video EEG recording in the diagnosis of non-epileptic seizures: a randomised controlled trial of simple suggestion techniques. J Neurol Neurosurg Psychiatry 72: 549–551.

Meissner K, Hofner L, Fassler M et al. (2012). Widespread use of pure and impure placebo interventions by GPs in Germany. Fam Pract 29: 79–85.

Mercado R, Constantoyannis C, Mandat T et al. (2006). Expectation and the placebo effect in Parkinson's disease patients with subthalamic nucleus deep brain stimulation. Mov Disord 21: 1457–1461.

Miresco MJ, Kirmayer LJ (2006). The persistence of mind–brain dualism in psychiatric reasoning about clinical scenarios. Am J Psychiatry 163: 913–918.

Moerman DE, Jonas WB (2002). Deconstructing the placebo effect and finding the meaning response. Ann Intern Med 136: 471–476.

Monzoni CM, Duncan R, Grunewald R et al. (2011). How do neurologists discuss functional symptoms with their patients: a conversation analytic study. J Psychosom Res 71: 377–383.

Nielsen G, Ricciardi L, Demartini B et al. (2015). Outcomes of a 5-day physiotherapy programme for functional (psychogenic) motor disorders. J Neurol 262: 674–681.

Nowak DA, Fink GR (2009). Psychogenic movement disorders: aetiology, phenomenology, neuroanatomical correlates and therapeutic approaches. Neuroimage 47: 1015–1025.

Park LC, Covi L (1965). Nonblind Placebo Trial: an exploration of neurotic patients' responses to placebo when its inert content is disclosed. Arch Gen Psychiatry 12: 36–45.

Petrovic P, Kalso E, Petersson KM et al. (2002). Placebo and opioid analgesia – imaging a shared neuronal network. Science 295: 1737–1740.

Purtilo R (1993). Ethical dimensions in the health care professions, WB Saunders, Philadelphia.

Rommelfanger KS (2013a). Attitudes on mind over matter: physician views on the role of placebo in psychogenic disorders. Am J Bioeth Neurosci 4: 9–15.

Rommelfanger KS (2013b). Opinion: a role for placebo therapy in psychogenic movement disorders. Nat Rev Neurol 9: 351–356.

Salinsky M, Spencer D, Boudreau E et al. (2011). Psychogenic nonepileptic seizures in US veterans. Neurology 77: 945–950.

Sandler AD, Glesne CE, Bodfish JW (2010). Conditioned placebo dose reduction: a new treatment in attention-deficit hyperactivity disorder? J Dev Behav Pediatr 31: 369–375.

Schafer SM, Colloca L, Wager TD (2015). Conditioned placebo analgesia persists when subjects know they are receiving a placebo. J Pain 16: 412–420.

Shamy MC (2010). The treatment of psychogenic movement disorders with suggestion is ethically justified. Mov Disord 25: 260–264.

Sharpe M, Stone J, Hibberd C et al. (2010). Neurology outpatients with symptoms unexplained by disease: illness beliefs and financial benefits predict 1-year outcome. Psychol Med 40: 689–698.

Sherman R, Hickner J (2008). Academic physicians use placebos in clinical practice and believe in the mind–body connection. J Gen Intern Med 23: 7–10.

Singer EA (2004). The necessity and the value of placebo. Sci Eng Ethics 10: 51–56.

Stagno SJ, Smith ML (1997). The use of placebo in diagnosing psychogenic seizures: who is being deceived? Semin Neurol 17: 213–218.

Stone J, Edwards M (2012). Trick or treat? Showing patients with functional (psychogenic) motor symptoms their physical signs. Neurology 79: 282–284.

Thomas M, Jankovic J (2004). Psychogenic movement disorders: diagnosis and management. CNS Drugs 18: 437–452.

Tilburt JC, Emanuel EJ, Kaptchuk TJ et al. (2008). Prescribing "placebo treatments": results of national survey of US internists and rheumatologists. BMJ 337: a1938.

Van Nuenen BF, Wohlgemuth M, Wong Chung RE et al. (2007). Acupuncture for psychogenic movement disorders: treatment or diagnostic tool? Mov Disord 22: 1353–1355.

Wager TD, Rilling JK, Smith EE et al. (2004). Placebo-induced changes in FMRI in the anticipation and experience of pain. Science 303: 1162–1167.

Wager TD, Scott DJ, Zubieta JK (2007). Placebo effects on human mu-opioid activity during pain. Proc Natl Acad Sci U S A 104: 11056–11061.

Wendt L, Albring A, Benson S et al. (2014). Catechol-O-methyltransferase Val158Met polymorphism is associated with somatosensory amplification and nocebo responses. PLoS One 9: e107665.

Whitehead K, Reuber M (2012). Illness perceptions of neurologists and psychiatrists in relation to epilepsy and nonepileptic attack disorder. Seizure 21: 104–109.

Whitehead K, Kandler R, Reuber M (2013). Patients' and neurologists' perception of epilepsy and psychogenic nonepileptic seizures. Epilepsia 54: 708–717.

Zubieta JK, Bueller JA, Jackson LR et al. (2005). Placebo effects mediated by endogenous opioid activity on mu-opioid receptors. J Neurosci 25: 7754–7762.

Handbook of Clinical Neurology, Vol. 139 (3rd series)
Functional Neurologic Disorders
M. Hallett, J. Stone, and A. Carson, Editors
http://dx.doi.org/10.1016/B978-0-12-801772-2.00050-3

Chapter 50

Transcranial magnetic stimulation and sedation as treatment for functional neurologic disorders

T.R.J. NICHOLSON[1]* AND V. VOON[2]

[1]*Section of Cognitive Neuropsychiatry, Institute of Psychiatry, Psychology and Neuroscience, King's College London, London, UK*

[2]*Department of Psychiatry, Behavioural and Clinical Neurosciences Institute, University of Cambridge, Cambridge, UK*

Abstract

Functional neurologic disorder (FND), also known as conversion disorder, is common and often associated with a poor prognosis. It has been relatively neglected by research and as such there is a conspicuous lack of evidence-based treatments. Physical and psychologic therapies are the main treatment modalities, over and above reassurance and sensitive explanation of the diagnosis. However there are two other historic treatments that have seen a recent resurgence of interest and use.

The first is electric stimulation, which was initially pioneered with direct stimulation of nerves but now used indirectly (and therefore noninvasively) in the form of transcranial magnetic stimulation (TMS). The second is (therapeutic) sedation, previously known as "abreaction," where it was mostly used in the context of psychologic investigation and treatment, but now increasingly advocated during rehabilitation as a way to therapeutically demonstrate reversibility of symptoms.

This chapter introduces the background of these treatment modalities, their evolution into their current applications before critically evaluating their current evidence base and exploring possible mechanisms of action. It also tentatively suggests when they should be considered in current practice and briefly considers their future potential. In summary there is encouraging preliminary evidence to suggest that both TMS and sedation may be effective treatments for FNDs.

INTRODUCTION

Functional neurologic disorder (FND), also known as conversion disorder, refers to neurologic symptoms that are not explained by organic (neurologic) disease. FND is as common as both Parkinson's disease and multiple sclerosis (Stone et al., 2011) and associated with similar levels of disability and distress (Carson et al., 2011) and long-term outcomes are poor (Gelauff et al., 2014). It has been a neglected area of research and consequently the evidence base for treatments is lacking, apart from preliminary evidence for the efficacy of cognitive-behavioral therapy (CBT), particularly for the seizure variant of FND (Goldstein et al., 2010; LaFrance et al., 2014) (see Chapter 46).

Compassionate explanation of the diagnosis – tailored to the individual patient – along with reassurance are often considered critical parts of recovery and sometimes all that is required (Stone, 2014; Chapter 44). Cases not showing a significant trajectory of recovery a few weeks or months after symptom onset often require consideration for psychologic therapies such as CBT. For those with amenable symptoms (e.g., weakness) physical therapies – also known as physiotherapy in countries such as the UK – can be critical to help relearn and restore normal function (Nielsen et al., 2013; Chapter 45), especially if secondary problems have developed, such as deconditioning or, in severe cases, contractures.

However there are two other treatment modalities, both with long histories as treatments for FND, that have

*Correspondence to: Dr. Timothy R.J. Nicholson, Section of Cognitive Neuropsychiatry, Institute of Psychiatry, Psychology and Neuroscience, King's College London, London, UK. Tel: +44-207-848-5136, E-mail: Timothy.nicholson@kcl.ac.uk

seen a recent resurgence of interest in their use, albeit in modified forms to those originally used. The first is electric stimulation, which was initially pioneered with direct stimulation of affected nerves but now used indirectly (and noninvasively) in the form of transcranial magnetic stimulation (TMS). The second is (therapeutic) sedation, previously known as abreaction, where it was mostly used in the context of psychologic investigation and treatment, but now increasingly advocated as a way to restart normal function and demonstrate the reversibility of symptoms such as dystonias.

TRANSCRANIAL MAGNETIC STIMULATION

Something old, something new – electric stimulation for FND

There is a long history of electric stimulation being used therapeutically for FND, dating as far back as the 18th century (see McWhirter et al., 2015, for a comprehensive review of the topic). At this time dysfunctional parts of the nervous system, due to both "organic" disease and FND, were treated with direct electric stimulation using primitive batteries (e.g., Leyden jars). This resulted in mixed, but generally positive, results such that mainstream medical texts at the time often advocated its use for FND, or hysteria, as it was then known. Even during these early times the role of suggestion, what we now call placebo, was acknowledged by many practitioners and was considered by some to be a large, and possibly the only, reason for its efficacy. Further controversies arose with the widespread use of direct electric stimulation to treat the epidemic of FND that arose in World War I, as part of the shell shock syndrome, when it was often deliberately used at levels of stimulation known to be painful, thereby adding an aversive "punitive" effect. Understandably this resulted in a backlash against the treatment, amongst both the public and the medical profession, and consequently its use notably reduced after the war.

Despite falling out of mainstream use, such direct electric stimulation continued to be advocated by a small number of clinicians with occasional reports of high levels of efficacy, the most recent being a case report in 1988 (Khalil et al., 1988). However, at around this time TMS was developed: this is an indirect, and consequently better-tolerated (i.e., less painful), method of neurostimulation. TMS works via magnetic coils, placed on the scalp, which induce electric stimulation of underlying brain tissue. Initially TMS was principally used as a neurophysiologic tool for both clinical diagnostics and research into brain function. Stimulating the underlying cortex can probe function of specific areas as well as assess cortical excitability and even connectivity with other areas (Rossini et al., 2015) and has been used to investigate the pathophysiology of FND (Geraldes et al., 2008; Liepert et al., 2011).

Therapeutic applications soon followed across a wide spectrum of disorders over the whole of clinical neuroscience. Initially it was used mostly for neurologic disorders, particularly movement disorders and stroke, but it has found increasing application for psychiatric disorders. It has been studied extensively for treatment of depression, for which it now has level "A" evidence of efficacy (Rossini et al., 2015), but it has also been used for a range of other psychiatric disorders, including schizophrenia, anxiety disorders, and substance abuse disorders (Lefaucheur et al., 2014). Most therapeutic applications have used repetitive TMS (rTMS), which is when sequences of pulses are delivered together in specific combinations of strength and timing. This can induce lasting changes in cortical excitability which are similar to the long-term potentiation and long-term depression effects seen after direct neuronal stimulation in experimental animals (Edwards et al., 2008).

Importantly, it has also been established that it is a safe and well-tolerated treatment if the TMS parameters are kept within certain limits, as defined by the International Federation of Clinical Neurophysiology (IFCN), who have published guidelines for TMS use and a review of the safety data (Rossi et al., 2009). Historically the principal safety concern has been seizure induction, but it is now clear that this is extremely rare and has largely occurred in the context of rTMS protocols exceeding IFCN guidelines or in those patients taking drugs that lower seizure threshold. The main side-effects are pain over the site of stimulation and a risk of headache. Whether pain is experienced, and its intensity, varies according to several methodologic factors, including coil design as well as the location, intensity, and frequency of stimulation, but individual susceptibility also plays a major role. A meta-analysis of rTMS depression trials reported 39% of patients experienced pain compared to 15% with placebo (Loo et al., 2008). For the majority of cases the pain rapidly vanishes after TMS application and, even in trials using high stimulation intensities and frequencies, less than 2% of patients discontinue due to pain. Headache shows similar variability and, although it is less frequently reported (28% with rTMS compared to 16% with placebo), it may occasionally persist.

Evidence for the efficacy of TMS

There has been a steady accumulation of evidence over the last decade to support TMS as a treatment for FND. To date, 10 case series, i.e., studies with control groups for comparison, have been published and once

Table 50.1

Published data of transcranial magnetic stimulation (TMS) treatment for functional neurologic disorders (FND)

Study	Patients (symptoms)	Target	Protocol	Effects (outcome measure)	Follow-up
Case series					
Jellinek et al. (1992)	1 (paresis)	Vertex	Single-pulse TMS (F8c) • "Supra" MT intensity; no other details given	Effective 1/1: full recovery at 1 week (clinical examination)	Sustained at 1 month
Schonfeldt-Lecuona et al. (2006)	4 (paresis)	MC	rTMS (F8c) • HF (15 Hz, 4000 pulses/session) • 110% MT, then 90% after 2 weeks • 1 session/day for 4–12 weeks	Effective 3/3 with FND • 2 complete recovery and 1 major improvement at 4–12 weeks • 1 patient did not improve but was diagnosed with malingering (clinical examination)	Sustained at 6–12 months
Deftereos et al. (2008)	1 (paresis)	MC	Single-pulse TMS (F8c) • 100% stimulator output • 1 session	Ineffective: but patient rediagnosed as malingering (clinical impression)	N/A
Chastan et al. (2009)	1 (aphonia)	MC (and PFC)	rTMS (Cc) • LF (0.33 Hz, 50 pulses) • 100% stimulator output (2.5 T) • 2 sessions 1 week apart (1st session to left PFC, 2nd session to right MC)	Effective 1/1: dramatic improvement within few days after MC stimulation only (clinical impression)	Sustained at 6 months
Chastan and Parain (2010)	70 (paresis)	MC	rTMS (Cc) • LF (0.2–0.25 Hz, 30 pulses) • 100% stimulator output (2.5 T) • 1 or 2 sessions on 1 day (2nd given if incomplete recovery after 1st)	Effective in 62/70 • Total recovery in 53 • Dramatic improvement in 9 (clinical impression)	8/62 who improved relapsed at mean of 156 days; 6 of these responded to further treatment
Kresojevic et al. (2010)	2 (1 × paresis 1 × MD)	Vertex	Single-pulse TMS (Cc) • 30–80% of stimulator output • 12 pulses	Effective in 2/2: • Complete recovery in 2 (clinical impression)	Recurrence of mild symptoms at 6 months
Dafotakis et al. (2011)	11 (MD)	MC	rTMS (F8c) • LF (0.2 Hz, 30 pulses) • 120% MT for 15, then 140% for 15 • 1 session	Effective in 11/11: • Mean of 97% immediate reduction in tremor (kinematic motion analysis)	7/11 relapsed and 4/11 recovery sustained at 8–12 months

Continued

Table 50.1

Continued

Study	Patients (symptoms)	Target	Protocol	Effects (outcome measure)	Follow-up
Garcin et al. (2013)	24 (MD)	MC	rTMS (Cc) • LF (0.25 Hz, 20 pulses) • 120% MT for 250 μs • 1 session	Effective in 24/24: • Improved >50% in 18 • "Cured" in 3 (AIMS/BFMS, CGI)	17/24 still improved at median 20 months and 12/24 CGI-I score of 1 or 2
Parain and Chastan (2014)	10 (visual loss)	Midline and occipitoparietal area	rTMS (Cc) • LF (approx. 1 Hz, 60 pulses) • '50% intensity' (unclear if of machine output or MT) • 2 sessions (1st & 2nd days after communication of diagnosis)	Effective in 9/10: • Immediate total recovery in 6 • Dramatic improvement in 3 (clinical impression)	2/9 who improved relapsed "some months later" but responded to further treatment
	12 (sensory loss)	Centroparietal area (midline or contralateral to symptoms)	rTMS (Cc) • LF (approx. 1 Hz, 60 pulses) • "Above" MT • 1 session	Effective in 9/12: • Immediate total recovery in 6 • Dramatic improvement in 3 (clinical impression)	Not stated
	45 (seizure)	Frontocentral area in midline	rTMS (Cc) • LF (approx. 1 Hz, 60 pulses) • "Above" MT • Multiple sessions: all had 2 sessions (1st and 2nd days after communication of diagnosis) with extra sessions if symptoms had no initial effect or relapse (max. 8 sessions/month for 3 months)	Effective in 40/45: • 2 months symptomfree in 34 (80%) • 50% reduction in seizures in 40 (seizure frequency)	Improvements sustained at 6- and 12-month follow-up 4/40 who improved relapsed but responded to further treatment
Shah et al. (2015)	6 (MD)	MC then PMC	rTMS (F8c) • LF (0.33 Hz, 50 pulses) • 90% MT • 5 sessions over 5 consecutive week days to MC then repeated to PMC • N.B.: Protocol included suggestion of recovery	Unclear if effective: • Significant improvement in physical (but decrease in psychological QOL) domain after PMC (but not MC) stimulation 2 weeks posttreatment • No clear change in CGI (WHOQOL-BREF, CGI)	None

Table 50.1

Continued

Study	Patients (symptoms)	Target	Protocol	Effects (outcome measure)	Follow-up
Controlled trials					
Broersma et al. (2015)	11 (paresis)	MC	rTMS (F8c) Active treatment: • HF (15 Hz, 4000 pulses/session) • 1 session/day for 2 blocks of 5 consecutive days (with 2 rest days in between) Control treatment: sham with above protocol Primary outcome: objective strength (dynamometry) immediately before and after	Objective strength*: significant ($p < 0.04$) higher increase in active (24%) > control (6%) Subjective strength: nonsignificant higher increase in active (7%) > control (1%)	None

AIMS, abnormal involuntary movement scale; BFMS, Burke–Fahn–Marsden scale; Cc, circular coil; CGI, Clinical Global Impression; F8c, figure-of-eight coil; HF, high frequency; LF, low frequency; MC, (primary) motor cortex; MD, psychogenic movement disorder; MT, motor threshold; N/A, not applicable; PFC, prefrontal cortex; PMC, premotor cortex; QOL, quality of life; rTMS, repetitive TMS; WHOQOL-BREF, World Health Organization Quality of Life Brief scale.

*Measured using dynamometer.

abstracts and studies reporting the same data are removed there are a total of 185 patients with FND who have been reported to have this treatment. The first randomized controlled trial (RCT) – explicitly a small "proof-of-principle" (feasibility) study – has also recently been published (Broersma et al., 2015). The data from these will be reviewed in turn and are all summarized in Table 50.1.

Case series

The 10 studies have generally been of small numbers of patients – three are single case reports (Jellinek et al., 1992; Deftereos et al., 2008; Chastan et al., 2009), one is of 2 patients (Kresojevic et al., 2010), with only two studies being of more than 24 patients. The vast majority (9/10) have treated patients with motor symptoms – totaling 78 patients with weakness (including a single case of aphonia) and 42 with movement disorders (e.g., tremor, dystonia, or myoclonus). One study reported results on 22 patients with sensory symptoms (10 visual and 12 peripheral sensation) and on 45 patients with seizures (Parain and Chastan, 2014). It should be noted that many patients, when such detail is provided, also had other FND symptoms along with the "primary" symptom. Two studies each included a subject eventually diagnosed with malingering (Schonfeldt-Lecuona et al., 2006; Deftereos et al., 2008), but as definitively establishing such a diagnosis can be problematic (Nicholson et al., 2011), and the authors of these studies explicitly interpret the response of these patients for comparison to FND, these subjects have been kept in this review.

There is a wide heterogeneity in the methodology used, with no two studies having used exactly the same TMS protocols. The majority (seven of 10) have used rTMS, with only three of the smaller studies (totaling just 4 patients) using single-pulse TMS. The majority of the rTMS studies have used "low-frequency" ($\leq$1 Hz) stimulation parameters which are generally considered inhibitory. Three studies by the same group have used similar stimulation protocols but with varying anatomic targets (Chastan et al., 2009; Chastan and Parain, 2010; Parain and Chastan, 2014). Two other studies, this time by different groups, also used similar protocols (Schonfeldt-Lecuona et al., 2006; Shah et al., 2015) and are the only studies to date using "high-frequency" ($\geq$5 Hz) parameters which are generally considered excitatory. The majority (seven of 10) of studies have targeted the primary motor cortex (MC) (one also targeting the prefrontal cortex and one also targeting the premotor cortex (PMC)), two of 10 targeted the vertex, and one targeted different locations according to symptoms (Table 50.1). A wide variety of outcome measures were used and most were subjective, apart from one study which used tremor frequency on kinematic motion analysis (Dafotakis et al., 2011). In most other disorders objective outcome measures are generally considered optimal to reduce rater bias, but in FND – due to the nature of the disorder – it is possible that functional outcomes (such as activities of daily living) might be more informative, despite the tradeoff of such potential bias.

A recent systematic review of this area developed scores to assess both overall study and TMS method quality score to help interpret data and, perhaps more importantly, allow reproducibility of treatments (Pollak et al., 2014). Many of the earlier studies had low scores on one or both of these ratings, such that at the time of Pollak et al.'s review, only one study (Dafotakis et al., 2011) achieved over 50% (6/12) on overall study quality and full marks (8/8) on TMS method score. The three publications since then have scored better, particularly with regard to TMS method reporting, with two scoring 8/8 (Garcin et al., 2013; Shah et al., 2015) and one 6/8 (Parain and Chastan, 2014).

In terms of the results, nine of these studies reported data on individual response, and 162 of 179 (91%) patients with FND were reported as having "improved." As above, there was a wide variety of methods used to assess response and it should be acknowledged that the majority of these were clinical impression – either informally or formally (e.g., using Clinical Global Impression scores: Guy, 1976). Many were reported as "large" or "dramatic" improvements and even some resulting in "complete recovery" or "cure" (Table 50.1). It is worth noting that, for the majority of those followed up, with the exception of 7 of 11 patients in one study (Dafotakis et al., 2011), the clinical benefit lasted the duration of follow-up (range 1–12 months).

One study of good methodologic quality (Shah et al., 2015) did not give details of individual scores on the primary outcome (quality of life) for the 6 patients recruited. It reported no significant group changes to primary MC stimulation but "dissonant" findings to PMC stimulation in that physical health scores significantly increased but psychologic scores decreased. On the secondary outcome of global impression of change, only 1 of the patients self-rated as improved after TMS ("minimally improved" after MC and "much improved" after PMC stimulation), and clinician ratings showed no clear change with TMS (1 patient minimally improved after both MC and PMC stimulation and 1 only after PMC stimulation). It is worth noting that this was the only study to explicitly include a standardized (scripted) suggestion of benefit as part of the study protocol. It should also be noted that this study only assessed patients at 2 weeks after MC and then again 2 weeks after PMC treatment.

When all these results are taken together and interpreted at face value, TMS appears to be a highly effective treatment. However, it is clearly hard to interpret data from uncontrolled case series, especially when methodologic reporting is suboptimal, as it is in the majority of these studies. Also, given that placebo is likely to play an important role in this intervention, and possibly also more generally in this disorder, these results must be interpreted with particular caution. It is also possible that publication bias of positive results might account, at least in part, for the apparent efficacy.

One final issue is that many of these studies also provided other treatments to patients at the same time as TMS such as physical rehabilitation and explanation (Chastan et al., 2009; Garcin et al., 2013) meaning that its hard to know which element of treatment was therapeutic. It will be critical to control for these differences and standardize explanation in future studies.

Controlled trials

There has only been one published controlled RCT – a single-blind two-period cross-over trial of high-frequency rTMS (Broersma et al., 2015). Eleven patients with paralysis of at least one hand were randomized to either active or placebo treatment before having the other treatment 2 months later. Active treatment was 15 Hz rTMS at 80% of resting motor threshold (train length 2 seconds and intertrain interval 4 seconds) to the primary MC contralateral to the affected limb (or most affected if there was bilateral dysfunction). As such the treatment was "subthreshold" in terms of stimulating the MC and creating movement (although a suprathreshold stimulation must have been given at least once, and probably at least several times, to each individual to determine motor threshold). The primary outcome was objective grip strength assessed using dynamometry measured by a blinded clinician.

Placebo treatment was sham TMS, using a real electromagnetic placebo (REMP) device placed in front of the real TMS coil (which is not used) so, apart from this addition, the equipment is identical. REMP stimulates the underlying scalp and makes the same sound as a "real" TMS coil, but produces no intracranial stimulation. The authors report that patients "could not differentiate the active from the placebo condition when asked," which is reassuring, although it is not clear what this conclusion is based on, i.e., exactly what responses subjects gave to the question asked ("Did you notice which condition was the real and which was the fake treatment?"). It perhaps would have been more informative to have asked patients to guess which treatment was active and which was placebo and analyze the accuracy of these responses.

There are several other potential weaknesses with this study, in that the randomization procedure was predictable to clinicians (allocation by odd/even patient number), allowing for possible bias, but perhaps more importantly, there is a potentially significant problem with using cross-over trial designs in this setting. This is because both active and placebo TMS treatment effects may – and probably do – persist beyond any washout period, resulting in "carry-over" effects that can contaminate the second arm of the study.

However, despite these limitations, it was able to achieve its aim as a "proof-of-principle" study and, even with such small numbers, a significantly larger median increase was detected in objective strength after active compared to sham TMS (24% vs. 6%, $p < 0.04$) for the 8 patients who received both treatments. No significant equivalent difference was found for subjective strength, although the study was clearly underpowered to detect anything but a very large effect. This mismatch between objective and subjective strength change is interesting and the authors postulate that objective muscle strength is perhaps not the core symptom: subjective strength and therefore disability, and by extension combining TMS with behavioral approaches to treatment, might be of more importance.

Potential mechanism(s) of action

There are several possible mechanisms that could account for the effects of TMS that could occur either independently or in combination.

Placebo

Of course, placebo can account for a significant proportion of the treatment effect of any intervention, but this could be expected to be particularly significant with TMS – an intervention that involves visiting a "high-tech" lab where a device is placed over the brain (which is highly salient to the patient in terms of mechanism) and can be felt, sometimes painfully. Furthermore, there is some evidence of elevated rates of suggestibility in FND (Bell et al., 2011; Chapter 9). Although most of this evidence is anecdotal, there are some striking examples of this effect, most notably reports of instant recovery of chronic and severe FND dystonias following botulinum toxin injection, which takes at least 72 hours to have an effect (Edwards et al., 2011), and the success of diagnostic induction procedures for FND seizures (Chapter 26).

"Possibility of symptom improvement"

This is where the transient restoration of normal function (movement of a paralyzed limb or interruption of a tremor) caused by TMS is the critical factor (Pollak et al., 2014). Such temporary return of function could lead to longer-lasting recovery in several ways, which are of course not mutually exclusive: by presenting the cognitive and/or higher motor system with an opportunity to relearn normal function, by facilitating insight into the fact that the nerves are intact and, hence recovery is possible, or, controversially, by creating a face-saving opportunity for recovery.

Neuromodulation

As detailed above, TMS can change, and therefore theoretically normalize, motor function cortically, for example by changing the threshold for stimulation of the MC, known as resting motor threshold. None of the studies of TMS for FND to date have described protocols that would normally be expected to bring about significant neuromodulation. However, there are some neurophysiology studies of the motor system, again detailed above, that have used TMS experimentally rather than therapeutically and found abnormalities in FND which could theoretically be normalized by therapeutic TMS.

FUTURE DIRECTIONS

Randomized controlled trials of TMS

Clearly RCTs are needed to establish if TMS is actually an effective treatment and what the optimal methodology is. However, there are many complexities to studying this treatment in FND – both methodologically, such as choice of control intervention and outcome measure, and ethically, such as whether to knowingly use any placebo effect and whether this should be explicitly mentioned to patients.

Regarding the choice of control intervention, sham coils have become the standard control intervention in rTMS trials. Sham coils look and sound similar to a real coil but emit no magnetic pulse. More recent versions are also able to create a sensation on the scalp that does not affect underlying brain function to minimize any different feeling on success of blinding. However, there is mixed evidence regarding the success of sham coils (Broadbent et al., 2011; Berlim et al., 2013) so other control methods should be considered, such as "waiting list" or "treatment as usual" controls. Subthreshold TMS could also be used, i.e., real TMS but given at intensities not known to create any physiologic response. The ideal outcome measure(s) for trials of TMS, and for that matter other treatments, in FND, is not clearly established and no scales have been specifically designed for FND. As discussed above, there are complexities to FND that make functional outcomes of more potential importance than objective measures, which are generally considered optimal to reduce rater bias. Another issue in any future trial design will be length of follow-up and ensuring this is sufficient to exclude premature conclusions of sustained improvement.

Regarding the ethical issues of using placebo, it has been coherently argued that this is justified in FND (Shamy, 2010). In terms of the dilemma of whether or not to fully disclose treatment methods and intentions, the evolution of induction procedure for FND seizure diagnosis perhaps shows a way forward – initial concerns about nondisclosure to patients evaporated when it was found that full disclosure did not reduce efficacy and recently there has even been some evidence that rates of seizure induction may actually be higher if the clinician is explicit about the method (Hoepner et al., 2013). This counterintuitive phenomenon has also been found more generally for placebos in that it works, even when clearly labeled as such (Kaptchuk et al., 2010), and it is perhaps relevant that this study was in irritable-bowel syndrome – a functional gastrointestinal disorder.

Finally it is possible that TMS can work synergistically with other treatment modalities, such as physical therapy and CBT. For example, physical therapy immediately after TMS could quickly build on any initial symptomatic gains (especially in cases of complete paralysis, where physical therapy would have not previously been possible) and a CBT therapist being present during a TMS session could provide very helpful topics of discussion during subsequent CBT sessions.

A double-blind RCT (Paralystim) is under way in France (https://clinicaltrials.gov/ct2/show/study/NCT01352910). This trial aims to randomize 94 FND patients with paralysis to either active rTMS (120 pulses over 2 days to the MC at 2 Hz) or to sham rTMS. The results of this and other trials should help determine whether TMS is an effective and safe treatment that could be put into routine clinical use. Once this primary question is addressed, RCTs will be needed to develop the optimal protocols as well as define which types of patients the therapy might be most effective for.

Other stimulation methods

The last decade has seen the development and increasing therapeutic application of other noninvasive brain stimulation techniques, particularly transcranial direct-current stimulation (tDCS), although other methods exist, such as cranial electrotherapy stimulation (CES) or reduced-impedance noninvasive cortical electrostimulation (RINCE). tDCS has been used therapeutically for a similar range of neurologic and psychiatric conditions as TMS (Tortella et al., 2015). As yet, there are no reports of its use for FND, but it has been used for fibromyalgia (Marlow et al., 2013), complex regional pain syndrome (Dufka et al., 2015), and chronic pain more widely. A Cochrane review of 14 trials concluded that tDCS was not an effective treatment for chronic pain (O'Connell et al., 2014), despite earlier reviews indicating possible efficacy. Although tDCS is increasingly being marketed directly to the public as a safe tool to increase alertness and/or cognitive function, there is also evidence that it might have negative effects on cognition (Sellers et al., 2015).

Although the placebo effect of tDCS is likely to be similar to TMS, it would not create brief involuntary movements of paralyzed limbs, if this was important for efficacy as a way of illustrating potential for recovery or enabling the relearning of normal function, as above. There are also other potentially important differences between tDCS and TMS, particularly its anatomic specificity and more generally its effects on brain networks and function.

Conclusion

There is an accumulating evidence base to support TMS as a safe, well-tolerated, and possibly effective treatment for a wide range of FND symptoms. However, this is largely based on case series with inadequate reporting of TMS methods. The role of placebo effects in series reporting efficacy is likely to be significant and, until placebo-controlled optimally randomized trials are performed, these results should be viewed with caution. However, even if placebo accounts for a large part of the treatment effect, this does not mean that TMS should not be used to help stimulate recovery in a disorder with few proven treatments and for which chronic severe disability is common. Finally, other noninvasive indirect electric stimulation methods may also soon be applied therapeutically in FND for which the same challenges of establishing efficacy beyond placebo effect will apply.

SEDATION

Pharmacologically induced sedation has a long history of use in the management of FND and was first developed to enhance suggestibility without using hypnosis (Horsley, 1943). It was subsequently also used both in the form of abreaction (also known as narcoanalysis) in which psychotherapy is facilitated with a change in consciousness and as an aid to rehabilitation.

Abreaction

A systematic review of abreaction identified a total of 116 FND patients from 55 studies, of which 79% recovered (Poole et al., 2010). The studies were predominantly case reports or series ($n=52$), or open-label trials ($n=4$), and none included placebo controls. Barbiturates (e.g., sodium amytal, thiopentone) were the main drugs used and benzodiazepines less commonly, with the occasional use of comorbid stimulants to enhance emotional catharsis (release of strong or repressed emotions) via hyperexcitability. The techniques used while under sedation included suggestion (verbal communication that a specific nonvolitional response will be experienced, 41%), emotional catharsis (or abreaction, 27%), exploration (72%), and rehabilitation (manipulation of the limb under sedation, 13%). Both suggestion and emotional catharsis appeared beneficial, with recovery rates of 92% and 94% respectively, with somewhat lower rates with exploration (81%) and rehabilitation (67%). The state of sedation along with an elaborate procedure is believed to enhance suggestibility and expectancies, an underlying mechanism that is believed to play a role in FND (Chapters 47 and 48).

In this review, the experience of "emotional catharsis" with retrieval of a repressed memory also appeared to be associated with high improvement rates. The act of retrieval of a repressed memory may, similar to that of posttraumatic stress disorder, decrease the anxiety associated with avoidance of a traumatic memory by exposure resulting in habituation. In the systematic review, there appeared to be worse outcome with a comorbid psychiatric disorder but no clear effect of symptom duration of greater than 6 months. Notably, these reports are limited by their lack of controls, small sample size, likely publication bias (i.e., publication of positive but not negative results), and lack of blinding, such that interpretation of effects could be based on the biases of the clinician.

Rehabilitation

A recent retrospective case series of 11 FND patients describes the use of sedation using propofol (Stone et al., 2014), which has rapid onset and offset and pleasant anxiolytic properties. Here the goal of sedation was to focus on movement and rehabilitation with an accompanying video used to aid recovery. Five of the 11 patients had major improvements or cessation of symptoms with sedation. The cases selected were chronic (median duration 14 months) and patients' symptoms could not be temporarily reversed during physical examination. The authors suggest possible therapeutic mechanisms, to include the demonstration of reversibility to persuade the correctness of the diagnosis or the potential for recovery; the role of suggestion; and that chemical alteration may interrupt abnormal neural pathways involved in cognitive, motor, and behavioral pathways. The drug may interfere with learned responses, disrupt excessive inhibition, or decrease anxiety. A guide to suitable patients, the procedure, and patient explanation is provided. Suitable patients, as described in the case series, include those with FND, a severe deficit such as dystonia or paraplegia whose reversibility cannot be shown during a normal clinical exam, good doctor–patient relationship, good patient confidence in the diagnosis, and good patient motivation. Transparency regarding the procedure was emphasized, including the possibility that the procedure may be a form of suggestion. The purpose was explained to the patient as a means to "kick start" movement or to normalize a position of an affected limb.

Conclusion

The use of sedation in the management of FND has a long history. Its intended purpose reflects underlying theories of mechanisms, with a long history of use for the purposes of abreaction and suggestion, with a more recent resurgence in interest focusing on rehabilitation and suggestion. Although the literature is without controlled trials, its use with carefully selected patients for well-defined purposes appears to have some efficacy.

ACKNOWLEDGMENTS AND FUNDING

Dr Tim Nicholson is funded by a National Institute for Health Research (NIHR) Clinician Scientist Fellowship award in the UK. This article presents independent research funded by the NIHR. The views expressed are those of the author and not necessarily those of the NHS, the NIHR or the Department of Health.

References

Bell V, Oakley DA, Halligan PW et al. (2011). Dissociation in hysteria and hypnosis: evidence from cognitive neuroscience. J Neurol Neurosurg Psychiatry 82: 332–339.

Berlim MT, Broadbent HJ, Van den Eynde F (2013). Blinding integrity in randomized sham-controlled trials of repetitive transcranial magnetic stimulation for major depression: a systematic review and meta-analysis. Int J Neuropsychopharmacol 16: 1173–1181.

Broadbent HJ, van den Eynde F, Guillaume S et al. (2011). Blinding success of rTMS applied to the dorsolateral prefrontal cortex in randomised sham-controlled trials: a systematic review. World J Biol Psychiatry 12: 240–248.

Broersma M, Koops EA, Vroomen PC et al. (2015). Can repetitive transcranial magnetic stimulation increase muscle strength in functional neurological paresis? A proof-of-principle study. Eur J Neurol 22: 866–873.

Carson A, Stone J, Hibberd C et al. (2011). Disability, distress and unemployment in neurology outpatients with symptoms "unexplained by organic disease". J Neurol Neurosurg Psychiatry 82: 810–813.

Chastan N, Parain D (2010). Psychogenic paralysis and recovery after motor cortex transcranial magnetic stimulation. Mov Disord 25: 1501–1504.

Chastan N, Parain D, Verin E et al. (2009). Psychogenic aphonia: spectacular recovery after motor cortex transcranial magnetic stimulation. J Neurol Neurosurg Psychiatry 80: 94.

Dafotakis M, Ameli M, Vitinius F et al. (2011). Transcranial magnetic stimulation for psychogenic tremor – a pilot study. Fortschr Neurol Psychiatr 79: 226–233.

Deftereos SN, Panagopoulos GN, Georgonikou DD et al. (2008). Diagnosis of nonorganic monoplegia with single-pulse transcranial magnetic stimulation. Prim Care Companion J Clin Psychiatry 10: 414.

Dufka FL, Munch T, Dworkin RH et al. (2015). Results availability for analgesic device, complex regional pain syndrome, and post-stroke pain trials: comparing the RReADS, RReACT, and RReMiT databases. Pain 156: 72–80.

Edwards MJ, Talelli P, Rothwell JC (2008). Clinical applications of transcranial magnetic stimulation in patients with movement disorders. Lancet Neurol 7: 827–840.

Edwards MJ, Bhatia KP, Cordivari C (2011). Immediate response to botulinum toxin injections in patients with fixed dystonia. Mov Disord 26: 917–918.

Garcin B, Roze E, Mesrati F et al. (2013). Transcranial magnetic stimulation as an efficient treatment for psychogenic movement disorders. J Neurol Neurosurg Psychiatry 84: 1043–1046.

Gelauff J, Stone J, Edwards M et al. (2014). The prognosis of functional (psychogenic) motor symptoms: a systematic review. J Neurol Neurosurg Psychiatry 85: 220–226.

Geraldes R, Coelho M, Rosa MM et al. (2008). Abnormal transcranial magnetic stimulation in a patient with presumed psychogenic paralysis. J Neurol Neurosurg Psychiatry 79: 1412–1413.

Goldstein LH, Chalder T, Chigwedere C et al. (2010). Cognitive-behavioral therapy for psychogenic nonepileptic seizures: a pilot RCT. Neurology 74: 1986–1994.

Guy W (1976). ECDEU Assessment Manual for Psychopharmacology, U.S. Department of Health, Education and Welfare, Rockville, MD.

Hoepner R, Labudda K, Schoendienst M et al. (2013). Informing patients about the impact of provocation methods increases the rate of psychogenic nonepileptic seizures during EEG recording. Epilepsy Behav 28: 457–459.

Horsley JS (1943). Narco-analysis. A New Technique in Short-cut Psychotherapy: A Comparison with other Methods and Notes on the Barbiturates, Oxford University Press, Oxford.

Jellinek DA, Bradford R, Bailey I et al. (1992). The role of motor evoked potentials in the management of hysterical paraplegia: case report. Paraplegia 30: 300–302.

Kaptchuk TJ, Friedlander E, Kelley JM et al. (2010). Placebos without deception: a randomized controlled trial in irritable bowel syndrome. PLoS One 5: e15591.

Khalil TM, Abdel-Moty E, Asfour SS et al. (1988). Functional electric stimulation in the reversal of conversion disorder paralysis. Arch Phys Med Rehabil 69: 545–547.

Kresojevic N, Petrovic I, Tomic A et al. (2010). Transcranial magnetic stimulation in therapy of psychogenic neurological symptoms: two case reports. Mov Disord 25: S220.

LaFrance Jr WC, Baird GL, Barry JJ et al. (2014). Multicenter pilot treatment trial for psychogenic nonepileptic seizures: a randomized clinical trial. JAMA Psychiatry 71: 997–1005.

Lefaucheur J-P, André-Obadia N, Antal A et al. (2014). Evidence-based guidelines on the therapeutic use of repetitive transcranial magnetic stimulation (rTMS). Clin Neurophysiol 125: 2150–2206.

Liepert J, Hassa T, Tuscher O et al. (2011). Motor excitability during movement imagination and movement observation in psychogenic lower limb paresis. J Psychosom Res 70: 59–65.

Loo CK, McFarquhar TF, Mitchell PB (2008). A review of the safety of repetitive transcranial magnetic stimulation as a clinical treatment for depression. Int J Neuropsychopharmacol 11: 131–147.

Marlow NM, Bonilha HS, Short EB (2013). Efficacy of transcranial direct current stimulation and repetitive transcranial magnetic stimulation for treating fibromyalgia syndrome: a systematic review. Pain Pract 13: 131–145.

McWhirter L, Carson A, Stone J (2015). The body electric: a long view of electrical therapy for functional neurological disorders. Brain 138: 1113–1120.

Nicholson TRJ, Stone J, Kanaan RAA (2011). Conversion disorder: a problematic diagnosis. J Neurol Neurosurg Psychiatry 82: 1267–1273.

Nielsen G, Stone J, Edwards MJ (2013). Physiotherapy for functional (psychogenic) motor symptoms: a systematic review. J Psychosom Res 75: 93–102.

O'Connell NE, Wand BM, Marston L et al. (2014). Non-invasive brain stimulation techniques for chronic pain. Cochrane Database Syst Rev 4: CD008208.

Parain D, Chastan N (2014). Large-field repetitive transcranial magnetic stimulation with circular coil in the treatment of functional neurological symptoms. Neurophysiol Clin 44: 425–431.

Pollak TA, Nicholson TR, Edwards MJ et al. (2014). A systematic review of transcranial magnetic stimulation in the treatment of functional (conversion) neurological symptoms. J Neurol Neurosurg Psychiatry 85: 191–197.

Poole NA, Wuerz A, Agrawal N (2010). Abreaction for conversion disorder: systematic review with meta-analysis. Br J Psychiatry 197: 91–95.

Rossi S, Hallett M, Rossini PM et al. (2009). Safety, ethical considerations, and application guidelines for the use of transcranial magnetic stimulation in clinical practice and research. Clin Neurophysiol 120: 2008–2039.

Rossini PM, Burke D, Chen R et al. (2015). Non-invasive electrical and magnetic stimulation of the brain, spinal cord, roots and peripheral nerves: basic principles and procedures for routine clinical and research application. An updated report from an I.F.C.N. Committee. Clin Neurophysiol 126: 1071–1107.

Schonfeldt-Lecuona C, Connemann BJ, Viviani R et al. (2006). Transcranial magnetic stimulation in motor conversion disorder: a short case series. J Clin Neurophysiol 23: 472–475.

Sellers KK, Mellin JM, Lustenberger CM et al. (2015). Transcranial direct current stimulation of frontal cortex decreases performance on the WAIS-IV intelligence test. Behav Brain Res 290: 32–44.

Shah BB, Chen R, Zurowski M et al. (2015). Repetitive transcranial magnetic stimulation plus standardized suggestion of benefit for functional movement disorders: an open label case series. Parkinsonism Relat Disord 21: 407–412.

Shamy MCF (2010). The treatment of psychogenic movement disorders with suggestion is ethically justified. Mov Disord 25: 260–264.

Stone J (2014). Functional neurological disorders: the neurological assessment as treatment. Neurophysiol Clin 44: 363–373.

Stone J, Carson A, Duncan R et al. (2011). Who is referred to neurology clinics? The diagnoses made in 3781 new patients. Clin Neurol Neurosurg 112: 747–751.

Stone J, Hoeritzauer I, Brown K et al. (2014). Therapeutic sedation for functional (psychogenic) neurological symptoms. J Psychosom Res 76: 165–168.

Tortella G, Casati R, Aparicio LVM et al. (2015). Transcranial direct current stimulation in psychiatric disorders. World J Psychiatry 5: 88–102.

Handbook of Clinical Neurology, Vol. 139 (3rd series)
Functional Neurologic Disorders
M. Hallett, J. Stone, and A. Carson, Editors
http://dx.doi.org/10.1016/B978-0-12-801772-2.00051-5

Chapter 51

Inpatient treatment for functional neurologic disorders

D.T. WILLIAMS[1]*, K. LAFAVER[2], A. CARSON[3], AND S. FAHN[4]

[1]*Movement Disorders Division, Columbia University Medical Center and Department of Psychiatry, Columbia College of Physicians and Surgeons, New York, NY, USA*

[2]*Movement Disorders Clinic, University of Louisville, Louisville, KY, USA*

[3]*Departments of Clinical Neurosciences and of Rehabilitation Medicine, NHS Lothian and Centre for Clinical Brain Sciences, University of Edinburgh, Edinburgh, UK*

[4]*Department of Neurology, Columbia University Medical Center, New York, NY, USA*

Abstract

Patients with functional neurologic disorders present to clinicians with a variety of symptomatic manifestations, with various levels of severity, chronicity, and comorbidity, as well as with various degrees of past adversity, intrinsic resilience, and available external support. Clearly, treatment must be individualized. For those patients who have been severely or chronically impaired, especially if adequate prior outpatient treatments have failed, inpatient treatment that integrates the various modalities outlined here provides a rational route of rescue from a course otherwise potentially characterized by protracted dependence and disability. Based on the data currently available, we believe this treatment approach is worthy of further study to refine the component treatment strategies and enhance the potentially most effective ingredients. For patients with severe levels of disability, who could be managed in a multimodal day-treatment program, that approach also warrants further consideration.

It may appear that having inpatient treatment as the last chapter in the section on treatment in a book on functional neurologic disorders (FNDs) implies that it is the treatment approach of last resort when all other interventions, first tried on an outpatient basis, have failed. That is not necessarily so. In a significant number of cases, the patient with an FND is admitted to an inpatient medical unit via the emergency department by virtue of having presented acutely with paralysis (including apparent "stroke"), apparent status epilepticus, or a dramatically disabling movement disorder, and it is not until careful neurologic evaluation has been completed on the inpatient unit that the diagnosis of a functional disorder is established with some level of confidence. It would be helpful to distinguish between such acute inpatient situations and the alternate scenario of an elective admission to hospital after the diagnosis is reasonably confidently established on an outpatient basis, but, by virtue of the symptom chronicity or number of prior failed treatment trials, a more intensive inpatient neuropsychiatric re-evaluation and treatment course is nevertheless recommended. The available clinical literature generally does not distinguish effectively between these rather different circumstances (Koelen et al., 2014). Consequently, we will address this topic as informed in part by the available literature and in part by our clinical experience.

A number of different inpatient treatment models for FND have been reported on by different groups. Not surprisingly, the roles of different practitioners vary between differing inpatient treatment models. In the first part of this chapter we describe these different models, and their supporting evidence base, and in the second part we highlight some of the issues that arise theoretically and practically for different healthcare practitioners in treating such patients. One theme that does emerge from all

*Correspondence to: Daniel T. Williams, M.D., 2001 Marcus Ave. Suite 218 North, New Hyde Park, New York NY 11042, USA. Tel: +1-516-488-3636, E-mail: dtw1@columbia.edu

the differing models is that a significant proportion of patients improve following an inpatient admission, even if they have had chronic and severe symptoms.

PIONEERING INPATIENT TREATMENT OF PSYCHOGENIC (FUNCTIONAL) MOVEMENT DISORDERS (PMDs)

Insofar as the vast majority of movement disorders are not perceived as being acutely dangerous, they are less often the basis of emergent hospital admission and patients with movement disorders present more often to neurologists initially as outpatients. Furthermore, insofar as most movement disorders, with the exception of tremors, myoclonus, and startle, do not have diagnostically specific electrophysiologic markers, they do not lend themselves to standard advocacy for admission to an inpatient neurology service, such as an epilepsy monitoring unit, for technologically informed neurologic diagnostic confirmation.

The challenge of diagnosing PMDs is formidable, as reflected by the fact that it is only in the past 35 years that neurologists have developed criteria to recognize and differentially diagnose these disorders (Fahn et al., 1983; Fahn and Williams, 1988; Fahn, 2011). Indeed, by virtue of the general lack of confirmatory laboratory, radiologic, or definitive electrophysiologic diagnostic tests, it requires a neurologist with substantial experience in evaluating movement disorders based on knowledge of the natural history and specific findings on careful neurologic exam to effectively establish a definitive diagnosis. One of the consequences of this is that patients with PMDs often carry the mistaken, discouraging diagnosis of a static or degenerative neurologic disorder for lengthy periods, sometimes years, before a correct diagnosis of a PMD is made. Patients may come burdened with a combination of chronic disability, inappropriate treatment, sometimes including not only inappropriate medication, but even misguided surgical intervention, as well as an iatrogenically reinforced conviction regarding their erroneous diagnosis.

Faced with this constellation of burdens, it is not surprising that, when presented with the correct diagnosis of a PMD by a sophisticated neurologist who appears late in the clinical course, the patient and concerned family members often responded with shocked disbelief and departed without accepting a justified referral for psychiatric evaluation, searching rather for another specialist who will find the "true organic basis" of the chronic, impairing disorder. Because of this repeatedly observed pattern, Fahn and Williams developed an informal protocol, implemented with significant positive results before the advent of "managed care constraints," to admit these patients to hospital for a more extended opportunity for collaborative neuropsychiatric evaluation and treatment.

In the initial clinical approach to PMD patients, the movement disorder neurologist, with varying levels of diagnostic confidence regarding a PMD at time of initial consultation, nevertheless withheld judgment regarding a definitive diagnosis and recommended to the patient an admission to the inpatient neurology service for further evaluation and treatment. A preliminary, tentative admitting diagnosis, based on the presenting phenomenology, was presented to the patient, e.g., dystonia, tremor, gait disorder, with the associated explanation to the patient that stress, often on an unconscious basis, may be contributory to the symptoms. It would be clearly explained that the planned 5–10-day admission would include repeated observational assessment and repeated examinations by the neurologist, extended evaluations by the team psychiatrist to explore possibly relevant stress issues, as well as possible physical therapy (for strengthening, "desensitization," and "retraining"), occupational therapy (for improving fine motor control) and possible pharmacotherapy, with a preliminary treatment plan formulation based on the combined ongoing assessments of the various members of the team.

Admissions were scheduled for Sunday evening, and after 2 days of intensive assessments, a conjoint meeting would be held, involving the patient and any authorized family member(s), the neurologist(s), the psychiatrist, and any other involved team members, including the staff nurse, whose clinical observations and supportive participation in the treatment were often valuable. If, by that time, a sufficient level of diagnostic consensus and confidence regarding the presence of a PMD had been established, this would be presented supportively to the patient and the family in two segments.

First, the neurologist outlined the patient's phenomenology as clinically significant, coupled with the good news that the assessment had ascertained that it was not part of a degenerative neurologic disorder, but rather the byproduct of a neurophysiologically based stress reaction, which was described either as a "psychogenic" movement disorder (to distinguish it from a neurologically based degenerative disorder), or as a "conversion disorder," based on the (presumptive) unconsciously based conversion of stress into physical symptoms. To help patients and family members digest this news conceptually and emotionally, supportive analogies commonly recognized by the lay public were used illustratively, such as stress-induced hypertension, headaches, or gastrointestinal symptoms. A proposed treatment plan would be outlined, including psychotherapy, physical therapy, and, if indicated, pharmacotherapy as clinically warranted. The neurologist noted that what was being offered was an opportunity for an intensive clinical intervention trial of multimodal therapy based on substantial clinical experience, with positive published results, in the face of often multiple prior failed interventions. The neurologist emphasized further that the patient's clinical outcome was highly contingent on the patient's active participation in all components of the multimodal treatment.

The psychiatrist's role at this debriefing meeting was to supportively present a formulation, based on the diagnostic framework outlined by the neurologist, to give detailed support to its relevance based on the stressors and sensitivities that had been elicited from the patient (sometimes with input from family members). The prospect of enhancing the patient's capacity to cope with the designated stressors and sensitivities with the help of relevant psychotherapeutic, physical therapy, and pharmacotherapy measures was delineated. Observations were made regarding the favorable response rate to this intensive treatment plan, which included some patients having made full functional recoveries, even after years of protracted disability. Patients who made rapid gains of clinical improvement were slated for discharge by Friday of the first week, with the longest duration of stay being Friday of the following week (maximum of 10 week days).

Detailed reports of the response rates both at discharge and follow-up are available elsewhere (Ford et al., 1994; Williams et al., 1995, 2011). It is noteworthy that, although these reports are retrospective and represent an incomplete sampling, the global self-assessment of movement disorder symptom status in follow-up in our most recent study (Williams et al., 2011) included 36% of patients with symptoms totally resolved; 25% markedly better; 14% moderately better; 7% unchanged; 4% moderately worse; and 4% markedly worse. Quality-of-life self-assessment at follow-up closely paralleled the degree of improvement in movement symptoms.

Insofar as these patients represented severely and often chronically impaired patients with PMDs, the results, despite being uncontrolled and retrospective, represent a useful clinical model to consider for patients who have failed prior efforts at outpatient treatment.

With the advent of "managed care" restrictions on reimbursement for inpatient treatment (in the USA), the above model was frequently problematic. Elective admissions often required "preauthorization," generally by a clerical agent following an algorithm on which inpatient multimodal treatment of PMDs did not appear. Efforts by the neurologist to arrange inpatient admission after initial office consultation, with explanatory verbal or written reports to the insurance company, were sometimes rebuffed. This led to the development of an outpatient preadmission psychiatric consultation that provided two advantages. First, it was found that some patients who were denied inpatient admission by their insurance company were willing to work with the psychiatrist and neurologist on an outpatient basis once it became clear that there was a collaborative team approach and the patient was not being "dismissed" to the psychiatrist, but followed conjointly in a format that was palatable and often effective.

For those patients where the severity and chronicity of their impairment or their geographic lack of access to appropriate integrated care on an outpatient basis precluded this, the team was in a position, after having both neurologic and psychiatric consultation reports, to appeal more effectively to insurance companies for a review of the merits of an inpatient admission. The rationale provided, based on these two reports, as well as copies of relevant clinical published studies, sometimes persuaded an insurance company that it would be more economically advantageous for them to support short-term intensive inpatient treatment that had a better prospect for substantial, cost-saving clinical improvement than the perpetuation of ongoing, expensive, and ineffectual outpatient treatment for a chronically disabled patient (Konnopka et al., 2013).

A REHABILITATION MODEL FOR CONVERSION PARALYSIS

An alternate approach to inpatient treatment of conversion disorder is described by Heruti and colleagues (2002). It needs to be treated with caution, in that they describe outcomes by anecdote rather than audit, but it was a notable review in regard to its enthusiasm for multimodal rehabilitation delivered within a neurorehabilitation service. "The preferred setting is hospitalization in a rehabilitation ward in order to observe the patients in all activities."

Their approach is notably different from Fahn and Williams (1988), in that they adopt a more agnostic symptom reduction model to treatment. They argue that a patient with paralysis should be rehabilitated in the same setting as other patients with paralysis, regardless of underlying mechanism, and that "those disabled due to conversion have many similarities to those with an organic basis for the disability, with regard to effects on physiology, social and occupational consequences." Treatment should begin as early as possible before secondary complications develop and should consist of three main components: behavior modification, psychotherapy, and physical therapy. Perhaps the most controversial aspect of their treatment is the issue of explanation. In contrast to the Fahn and Williams approach, they recommend adopting a deliberate vagueness and tend not to be explicit with this patient what is wrong – they will comfortably use euphemisms such as "spinal concussion," but with an emphasis on reversibility. Whilst this approach can easily coalign with physical therapy delivered along traditional lines, it is less clear how the rationale for psychologic aspects of treatment is explained to the patient. These treatments are also delivered in a traditional fashion with behavior modification, adopting a positive reinforcement of desirable adaptive behaviors that promote function and minimize disability, and psychotherapy directed towards a cathartic approach to underlying conflicts. One is left wondering how this "diagnostic fudge" can be satisfactorily maintained in both patients doing well and those who fail to progress.

STRATEGIC INTERVENTION IN INPATIENT REHABILITATION OF SEVERE FUNCTIONAL/FACTITIOUS DISORDERS

The issue of how open and honest to be with patients over their diagnosis is taken to a different level of ethical debate in an approach described by Shapiro and Teasell (2004) in which they explicitly advocate deceiving the patient. They report on a paradoxic intervention, the core element of which involved telling patients that, although full recovery constituted proof of a physical etiology, failure to recover constituted conclusive evidence of a psychiatric etiology. This was communicated by the attending physician based upon a detailed script that also included instructions for all team members on implementing their part of the program. They claim dramatic improvement rates, with 13 of 21 chronic patients making a complete recovery. By contrast, typical behavioral therapies, in a nonrandomized chart review group, had led to improvements in only 1 of 28 patients. The outcome measurement was weak and consisted of an observer-rated Clinical Global Impression measurement made independently by the two authors. The possibilities of both conscious and unconscious biases must lead to questions over the reliability of the results and independent replication of the results would be essential. However, even allowing the claimed astonishing efficacy of the treatment, we would strongly question whether the ethics of deliberately distorting the truth could justify such a method, even if it was efficacious. This proposed approach, furthermore, goes beyond simply enhancing a placebo effect and into the realms of frank deceit. It also seems inherently unlikely to stand the test of time once knowledge of the approach is "out there" among patients, who have far better access to health information than they did at the time of this study's publication.

A MULTIMODAL PROGRAM-BASED INPATIENT APPROACH

Saifee et al. (2012) report outcomes from a multimodal approach that has developed over a number of years at the National Hospital for Neurology and Neurosurgery in London. Like Heruti et al. (2002), they make considerable use of physical therapies and psychologic therapies, but move from a psychodynamic model viewing FND as a response to repressed psychologic conflicts to a cognitive-behavioral therapy (CBT) model emphasizing illness beliefs and coping strategies.

Like Fahn and Williams, they start from the perspective of a secure neurologic diagnosis, but they recommend being clear about that diagnosis prior to admission if further tests are required. These are completed prior to any discussion of inpatient assessment. Patients are then invited to an assessment clinic for the program, where they meet the rehabilitation team and the diagnosis and treatment program are fully explained. Patients who are not accepting of either diagnosis or the treatment rationale are not progressed.

> *Treatment has common components, but is tailored to the individual. The common components of the programme are neurophysiotherapy, occupational therapy, cognitive behavioural therapy, nursing from staff with a mental health nursing background, neuropsychiatry assessment and input (1 consultant neuropsychiatrist, 2 psychiatry trainees), and neurology input as required (2 neurology trainees, plus consultant neurology input as required) (Saifee et al., 2012).*

It is delivered 5 days a week over a 4-week program subject to making progress.

> *The general approach to functional symptoms is that they are genuine symptoms that are reversible via rehabilitation. The rationale for using combined cognitive and physical rehabilitation is that cognitive/psychological factors are important in the way symptoms are produced and therefore in how they can be treated. From the cognitive perspective, there is an emphasis on developing coping strategies and changing illness beliefs, and from the physical rehabilitation perspective, distraction techniques and error-based learning techniques are employed (Saifee et al., 2012).*

Psychodynamic approaches of exploring psychologic conflicts or a history of trauma or aversive events are generally not used unless particularly relevant to an individual case. The program is particularly notable for the sophisticated physiotherapy models used (see Chapter 45 and Nielsen et al., 2015).

The authors report on follow-up approximately 2 years after admission and found significant self-reported improvement in 58% of patients who also reported an improvement in their functioning, but unfortunately there was little translation of this improvement into work status or levels of receipt of health-related benefits. One feature of note is the enthusiasm patients reported for the treatment program and, in particular, the endorsements they made of the usefulness of allied health professionals and the helpfulness of physiotherapy, occupational therapy, and CBT. The same team later conducted a prospective cohort study of patients going through their service and found broadly similar results (Demartini et al., 2014). One notable feature of this study was that they found that improvements on the clinician-rated Health of the Nation Outcome Scale (Wing et al., 1998) correlated most closely with patient-rated improvement.

A NEUROPSYCHIATRY-LED MULTIMODAL INTERVENTION

Although adopting a broadly similar etiologic outlook to Saifee et al. (2012), the Maudsley Hospital in London also offers an intensive inpatient rehabilitation course for patients with severe FNDs. The treatment differs from most others described in that it is psychiatrically led and without neurologic involvement. One also senses, reading their description, that the treatment has more emphasis on CBT-based psychotherapy, in contrast to the physiotherapy emphasis in Jordbru et al. (2014; see below) and Saifee et al. (2012).

Neuropsychiatrists took on the role of diagnostic explanation, including explaining to patients why more tests were not going to be conducted, and liaising with medical colleagues over diagnostic security as required. They also assessed and treated psychiatric comorbidities and guided any pharmacologic interventions. Psychologists progressed treatment on a largely CBT-based model, but with elements of psychoeducation and relapse prevention strategies included. The core components of CBT were to:

> *challenge any cognitive distortions that might affect a patient's motivation, determination or ability to engage on an interpersonal level. The therapist works to build insight into a more psychological understanding of symptoms and assists in shifting the locus of control from 'external' (eg, a dependence on medications or care takers) to 'internal', by fostering insight and assertiveness. If thought important, the patient is assisted to discover links between past or present experience and physical symptoms although this is not essential. Techniques may include mood and thought diaries (the patient then trying to link these moods and thoughts with environmental exposures), relaxation techniques (particularly if the patient has fears and expectations around improvement) and graded exposure (if avoidance is employed as a coping strategy), along with homework and tasks decided upon in collaboration with the patient (Saifee et al., 2012).*

In the case series they describe, 28 of 33 cases (84.9%) had CBT – the rest declined treatment or were not suitable. Physiotherapy and occupational therapy were also involved but generally at a less intensive level than in the other programs described – usually twice a week and with relatively nonspecific approaches. The whole program was delivered in a positive, nonjudgmental fashion.

Given the severity of the patient group (61% wheelchair-bound at admission), the degree of improvement was encouraging, with two-thirds no longer requiring their chair at discharge and the percentage walking completely unaided rising from 15% to 42%.

A UNIQUE RANDOMIZED TRIAL OF INPATIENT PHYSICAL REHABILITATION THERAPIES

Jordbru et al. (2014) reported on a randomized trial of physical therapy for patients with severe psychogenic gait impairments. There are a number of methodologic issues which a trials purist would be concerned about, such as the actual randomization techniques, but it nonetheless represents a fascinating first attempt at evaluating inpatient treatment properly. It is also pleasing to read a paper on rehabilitation in which the nature of the treatment is clearly articulated.

The authors follow Heruti's model and do not apply any diagnostic label on admission, simply saying that there is no exact explanation for a patient's symptoms but serious illness has been ruled out, and such disconnections between the nervous system and muscles frequently follow stressful life events. The idea of reversibility is emphasized and patients are told that attending to multiple activities helps reconnection.

The treatment itself was very oriented to physical activity rather than clinical physiotherapy with "an emphasis on daily adapted sport activities, such as riding a bicycle, ball activities, outdoor canoeing, and indoor climbing, and patients were helped to shift focus from disability to mastering of activities" (Jordbru et al., 2014). Any improvement in function or distraction form disability was responded to by marked positive reinforcement by staff. By contrast, staff gave minimal attention and tried to ignore impairments, disability, and nonparticipative behaviors. Ultimately, patients failing to progress were discharged early.

The majority spent at least the first weekend at the hospital. Encouraging and reinforcing normal function was also a joint treatment strategy when patients were not in training situations. This made the institution a round-the-clock arena for treatment. Thus, "we tried to convey a clear message that a person can get better by training, with focus on activities they can do in spite of their dysfunction."

It can be seen, as the authors openly acknowledge, that, although described as a physical therapy, treatment is in fact heavily based on behavioral therapy principles. What might be less apparent was the sheer physical beauty of the hospital setting: the nonspecific engagement effects of canoeing in a Norwegian fjord may not be replicated during physiotherapy on a treadmill in a highly urban setting.

Sixty patients were randomized, with an average symptom duration of 10 months. Notably, 54 were excluded, the majority for being symptomatic for over 5 years, but 8 for lacking motivation. These limitations aside, the 3-week program led to substantive gains in function measured on observer-rated scales – the Functional Independence Measure (11 units) and the self-report Short Form 12 (SF12: 14 units). Perhaps a more telling indication of outcome was that 25% were wheelchair-bound and a further 38% used walking aids at baseline, but none used them at follow-up. The authors also report, but don't provide actual data, that many patients returned to work.

AN EXEMPLAR OF A VERY BRIEF MULTIDISCIPLINARY INPATIENT REHABILITATION PROGRAM

At the University of Louisville, KY, patients with a functional movement disorder with sufficient severity to impact their ability to work or perform activities of daily living are offered admission to a rehabilitation hospital for a 1-week inpatient motor retraining (MoRe) program. Prior to admission, patients undergo a detailed evaluation by a movement disorder specialist, physical therapist, and psychologist to confirm their diagnosis, determine psychiatric comorbidities, and prepare them for the treatment week. The program is aimed at improving patients' motor symptoms, gaining insight into disease mechanisms, regaining control over abnormal movements, and learning better coping strategies. Patients are scheduled for daily sessions with physical, occupational, and speech therapy as well as a 1-hour session with a psychologist. Psychologists work with a validated treatment manual for treatment of functional neurologic symptoms (Sharpe et al., 2011) and also incorporate mental imagery training into the session (de Lange et al., 2008; Malouin et al., 2013). A supportive environment is provided by the physiatrist overseeing the treatment week, therapists and nurses, with daily positive reinforcement of treatment success. Patients are videotaped on the first and last day of therapy to document treatment outcomes and self-rated symptom questionnaires are completed before and after the program as well as after a 6-month follow-up period. Patients are given exercises to perform at home to maintain treatment success and are referred for appropriate outpatient follow-up. A retrospective analysis of 22 patients completing the program showed an excellent outcome with minimal to no abnormal movement symptoms in 45.5%, a good outcome with significant reduction in abnormal movements in 45.5%, and unchanged symptoms in 9%, and treatment benefit was largely maintained on 6-month follow-up (unpublished data).

PRINCIPLES OF THERAPY WITHIN THE MoRe PROGRAM

1. The diagnosis of a functional movement disorder is communicated by the neurologist after completing an appropriate comprehensive workup, before the patient is referred to the treatment program.
2. There is consistency among all members of the therapy team in communication and treatment goals.
3. Motor dysfunction is described in functional rather than psychologic terms, avoiding pejorative implications. It can be helpful to use analogies, e.g. having a computer "software" rather than "hardware" problem. The term "functional movement disorder" is preferred over "psychogenic" or "conversion disorder," as these imply a purely psychologic etiology of the movement disorder. Attributing symptoms to "stress" can be unhelpful, as patients will often state they are no longer experiencing stress but symptoms persist.
4. The principle of "motor retraining" (MoRe) is relearning of normal movements analogous to treatment of other neurologic conditions (e.g., hemiparesis, paraplegia, or ataxia) with the stated goal of neurologic normality.
5. Mental practice is used at the beginning of the first therapy session every day. Patients are guided to imagine their goal activity, e.g., walking down a corridor with a normal gait pattern or eating with a fork and knife without tremor. Patients are asked to recall their mental imagery during therapy sessions and given encouragement that they will be able to relearn normal movements. Patients are instructed to perform mental practice on their own every morning and every evening.
6. Treatment begins with establishing very elementary movements in the affected limb or body region, and

building on those. As simple movements are satisfactorily performed, appropriate motor complexity is added. More complex movements are only introduced after simple movements are performed successfully.

7. Emphasis is placed on the quality of movement instead of the quantity of movement. The patient receives verbal cueing to regain control of his or her motor performance and focuses on the quality of the movement instead of the speed or distance.
8. Ample opportunity for rest is provided. The patient is asked to focus on breathing or relaxing imagery when feeling overwhelmed. Pushing the patient too hard too soon can lead to regression of skills and worsening of symptoms.
9. Positive gains are verbally reinforced. Abnormal movements are ignored, although major and frequent adventitious intrusions may suggest the need to rest. Repetition is important to lock in the gains.
10. Assistive devices are removed as soon as possible.

PEDIATRIC INPATIENT SERVICES

Kozlowska et al. (2012) describe what they call "Multimodal rehabilitation: a mind–body, family-based intervention for children." The paper is not easy to read and sometimes lacks clarity. The etiologic model used is a unique one to the service but based loosely around the view that symptoms represent somatized distress, emphasizing the role of physiologic arousal. The essence of this complex intervention is a number of stages. The assessment process is described as having four stages: (1) completion of medical investigations; (2) family systems assessment; (3) "co-constructing a formulation with the family: a clear explanation that makes sense of the child's symptoms in the context of the family story"; and (4) providing a clear outline of treatment options.

The rehabilitation itself is delivered within a general medical ward over a 2-week period. A daily timetable is provided; physiotherapy, individual therapy, hospital school, adolescent group programs, and family meetings are all included, as well as free time. Family visiting times are limited to 2–3 hours at the end of the day and parents are given a designated contact person. Physiotherapy is based around trying to build up overall body strength rather than focusing on the specific therapy. Surprisingly, alternative medical strategies are encouraged. Pharmacotherapy for mood, sleep, and pain is used, the latter being simple analgesics; opiates, if already prescribed, are gradually withdrawn. Individual therapy focuses on managing physiologic arousal, addressing concerns not articulated in family sessions, and helping children deal with psychologic traumas. Family therapy has three goals: (1) to give feedback on progress; (2) to address family or systems issues contributing to the child's presentation; and (3) to empower family members to continue the intervention on their return home. Outcomes are described by case examples.

A MOVE TO DAY-PATIENT TREATMENT?

An alternate scenario that may provide a viable, yet cost-effective, option for some of these patients is an intensive, multimodal treatment program in a day-hospital setting. Logan et al. (2012) studied a day-hospital interdisciplinary rehabilitation approach for children and adolescents with complex regional pain syndromes that have failed to improve with outpatient treatment. This study incorporated physical, occupational, and CBT with medical and nursing services. It demonstrated in a systematic open clinical trial, with follow-up, that their program was effective in reducing disability and improving physical and emotional functioning as well as occupational performance.

Nielsen et al. (2015a,b) studied a 5-day physiotherapy rehabilitation program for patients with FNDs which was offered in a day-hospital. The treatment incorporated psychoeducation and movement retraining based on a pathophysiologic model for FNDs that stressed the importance of self-focused attention and illness belief. At the end of the treatment week, 65% of patients reported self-rated significant improvement, which was maintained in 55% of patients at 3-month follow-up. The program demonstrated, furthermore, improvement in self-reported quality-of-life measures and objective assessments of motor function in a cohort of patients with symptom duration of over 5 years and a high rate of patients receiving disability benefits.

SOME CONSIDERATIONS ON PSYCHOGENIC NONEPILEPTIC SEIZURES (PNES)

We are unaware of any specific reports from individual groups on the efficacy of inpatient treatment regimes for patients with PNES. However, a significant proportion of patients start their treatment in an inpatient setting, as best-practice diagnosis should include video-electroencephalography (video-EEG: video telemetry) for each patient with suspected PNES. This traditionally requires an inpatient admission, although more recently outpatient-induced telemetry has been increasingly adopted (LaFrance et al., 2007). A recent survey of 97 US epilepsy centers found that just under half of them utilized inpatient psychiatric consultation routinely for patients newly diagnosed with PNES (Acton and Tatum, 2013). Based on a small sample at a single center, studied retrospectively, these authors found that there was not a significant difference between the mood or anxiety disorders diagnosed by inpatient psychiatric consultation and those self-reported by the patients (Acton and Tatum, 2013). Based on these study results, the authors suggest that routine inpatient psychiatric consultation is not necessary in patients newly diagnosed with PNES and that a case-by-case evaluation by a nonpsychiatrist would presumably ensure that the minority of patients with acute psychiatric risks receive timely diagnosis and treatment. In our view, and that of others in the field, this is a failed understanding of the role of the psychiatric consultation, which is not only about treating mood disorders but, more importantly, about diagnosing and formulating treatment of the PNES itself. Furthermore, even if one accepts the authors' narrow view, the literature on screening of mood disorders in general hospital settings is clear that screening alone has no added benefit if it is not embedded into a system for treatment delivery. The case-by-case evaluation approach suggested by these authors introduces hazards of minimizing attention to evaluating relevant psychopathology in the patient prior to discharge from an epilepsy monitoring unit and undermines the capacity for an adequate understanding by both the patient and staff that is needed to inform appropriate treatment plan formulation. Support for a more thorough inpatient psychiatric assessment to direct treatment to increase patient and staff capacity to grasp the complexities and implications of a PNES diagnosis and thereby improve capacity to respond to treatment recommendations should be considered mandatory. Similar opinions are reflected in Baslet (2012) and LaFrance et al. (2013), based both on extensive clinical experience and detailed reviews of the relevant literature.

Insofar as diagnostic issues in distinguishing between epileptic seizures and PNES have been addressed in earlier chapters of this volume, consideration will be given here to inpatient management and treatment issues, following the consensus guidelines delineated by the International League Against Epilepsy (LaFrance et al., 2013).

Formal psychiatric assessment by a psychiatrist familiar with the management of PNES should be arranged and performed

This is warranted for all of the reasons outlined above, in terms of enhancing diagnostic understanding of relevant psychopathology as a prelude to effective treatment planning. A history of trauma or abuse may be found in a large percentage of patients with FND in general and PNES in particular (Bowman and Markland, 1996; Ozcetin et al., 2009). A patient is more likely to disclose this relevant history in an examination where current and past stressors are assessed in a systematic and empathetic manner. In selected cases, where there is evidence suggesting possible cognitive impairment impacting on school, work, or social adjustment, formal neuropsychologic evaluation may be additionally helpful in clarifying this issue, although the reliability and validity of standard psychometric testing are questionable in functional patients and effort testing should in our opinion be mandatory in such assessments (see Chapter 35).

Predisposing, precipitating, and perpetuating factors should be explored as a prelude to delineating appropriate psychotherapeutic interventions

The inclusion of relevant family members in helping delineate these factors, which may be beyond the capacity of the patient to recall or express, can often be helpful in enhancing understanding of the evolution of the relevant psychopathology. The enhanced understanding of family communication patterns may also be helpful in formulating psychotherapeutic strategies with a relative's participation, if possible, or to help improve the patient's strategies for coping with family psychopathology. Examples of such relevant pathology may include relatives either enabling the patient's disability by misguided encouragement of the patient's dependent state, or actually abusively generating and perpetuating it.

Psychotherapy should be implemented when possible

This recommendation is generally made in guidelines in all cases of FND, including those of PNES. However, it should be noted that the actual evidence base to support it is related more to theoretic models of the etiology of FND (see Chapter 10) and there is a notable lack of clinical trials to demonstrate efficacy (see Chapter 46). Two further points are worthy of consideration. First is which type of psychotherapy should be initiated. The two trials to date in PNES (Goldstein et al., 2010; LaFrance et al., 2014) both utilize CBT models, but that is not to say that psychodynamic treatments lack efficacy; simply there are no trials at present to give guidance either way (Martlew et al., 2014). The CODES trial, a large randomized controlled trial of treatment of PNES with CBT, should provide some clarity (Goldstein et al., 2015). Second, as noted above, this recommendation is not always accepted by patients.

What is clear is that simply explaining to patients that their events are psychogenic or nonepileptic in origin is not sufficient to generate cessation of their seizures in the majority of patients. Indeed, the majority of studies show that PNES persist in at least two-thirds of patients in long-term follow-up (Reuber et al., 2003). In the absence of other viable treatments there is reason to encourage the initiation of a psychotherapeutic process on the inpatient service so that, if a positive connection is made that provides meaningful hope for symptom attenuation and better adaptive functioning, the patient has a basis of encouragement to persevere with this process after discharge.

Pharmacologic treatment of patients

The pharmacologic treatment of patients should begin with early tapering and discontinuation of antiepileptic drugs (AEDs), which are an ineffective treatment for people with exclusive PNES, unless a specific AED has a documented beneficial psychopharmacologic effect in an individual (e.g., use for bipolar disorder or as a treatment for migraine) (LaFrance et al., 2013). Safe, gradual tapering of unneeded antiepileptic medications is often initiated early in the course of inpatient video-EEG monitoring, first as a diagnostic aid, to verify that its removal does not "unmask" an underlying epileptic seizure disorder and, concomitantly, by suggestion, to enhance the likely emergence of PNES that will be of confirmatory diagnostic value during EEG monitoring. When accompanied by the supportive diagnostic debriefing and the concomitant initiation of appropriate psychotherapeutic intervention, removing the burden of unneeded antiepileptic medications can be liberating both emotionally and by removal of cognitive as well as other pharmacologic side-effects.

Initiate psychopharmacologic agents to treat comorbid mood, anxiety, obsessive compulsive disorder, or psychotic disorders

In addition to the specific benefits to be obtained from effective psychopharmacologic treatment of relevant psychopathology, some patients may be reassured by the prescription of an appropriate active medication if they have difficulty in grasping the capacity of exogenous stressors and intrinsic psychologic vulnerabilities to generate seizures on a psychophysiologic basis. For some, a supportive explanation of "a different physiologic mechanism in the brain" generating these nonepileptic seizures may be conceptually more fathomable or more aesthetically palatable. In some cases, medication may serve as the "sugar that helps the psychotherapy go down."

THE INTERDIGITATING ROLES OF THE NEUROLOGIST AND MENTAL HEALTH PRACTITIONER (MHP) IN DIAGNOSTIC ASSESSMENT AND TREATMENT OF INPATIENTS WITH FND

When an inpatient on a medical ward presents with clinical features that point to the apparent implausibility of an organic neurologic diagnosis, an MHP is often called on to assist with the differential diagnosis and collaboration in formulating a treatment plan. Earlier chapters in this book have dealt with the multiple considerations associated with the generally relevant diagnostic challenges, both neurologic and psychiatric. What should be emphasized in the inpatient setting, however, is the advisability of calling in the MHP to assist in the diagnostic process as soon as the question of an FND generates serious consideration in the mind of the neurologist; even an experienced MHP needs time to adequately evaluate the frequently complex developmental course and the multiple factors maintaining the maladaptive aspects of the FND that led to the hospital admission. The frequent resistance of patients with somatizing disorders, including FND, to accept a straightforward diagnostic debriefing has been documented (Peckham and Hallett, 2009). This potential resistance can often be attenuated if the MHP consultation is initiated early, as part of a broad-based diagnostic assessment of possible physical and psychologic contributory factors to the patient's symptoms, including physical illness, external stressors, and intrinsic individual sensitivities. Having a "routine" MHP consultation earlier in the hospital course is more likely palatable than a hastily arranged MHP consultation on the day of discharge, when the patient is presented with an FND diagnosis peremptorily and feels "dismissed."

This advice however places a burden on the neurologist to initiate explanation of the potential diagnosis early and explain why psychiatric colleagues are being consulted. Even if the psychiatrist appears on the scene early, as part of the "evaluative team," the question remains as to when in this process the neurologist should address the putative diagnosis with the patient. We would argue that it should be openly discussed as a possible explanation from the time that it is suspected, in an open and collaborative manner, and finalized at the point when assessment is complete. This gives the patient, family, and treatment team time to work through the complex task of conceptual and emotional reformulation of the diagnosis and treatment plan. Others take the view (see above, which we strongly dispute) that a diagnosis should not be formally made and they maintain a diagnostic vagueness even during rehabilitative therapies. A third approach is the delivery of a definitive diagnosis at the end of the period of assessment prior to the delivery of treatment but without any prior "warming the patient up" to the possibility of such an explanation for the symptoms. The choice of approach may in part depend on the clinician's sense of the patient's cognitive and emotional capacities, which ideally, should influence the treatment modality to be used. If the patient is to be offered a program that is more physiotherapy-based and delivered within a neurorehabiltation center, it is probably practically possible to maintain a diagnostic vagueness, but if the program of treatment is going to be wholly or even largely psychotherapeutic, it is hard to understand how one could sell such an approach to the patient without being explicit about the diagnosis.

While allowing for variations in style and timing of communicating the diagnosis to the patient and family members, the authors emphasize our view that a thorough psychiatric evaluation to allow adequate diagnostic understanding or relevant psychopathology is an important prerequisite to inform adequate treatment plan formulation. It is a comparable disservice to misunderstand relevant psychopathology as it would be to overlook an undiagnosed neurologic condition.

The issues surrounding what one actually says in diagnostic explanation are dealt with in detail in Chapter 44. This does not need to change because explanation occurs in an inpatient setting. Further guidance can be seen in Carson et al. (2016). However, it can be seen (above) that there is a lack of consensus among groups reporting inpatient programs on terms used; some groups simply say there is no serious neurologic condition and that with rehabilitation reversibility is possible (above), whereas others are explicit that the condition is psychogenic (Edwards et al., 2014; Fahn and Olanow, 2014a b; Ganos et al., 2014; Jankovic, 2014) and others emphasize a functional model (Sharpe and Carson, 2001). In the absence of data, one can argue over the merits of different descriptions but no one term can claim superiority – indeed, one suspects that it is not only what is said but also how it is said that may be of equal value.

However, what does differ in an inpatient setting compared to an outpatient consultation is the range of different sources of clinical contact. A patient may well seek information from the consultant, the junior medical staff, various members of nursing staff, physiotherapy, occupational therapy, psychology, or even social work. Even different terminology pointing to the same diagnosis can sew the seeds of confusion, particularly if the patient has prominent health anxiety. Thus, a consultant explaining a "functional neurological disorder," juniors referring to "somatization," nursing staff saying it is "stress-related," and the social worker implying it is secondary to an abusive domestic relationship may not be integrated as a unitary concept by the patient and may leave the individual with the feeling that nobody knows what is wrong. We would recommend not just writing the diagnosis in the case records but also giving a brief note on the actual explanation used and then working within staff training on all using the same terminology, whatever might be the chosen term.

CONCLUSIONS

Patients with FNDs present to clinicians with a variety of symptomatic manifestations, with various levels of severity, chronicity, and comorbidity, as well as with various degrees of past adversity, intrinsic resilience, and available external support. Clearly, treatment must be individualized. For those patients who have been severely or chronically impaired, especially if adequate prior outpatient treatments have failed, inpatient treatment that integrates the various modalities outlined here provides a rational route of rescue from a course otherwise potentially characterized by protracted dependence and disability. Based on the data currently available, we believe this treatment approach is worthy of further study to refine the component treatment strategies and enhance the potentially most effective ingredients. For patients with severe levels of disability who could be managed in a multimodal day-treatment program, that approach also warrants further consideration.

References

Acton EK, Tatum WO (2013). Inpatient psychiatric consultation for newly-diagnosed patients with psychogenic nonepileptic seizures. Epilepsy Behav 27: 36–39.

Baslet G (2012). Psychogenic nonepileptic seizures: a treatment review. What have we learned since the beginning of the millennium? Neuropsychiatr Dis Treat 8: 585–598.

Bowman ES, Markland ON (1996). Psychodynamics and psychiatric diagnoses of pseudoseizure subjects. AJP 153: 57–63.

Carson A, Lehn A, Ludwig L et al. (2016). Explaining functional disorders in the neurology clinic: a photo story. Pract Neurol 16: 56–61.

de Lange FP, Roelofs K, Toni I (2008). Motor imagery: a window into the mechanisms and alterations of the motor system. Cortex 44: 494–506.

Demartini B, Batla A, Petrochilos P et al. (2014). Multidisciplinary treatment for functional neurological symptoms: a prospective study. J Neurol 261: 2370–2377.

Edwards MJ, Stone J, Lang AE (2014). From psychogenic movement disorder to functional movement disorder: it's time to change the name. Mov Disord 29 (7): 849–852.

Fahn S (2011). Psychogenic movement disorders: Phenomenology, diagnosis and treatment. In: S Fahn, J Jankovic, M Hallett (Eds.), Principles and Practice of Movement Disorders, 2nd edn. Elsevier, New York, pp. 513–527.

Fahn S, Olanow CW (2014a). "Psychogenic movement disorders": they are what they are. Mov Disord 29 (7): 853–856.

Fahn S, Olanow CW (2014b). Reply to: Psychogenic movement disorders: What's in a name? Mov Disord 29 (13): 1699–1701.

Fahn S, Williams D (1988). Psychogenic dystonia. In: S Fahn, C Marsden, D Calne (Eds.), Dystonia 2, Raven Press, New York, pp. 431–455.

Fahn S, Williams D, Reches A et al. (1983). Hysterical dystonia, a rare disorder: report of five documented cases. Neurology 33 (suppl 2): 161.

Ford B, Williams DT, Fahn S (1994). Treatment of psychogenic movement disorders. In: R Kurlan (Ed.), The Treatment of Movement Disorders, JB Lippincott, Philadelphia, PA, pp. 475–485.

Ganos C, Erro R, Bhatia KP et al. (2014). Comment on psychogenic versus functional movement disorders. Mov Disord 29 (13): 1696–1697.

Goldstein LH, Chalder T, Chigwedere C et al. (2010). Cognitive-behavioral therapy for psychogenic nonepileptic seizures: a pilot RCT. Neurology 74 (24): 1986–1994.

Goldstein LH, Mellers JDC, Landau S et al. (2015). Cognitive behavioural therapy vs standardised medical care for adults with dissociative non-epileptic seizures (CODES): a multicentre randomised controlled trial protocol. BMC Neurol 15 (1): 98.

Heruti RJ, Levy A, Adunski A, Ohry A (2002). Conversion motor paralysis disorder: overview and rehabilitation model. Spinal Cord 40: 327–334.

Jankovic J (2014). "Psychogenic" versus "functional" movement disorders? That is the question. Mov Disord 29 (13): 1697–1698.

Jordbru AA, Smedstad LM, Klungsøyr O, Martinsen EW (2014). Psychogenic gait disorder: a randomized controlled trial of physical rehabilitation with one-year follow-up. J Rehabil Med 46: 181–187.

Koelen JA, Houtveen JH, Abbass A et al. (2014). Effectiveness of psychotherapy for severe somatoform disorder: meta-analysis. Br J Psychiatry 204: 12–19.

Konnopka A, Kaufmann C, König H-H et al. (2013). Association of costs with somatic symptom severity in patients with medically unexplained symptoms. J Psychosom Res 75: 370–375.

Kozlowska K, English M, Savage B et al. (2012). Multimodal rehabilitation: a mind–body, family-based intervention for children and adolescents impaired by medically unexplained symptoms. Part 1: The program. Am J Fam Ther 40: 399–419.

LaFrance Jr WC, Blum AS, Miller IW et al. (2007). Methodological issues in conducting treatment trials for psychological nonepileptic seizures. J Neuropsychiatry Clin Neurosci 19: 391–398.

LaFrance WC, Reuber M, Goldstein LH (2013). Management of psychogenic nonepileptic seizures. Epilepsia 54: 53–67.

LaFrance Jr W, Baird GL, Barry JJ et al. (2014). Multicenter pilot treatment trial for psychogenic nonepileptic seizures: a randomized clinical trial. JAMA Psychiatry 71: 997–1005.

Logan DE, Carpino EA, Chiang G et al. (2012). A day-hospital approach to treatment of pediatric complex regional pain syndrome: initial functional outcomes. Clin J Pain 28: 10.1097.

Malouin F, Jackson PL, Richards CL (2013). Towards the integration of mental practice in rehabilitation programs. A critical review. Front Hum Neurosci 7: 576.

Martlew J, Pulman J, Marson AG (2014). Psychological and behavioral treatments for adults with non-epileptic attack disorder. Cochrane Database Syst Rev.

Nielsen G, Ricciardi L, Demartini B et al. (2015). Outcomes of a 5-day physiotherapy programme for functional (psychogenic) motor disorders. J Neurol 262: 674–681.

Nielsen G, Ricciardi L, Demartini B et al. (2015a). Outcomes of a 5-day physiotherapy program for functional (psychogenic) motor disorder. J Neurol 262: 674–681.

Nielsen G, Stone J, Matthews A et al. (2015b). Physiotherapy for functional motor disorders: a consensus recommendation. J Neurol Neurosurg Psychiatry 86 (10): 1113–1119.

Ozcetin A, Belli H, Esteem U et al. (2009). Childhood trauma and dissociation in women with pseudoseizure-type conversion disorder. Nord J Psychiatry 63: 462–468.

Peckham EL, Hallett M (2009). Psychogenic Movement Disorders. Neurol Clin, Mov Disord 27: 801–819.

Reuber M, Pukrop R, Bauer J et al. (2003). Outcome in psychogenic nonepileptic seizures: 1 to 10-year follow-up in 164 patients. Ann Neurol 53: 305–311.

Saifee TA, Kassavetis P, Pareés I et al. (2012). Inpatient treatment of functional motor symptoms: a long-term follow-up study. J Neurol 259: 1958–1963.

Sharpe M, Carson A (2001). "Unexplained" somatic symptoms, functional syndromes, and somatization: do we need a paradigm shift? Ann Intern Med 134 (9_Part_2): 926–930.

Shapiro P, Teasell RW (2004). Behavioural interventions in the rehabilitation of acute *v.* chronic non-organic (conversion/factitious) motor disorders. Br J Psychiat 185 (2): 140–146.

Sharpe M, Walker J, Williams C et al. (2011). Guided self-help for functional (psychogenic) symptoms: a randomized controlled efficacy trial. Neurology 77: 564–572.

Williams DT, Ford B, Fahn S (1995). Phenomenology and psychopathology related to psychogenic movement disorders. In: WJ Weiner, AE Lang (Eds.), Behavioral Neurology of Movement Disorders, Advances in Neurology Series, Vol. 65. Raven Press, New York, pp. 231–257.

Williams DT, Dyakina N, Fisher P et al. (2011). Inpatient treatment of psychogenic movement disorders. In: M Hallett, A Lang, J Jankovic et al. (Eds.), Psychogenic Movement Disorders and Other Related Conversion Disorders. Cambridge University Press, Cambridge, pp. 302–309.

Wing JK, Beevor AS, Curtis RH et al. (1998). Health of the Nation Outcome Scales (HoNOS). Research and development. Br J Psychiatry 172: 11–18.

Index

NB: Page numbers in *italics* refer to figures, tables and boxes.

G

N

Edwards Brothers Malloy
Ann Arbor MI. USA
November 26, 2016